AF758352

HANDBOOK OF THE SCIENCE OF EXISTENTIAL PSYCHOLOGY

Also Available

Handbook of Mindfulness:
Theory, Research, and Practice, Third Edition
Kirk Warren Brown, J. David Creswell, and Richard M. Ryan, Editors

Self-Determination Theory: Basic Psychological Needs in Motivation, Development, and Wellness
Richard M. Ryan and Edward L. Deci

Handbook of the Science of Existential Psychology

Edited by
Kenneth E. Vail III
Daryl R. Van Tongeren
Rebecca J. Schlegel
Jeff Greenberg
Laura A. King
Richard M. Ryan

THE GUILFORD PRESS
New York London

Copyright © 2026 The Guilford Press
A Division of Guilford Publications, Inc.
www.guilford.com

All rights reserved

No part of this book may be reproduced, translated, stored in a retrieval system, or transmitted, in any form or by any means, electronic, mechanical, photocopying, microfilming, recording, or otherwise, without written permission from the publisher.

Printed in the United States of America

This book is printed on acid-free paper.

For product and safety concerns within the EU, please contact *GPSR@taylorandfrancis.com*, Taylor & Francis Verlag GmbH, Kaufingerstraße 24, 80331 München, Germany.

Last digit is print number: 9 8 7 6 5 4 3 2 1

Library of Congress Cataloging-in-Publication Data

Names: Vail, Kenneth E. editor | Van Tongeren, Daryl R. editor | Schlegel, Rebecca editor | Greenberg, Jeff, 1954– editor | King, Laura A. (Laura Ann) editor | Ryan, Richard M. editor
Title: Handbook of the science of existential psychology / edited by Kenneth E. Vail III, Daryl R. Van Tongeren, Rebecca J. Schlegel, Jeff Greenberg, Laura A. King, Richard M. Ryan.
Description: New York : The Guilford Press, [2026] | Includes bibliographical references and index.
Identifiers: LCCN 2025035445 | ISBN 9781462560226 cloth
Subjects: LCSH: Existential psychology | BISAC: PSYCHOLOGY / Movements / Existential | PSYCHOLOGY / Experimental Psychology
Classification: LCC BF204.5 .H348 2026 | DDC 150.19/2—dc23/eng/20260106
LC record available at *https://lccn.loc.gov/2025035445*

About the Editors

Kenneth E. Vail III, PhD, is Associate Professor of Psychology and Director of the Social Psychology and Existential Attitudes Research Laboratory at Cleveland State University (CSU). Dr. Vail's research focuses on existential psychology, including the consequences of humans' awareness of their own mortality, autonomy, and choice freedom, and the influence of these existential concerns on cultural activity, personal growth, and both physical and mental health. He is cofounder and president of the International Society for the Science of Existential Psychology. Dr. Vail is a recipient of the Rising Star Award from the Association for Psychological Science, as well as research, teaching, mentoring, and service awards from CSU.

Daryl R. Van Tongeren, PhD, is Associate Professor of Psychology and Director of the Frost Center for Social Science Research at Hope College. He addresses "big questions" humans face by conducting multimethod research from an existential perspective. His recent research foci include the causes and consequences of religious deidentification and the costs and benefits of intellectual humility in the face of existential challenges. With over 200 publications, Dr. Van Tongeren is a recipient of the Rising Star Award from the Association for Psychological Science and of Early Career Awards from the Society for the Psychology of Religion and Spirituality (Division 36 of the American Psychological Association) and the International Society for the Science of Existential Psychology.

Rebecca J. Schlegel, PhD, is Professor in the Department of Psychological and Brain Sciences at Texas A&M University (TAMU), Co-Principal Investigator in the TAMU Existential Psychology Collaboratory, and Interim Director of the TAMU Institute for Technology-Infused Learning. Her research focuses on issues related to self/identity, authenticity, and meaning in life, particularly on the idea of a "true self" and the ways in which people use beliefs surrounding their avowed true self to imbue their life with meaning. In recent years, Dr. Schlegel has worked with education researchers, computer scientists, and engineers in an interdisciplinary effort to develop and test interventions that aim to foster an academic sense of self among students in elementary, middle, and high school.

Jeff Greenberg, PhD, is Regents Professor of Psychology and College of Science Fellow at the University of Arizona. His work has contributed to understanding self-serving biases, how motivation affects cognition, the effects of ethnic slurs, the role of self-awareness in depression, cognitive dissonance, existential isolation, and how concerns about death contribute to prejudice, self-esteem striving, and many other aspects of social behavior. Co-creator of terror management theory, Dr. Greenberg is a recipient of honors including the Distinguished Career Contributions Award from the International Society for the Science of Existential Psychology, the Career Contribution Award from the Society for Personality and Social Psychology, and the Outstanding Lifetime Career Award from the International Society for Self and Identity.

Laura A. King, PhD, is Curators' Distinguished Professor of Psychology and Director of the Personality Dynamics Lab at the University of Missouri–Columbia. Her research focuses primarily on the experience of meaning in life, embedding that experience in everyday life. She has also examined the existential benefits of worldviews, such as right-wing authoritarianism, and the existential challenge of pluralism. Dr. King is a recipient of the Jack Block Award for Distinguished Research in Personality from the Society for Personality and Social Psychology, among other research and teaching awards. She has served in many editorial and leadership roles in personality and social psychology. A member of the LGBTQ+ community, Dr. King has advocated for diversity and inclusion in these various roles.

Richard M. Ryan, PhD, is Professor at the Institute for Positive Psychology and Education at the Australian Catholic University. He is also Distinguished Professor in the College of Education at Ewha Womans University, Republic of Korea; Professor Emeritus of Psychology at the University of Rochester; and Visiting Professor at Imperial College London, United Kingdom. The co-developer of self-determination theory, Dr. Ryan is a therapist, consultant, and cofounder of Motivation Works, an organizational research and intervention firm. He is the most-cited psychologist in the world today and has authored over 450 papers and books. Dr. Ryan has been honored with four lifetime achievement awards for his work on motivation, personal meaning, self and identity, and existential psychology.

Contributors

Kevin Aho, PhD, Department of Communication and Philosophy, Florida Gulf Coast University, Fort Myers, Florida

Benjamin J. Anjewierden, MA, Department of Psychology, Cal Poly Humboldt, Arcata, California

Jamie Arndt, PhD, Department of Psychological Sciences, University of Missouri, Columbia, Missouri

Stephanie A. Barrientos, MS, Department of Psychology, Virginia Commonwealth University, Richmond, Virginia

Jack J. Bauer, PhD, Department of Psychology, University of Dayton, Dayton, Ohio

Roy F. Baumeister, PhD, Department of Psychology, Constructor University Bremen, Bremen, Germany

Elif Bilal, MS, Department of Psychology, Montana State University, Bozeman, Montana

Karolina Bonarska, MA, Doctoral School in Social Sciences and Philosophy Faculty, Institute of Psychology, Jagiellonian University, Krakow, Poland

Adam Buben, PhD, Leiden University College, Leiden University, The Hague, The Netherlands

Jakub Cacek, MA, Doctoral School in Social Sciences and Philosophy Faculty, Institute of Psychology, Jagiellonian University, Krakow, Poland

Nathan N. Cheek, PhD, Department of Psychology, University of Maryland, College Park, Maryland

Thomas B. Coulson II, MA, Division of Behavioral and Organizational Sciences, Claremont Graduate University, Claremont, California

Emily P. Courtney, PhD, Department of Psychology, University of South Florida, and Department of Health Outcomes and Behavior, Division of Population Science, H. Lee Moffitt Cancer Center and Research Institute, Tampa, Florida

Philip J. Cozzolino, PhD, Department of Psychiatry and Neurobehavioral Sciences, Division of Perceptual Studies, University of Virginia School of Medicine, Charlottesville, Virginia

Michael A. Day, BS, Department of Psychological and Brain Sciences, Texas A&M University, College Station, Texas

Isabella L. Di Lauro, MA, Department of Psychology, Virginia Commonwealth University, Richmond, Virginia

Jonathan Dinsmore, MS, Department of Psychology, University of Arkansas, Fayetteville, Arkansas

Gerald Echterhoff, PhD, Department of Psychology, University of Münster, Münster, Germany

Megan E. Edwards, PhD, Duke Social Science Research Institute, Duke University, Durham, North Carolina

Julie J. Exline, PhD, Division of Perceptual Studies, Department of Psychiatry and Neurobehavioral Sciences, University of Virginia, Charlottesville, Virginia

Christopher M. Falco, MA, Division of Behavioral and Organizational Sciences, Claremont Graduate University, Claremont, California

Roxanne N. Felig, PhD, Department of Psychology, University of South Florida, Tampa, Florida

Kevin Flores, BA, Department of Psychology, California State University, Bakersfield, California

Natalie Fraser, DCPsych, private practice, London, United Kingdom

Immo Fritsche, PhD, Wilhelm Wundt Institute for Psychology, Leipzig University, Leipzig, Germany

Amber M. Gaffney, PhD, Department of Psychology, Cal Poly Humboldt, Arcata, California

Luke W. Galen, PhD, Department of Psychology, Grand Valley State University, Allendale, Michigan

Madhwa S. Galgali, MA, Department of Psychological Sciences, University of Missouri, Columbia, Missouri

Alexis N. Goad, MA, Psychology Department, University of Arizona, Tucson, Arizona

Timothy J. Golden, JD, PhD, Visiting Professor of Philosophy, Whitman College, Walla Walla, Washington

Jamie L. Goldenberg, PhD, Department of Psychology, University of South Florida, Tampa, Florida

Jeffrey D. Green, PhD, Department of Psychology, Virginia Commonwealth University, Richmond, Virginia

Jeff Greenberg, PhD, Department of Psychology, University of Arizona, Tucson, Arizona

Bruce Greyson, MD, Department of Psychiatry and Neurobehavioral Sciences, Division of Perceptual Studies, University of Virginia School of Medicine, Charlottesville, Virginia

Jenny M. Groarke, PhD, School of Psychology, University of Galway, Galway, Republic of Ireland

Roosa Haimila, PhD, Department of Cultures, University of Helsinki, Helsinki, Finland

Andrew H. Hales, PhD, Department of Psychology, University of Mississippi, Oxford, Mississippi

Joseph Hayes, PhD, Department of Psychology, Acadia University, Wolfville, Nova Scotia, Canada

Steven J. Heine, PhD, Department of Psychology, University of British Columbia, Vancouver, British Columbia, Canada

Peter J. Helm, PhD, Department of Psychology, Montana State University, Bozeman, Montana

Fabian M. Hess, MSc, Institute of Psychology, Friedrich Schiller University Jena, Jena, Germany

Joshua A. Hicks, PhD, Department of Psychological and Brain Sciences, Texas A&M University, College Station, Texas

Sophie Höfer, MA, Department of Metaphysics and Philosophical Anthropology, Radboud University, Nijmegen, The Netherlands

Louis Hoffman, PhD, Rocky Mountain Humanistic Counseling and Psychological Association, Colorado Springs, Colorado

Ian Hohm, MA, Department of Psychology, University of British Columbia, Vancouver, British Columbia, Canada

Erica A. Holberg, PhD, Department of Psychological Sciences, University of Missouri, Columbia, Missouri

Ralph W. Hood, Jr., PhD, Department of Psychology, University of Tennessee at Chattanooga, Chattanooga, Tennessee

Gabrielle C. Ibasco, BA, Department of Psychology, University of British Columbia, Vancouver, British Columbia, Canada

Eric R. Igou, PhD, Department of Psychology, University of Limerick, Limerick, Republic of Ireland

Joshua J. Jackson, PhD, Department of Psychological and Brain Science, Washington University in St. Louis, St. Louis, Missouri

Theopia R. Jackson, PhD, Humanistic Clinical Psychology Department, Saybrook University, Pasadena, California

Elizabeth A. Janey, MA, Psychology Department, University of Chicago, Chicago, Illinois

Stephen Kearns, DPhil, Department of Philosophy, Florida State University, Tallahassee, Florida

Lucas A. Keefer, PhD, Department of Psychology, University of Southern Mississippi, Hattiesburg, Mississippi

Amy P. Kenny, BS, Psychology Department, University of Kansas, Lawrence, Kansas

Kathryn M. Kincaid, MS, Department of Psychology, University of Alberta, Edmonton, Alberta, Canada

Laura A. King, PhD, Department of Psychological Sciences, University of Missouri, Columbia, Missouri

Małgorzata Kossowska, PhD, Philosophy Faculty, Institute of Psychology, Jagiellonian University, Krakow, Poland

Jaime L. Kurtz, PhD, Department of Psychology, James Madison University, Harrisonburg, Virginia

Mark J. Landau, PhD, Psychology Department, University of Kansas, Lawrence, Kansas

Caroline C. Lapish, BS, Department of Psychology, Cleveland State University, Cleveland, Ohio

Uri Lifshin, PhD, Department of Psychology, The Hebrew University of Jerusalem, Jerusalem, Israel

Sarahi Lopez Amaro, BA, Department of Psychology, California State University, Bakersfield, California

Paul K. Lutz, MA, Department of Psychology, Carleton University, Ottawa, Ontario, Canada

Dylan R. Marsh, MS, Psychology Department, Colorado State University, Fort Collins, Colorado

Frank Martela, PhD, School of Science, Aalto University, Aalto, Finland

Andre Martinez, BA, Department of Psychology, California State University, Bakersfield, California

Matteo Masi, PhD, Department of Psychology, University of Münster, Münster, Germany, and Department of Psychology, University of Milano-Bicocca, Milano, Italy

Michael B. Mask, BA, Department of Psychology, University of British Columbia, Vancouver, British Columbia, Canada

Molly Maxfield, PhD, Edson College of Nursing and Health Innovation, Arizona State University, Phoenix, Arizona

Dan P. McAdams, PhD, Department of Psychology, Northwestern University, Evanston, Illinois

Ian McGregor, PhD, Department of Psychology, University of Waterloo, Waterloo, Ontario, Canada

Phoebe E. McKenna-Plumley, PhD, Queen's University Belfast, Belfast, United Kingdom

Alfred R. Mele, PhD, Department of Philosophy, Florida State University, Tallahassee, Florida

Rachel E. Menzies, PhD, School of Psychology, University of Sydney, Sydney, Australia

Mario Mikulincer, PhD, Department of Psychology and Israel Center for Addiction and Mental Health, The Hebrew University of Jerusalem, Jerusalem, Israel

Raffaella Misuraca, PhD, Atkinson Graduate School of Management, Willamette University, Salem, Oregon

Sarah Mohammadi, MSc, Department of Psychology, University of Mississippi, Oxford, Mississippi

Andrew B. Moynihan, PhD, Department of Psychology, University of Limerick, Limerick, Republic of Ireland

Ryan Murphy, BS, Department of Psychology, James Madison University, Harrisonburg, Virginia

Lydia M. Needy, MS, Department of Psychological and Brain Sciences, Texas A&M University, College Station, Texas

David B. Newman, PhD, Department of Psychology, Loma Linda University, Loma Linda, California

Georg Northoff, PhD, MD, Department of Medicine, Institute of Mental Health Research, University of Ottawa, Ottawa, Ontario, Canada

Ed O'Brien, PhD, Booth School of Business, University of Chicago, Chicago, Illinois

Julianna Ochoa-Peralta, BA, Department of Psychology, California State University, Bakersfield, California

Muireann K. O'Dea, PhD candidate, Department of Social, Environmental, and Economic Psychology, RPTU University of Kaiserslautern-Landau, Kaiserslautern-Landau, Germany

Gabriele Oettingen, PhD, Department of Psychology, New York University, New York, New York

Shigehiro Oishi, PhD, Department of Psychology, University of Chicago, Chicago, Illinois

Roman Palitsky, PhD, Emory Spiritual Health, Emory University, Atlanta Georgia

Kenneth I. Pargament, PhD, Department of Psychology, Bowling Green State University, Bowling Green, Ohio

Crystal L. Park, PhD, Department of Psychological Sciences, University of Connecticut, Storrs, Connecticut

Derk Pereboom, PhD, Department of Philosophy, Cornell University, Ithaca, New York

Tom Pyszczynski, PhD, Department of Psychology, University of Colorado at Colorado Springs, Colorado Springs, Colorado

Markus Quirin, PhD, Department of Medicine and Health, TU Munich, Munich, Germany, and Department of Psychology, PFH Göttingen, Göttingen, Germany

David E. Rast III, PhD, Department of Psychology, University of Alberta, Edmonton, Alberta, Canada

Elena Reutskaja, PhD, Marketing Department, IESE Business School, Barcelona, Spain

Grace N. Rivera, PhD, Department of Psychology, University of Mississippi, University, Mississippi

Tomi-Ann Roberts, PhD, Department of Psychology, Colorado College, Colorado Springs, Colorado

Benjamin D. Rosenberg, PhD, Psychology Department, Dominican University of California, San Rafael, California

Zachary K. Rothschild, PhD, Psychology Department, Bowdoin College, Brunswick, Maine

Pninit Russo-Netzer, PhD, Department of Psychology, Achva Academic College, Israel

Richard M. Ryan, PhD, Institute for Positive Psychology and Education, Australian Catholic University, North Sydney, Australia, and College of Education, Ewha Womans University, Seoul, South Korea

William S. Ryan, PhD, Department of Psychology, University of Toronto, Toronto, Ontario, Canada

Carol D. Ryff, PhD, Department of Psychology and Institute on Aging, University of Wisconsin–Madison, Madison, Wisconsin

Young-Ju Ryu, MA, Psychology Department, University of Kansas, Lawrence, Kansas

Rebecca J. Schlegel, PhD, Department of Psychological and Brain Sciences, Texas A&M University, College Station, Texas

Toni Schmader, PhD, Department of Psychology, University of British Columbia, Vancouver, British Columbia, Canada

Harrison J. Schmitt, PhD, Department of Psychology, Skidmore College, Saratoga Springs, New York

Kirk J. Schneider, PhD, Existential Humanistic Institute, San Francisco, California, and Saybrook University, Pasadena, California

Stefan E. Schulenberg, PhD, Department of Psychology, University of Mississippi, University, Mississippi

Constantine Sedikides, PhD, School of Psychology, University of Southampton, Southampton, United Kingdom

Ashley D. Seeling, MA, Department of Psychology, Cleveland State University, Cleveland, Ohio

Elizabeth Seto, PhD, Department of Psychology, Colby College, Waterville, Maine

Phillip R. Shaver, PhD, Department of Psychology, University of California, Davis, California

Kennon M. Sheldon, PhD, Department of Psychological Sciences, University of Missouri, Columbia, Missouri

Sara A. Showalter Van Tongeren, MSW, LCSW, Private Practice, The Flourishing Collective, Holland, Michigan

Jason T. Siegel, PhD, Division of Behavioral and Organizational Sciences, Claremont Graduate University, Claremont, California

Lauren K. M. Smith, PhD, School of Environment and Sustainability, Royal Roads University, Victoria, British Columbia, Canada

Sheldon Solomon, PhD, Department of Psychology, Skidmore College, Saratoga Springs, New York

Michael F. Steger, PhD, Department of Psychology, Center for Meaning and Purpose, Colorado State University, Fort Collins, Colorado, and Optentia Research Programme, North-West University, Vanderbijlpark, South Africa

Daniel Sullivan, PhD, Department of Psychology, University of Arizona, Tucson, Arizona

Stylianos Syropoulos, PhD, Department of Psychology and Neuroscience, Boston College, Boston, Massachusetts

Ewa Szumowska, PhD, Institute of Psychology, Jagiellonian University, Krakow, Poland

Natasha A. Tassell-Matamua, PhD, School of Psychology, Centre for Indigenous Psychologies, Massey University, Aotearoa, New Zealand

Jessica L. Tracy, PhD, Department of Psychology, University of British Columbia, Vancouver, British Columbia, Canada

Robert W. G. Tupper, MSc, Department of Psychology, Acadia University, Wolfville, Nova Scotia, Canada

Sebnem Ture, MSc, Department of Psychology, Northwestern University, Evanston, Illinois

Kenneth E. Vail III, PhD, Department of Psychology, Cleveland State University, Cleveland, Ohio

Patty Van Cappellen, PhD, Social Science Research Institute, Duke University, Durham, North Carolina

Wijnand A. P. van Tilburg, PhD, Department of Psychology, University of Essex, United Kingdom

Daryl R. Van Tongeren, PhD, Department of Psychology and Frost Center for Social Science Research, Hope College, Holland, Michigan

Matthew Vess, PhD, Department of Psychological and Brain Sciences, Texas A&M University, College Station, Texas

Sydney G. Wicks, MA, Department of Psychology, University of Mississippi, Oxford, Mississippi

Tim Wildschut, PhD, School of Psychology, University of Southampton, Southampton, United Kingdom

Yuji K. Winet, PhD, Fuqua School of Business, Duke University, Durham, North Carolina

Sarah E. Wolfe, PhD, School of Environment and Sustainability, Royal Roads University, Victoria, British Columbia, Canada

Jake Womick, PhD, Department of Psychology, California State University, Bakersfield, California

Natasha R. Wood, PhD, Institute of Security and Global Affairs, Leiden University, The Hague, The Netherlands

Muchen Xi, MA, Department of Psychological and Brain Science, Washington University in St. Louis, St. Louis, Missouri

Xiaobo Xu, PhD, School of Psychology, Shanghai Normal University, Shanghai, China

Isaac F. Young, PhD, Psychology Department, Beloit College, Beloit, Wisconsin

Natalie Zarzeczna, PhD, Department of Psychology, University of Essex, Colchester, United Kingdom

Xin Zhao, PhD, Department of Educational Psychology, East China Normal University, Shanghai, China

Contents

SECTION II. Death, Aging, and Time

SECTION III. Freedom, Authenticity, and Moral Responsibility

SECTION IV. Isolation, Uncertainty, and Shared Reality

Chapter abstracts are available on the companion website at *www.guilford.com/vail-materials*.

Introduction

Kenneth E. Vail III, Daryl R. Van Tongeren, Rebecca J. Schlegel, Jeff Greenberg, Laura A. King, *and* Richard M. Ryan

One of the most engaging aspects of psychological science is the challenge to better understand the fundamentally existential issues involved in human *being* and *becoming*. Throughout our lives, we each continuously navigate psychological experiences that are ultimately about the nature of our existence. We comprehend the passing of time, aging, and death. We grapple with freedom, authenticity, and moral responsibility. We struggle with isolation, uncertainty, and shared reality. We participate in culture and develop selves and identities. We yearn for meaning and purpose. We may believe in souls, gods, and afterlives. We strive for the "good life." And each of these existential concerns are no doubt interrelated in complex ways, with rich implications for better understanding human nature.

Building on recent theoretical and methodological advances in modern psychological science, a large and growing number of researchers around the world have begun to rigorously and systematically study the roles of various existential concerns in an increasingly broad range of the human experience. This *Handbook of the Science of Existential Psychology* is unique for being among the first handbooks covering this exciting and newly emerging field. As the field has been developing and growing over the past 40-plus years, this handbook offers an expansive coverage of the topic—with 65 chapters, authored by roughly 150 of the world's leading experts, showcasing the cutting-edge research that has been taking shape over the past several decades. The result is a text that we hope will usefully serve students, professionals, and scholars for years to come. Below, we outline some of the background of the field and provide an overview of the theory and research discussed in the various sections and chapters of this handbook.

PHILOSOPHICAL SEEDS: EXISTENCE PRECEDES ESSENCE

The broad range of existential concerns about the nature of being and becoming have been at the heart of many of humankind's richest reflections on ourselves and the world around us. Such reflections include religious teachings and scriptures from the Bible to the Bhagavad Gita, epics from Gilgamesh to Tolkien, meditations from Confucius to James Baldwin, poems and songs from Omar Khayyam to Bob Dylan, and even the moralistic folk tales, fables, and parables of Aesop and The Brothers Grimm.

These and mountains of other works represent some impressive efforts to better understand the human condition and collectively equip ourselves for a brighter future.

Adding to this chorus, direct philosophical considerations have tried to understand the nature of human existence. One common way of approaching the topic has been to assume that essence precedes existence. For many objects, that is certainly the case. People want to cut food for their meals, so a smith makes a chef's knife. People want to play and listen to music, so a luthier crafts a violin. Likewise, it can be tempting to assume that each of us humans also have an essential purpose that is the reason for our existence—the answer to questions like "Why am I here?" and "What is my purpose?" From that approach, discovering an object's essential purpose would be an important step both toward understanding it and toward achieving its optimal state of being, whether the object is a chef's knife, a violin, or oneself.

However, although essentialist conceptualizations of human nature are intuitive and common, some philosophers began to challenge the idea that we humans exist to fulfill some mysterious essential purpose. They turned the wisdom of essentialism on its head, arguing instead that *existence precedes essence*—that we exist first and then any essential purpose in life that we may perceive emerges because we humans, collectively and individually, create it for ourselves. From that view, it would not make sense to try to understand human nature by "discovering" some predefined essential purpose, nor that one ought to pursue it to achieve some predefined optimal state of being. Instead, the existentialist perspective redefined human nature as the *dynamic process* of navigating the ultimate concerns of *being* and *becoming*, contextualized by time and place, to fashion a sense of meaning and purpose in life.

In that regard, the existentialist philosophical movement was never about producing a coherent systematic ethic to prescribe who to be, what to do, how, and why. Rather, it has often been described as more focused on exploring the existential dynamics involved in human being and becoming and understanding the process of navigating them. Thinkers explored existential challenges such as time, aging, and death; freedom, authenticity, and moral responsibility; isolation, uncertainty, and shared reality; culture, self, and identity; meaning and purpose; religion and spirituality; and awe, personal growth, and the good life. Thus, the existential philosophical movement put existential dynamics "on the map," so to speak, and offered myriad ideas about how those experiences might unfold.

THE SCIENCE OF EXISTENTIAL PSYCHOLOGY: A BRIEF HISTORY OF THE TRADITION

The existentialist philosophical movement is often considered to have begun nearly two centuries ago, in the 1840s, when Søren Kierkegaard put his ideas to paper. His work was followed in the late 1800s by those of Fyodor Dostoyevsky and Friedrich Nietzsche, and in the 1900s by Martin Heidegger, Jean-Paul Sartre, Albert Camus, and various others throughout Europe. The central focus of existentialist philosophy spread quickly during that time, and many existentialist theoretical lenses were developed and applied across a variety of academic domains and therapeutic disciplines such as theology (e.g., Tillich; Buber), sociology (e.g., Émile Durkheim; Berger & Luckmann), and cultural anthropology (e.g., Ernest Becker), among others, but most directly and thoroughly to psychology (e.g., William James; Otto Rank; Erich Fromm) and psychotherapy (e.g., Viktor Frankl; Rollo May; Irvin Yalom).

The application of the scientific method, however, was held back in the early- and mid-1900s for two main reasons, both of which were related to the methodological limitations of psychology at the time. First, partly as a rejection of the Freudian "depth psychology," the dominant behaviorist views of scientific psychology placed strict emphasis on direct observations. However, the lack of sophisticated research methodologies in those early days meant internal mental experiences—such as the cognitive and emotional handling of existential concerns—were simply beyond the reach of the objective research methods available. Second, although humanistic psychology broke from both Freudian theory and behaviorism and was influenced by existentialist philosophy in carving out a "third way," its proponents objected to scientific research methods as reductionist and generally inadequate for studying the rich complexities and nuances of human being and becoming. In those early days of lever-pressing pigeons and simple reward–punishment schemes, that was perhaps a reasonable objection.

But by the 1970s and 1980s, following the successes of the cognitive revolution, researchers in mainstream psychological science had developed techniques to objectively study subjective experiences, inner mental processes, and their behavioral indicators. Thus, equipped with the newly emerging methods, some of those researchers began conducting some of the first scientific studies establishing that it was indeed possible to apply the scientific method to productively study existential psychological dynamics in everyday life. As a result, interest in the science of existential psychology spread throughout the 1980s and 1990s, during which researchers began developing novel theoretical perspectives and innovative research methods to better understand the roles of various existential concerns in an increasingly broad range of the human experience.

In 2001, researchers held an International Conference on Experimental Existential Psychology in Amsterdam, which led to the *Handbook of Experimental Existential Psychology* (Greenberg et al., 2004) and an article introducing the field in *Current Directions in Psychological Science* (Koole et al., 2006). Since then, interest in the science of existential psychology has continued to grow. An increasing number of researchers have been using diverse methods—qualitative and quantitative—to rigorously and systematically explore and document the roles of various existential concerns in human mental and social functioning. A growing number of major peer-reviewed research journals began hosting "special issues" focused exclusively on existential psychology topics, and a growing number of handbooks began summarizing research on existential psychological topics (e.g., authenticity, meaning, religiosity).

Flash forward two decades, and the field had grown to the point that it warranted organizational support. In 2019, researchers began what is now an annual conference on the science of existential psychology. Soon after, in 2020, researchers founded the International Society for the Science of Existential Psychology (*issep.org*), which gives awards to recognize excellent contributions to the field, disburses grant funding to stimulate further research advances, runs a dedicated peer-reviewed journal, organizes the field's annual conference, curates pedagogical resources for teaching and learning about existential psychology research, and communicates the science of existential psychology to the general public through an e-magazine program, among a variety of other resources offered.

Thus, the science of existential psychology of today is unique in tradition, method, and scope. Whereas the existential–humanistic tradition, which sprouted in the early 1900s, developed an excellent body of scholarship on existential psychotherapy, it has remained almost entirely limited to therapy and continues to largely resist the application of modern scientific research methods. The science of existential psychology did not stem from that tradition. Rather, it stemmed from the mainstream psychological science tradition, with researchers gaining the methodological sophistication to expand their reach to existential psychological topics. As a result, the field actively applies the methods of modern psychological science to develop an improved understanding of existential dynamics in human functioning and broadly explores those dynamics in all aspects of life. We turn now to a brief overview of some of the more common methodological approaches employed, followed by an illustrative sampling of the scope of theory and research in the field.

RESEARCH METHODS IN THE SCIENCE OF EXISTENTIAL PSYCHOLOGY

One of the things that makes the science of existential psychology new and unique is its embrace of the full range of the research methods available in modern psychological science. Here, the field participates in the traditional scientific process of acquiring knowledge and understanding through observation, evaluation, interpretation, and theoretical explanation, and it does so through the application of rigorous scientific research methods—systematic techniques to acquire, update, or integrate knowledge about the roles of existential psychological phenomena in everyday life. Though a full treatment of the details of psychological science research methods is of course beyond the scope of this introduction, here we highlight some of the relevant issues: defining and measuring variables, considering levels of processing, and gathering and analyzing qualitative and quantitative data.

A Foundation of Objective and Replicable Observation

As with the rest of psychological science, the goals of the science of existential psychology are to understand the roles of existential psychological dynamics so well that they can be described, explained, predicted, and even controlled. What are the relevant existential concerns? How do they work; what are their causes, mechanisms, and consequences? Can we anticipate when they will emerge and how they will impact our thoughts, feelings, and behaviors? If so, can we control the conditions necessary for them to occur or not occur, or to impact one outcome or another? Progress toward these goals requires the gathering of valid and reliable information, and the continual organization and reorganization of that information in a cumulative way. In that regard, the collection of information can lead to the development of scientific theories to understand that existing cumulative body of information, and hypothesis testing can further interrogate any lingering questions about the implications of theoretical ideas.

The foundation of scientific advances in understanding existential dynamics, as in the rest of modern psychological science, is objective and replicable observation. This stands in contrast to the subjective and nonreplicable methods typical of (nonbehaviorist) psychology in the early 1900s, when it was not uncommon for a researcher to "study" a phenomenon (in themself or another person) and then publish a report describing their interpretation of the relevant process. In that approach, the "empirical data" was the *researcher's subjective* description or interpretation of the participant's lived experience. Although sometimes impressive, such reports were largely unverifiable; nobody else could examine whether the "results" were valid (because they were the original researcher's subjective interpretations) nor could they rerun the study to see if the results could be reliably reproduced under similar circumstances (because the observational "instrument" was the original researcher).

But researchers eventually became aware of and addressed these problems, and in the second half of the 1900s they began developing sophisticated techniques to observe *subjective mental experiences* in *objective* and *replicable* ways. To be objective, the observation technique must be impartial, independent of any given researcher's personal opinions and biases. To be replicable, the observation technique must be able to be repeated by any researcher in the same way. These strictures make it important to clarify theoretical constructs and operational definitions of observed variables. A construct is a conceptual variable that is known or thought to exist but cannot be directly observed, whereas an operational definition is a specific expression of the construct that can be indirectly observed.

For example, George and Park (2017) conceptualized meaning in life as a tripartite construct involving the sense of coherence (life makes sense, things are clear and seem to fit together), purpose (overarching life goals, a reason for being), and significance (one's existence matters in profound and lasting ways). They operationally defined it as agreement, on a 7-point Likert-type scale (1 = Strongly disagree, 7 = Strongly agree), with 15 statements, such as "I can make sense of the things that happen in my life" (coherence), "I have overarching goals that guide me in my life" (purpose), and "I am certain that my life is of importance" (significance). Although meaning in life is a subjective mental experience, the observation technique is objective because the response scores are recorded objects that can be analyzed independent of any given researchers' opinions and biases, and replicable because this technique can be repeated by other researchers. Thus, the data and their interpretation is now verifiable—other researchers can independently analyze the original data objects (in this case, survey response scores) and even rerun the study to see if the same results can be reliably reproduced under similar circumstances.

Level/Depth of Processing

Throughout the science of existential psychology, researchers give much attention to considering the relevant level(s) of processing—behavioral, conscious, nonconscious, physiological—and tailor research methods accordingly. A useful (but imperfect) metaphor is to think of the body and mind as one might think of computer hardware and software; the hardware is the body/brain that creates the software experiences of the mind, with some software programs that the user consciously operates and some that automatically run in the background, all of which may contribute to behavioral outcomes. When studying an aspect of existential dynamics within participants' conscious awareness, the door is open to direct methods such as interviews or surveys. But when studying behaviors or experiences that might be outside conscious awareness, or that participants might like to avoid or deny (even to themselves), more indirect methods would be appropriate.

Qualitative Methods

Qualitative research is often about gathering information for the arts and humanities disciplines, but it can also play a role in the scientific process. Qualitative research typically gathers data from "natural settings" where people live their lives and typically involves written transcripts of spoken interviews, but might also include notes about observed behaviors, documents, and/or audiovisual media. The researcher then examines the data gathered and functions as the analytic "instrument" to identify, interpret, and report what they see as important patterns in the data. Thus, it is important to keep in mind that the level of analysis is typically limited to thoughts, feelings, and behaviors that can be consciously experienced and reported by participants and consciously noticed and described by researchers; participants cannot report and researchers cannot observe the mountains of nonconscious mental or biological processes that might be occurring. Thus, qualitative research is most effective when it is done to provide a detailed, complex, and holistic description of conscious cognitive or emotional experiences or overt behaviors.

There are many types of qualitative research, but we highlight three of the most relevant: phenomenology, grounded theory, and narrative. Phenomenological research draws heavily from Edmund Husserl and those he influenced, such as Heidegger, Sartre, and Merleau-Ponty, and aims to be atheoretical in describing conscious lived experiences rather than explaining them. In a phenomenological study, the researcher identifies a phenomenon of interest (e.g., grief, authenticity, awe), typically interviews several participants who have experienced that phenomenon, and then seeks to identify, describe, and interpret the common aspects of their experience. In grounded theory research, the goal is to inductively develop a testable theory about the processes and actions surrounding an experience. The researcher typically interviews several participants, often multiple times, to identify and describe the core phenomenon as well as possible causal or mitigating conditions, mechanisms, and outcomes. Narrative research is similar but focuses on individuals lived and told stories, with sensitivity to contextual factors, longitudinal chronology, and story turning points. Researchers can employ these methods in scientific ways by, for example, developing detailed codebooks, doing negative case analysis, and soliciting third-party coding reviews, such that the analyses become more objective and replicable.

For example, Maxfield, Peckham, and James (2024) conducted a thematic analysis of the experiences, context, and phenomena associated with dementia-related anxiety. The researchers conducted semi-structured interviews with 50 community-dwelling adults, ages 58–89, without dementia diagnoses, about their thoughts, feelings, and reactions to the possibility of being diagnosed with dementia. Researchers identified seven themes suggesting participants (1) considered dementia anxiety-provoking, with negative emotions and catastrophic thinking; (2) worried about how they might be treated by others; (3) worried about losing their self and becoming dehumanized; (4) worried about a loss of freedom, self-determination, and control; (5) worried about becoming a burden on others; (6) worried about risk from family history; and (7) worried more about dementia than about decline in physical health. Concerning dementia's implication for sense of self, one participant said, "It's scary to think of losing yourself . . . who you are . . . your soul"; another said, "I'll be gone, and I'll not be coming back"; and another said, "You are no longer you . . . you might as well be dead." Concerning the implications for freedom and self-determination, one said, "If I were to get it . . . losing control . . . that would just terrify me"; another said, "I would hate to give up my ability to choose what I do, when I can do it"; and another said, "I don't want to lose control . . . fear . . . terror is a better word." This analysis highlights some of the intense and complex existential dynamics in the process of adult development and aging.

Quantitative Methods

The bulk of research in the science of existential psychology, as in the rest of mainstream psychological science, employs quantitative methodologies. These methods entail a highly rigorous and systematic approach to the collection and analysis of numerical data with a strong emphasis on objective and replicable observation and the ability to study systematic relationships between variables, including possible causal relationships.

At the heart of quantitative methods is the numeric measurement and analysis of human functioning. Quantitative data can address all levels of human functioning—behavioral, conscious, nonconscious, and physiological—and can be collected from natural settings or from tightly controlled laboratory settings. To illustrate, consider just a few of the measurement techniques used by researchers studying death-related concerns and their mechanisms and consequences.

- *Behavioral.* Researchers studying health/fitness-related self-esteem striving had participants squeeze a hand-dynamometer and recorded strength output in pounds per square inch (Peters et al., 2005), and researchers studying cleaning behavior among people with obsessive–compulsive disorder recorded the duration of handwashing (in seconds), amount of soap used (in milliliters), and number of paper towels used (Menzies & Dar-Nimrod, 2017). Quantitative measurement of such overt behaviors is important because any systematic changes are likely subtle but could be deeply informative.
- *Conscious thoughts and feelings.* Surveys can be used when participants might be consciously aware of, and willing to honestly report, cognitive and emotional experiences. For example, researchers studying death anxiety (Lester, 1994) might ask "How disturbed or made anxious are you by the following aspects of death and dying?" and numerically measure, on a 5-point scale (1 = Not at all, 5 = Very much), responses to 36 aspects, such as "The shortness of life," "The pain involved in dying," "Losing someone close to you," and "Watching a dying person suffer from pain."
- *Nonconscious thoughts and feelings.* Many important existential dynamics may take place nonconsciously, such that participants cannot consciously report on them and researchers cannot directly observe them. Thus, researchers devise indirect indicators of nonconscious cognitive and affective phenomena. For example, researchers have devised both analog and computerized techniques to measure the nonconscious activation of death-related cognition (Cox et al., 2019). In the word-stem completion task, participants complete 36 partially completed words (e.g., GRA_ _), 12 of which can be completed in either neutral (e.g., GRANT) or death-related ways (e.g., GRAVE). The sum of the death-related word-stem completions indicates the accessibility of death-related cognitions. In the lexical decision task, a computer screen shows a series of 70 letter strings, 30 of which are words and 40 of which are gibberish nonwords (e.g., *zudric*, *mablko*), and participants use two buttons to categorize the strings as words or non-

words as quickly and accurately as possible. The computer measures the response latencies, in milliseconds, of correctly categorized strings. Of the 30 words, 18 are neutral (e.g., cloak, bottle), 6 are negative (e.g., suffer, fail), and 6 are death-related (e.g., dead, killed). The average latency on the death-related (neutral vs. negative) strings indicate the relative direction and magnitude of nonconscious death-thought accessibility.

- *Psychophysiological processes.* Deeper still are psychophysiological processes. Eye-tracking technology, for example, can measure attentional biases toward or away from death-related stimuli, presenting a series of image arrays and recording the location, number, and duration (in milliseconds) of gaze fixations on death-related images (Chen et al., 2022). Other "existential neuroscience" research focuses more directly on measuring brain activity during the conscious and nonconscious processing of existential concerns, using techniques such as cranial electroencephalogram (EEG) and functional magnetic resonance imaging (fMRI). With cranial EEG, electrodes are placed on standard scalp locations adjacent to various cortical structures and electrical waveforms are recorded (in milliseconds) at each location throughout the duration of the experience, such that existential event-related changes in amplitudes at particular locations indicate changes in the activity of corresponding brain regions (Henry et al., 2010). With fMRI, magnetic fields are applied and radio frequency images of sequential slices of the brain are captured at regular intervals to measure hemodynamic changes in specific brain locations as existential psychological dynamics unfold (Chapter 12). Electrical techniques such as cranial EEG offer high temporal but low spatial precision, whereas hemodynamic techniques such as fMRI offer low temporal but high spatial precision.

Sometimes researchers study just one variable, analyzing its descriptive statistics. But typically, researchers study more complex relationships between two or more variables, analyzing their inferential statistics. Such studies might use correlation-based designs to calculate the direction and strength of the relationship. For example, George and Park (2017) found meaningful comprehension of the world was correlated with greater life satisfaction and lower depression, anxiety, and stress. More sophisticated statistical techniques can go beyond simple zero-order correlations to more complex models capable of controlling for confounds and isolating analyses to the relationships of interest. However, correlation is not causation, and no amount of statistical sophistication can change the fact that the variables were merely measured; we cannot know whether or how they might be causally related. Comprehension might have caused greater life satisfaction, or vice versa, or some third variable might have caused both to rise and fall together.

Experiments, however, can test a hypothesized causal relationship. Consider the hypothesis that death awareness causes religious believers to strengthen their faith (Chapter 52). To test that idea, researchers would first select/develop a technique to manipulate the presumed causal variable: the awareness of death. In a mortality salience condition participants might be prompted to think about death, whereas in a comparison condition they might be prompted about dental pain (a non-death-related topic). Second, researchers would randomly assign religious believers into one of those manipulated conditions, so the manipulated variable changes independent of other variables (e.g., age, political orientation) and any preexisting differences among participants would be evenly spread across conditions. Third, researchers would measure the outcome variable in all participants, such as by having participants use a 10-point scale to indicate their strength of religious faith. Finally, researchers would statistically analyze the religious faith score distributions in the two conditions. If the distribution in the mortality salience condition is higher than in the control condition, then the experiment indicates the awareness of death caused religious believers to increase their religious faith.

Integrative Methods

Researchers in the science of existential psychology also employ a variety of integrative methods. Mixed methods, for example, employ both qualitative and quantitative methods within a single study, allowing researchers to report the rich descriptions of conscious phenomena and the precise numeric trends of relevant dynamics at various levels of processing. A variant on the mixed-methods technique is to convert qualitative into quantitative data and analyze it statistically. Raw narrative data, for instance, might be transcripts of personal stories; but researchers might then develop sophisticated manuals for quantifying the narratives, for example, giving numeric values to the presence, magnitude, and valence of significant themes and turning points in those stories, and then analyzing the statistical patterns of those characteristics in participant narratives (Chapters 40, 59).

Researchers also conduct systematic reviews and meta-analyses that synthesize findings—sometimes hundreds of studies conducted over decades—to learn from the whole of the field's accumulated research. Systematic reviews follow rigorous protocols to gather and organize relevant prior studies on a topic, and meta-analyses statistically combine and analyze findings from those previous studies to identify overall patterns and variations. Lastly, just as no single piece of a puzzle shows the overall picture, no single study can fully capture the complexity of any one individual's experience nor the entirety of any existential dynamic. Rather, each study represents one piece of the larger puzzle. As the field accumulates more pieces, researchers can learn more about how those pieces fit together to illustrate an increasingly complete overall picture.

SCOPE OF THE SCIENCE OF EXISTENTIAL PSYCHOLOGY

To provide an illustrative sampling of the scope of theory and research in the field, we turn now to an overview of the contents of this handbook. Authored by roughly 150 of the world's leading experts, this handbook includes 65 chapters arranged in eight parts. After laying a broad topical foundation in the first section, the remaining seven sections provide in-depth coverage of research exploring how various existential dynamics impact mental and social life.

Section I: Philosophical Roots, Scientific Methods

Section I covers some key topics relevant to existential philosophy and how researchers have begun to address existential psychological questions using the broad range of research methods available in modern psychological science.

In Chapter 1, Höfer and Buben discuss some of Kierkegaard's ideas about the importance of death in life. For Kierkegaard, and many he inspired, one is not born with meaningful conceptualizations of one's self. Rather, crafting a meaningful sense of self is something that unfolds throughout one's daily lived experiences. The challenge, he noted, is that it can be all too easy to simply go along with activities in life that are, in the grand scheme of things, rather unimportant. In that regard, he pointed to death as the ultimate taskmaster in helping us stay grounded in crafting a self that is more squarely based in meaningful life projects. One complication, however, is that people may not give death its due—either because it is uncomfortable to think about or because they neglect to see death as self-relevant until their final hour, or both. People may engage in some form of motivated death denial, to push death thoughts out of the mind as much as possible, or they might understand death in objective terms that apply to others (e.g., cancer patients, soldiers, elderly) rather than themselves.

In contrast, Kierkegaard argued for an "earnest" recognition of the relevance of death to one's own subjective experiences, recognizing that death is both certain and uncertain. Death will undoubtedly come, but with unknown time and place—decades from now, next week, or this afternoon—which should serve as a wake-up call for our self, our life goals, and our daily actions. The earnest thought of death involves an awareness of the scarcity of time in which every moment is precious and should not be wasted. What becomes crucial, then, is to develop a sense of self oriented toward meaningful goals and life projects that are valuable regardless of whether they are completed in one's lifetime or not.

Indeed, a central theme in existentialist thought is that a limited time frame, which comes with the human awareness of mortality, is what orients us to engage our freedom—motivating us to want to be our most authentic self in any given moment. There are seemingly infinite paths in the world; countless career paths to join, clothing styles to adopt, people to befriend, and so on. If we knew we had unlimited time, we would not need to choose—we could engage with all of them. But we know that our time is limited; we know we are mortal; and so we can only engage with a few of them. Thus, the question is whether we allow our lives to be shaped by external forces (e.g., parents, employers, cultural norms) or by our own self-determined expression of ourselves.

In Chapter 2, Kearns and Mele consider various conceptualizations of free will, found in contemporary analytic philosophy, alongside Sartre's existentialist account of freedom. Four of the most common ways of understanding freedom are that an agent acts freely when they are able to choose an action from a variety of options (leeway), when they are the origin of their actions independent of external forces (sourcehood), when they have the capacity to act on good reasons for an action (reason), or when their action expresses what they truly value, reflectively endorse, or who they truly are (deep self). The experience of each of these conceptualizations of free will bears important implications for moral responsibility for one's actions and even the meaning of one's life, more broadly. If one does not have any leeway ("I had no choice"), sourcehood ("my boss made me do this"), capacity to follow good reason ("I didn't know about that"), or deep self-expression ("that doesn't reflect my true self"), then one would hardly be responsible for their actions and life experiences.

Thus, one important question is: Do we have free will? The primary threat to free will is determinism: the idea that any given state of the universe, following the laws of nature, determines every subsequent state of the universe. There is no special exception for human agency. If determinism is true, then all our actions are controlled by the systematic unfolding of external forces stretching back to the Big Bang. Some view determinism as incompatible with free will, as it seems to undermine the genuine ability to have done otherwise (leeway) and means we are not the true authors of our actions (sourcehood). But others accept that we have free will, either by viewing free will in a way that is compatible with determinism (even if no leeway or sourcehood, action can be freely chosen if people act on reasons or express their deep/true self) or by rejecting the constraints of determinism on human agent-determined (libertarian) free will.

Here, it is worth recalling that there is no one existential philosophical view. Individual philosophers certainly advocated for one or another theoretical perspective, but thinkers often had substantial differences of opinion. Nietzsche contributed to existentialist thought as a hard determinist free will skeptic, whereas Sartre contributed as an agent-deterministic libertarian. In an important way, the science of existential psychology is not interested in the philosophical debate about the metaphysics of free will. Instead, the point is to better understand the *psychology* of free will. People can experience situations and make decisions that guide thoughts, feelings, and behaviors; they can appraise those phenomena in ways ranging from determined to freely chosen; and those appraisals matter. A thought, feeling, or behavior could be "truly" metaphysically determined or free, or mistaken as determined or free; that doesn't matter. What matters, in either case, is the psychological experience of freedom and responsibility, and researchers can take steps to better understand the *psychological* dynamics involved.

At one end of the spectrum, Chapter 2 explores some of the dynamics associated with Sartre's account of free will. In Sartre's view, one might feel anguish about any course of action if one perceives it as only possible, rather than determined. He also devoted considerable attention to exploring the connections between the experiences of freedom and nothingness (the mental separation of oneself from things that already exist in the world). Such processes as imagination, expectation, doubt, and questioning (will Pierre be at the café?) all involve a possibility of what might *not be*, which suggests a freedom to understand situations and act independent of—and thus not determined by—what already *is*. Sartre also highlighted the importance of our fundamental life projects, or who we aim at being or becoming. Our fundamental projects are a sort of ideal self that gives shape to ends, animates means, and breathes life into reasons and motives. Sartre acknowledged the presence of limiting external forces, such as family, race, class, or nation, but he argued that we are nevertheless free to choose any fundamental life projects, and pursue any ends, and are thus ultimately responsible for our own frustrations or joys and for the meaninglessness or meaningfulness of our lived experiences.

Toward the other end of the spectrum, in Chapter 3, Pereboom adopts a determinist perspective, closer to Nietzsche's view, to explore the dynamic tension between our facticity (e.g., our limitations as mortal creatures) and our ability to transcend that facticity. This view leads to a somewhat different question about this existential dynamic: If our deliberations and choices seem determined by factors beyond our control, then how can we transcend our facticity to make a meaningful impact in our lives and in the world? It may be rather difficult to believe that our deliberations and choices matter while also believing that our path in life is causally determined by factors beyond our control. However, even lacking freedom, our (determined) choices still exert power over ourselves and our environments. Thus, one could reject a life of resentful resignation and (in Nietzschean terms) assert one's "will to power," embracing one's control despite the limitations of one's facticity. In his own twist, Pereboom suggests important implications for our emotional experiences (e.g., letting go of anger), cultural institutions (e.g., criminal justice, public safety), and hope for progress over suffering.

In Chapter 4, Golden discusses the unique set of ideas associated with Black existential thought. The chapter first covers some foundational phenomenological and existential ideas and then builds on the thought of Frederick Douglass, W. E. B. Dubois, Frantz Fanon, Lewis Gordon, George Yancy, Derrick Bell, and others to explore the application of existentialist ideas to better understanding the challenges of the Black experience across a variety of contexts (e.g., Afro-European, Afro-Caribbean, Afro-American). The problems of both hostile and systemic anti-Black racism, for example, can be understood through Sartre's notion of "bad faith." Although anti-Black racism is either perpetrated or permitted by the majority-White population, Whites might nevertheless live in "bad faith" by failing to appreciate or even lying to themselves about their freedom and responsibility in accepting it—consider some resigned or self-deceptive excuses: "that's just how it is" (leeway), "*I* don't do it" (sourcehood), "I don't think it's really a problem" (reason), or "that's not who I am" (deep self). A related issue of the bad-faith White gaze is the objectification and dehumanization of Black bodies, making it easier for Whites to attempt control or ownership (if viewed as chattel) or policing or death (if viewed as dangerous).

Black individuals, thus, may often experience an elevated sense of existential threat to life and limb, even during the most quotidian of activities (e.g., visiting a grocery store, going for a jog, being asleep in bed). Additionally, one may experience a state of double consciousness—an awareness of two very different views of oneself. The first is what would otherwise be one's own subjectively crafted self, oriented toward meaningful fundamental projects that might focus, for example, on being or becoming an excellent American, son, engineering student, artist, and so on. The second, however, is the view from the bad-faith White gaze, laden with all the associated stereotypes, prejudices, and suspicions. The latter introduces contradictions that threaten the development of coherent life projects and meaningful lived experiences. However, the chapter considers that, even if the limiting circumstances are bleak and difficult to change, one might find the strength to craft a meaningful life despite the circumstances and/or adopt into one's fundamental project the goal of changing the circumstances themselves. Either way, one might adopt an orientation to the world that fills life with meaning and makes it worth living.

In Chapter 5, Vess discusses the application of some of the research methods of modern psychological science to better understand existential psychological dynamics. He emphasizes the importance of clear theoretical conceptualization, thoughtful operational definitions, and building theory through incremental gains in evidence across multiple studies. Then, he outlines the application of various research methodologies—including qualitative, correlational, longitudinal, and experimental—and highlights how each can contribute to better understanding existential experiences. He discusses the value of integrative methods, such as mixed methods and meta-analyses, for synthesizing findings and refining theory. He also considers judgment calls, such as whether to build upon prior measurement or manipulation techniques or to develop new ones and whether to collect data in the natural setting, in the lab, or online. Lastly, he concludes by considering best practices in psychological science more broadly.

Section II: Death, Aging, and Time

Section II focuses on mortality awareness, near-death experiences, suicide, limited time perspectives, nostalgia, and adult development and aging.

Three chapters consider death-related dynamics. In Chapter 6, Solomon and colleagues provide an overview of roughly 40 years of research on terror management theory (TMT), which posits the awareness of mortality motivates investment in cultural worldviews and pursuit of self-esteem. The authors outline TMT's development, empirical support, applications, criticisms, and refinements, and highlight its relevance to politics, health, mental illness, and culture. In Chapter 7, Lifshin and colleagues further apply TMT to consider how our interaction with nature—including the environment, animals, and our own bodies—can provoke complicated death-related existential dynamics, with implications for animal welfare, intergroup relationships, psychological well-being, and spirituality. In Chapter 8, Tassell-Matamua and colleagues discuss near-death experiences, highlighting their transformative impact on self-concepts, worldviews, and meaning. Near-death experiences often lead to reduced death anxiety, increased spirituality, and a deeper sense of purpose. The authors consider neurological and psychological explanations and highlight implications for promoting personal growth and reflection.

Three chapters consider TMT's implications for mental and physical health, including suicide. In Chapter 9, Menzies describes evidence that death anxiety is a transdiagnostic factor underlying various mental health disorders, including anxiety, mood, obsessive–compulsive, and trauma-related conditions. Drawing on TMT, she emphasizes the need for psychological treatments that directly target death anxiety, highlighting therapeutic approaches such as cognitive-behavioral therapy, acceptance and commitment therapy, and existential psychotherapy. In Chapter 10, Courtney and colleagues describe research on the terror management health model, which explains how mortality awareness influences physical health behavior. When death is consciously salient, people adopt "proximal" defenses, either health-promoting or threat-denying. When death thought is nonconsciously accessible, "distal" defenses guide behavior toward cultural values and self-esteem. The authors consider how culturally meaningful, esteem-based framing can promote better engagement with healthy behaviors. In Chapter 11, Hayes and Tupper consider why people die by suicide. As people are aware the goal to continue living is inevitably futile, the propensity to withdraw from that goal is ever-present. The pursuit of symbolic permanence can promote engagement with life, but obstructions and failures can lead to hopelessness and suicidal withdrawal. The authors discuss implications for suicide prevention and therapeutic intervention.

In Chapter 12, Quirin and Northoff review research on the neuropsychological basis of various existential psychological dynamics related to death, but also uncertainty, freedom, identity, authenticity, love, self-connectedness, meaning, and will or volition. Adopting a monistic brain-mind perspective, this chapter integrates psychological and neuroscience perspectives to better understand how existential experiences arise from brain activity. Brain structures such as the medial prefrontal cortex, anterior insula, amygdala, and the ventral striatum operate during existential experiences involving uncertainty, mortality salience, and latent angst; the ventral and dorsomedial striatum, medial prefrontal cortex, and amygdala are involved in love, attachment, and isolation; the medial prefrontal cortex, posterior cingulate cortex, precuneus, right anterior insula, and ventral striatum are involved in self and identity development and authenticity; the superior temporal gyrus, medial and dorsolateral prefrontal cortex, amygdala, anterior cingulate cortex, anterior insula, and precuneus are involved in absurdity and meaning making; and the medial prefrontal and dorsolateral prefrontal cortices are involved in will. The authors consider the implications and discuss future directions.

Three chapters cover savoring limited time, nostalgia, and aging. In Chapter 13, Kurtz and Murphy explain how perceived temporal scarcity can increase motivation to appreciate positive moments and savor experiences, with implications for happiness, sociability, and well-being. In Chapter 14, Sedikides and Wildschut tackle nostalgia—the sentimental longing for the past—and research showing it fosters meaning, social connectedness, and engagement in culture; impacts motivation and behavior; and buffers against death-related thoughts and emotions. In Chapter 15, Maxfield considers research on general perceptions of aging and older adults, age-related variations in how people handle the awareness of mortality, shifts in existential concerns over the lifespan, and how life experiences and existential concerns impact attitudes toward end-of-life planning and care.

Section III: Freedom, Authenticity, and Moral Responsibility

Section III focuses on experiences of autonomy and authenticity, choice and choosing, and the role of free will beliefs in perceiving agency, moral responsibility, and self-conscious emotions such as guilt, shame, and pride.

Five chapters focus on free will, autonomy, and authenticity. In Chapter 16, Zhao discusses cross-cultural developmental research on children's understanding of choice and beliefs about free will. In Chapter 17, Baumeister considers theory and research on free will, focusing on the evolved capacity for humans, as conscious and cultural animals, to effectively navigate complex social situations by exerting self-control and rational choice. These features are either free will or what is mistaken for free will; either way, he argues, they create the experience of existential agency. In Chapter 18, Ryan and Ryan discuss self-determination theory (SDT) and its relations with core existential themes and issues, including the phenomenology of autonomy, the role of awareness in self-regulation and wellness, authenticity in relationships, fulfilling and nonfulfilling life goals, and existential buffers to death anxiety. SDT research suggests that the key to eudaimonic living lies in reflectively addressing internal and external values and selectively embracing those that satisfy basic psychological needs for autonomy, competence, and relatedness. In Chapter 19, Sheldon considers the experience of authenticity, as an integration of conscious and nonconscious information processing, and the selection and pursuit of self-concordant goals. In Chapter 20, Schlegel and Rivera consider the role of the "true self" concept in authenticity and meaning. Although unlikely that a "true self" exists, in an ontological sense, people believe it is one's "essence" and is stable over time, causally powerful, and morally good. Thus, research suggests perceived authenticity is perhaps less about self-consistency and more about expressing self-enhancing, aspirational, or meaningful behaviors.

The next three chapters explore too little, too much, and a "happy medium" of freedom of choice. In Chapter 21, Rosenberg and colleagues cover research showing that perceived restrictions of personal freedom trigger reactance—the anger-based motivation to restore autonomy, often through oppositional defiance. The authors review foundational theory and research, measurement, and applications to clinical psychology, communication, and health interventions, and discuss strategies for managing or leveraging reactance, such as inoculation, providing compliance options, and triggering reactance as a persuasive strategy (colloquially known as "reverse psychology"). In Chapter 22, Cheek covers theory and research finding that too many options can create choice overload; too many choices can create decision fatigue; and too many types of choices can create self-uncertainty and a burden of self-expression. In such situations, freedom can be unpleasant and can motivate efforts to "escape" it such as by reducing self-awareness or delegating one's decision-making responsibility to surrogates. In Chapter 23, Reutskaja and Misuraca highlight research on benefits and costs of choice and the "inverted-U" model—finding that too few or too many options can be problematic, whereas a moderate "happy medium" number of choices is motivating, yields the best decision-making outcomes, and is most satisfying.

Two chapters then focus on free will beliefs and moral responsibility. In Chapter 24, Seto discusses research on the definition and function of free will beliefs among lay people. Free will is typically understood as the ability to make a choice and pursue an outcome when one could have done otherwise. Belief in free will is widespread, and research shows it is important for holding people morally responsible for their actions and for motivating personal agency. In Chapter 25, Tracy and colleagues consider self-conscious emotions, which rise and fall as the standards of one's moral identity are met or surpassed (pride) or violated (guilt, shame), and which motivate behavior to either continue or rectify the situation. Research finds people feel guilt about negative outcomes of their behavior, shame about negative aspects of themselves, and authentic pride about individual or group achievements or prosocial actions congruent with their moral identity. The authors also consider other emotions such as envy, anger, gratitude, and awe.

Section IV: Isolation, Uncertainty, and Shared Reality

Section IV focuses on isolation and the role of social connection in the struggle to maintain a confident perception of truth and reality.

Two chapters explore existential isolation and shared reality. In Chapter 26, Bilal and Helm distinguish the objective self (tangible attributes) from the subjective, agentic self who perceives, interprets, and reacts to the world. Feeling alone in one's subjective experience can make it seem difficult to know, for certain, whether one is accurately perceiving and interpreting reality as it "truly" is, and whether one is "truly" connected with others in a common shared experience. Research finds that existential isolation experiences are commonplace, especially among members of minority groups, and related to a host of epistemic and social processes. In Chapter 27, Masi and Echterhoff review research finding that maintaining a shared reality with others—co-constructing reality and validating each other's experiences—serves important epistemic and affiliative needs and provides a foundation for healthy and meaningful engagement in the world. Sharing subjective experiences reduces uncertainty in beliefs about people and the world, helps people interpret and understand events, and brings sharers closer and improves relationship quality.

Three chapters consider the motivations to reduce epistemic uncertainty at the intrapersonal, interpersonal, and group levels. In Chapter 28, Bonarska and colleagues first discuss research on motivations for knowledge acquisition and cognitive closure, shaping the formation of attitudes and impressions, social judgments, and social processes such as empathy, communication, and persuasion. Then they cover research on the mechanisms of epistemic uncertainty reduction, such as information relevance and the availability of cognitive processing resources. Finally, they describe research on social factors affecting the process, such as perceived epistemic authority of the communicator and the inertia of one's prior belief. In Chapter 29, Anjewierden and colleagues explore research suggesting that motivation for epistemic uncertainty reduction, especially uncertainty about one's self-concept and identity, has major societal implications. The authors review research showing people can effectively reduce uncertainty through identification with groups, clarifying the characteristics of uncertainty-reducing groups, and exploring the consequences for leadership, social influence, polarization, and extremism. In Chapter 30, McGregor offers a neuromotivational account of how uncertainty might sometimes lead to hostile extremism by triggering reactive approach motivation.

Three chapters address the existential dynamics of social connections and isolation. In Chapter 31, Mikulincer and Shaver cover research on three core existential dynamics of interpersonal attachment. First, people respond to existential stressors by seeking the proximity and support of competent and benevolent others. Second, the availability of loving support from others, and the resulting security, helps people navigate existential distress. And third, such security allows people to experience autonomy, self-continuity, meaning, and personal growth. In Chapter 32, Wicks and colleagues present research showing ostracism (being ignored and excluded) aggravates existential concerns and triggers responses in three distinct stages. First, a reflexive stage involves immediate and strong negative thoughts and painful feelings. Second, the reflective stage involves appraisals and attempts to repair the relationship or otherwise restore affiliation. If prolonged, people may enter the third stage of resignation. In Chapter 33, McKenna-Plumley and Groarke discuss research showing that existential loneliness, which is distinct from social and emotional loneliness, involves a feeling of profound separation from others and can generate feelings of deep emptiness, sadness, and longing. The chapter focuses on how existential loneliness is experienced at a range of stages across the lifespan.

Section V: Culture, Self, and Identity

Section V explores how culturally shared existential dynamics shape self and identity, how existential dynamics of self and identity shape sociocultural phenomena, and the self-construction of identity and personality.

Three chapters address culture, self, and meaning. In Chapter 34, Heine and Mask cover research showing that meaning, in general, is about the perception of coherent relationships among objects and events in the world, and that people live in shared (cultural) ecologies of meaning. Likewise, meaning in life is shaped by connections with other people, with one's work, and with broader transcendent concepts. The authors cover cross-cultural differences, but also similarities, in sources of meaning in life. In Chapter 35, Landau and colleagues note that important existential concerns are conceptually abstract and difficult to grasp, so people cultivate metaphors to construct a meaningful understanding of themselves and the world around them. They describe conceptual metaphor theory and research, addressing the influence of metaphor target and source framing, with an emphasis on self-continuity, self-esteem, and authenticity. In Chapter 36, Sullivan and colleagues discuss theory and research in cultural–existential psychology, organized around two major ideas. First, cultures represent shared definitions about which experiences and events are existentially threatening. Second, cultures represent shared approaches to interpreting and responding to existential threats, such as by prioritizing collective meaning at the expense of guilt or individual esteem at the expense of uncertainty.

Three chapters explore the bidirectional relationship between self-identity and cultural context. In Chapter 37, Rothschild and Keefer review research finding people can manage existential concerns about uncontrollable chaos and death by using moral outrage to construct a heroic moral identity. By identifying clear villains and expressing righteous anger in the name of justice, sometimes through scapegoating and localized enemyship, people can cultivate a sense of moral clarity, tractable agency, and a sense of enduring value and significance. In Chapter 38, Goldenberg and colleagues offer a feminist existential perspective on the objectification of women. They review research finding that women's bodily functions (e.g., menstruation, pregnancy, lactation) represent "creaturely" reminders of human corporeality, raising death-related existential motivation to control women's bodies and prioritize a contrived "Barbie-like" appearance. The chapter explores feminist ideas about the self-determined reclamation of the creaturely, mortal body. In Chapter 39, Sedikides and Schmader describe research on the state authenticity as fit to the environment (SAFE) model, finding that people feel authentic based on self-perceptual fluency (self-concept fit), motivational fluency (goal fit), and interpersonal fluency (social fit). Fit motivates engagement with situations, whereas misfit promotes disengagement, which may culminate in cultural self-segregation even in the absence of overt bias and discrimination.

Two chapters address the existential dynamics involved in the self-construction of identity. In Chapter 40, McAdams and Ture discuss narrative identity, the internalized and evolving story of the self, in which people construct meaningful interpretations of self and address concerns about death and freedom. They cover major theory and research advances through the lens of Sartre's "true novel," Becker's ideas about generativity, and Camus' ideas about life stories of acceptance. In Chapter 41, Xi and Jackson address existential themes of authenticity and self-creation in the tension between personality continuity and change. The chapter highlights key types of personality change, such as rank-order stability, mean-level change, structural changes, ipsative consistency, and idiographic changes. Importantly, mechanisms for personality development include intentional changes, such as when people consciously align their behaviors with evolving goals, values, and circumstances.

Section VI: Meaning and Purpose

Section VI focuses on the commonplace experience of meaning in everyday life, the experiences of aspects of meaning (coherence, purpose, significance) in various life domains, and the processes of maintaining, restoring, or searching for meaning.

Two chapters explore commonplace meaning in everyday life. In Chapter 42, Holberg and King define meaning in life and its facets (coherence, purpose, significance) and then review research on the way each facet is supported by common experiences in everyday life. They also consider how the three facets of meaning are intertwined (e.g., coherent understanding might energize purpose which might facilitate significance), and potentially interchangeable, before considering modern threats to meaning. In Chapter 43, Newman and Lutz describe research employing ecological momentary assessment, which measures meaning in-the-moment (vs. global or long-term recall assessments, influenced by memories of "peak" experiences) and illuminates within-person (vs. between-person/group) processes. This research suggests, for example, that people view their life as more meaningful when assessing it globally but perhaps less so during mundane lived experiences.

Four chapters more closely explore coherence, significance, and purpose in various life domains. In Chapter 44, Womick and colleagues review research finding that right-wing political beliefs, including conservativism, system justification, just-world beliefs, and right-wing authoritarianism, are largely about enhancing a sense of significance rather than coherence or purpose. Interestingly, research does not find a similar pattern among left-wing political views, raising important questions about how coherence, purpose, and significance manifest in left-leaning political orientations. In Chapter 45, Zarzeczna and Haimila explore how religion and science function as important meaning-making tools, and review research finding their incompatibility stems from their different answers to the same ontological and epistemological questions. Further, religion and science likely exert non-overlapping psychological leverage, in terms of coherence, purpose, and significance, such that their perceived incompatibility can negatively impact believers and lead to science rejection. In Chapter 46, Needy and colleagues review research distinguishing sociocultural significance (lasting impact on the world) and experiential significance (valuable/fulfilling activities). They review factors influencing the detection/overlooking of significance as well as frequent elicitors of significance, such as positive affect, epistemic emotions (curiosity, wonder, awe), creativity, mindfulness, nostalgia, care, prosociality, and authenticity. Last, they consider the interplay and balance of developmental, sociocultural, and intrapersonal factors. In Chapter 47, Oettingen explains how a self-regulatory process of mental contrasting affects purpose and goal pursuit, a process involving identifying a desired future outcome contrasted against anticipated present and future obstacles. Unfeasible goals are dropped, whereas feasible goals are retained. Combined with implementation intentions (if–then plans), the pursuit of such goals can imbue life with a meaningful sense of purpose.

Four chapters explore the ways people typically maintain meaning, restore meaning in adversity, and generally search for meaning. In Chapter 48, Igou and colleagues address boredom, the aversive experience of being unable or unwilling to allocate attention to subjectively meaningless activities. Research finds boredom triggers self-regulatory mechanisms to prevent inaction, avoid meaningless action, and enhance meaningful action. In Chapter 49, Russo-Netzer and Schulenberg consider a variety of strategies for constructing and maintaining micro- and macro-level meaning, including motivational, narrative, therapeutic, and cross-cultural influences. In Chapter 50, Park discusses research finding that when stressful events occur (e.g., unemployment, illness, natural disaster) people appraise its situational meaning, evaluate its magnitude of violation of global meaning, engage in a compensatory meaning-making process, and potentially restore meaning or adopt new meanings. Park reviews the nuances of each step and implications for resilience to adversity. In Chapter 51, Steger and Marsh provide a major review of theory and research on the search for meaning. The chapter provides definitional clarity, reviews research substantiating the absence-to-search and search-to-presence models, and—in terms of functional well-being—finds that search for meaning may be negative, neutral, or positive depending on the context (e.g., age, culture).

Section VII: Religion and Spirituality

Section VII focuses on the roles of death and freedom in religion, nonreligious existential dynamics, and religious/spiritual struggles and anomalous experiences.

Two chapters cover the roles of death and freedom in religion. In Chapter 52, Vail and colleagues review research finding that death awareness motivates faith in core religious supernatural concepts (e.g., souls, gods, afterlife) and worldview defense such as supporting fellow believers, rejecting heathens, accommodating alternatives, assimilating converts, and annihilating threatening others. Research also finds these processes are impacted by skepticism (e.g., atheism) and faith orientations that vary in form and function (e.g., intrinsic/extrinsic, fundamentalism, quest). In Chapter 53, Green and colleagues explore the complexity of free will in religious faith. Religious believers typically have stronger belief in free will than less religious people have, but also selectively defer responsibility to their deity. Attributing responsibility to a deity may reduce one's perceived agency in exchange for reduced incoherence (divine plan), a sense of divine purpose, and a sense of divine significance.

Two chapters address nonreligious existential dynamics. In Chapter 54, Van Tongeren considers religious deidentification and various nonreligious identities, and reviews research on "religious residue," which is the persistence of cognitive, emotional, and behavioral patterns after religious deidentification among the formerly religious. Leaving religion can trigger new existential banes (e.g., angst, dread) but also boons (e.g., freedom, awe). In Chapter 55, Galen covers research finding nonreligious people can cultivate secular ways of life that guide their choices and inform their sense of moral responsibility, manage death-related concerns, bolster shared reality, build culture and identity, and promote meaning and purpose. Galen also argues the presumed existential benefits of religion for well-being and prosociality are often due to basic sociocultural factors, rather than belief content, which could be leveraged by secular cultures as well.

Two chapters consider religious/spiritual struggles and anomalous experiences. In Chapter 56, Exline and Pargament consider the existential dynamics of religious/spiritual struggles, such as difficulty with choices and following moral principles (freedom/moral struggle); confusion about beliefs (doubt struggle); anger or conflict within religious communities (social struggle); feeling attacked by the devil (demonic struggle); feeling angry or fearful about God (divine struggle); and whether one's life has any ultimate purpose (meaning struggle). The chapter addresses measurement, prevalence, and implications for mental and physical well-being, as well as the question of whether religious/spiritual struggles lead to growth. In Chapter 57, Hood and Dinsmore discuss anomalous or mystical experiences. As in this chapter, the topic is often addressed in ways that flout modern science to remain open to the possibility that such experiences might be "true glimpses" of another world. Nevertheless, the chapter briefly describes the importance and history of anomalous experiences—which we hope will put the topic on the map for more objective study by the science of existential psychology.

Section VIII: Awe, Growth, and the Good Life

Section VIII focuses on awe and personal growth, the good life, and existential psychotherapy.

Three chapters consider existential awe and growth dynamics. In Chapter 58, Edwards and Van Cappellen cover theory and research on awe—the perception of vastness that challenges and expands one's existing conceptualizations of the world, ranging in experience from negative and self-diminishing to positive and grounding. Awe can lead to a quiet and transcendent self, both existential isolation and connection, and can influence one's sense of coherence, purpose, and significance. In Chapter 59, Bauer explores the narrative identity of the transformative self, which features elements of narration (tone, theme, structure) that cultivate humanistic qualities of a good life—such as purpose, well-being, and wisdom. Although transformative self-narratives come in countless forms, they share features of thematic motives directed toward engaged experiencing and curiosity-driven reflection for oneself and others. In Chapter 60, Winet and O'Brien review research on repeat consumption of familiar, rather than novel, experiences, such as revisiting one's favorite movies, music, books, or cafés again and again. Repeat consumption can lead to growth through novel appreciation of the experience itself (e.g., seeing new connections in a book plot) and of oneself (e.g., shaping new self-concepts, identities, beliefs and values).

Two chapters consider existential dynamics of the good life. In Chapter 61, Martela considers the pursuit of happiness. Research finds that although happiness is generally associated with good things, the *pursuit* of happiness can, ironically, lead to reduced positive affect and even depressive symptoms. Martela notes that existential approaches to happiness typically regard it as the possible side-effect of the pursuit of meaning in life and a life well lived. In Chapter 62, Janey and Oishi review a broad swath of research suggesting the good life entails more than just hedonic well-being (e.g., happiness) and eudaimonic well-being (e.g., meaning in life); it also includes psychological richness—diverse, interesting experiences. Thus, the good life may be composed of happiness, meaning, and novelty.

The final three chapters consider the philosophy, research, and practice of existential psychotherapy. In Chapter 63, Aho and colleagues first cover the historical context and core philosophical ideas. Then, they describe research on eudaimonic well-being, purposeful life engagement, and the realization of personal potential. Next, they discuss Global Existential Summits, which focus on lived experiences in diverse contexts. Finally, they offer some critical reflections about the field. In Chapter 64, Schneider and colleagues describe existential–humanistic and existential–integrative psychotherapies. They cover the roots, basic principles, and expanded applications to therapy, multicultural diversity, and social crises. They also identify some relevant areas for research, such as existential psychotherapeutic intervention components, mechanisms, and outcomes. In Chapter 65, Van Tongeren and Showalter Van Tongeren offer a novel model of existential hope for working with clients who are suffering: an approach that is humble (engages honestly with reality), optimistic (anticipates positive outcomes), participatory (promotes meaningful engagement), and existential (engages with existential concerns). They also identify testable hypotheses and discuss practical clinical applications of the approach.

GOALS OF THIS HANDBOOK

Many of the field's initial advances were discussed in the *Handbook of Experimental Existential Psychology* (Greenberg et al., 2004). But in the 20-plus years since its publication, an enormous amount of new theory has been developed and new research conducted. Yet, over these two decades no handbook has attempted to cover the breadth and depth of those exciting advances. Thus, a new anthology providing an update on the state of the field's theory and research is not only necessary—it's long overdue.

Additionally, given that the previous anthology on the topic was produced when the field was still just emerging, casual observers may be under the impression that the science of existential psychology is still an emerging, small, niche, or "specialty" topic. However, as can be seen in this handbook, that is not the case anymore. The field has grown into a robust and expansive enterprise over the past several decades. Researchers are now studying existential psychological dynamics across a broad range of many areas—social and personality, developmental, cognitive, affective, neuroscience, health, clinical/counseling, and many others. Indeed, existential psychological dynamics are of broad importance across nearly all areas of psychological science.

Thus, the goals of the present handbook are to provide a much-needed update on the state of the field, while demonstrating that the science of existential psychology has an incredibly broad relevance across many important areas of contemporary psychological science. We hope the volume encourages readers to see the value of studying existential psychological dynamics, recognize those dynamics can be studied using the full force of mainstream qualitative and quantitative research methods available in modern psychological science, and build on the recent advances described here to help push the science of existential psychology forward in productive new directions.

REFERENCES

Chen, J., Sedikides, C., & Cai, H. (2022). Self-affirmation reduces vigilance to mortality threat: An eye-tracking study. *Asian Journal of Social Psychology, 25,* 219–226.

Cox, C. R., Darrell, A., & Arrowood, R. B. (2019). The method behind the science: A guide to conducting terror management theory research. In C. Routledge & M. Vess (Eds.), *The handbook of terror management theory* (pp. 85–132). Elsevier.

George, L. S., & Park, C. L. (2017). The Multidimensional Existential Meaning Scale: A tripartite approach to measuring meaning in life. *Journal of Positive Psychology, 12*(6), 613–627.

Greenberg, J., Koole, S. L., & Pyszczynski, T. (Eds.). (2004). *Handbook of experimental existential psychology.* Guilford Press.

Henry, E. A., Bartholow, B. D., & Arndt, J. (2010). Death on the brain: Effects of mortality salience on the neural correlates of ingroup and outgroup categorization. *Social Cognitive and Affective Neuroscience, 5,* 77–87.

Koole, S. L., Greenberg, J., & Pyszczynski, T. (2006). Introducing science to the psychology of the soul: Experimental existential psychology. *Current Directions in Psychological Science, 15,* 212–216.

Lester, D. (1994). The Collett–Lester Fear of Death Scale. In R. A. Neimeyer (Ed.), *Death anxiety handbook: Research, instrumentation, and application* (pp. 45–60). Taylor & Francis.

Maxfield, M., Peckham, A., & James, D. L. (2024). "Terror is a better word": A qualitative analysis of dementia-related anxiety. *The Gerontologist, 64*(5), gnad146.

Menzies, R. E., & Dar-Nimrod, I. (2017). Death anxiety and its relationship with obsessive-compulsive disorder. *Journal of Abnormal Psychology, 126,* 367–377.

Peters, H. J., Greenberg, J., Williams, J. M., & Schneider, N. R. (2005). Applying terror management theory to performance: Can reminding individuals of their mortality increase strength output? *Journal of Sport and Exercise Psychology, 27,* 111–116.

SECTION I

PHILOSOPHICAL ROOTS, SCIENTIFIC METHODS

CHAPTER 1

The Role of Death in Becoming Subjective and Cultivating Meaning in Kierkegaard

Sophie Höfer *and* Adam Buben

As a thinker of death and meaning in life, Søren Kierkegaard has a profound influence on 20th-century existentialism, most notably inspiring Martin Heidegger's account of authentic Being-toward-death in *Being and Time*.[1] Kierkegaard's authorship discusses the themes of mortality and death in various places, and the variety of these discussions reflects "his remarkable, lifelong preoccupation with death, dying, and the dead" (Stokes & Buben, 2011, p. 1). These themes appear in both his pseudonymous and signed works, in more and less explicitly religious contexts, and in both literal and metaphorical senses, all of which contributes to the difficulty of understanding his thoughts on them.[2] In order to keep things manageable (and broadly relevant) in this chapter, while also touching on death's place in Kierkegaard's influential notion of cultivating subjectivity, or meaningful selfhood, it will help to focus on just two works, most importantly the discourse "At a Graveside."[3] This discourse contains his clearest, least explicitly religious, and most sustained elaboration on the topic of mortality, and it has been considered "one of the high points of European thinking about death" (Theunissen, 2006, p. 321). Part of a collection named *Three Discourses on Imagined Occasions*, the graveside discourse was published in 1845, just a year before Kierkegaard makes mortality a central element in the discussion of "becoming subjective" in his pseudonymous magnum opus, *Concluding Unscientific Postscript to "Philosophical Fragments"* (henceforth *Postscript*). For Kierkegaard, like many of the later so-called existentialists he inspires, humans are not born selves or subjects in any meaningful sense; authentic subjectivity is something one must work at throughout life, and death will be perhaps the greatest taskmaster one encounters along the way. To illustrate why the right sort of reflection on death is so impactful, we begin with a literary example of the perils of ignoring such reflection.

NOT GIVING DEATH ITS DUE

It is not unusual to see "At a Graveside" put into conversation with Lev Tolstoy's *The Death of Ivan Ilyich*, given the temporal proximity of their origins and some clearly overlapping existential themes. However, since this comparison has already been done to death (pun definitely intended), we thought it might be worthwhile to put Kierkegaard in touch with a similarly relevant, but lesser-known, 19th-century work of fiction. Hugo von Hofmannsthal's lyrical drama *The Fool and Death* (*Der Tor und der Tod*) was published in 1893 and depicts the aesthete Claudio's encounter with his own death. The story has a hint of autobiography to it in that it reflects the Austrian writer's own inability to create a unity between his artistic activity and his personal life (Porter, 1972, pp. 20–21). The drama begins with a scene in which Claudio laments his "missed life" (Hofmannsthal, 2015, p. 8).[4] He describes his own existence as a "dream" and "semblance" and himself as "born mute on the inside," and even though he leads an apparently carefree life, he has always failed to immerse himself in the world in the same way as those around him (p. 12): "What am I supposed to know about human life? / Surely, I seem to have stood in it, / But I have understood it at best, / Could never weave myself into it. / Have never lost myself in it" (p. 9). While ordinary people delight in nature, work, and each other's company, Claudio, having "never drunk the true potion of life," can only yearningly observe them from a distance (p. 9). The cause of his alienation and fragmentation is his artistic activity, which has put him at an aesthetic distance from true life: "I have lost myself in artificiality in such a way, / That I saw the sun with dead eyes / And heard nothing more than through dead ears" (p. 12). He knows he must change something about his life, but he cannot get himself to do it.

Claudio's melancholic reflections are interrupted by the arrival of Death, who appears personified as a male figure with a violin and comes to see him in his room. As soon as Claudio recognizes him, he is seized by dread and commands Death to leave. Death reveals to him that his final hour has struck, whereupon Claudio responds that he is not ready yet: "For me it's still a while away! . . . I haven't lived! . . . So my young days slipped away / And I never knew that this is already what it means to live" (p. 19). Death, however, is unimpressed with Claudio's attempt to delay the matter, explains to him that he was granted the same chance to make something of his life as everyone else, and chastises him: "Woe to you if I have to be the one to tell you that!" (p. 20). When Claudio realizes that he is actually about to die, he is torn from the melancholic inactivity that had hitherto characterized his life. Panic takes hold of him, and he desperately tries to negotiate with Death: "But I am not ripe, so leave me here. / I will no longer complain foolishly, / I will cling to this clod, / The deepest longing for life is crying out within me. / The highest fear tears the old spell; / Now I feel—leave me—that I can live!" (p. 20). In the moment of his death, Claudio is being seized by an unprecedented desire for life. He can finally break free from his aesthetically distant contemplation of the world and fully devote himself to his existence. Determinedly, he resolves to change his life at this very moment and implores Death to give him a little more time to put his plan into action. Death, however, gets angry and decides to teach Claudio a lesson by showing him the consequences of his wasted life: "You fool! You insolent fool, I shall teach you / To honor life for once before it is over. / . . . And learn that all the others / Have sprung from this clod with a loving earthly spirit, / And only you yourself are boastingly loud and empty" (p. 22). Subsequently, he summons three people from Claudio's life who have already passed away—his mother, his lover, and a childhood friend—and makes him painfully aware of the suffering that Claudio caused them with his cold-heartedness and indifference. When he realizes that, in his entire life, he has not felt any genuine love or care for another person and that there is no way to make up for it, Claudio repents of his selfishness: "Why, o Death / Must you be the one to teach me how to see life, / Not as though through a veil, awake and whole, / And pass by like this, generating something?" (p. 29). His death pushes him toward resolution and activity, and before he falls dead to the ground, Claudio cries out: "Since my life was dead—be thou my life, o Death!" (p. 30). Even though he is aware of his own estrangement and disconnection before encountering his death, it is only dying that truly brings him back to life.

Hofmannsthal's drama provides an insightful illustration of what it means to relate ourselves to our own mortality, and one that (as we will see) has many parallels with what Kierkegaard says about this relationship. When confronting death, the aesthete realizes that he has wasted his life, and Death becomes the judge that weighs the value or meaning of his existence up to this moment. The terror that Claudio experiences upon encountering Death is not to be interpreted so much as a fear of death, but rather as the sorrow and remorse that comes with understanding he has lived his life in the wrong way. Paradoxically, the hour of death becomes an hour filled with vitality that urges him to live fully. The tragic element of the story, then, lies in the fact that Claudio cannot change anything about his life anymore. While he wants to put his newfound resolutions immediately into action, death makes this impossible—his repentance comes too late. His failure to confront his mortality during his lifetime takes a toll at the moment of death and Claudio must die unreconciled with the knowledge that he has lived a misguided life. This is precisely the scenario that Kierkegaard means to help his readers avoid.

DEATH AS A SUBJECTIVE PROBLEM OF EXISTENCE

Kierkegaard's thought on mortality is characterized by a blurring of the usual strict distinction between life and death. Rather than being an event waiting for us in some more or less distant future that has no impact whatsoever on the present, Kierkegaard considers death a meaningful part of our existence that is intimately tied up with our everyday activities. In *Postscript*, one's own mortality is presented as an existence problem with which the aspiring subjective thinker must grapple before being able to move on to more abstract and theoretical endeavors. According to Kierkegaard's (1992, pp. 165–166) pseudonym Johannes Climacus, objective, factual, and speculative thinking are all insufficient to grasp what death actually means:

> On that topic [of death] I know what people ordinarily know: that if I swallow a dose of sulfuric acid I will die, likewise by drowning myself or sleeping in coal gas etc. I know that Napoleon always carried poison with him, that Shakespeare's Juliet took it; that the Stoics regarded suicide as a courageous act and others regard it as cowardice. . . . However, despite this almost extraordinary knowledge or proficiency of knowledge, I am by no means able to regard death as something I have understood.

None of those facts explain what is at stake in the question of death, and whatever we might ordinarily know about death as a general phenomenon has nothing to do with the kind of existential grappling with our own mortality that Climacus (and Kierkegaard more broadly) envisions. For the task of subjectivity—"the highest task assigned to a human being"—it is necessary that we understand ourselves in relation to our mortality, which is an intrinsic feature of our existence (Kierkegaard, 1992, p. 129). In order to do so, we must think about death not in general terms, but as our own death, since "*my* dying is by no means something in general" (Kierkegaard, 1992, p. 167). Climacus goes on to demonstrate that understanding one's own death along subjective rather than objective lines is an incredibly protracted and complex task:

> there is the question about what death is and what it is for the living person, how the idea of it must change a person's whole life if he . . . must think it every moment in order thereby to prepare himself for it. Then there is the question about what it means to prepare oneself for it. . . . And then there is the question of an ethical expression for the meaning of death, a religious expression for vanquishing it. (Kierkegaard, 1992, pp. 168–169)

In *Postscript*, these fundamental questions are raised but not answered, and just like all problems of existence Climacus discusses, it remains the task of the reader to reflect about them on their own. What is important about the discussion of death in *Postscript* is that by indicating the insufficiency of objective knowledge about death, Climacus displaces the focus on death as a factual event and replaces it with existing in the light of finitude. Thus, his critique of factual approaches to death modifies the original object of the enquiry. A more elaborate, albeit still tentative, exploration of what mortal life means is found in "At a Graveside."

"At a Graveside" aims to alert its reader—or listener, as Kierkegaard addresses us—to the certainty of their death and to the necessity of relating to it in the right way. In a discourse that is primarily intended for edification, or more literally "upbuilding" (*opbygge*), Kierkegaard urges his listener to take on what he calls an earnest attitude toward death.[5] The most important feature of earnestness about death is thinking about one's own particular death and living in accordance with that thought. Thus, the earnest thought of death is essentially related to the subject thinking it. Kierkegaard (1993, p. 75) holds that we should approach death in such a way "that you think death, and that you are thinking it as your lot, and that you are then doing what death is indeed unable to do—namely, that you are and death also is." With this sideswipe at Epicurus, who famously claimed that death was nothing to fear since our life and our death never coincide, Kierkegaard pushes us to think about death as our own condition. According to him, Epicurus's (1994, p. 29) remark about death—"when we exist, death is not yet present, and when death is present, then we do not exist"—is nothing but a "jest" meant to mitigate the dread that comes with imagining his own death (Kierkegaard, 1993, p. 73).[6]

Kierkegaard clearly recognizes the varied strategies human beings employ to put death at a distance. Most of us avoid the uncomfortable thought of death altogether, and if we do consider it, we might just think about it as a necessary feature of biological life, or as the price we all have to pay for being alive. However, thinking about death in such objective terms is insufficient for a subjective engagement with *my own death* as the end of *my very particular existence*, which cannot be captured in abstractions and generalizations.[7] As already indicated in the *Postscript* passages above, as well as in Kierkegaard's dismissal of the Epicurean approach, such a detached understanding of death is deeply misleading and often unproductive. Kierkegaard (see 1993, p. 73) considers it insufficient to think about death as an abstract phenomenon that does not affect oneself, or as the general human condition without at the same time realizing that this condition also applies to oneself. Our tendency to evade thinking about our mortality is even present when we are forcefully confronted with it. "Even in the moment of death," Kierkegaard (1993, p. 79) notices, "the dying person thinks that he still might have some time to live" (consider, for example, Hofmannsthal's Claudio). However, in order for death to have a meaningful impact on our lives, we need to be shaken out of indifference and false comfort with respect to it. Rather than distracting or deceiving ourselves, we need to become aware of our own death as an inescapable truth about existence: "to be wide awake and to think death, . . . to think that all was over, that everything was lost along with life, in order then to win everything in life—this is earnestness" (p. 76).

Throughout the graveside discourse, Kierkegaard develops a distinction between earnestness and moods, which are nonearnest ways of engaging with death. Here it also becomes clear that, for Kierkegaard, the way a person views death is indicative of the way they approach life: Moods often contain a self-deceptive component and serve to neutralize and diminish some of the disruptive, yet upbuilding, power of death within one's life. In moods, we either fail to think about our own specific death, as is the case with the objective-speculative thinker in *Postscript*, or we appropriate this thought in the wrong way, as in a Romantic longing for death.[8] The former failure is perhaps somewhat controversial, as Kierkegaard (1993, pp. 73–75) quite radically claimed that if we experience someone else's death, as long as we do not think about it as our own condition, we will remain caught up in mood. The loss of a loved one, the witnessing of a catastrophe involving casualties, or even the daily experience of war are by themselves insufficient to qualify as earnest engagements with death. Such experiences may cause grief, pain, and sorrow, but not earnestness, although it has been argued that they may well catalyze an earnest relation with death.[9] Nonetheless, the inherent severity and gravity of the event of someone else's death, no matter how important that person might have been for someone, is simply not enough to be considered earnest (see

Kierkegaard, 1993, p. 75). For Kierkegaard, what matters is that the individual appropriates the thought of *their own death* in such a way that they understand themselves in light of their mortality.

Kierkegaard's discussion of moods covers a wide range of inappropriate, ineffective, inaccurate, and self-deceptive ways of thinking about and approaching death, but some of the most important examples seem to fall into the category that psychologists and social scientists talk about in terms of the denial of death awareness. As suggested above, Kierkegaard (1967, p. 335) thinks humans mostly "want to shove away the thought of death and shove death out of life as much as possible. Men desire to live as if there were no death." The two most prominent of the common "shoves" he notices involve the aforementioned swapping of a genuinely personal, subjective appropriation of one's own mortality for an impersonal, objective, or outsider's understanding of death, and putting off coming to terms with one's own death because one always feels like there will be more time. This procrastination or postponement is treated further in the following section, but these are hardly the only ways humans frequently fail to be honest with themselves about their own mortality and thereby end up living frivolous, unreflective, and superficial lives. Another one discussed below is the tendency for struggling individuals to convince themselves that death does not sound so bad in comparison with the trials and tribulations of life. This form of self-pity and self-deception, like thinking only objectively about mortality or putting it off altogether, is a clear sign that one is denying oneself a proper life-changing death awareness, that one is not thinking earnestly about death.

LIVING WITH THE EARNEST THOUGHT OF DEATH

An earnest approach to death, Kierkegaard believes, should profoundly transform the way we go about our lives. His call to think our own death is to be understood not as a speculative thought experiment or a melancholic dwelling on thoughts of death but as a driving force that compels us to action. In *Postscript*, Climacus emphasizes that

> for the subject it is an *act* to think his death . . . because the development of subjectivity consists precisely in this, that he, acting, works through himself in his thinking about his own existence, consequently that he actually thinks what is thought by actualizing it, consequently that he does not think for a moment: Now, you must keep watch every moment—but that he keeps watch every moment. (Kierkegaard, 1992, p. 169, emphasis added; cf. 1993, p. 83)

Ethical subjectivity is always an action and expresses itself in the *actualization* of a specific understanding. As all problems of subjective existence, the act of thinking death is not something we can ever be done with: "To be finished with life before life is finished with one is not to finish the task at all" (Kierkegaard, 1992, p. 164). Death needs to be thought into every moment of one's life; considering it only once in a while when the transience of life becomes the most obvious—for instance on the occasion of someone else's death or as a New Year's resolution—"is not to think it at all" (p. 166).[10] Rather, it is a task for one's whole life to which the subjective, earnest person must commit their whole way of being.

In order for death to gain actuality in one's life, certain aspects of death must be understood and appropriated in a correct way. A first necessary realization for an earnest existence is that death is both certain and uncertain: It will undoubtedly come, but when exactly and under what circumstances cannot be known (Kierkegaard, 1993, p. 93). While we might rely on statistical probabilities, youth, and health to convince ourselves that an imminent death is unlikely for us, the sense of security we gain from such calculations is false and essentially self-deceptive (p. 79).[11] There is no guarantee that death will wait for as long as we think it will, and we are lying to ourselves if we think we can postpone grappling with our own mortality for that reason. The uncertainty of death is something that should unsettle us, alert us, and serve as a wake-up call to action. When considered in a dialectical relationship to death's certainty, it becomes a uniquely profound guide for an earnest existence (much as Death becomes Claudio's teacher and judge): "No teacher is able to teach the pupil to pay attention to what is said the way the uncertainty of death does when it points to the certainty of death; and no teacher is able to keep the pupil's thoughts concentrated on the one object of instruction the way the thought of the uncertainty of death does when it practices the thought of the certainty of death" (p. 95). Further discussion of this matter is found in *Postscript*, where Climacus writes that the earnest thinker needs to make the "enthusiastic purpose for the whole life . . . dialectical in relation to the uncertainty of death" (Kierkegaard, 1992, p. 166). This means that all actions we plan to take must be evaluated in light of the fact that death—"suppose [it] were insidious enough to come tomorrow!"—could at any moment interrupt the activities we are engaged in, regardless of what point in our lives we are at (p. 166). This is why we should commit ourselves to projects that are intrinsically valuable, even if they remain uncompleted, and prioritize the manner in which we engage in our activities over their completion. In "At a Graveside," Kierkegaard (1941, pp. 106–107) writes:

> For with respect to the good use of time, it is not, in relation to the interruption of death, essential whether the time was long or short; and with respect to an essential activity, in relation to the interruption of death, it is not essential whether it was finished or only begun. . . . And so earnestness comes to consist in . . . choosing an activity which is not dependent upon whether a whole generation is granted to complete it well, or only a brief time to have begun it well.

Besides the certainty and uncertainty of death, "At a Graveside" discusses three further truths about death that the earnest individual needs to grasp. First, Kierkegaard (1993, p. 78) writes that death is "decisive." Throughout the discourse, he repeatedly emphasizes that with death, "all is over," and that earnestness means precisely "to think [death], to think that all is over, and that there comes a time when all is over" (p. 79). Death cannot be negotiated with, it cannot be postponed according to one's will, and it marks the end of human existence.[12] This shattering fact is not supposed to depress us, paralyze us, or—on the opposite side of the mood spectrum—awake in us a longing for death, but instead it should impel us forward in life:

> If it is certain that death exists, as it is; if it is certain that all is over in its finality . . . the earnest understanding is that if death is a night, then life is a day, and if it is not possible to labor in the night, then it is possible to work while it is day; and the brief but stimulating cry of earnestness is like death's brief cry: yet today. For when conceived in earnestness death gives energy to live as nothing else does; it makes a man awake and watchful as nothing else does. (Kierkegaard, 1941, p. 90)

Thus, earnestness recognizes that in death, "all is over"—but it also understands that this moment has not yet arrived, and that therefore "all is not over" (Kierkegaard, 1993, p. 85). As long as we can think death, we are still alive, and it is up to us to make something of our remaining time, especially because we do not know how long we have. The earnest thought of death gives meaning to life by creating a scarcity of time in which every moment, no matter how short, becomes infinitely valuable. The earnest thinker recognizes that they cannot afford to waste any more time and thus immediately acts instead of postponing essential tasks (p. 78). This recognition is what Claudio misses until the last minute when it is too late to act upon it. We can contrast him with the recently deceased shopkeeper Kierkegaard (p. 71) reminisces about at the very beginning of his discourse, who knew that he could not fulfil his religious duties after his death, and therefore made them a priority in his life. Important in this context is also Kierkegaard's (p. 83) argument that the earnest thought of death both urges us to act and simultaneously shows us what it is we should do: "the thought of death gives the earnest person the right momentum in life *and the right goal* toward which he directs his momentum" (our emphasis). Hence, there is always a double power in death: It shows which priorities to have and also teaches us to act upon these priorities. What becomes crucial here is the ethical relevance of the thought of death: One needs to act, but not for just anything—one needs to put one's life in service for the good.

Admittedly, outside of some scattered references to God, like the one just mentioned, Kierkegaard does not really specify what this good is in "At a Graveside." Rather, he focuses on the negative, disruptive element of the earnest thought of death; death highlights and shakes us out of the concerns we often uncritically get caught up in that simply do not matter. Given that time to complete projects cannot be guaranteed, as discussed previously, what we complete should not be the thing that matters most to us. Choosing tasks that are valuable regardless of whether or not they are completed is what brings true meaning to our lives on this account. But, of course, the nature of these tasks seems to vary according to individual interests, so it is possible we will learn some very different lessons about what specifically we should be doing from an earnest awareness of our mortality. For Claudio, love and intersubjective relationships stand in the center of his (too) late realization about a meaningful life, but this need not be the case. Thus, the guidance we get from Kierkegaard in "At a Graveside" is basically empty, and this is typical of existentialism, which tends to place an emphasis on the manner of relating to oneself and one's actions rather than the content of these actions—it is about the how and not the what (cf. Kierkegaard, 1992, pp. 199, 202–203). It is for this reason that earnestness, subjectivity, and related non-Kierkegaardian concepts like authenticity seem compatible with different attitudes and worldviews (including some questionable politics in Heidegger's case). The key point is that the earnest thought of death can pull us out of a thoughtless existence.

This is not to say Kierkegaard offers no specific content or guidance whatsoever, but for that one must look to later, more overtly religious texts, such as *Works of Love* and *Upbuilding Discourses in Various Spirits*, which follow not long after the graveside discourse (and come with all the standard qualms about relying on content from revealed religion). Even so, in contrast to some popular notions of where existentialism's supposed fixation on mortality leads, the decisiveness of death discussed in "At a Graveside" does not, for example, spark a nihilistic-hedonistic *carpe diem*-attitude centered around the maximization of pleasures in the here and now, in part because it still seems to belong to the ethical-religious sphere (cf. Kierkegaard, 1993, p. 83). As Patrick Stokes (2006, p. 409) puts it, "insofar as earnestness is therefore a feature of agency in which the self's will is fully and self-consciously collected into action . . . aesthetic earnestness would not, for Kierkegaard, have the self-conscious grounding necessary to qualify as earnestness at all."[13] In an earnest attitude toward our own deaths, we understand that death has an ethical claim on us in the here and now and strive to live up to the moral responsibility that it teaches us. This is how death acquires ongoing actuality in our ethical lives.

Another thing the earnest thinker must understand is that death makes everyone equal. Kierkegaard (1993, pp. 85–86) clarifies that the equality in question lies not in the fact that we are all going to die, since an equality that lies in annihilation would be no meaningful equality at all. Further, the thought of equality is not to be understood antagonistically, as in a spiteful anticipation of death because it will finally make the fortunate person equal to the one who had to suffer misfortunes in life. This attitude Kierkegaard (p. 87) calls a mood, "a cowardly craving of depression." Rather, death demonstrates to the earnest thinker that everyone is equal before God and teaches them to look beyond superficial differences (p. 89). In earnestness, comparison should not take place between people—who is more fortunate, richer, healthier—but between oneself and the task one still has to fulfil, which in turn again leads the earnest thinker to action: "No comparison has that impelling power and so reliably gives the urgent person the true direction as does the comparison the living person makes between himself and the equality of death" (p. 89). Summoning the earnest thought of death in the moments in which one is shattered and discouraged by life's dissimilarities will allow one to find comfort in the fundamental equality of every person before God that lies beneath all superficial differences (p. 90).

Lastly, earnestness needs to understand that death is inexplicable; it "itself explains nothing" (Kierkegaard, 1993, p. 96). All attempts to interpret death as having some meaning by itself, such that it is the best or worst thing that could happen to a person, are doomed to fail, since death marks the limits of our human understanding (p. 98).[14] Death does not tell us why it comes at this specific moment rather than at another one, or whether it is a good or bad thing that it came at this specific moment, or why it took hold of one person instead of another. Thus, the earnest person should be reluctant to have an opinion about death (p. 100). Since death itself is inexplicable, an objective or factual approach to death as ridiculed in *Postscript* is useless—death only has the interpretation we assign to it, and it therefore becomes a subjective problem. The only meaning of death is found in its relation to our life: "What is decisive about the explanation . . . is that it acquires retroactive power and actuality in the life of the living person; then death becomes a teacher to him" (p. 97). Kierkegaard (1941, p. 112) elaborates:

> The inexplicability is the boundary, and the significance of the utterance is to give the thought of death retroactive power, to make it impulsive in the life, because in the finality of death it is over, and because the uncertainty of death makes an inspection every moment. The inexplicability is therefore not a summons to guess riddles, an invitation to be ingenious, but the earnest admonition of death to the living: "I need no explanation, but do you consider that in this decision everything is over, and that it may at any moment be at hand; see, this is well worth your consideration."

Death's retroactive power is ultimately what makes it possible for us to integrate it into our existence. Michael Theunissen (2006, p. 350) calls this phenomenon the "material dialectic" of the graveside discourse: Death, not actually present when we still exist, only receives its power from the subject interpreting it in such a way that it gains actuality in their life. The earnest thought of death leads us back to ourselves, and our self-cultivation, by teaching us to take a close look at what we are doing and how we are doing it, and it is in this way that death can exercise its "impelling power" over our lives (Kierkegaard, 1993, p. 89).

CONCLUSION

Kierkegaard's work shows us the possibility of integrating death into our lives in a meaningful way. Through earnestness, the encounter with death can be anticipated and its lessons put into practice. The paralyzing regret in the moments before death, as experienced by Claudio in *The Fool and Death*, is thereby replaced with an active realization of life that one can consider meaningful. Instead of suppressing the thought of death, it is essential to keep it in mind throughout our lives in order to avoid the deeply tragic fate of Claudio. As he comes to understand too late, only death manages to show us the value of life, "Only when I die do I feel that I exist" (Hofmannsthal, 2015, p. 31). Like Kierkegaard, the message Hofmannsthal wants to convey is that "what gives life its meaning and beauty is the awareness of death throughout, not just in the last few moments" (Porter, 1972, p. 21). The constant presence of death in one's life is the constant call to self-reflect and take personal responsibility for oneself and the significance of one's choices and actions. In a passage one scholar uses to explain *The Death of Ivan Ilyich* but could just as well be used to discuss "At a Graveside" or *The Fool and Death*, "Death shows man the essence of his soul and teaches him to understand it; death compels man to review his life and to grasp its meaning. Death and the suffering preceding death are a means for knowing our own being, and through this we gain a consciousness of real existence" (Pachmuss, 1961, p. 80). For Kierkegaard, no less than for the authors of these other works, one must first confront one's own mortality and the fact that in death all will be over in order to then understand oneself as alive in the deepest meaning of the word.

NOTES

1. This is not to say that Heidegger considers himself to be an existentialist, which he does not, but he is often included in that group by later

commentators, who see a "family resemblance" in his discussion of topics such as anxiety, authenticity, facticity, freedom, and mortality. One of us has argued at length that the resemblance between Kierkegaard and Heidegger, especially when it comes to death and its impact on meaning and authenticity, is no mere coincidence. For a detailed analysis of how Heidegger appropriates Kierkegaard's ideas about these matters, see Buben (2013, 2016).

2. Kierkegaard (1992, p. [627]) makes use of pseudonyms in a peculiar way, and he asks that his readers recognize them and not himself as the authors of the texts he assigns to them. Because there are some perspectives and attitudes that Kierkegaard (1992, p. [625]) does not believe he can consistently inhabit and represent himself, he creates "poetically actual" personalities that possess the "psychological consistency," and embody the "life-view[s]," he does not. This idiosyncratic employment of pseudonymity creates many difficulties for interpreters of Kierkegaard's work. Fortunately, outside of honoring his request that the pseudonyms be treated as the authors of the works assigned to them, there should not be much related confusion in this chapter, as the main pseudonym discussed here (Johannes Climacus) is often seen as holding views not so far removed from Kierkegaard's own, and this seems especially true on the topic of death.

3. When quoting from this text, we are working with two different translations to avoid overreliance on one that would lead to copyright issues. For discussion of the topic of death in other works by Kierkegaard, most notably the pseudonymous *Either/Or*, see, for example, Stewart (2023, pp. 205–222) and Watkin (1990, pp. 66–75).

4. All quoted passages from Hofmannsthal's story are original translations by Sophie Höfer.

5. The Danish term *Alvor* that Kierkegaard employs here can be translated as "earnestness," "seriousness," or "gravity."

6. See Buben (2013, pp. 976–984; 2016) for a more elaborate explanation of how Kierkegaard breaks with the Epicurean tradition.

7. For a striking illustration of the difference between a generalized understanding of death and the thought of death applied to oneself, see the famous passage from *The Death of Ivan Ilyich*: "All his life the example of a syllogism he [Ivan] had studied in Kiesewetter's logic—'Caius is a man, men are mortal, therefore Caius is mortal'—had seemed to him to be true only in relation to Caius but in no way to himself. There was Caius the man, man in general, and it was quite justified, but he wasn't Caius and he wasn't man in general, and he had always been something quite, quite special apart from all other beings. . . . *And Caius is indeed mortal and it's right that he should die, but for me, Vanya, Ivan Ilyich, with all my feelings and thoughts—for me it's quite different. And it cannot be that I should die. It would be too horrible*" (Tolstoy, 2014, p. 77).

8. Recent scholarship suggests that the distinction between mood and earnestness does not have to be so rigid after all; there seems to be some ambiguity in Kierkegaard's work that might not be immediately evident in looking only at "At a Graveside." Michael Strawser (2023, p. 145), for instance, argues that earnestness can be intermixed with moods such as jest or nihilistic weakness. In a similar vein, David Law (2021, p. 63) points out that there might be room for—in Heideggerian terminology—"authentic moods," which can spark an earnest engagement with death, and he also notes that at various points in his authorship, Kierkegaard seems to consider earnestness itself a mood.

9. Kierkegaard's account of death has been criticized as overly individualistic, solitary, and self-obsessed. Theunissen (2006, p. 336), for instance, refers to Kierkegaard's treatment of the death of others in the graveside discourse as a "denigration of the dying of others," and multiple other commentators have noted the absence of relational aspects connected with death and dying, such as loss and mourning. Gordon Marino criticizes Kierkegaard for suggesting that we cannot learn anything meaningful from someone else's death. According to Marino (2011, p. 152), Kierkegaard neglects the fact that "moods, the grief and terror, can also be revelatory—can also be teachers." Drawing an unfavorable comparison with *The Death of Ivan Ilyich*, which does make a point of death's interpersonal side, Marino (p. 156) suggests that the thought of death can "humanize" us and that "a death awareness ought to have a positive impact on our relationship with other humans, making us better neighbors and more responsive to others." In the graveside discourse, however, "there is scarcely a word about the relationship between our death awareness and the ties that bind us," and Marino concludes that "for all of its brilliance, the discourse seems inhuman" (p. 158). Against Marino, one of us has argued elsewhere (Höfer, 2024) that the ethical tone of the graveside discourse, discussed briefly later in this chapter, has been neglected in criticisms like his, and that the earnest thought of death is more humanizing than he suggests. Furthermore, reading "At a Graveside" alongside a text like *Works of Love* makes it clear that Kierkegaard believes death can bring us closer together, and that it is deeply intertwined with neighborly love in his thought.

10. Climacus's encouragement to think death into every moment poses various questions that are left unanswered in *Postscript*, such as what exactly such a reflection looks like, how it is possible to conceive of our own nonexistence while we still exist, and how we can still act or think about other things if we are constantly supposed to have death on our minds. It is very well imaginable that such an awareness would simply paralyze us. Interpretive attempts to answer these questions have been made, for instance, in Mooney (2011), Muench (2011), Possen (2011), and Westphal (1996). Drawing on these four accounts, we understand Climacus's idea of the thought of death not as one that we necessarily have to be conscious of all the time, but rather as a background condition of our lives that guides the decisions we make.

11. This works the other way too. Perhaps, one might think, there is more certainty in the timing and circumstances of a planned death, such as a suicide or an execution, but there is also a risk of self-deception in this thought. Even a well-organized suicide attempt can fail to meet its objective, and the governor might always come through with an unexpected last-minute pardon (cf. Sartre, 1992, pp. 690–691). It seems the uncertainty of death is ineliminable.

12. The fact that neither "At a Graveside," nor the section on death in *Postscript* discusses the possibility of a Christian afterlife does not mean that Kierkegaard personally does not believe in it (and, it must be noted, that section in *Postscript* is immediately followed by a section on the meaning of being immortal). In line with his Lutheran upbringing, Kierkegaard has faith in a transcendent posthumous survival, but he refuses to find certainty and comfort in such a thought. Acknowledging that nothing can be said about an afterlife with certainty, his works avoid metaphysical speculation, discuss death as the end of all conscious activity, and focus on what this means to us as long as we are still alive (cf. Stokes, 2015, p. 202). In this way, Kierkegaard prevents the possibility of an afterlife from distracting us from our present tasks (even the aforementioned discussion of the meaning of being immortal in *Postscript* is aimed entirely at taking responsibility for one's present existence and activities). It is this immanentism that makes Kierkegaard's account of death so compelling also for nonreligious readers. For a more thorough consideration of Kierkegaard's views on the afterlife, see Marks (2011) and Watkin (1990).

13. In this chapter, we do our best to avoid the thorny topic of Kierkegaard's early pseudonymous discussion of the three stages or spheres of existence. Few topics in Kierkegaard studies have received as much scholarly attention as the nature of these stages and the relationship between them. Briefly, an aesthetic existence (like the one Claudio seems to have embodied) is generally seen as immersed in superficial amusement and lacking the strong sense of personal responsibility and more comprehensive and cohesive sense of self-development found in the ethical and religious realms.

14. Much as he does explicitly with Epicurus toward the beginning of the discourse, Kierkegaard takes Socrates to task, albeit more subtly, in this passage toward the end. Although for Kierkegaard, and especially his pseudonyms, Socrates is something of a philosophical hero, Kierkegaard suggests in this case that the Socrates of Plato's *Apology* uses ironic detachment to dodge the fear of death and with it the beneficial disruptive quality Kierkegaard seeks in earnest thinking about it. Avoiding the fear of death just is not Kierkegaard's (cf. 1993, p. 88) priority, as it is for his ancient Greek predecessors. For a more detailed account of how Kierkegaard crafts his earnest thought of death in dialogue with Socrates and Epicurus, see Buben (2017).

REFERENCES

Buben, A. (2013). Heidegger's reception of Kierkegaard: The existential philosophy of death. *British Journal for the History of Philosophy, 21*(5), 967–988.

Buben, A. (2016). *Meaning and mortality in Kierkegaard and Heidegger: Origins of the existential philosophy of death.* Northwestern University Press.

Buben, A. (2017). Kierkegaard's philosophy of death: Between Socrates and Epicurus. In A. Burgess & W. McDonald (Eds.), *Acta Kierkegaardiana VII: Kierkegaard and classical Greek thought* (pp. 173–186). Central European Research Institute of Søren Kierkegaard and Kierkegaard Circle.

Epicurus. (1994). *The Epicurus reader* (B. Inwood & L. P. Gerson, Trans.). Hackett.

Höfer, S. (2024). Death as a teacher of love. *International Journal of Kierkegaard Research, 1*(1), 55–74.

Hofmannsthal, H. v. (2015). *Der Tor und der Tod.* Insel-Verlag.

Kierkegaard, S. (1941). *Thoughts on crucial situations in human life: Three discourses on imagined occasions* (D. F. Swenson, Trans.). Augsburg.

Kierkegaard, S. (1967). *Søren Kierkegaard's*

journals and papers (Vol. 1; H. V. Hong & E. H. Hong, Trans.). Indiana University Press.

Kierkegaard, S. (1992). *Concluding unscientific postscript to "Philosophical Fragments"* (Vol. 1; H. V. Hong & E. H. Hong, Trans.). Princeton University Press.

Kierkegaard, S. (1993). *Three discourses on imagined occasions* (H. V. Hong & E. H. Hong, Trans.). Princeton University Press.

Law, D. R. (2021). Learning to face death earnestly: Kierkegaard's critique of inauthentic conceptions of death in "At a Graveside." *International Journal on Humanistic Ideology, 11*(1), 49–87.

Marino, G. D. (2011). A critical perspective on Kierkegaard's "At a Graveside." In P. Stokes & A. J. Buben (Eds.), *Kierkegaard and death* (pp. 150–159). Indiana University Press.

Marks, T. M. (2011). Kierkegaard's understanding of the afterlife. In P. Stokes & A. J. Buben (Eds.), *Kierkegaard and death* (pp. 274–298). Indiana University Press.

Mooney, E. F. (2011). The intimate agency of death. In P. Stokes & A. J. Buben (Eds.), *Kierkegaard and death* (pp. 133–149). Indiana University Press.

Muench, P. (2011). Thinking death into every moment: The existence-problem of dying in Kierkegaard's *Postscript*. In P. Stokes & A. J. Buben (Eds.), *Kierkegaard and death* (pp. 101–121). Indiana University Press.

Pachmuss, T. (1961). The theme of love and death in Tolstoy's "The Death of Ivan Ilyich." *American Slavic and East European Review, 20,* 72–83.

Porter, M. (1972). Hugo von Hofmannsthal's "Der Tor und der Tod": The poet as fool. *Modern Austrian Literature, 5,* 14–29.

Possen, D. D. (2011). Death and ethics in Kierkegaard's *Postscript*. In P. Stokes & A. J. Buben (Eds.), *Kierkegaard and death* (pp. 122–132). Indiana University Press.

Sartre, J.-P. (1992). *Being and nothingness* (H. E. Barnes, Trans.). Washington Square Press.

Stewart, J. (2023). *A history of nihilism in the nineteenth century.* Cambridge University Press.

Stokes, P. (2006). The power of death: Retroactivity, narrative, and interest. In R. L. Perkins (Ed.), *International Kierkegaard commentary: Vol. 9. Prefaces and writing sampler, and Vol. 10. Three discourses on imagined occasions* (pp. 387–418). Mercer University Press.

Stokes, P. (2015). *The naked self: Kierkegaard and personal identity.* Oxford University Press.

Stokes, P., & Buben, A. (2011). Introduction. In P. Stokes & A. J. Buben (Eds.), *Kierkegaard and death* (pp. 1–20). Indiana University Press.

Strawser, M. (2023). Between mood and spirit: Kierkegaard's conception of death as the teacher of earnestness. *Kierkegaard Studies Yearbook, 28*(1), 143–160.

Theunissen, M. (2006). The upbuilding in the thought of death: Traditional elements, innovative ideas, and unexhausted possibilities in Kierkegaard's "At a Graveside" (G. Pattison, Trans.). In R. L. Perkins (Ed.), *International Kierkegaard commentary: Vol. 9. Prefaces and writing sampler, and Vol. 10. Three discourses on imagined occasions* (pp. 321–358). Mercer University Press.

Tolstoy, L. N. (2014). *The death of Ivan Ilyich* (P. Carson, Trans.). Liveright.

Watkin, J. (1990). Kierkegaard's view of death. *History of European Ideas, 12*(1), 65–78.

Westphal, M. (1996). *Becoming a self: A reading of Kierkegaard's* Concluding Unscientific Postscript. Purdue University Press.

CHAPTER 2

A Sense of Freedom

Free Will in Contemporary Analytic Philosophy and Sartre's Being and Nothingness

Stephen Kearns *and* Alfred R. Mele

Existential psychology focuses on our experience of existence, including our sense of freedom, agency, limited time, and meaning. It examines how individuals make sense of their existence in the world, their own actions, and the actions of others. Free will is a central concept in existential psychology, and it is closely tied to moral responsibility. Together, the concepts of free will and moral responsibility form the foundation of existential psychology and its endeavor to understand the human experience of existence. In this chapter we discuss various philosophical perspectives on free will and moral responsibility, including contemporary perspectives in analytic philosophy and influential work by Jean-Paul Sartre. We also consider how the science of existential psychology can help us better understand how people navigate the complexities of their existence.

TWO QUESTIONS ABOUT FREE WILL

What is free will? Do we have it? When presented with such questions, one may be tempted to wax lyrical about immaterial souls impinging unbidden on the physical world, or, on the contrary, take a hard-headed physicalist stance against such metaphysical speculation and reject free will as a fairytale. In contemporary philosophy of free will, many would now consider both such stances to be assuming something false about what free will requires. In other words, many people now accept that a picture that rejects immaterial souls, or even a special faculty that we may call "the will," is compatible with our having free will. Rather, one has free will if *one acts freely* (or is able so to act).

Of course, this raises the question of what it takes to act freely. Several answers have been given to this question. Here are basic versions of four of the more popular answers:

- (Leeway) An agent acts freely when they are able to do otherwise than they do (they have multiple alternatives available to them from which to pick).
- (Sourcehood) An agent acts freely when they are the source or origin of their actions (their actions are sufficiently independent of various external influences).
- (Reason) An agent acts freely when they are sensitive to their reasons for action

(they manifest a regular pattern of reason-recognition and have the capacity to act on good reasons).
- (Deep Self) An agent acts freely when their actions express their deep self (their actions express what they truly value, what they reflectively endorse, or who they truly are).

Such answers need not be considered mutually exclusive—perhaps free will is best captured by some combination of the above views.

There are various reasons one might be attracted to one or more of the above views of free will. One of the most important such reasons emphasizes the link between free will and *moral responsibility*. Roughly, an agent is morally responsible for an action if and only if it is appropriate to hold them to account for it. Thus, if an agent is morally responsible for acting wrongly, they are blameworthy for so acting. If they are morally responsible for acting rightly, they are praiseworthy for doing so. Many now accept the highly plausible claim that moral responsibility requires free will (i.e., an agent is morally responsible for some of their actions only if they sometimes act freely). In light of this idea, we may ask ourselves what kind of thing free will must be to be necessary for moral responsibility.

Interestingly enough, there is a case to be made that each of the above views spells out a requirement for moral responsibility—we are responsible for an action only if we could have done otherwise, or only if we are the genuine author of this action, or only if we are suitably sensitive to the reasons for and against this action, or only if this action truly expresses who we are. Think of the excuses one might hear from someone trying to avoid responsibility for an action—"I couldn't help it"; "They made me do it"; "I didn't know it was wrong"; "It doesn't reflect who I really am"—these invoke, even if obliquely, each of the above ideas of freedom in turn.

Another source of evidence concerning the nature of free will is *experience*. That is, we might be said to know what free will is like precisely by experiencing it. Thus, consider Tim O'Connor's attempt to describe our experience of making a (free) decision:

> A natural way of characterising our typical experience of making decisions and acting upon them . . . goes something like this: When I decide, say, to go for a walk on a cool autumn evening, I am conscious of various factors at work . . . motivating me either to do so or do something else instead. . . . It seems for all the world to be *up to me* to decide which particular action I will undertake. The decision I make is no mere vector sum of internal and external forces acting upon me during the process of deliberation. (2003, p. 257)

Insofar, then, as we experience free will, we presumably have some insight into what it is. O'Connor's characterization of our experience may lead us to embrace one account of free will (the first two above views of free will, Leeway and Sourcehood, seem to best capture the above description), while another characterization, which emphasizes different aspects of our experience, may lead us to embrace another.

Alternatively, one may describe experiences not of free will but of those occasions when freedom seems to slip away. For example, Gary Watson drew our attention to the arising of desires that are not freely chosen or endorsed: "Consider the case of a woman who has a sudden urge to drown her bawling child in the bath; or the case of a squash player who, while suffering an ignominious defeat, desires to smash his opponent in the face with the racquet" (2003, p. 342). We may then learn something about free will by how it *contrasts* with such experiences. (Watson's examples are perhaps best captured by (one of) the *latter* two views of free will, Reason and Deep Self: Such urges are not free either because they are not sufficiently sensitive to the agents' reasons or they do not express agents' true values.)

Consider lastly the idea that we may get a better grasp on what free will is by considering the nature of various phenomena concerning action in general, such as intentional action, voluntary action, addiction, conscious action, control, ability, deliberation, and so forth. Helen Steward (2011), for example, took the very notions of agency and action to involve something akin to the second above characterization of free action: "Actions are the beginnings of causal chains which are initiated by their agents—and so where the initiation of such a chain lies elsewhere than with a given agent, what has occurred cannot be an action of that agent" (p. 149). John Fischer and Mark Ravizza (1998) theorized about free will by trying to uncover the type of *control* required for *moral responsibility*, thus invoking both agential and ethical notions in their investigation of free will (they ended up with a version of what we call "Reason" above).

Let's turn now to the question of whether we *have* free will. Just as we might attempt to find insight into what free will *is* by appeal to our experience, we might also think that our experience constitutes excellent evidence that we *have* free will. After all, we generally trust that things are as they appear to us to be (if you see a cat on a mat, you believe there's a cat on a mat)—if we experience freedom, then should we not conclude that we are free? In essence, that is right, but note that such a rule is *defeasible* (that is, though it is usually a good rule to trust one's experiences, there are occasions when this rule does not apply). In particular, if one has reason to think either that one's experience is unreliable or that the apparent phenomenon one seems to be experiencing is illusory, then one should *not* simply trust one's experiences. Furthermore, in the case of freedom, there is a long history of arguments that, in fact, free will does not exist.

One of the most common such arguments invokes the thesis of *determinism*. As is standard in the philosophy of free will, we understand determinism to be the claim that every total state of the universe at a time necessitates, in combination with the laws of nature, every subsequent state of the universe. Thus, for example, if our universe is deterministic, then, given the conditions of the universe just after the Big Bang and the laws that govern the development of the universe, there is only one possible way the future can unfold. Determinism makes no exceptions for human agency—if determinism is true, then all our actions are necessitated by past states and the laws of nature.

Unsurprisingly, many thinkers have found determinism incompatible with free will (such thinkers are thus called *incompatibilists*). This is especially so for those attracted to Leeway and Sourcehood accounts. Determinism seems both to rid us of genuine alternatives for our actions (if all of our actions are determined by states of the universe from billions of years ago in combination with the immutable laws of nature, how on Earth could we have done otherwise?) and strip us of the capacity to be the true authors of our actions (our actions become mere links in a deterministic chain winding all the way back to the Big Bang). Thus, if one accepts determinism, perhaps due to a sense that there is a sufficient reason for everything that happens (God does not play dice, as Einstein's words are often paraphrased), one must contend with a powerful reason to reject the existence of free will.

For those who *embrace* free will, there are two obvious ways to escape this threat—one may either reject determinism or accept a view of free will that is not imperiled by it. Those who take the latter path may point out that, while Leeway and Sourcehood conceptions of free will seem to put free will in conflict with determinism, Reason and Deep Self conceptions do not.

Consider Reason first. It seems perfectly possible for an agent to be sensitive to reasons even if everything they do is necessitated by the remote past and the laws of nature. What Reason demands of a free agent is not independence from the past or access to different possible futures, but rather a suitable set of capacities to recognize and act on reasons in various counterfactual scenarios. An A/C unit may be capable, in a wide range of counterfactual scenarios, of recognizing command inputs, measuring temperature within a wide spectrum, and producing desired room temperatures within such a spectrum, while still being a purely deterministic system. Similarly, a deterministic agent may be capable, in a wide range of counterfactual scenarios, of recognizing reasons and weighing their strengths, as well as acting on sufficient reasons in some such scenarios.

Consider also Deep Self. A deterministic agent, though necessitated by the past and laws in everything they do, may nevertheless have a *deep value system*. They may value honor, family, love, friendship, money, and so forth. Their values may form a (mostly) coherent whole, with partial rankings of their values and policies concerning in what conditions such values are pertinent. They may *reflectively endorse* many of these values or see them as essential aspects of their self-identity. Lastly, they may *manifest and express* such values in their actions, instead of acting on other motivations that they do not endorse or see the value in (such as, perhaps, cravings for cigarettes, or short-lived violent urges). For proponents of Deep Self views of free will, such an agent is free—they express their true self in their actions, even while living in a fully deterministic universe.

While free will, on the Reason or Deep Self conceptions, is likely compatible with determinism, some may see this precisely as a strong reason for *rejecting* such conceptions. They may claim that any compatibilist view of free will must be, as Immanuel Kant put it, a "wretched subterfuge"—such conceptions simply cannot do justice to true free will. Another way to (try to) escape the threat of determinism, then, is to maintain that determinism is false. We may point to common interpretations of quantum mechanics according to which reality is irreducibly probabilistic as evidence of this. Instead of claiming that the world is governed by strict deterministic laws that allow only one possible evolution of the universe from a given state, these interpretations tell us that there are several physically possible such evolutions that can further be assigned objective probabilities. Should the world turn out to work like this (and, in particular, should our *decisions* turn out to work like this), there are genuine alternatives open to us (as Leeway views require) and the decisions we make do not stem from external sources that necessitate them (as Sourcehood requires). Can free will, even on the more demanding accounts, be saved by such indeterminism?

The main worry facing this idea is that undetermined decisions, rather than striking us as *free*, seem to be *matters of luck*. If nothing at all determines what decision I make, then how can I exercise control over which option I choose? Just as we might judge that an indeterministic number generator—a machine that spits out random numbers determined by nothing at all—does not *control* which numbers are generated, we might similarly judge that undetermined choices are not truly *up to us*. As we put the thought in previous work:

> A philosopher may believe that having *control over whether* one *A*-s or does something else instead is required for directly freely *A*-ing and for being directly morally responsible for *A*-ing and believe that having such control requires that *A*-ing at *t* and doing something else instead at *t* are possible continuations of the past up to *t* for the agent. But the same philosopher may worry that these possible continuations are similar enough to possible continuations for the indeterministic number generator that whatever control the agent may have over whether he *A*-s or does something else instead falls short of what is required for directly free *A*-ing and for direct moral responsibility for *A*-ing. (Kearns & Mele, 2014, p. 11)

Thus, even if we think that free will *requires* indeterminism (because determinism rules out free will), this is no guarantee that indeterminism will prove to be any more hospitable to freedom than determinism is. So-called *libertarians* about free will embrace the existence of free will while also accepting its incompatibility with determinism. One of the main tasks for such libertarians, then, is to attempt to reconcile freedom with indeterministic agency (see Mele, 2006).

Still, it is determinism, and similar theses, that seem to worry most. Many other (supposed) threats to free will are more specific than the general thesis of determinism but are similar in significant respects. Thus, some worry that Benjamin Libet's (2004) experiments show that our conscious decisions are preceded by unconscious brain activity that determines what decisions we make. Others are concerned about the powerful impact our *genetics* have on our behavior. Similar points can be made about our upbringings, our social roles, and the situations we find ourselves in. These threats all have a similar form—something beyond our control determines (or at the very least highly influences) our behavior, rendering us unfree.

Some exhort us to embrace this conclusion—we are not free, nor are we morally responsible for our actions. Such skeptics might bemoan our lack of freedom, or instead embrace it, arguing that a world in which we accept there is no free will would be better in various respects (e.g., we would be rid of unfitting righteous anger at others; see Pereboom, 2001). Still, such skeptics face considerable tasks themselves, such as explaining the point of deliberation (doesn't deliberating assume multiple options from which to choose?), how to live without responsibility (is a world with no blame, no praise, no guilt, no pride possible, and is it worth it?), what meaning there can be in life without freedom (after all, freedom is central to how many make sense of their lives), and so forth.

Free will is, then, a challenging and important topic, on which there are several defensible viewpoints. In the next section, we explore an *existentialist* view of free will and its relation to our experience, our agency, our responsibility, and the meaning of our lives.

A SARTREAN ACCOUNT OF FREE WILL

In the preceding section, we asked two questions about free will—what is it, and do we have it? In this section, we examine an approach to these questions from within the existentialist tradition. There is, of course, no one existentialist view of free will. Indeed, there is no uncontested answer to who counts as an existentialist—if we include Friedrich Nietzsche, for example, then existentialism is a broad enough church to allow in a skeptic about free will. In this chapter, we concentrate on a view of freedom derived from relevant passages of Jean-Paul Sartre's *Being and Nothingness*. Simone de Beauvoir, in some of her work (e.g., *Pyrrhus and Cineas*), espoused a somewhat similar view (the extent to which Sartre and Beauvoir agreed or disagreed about freedom is a subject of some scholarly debate [see Kirkpatrick, 2023, for an overview]).

We can begin characterizing this view of free will (or "freedom," as Sartre's *liberté* is invariably translated into English) by addressing how it answers the above questions. Most straightforwardly, in answer to the second question, we certainly *do* have free will by Sartre's lights. Indeed, the idea that we are free is one of the central features of his philosophy.

Anguish

One way in which Sartre supported the idea that we are free is by providing vivid phenomenological descriptions of *anguish*. Sartre used this term to denote our consciousness of our own freedom (see 2018, p. 66).

Sartre distinguished two types of anguish—anguish in the face of the future and anguish in the face of the past. The former consists, roughly, in our consciousness that our present plans have no hold on our future selves. His most famous example of this concerns traversing a narrow path by a chasm. At first, this journey produces *fear*, which is a reaction to forces outside of one's control, such as accidentally falling, slipping on loose stones, and so forth (2018, p. 67).

In response to such fear, we formulate plans to avoid an accidental death. The possibilities of *accident* are replaced in our consciousness by the possibilities of *action*, and my fear of something happening outside of my control is replaced by a sense of the possibilities *within* my control. And precisely because they are within my control, it is not certain that I will follow any plan I formulate—the possibility of my traversing the path safely brings with it the possibility of intentionally flinging myself off the path, of not paying proper attention, and so forth (Sartre, 2018, p. 68). This sends us from the frying pan of fear into the fire of anguish—my initial horror and my subsequent careful route along the path occur against a backdrop of other options that I consciously apprehend as my possibilities. The choice to be careful does nothing, so it can strike us, to ensure that we do not change our minds in the future and instead embrace one of these other possibilities. We apprehend that our future behavior is not beholden to our present plans.

Anguish in the face of the *past* is one's consciousness that one's past has no hold over one's present behavior. Sartre illustrated such anguish with his example of a gambler who has yesterday resolved to stop gambling but finds his resolution useless when he approaches the green baize. The gambler realizes in anguish that he is perfectly free to gamble regardless of any past resolution he has made not to (2018, pp. 71–72). Just as we can become vividly conscious that our future selves may ignore or subvert our current plans, we can become vividly conscious that we may ignore or subvert our past plans.

Sartre was quite aware of the worry that such experiences, while perhaps indicating something about what free will is *or would be* like, do not constitute conclusive evidence that free will exists, because such experiences might be illusory. Indeed, he pointed out that some may account for the feeling of anguish in other ways (2018, p. 72). Sartre replied, in part, that, prior to his discussion of anguish, he had already shown that freedom must exist, as it is a necessary condition for our being the kinds of things we are (in particular, our capacity to question requires that we are free [p. 72]). Let us turn, then, to Sartre's prior case for freedom.

Freedom and Nothingness

Sartre's initial argument that we are free takes us to the heart of his philosophy. He claimed that certain capacities we have, such as our capacity to question, require the ability to "step back" from the world and escape its causal grip (2018, p. 59). In essence, humans can separate themselves from the world's influence. Though, in the above passages, Sartre emphasized *questioning* as a way of thus separating us from the world, there are a variety of such ways, including expectation, doubt, intention, measurement, imagination, and attention. All these ways involve a *nihilating activity* by the agent. That is, when we question, expect, doubt, and so forth, we apprehend the world as (potentially) *lacking* something, and it is precisely our attitude or activity that grounds the existence of this lack. When we expect to find Pierre in the café, and fail to see him, we are instead *conscious of Pierre's absence.* When we *question* the world (will Pierre be there?), we are open to the world's answering *negatively*. When we apprehend the *distance* between two things, we apprehend them as *separated*—that is, *not together.* When we *attend* to something, we separate it in consciousness from its surroundings, which become the background against which we apprehend the object. When we *imagine* something, we are conscious of it as *unreal.* According to Sartre, the only kind of being who can bring about negative phenomena such as these must itself be negative, or a *nothingness,* as he put it (2018, p. 58).

Given that *we humans*, then, can ground such negative phenomena as lacks, absences, distances, backgrounds, imaginary objects, and so forth, we must ourselves be in some respect *negative.* Applying Sartre's idea that the purely positive cannot determine the negative (2018, p. 572), we get the result that the world cannot determine our behavior. This, for Sartre, meant we are free.

Sartre's initial case for the existence of freedom also provides us with the outlines of his *conception* of freedom. Sartre's characterization is most straightforwardly taken as a Sourcehood account, given his emphasis on the idea that free agents are not determined by anything else. This said, we must be careful not to attribute to Sartre the idea that we are substantial selves who give rise to actions in accord with our natures. Though we are the authors of our actions, we are just as much the authors of *ourselves.* Freedom was, for Sartre, *self-creation.* This is in part what the famous idea that *existence precedes essence* is meant to capture. As Sartre put it in *Existentialism Is a Humanism*:

> What do we mean here by "existence precedes essence"? We mean that man first exists: he materializes in the world, encounters himself, and only afterward defines himself. If man as existentialists conceive of him cannot be defined, it is because to begin with he is nothing. He will not be anything until later, and then he will be what he makes of himself. (2007, p. 22)

Free will (i.e., freedom) is precisely this process of active self-creation. A contemporary philosopher who emphasized the importance of self-creation to freedom was Robert Kane, who told us:

> Often we act from a will (character, motives and purposes) already formed, but it is "*our own* free will," to the extent that we had a role in forming it by earlier self forming acts (SFAs) for which we could have done otherwise. If this were not so, *there would have been noth-*

ing we could have ever done differently in our lives to make our wills different than they are; and we would never act "of our own free will" in the sense of a will that is to some degree "of our own free-making." (2019, p. 147; original emphasis)

For both Sartre and Kane, should we only ever act from motives we had no role in forming, we would not be truly free.

Although the Sourcehood category is the most comfortable fit for Sartre's view of free will (at least out of the four options above), there are elements of all four conceptions of freedom in *Being and Nothingness*. We can bring this out by outlining some elements of Sartre's philosophy of action.

Reasons, Motives, Ends

For Sartre, all genuine action was oriented around an *end*—something the world lacks that the agent apprehends and toward which their action is aiming. As ever, Sartre was keen to emphasize the way in which an end is *negative*—it is absent from the world and *to be pursued*. Thus, in his example of Constantine's intention to found a city that rivals Rome (2018, p. 570), Constantine's ends *make sense* of his subsequent actions—he goes about founding the city of Constantinople *in order to bring this desirable city into existence*, that is, to change its status from nonbeing to being. Here again we see echoes of Sartre's idea that the past cannot determine what we do because what we do is in part explained by that which is *not* (or, at least, *not yet*).

One might fairly wonder how an agent's *reasons and motives* fit into Sartre's picture of action. After all, we naturally explain actions in such terms—Bob's *motive* for giving to the ASPCA is his sympathy toward animals, while his *reason* is that many animals are suffering. Highlighting Bob's motive, or his reason, goes a considerable way toward *explaining* his action. Sartre accepted this. Indeed, he insisted that all intentional actions are performed for reasons (2018, p. 573). Still, we err in judging motives and reasons to exist *independently* of our ends. Rather, an agent's reasons, motives, and ends are inextricably tied together as different aspects of the agent's project to make real the unreal (p. 589). Let's examine this idea further.

Sartre's conception of a reason is relatively standard—a reason *justifies* an action (2018, p. 585)—but he took reasons to justify actions only relative to the agent's ends. Thus, the fact that animals are suffering is a reason for Bob to give money to the ASPCA only because Bob has certain ends that lend significance to this fact. One of Bob's projects is to help animals. The fact that animals are suffering, then, is, for Bob, *something to be rectified*. It has this status only in the light of Bob's ends. The point generalizes—reasons exist only in the light of an agent's ends and their pursuit of them (2018, p. 588). Sartre concluded that a reason is a consideration that justifies an action *as a means of pursuing some given end* (p. 586). Reasons do not preexist ends, then, but rather presuppose them (or, more accurately, a fact's *status* as a reason presupposes some end).

The story is similar with respect to motives. Consider Bob's sympathy for animals—this is his motive for helping them. Again, however, Sartre denied that such a motive exists apart from Bob's end of helping animals. Indeed, Bob's sympathy for animals is simply Bob's *project* of helping animals, manifested affectively. This motive also colors his consciousness—it is in virtue of his sympathy that he grasps the fact that animals are suffering *as a reason to help them*. As Sartre said about Clovis, the first king of the Franks, we ultimately cannot distinguish his deep ambition from his project of conquering Gaul—the motive simply *was* this project as Clovis lived it (2018, pp. 588–589). Reasons, motives, and ends, then, are not separable existences, one giving rise to the next, but rather essential and inextricable elements of action that arise together, united.

Fundamental Projects

Another important element of Sartre's philosophy of action was his notion of *a fundamental project*. According to Sartre, our multiple projects toward various ends form a united project toward an overarching end that encompasses these other ends—this ultimate end is *who we aim at being*—a kind of ideal self that makes sense of our actions while at the same time being sustained and explained by them (2018, p. 602).

Thus, for example, Bob's project to help animals is part of a larger project to relate to the world in a particular way—perhaps to be the kind of person who puts the needs of other sentient creatures before himself, which in turn is part of a larger project to be a person with goals that extend beyond him. It is worth noting that such a project, and its end, need not be *explicit*. Indeed, it will likely not be something that Bob's consciousness takes as an object. That said, Sartre did believe that such a project is conscious in a certain sense—its being conscious in this sense is what makes it possible for it to *become* an object of consciousness, and also what underlies how this project organizes Bob's consciousness of the world. It is part of the aim of existential psychoanalysis, as Sartre understood it, to uncover an agent's fundamental project.

Freedom as . . .

The above discussion helps us further categorize Sartre's view of freedom. We have already seen how it is a type of Sourcehood account. What of the other three accounts?

For Sartre, in everything we freely do, there is some objective aspect of the world—*our situation*—to which we are responding. Indeed, in the light of Sartre's notion of a fundamental project, Sartrean free agents will also manifest *regular patterns* of reasons-recognition and often act on good reasons. This is exactly how Reason views characterize free will. One major difference between usual Reason views (e.g., Fischer & Ravizza 1998) and Sartre's view is that a Sartrean agent's reasons have no existence independent of this agent's ends. Thus, good reasons will not be good because of how they relate to what is valuable independent of any aim, but because they are good *in the light of some given aims*. Another difference worth noting is that typical Reason views emphasize the importance of agents' capacities to respond to reasons in a variety of *counterfactual* scenarios—scenarios that do not, but could, occur. Sartre thought such scenarios are effectively irrelevant to our freedom—what matters is what we do in our actual situations, not what we have the capacity to do in other circumstances. As he put it in *Existentialism Is a Humanism*:

> For existentialists there is no love other than the deeds of love; no potential for love other than that which is manifested in loving. There is no genius other than that which is expressed in works of art; the genius of Proust resides in the totality of his works; the genius of Racine is found in the series of his tragedies, outside of which there is nothing. (2007, p. 37)

A more contemporary and analytic approach in this vein is Carolina Sartorio's (2016) own "actual sequence" Reasons view, which attempts to account for a free agent's sensitivity to reasons purely in terms of what the agent actually responds to (reasons and their absences), rather than what they might respond to in other circumstances.

We may also draw parallels between Sartre's view of freedom and Deep Self accounts of free will. Deep Self accounts posit a generally coherent evaluative system that can be expressed through action (see, e.g., Watson, 2003). This idea bears obvious similarities to Sartre's notion of a fundamental project—a significant aspect of the meaning of an action is given by the larger projects of which it is an element. However, there are also significant differences between the two views. First, Deep Self views think of these evaluative systems as preexisting and giving rise to free actions. Sartre maintained that an action not only manifests an agent's fundamental project but also sustains its existence—our fundamental projects exist only insofar as they are pursued in our individual actions. Second, Deep Self views often claim that our true values are those we reflectively endorse or explicitly identify with. Sartre rejected the idea that actions that stem from reflection or deliberation are any freer than those that do not. Indeed, for Sartre, our reflective "wills" dictate not our ends but simply the way in which we carry them out (2018, p. 592–593). The deeper freedom of the fundamental project is typically *not* something an agent reflectively endorses, or, indeed, takes as an object of consciousness at all.

What, finally, of Leeway views of freedom? It is clear from Sartre's descriptions of anguish that he thought that being free involves having multiple alternatives from which to choose. He further distinguished two types of choices open to us—those that are compatible with our fundamental projects, and those that reject or radically revise these projects. He described both types in reference to his giving in to his fatigue while hiking. In this example, his stopping is inevitable given his fundamental project. But, Sartre insisted, his stopping is not inevitable *tout court*, as it is always open to us to radically revise or even abandon our current fundamental projects (2018, pp. 607–608). On the other hand, *how* he stops is not thus dictated by his fundamental project. Should Sartre choose to collapse on the floor in exhaustion or instead make it slightly further to a nearby pub, either action may be perfectly in keeping with his general fundamental project (p. 615). In such cases, each option is possible to pursue and, in choosing one, we invent reasons and motives for whichever choice we make. Either way, then, we are always free to do otherwise, even when doing so involves rejecting many of our longstanding values and adopting new ones.

Sartre's account of free action, then, contains elements of all four of the views with which we started—free agents have multiple alternatives open to them; they are the authors of their actions; they systematically recognize and act on reasons; and their free actions express and manifest who they are. It also *diverges* from typical such views—free agents are not only free to *act* in multiple ways, but free to determine their reasons, motives, and ends; free agents are the authors not only of their actions but of *themselves*; free agents not only recognize but also *give rise* to the reasons they act on; and their free actions not only express but *create* who they are.

Responsibility

Like most philosophers, Sartre saw a deep link between freedom and responsibility (2018, p. 718). Given that Sartrean free agents are the authors of themselves, their responsibility is extensive. In fact, we are responsible not only for ourselves, but, in a certain sense, for *the world*. Indeed, even if a war breaks out, such a war is my responsibility not only because I could have avoided it (by committing suicide, or deserting), but because this war *is the war it is* in part because of the meaning I confer on it—my ends transform the war into something calamitous or welcome (pp. 719–720). Generalizing, the world is *my* world—I determine its significance for me by the choices I make.

Threats to Freedom

What would a Sartrean make of the threats to freedom that we mentioned in the previous section? While Sartre rejected a thesis he called "determinism," it is unclear whether Sartre meant the same thing we define. Still, given Sartre's emphasis on self-creation and our freedom to choose between alternatives, it is natural to think of him as a *libertarian* about free will. This is not to say that he did not see the force of apparent threats to free will—he was aware to what extent we are ostensibly the products of our upbringing, our inheritance, our society, and so forth (2018, p. 629).

Sartre devoted considerable space to trying to answer such worries. We focus here on the thrust of his response. Such external influences on us, rather than showing we are *not* free, are evidence that we *are* free. This is because whether they are limitations or obstacles to our free action is dependent on our freely chosen ends. A rock may strike me as unclimbable, and thus an obstacle to my path, but only because I choose to take such a path. Sartre took this point to generalize. For example, he said that while our pasts deeply influence us, they do so only in light of our present freely chosen ends—we decide on the meaning of our pasts precisely by projecting ourselves toward our future goals (2018, p. 649).

He combined this idea with a clarification concerning his understanding of freedom—we are not, of course, free to do anything at all (fly, jump to the Moon, become royalty, etc.), but are rather free with respect to the projects we *pursue*—Sartre's freedom is the freedom to *choose*, not the freedom to *succeed* (2018, p. 631). Thus, while Sartre's idea of freedom may seem radical, it is not as radical as it is sometimes made out to be. Indeed, he allowed that the ends we would succeed in obtaining might be highly limited. What is not so limited are the ends we are free to *pursue*.

What of the worry that, if our actions are not determined, they are mere matters of luck, and thus not free? Sartre agreed this is a problem for those who take reasons, motives, and ends to be separable, with the former failing to suffice for the latter (2018, p. 573). As we have seen, however, Sartre's view was that, in freely acting, agents create their reasons, motives, and ends in one fell swoop—each being able to make sense of, and to that extent *explain*, the others. Thus, for Sartre, our undetermined actions bring with them their own explanations in terms of reasons and motives. Had we performed different actions, which we are always able to do, we would thereby have had different reasons and motives. Whichever end we pursue, then, it is not a matter of luck that we pursue this end, as it can be explained by reference to reasons and motives that suffice for our doing so.

Absurdity, Being Condemned to Be Free, and Optimism

Sartre conceded that his picture, whereby our reasons and motives do not preexist the pursuit of our ends, renders our choices in some sense *absurd* (2018, pp. 625–626). Thus we are led again to anguish and angst—because we are free, we are the foundation of reasons and thus unjustifiable by anything external to us. And this is a condition we cannot escape (p. 577)—as we are negative creatures, nothingnesses, we forever flee the foundations we lay down and are obliged to take them up or reject them anew.

Though Sartre's tone here seemed pessimistic, he later assured us, in *Existentialism Is a Humanism*, that "no doctrine is more optimistic, since it declares that man's destiny lies within himself" (2007, p. 40). Our freedom can be a source of anguish and bad faith but embracing it with eyes open is the key to a fulfilling, authentic existence.

PARTING REMARKS

We are philosophers, not psychologists. Even so, we agreed to comment on how the science of existential psychology can help us better understand free will and its bearing on how people navigate the complexities of their existence.

One role for existential psychology in this connection is to examine various science-based arguments for the claim that free will is an illusion—arguments from neuroscience (Gazzaniga, 2011), social psychology (Wegner, 2002), and biology (Sapolsky, 2023), for example. If these arguments are found to be unconvincing, as we believe they are (Mele, 2009, 2014), that is good news for existential psychology. But if they are found to be convincing, existential psychologists and others should think hard about how to navigate a world without free will.

As one of us has explained elsewhere, science-based arguments for the nonexistence of free will tend to set a very high bar for free will, often claiming that our having free will depends on our having immaterial souls (Mele, 2009, 2014). There is some work in psychology and experimental philosophy on how nonspecialists conceive of free will (see, e.g., Vonasch et al., 2018). More work of that kind would be useful. If the free will people believe they have and value having is not the "free will" some scientists say they don't have, that is good news for these believers in free will.

Existential psychologists are well positioned to examine another important issue about free will—its phenomenology. How is the feeling of acting freely (or of one's own free will) best characterized? With an answer to that question in place, the next two questions are almost irresistible. What do we and our world need to be like if that feeling is to be veridical? And are we and our world that way? These questions are, of course, intimately bound up with the questions that opened the first section: What is free will, and do we have it? They are deep questions indeed, and they fall within the purview of many disciplines, including—prominently—existential psychology.

REFERENCES

Beauvoir, S. de. (2004). Pyrrhus and Cineas. In M. Simons (Ed.), *Philosophical writings* (pp. 77–150). University of Illinois Press.

Fischer, J. M., & Ravizza, M. (1998). *Responsibility and control*. Cambridge University Press.

Gazzaniga, M. (2011). *Who's in charge?: Free will and the science of the brain*. Ecco.

Kane, R. (2019). "The complex tapestry of free will." *Synthese, 196,* 145–160.

Kearns, S., & Mele, A. (2014). Have compatibilists solved the luck problem for libertarians? *Philosophical Inquiries, 2,* 9–36.

Kirkpatrick, K. (2023). Beauvoir and Sartre's "disagreement" about freedom. *Philosophy Compass*, 18, 1–14.

Libet, B. (2004). *Mind time.* Harvard University Press.

Mele, A. (2006). *Free will and luck.* Oxford University Press.

Mele, A. (2009). *Effective intentions: The power of conscious will.* Oxford University Press.

Mele, A. (2014). *Free: Why science hasn't disproved free will.* Oxford University Press.

O'Connor, T. (2003). Agent causation. In G. Watson (Ed.), *Free will* (2nd ed., pp. 257–284). Oxford University Press.

Pereboom, D. (2001). *Living without free will.* Cambridge University Press.

Sapolsky, R. (2023). *Determined: A science of life without free will.* Penguin Press.

Sartorio, C. (2016). *Causation and free will.* Oxford University Press.

Sartre, J.-P. (2007). *Existentialism is a humanism.* Yale University Press.

Sartre, J.-P. (2018). *Being and nothingness* (S. Richmond, Trans.). Washington Square Press.

Steward, H. (2011). Moral responsibility and the concept of agency. In R. Swinburne (Ed.), *Free will and modern science* (pp. 141–157). Oxford University Press.

Vonasch, A., Baumeister, R., & Mele, A. (2018). Ordinary people think free will is a lack of constraint, not the presence of a soul. *Consciousness and Cognition, 60,* 133–151.

Watson, G. (2003). Free agency. In G. Watson (Ed.), *Free will* (2nd ed., pp. 337–351). Oxford University Press.

Wegner, D. (2002). *The illusion of conscious will.* MIT Press.

CHAPTER 3

Determination and Transcendence

An Existentialist Account of Our Freedom to Shape Ourselves in a Deterministic World

Derk Pereboom

A core thesis of existentialism is that human life features a tension between our facticity (the constraints of being human that are independent of our control as agents, such as our embodiment and its accompanying vulnerability) and our transcendence (our ability to exercise that control, given those constraints, to give our lives meaning and purpose). Existentialists differ on the nature of that control. Sartre (1943/1956, 2001) argued that we have a free will that is independent of the laws of nature. Even if the laws that characterize nature are deterministic, we yet have the capacity to choose without being causally determined to choose. In this respect, in his terms, we are not just *being-in-itself*, his term for facticity, we participate in *being-for-itself*, his term for transcendence. As a result, we are fully responsible for our choices and, because we form who we are by those choices, we are fully responsible for who we are. Nietzsche's (1882/1974, 1887/1998; Leiter, 2007) position contrasted markedly with Sartre's, since he contended that in a core sense we lack free will. Nonetheless, he also maintained that we have the control required to reject a life of resentful disempowerment and its accompanying values, and to embrace what he called the will to power instead (Guignon & Pereboom, 1995, 2001).

My position on free will is closer to Nietzsche's than to Sartre's. With respect to the relation between facticity and transcendence, it is closer to Kierkegaard's (1846/1941) than to Sartre's, since in my view facticity and transcendence are in tension, while in Sartre the transcendent dominates. I'm particularly interested in how we should view our transcendence, given an account of our facticity that precludes the free will Sartre (2001) championed and comes closer to Nietzsche's denial of free will. There is, I argue, an account of transcendence that does not require a kind of free will incompatible with causal determination. Part of my objective in this chapter is to explain this notion. Furthermore, I argue that this notion of transcendence, whose precursors are Spinoza and the Buddhist philosopher Śāntideva, stands to encourage acceptance and compassion and recommends hope in a way congenial to human communal life.

FREE WILL AND DETERMINISM

In the historical debate, the term *free will* has several distinct senses. Two are especially relevant to the existentialist discussion and have a prominent role in Sartre's account. A first is alternative-possibilities free will. To have free will in this sense is to have more than one option for action: Free will is an agent's ability, at a given time, either to act or to refrain. That is, if an agent acts with free will, they instead could have refrained at that time from acting as they did. A second sense is connected to moral responsibility: Free will is an agent's ability to exercise the control in acting required to be morally responsible for the action. There are different senses of moral responsibility, and this difference plays a role in the ensuing discussion.

Causal determinism, according to which every event has causal antecedents that render it inevitable, has historically been taken to be the main threat to our having free will. Two prominent versions of determinism are theological determinism, in which the determining causal antecedent is the divine will, and naturalistic determinism, in which the antecedents are past events that causally determine succeeding events in accord with the laws of nature. The contestants in the free will debate traditionally divide with reference to whether causal determinism and free will are compatible. Compatibilists hold that our having free will is compatible with causal determinism—with all of our actions being causally determined by factors beyond our control, while incompatibilists maintain that our having free will is not compatible with causal determinism.

Incompatibilists further divide into those who hold that determinism is false and that we have free will (the libertarians), and those who maintain that determinism is true and that we lack free will (the hard determinists, also called free will skeptics). Incompatibilists about alternative-possibilities free will contend that if causal determinism were true, we would lack this sort of free will. Compatibilists (e.g., Hume, 1748/1999, Section 8) maintain that even if an action is causally determined by factors beyond our control, it still may be, at the time of the action, that we could have refrained from performing it. For even if determinism is true, it may still be that we would have acted otherwise than we did had we chosen to act otherwise, since there may have been no external physical constraints preventing us from doing otherwise. With respect to this sense of free will, Sartre is a libertarian of some kind, while Nietzsche is a hard determinist and thus a free will skeptic.

On the sense of free will linked to moral responsibility, virtually all participants in the debate agree that causal determinism is compatible with our having the control in action required for moral responsibility in *some* sense—for example, in a sense solely focused on forward-looking objectives such as the moral reform of a wrongdoer and reconciliation relationships (to be discussed). But they disagree about whether causal determinism is compatible with our having the control in action required for moral responsibility in a sense involving a resolutely backward-looking notion of desert, specifically *basic desert*:

> For an agent to be *morally responsible for an action in the basic desert sense* is for the action to be attributable to her such a way that if she was sensitive to its being morally wrong, she would deserve to be blamed or punished in a way that would be harmful, and if she was sensitive to its being morally exemplary, she would deserve to be praised or rewarded in a way that would be beneficial. The desert at issue here is basic in the sense that the agent, to be morally responsible in this sense, would deserve the harm or benefit just by virtue of having performed the action with sensitivity to its moral status, and not, for example, by virtue of consequentialist or contractualist considerations. (Pereboom, 2021, pp. 11–12)

We can add that the imposition of such basically deserved pain or harm, pleasure or benefit, is conceived as noninstrumentally good, since such imposition is not envisioned as good only insofar as it brings about a further good. Rather, it is conceived as good in itself (McKenna, 2019). Compatibilists about this sort of free will point out that the conditions held sufficient for basic desert responsibility in court cases, such as sanity and adequate understanding of the wrong done, are clearly compatible with determinism, and that the law courts do not suppose the truth or falsity of determinism to be relevant to their decisions. Incompatibilists claim that this is insufficient reason to think that determinism is in fact irrelevant to such responsibility, and that our practice in the courts may well presuppose and never question the falsity of determinism.

TRANSCENDENCE

Practical objections have been raised against skeptics about alternative-possibilities and moral-responsibility free will. Can we live without the belief that we have free will in these senses? Here I consider a challenge to any determinist, whether a free will skeptic or a compatibilist, that targets the possibility of transcendence. It concerns the efficacy of rational deliberation and choice in a deterministic world. If all rational deliberation and action are causally determined by factors beyond our control, then which option one selects is made inevitable by causal factors beyond one's control. The effects of that selection are also inevitable by virtue of such factors. Thus, how one deliberates and chooses, as well as the effects of those choices are beyond one's control. If so, how could we transcend our facticity to make a difference to our lives and to the world?

It's a theme of existentialism that the tension between our facticity and transcendence makes us ill at ease, and that in this respect we are apt to call what makes us distinctive into question. What can we say, specifically, about the resolution of the tension between facticity understood as causal determination and the transcendence required for control in action? First, it's generally accepted that given causal determinism, there remains a sense in which how we deliberate makes a difference to how we decide, which in turn makes a difference to our futures.

Sartre understood transcendence as the capacity to form what one is. He famously argued that existence precedes essence, by which he meant that I come to exist prior to what shapes me as an individual person, and that what shapes is my free choices. To expand on Sartre's example, imagine that you promise to join the resistance, but you consider breaking your promise and taking care of your ailing mother instead—a life-defining choice. Upon rational deliberation—considering and weighing reasons for each option—you decide to keep the promise and join the resistance. Suppose that it was causally determined that you deliberated as you did and decided to keep the promise, and that the resistance was as a consequence more effective than it would have been without you. Had you deliberated differently, you would have decided to stay with your mother instead, and the resistance would have been less effective. In this sense your deliberation made a difference to your decision and to the world outside of you.

This sort of difference-making control can be contrasted with what Eddy Nahmias calls *bypassing*—that "our rational, conscious mental activity is *bypassed* in the process of our making decisions and coming to act" (2011, p. 556). Bypassing would occur, for example, if a neuroscientist caused you to make a decision by direct neural stimulation without any deliberation on your part. But causal determination does not entail bypassing; you may be causally determined to deliberate about your options rationally and consciously, while your conscious deliberation causes and makes a difference for your decision.

Still, given naturalistic causal determinism, there are factors beyond your control—the distant past and the laws of nature—that rendered inevitable how you rationally and consciously deliberated, the choice to keep the promise that resulted, and the effects it had. So, the difference deliberation can make is in this sense limited. While causally determined deliberation can make a difference relative to other options being considered, the other options not coming about are made inevitable by factors beyond our control and beyond our causal reach.

Here there is a tension between facticity and transcendence that is challenging to resolve. Hegel held that such tensions can be overcome, while Kierkegaard argued that they constitute an existential paradox, that the tension can at best be affirmed and not resolved. I believe that this is a tension that resists, given human psychology, resolution. It is difficult for us to occupy at the same time the perspective that our decisions and actions make a difference and that they are causally determined by factors beyond our control, even though these perspectives are strictly speaking consistent.

But this dual perspective also has significant benefits. On the one hand it allows us to justifiably believe that our deliberation and actions, for instance on behalf of social justice, can make a difference in a robust sense. This is our transcendence. On the other hand, recognition of our facticity justifies compassion in the face of human frailty and the significant and sometimes seemingly intractable problems we face.

ANGER AND TRANSCENDENCE

A Sartrean account of transcendence poses the risk of discord with our developing view of ourselves as natural beings, and it also risks holding others to control in acting that both is unrealistic and detracts from an accepting and compassionate outlook. One existentialist perspective sets human beings against a world that does not meet their aspirations for equanimity and meaning in life, and to the extent that the deficiencies are human, anger is a paradigmatic response. An alternative perspective foregrounds a different aspect of transcendence: aspirations for ourselves and others tempered by an assessment of the limitations due to our nature and our ability to understand and accept these limitations.

Coming to terms with our facticity involves accepting that we are situated in a natural world of law-governed causes and effects. Our character and actions are conditioned by causes that we do not control—our genetic makeup, our basic neural endowment, and our physical environment. Given that we are components of a natural world, does it make sense to be angry as retribution when people act badly? Eighth-century Buddhist philosopher Śāntideva thought not, as he indicated in his poem *Bodhicaryāvatāra*:

> Why am I angry with sentient beings? They too have causes for their anger. Whatever transgressions and evil deeds of various kinds there are, all arise through the power of conditioning factors, while there is nothing that arises independently. Therefore, even if one sees a friend or an enemy behaving badly, one can reflect that there are specific conditioning factors that determine this, and thereby remain happy. If it is their very nature to cause others distress, my anger towards these unwise ones is as inappropriate as it would be towards fire for its nature to burn. (700/1995, pp. 52–53)

Śāntideva was expressing skepticism about human free will and counting this as a reason against being angry at all with people for the wrongs they have done.

Spinoza also advocated skepticism about free will, and a similar renunciation of anger. He contended that "in the mind there is no absolute, or free, will, but the mind is determined to will this or that by a cause which is also determined by another, and this again by another, and so to infinity" (1677/1985, *Ethics* II, Proposition 48, p. 483). The reason we don't have free will is that all occurrences are causally determined by preceding causes, resulting in chains of causes stretching to infinity. The ultimate deterministic cause of all that happens is the divine nature; but even God does not have free will: "all things have been predetermined by God, not from freedom of the will or absolute good pleasure, but from God's absolute nature, or infinite power" (1677/1985, *Ethics* I, Appendix, p. 439). Like Śāntideva, Spinoza maintained that the doctrine that we lack free will has beneficial consequences:

> It teaches us that we must expect and bear calmly both good fortune and bad. For everything that happens follows from God's eternal decree with the same necessity as it follows from the essence of a triangle that its three angles are equal to two right angles. This doctrine contributes to the social life by teaching us to hate no one, to disesteem no one, to mock no one, to be angry at no one, to envy no one. (1677/1985, *Ethics* II, Proposition 49, Discussion, p. 490)

Understanding that people lack free will counteracts hostile emotions we have toward others, and anger is prominently among them.

Genuine moral anger often comes with the retributive presupposition that its target basically deserves the imposition of pain or harm. If free will skepticism is true, the basic desert presupposition of moral anger is false, thus raising a general challenge to anger in its retributive form. Rather than confronting wrongdoing by blame suffused with retributive anger, we can turn to a forward-looking stance of moral protest instead. Pamela Hieronymi (2001) has proposed that blame should be understood as moral protest, and I follow her lead, with the difference that while in her view the negative reactive attitudes have an essential role in blaming, in my view they do not.

As I see it, moral protest is a psychological stance, a posture of mind that has certain aims or functions that are manifest as dispositions to act. It is a stance of opposition to specific immoral actions and their general type, whose aims include communication of this opposition to wrongdoing, together with reasons to refrain from it. I endorse such a model supposing that the objectives of blaming are forward-looking goals of the moral formation of wrongdoers, protection against wrongdoing, and reconciliation in relationships impaired by wrongdoing (Pereboom, 2014, 2021). With this model, it is the agent's responsiveness to reasons that is engaged in moral protest. In that process we may request an explanation with the intent of having the agent acknowledge a motivation to act wrongly, and then, if they have in fact so acted without excuse or justification, we may intend for them to come to see that the motivation issuing in the action is best eliminated. This change is produced by way of the agent's recognition of moral reasons to make it. More generally, it is a wrongdoer's responsiveness to reasons, together with the forward-looking aims, that explains why they are appropriately addressed by moral protest so characterized.

One might also take on a stance of moral protest in response to one's own immoral actions. One might view one's action as wrong, and one's motivations for it morally defective, and as a result take on a stance of opposition against oneself. In adopting this stance, one may aim at one's own moral formation or at reconciliation with someone one has wronged. If, for example, one has disrespected a friend, and one's relationship is impaired as a result, one might assume a stance of protest against that past action with the aims of eliminating such motivations and actions and of reconciliation with the friend. This may be accompanied by regret, a pained recognition that one has done wrong, but that, unlike guilt, doesn't involve the belief that one basically deserves to impose that pain upon oneself or have it imposed on oneself by another.

One might argue, however, that expression of moral anger can often be valuable, for instance in communication of wrongdoing. Calm communication may often not be effective, while an angry expression stands to have the requisite clarity and impact for success (Shoemaker, 2018; Wolf, 2011). Samuel Reis-Dennis (2019) argued that when a victim of wrongdoing aims to fight back, expression of anger is well suited to communicate that intention. Our disposition to be angry in these contexts is a feature of our facticity to be valued and not overridden by our capacity for transcendence.

Can such expressions of anger be justified given the rejection of basic desert? The free will skeptic calls into question the role of moral anger in our practice of holding someone morally responsible, insofar as that anger features a presupposition that the wrongdoer basically deserves an imposition of the harm or pain of an expression of such anger. Cognitivists about the emotions maintain that emotions generally have presuppositions as components—they may be judgments, thoughts, appraisals, or, arguably, beliefs held with some degree of confidence, that is, credences (e.g., Nussbaum, 1997, 2016). Such components are cognitive since they can be true or false, by contrast with, say, taste or odor sensations on typical accounts. On the cognitivist conception, an instance of fear features a cognitive appraisal about the presence of danger, conceived as a threat to the agent's objectives. Anger at least often includes the cognitive appraisal that its target deserves blame or punishment that imposes harm or pain.

It is possible, however, to be angry with wrongdoers because they did wrong, and while that anger initially has a basic desert appraisal as a component, one may remain morally angry while rejecting that appraisal. In Robert Roberts's (2003, 2013) cognitivist theory of the emotions, the cognitive element of an emotion is a "concerned construal," which represents its target as having a feature that calls for a response. Yet a subject who has the emotion can avoid affirming that the target is correctly represented in this way. The emotion has a component that is analogous to a judgment that the subject of the emotion does not necessarily share, even if the subject does share it in typical cases. In one of his examples, someone who was raised in a strict religious household but has since become more worldly may feel guilty for going to the movie theater, but not affirm that they have done something wrong, which is nonetheless a component of their emotion of guilt. On this account, one can be morally angry, and that anger has, as a component, the appraisal that its target basically deserves to be the recipient of a harmful or painful expression of that anger, while rejecting that appraisal. So moral anger may include a basic desert presupposition, which its subject might not endorse.

The free will skeptic would emphasize the importance of rejecting the retributive appraisal that the anger justifies targeting the wrongdoer with a painful or harmful expression of that anger conceived as basically deserved. But once that appraisal is rejected, on balance the resulting anger may be valuable in the ways recounted above, as facilitating clear and direct communication of wrongdoing and a willingness to fight. Myisha Cherry, in *The Case for Rage* (2021), argued for the value of anger specifically in the fight for racial justice, targeted at those who are complicit in and perpetrate such injustice. When this anger is calibrated so that it is most effective, it is shorn of any retributive element, and instead informed by an inclusive and liberating perspective, whereupon it can motivate productive action and build resistance. Cherry specified that the type of anger she defends does not aim at harm and is compatible with compassion and empathy. To this we can add, as Annette Zimmerman pointed out (in conversation), that such anger can have a benefit for oppressed people who have been socialized into a regime of oppression. Their anger in particular cases of oppression may awaken them to the knowledge that how they are treated, and the regime of oppression more broadly, is unjust.

TRANSCENDENCE AND EMOTIONAL SELF-FORMING

As noted, an important theme of existentialism is the possibility of self-shaping. Again, one might think that self-shaping choices have no role in a deterministic scheme, but this is not so. First, as we've seen, given determinism our choices can make a difference to our lives, despite the fact that how they make a difference is fixed by factors beyond our control. Second, the difference our choices make can shape the core features of ourselves—our life trajectories, but also our emotional natures.

There is a common perspective on which the core human emotional character is fixed. For instance, in a common universalist conception of the practice of holding oneself and others morally responsible, this practice is an expression of human beings universally as constituted by their relatively fixed nature, thus conceived as an aspect of human facticity. At the core of the practice lie the emotions of resentment, indignation, guilt, and gratitude, expressed in a certain range of ways. It is a valuable practice functioning well in regulating human actions, attitudes, and dispositions universally to the benefit of all. There is some freedom to change in this practice, but justified change is decidedly limited. A significantly different practice would be worse, and indeed practically impossible for us to adopt.

My challenge to this universalism has two components. The first is that this practice as universalists conceive it is not universal; there is significant cultural variation among practices of holding people morally responsible. The second is that there are valuable modes of emotional being in various cultures, which we can adopt to change the way we take them on and thereby shape who we are, and thus it's possible for us to transcend what in effect the universalist conception counts as human emotional fixed nature.

When it comes to angry blame, there is considerable variation among cultures, much more than is supposed on a universalist view (De Leersnyder et al., 2013; Flanagan, 2016; Mesquita, 2022). In her book *Between Us*, Batja Mesquita (2022) discussed many studies that document cultural variability for anger. In a summary of findings, she wrote that in the United States, "in close relationships, it is thought to help individuals protect their needs and expectations, and in work settings, it sets clear boundaries. In puberty, it helps adolescents gain independence." But while measured anger is considered right and healthy in U.S. contexts, "this is not true everywhere." Buddhist Tibetans regard anger as "a fundamentally destructive sentiment, equally harmful to self and others." The Polynesian Ifaluk, studied by Catherine Lutz (1988), similarly condemn anger: "frustration building up over the succession of minor unwanted things, or annoyance at relatives not living up to their obligations . . . these varieties of anger were perceived to be immoral and undignified." In Japan, "anger is considered to be a destructive emotion, better to be avoided." More radically, adults in the Utkuhiksalingmiut,[1] an Inuit community of the west coast of Hudson Bay in Canada, avoid angry blame altogether, and raise their children to avoid it, as Jean Briggs recounted in her study *Never in Anger: Portrait of an Eskimo Family*. The generalization she drew is that "where relational harmony is prioritized over the individual autonomy, anger is considered to be wrong."

One might argue on the basis of the widely endorsed biocognitive model for the emotions (Levenson, 1994, 1999) that our basic emotional nature is fixed by our genetic and neural endowment and is thus a feature of our facticity. But this model in fact accommodates very significant cultural diversity. The model begins with the idea that the emotions are responses shaped by both evolution and culture to perceived threats and opportunities. A culture is defined as a socially shared and transmitted pattern of ideas (values, norms, and beliefs) that are instantiated in everyday practices, institutions, and artifacts (Kroeber & Kluckhohn, 1952). An emotion such as anger, fear, or happiness is a motivational response to a perception of a threat or opportunity with attentional, physiological, expressive, motor, and cognitive behavioral routines that result from two systems: a biologically hardwired "core" system and a more flexible, cognitive, and culturally shaped "control" system. At the center of the emotion system is a durable, simple, and efficient processor, designed early in evolution as a response that motivates effectively solving very basic, ubiquitous problems in time-tested, highly predictable, and automatic ways. This part may not be malleable, but supplementing the core system is a more recently evolved, flexible, and less predictable set of control mechanisms that influence the responses of the core system. While the core system is largely hardwired and not capable of major modification in response to experience, the control mechanisms are sensitive to learning, fine-tuning their operating parameters (Kurth, 2023, summary; Levenson, 1994, 1999).

The biocognitive model has been disputed, for example by Lisa Feldman Barrett (2017) and Mesquita (2022). They have argued that (at least given typical ways in which the model is represented) the core system bears the weight for the identity of an emotion, while the control system is peripheral, and so the model doesn't accommodate robust cultural variation for emotions. But as Ron Mallon and Steven Stich (2000) pointed out, this dispute is arguably semantic and not substantive, since we may tie emotion terms such as *fear* and *anger* to either thin descriptions that factor out the culturally variable control mechanisms or thick descriptions that factor them in.

Cultural variability serves to indicate that aspects of our own cultural emotional profile are subject to change. For evidence of malleability, we can turn to anthropologist Briggs's (1970) study of the Utkuhiksalingmiut, who, again, rarely express anger. While the very young in this culture display familiar outbursts of angry emotion, children are educated by community role modeling and calm parental exhortation to avoid displays of anger. The process is generally successful, and the resulting dispositions persist and are ubiquitous in the community. This example illustrates how cultural regulation of emotion, understood as a process that results in the alignment of emotion with cultural values, objectives, and concerns (De Leersnyder et al., 2013), can make a significant difference for the expression and arguably for the occurrence of anger. On Briggs's proposal, closeness and harmony is the cultural goal that underlies this case of emotional regulation, occasioned by the potential destructive effects that divisiveness would have in the harsh Arctic climate. Perhaps our global situation is analogously harsh, and similar cultural regulation of anger would be to our advantage.

Further techniques for malleability are indicated by communal monastic Buddhist practice (Chadha & Nichols, 2024). Buddhists maintain that anger is based on a false presupposition of the self and contributes to suffering, and on this basis encourage practitioners to extirpate anger. But this tradition recognizes that it is insufficient simply to eliminate anger with no other adjustments, precisely because that anger also has valuable social functions. One method in use is the inculcation of feeling anticipatory guilt and fear at the prospect of wrongdoing. Another is the development of patience and forbearance that allow practitioners to respond calmly rather than angrily to wrongdoing. In addition, the practice features a set of vows, recited fortnightly, against performing the kinds of actions that lead to angry reactions, together with vows against angry reactions themselves. Repeated expressions of anger are regarded as a serious offense, leading to temporary suspension—also a response in the withdrawal category. These practices have persisted in Buddhist monastic communities for many centuries, and overall, they satisfy the criteria for an equilibrium of a valuable sort.

Indeed, there are examples of changes over the past century in our practice of holding responsible and the emotions that this practice features that confirm malleability. It was once considered legitimate to angrily blame people for being mentally ill, and in particular for behavior that manifests mental illness; to angrily blame and punish people for being gay or lesbian and specifically for gay or lesbian behavior; to angrily discriminate against and harm people on the basis of race or ethnicity; for husbands to beat their spouses and for parents to beat their children; for teachers to express rage in the classroom and subject pupils to violence; for criminals to be severely harmed, physically and mentally. Humanity has made significant inroads against all of this, which indicates that the tendencies to negative emotions at work in the practice are changeable, and that in this respect we can also manifest our transcendence.

SUFFERING AND TRANSCENDENCE[2]

A further existentialist theme concerns how we see our place in the great scheme of things, given the existence of threats to our well-being, both moral and natural. Theistic religions have provided answers to this question, as have nontheistic views such as Buddhism and modern descendants of orthodox theisms whose conception of the divine is impersonal. A shared theme is that such conceptions provide for greater equanimity in our lives, specifically in view of the suffering caused by wrongdoing and by natural causes, and that this equanimity results from understanding the scheme and our place in it In the theistic religions the conception often features divine providential governance. That is, whatever happens accords with a divine plan that aims at the good, and this provides us with equanimity and meaning in life (Pereboom 1994).

Conceptions of divine providence, whether or not they endorse freedom of the will, are challenged by the presence of evil, both moral and natural, that we cannot view as justified by any good to which they contribute. If an all-powerful, wholly benevolent and providential being exists, then that being would have the power and the will to prevent all such evil. Yet such evil does exist. Existentialists, theistic or nontheistic, are united in their pessimism for establishing a decisive and compelling justification for the evil in this world. An alternative, one that is in accord with existentialist uncertainty about the justification of evil, involves the attitude of hope. Hope is validated when our interest lies in an unknown outcome due to factors completely beyond our control, as is the case if the future is rendered inevitable by theological determinism or else by the past and the laws of nature. On either the theistic or a naturalistic conception, we can aspire to a hope on the model of John Dewey's (1934) "common faith," a hope in the progress of humanity in our environment.

What is it to hope for an outcome? Those who have considered this question agree that it involves a desire that the expressed outcome will come about, and a belief that it's possible that it will. Andrew Chignell (2014) pointed out that Immanuel Kant (1781/1987) famously asked: "What *may* I hope?" and that this question expresses apprehension about rational justification, unease that the desire for the outcome or the belief in its possibility might be irrational, whereupon the hope would also be irrational. This suggests hope for an outcome only if one rationally desires it and rationally believes that it indeed can come about (Chignell, 2014).

A potential fix is that rational hope depends on some degree of rational credence that the outcome will come about (e.g., Milona, 2019). Michael Milona (2019) argued that hope does not require that one's rational credence be very high. But the outcome also can't be certain; as J. M. O. Wheatley (1958) pointed out, "to hope, regarding the future, is in part to expect but not to be sure." Accepting Wheatley's restriction, I've proposed that the more a hope has a significant and rational effect on one's actions—the more it is what I'll call a *substantial hope*—the higher the credence needs to be, all else equal (Pereboom, 2021). Defending rational hope in the progress of humanity in our environment, if it is to be a substantial hope, requires some evidential support, which I believe is available.

In the late 18th and early 19th centuries, humanity widely came to be viewed as a force for inevitable and sustained progress on multiple fronts. This theme is pursued by the German idealists, of which Hegel is representative. One Hegelian idea in particular is crucial in this context. He proposed a deterministic process of human rational development over the span of history, revising the providential aspect of traditional theism by conceiving human rational development itself as in a sense divine. For Hegel the divine was a historical process of realizing an ideal, and human beings and their history were a central component. This historical process is structured in a dialectical way that is multifaceted: It realizes potential in the sciences, the arts, and the humanities; and in social and political development, of which we become conscious through philosophical reflection. Philosophical reflection on this development of human history reveals it as a theodicy, demonstrating how it is providential despite apparent evil. At the end of his *Philosophy of History*, Hegel wrote:

> our mode of treating the subject is, in this aspect, a theodicy—a justification of the ways of God—which Leibniz attempted metaphysically in his method, i.e., in indefinite abstract categories,—so that the ill that is found in the world may be comprehended, and the thinking Spirit reconciled with the fact of the existence of evil. Indeed, nowhere is such a harmonizing view more pressingly demanded than in universal history. (1824/1956, p. 48)

Hegel's notion of the progress of human history as a theodicy encountered strong resistance in the 20th century by existentialists and those influenced by them. Theodor Adorno's response of "No universal history leads from savagery to humanitarianism, but there is one leading from the slingshot to the megaton bomb" (Adorno, 1970, p. 312) is characteristic. But the theme that continued to have influence is Hegel's notion of religion as focused on progress in history. This idea was developed in the 19th century by American transcendentalists such as Ralph Waldo Emerson and Henry Thoreau, and later by pragmatists such as John Dewey in the first part of the 20th century. Dewey proposed a "common faith," a religious attitude broader than traditional theism, whose leading feature is a "sense of nature as the whole of which we are parts, while it also recognizes that we are parts that are marked by intelligence and purpose, having the capacity to strive by their aid to bring conditions into greater consonance with what is humanly desirable" (Dewey, 1934, p. 25). Here Dewey (1934) echoed a theme of the transcendentalists with an idea of progress not solely focused on human beings, but on a human community embedded in a natural environment, "the enveloping world that the imagination feels is a universe" (p. 53).

To claim actual knowledge of human progress in our environment is ambitious. The rationality of substantial hope in this outcome, however, can be defended. We might indeed aim to secure this hope in a world in which human beings do not ultimately exercise control. Given determinism, the history and future of humanity is made inevitable by causal factors beyond our control, by the states of the universe that precede humanity's existence in accord with the laws of nature. In this context, hope is the right attitude to invoke for humanity's progress in our environment, since hope is appropriate in contexts in which we are dependent on how factors beyond our control turn out. As Katie Stockdale (2019) affirmed, hope reminds us of "the kinds of creatures we are: we are creatures who, because of the constraints we necessarily and contingently face as agents, must depend on factors external to ourselves for many of our desires to be fulfilled."

Some of our hopes are personal and are partial for our own well-being. The hope for humanity is, by contrast, impartial. One may ask whether such impartial hope is easy or difficult for us to attain. Martha Nussbaum (2001) had a similar question for compassion; we are more likely to feel compassion for those close to us than for people we don't know at all. A parallel problem has been raised for related notions such as empathy and sympathy (recently by Paul Bloom, 2017). David Hume, in his *Treatise of Human Nature* (1739), expressed this concern as an objection to his claim that moral judgment is founded in sympathy:

> But as this sympathy is very variable, it may be thought that our sentiments of morals must admit of all the same variations. We sympathize more with persons contiguous to us, than with persons remote from us: With our acquaintance, than with strangers: With our countrymen, than with foreigners. (Book III, Part III, Section I)

But he then remarked:

> Notwithstanding this variation of our sympathy, we give the same approbation to the same moral qualities in China as in England. They appear equally virtuous and recommend themselves equally to the esteem of a judicious spectator. (Book III, Part III, Section I)

Hume then set out an influential solution:

> In order, therefore, to prevent those continual contradictions, and arrive at a more stable judgment of things, we fix on some steady and general points of view; and always, in our thoughts, place ourselves in them, whatever may be our present situation. (Book III, Part III, Section I)

Elevating oneself to such an impartial point of view affords an elegant solution and is a further feature of transcendence. We can similarly endorse a transcendent substantial hope for the progress of humanity in our environment.

Can we secure the rational credence required for such substantial hope? Theodore Parker, American transcendentalist, expressed the idea of continued human progress in its moral dimension in his reflections on the abolition of slavery, using a now-familiar metaphor:

> We cannot understand the moral Universe. The arc is a long one, and our eyes reach but a little way; we cannot calculate the curve and complete the figure by the experience of sight; but we can divine it by conscience, and we surely know that it bends toward justice. Justice will not fail, though wickedness appears strong, and has on its side the armies and thrones of power, the riches and the glory of the world, and though poor men crouch down in despair. Justice will not fail and perish out from the world of men, nor will what is really wrong and contrary to God's real law of justice continually endure. (1853, pp. 84–85)

In his speeches, Martin Luther King, Jr. also encouraged us to envision, quoting Parker, that "the arc of the moral universe is long, but it bends toward justice." Here Parker claimed knowledge, but transcendent hope is less demanding and more accessible, even if it is substantial and accordingly has a significant effect on how we act.

What evidence do we have to support Parker's optimism? In the last century alone humanity has faced extremely serious challenges: global wars, mass genocide, terrorism, and epidemics. But we repeatedly confronted these challenges with hard-won but nonetheless impressive success. Medical science has made amazing progress, technology has advanced remarkably, and knowledge in many fields has witnessed immense, astonishing expansion. International politics is more challenged but has at the same time featured impressive success. On balance, challenges were effectively confronted, and progress was achieved.

Consider the threat of climate change to our natural environment and to the flourishing of humanity, with the prospect of melting polar ice inundating land, and the planet becoming too hot to sustain the life of many of its current inhabitants, a threat which resulted at least in part from failure of stewardship. Hope can be grounded in the growth of climate awareness, affirmation of international agreements, the advancement of reforestation and climate-friendly methods in agriculture, and the distinct possibility of feasible direct carbon capture. Human resolve in these cases provides evidence to ground the rationality of the hope that we will be successful in overcoming such challenges more generally.

So what may we hope? We may hope that human intelligence, skill, and moral resolve is sufficient for overcoming the challenges we will face to ourselves and our environment. The feature of this conception that provides inspiration and comfort is that we, embedded in our natural world, form a system whose future is survival and progress, and whose arc tends toward justice. Human experience, despite the irrationality and injustice that we see, secures the rationality of this transcendent hope.

NOTES

1. The name means "the people of the place where there is soapstone."

2. See Pereboom (2021, Chap. 7) for further development of themes in this section.

REFERENCES

Adorno, T. W. (1970). *Negative dialektik*. Suhrkamp.

Barrett, L. F. (2017). *How emotions are made: The secret life of the brain*. HarperCollins.

Bloom, P. (2017). *Against empathy: The case for rational compassion*. Random House.

Briggs, J. L. (1970). *Never in anger: Portrait of an Eskimo family*. Harvard University Press.

Chadha, M., & Nichols, S. (2024). Living without anger. In D. Shoemaker (Ed.), *Oxford studies in agency and responsibility* (Vol. 9). Oxford University Press.

Cherry, M. (2021). *The case for rage*. Oxford University Press.

Chignell, A. (2014). Rational hope, possibility, and divine action. In G. Michalson (Ed.), *Kant's religion within the bounds of mere reason: A critical guide* (pp. 98–117). Cambridge University Press.

De Leersnyder, J., Boiger, M., & Mesquita, B. (2013). Cultural regulation of emotion: Individual, relational, and structural sources. *Frontiers in Psychology, 4*, Article 55.

Dewey, J. (1934). *A common faith*. Yale University Press.

Flanagan, O. (2016). *The geography of morals: Varieties of moral possibility*. Oxford University Press.

Guignon, C., & Pereboom, D. (1995). *Existentialism: Basic writings, an anthology, with introductions*. Hackett. (2nd [expanded] ed. 2001)

Hegel, G. W. F. (1956). *The philosophy of history* (J. Sibree, Trans.). Dover. (Original work published 1824)

Hieronymi, P. (2001). Articulating an uncompromising forgiveness. *Philosophy and Phenomenological Research, 62*, 529–555.

Hume, D. (1978). *Treatise on human nature*. Oxford University Press. (Original work published 1739)

Hume, D. (1999). *An enquiry concerning human understanding*. Oxford University Press. (Original work published 1748)

Kant, I. (1987). *Critique of pure reason* (P. Guyer & Allen Wood, Trans.). Cambridge University Press. (Original work published 1781/1787)

Kierkegaard, S. (1941). *Concluding unscientific postscript* (W. Lowrie, Trans.). Princeton University Press. (Original work published 1846)

Kroeber, A. L., & Kluckhohn, C. (1952). Culture: A critical review of concepts and definitions. *Papers. Peabody Museum of Archaeology & Ethnology, Harvard University, 47*(viii), 223.

Kurth, C. (2023). *The anxious mind*. MIT Press.

Leiter, B. (2007). Nietzsche's theory of the will. *Philosophers' Imprint, 7*, 1–15.

Levenson, R. W. (1994). Human emotion: A functional view. In P. Ekman & R. J. Davidson (Eds.), *The nature of emotion: Fundamental questions* (pp. 123–126). Oxford University Press.

Levenson, R. W. (1999). The intrapersonal functions of emotion. *Cognition & Emotion, 13*(5), 481–504.

Lutz, C. (1988). *Unnatural emotions*. University of Chicago Press.

Mallon, R., & Stich, S. (2000). The odd couple: The compatibility of evolutionary psychology and social construction. *Philosophy of Science, 67*(1), 133–154.

McKenna, M. (2019). Basically deserved blame and its value. *Journal of Ethics and Social Philosophy, 15*, 255–282.

Mesquita, B. (2022). *Between us: How cultures create emotions*. W. W. Norton.

Milona, M. (2019). Finding hope. *Canadian Journal of Philosophy, 49*(5), 710–729.

Nahmias, E. (2011). Intuitions about free will, determinism, and bypassing. In R. Kane (Ed.), *The Oxford handbook of free will* (2nd ed., pp. 555–576). Oxford University Press.

Nietzsche, F. (1974). *The gay science* (W. Kaufmann, Tans.). Viking. (Original work published 1882)

Nietzsche, F. (1998). *On the genealogy of moral-*

ity (M. Clark & A. Swensen, Trans.). Hackett. (Original work published 1887)

Nussbaum, M. C. (1997). Emotions as judgments of value and importance. In P. Bilimoria & J. Mohanty (Eds.), *Relativism, suffering and beyond* (pp. 271–283). Oxford University Press.

Nussbaum, M. C. (2001). *Upheavals of thought: The intelligence of emotions.* Cambridge University Press.

Nussbaum, M. C. (2016). *Anger and forgiveness.* Oxford University Press.

Parker, T. (1853). Of justice and the conscience. In *Ten sermons of religion by Theodore Parker.* Crosby, Nichols and Company.

Pereboom, D. (1994). Stoic psychotherapy in Descartes and Spinoza. *Faith and Philosophy, 11,* 592–625.

Pereboom, D. (2014). *Free will, agency, and meaning in life.* Oxford University Press.

Pereboom, D. (2021). *Wrongdoing and the moral emotions.* Oxford University Press.

Reis-Dennis, S. (2019). Anger: Scary good. *Australasian Journal of Philosophy, 97*(3), 451–464.

Roberts, R. C. (2003). *Emotions: An essay in aid of moral psychology.* Cambridge University Press.

Roberts, R. C. (2013). *Emotions in the moral life.* Cambridge University Press.

Śāntideva. (1995). *The Bodhicaryāvatā]ra* (K. Crosby & A. Skilton, Trans.). Oxford University Press, 1995. (Original work published 700)

Sartre, J.-P. (1956). *Being and nothingness* (H. E. Barnes, Trans.). Philosophical Library. (Original work published 1943)

Sartre, J.-P. (2001). Existentialism is a humanism. In C. Guignon & D. Pereboom (Eds.), *Existentialism: Basic writings* (2nd ed.). Hackett.

Shoemaker, D. (2018). "You oughta know!: Defending angry blame. In M. Cherry & O. Flanagan (Eds.), *The moral psychology of anger.* Lanham, MD: Rowman & Littlefield.

Spinoza, B. (1985). *The collected works of Spinoza* (Vol. 1; E. Curley, Ed. & Trans.). Princeton University Press. (Original work published 1667)

Stockdale, K. (2019). Social and political dimensions of hope. *Journal of Social Philosophy, 50,* 28–44.

Wheatley, J. M. O. (1958). Wishing and hoping. *Analysis, 18,* 121–131.

Wolf, S. (2011). Blame, Italian style. In R. J. Wallace, R. Kumar, & S. Freeman (Eds.), *Reasons and recognition: Essays on the philosophy of T. M. Scanlon* (pp. 332–347). Oxford University Press.

CHAPTER 4

The Failure of Science and the Science of Failure

Toward a Black Existential Psychology

Timothy J. Golden

Twentieth-century philosopher Emmanuel Levinas, in the first sentence of the preface of his magnum opus, *Totality and Infinity* (1961), wrote that it was of the utmost importance to know whether we had been "duped" by morality. The same can be said of law: Are we duped by jurisprudence? Is law an a priori science that guarantees predictable outcomes? Is the resolution of litigation simply a matter of a formulaic application of the law to a set of facts? Or, does the supposed a priori nature of law conceal something based on experience rather than the intellect? What are we to make of the claims that law is a priori, considering the peculiar relationship of law to racial oppression? This is especially relevant in the United States, a country that has deployed law in the service of unjust treatment of African Americans. Again, has the "science" of jurisprudence duped us? There is ample evidence that we have been so duped.

THE LEGAL CONTEXT: JURISPRUDENCE AS A FAILED SCIENCE

From racial profiling in constitutional criminal procedure under the Fourth Amendment of the U.S. Constitution (Alexander, 2010), to the denial of voting rights under federal law (*Shelby County, Alabama v. Holder*, 2013) to the declarations of unconstitutionality directed at remedial measures for past injustices under the Fourteenth Amendment's Equal Protection Clause (*Students for Fair Admissions, Inc. v. President and Fellows of Harvard College*, 2023), jurisprudence can be viewed more as the failure of a science than as a legitimate scientific endeavor on the order of physics, chemistry, biology, or psychology. Consider the complicity of the U.S. Supreme Court in perpetuating Jim Crow for nearly 100 years after Reconstruction with its restrictive, abstract interpretation of the Civil War Amendments. Did not the Supreme Court disregard the will of Congress when, rather than allowing the Reconstruction Amendments to protect newly emancipated African Americans, the Court disingenuously ruled that those Amendments only applied to encroachments of the federal government on the rights of African Americans and not to the states (*Slaughterhouse Cases*, 1872)? Such a ruling from the Court is especially troubling since the social reality of the time was that newly freed slaves were more in danger from state governments than from the federal government that was vigorously trying to protect them from racial violence. The history of law in the United States, then, when juxtaposed to the supposed a priori nature of law, demonstrates jurisprudence as a failure of science driven more by racial animus than by any neat, formulaic application of the law.

What are we to make of this failure of law as a science? That is, if law represents, at least in the case of the United States—and arguably other countries that have long histories of injustice toward their citizens—a failure of science, do we not need a science of failure? Due regard to the human interests of those whom law has wronged demands some way of tending to the damage done to such persons. Do we not need a scientific intervention to address the deep psychological and emotional needs of those who receive unjust treatment from the failed science of law? Indeed, we do. Recent social science research has argued that the psychological harm of aggressive policing is both significant and underexamined (Bandes et al., 2019). Consider the example of stop and frisk in the context of constitutional criminal procedure. The phrase *stop and frisk* is derived from a landmark U.S. Supreme Court decision (*Terry v. Ohio*, 1968) that allows for the detention and physical pat-down of a criminal suspect if police and prosecutors can meet a rigorous, two-pronged legal threshold, premised upon the legal standard of "reasonable suspicion." Police have a reasonable suspicion if they have specific and articulable facts, which, when taken together with the rational inferences from those facts, lead them to believe two things: (1) that the suspect is engaged in criminal activity (that criminal activity is afoot) and (2) that the suspect is armed and presently dangerous (*Terry v. Ohio*, 1968). Constitutional justification for a stop in Fourth Amendment law is distinct from constitutional justification for a frisk. Moreover, the scope of both is limited. A stop is limited to a request for identification and minimal questioning related to the nature of the stop. For example, if police want to stop someone for burglary, the officer must be able to point to specific and articulable facts that lead them to conclude that the suspect may be involved in a burglary. A generalized suspicion is insufficient. Assuming the officer can point to such specific and articulable facts, the stop is limited to a request for identification and basic questions regarding the suspect's location and purpose at that location, nothing more. A stop is not an interrogation, it is a brief investigative detention and can only last as long as necessary to dispel the reasonable suspicion. And the same is true of a frisk, which is not a probing search of bodily cavities, but rather is restricted to a pat-down of the suspect's outer clothing to detect weapons that can be of danger to the officer. Again, there must be a reasonable suspicion (specific and articulable facts) that lead the officer to conclude that the suspect is armed and presently dangerous (*Terry v. Ohio*, 1968).

These legal standards, however, are not always followed. Racial profiling effectively jettisons constitutional criminal procedure in favor of implicit racial bias that becomes problematic. Indeed, some authors have pointed out that in the context of stop and frisk, not only are constitutional legal standards ignored but also their disregard results in serious psychological harms to members of marginalized communities (Bandes et al., 2019). Consider the psychological harm done to an African American man in his 50s who was stopped 30 times in less than 4 years, without any of the stops resulting in either a citation or a criminal charge and that African Americans amounted to 95% of the 410 people stopped at least 10 times over a 5-year period (United States Justice Department Civil Rights Division, 2016). The disregard of constitutional standards, then, is the failure of science (law or jurisprudence). And the need to address the psychological harms done to people, many of them Black, generates a need for the science of that failure in the form of a Black existential psychology.

This chapter addresses that psychological need using some of the principles and thinkers of Black existentialism, a philosophical subfield associated with the psychologically oriented subfields of phenomenology and existentialism. Concerned with the consciousness of the human person, both the existential and phenomenological philosophical traditions incline toward humanity rather than traditional scientific objectivity, and thus, I argue, pave the way for a Black existential psychology that can uniquely address the emotional and psychological harm done to Black people. This chapter, then, has as its point of departure jurisprudence as a failure of science. From the failure of science, I move toward a science of the effects of that failure: a Black existential psychology that can meet the deep psychological and emotional needs of Black people harmed by certain legal principles, practices, and outcomes in American law.

The chapter proceeds in three phases. First, the chapter elucidates the existential and phenomenological tradition and situates Black existentialism's basic principles and some major thinkers within that broader tradition. Second, it draws upon Frantz Fanon's Afro-European (Black) existential and psychological insights from *Black Skin, White Masks* and *The Wretched of the Earth.* Third, using these insights from Fanon, the chapter turns to an African American iteration of Black existentialism in the context of American law, interpreting W. E. B. DuBois's (1986) notion of double consciousness as an existentially absurd formation of the Black self descended from American legal institutions in which the African American originated as a slave that was both person and property. Frederick Douglass's accounts of time and the imagination are, I argue, viable Black existential resources for dealing with the harmful effects of DuBois's account of the Black self on the human psyche.

The discussion of Blacks before the bar of justice in American law shows what I believe are profound implications for Black existentialism and psychology: The failure of jurisprudence to function as an a priori science of law shows the ways in which that failure demands, in the name of Black humanity, its own science of an existential psychology comprehensive enough to be attuned to the anxiety, radical freedom, responsibility, absurdity, paradox, and so forth of Black subjects who stand before the law, both in America and throughout the world.

PHENOMENOLOGY TO BLACK EXISTENTIALISM: KEY THINKERS AND BASIC PRINCIPLES

The philosophical subfields of existentialism and phenomenology can be characterized as reactions against certain tendencies in modern philosophy. These tendencies emerge from an enlightenment-oriented modern philosophy—from Francis Bacon, Thomas Hobbes, and René Descartes, through Immanuel Kant—that, in its valorization of reason and high regard for the importance of the natural sciences, developed a certain epistemological point of view that posits a subject standing over and against a world of objects. These objects are there to be studied, analyzed, and known in the interest of a better understanding of the world—a world of objects, an "objective" world. It is from within this epistemological point of view, this paradigm of knowledge, so to speak, that modern philosophy becomes object-centered ("objective") in its orientation: In furthering the cause of enlightenment science to enable a better understanding of the external world through the use of reason alone, independent of any authority external to the subject, the human self becomes its own epistemic foundation (Descartes, 1993) who can know the objective world. The existential and phenomenological philosophical traditions generally resist these tendencies toward objectivity in favor of a more robust understanding of subjective, human life.

Black existentialism is part of a broader existential and phenomenological philosophical tradition. Here, I discuss four philosophers from that broader European tradition to lay the foundation for my discussion of some of Black existentialism's principal ideas and thinkers (Lewis Gordon, George Yancy, and Derrick Bell), their readings of Black thinkers such as Frederick Douglass, and their appropriations of phenomenology (Gordon and Yancy). The philosophers I discuss from the broader European tradition are Søren Kierkegaard (1813–1855), Albert Camus (1913–1960), Jean-Paul Sartre (1900–1980), and Edmund Husserl (1859–1938). There are, of course, other philosophers from within this tradition. I discuss these particular thinkers for two reasons. First, because they all represent a movement away from the objectivity of modern philosophy and toward a depth of engagement with the human person (something that can, again, generally be said of all philosophers in the existential and phenomenological traditions). And second, I choose these philosophers because I think they best represent the existential and phenomenological concepts of anxiety, the absurd, radical freedom, and responsibility that are both prominent and influential themes in works of Black existentialism and phenomenology. A final word of caution about the existential and phenomenological philosophical tradition is that none of its thinkers reject science per se. To make such an assertion would be a straw man. Rather, the existential and phenomenological philosophical tradition emphasizes a relative imbalance of concern tilted in favor of objectivity at the expense of humanity. So, existentialism and phenomenology are not hostile to science but, rather, are oriented toward the subject rather than the object. Indeed, my point in this chapter is to show how Black existentialism turns toward psychology as a rigorous, empirical, scientific discipline, becoming a "science of failure" and thus helps develop a Black existential psychology to address the human effects of law's failure as a science.

Kierkegaard, Camus, Sartre, and Husserl

Existentialism as a thematic philosophical subfield arguably originates in the nineteenth century with the Danish philosopher Søren Kierkegaard (1813–1855). Kierkegaard argued that the modern epistemological paradigm of subject–object and its attendant disposition to objectivity was wholly inappropriate to evaluate the inner life of the human person, in particular, the religious (Christian) life. Writing such works as *The Concept of Anxiety* (1980), Kierkegaard, through his literary use of pseudonyms, decried the application of scientific concepts to religious life, arguing vociferously that religion was not a matter of science at all, but rather a matter of deep psychological significance and personal importance to the human being, whom modern philosophy's objective orientation overlooked altogether. For example, in *The Concept of Anxiety*, Kierkegaard, through his pseudonym, Vigilius Haufneinsis (the watcher of Copenhagen), argued that Christians had been so enchanted—indeed bewitched—by modernity's scientific tendencies that they utterly ignored the complex psychology of moral deliberation and its accompanying anxiety over the possibility of human freedom. Instead of grappling with the complexities of anxiety and freedom in moral psychology, too many Christians rather deployed the theological doctrine of original sin to provide an "answer" for the presence of our moral shortcomings at the expense of psychological insights about anxiety and freedom that provided great depth and meaning (Kierkegaard, 1980). For Haufneinsis, then, Christians began to treat their religion as a science. And it is this misapplication of modernity's scientific principles to religion that results in a woefully underexamined human self. With Kierkegaard, we thus see the first movement away from objectivity and toward the human subject with his discussion of the concepts of anxiety and freedom, two themes of great import for African Americans and their interactions with American law in Black existentialism.

The 20th century brought existentialism even closer to the subject through the work of Albert Camus, who argued in *The Myth of Sisyphus* (1991) that life is fundamentally absurd and thus meaningless, resulting in his conclusion that the only serious philosophical question is that of suicide. In other words, the theoretical questions of modern philosophy's emphasis on physics and mathematics lack the significance of questions of life and death (Camus, 1991). Camus pointed out that even Galileo recanted his scientific observations when confronted with the life-and-death decision facing him before the Inquisition. For Camus, the most urgent concerns were fundamentally related to and reducible to one question: How does one make life worth living in an absurd world? Human life, according to Camus, is beset by a contingency that we attempt to mask with quotidian routines that invest a certain sort of regularity and thus meaning to life. We invest this meaning to life because of our rational desire to make sense of the world, but the world does not provide this sort of meaning in response to our desire. Despite the myriad philosophical attempts, for example, to present reality as a unified whole that can be rationally understood, we fall short of such a rational explanation for the world and thus lapse into a world without meaning. But just because life is meaningless does not mean it is not worth living. Indeed, Camus fashioned a heroic archetype, the absurd hero, who confronts the absurdity of life and yet determines to live both passionately and courageously. It is this archetype of the absurd hero, Sisyphus (discussed later in this section), that becomes a central figure in Black existentialism.

Jean-Paul Sartre's existentialism is important for its contributions to radical freedom and responsibility, which are major themes within the existential and phenomenological traditions. Sartre's philosophy was, in part, at least, in response to the objectivity of modern philosophy discussed at the beginning of this section. Recall that philosophy has an epistemological preoccupation oriented externally toward the "objective" world. Classical metaphysical formulations in philosophy posit that for everything, there is some preordained purpose: A knife is designed for cutting, a clock is designed for keeping time, a car is designed to drive, and so forth. For Sartre, it was dehumanizing to assume the same thing about human beings. To suggest that human beings are patterned after some preordained plan (one that God establishes, for example) is to deny human beings the radical freedom to be something other than they were created to be, hence Sartre's thoroughgoing atheism. Sartre's point here was that instead of one having an essence that precedes one's existence, one's existence precedes one's essence, and one creates one's essence through the power of one's choice, understood as being made free from any preordained essence. Sartre was arguing that we are not only radically free but also radically responsible for our lives through the choices we make in that radical freedom. The world is as it is, our lives are as they are precisely because of the choices we have made. To deny that one is free is to engage in a process of self-imposed metamorphose that Sartre called "bad faith," which is a lie to oneself about the reality of one's freedom. Through several examples in his magnum opus, *Being and Nothingness*, Sartre showed how people often would rather transform themselves into objects bereft of freedom than embrace their radical freedom and live more responsibly. One must be careful appropriating Sartre in Black existentialism, as Sartre's model of radical freedom and responsibility does not account for external forces that limit choice, such as American chattel slavery. Nevertheless, Sartre's notions of radical freedom and bad faith have been constructively and compellingly used in Black existentialism and phenomenology, as discussed below.

Lastly, Edmund Husserl (1859–1938), the founder of phenomenology, maintained an ongoing critical engagement with the objectivity of modern philosophy. For Husserl, modern philosophy created a scientific approach to the world that, in his words, is so highly "mathematized" that it has forgotten the human subject altogether. And it is this forgetfulness that Husserl believed led to what he called a "crisis of the European sciences": On one hand, enlightenment science, through the use of reason, was supposed to lead to a more civilized world, liberated from superstition, but on the other hand, enlightenment science and its relentless quest for objectivity produced a world in the 20th century on the brink of nuclear annihilation. The etymology of the word *crisis* is instructive here in that the Greek word *krinein* means "to decide." Husserl believed that decisions must be made about the viability of living in a world in which scientific objectivity almost entirely eclipsed the importance of personhood. To address this crisis, this need for decision-making, Husserl developed a method designed to redirect attention from the objectivity of modern science to the subjectivity of human life. Husserl referred to his philosophical method as "phenomenology," which literally means "the study of that which appears." What Husserl wanted to show is that there are two ways of seeing the world. The first of these ways is a theory-laden view of the world that essentially separates human subjectivity from a connection to the world. On this view all things in the world transcend the human subject: clocks, books, cars, houses, and so forth are all objects that we theoretically understand as having certain purposes and that are numerically distinct from us. Husserl referred to this way of seeing the world as "the natural attitude," and it is this way of seeing the world that is the way of modern philosophy and enlightenment "Galilean" science.

The problem for Husserl was that the natural attitude obscures humanity's real connection to the world. In automatically viewing the world as separate from us, we impede our ability to fully comprehend our connection to it. Husserl thus called for a suspension of the natural attitude through what he termed the *epoché*, which is a bracketing of the natural attitude that enables us to see our true connection to the world. For instance, viewing a set of keys in the natural attitude may give me a theoretical understanding of what keys are—implements to unlock doors and provide access to certain spaces—but it does not provide any meaning beyond such a theoretical understanding. But suppose I suspend that theoretical view of the keys and instead recognize the set of keys in terms of how I intend to use them. On this account, the keys are not separated from me as in the natural attitude but, rather, are connected to me (or I to them) because of how I intend to use them. In suspending the natural attitude, the transcendence of modern philosophy becomes the immanence of phenomenology. Through understanding my intentional relationship to the keys, I become responsible for both them and the places to which those keys provide access. The lynchpin of Husserl's phenomenology was his thesis of intentionality. Appropriated from Franz Brentano, Husserl's emphasis on intentionality transforms the moral distance associated with a world of theoretical "things" into a sense of moral urgency associated with a world of responsibility. It is this sense of responsibility, this connectedness to the world, that can help curb its objectification and turn us back toward human subjectivity in a way that we can learn more about ourselves, or what Husserl called the *lebenswelt*, or "life world." Opposed to the world of science, the life world is a pretheoretical realm of lived experience in which human beings have intersubjectivity without the theoretical demands of modern science, experiencing things as they are in themselves, rather than as theoretically understood as "objects." Indeed, for Husserl, the life world lay at the foundation of science itself. Philosophical analogues to Husserl's phenomenology include Plato's "Allegory of the Cave" in book VII of *Republic*, and Descartes's *Meditations on First Philosophy*, both of which articulate two distinct ways of seeing the world. Plato portrayed truth as fundamentally obscured by fetters that only enable us to see shadows that we mistake to be real. Were the fetters removed, we could see the world as it actually is, rather than as mere shadows. And Descartes argued that the truth is obscured by false beliefs, which are expunged through his method of hyperbolic doubt that assumes all to be false in order to arrive at what is true. Like Plato and Descartes, Husserl urged a departure from seeing the world theoretically to seeing it as actually lived. Indeed, Husserl himself argued that Descartes came closest to his phenomenological method. Husserl's phenomenological method figures prominently in Black existentialism, as discussed below.

Black Existentialism via Gordon, Yancy, and Bell

The philosophical subfield of Black existentialism and its themes of anxiety, the absurd, radical freedom, and responsibility exist against the philosophical backdrop articulated to this point. Black existentialism is a philosophical subfield that has developed over the last 32 years or so from prominent Black philosophers reading Black thinkers typically associated with other academic disciplines. With this in mind, it is important to distinguish between the Black existentialist philosophers who interpret Black thinkers and the Black thinkers they interpret. Of the latter group, there are Black thinkers such as Maria Stewart, Ida B. Wells, Frederick Douglass, Frantz Fanon, and W. E. B. DuBois. And of the former group are contemporary Black philosophers such as Lewis R. Gordon and George Yancy. Another Black thinker, not traditionally considered a Black existentialist but one whose work is especially pertinent for this chapter, is African American legal theorist Derrick Bell. Neither of these groups mentioned here—those Black thinkers interpreted or those Black philosophers doing the interpreting—are intended to be exhaustive, for there are many Black thinkers who can be interpreted as doing existential and phenomenological thought, as there are many Black philosophers who develop their interpretations into the philosophical insights that comprise Black existentialism. One cannot, of course, articulate all such thinkers and philosophers in one chapter, so some selectivity is necessary. With this in mind, I present in this subsection the basic ideas and concepts of Black existentialism as presented in the works of Gordon, Yancy, and Bell, as thinkers who do the interpreting, and in the next two sections, I discuss Fanon and DuBois as Black thinkers who have been interpreted in existential and phenomenological terms. As is the case with the selection of Black existential philosophers, so it is with their individual works: the oeuvres of Gordon, Yancy, and Bell are extensive, so selectivity is necessary. The works of each thinker discussed here are thus not intended to be exhaustive but rather are presented as being representative works that will familiarize the reader with basic existential and phenomenological concepts and themes essential to understanding the subject of this chapter, which is the need for a Black existential psychology.

The claim that Gordon's work is formative of Black existentialism is no exaggeration. Through a series of works, beginning with his 1995 text, *Bad Faith and Anti-Black Racism*, Gordon has engaged the existential and phenomenological philosophical tradition, presenting highly original analyses of existential and phenomenological concepts from the standpoint of Black life. Recall in the above discussion that Sartre's notion of bad faith is a lie told to oneself to avoid the responsibility of radical freedom. Gordon argued that anti-Black racism is an expression of bad faith in that dehumanizing beliefs about Black people represent attempts to avoid responsibility for treating Black people as human beings. Philosophical anthropologies that attempt to scientifically develop theories of human nature are thus made more difficult because of existential bad faith: If one's theories of humanity are beset by a dehumanization of other human beings (in this case, Black people) in the interest of an evasion of moral responsibility, then such theories are inherently unreliable at best (Gordon, 1995a).

Gordon furthered his work on existential bad faith and drew from the phenomenological tradition in another of his 1995 works, *Fanon and the Crisis of European Man: An Essay on Philosophy and the Human Sciences*. In this work, Gordon argued that the European sciences have anti-Black, anticolonial assumptions at their core that function as a sort of bad faith that perpetuates the oppression of colonized people. For Gordon, the very enterprise of European knowledge production was predicated upon the aim of a European racial hierarchy with Whites atop it, deploying "knowledge" and "science" in the interest of racial subjugation. So it is that from racial taxonomy to world "exploration," anti-Black and colonial logics are presupposed (Gordon, 1995b). Reading the works of Frantz Fanon, Gordon did in this work something similar to what Husserl was doing in phenomenology: Whereas for Husserl, the crisis of the European sciences was one of a forgetfulness of humanity, for Gordon the crisis of the European sciences was its unrecognized yet highly functional and bad faith dehumanization of colonized people. Gordon wrote: "Husserl's complaint is that practitioners of the human sciences, philosophy, and cultural criticism often identify the symptoms, but they shrink cowardly from the task involved in identifying the disease" (1995b, p. 7) and that "Whereas for Husserl there was a nightmare of disintegrated reason, for Fanon there was the nightmare of racist reason itself—reason that leaves him out in the cold" (p. 8). Gordon thus concluded that it is not enough to study "social phenomena" such as ghettos, for example, but rather we need to identify their causes, which, through the works of Fanon, Gordon identified in the structural logic of the European sciences. That Gordon engaged with Fanon in this text is significant for this chapter, as Fanon's work on the psychological effects of colonization on colonized people is necessary to move toward a Black existential psychology. Fanon is discussed in this way in the next section.

In Gordon's landmark text, *Existensia Africana: Understanding Africana Existential Thought*, he articulated some problems interpreting Black thinkers existentially and phenomenologically. In his essay "A Problem of Biography in Africana Thought," he argued that readings of such Black thinkers by Black philosophers liberates Black thinkers from what Gordon called "epistemic closure," a phenomenon in which a Black thinker becomes so overly associated with either a genre or a discipline that they cannot be considered "philosophical." For Gordon, this resulted in an undertheorization of Black thought. Gordon (2000) thus pointed out that Phillis Wheatley was more than a poet, and that Frederick Douglass wrote and thought about more than just the abolition of American chattel slavery. With Black thinkers thus freed from such constraints that truncate their identity and the full measure of their contributions to human thought, they become "thinkers" in the broadest sense, and this breadth includes theorizing them as philosophers. But Gordon (2006) even cautioned the philosopher to beware; for a hazard of philosophy is that it can, due to what he called "disciplinary decadence," end up reimprisoning Wheatley and Douglass by regarding them as philosophers to the exclusion of other ways to read them.

It is precisely this overcoming of epistemic closure that enabled Gordon to theorize Douglass as an existentialist. In his essay, "Frederick Douglass as an Existentialist," Gordon read Douglass with existentialist themes of anxiety, freedom, and responsibility—analyzing Douglass's journey from slavery to freedom, in particular his fight with the overseer, Edward Covey, and Douglass's attainment of literacy. As for Covey, Gordon (2000) pointed out that Douglass "became" a human being through his fight with Covey, and that, through a study of existential themes in Douglass's thought, "we find what is in the annals of existential thought a portrait that foreshadows some of the best of Richard Wright's and Frantz Fanon's reflections on struggle and freedom" (p. 45). Douglass embraced his radical freedom in his fight with Covey, his overseer. Recall that for Sartre, the traditional philosophical paradigm of an essence preceding a thing's existence is unacceptable for human beings. Instead, Sartre embraced the notion of radical existential freedom by arguing that one's essence is created through one's choices, such that one's existence precedes one's essence. Applying this principle to Douglass, Gordon argued that Douglass rejected the essence of slave in favor of freely choosing an essence of human. And on the point of Douglass's attainment of literacy, Gordon noted that "Reading exemplified a transgression: it exemplified being able to do what was both denied and forbidden. But the moment the possibility that it could be achieved was raised, Douglass was thrown into a process of imagining himself beyond his condition" (p. 51). Recall that Kierkegaard, through his pseudonym, Vigilius Haufneinsis, was trying to recapture the psychological complexities of moral choice from an oversimplified brand of the Christian religion, which has wrongly been treated as scientific. With his existential analysis of Douglass's transgression of his prohibition on literacy, Gordon uncovered the complexities of Douglass's existential freedom, especially his anxiety of being able not only to imagine his capabilities as those belonging to a human being, but to act on those capabilities, moving from possibility to actuality in a psychological context beset with deep existential anxiety. Through Gordon's work, then, Black existentialism emerges with trenchant critiques of science based on bad faith, and through radical freedom and responsibility.

Husserl's work has been profoundly influential, reaching through the 20th century and, with Yancy's work, now into the 21st century. Among those whom Husserl influenced are the French philosopher, Maurice Merleau-Ponty (1908–1961), whose work centered on a phenomenology of the human body, and what the body is "as-experienced" by oneself, rather than as a scientifically defined anatomical being composed of fluid, bones, and tissue. Yancy's work took Merleau-Ponty's further in that Yancy, while interested in a phenomenological account of the body, was interested in a peculiar type of body: the racialized Black body. Yancy's work can thus be characterized as a phenomenology of racial embodiment. Drawing from the work of Merleau-Ponty, Yancy's work articulated a phenomenology of what it means to be a raced-body, in particular, a Black body. Yancy's work discussed what it means to be a Black body in a culture with a history saturated with anti-Black racism. What does it mean, then, Yancy asked, to experience life as a "nigger"? Yancy probed this question in his landmark text, *Black Bodies, White Gazes: The Continuing Significance of Race*. With this inquiry as his point of departure, Yancy, in another of his works, *White Self-Criticality beyond Anti-Racism: How Does It Feel to Be a White Problem?* (2015), described his work as a "density" project, engaged in the complex, messy thicket of Husserl's pretheoretical life world; a life world, in the case of the Black body, of racial violence, terror, and existential and phenomenological subjugation. Yancy was not interested in theoretical "solutions" to the problems of anti-Black racism any more than Husserl was interested in theoretical explanations for objects in the world. Yancy, understanding a crisis to imply a decision, thus calls for us to decide to suspend our theorizations about anti-Black racism—to be, in his words, "un-sutured," long enough to experience the life world of the Black body; a pretheoretical world in which there are devastating effects on Blacks, whose lived experience is horrific in its occurrence of what Yancy would call the "quotidian." Here one can consider the compelling work of Black existentialist thinker, Saidiyah Hartman, who argued that rather than engage the overtly horrific instances of American chattel slavery, she wanted to emphasize the more mundane aspects of Black life as slaves. In this way, Yancy's work is compelling because it requires us to pay attention to daily interactions rather than dramatic incidents.

Yancy's notion of the quotidian has serious psychological implications for Black people. Consider that horror, as a cinematic genre, brings to mind images of dark nights, of ghosts and paranormal "energies" that inhabit decrepit houses. There are high levels of artistic license and creativity indulged in the making of horror films. In contrast, to experience the horror of racial embodiment as a Black body requires no such artistic creativity; for to experience the horror of the Black body, one need not be in a haunted house or in a dark alley on a foggy night. Indeed, taking Yancy's notion of the quotidian seriously, a Black body can meet its demise on a bright sunny day, picking the kids up from school midafternoon or taking a ride to run errands. For Yancy, the Black body is always already at risk, vulnerable, and dangerously ahead of itself. The real horror of racial embodiment at the level of the quotidian is almost something supernatural: The Black body, as the *imago* of the White gaze, is present even when absent, such that when a Black body is present, it is tragically brought within racist conceptual schemes, truncated, and marked for death—even at 2:00 P.M. while taking a jog on a bright, warm, sunny, spring afternoon. Yancy's work demands that Whites assume responsibility for these quotidian interactions, again, by remaining unsutured, being willing to dwell in the phenomenological life world of Black racial embodiment and not inauthentically retreat into theorized "reasons," constituted as "solutions" to the problems attendant to racial violence against Black bodies. Such retreats to theorizations are, according to Yancy's work, morally, existentially, and phenomenologically speaking, unacceptable. To remain in the life world is to remain in a pretheorized quotidian realm of profound responsibility and freedom, something that many Whites refuse to do, retreating into the abstractions of hypotheticals and such musings as necessary to avoid the responsibility of the life world. Yancy's work, then, through its emphasis on responsibility, freedom, and the lived, pretheoretical experience of the Black body, is a major, highly original, and formative contribution to Black existentialism.

Gordon's and Yancy's Black existentialism engages with anxiety, radical freedom, and responsibility. Bell's Black existentialism engages with Camus's notion of the absurd, and it does so in ways that are directly related to this chapter's aim of moving toward a Black existential psychology because Bell, a Black legal theorist, developed an existentialism that emphasizes the impact of American law and American legal systems on Black people. In Bell's important book, *Faces at the Bottom of the Well: The Permanence of Racism*, Bell advanced his thesis of racial realism, which is composed of two seemingly contradictory theses. First is the thesis that anti-Black racism is a permanent feature of American legal institutions and American life (the permanence thesis). Bell flatly rejected the notion that African Americans will ever gain full equality in America. Second is the thesis that despite the permanence of anti-Black racism, every person of good will is morally obliged to resist it (the resistance thesis). The antagonism between these two theses is significant, for what sense does it make for one to resist that which is inevitable or permanent? Indeed, what meaning can be derived from such futility? Bell himself cited Camus and Fanon, arguing that political resistance is an essential feature of his racial realism. Bell wrote that Camus "saw the need for struggle even in the face of certain defeat" (1992, p. x) and that Camus "sees incredible courage and even liberation" in resistance to oppression (1994, p. 161). Bell argued that "Fanon argued two seemingly irreconcilable points, and insisted on both. On the one hand, he believed racist structures to be permanently embedded in the psychology, economy, society, and culture of the modern world. . . . But, on the other hand, he urged people of color to resist psychologically the inheritance they had come into" (1992, p. x).

Bell thus demanded that in the face of this absurd reality of racism's permanence and the moral obligation to resist it, we all become absurd heroes, determined to resist a legally imposed and permanent anti-Black racism with passion and courage, much like Sisyphus. Bell adopted Camus' argument from *The Myth of Sisyphus* here. Bell wrote of Camus, in his book *Confronting Authority: Reflections of an Ardent Protestor*, that, in the context of political protest:

> Often, the lone protestor—abandoned (or worse) by associates and unable to reach his or her goal—will feel less like a teacher than the mythical Sisyphus, forever pushing to the top of the mountain the rock that, upon nearing the heights, only rolls back down to the bottom. At a first reading of Sisyphus, it is hard to escape the despairing, existential angst that accompanies any realization of the futility of struggle. But . . . Camus puts a different face upon Sisyphus's tragic fate. Rather than hopelessness, Camus sees incredible courage and even liberation in this timeless story. He sees strength in Sisyphus' course, not because Sisyphus continues to push the rock to the mountain's top, but because he returns to the bottom to retrieve it-knowing he will never get to the top. (1994, p. 161)

Even amid the existential absurdity, then, for Bell, a meaningless life was not necessarily a life not worth living. To the contrary, Bell, with Camus, found great meaning in the struggle against anti-Black racism, despite the futility of that struggle. The psychological implications of Bell's Black existentialism are worthy of serious consideration, especially as one moves toward a Black existential psychology, examined in this chapter in the context of American law and racial oppression. How can psychology draw from Bell's racial realism to treat instances of depression in the face of those confronting social injustice? Can therapeutic interventions, structured on the notion of the absurd hero in Bell's iteration of Black existentialism provide meaning to people suffering psychological harm from racial oppression?

FANON: THE PSYCHOLOGICAL OPPRESSION OF RACIAL OBJECTIFICATION

Fanon's *Black Skin, White Masks* and *The Wretched of the Earth* are texts central to Black existentialism because of their articulation of both the daily life of racial embodiment and the need for psychological interventions to address the problems arising from that same daily life. Fanon, a psychiatrist by training, was keenly interested in the problems attending both anti-Black racism and colonization and emphasized that anti-Black racism adversely affected both Blacks and Whites. For Fanon, there was a constant throughout his work. In *Black Skin, White Masks*, he wrote that the book was "the sum of the experiences and observations of seven years; regardless of the area I have studied, one thing has struck me: The Negro enslaved by his inferiority, the White man enslaved by his superiority alike behave in accordance with a neurotic orientation" (1967, p. 60). The colonial situation, undergirded by anti-Black racism is thus reciprocally pathological, producing an "obsessive, neurotic type" in Black people and a phobic type in Whites (Fanon, 1967).

Through fear in Whites and neurotic instability in Blacks, psychological pathologies are prominent in the everyday life of colonial situations. The well-known example from *Black Skin, White Masks* is when Fanon heard a White child say to his White mother, "Look, a Negro! Mama, see the Negro! I'm frightened!" (1967, p. 111). With this utterance, the phobic pathology of Whites is best exemplified. Fanon pointed out that this phobic pathology is a mythology that European science itself perpetuates—as Gordon has argued. Fanon wrote that "For several years certain laboratories have been trying to produce a serum for "denegrification"; with all the earnestness in the world, laboratories have sterilized their test tubes, checked their scales, and embarked on researches that make it possible for the miserable Negro to whiten himself and thus to throw off the burden of that corporeal malediction" (p. 111). This "science" is an attempt to theorize a "corporeal schema"—something metaphysically real and epistemologically verifiable that Whites can deploy to "scientifically" justify their phobic pathology. Hence, the bad faith and overall crisis of the European sciences that Gordon, through his reading of Fanon, has argued renders a responsible account of the European human sciences impossible without a complete rethinking of what it means to be human. Interestingly, for Fanon, beneath the attempts to create this "corporeal schema" is a far more sinister "historico-racial schema," produced not by any perceptions of his own, but rather by the White gaze, for when the White child proclaims fear of the Negro, Fanon was constituted and known, but not by his own agency. Instead, it was a historically, racially charged gaze of the White child that constituted Fanon, who had, in the moment of exclamation, woven Fanon "out of a thousand details, anecdotes, stories" (p. 111). He was, all at once, "responsible at the same time for my body, for my race, for my ancestors. I subjected myself to an objective examination, I discovered my blackness, my ethnic characteristics; and I was battered down by tom-toms, cannibalism, intellectual deficiency, fetichism, racial defects, slave-ships, and above all else, above all: 'Sho' good eatin'" (p. 112). Yancy's connection to Fanon is prominent here in what Yancy called the "confiscation" of the Black body. Constituted by a pathological White gaze, a further pathology was created in Fanon, as his identity was stripped from him, distorted into a "nigger," and then returned to him.[1] After the White child exclaimed "Look at the Nigger! . . . Mama, a Negro! . . . Hell, he's getting mad . . . Take no notice, sir, he does not know that you are as civilized as we. . . ." (p. 113), Fanon wrote that:

> My body was given back to me sprawled out, distorted, recolored, clad in mourning in that white winter day. The Negro is an animal, the Negro is bad, the Negro is mean, the Negro is ugly; look, a nigger, it's cold, the nigger is shivering, the nigger is shivering because he is cold, the little boy is trembling because he is afraid of the nigger, the nigger is shivering with cold, that cold that goes through your bones, the handsome little boy is trembling because he thinks that the nigger is quivering with rage, the little white boy throws himself into his mother's arms: Mama, the nigger's going to eat me up. (pp. 113–114)

For Fanon, this sort of occurrence was daily, which was what made it so frightening. The emphasis on the ordinary social interactions of daily life as sites of anti-Black racism in the form of bigoted individual acts, acts of institutionalized racism, and the combination of the two—such as when a bigoted White individual's neurosis calls the police and sets in motion the entire history of American anti-Black racism implicated in contemporary policing—is both significant and an important part of the Black phenomenological and existential philosophical tradition.

Indeed, Saidiyah Hartman, whose landmark text, *Scenes of Subjection: Terror, Slavery, and Self-Making in Nineteenth Century America* (1997), amplifies the importance of the quotidian between Fanon and Yancy, problematizes the spectacular, writing that it has a tendency to make us "voyeurs" of "the ghastly and the terrible" (pp. 3, 4). Hartman's aim, like Fanon's, was to "defamiliarize the familiar . . . to illuminate the terror of the mundane and the quotidian rather than exploit the shocking spectacle" (p. 4). What was at stake for Hartman was the psychological importance of empathy, which is compromised by how we ingest spectacular acts of anti-Black racial violence:

> At issue here is the precariousness of empathy and the uncertain line between witness and spectator. Only more obscene than the brutality unleashed at the whipping post is the demand that this suffering be materialized and evidenced by the display of the tortured body or endless recitations of the ghastly and terrible. In light of this, how does one give expression to these outrages without exacerbating the indifference to suffering that is the consequence of the benumbing spectacle or contend with the narcissistic identification that obliter-

ates the other or the prurience that too often is the response to such displays? (p. 4)

Yancy, like both Fanon and Hartman, is more interested in the ordinary, everyday, "quotidian" instances of racism than he was in spectacular displays of racial oppression, as with George Floyd's death, which can benumb empathetic sensibilities, leading to an indifference to human suffering.

Another reason for Fanon, Hartman, and Yancy emphasizing the quotidian is that it is much easier for Whites to oppose the spectacle of a police officer with his knee on a Black man's neck for nearly 10 minutes. Although some Whites tried to support Officer Chauvin—which is problematic for other reasons—many Whites, exclaiming how awful a spectacle it was, acquitted themselves of any charge of racism. Thus, many Whites find it easier to comfort themselves from within the spectacular as not being racist. But it is much more difficult for Whites to confront their pathological neurosis in ordinary, daily situations. The difficulty is ultimately a difficulty of self-criticism, a sort of incessant self-reflection that demands Whites be always already aware of their neurosis so as to help heal themselves of it through daily self-correction. The quotidian, then, for Black phenomenology and existentialism in general—and for Fanon, Hartman, and Yancy in particular—is a sort of laboratory in which White pathology is diagnosed, confronted, and treated.

Further, what do we make of such quotidian distortions of human identity from a psychological standpoint? What happens when the pathological White gaze is not from a child, as it is with Fanon, but from a police officer with a gun and a badge or from a child's gaze that summons the police officer with a gun and badge? These questions from Black existential and phenomenological philosophical reflection are indeed troubling and indicate a need to address the psychological harms of legally institutionalized racial oppression, a need which Fanon addressed in detail in *The Wretched of the Earth*. As the recent psychological research from the introduction to this chapter suggests, such psychological harms are in need of treatment today.

DUBOIS AND DOUGLASS: THE PROBLEM OF DOUBLE CONSCIOUSNESS AND THE ROLE OF IMAGINATION AS AN EXISTENTIAL INTERVENTION

Bell addressed the absurd in light of a need for an absurd, Sisyphus-like hero to make resistance to oppression meaningful. DuBois's existential insights take the absurd even further, relating it to a core of Black identity such that a paradox of almost mystical proportions plagues the Black self. Reading DuBois with Bell and Fanon, then, leads to a regularity of disruptions (Fanon) that force Black people to wonder who they really are, especially in America (DuBois), and it is in this context that the Black self is morally obligated to strive for meaning, despite how American law and legal systems legitimize its oppression (Bell). Fanon's analysis of European colonization and its attendant dehumanization finds its American counterpart in DuBois's work, *The Souls of Black Folk*. DuBois, comparing African Americans to other racial and ethnic groups, made the observation that:

> The Negro is a sort of seventh son, born with a veil, and gifted with second-sight in this American world—a world which yields him no true self-consciousness, but only lets him see himself through the revelation of the other world. It is a peculiar sensation, this double-consciousness, this sense of always looking at one's self through the eyes of others, of measuring one's soul by the tap of a world that looks on in amused contempt and pity. One ever feels his two-ness—an American, a Negro; two souls, two thoughts, two unreconciled strivings; two warring ideals in one dark body, whose dogged strength alone keeps it from being torn asunder. (1986, pp. 364–365)

Like Fanon, DuBois articulated an existential situation of an embodied contradiction that comes from the White gaze: He was, on the one hand, what he hoped to be (an American), and on the other hand, he was what Whites saw him as—a Negro. Utterly bereft of agency, a contradiction in his identity was foisted upon him and demanded that he hold such contradictions in tension with one another. Such a feat requires nothing less than "dogged strength" that kept him from being "torn asunder." Add to this psychological stress the impact of legalized racial oppression that only recognizes Black bodies as criminal and suspicious, and the need for a psychological intervention comes into sharper focus: A Black existential psychology is badly needed.

DuBois articulated an inheritance bequeathed to African Americans from the American founding, which is Black identity as part person, part property. Among the compromises that led to the founding of the American republic was a compromise that reduced slaves to a subhuman status by counting them, for purposes of population and taxation, as only 60% of a person. What DuBois referred to as the identity thrust upon him by the view of Whites is a view of Black identity that had been long-established in both social life and legal doctrine.

Is such long-established American legal doctrine determinative of Black identity? Or can one, through some sense of existential self-determination, view one's Black self otherwise? Frederick Douglass certainly thought so. Douglass is well known for his changed stance on the U.S. Constitution. After escaping from slavery, Douglass joined with a White abolitionist group led by William Lloyd Garrison. This group believed that the Constitution was a proslavery document, and that to participate in its form of government, in any way, was to further the document's proslavery objectives. The corollary of this was that Douglass and the Garrisonians, as they were known, advocated complete withdrawal from American political life. The Garrisonians held this view because of four provisions of the Constitution that they believed unquestionably supported slavery: (1) Article I, Section 2, which contained the infamous three-fifths clause referenced above; (2) Article I, Section 8, which permitted Congress to use military force to "suppress insurrections and repel invasions"; (3) Article I, Section 9, which forbade Congress from ending the slave trade prior to 1808; and (4) Article IV, Section 2, which required anyone who escaped from service due to another to be returned, known as the "fugitive slave clause" within the Garrisonian abolitionist community.

The psychological impact of a proslavery view of the Constitution was likely devastating for Blacks. Enslaved and without any hope of being ever treated as social and political equals, the "black and white, letter of the law" in the Constitution doomed Blacks to a permanent subhuman status. Again, the psychological damage to one's self-concept from this political view is, I think, significant. But Douglass, as a political activist with maturing views that were independent of the Garrisonian abolitionists, began to see things otherwise.

Douglass, through his political activism, came to understand that real political hope for the abolition of slavery and for the well-being of Black people beyond slavery would lie in an America engaged, not an America ignored. In other words, the withdrawal strategy of the Garrisonians brought with it the lack of an opportunity to hope in a struggle. Indeed, there could be no struggle because, for the Garrisonians, the struggle simply was not an option. The only option was America starting over again. But with the country on the brink of the Civil War, this did not bode well for Black people. So, Douglass, according to the exigencies of the historical moment, understood time as politically and psychologically dictating the use of his imagination to see the Constitution as anti-slavery. Douglass argued that the three-fifths clause did not show that the Constitution was proslavery, it showed that the south had compromised itself on representation in Congress, therefore motivating its slave states to become free states; he argued that Congress quelling insurrections could also imply that slavery itself was an insurrection against natural law and thus lead to the abolition of slavery; that prohibition on abolishing slavery prior to 1808 at least implied that the American founders foresaw an end to slavery; and that the so-called fugitive slave clause did not apply to slaves at all, but rather to a group of White European immigrants, known as Redemptioners who were bound to American ship captains for a term of service in exchange for transportation from Europe to America (1985, pp. 351–356).

The relative strengths and weaknesses of Douglass's arguments about the Constitution being anti-slavery, as a logical matter, are, frankly, irrelevant. What is relevant, however, is that Douglass, understanding the exigencies of the historical moment, heeded the temporal imperative to use his imagination: He was able to see things not as they were, but rather as they could become. This is not a quixotic encounter with windmills from the pages of Cervantes. No, this is the robust existential psychology of a Black self and political activist who understood that viewing the Constitution as anti-slavery meant that slavery would always be wrong; it meant that Black people were human regardless of whatever legislative and judicial pronouncements would be made, and, perhaps most importantly, it meant that America belonged as much to Black people as it did to anyone else.

It is these sorts of conclusions that again, however logically weak or strong, brought forth in the existential reflection on what it means to be a Black self, make the political struggle that Bell deemed so meaningful possible in the first place. For, without an imaginative capacity to bridge the gap from the actuality of Black dehumanization to the possibility of equality, Blacks can never participate in the America in which they live—even if that participation only allows a meaningful struggle for racial equality rather than equality itself. The struggle must at least be possible. Douglass's imagination enabled him to at least see that struggle, and Bell made that struggle meaningful.

DuBois and Douglass, then, gave us a problem and a meaningful therapeutic intervention from a Black existential psychology. The troubles of racial oppression are indeed real. But so is the capacity of the human imagination, which, when trapped by racist logics, can see beyond such logics to create new, transformative possibilities. DuBois understood this himself, doing serious empirical work as a trained sociologist, but also writing exquisite literary works (Lloyd, 2016, pp. 58–59). Black people are not 60% human; Black people are fully human with "souls," as DuBois put it, that are composed of both intellect and inspiration. A Black existential psychology must encourage Black people to develop the complexities of their Black souls, in all of their intellectual, inspirational, and imaginative dimensions.

CONCLUSION

Black existentialism has the intellectual resources necessary for the development of Black existential psychology. The failure of science is evident from uneven law enforcement tactics that reinforce anti-Black racist practices in ways that are psychologically harmful to Black people. This much is recognized in recent literature (Bandes et al., 2019). Any responsible Black existential psychology ought to treat the law's failure as an a priori science as an opportunity to address such failure with a scientifically sound, psychological approach that will address the harm done to those on the receiving end of oppression from American law and legal systems, and will address that harm therapeutically through encouraging meaningful political associations with others and through emphasizing the imaginative capacities of the Black self. It is also important to note that this chapter is an articulation of *one way* to develop and utilize a Black existential psychology. There are other ways to understand the scientific applications for a Black existential psychology; this I leave to others. Here, however, I have tried to begin that conversation.

NOTE

1. Quotes from Fanon are verbatim from the original source. We believe it is important to keep all the words in the quotes as in the original source.

REFERENCES

Alexander, M. (2010). *The New Jim Crow: Mass incarceration in the age of colorblindness.* The New Press.

Bandes, S., Pryor, M., Kerrison, E., & Goff, P. (2019). The mismeasure of *Terry* stops: Assessing the psychological and emotional harms of stop and frisk to individuals and communities. *Behavioral Sciences and the Law, 37*(2), 176–194.

Bell, D. (1992). *Faces at the bottom of the well: The permanence of racism.* Basic Books.

Bell, D. (1994). *Confronting authority: Reflections of an ardent protestor.* Beacon Press.

Camus, A. (1991). *The myth of Sisyphus* (J. O'Brien, Trans.). Vintage Books.

Descartes, R. (1993). *Meditations on first philosophy* (D. Cress, Trans.). Hackett.

Douglass, F. (1985). The American Constitution and the slave. In J. W. Blassingame (Ed.), *The Frederick Douglass papers* (pp. 340–366). Yale University Press.

DuBois, W. E. B. (1986). *The souls of Black folk* (N. Huggins, Ed.). Library of America.

Fanon, F. (1961). *The wretched of the earth* (R. Philcox, Trans.). Grove Press.

Fanon, F. (1967). *Black skin, White masks* (C. Markman, Trans.). Grove Press.

Gordon, L. (1995a). *Bad faith and anti-Black racism.* Humanity Books.

Gordon, L. (1995b). *Fanon and the crisis of European man.* Routledge.

Gordon, L. (2000). *Existentia Africana: Understanding Africana existential thought.* Routledge.

Gordon, L. (2006). *Disciplinary decadence: Living thought in trying times.* Paradigm.

Hartman, S. (1997). *Scenes of subjection: Terror, slavery, and self-making in nineteenth century America.* Oxford University Press.

Kierkegaard, S. (1980). *The concept of anxiety* (R. Thomte & A. Anderson, Trans.). Princeton University Press.

Levinas, E. (1961). *Totality and infinity* (A. Lingis, Trans.). Duquesne University Press.

Lloyd, V. (2016). *Black natural law.* Oxford University Press.

Plato. (1997). *Republic* (J. Cooper, Trans.). Hackett.

Shelby County, Alabama v. Holder, 570 U.S. 529 (2013).

Slaughterhouse Cases, 83 U.S. 36 (1872).

Students for Fair Admissions, Inc. v. President and Fellows of Harvard College, 600 U.S. (2023).

Terry v. Ohio, 392 U.S. 1 (1968).

United States Justice Department Civil Rights Division. (2016). Investigation of the Baltimore City Police Department.

Yancy, G. (2015). *White self-criticality beyond anti-racism: How does it feel to be a White problem?* Lexington Books.

Yancy, G. (2016). *Black bodies, White gazes: The continuing significance of race.* Rowman & Littlefield.

CHAPTER 5

Research Methods in the Science of Existential Psychology

Matthew Vess

Writing a research methods chapter for the science of existential psychology is probably a lot like putting together a "new" presentation of sheet music for Beatles songs. Users likely possess a general familiarity with the topics and the utility of the work depends on a certain degree of foundational knowledge. This is not to say that executing a methodologically sound existential psychology study requires a degree of skill on par with the musical aptitude of John Lennon, nor is it meant to suggest that existential psychological science is to psychology what the Beatles are to music; rather, it is meant to convey that the science of existential psychology is built upon the same foundation of methodological principles that guides all psychological science. The Beatles didn't create new musical notes, and pioneering scholars in the field of existential psychological science didn't create entirely new methodological principles. They simply leveraged existing principles to empirically address questions and concepts that have a more existential bent to them.

This translation was not trivial, however. It ushered in a new way of examining existential topics that has helped elucidate how existential issues connect to the basic psychological processes that govern wide amounts of people's thoughts, feelings, and actions. By using the methodological toolbox germane to psychological science, researchers have advanced novel inquiries into the nature of existential concerns and have generated a different kind of understanding than previously existed. Existential psychological scientists have, among other things, developed measures that quantify subjective construals of existential concepts (e.g., meaning in life); they have implemented longitudinal studies that probe trajectories of existential experiences across time; they have identified the neural underpinnings of existential concerns using techniques that measure brain activity; they have developed approaches that detect correlations between existential experiences and other important outcomes (e.g., physical health); and, perhaps most importantly, they have developed techniques to experimentally probe existential experiences in ways that can inform *causal* psychological processes. Underlying all of these approaches are principles inherent in the psychological science tradition, namely a prioritization of empiricism, objectivity, and the essential importance of utilizing rigorous methodologies to draw valid conclusions.

The emergence of an existential psychological science also necessarily brought with it a quantitative orientation. This notably departs from the humanistic traditions that have tended to utilize qualitative inquiries (e.g., case studies, qualitative interviews).

These qualitative approaches have no doubt been important and possess the notable strength of being positioned to effectively probe the richness of an individual's existential experience. To that point, a common critique of existential psychological science is that a single quantitative study fails to accurately capture a person's entire subjective experience in the way that a qualitative inquiry from the humanistic tradition might. That critique may, at least to some extent, originate from a misconception about the goals of a psychological science quantitative approach. Existential psychological science is not really focused on—and certainly not always positioned to—capture and describe the fullness of an individual's existential experience in a single study. Rather, existential psychological science is focused on elucidating general psychological processes that are tethered to specific aspects of people's existential experiences (e.g., authenticity). It does so quantitively and systematically. Existential psychological scientists make predictions about how constructs relate (e.g., how does a sense of purpose in life relate to longevity; Martela et al., 2024); they systematically (i.e., in an unbiased fashion) collect large amounts of data to quantitatively represent those constructs; they subject those data to statistical tests to assess whether (and how strongly) the predictions are supported by the data; and they use those quantitative results to develop and refine theories about distinct psychological processes. The ultimate goal is to build explanatory models for various aspects of people's existential experiences (e.g., authenticity, meaning in life) that can be tested in an unbiased fashion, generalized across people and contexts, and used to make more accurate predictions about people's thoughts, feelings, and behaviors. A quantitative approach facilitates progress toward that goal in ways that other approaches do not, and thus complements (rather than competes with) more qualitative methods that focus on describing and documenting the content of an individual's subjective lived experience.

In particular, an approach to existential topics that is grounded in a more quantitative psychological science tradition allows for the development of general theories and frameworks that can be empirically evaluated in an incremental fashion. Psychological scientists develop theories from the empirical observations they make across many, many independent studies. Rather than describing the content of a single person's entire subjective experience, psychological scientists' studies largely focus on distinct aspects of those experiences (operationalized as systematically measured variables) that may be common features of a broader population of people. They conduct many studies to test how those variables relate to other variables and use statistical inferences about the strength of those observed associations to generate broad explanations (theories) about the psychological nature of existential experiences/concerns. Confidence in the accuracy of those theories is built incrementally through multiple studies and large amounts of convergent empirical data. And, somewhat similarly, an understanding of the full range of people's existential experiences—at least in terms of how they connect to basic psychological processes (e.g., motivation, self-regulation)—is approached through the development of multiple theories for specific existential issues (e.g., authenticity, meaning in life). A broader depiction of the psychology of existential concerns is thus achieved not by focusing on a single data point, but instead through the integration of multiple theories grounded in an aggregate assessment of myriad observable data points.

This chapter presents a broad overview of the methodological approaches that are used by existential psychological scientists to build this integrative and systematic understanding of the ways that people's existential experiences shape their lives. Because the field emerged when basic psychological scientists began to apply their methodologies to existentially informed questions, the foundation for existential psychological science rests firmly in the basic methods that all psychological scientists employ. There are many, many excellent resources that describe these basic methods and the scope of this chapter does not really permit a full presentation of them. Indeed, entire advanced handbooks (e.g., the *Handbook of Research Methods in Social and Personality Psychology* [Reis & Judd, 2000]) and introductory textbooks (including some that are open access) already exist, and readers hoping to gain an introduction to psychological science methods should look to those excellent resources. I saw very little need to reproduce the "wheel," so to speak. Instead, with this chapter, I endeavored to do two specific things. First, I aimed to provide a resource that highlights methodological issues germane to existential psychological science that scholars should be cognizant of when designing, analyzing, and interpreting their studies. Second, I attempted to provide a narrative account of how specific kinds of research projects might unfold. The hope for this chapter is that it will become a resource for scholars who need some initial guidance in designing and implementing a study to address an existential psychology research question. It is meant to be a road map of sorts that organizes relevant methodological issues and highlights existing approaches in the literature that can serve as guideposts for designing and implementing effective studies.

Before turning to these aims, though, I would like to revisit the Beatles sheet music analogy in order to voice a word of caution (or, perhaps, perspective). No one would realistically conclude that the possession of a Beatles sheet music book provides all one needs to know to create music equivalent to the Beatles' long list of hits. The book equips one to approximate the sounds, but capturing the exact expression of the music may require insights and instruction that only the Beatles, themselves, could provide. Similarly, a methods chapter in a psychological science handbook is limited in that it cannot replace the hours of meaningful training that goes into being an expert in a particular area of scholarship. Such chapters can, of course, provide examples of effective measures, manipulations, and approaches to utilize, but I caution readers against assuming that effective existential psychological science only requires knowing what measures and manipulations have been deployed. Existing measures and manipulations were often developed in specific contexts under specific conditions, and ignoring that fact may produce unanticipated consequences. One example of this might be failing to consider how the inclusion of one kind of measure in a study can undermine the very experimental effect that one intends to examine (see, e.g., Hayes & Schimel, 2018). While I view this chapter as a useful starting point, I urge scholars who may be new to existential psychological science to reach out to other active scholars in this research area for advice and suggestions. Sometimes simply talking through a research design question with an experienced scholar can highlight issues that authors of a methods chapter cannot anticipate or find space to elaborate on.

DEVELOPING RESEARCH IDEAS IN EXISTENTIAL PSYCHOLOGICAL SCIENCE

Understanding What You Intend to Study

My path to existential psychological science started in the fall semester of my junior year at Ohio University. I was simultaneously taking existential philosophy and social psychology courses and, though I enjoyed both courses immensely, I was drawn more to the empirical nature of social psychology and its potential to directly test questions about human experience. I naively viewed existential philosophy mostly as a collection of incredibly interesting and thought-provoking ideas that need not be subjected to the scrutiny of an empirical approach. That view changed when Dr. Keith Markman, my social psychology instructor at the time, gave a 15-minute overview of terror management theory (TMT; Greenberg et al., 1986). That lecture revealed the utility of enrichening social psychological science with formally developed theorizing from the humanities, particularly those originating in existential philosophy. The presence of TMT as a viable social psychological theory was, for me at the time, a revealing illustration of how conceptual ideas developed in philosophy can be represented in the operational variables featured in social psychological inquiry. It was a tremendously exciting revelation that was, fortunately, quickly replaced with a much more realistic understanding and appreciation of the many challenges that complicate the existential philosophy–psychological science interface.

The first of these challenges is recognizing and appreciating the "concept loss" that occurs when attempting to translate an abstract concept into a concrete and observable operational variable. Existential psychological science often wrestles with conceptual variables that exist at a relatively high level of abstraction. Meaning, authenticity, responsibility, freedom, death anxiety, and the like are all inherently complex ideas and subjective experiences. As such, there will likely always be some degree of tension between the ideas that we want to empirically examine and the methods that we develop to do so. The strength of any existential psychological science study is fundamentally linked to how well it has translated theoretical concepts into the measures and manipulations in the study. The starting point for maximizing the effectiveness of this translation is developing a strong and coherent understanding of the conceptual variable of interest.

The most direct way to optimally understand a targeted concept would be to leverage existing theoretical perspectives. Such perspectives need not be grounded in psychological science, of course, but they should provide a clear and coherent depiction of what exactly the "thing" of inquiry is thought to be. There are many excellent examples of this kind of theoretical development in the existential psychology literature, with many commonly appearing in articles that present a new measure for a psychological construct. Kernis and Goldman's (2006) classic work on trait authenticity readily comes to my mind as something to strive for. In that work, the authors spend a significant amount of time documenting how they arrived at their conceptualization of authenticity and how that conceptualization pulls from a rich intellectual history of relevant theorizing (e.g., Heidegger, Descartes, Rogers). Their operationalization reflects a synthesis of this theorizing, thereby making it possible to critically evaluate whether their measure of authenticity captures the authenticity concept as they construe it. Scholars can (and will) obviously quibble with whether or not their conception of authenticity is accurate, but the fact that their measure is grounded in a well-developed conceptualization means that there is a clear link between the abstract and the concrete.

We can also, of course, consider the problems that might manifest if one doesn't fully understand the theoretical or conceptual grounding of their constructs. It is (thankfully!) quite common for advanced undergraduate students and early-stage graduate students to become interested in a construct featured in an empirical article that they've been assigned to read. They then generate research questions about how that construct might relate to other constructs that they have learned about. So far, so good. However, oftentimes the "construct" that a student is referring to is the measure or operationalization featured in the study. When pressed to explain why their favored construct, and not something else, might be operative or most central, confusion quickly sets in because such questions focus on the abstract conceptual variable that the measure is meant to assess. Particularly assertive students might contend that such theoretical elaboration is unnecessary to test the hypothesis that a measure of x will correlate with a measure of y when valid measures of x and y already exist in the literature. Given the significant empirical and conceptual overlap of many variables in psychological science, this type of thinking can be problematic. It can, at the very least, lead researchers to neglect other constructs that might better explain specific aspects of their research questions.

A related issue can also arise when one fails to consider that psychological processes, including existential ones (Pyszczynski et al., 1999), operate on both conscious (explicit, intentional, verbal) and nonconscious (implicit, automatic, nonverbal) levels. A great deal of research in psychology indeed indicates that psychological phenomena can be influenced differentially by deliberate (conscious) and automatic (nonconscious) processes and failing to consider that distinction can lead to an incomplete understanding of the broader phenomena of interest. A good example of this is the examination of existential concerns about mortality that is central to TMT. Someone interested in the ways that death concerns relate to social behavior might reasonably assume that conscious reports of death anxiety would be a good construct to target in examining the role that mortality concerns play in human social life. And, the relatively low levels of death anxiety that people generally explicitly report in studies might lead to a conclusion that death anxiety might not be all that significant or consequential. This would, of course, be an incomplete conclusion caused by an incomplete conceptualization of the construct of interest. As years of TMT research has revealed, death concerns impact wide amounts of human behavior, but they do so largely via nonconscious processes that are revealed through operations that specifically capture nonconscious constructs (see Hayes et al., 2010). Thus, shoring up a conceptual understanding of the psychological process or construct of interest, including whether it might operate through conscious and/or nonconscious means, is a critical early step in the research process.

TAKING THE TIME TO CONSIDER AND DEVELOP THEORY

Once the conceptual grounding of the construct or constructs of interest is developed and understood, it becomes much easier to generate plausible and testable hypotheses. Part of the reason for this is that conceptual grounding provides the information that might be needed to predict or explain how conceptual variables relate. For example, explaining why a concept like meaning in life might positively correlate with routines is easier when one understands that meaning in life consists of a sense of coherence and that routines represent consistent and predictable ways of behaving. Because predictability is a component of coherence, the prediction that measures of routines will positively correlate with measures of meaning in life aligns with a plausible theoretical explanation. Proceeding with a study to test that hypothesis would obviously make sense with such a strong theoretical grounding—as it did for Heintzelman and her colleagues (Heintzelman & King, 2019; Mohideen & Heintzelman, 2023).

One might wonder, though, if theoretical plausibility is necessary to conduct a study to test hypotheses about the ways that measures relate? It's a reasonable question. I've certainly had the experience of frustrating more than a couple of students by not agreeing to move forward with a study until they were able to explain the theoretical plausibility of their predictions. Scholars will likely land on different sides of this question/issue and there is a place for exploratory atheoretical work in existential psychological science.

I would contend, though, that taking a bit of time to assess the theoretical plausibility of a particular hypothesis or answer to a research question is a worthwhile endeavor. Gray (2017) pointed out that the development of sound theory around a particular research question is essential for sound methodology and science. He introduced a metaphor that likens scientific progress to the construction of a building. Individual studies are viewed as bricks, and theory represents the bonding that effectively holds those bricks together. Just as the possession of strong bricks is not in itself sufficient to guarantee a structurally sound building, the utilization of reliable research methods is not in itself sufficient to guarantee sound scientific understanding. Theory is necessary to "put the pieces together" in a meaningful way.

It can therefore be useful to situate research questions into a broader "theory map" (see Gray, 2017) in order to better understand the particular question and/or prediction that is being raised. For example, my colleagues and I (Vess et al., 2016) were interested in the possibility that instances of mind wandering might correlate with the subjective experience of authenticity. At the time, reliable measures of mind wandering and authenticity existed, which made it potentially easy to implement a study that collected the data necessary to explore that association. Thinking through a "theory map," however, provided greater conceptual clarity around our predictions and inspired more informative research designs.

We started by identifying the core components of authenticity and mind wandering as articulated in existing theoretical and empirical work. Authenticity comprises multiple components (Wood et al., 2008) and we reasoned that self-alienation—defined as a subjective experience of disconnect between consciousness and actual experience—may be particularly relevant to mind wandering because mind wandering reflects an instance of conscious thought being directed toward something other than the present environment. This consideration of the conceptual aspects of these constructs enabled us to make plausible predictions about the link between mind wandering and a specific facet of authenticity (self-alienation), and to explain why that facet of authenticity seemed most important.

Next, we considered the nomological net (Cronbach & Meehl, 1955) of self-alienation and identified a number of empirically and theoretically connected constructs. These included self-concept clarity, self-esteem, neuroticism, affect, and other constructs that share some degree of overlap with the abstract experience of self-alienation. This consideration helped us identify theoretically important constructs to measure in our study in order to better establish the validity of our focal hypothesis tests. That is, measuring these conceptually and empirically connected variables allowed us to employ statistical techniques to account for the overlap. As a result, our first two studies (Vess et al., 2016) tested our primary hypothesis *and* ruled out plausible alternative hypotheses that were informed by our a priori theorizing about related constructs.

Theorizing does not, however, stop once the study is designed and the data are analyzed. Our initial data supported our prediction that self-alienation would be positively associated with mind wandering. It did not test why that is the case. Our theoretical mapping suggested that the association was plausible given the overlapping conceptual features of the two constructs, but this theoretical mapping also fell short of a real theoretical explanation. Vess and Maffly-Kipp (2022) went further in their theorizing by specifying that experiences of self-alienation may—to some extent—emerge when people no longer experience ownership over their psychological experiences. That is, a lack of intentionality and agency might be a particularly important component of self-alienation. This kind of deeper theorizing had important methodological implications for the study of self-alienation and mind wandering. It highlighted an untested theoretical assumption and a need to design a study that might better test the importance of intentionality or ownership. Fortunately, after Vess and colleagues (2016) was published, a methodological and theoretical development in the mind-wandering literature distinguished between intentional and unintentional mind wandering (Seli et al., 2019). Demonstrating that self-alienation negatively predicted intentional mind wandering and positively predicted unintentional mind wandering, which Vess and Maffly-Kipp did, thus extended the previous empirical work *and* provided support for a new conceptual understanding of the phenomena.

Such progression may, to many scholars, seem like a natural trajectory for science that is not particularly remarkable. I agree that good science does tend to progress in this way and that there is nothing particularly remarkable about what we did in this program of research from a meta-science innovation standpoint. However, what I hope to impress upon readers is that the development of a theoretical map or framework for organizing a program of research is incredibly useful. It helps connect the conceptual ideas that underlie a particular research question and highlights specific assumptions that need to be placed under intentional, rather than arbitrary post-hoc, empirical scrutiny. Taking the time to develop theory can therefore better inform the types of studies that one might conduct, the types of data that one might collect, and the specific hypotheses that should be prioritized in one's program of research.

STUDY DESIGNS IN EXISTENTIAL PSYCHOLOGICAL SCIENCE

Cross-Sectional Correlation Designs

Although often undervalued, studies that are positioned to test basic cross-sectional correlations between two or more constructs have made substantial contributions to existential psychological science. For example, many of these studies have offered initial support for complex structural relationships among existential outcomes (e.g., meaning in life, authenticity) and personality (e.g., Schnell & Becker, 2006), emotion (e.g., Abeyta et al., 2015; Hicks et al., 2012; Routledge et al., 2011; Yang et al., 2024), fantasy (Maffly-Kipp & Vess, 2024), daydreaming (Williams & Vess, 2016), nature involvement (Yang et al., 2024), routines (e.g., Heintzelman & King, 2019), and mental illness (e.g., Menzies et al., 2019). The strongest exemplars of these kinds of studies are those that include psychometrically sound measures that effectively operationalize the conceptual variables of interest (e.g., they possess high criterion validity). Sample sizes that provide adequate power to detect typical psychology effect sizes (see Schönbrodt & Perugini, 2013) in a single study or packages that include meta-analyses of multiple samples (e.g., Maffly-Kipp & Vess, 2024) are also notable. Typically, cross-sectional correlation studies appear as early studies in a programmatic series that includes additional kinds of designs (e.g., experiments, longitudinal studies) to address the obvious inferential limitations of the basic cross-sectional correlation (see Routledge et al., 2011; Yang et al., 2024). Regardless, in many situations in existential psychological science, a basic cross-sectional correlation design can provide important information to build upon.

Longitudinal Correlation Designs

Existential psychological science has also benefited from studies that employ repeated measurements of individuals across time. Time lags between measurements can range from many years (e.g., Hill & Weston, 2019), to weeks (Maffly-Kipp et al., 2023), to days (Newman et al., 2018), to hours (e.g., Landa & English, 2022). The type of design is obviously dictated by the focal question, but researchers need to consider what measurement lag makes sense for the kind of question they are asking. They also need to ensure that the measurements are framed or locked to the interval under scrutiny. For example, my colleagues and I (Vess et al., 2019) intended to examine prospective relationships between mind wandering and self-alienation using Random Intercepts Cross-Lagged Panel Modeling Analyses (Hamaker et al., 2015) on data collected across four separate occasions. This kind of longitudinal analysis can be very helpful for elucidating the temporal ordering of correlated constructs. However, in our Study 1, the self-alienation and mind-wandering measures asked participants to respond to questions based on how they generally felt and our lags between measurement occasions were quite long (3–4 weeks). We failed to detect any prospective associations in this study that were independent of the between-person trait-level effects. Although this could have meant that no such relationships existed, we reasoned that the null effects could have been due to methodological artifact. Study 2 tied participants' responses to the time frame under scrutiny (24 hours) and measurement lags were significantly shorter than in Study 1. Our second study detected significant prospective associations, which illustrates the importance of considering how the measurement interval might affect the ability to detect significant longitudinal associations in a longitudinal design.

Experiments

The psychology experiment is, in many respects, the backbone design in existential psychological science. Well-designed and -implemented experiments can yield strong conclusions about the causal processes that underlie people's existential concerns and the ways that people manage them. Excellent resources on experimental design already exist (see, e.g., *Handbook of Research Methods in Social and Personality Psychology* and *Methods of Research in Social Psychology*) and, as I noted at the outset, I do not intend to regurgitate the information that already exists on the topic. I do, however, want to highlight a challenge in developing effective experimental manipulations in existential psychological science that may be underappreciated.

In addition to effective random assignment and appropriate sample size, the validity of an experimental effect is fundamentally tied to the validity of the manipulations employed. It is precisely the ability to manipulate the psychological construct of interest, while holding everything else constant, that grants experiments the power that they possess for elucidating causal relations. This can be a relatively straightforward task in many areas of psychology. In existential psychological science, however, efforts to isolate a particular construct via manipulation can prove challenging. The mortality salience manipulation in TMT research (Cox et al., 2019) is a good illustration of this. The manipulation asks participants to reflect on the prospect of their own death and to describe the emotions that their deaths arouse. On the surface, this seems like a very straightforward and valid way to induce death-related ideation. Some of the early TMT studies, however, contrasted this manipulation with a control condition focused on the experience of watching television (e.g., Greenberg et al., 1994). It is fairly easy to see that this particular set up fails to isolate death-focused ideation because the control condition also differs from the mortality salience condition in a number of important ways (e.g., valence). However, deeper reflection on this issue also illuminates the fact that death-focused ideation may include the arousal of a number of distinct existential concerns, including uncertainty, meaning, and isolation. Such a reality likely explains, at least in part, why alternative explanations for TMT effects centered on other specific existential concerns (e.g., meaning—Proulx & Heine, 2006; uncertainty—van den Bos, 2009) emerged. To address these alternative explanations, researchers programmatically examined TMT hypotheses with control conditions that independently targeted other distinct existential concerns like meaninglessness and uncertainty (see Martens et al., 2011). Such inquiry lent confidence to the conclusion that death-related concerns trigger psychological responses that cannot entirely be explained by other specific concerns. Indeed, it likely suggests that death-focused concerns likely reflect a multi-faceted existential experience that cannot be reduced to a single worry/threat.

Methodologically, though, the case of the mortality salience manipulation highlights an issue that may be somewhat common in existential psychological science. Existential constructs exist at a relatively high level of abstraction and may be difficult to isolate entirely via manipulation. Trying to induce authenticity, for example, is incredibly difficult to do without affecting other related constructs (e.g., self-esteem, positive affect). This makes the selection of a control or comparison condition incredibly important and reaffirms the ways that theorizing can aid in effective study design. A theoretical account of the construct of interest should include articulation of how it relates to other constructs and how/why its effects on a psychological outcome might differ from those constructs. Knowing which other constructs offer viable alternative explanations is crucial for identifying what kinds of control and comparison conditions will be most informative for the focal research question. At the very least, researchers should appreciate that existential constructs are often quite complex and make efforts to consider this complexity when interpreting their experimental findings.

Neuroscience Studies

As existential psychological science has grown, an interest in moving to lower levels of analysis naturally emerged in the literature. This is probably not surprising given that the accumulation of existential psychology research coincided with important advancements in the collection of neuroscience data. To me, and I'm sure some will push back on this, neuroscience studies are not qualitatively different from correlation studies or experiments. It is a measure that makes a study a neuroscience inquiry, but studies that utilize neuroscience measures are still classified as correlational or experimental in type. For example, Waytz and colleagues (2015) used neuroimaging data to show that neural activation patterns in the default mode network positively correlated with meaning in life in a bivariate cross-sectional correlation design and Klackl and colleagues (2014) found that self-esteem moderated specific patterns of neural activation in response to an experimental manipulation that focused participants on death-related or death-unrelated sentences. The specific kinds of neuroscience measures and methods employed in existential psychological science are varied, but, to me, the benefit of an "existential neuroscience" (Quirin et al., 2019) is that it affords opportunities to test theoretical predictions in ways that provide key convergent validity information. As an illustration, consider the TMT account that self-esteem buffers individuals from the potential threat of mortality awareness (Pyszczynski et al., 2004). Evidence showing that self-esteem boosts eliminate increases in self-reported death anxiety following reminders of death (Abeyta et al., 2014), that self-esteem reduces defensiveness following reminders of death (Schmeichel et al., 2009), and that self-esteem predicts deactivation of specific brain areas thought to be involved in the "global emotional moment" of death-focused thought (Klackl et al., 2014) all converge to support the TMT analysis. The addition of neuroscience methods, however, goes farther than the self-report data by grounding these processes in biological systems, thereby potentially informing a more thorough understanding of the existential phenomenon that transverses multiple levels of analysis. Neuroscience studies have thus emerged as an exciting and important addition to existential psychological science.

Narrative and Purely Qualitative Methods

In contrast to the lower-level analysis afforded by neuroscience techniques, researchers have also developed useful methods for probing processes that occur at a much higher level of abstraction and/or psychological integration. The narrative-identity literature (McAdams & McClean, 2013), for example, provides participants an opportunity to freely respond to a prompt to describe an experience in their lives (for a great primer on these methods, see Adler et al., 2017). The specific nature of the prompt is tailored to elicit the kind of psychological process under scrutiny, and responses broadly reflect an emergent property or theme of their psychological experiences. The approach is—for lack of a better word—a sort of hybrid that mixes characteristics of qualitative and quantitative methods. The quantitative piece derives from the fact that qualitative responses are quantified on the basis of some "coding" scheme. These "codes" reflect quantitative transformations of the qualitative data that can be utilized in quantitative analyses. The benefit of this approach is that these narrative (or open-ended) methods often allow researchers to detect psychological processes that may remain obscured by a purely quantitative (e.g., fixed-response questionnaire) measure. For example, there is substantial evidence that common features detected in people's life narratives (e.g., an arc of redemption in the life story) reliably predict well-being over and above other kinds of measures (e.g., personality scales; Adler et al., 2016). This indicates that narrative measures do more than simply measure familiar constructs in a different way; instead, they enable scholars to assess distinct constructs that might otherwise be missed.

In addition, and although existential psychological science is fundamentally undergirded by a quantitative approach, there are examples of purely qualitative measures being used to describe and inform existential psychological processes. In some ways, the utilization of this methodological approach connects to the methods traditionally utilized by humanists to probe the nature of people's subjective experiences. Work guided by this approach can consider various kinds of information, including responses to formal interviews and observations contained in archived collections, to better understand a specific kind of existential experience. As an example, McKenna-Plumley and colleagues (2023) theorized that people may experience different kinds of loneliness and that existential loneliness—which they defined as a sense of deep disconnection from the world and others—may not be accurately captured by unidimensional measures of loneliness that dominate the research literature. To address this gap, they asked people to define what existential loneliness means to them and to give a description of their existential loneliness experiences. The responses were subjected to reflexive thematic analysis in which responses are read closely and iteratively coded based on the thematic content they are perceived to possess. Rather than a descriptive or inferential analysis of any quantities of the thematic content, the *qualities* of these common themes (e.g., it's different from social isolation) is finally organized and presented to the field in the form of a coherent verbal description of the qualities of the construct, which is the outcome of the study. The ultimate goal of this type of research is to distill people's qualitative data into themes that describe a subjective experience. Although such thematic content cannot be leveraged in the same ways that quantitative measures can (e.g., they don't afford the opportunity to test mechanistic accounts of psychological processes), they can help inform the development of theory and methods to do so (see, e.g., McKenna-Plumley et al., 2024) by shedding light on the subjective ways that people report experiencing existential phenomena.

Meta-Analyses

Due to its incremental nature, psychological science can benefit from statistical inferences based on many, many studies across an entire research literature. This meta-analytic approach enables scholars to assess the relative strength of evidence for a particular phenomenon in aggregate, and to detect meaningful patterns that might exist within the entire corpus of findings focused on that phenomenon. Meta-analyses have become particularly important in the midst of contemporary concerns about research replicability and reproducibility in psychological science (e.g., Nosek et al., 2022), and useful resources for effectively conducting meta-analyses are not difficult to find (Moreau & Gamble, 2022).

Briefly, the process for conducting an effective meta-analysis begins with an effort to formally develop the question that the meta-analysis will address. This might be a question about the size of the effect of a particular intervention, a question about whether a certain existential concern (e.g., authenticity) robustly relates to another psychological variable (e.g., well-being), or some other question that can be informed by an aggregate assessment of available findings in the literature. From there, a thorough search for published research and an effort to acquire all unpublished data relevant to the question is carried out. Efforts to find unpublished data are quite important because publication biases can lead to an overestimated meta-analytic effect if the analysis is solely based on published findings (though methods for detecting and controlling publication bias exist; Ferguson & Brannick, 2012). Once the group of available studies has been identified, data from those studies (e.g., effect sizes) are saved and used in a formal meta-analysis that enables statistical inferences relevant to the research question under scrutiny. These inferences often serve as summary interpretations of a research literature as a whole, which may carry important theory implications.

For example, a meta-analysis of findings in the TMT literature (Martens et al., 2011) focused on comparing the effects of thinking about death to the effects of thinking about meaninglessness and uncertainty. These comparisons were important for theory because other frameworks have emphasized that the effects typically observed in TMT studies are due to meaning and/or uncertainty, rather than death (as TMT argues). The meta-analysis revealed that all three kinds of threats reliably (relative to a control condition) increased defensiveness, as would be predicted by their relative theoretical frameworks. However, because the meta-analysis permitted a test of whether these effects varied by the delay between the manipulation and the primary measure of defensiveness, a distinction between these threats was possible to assess. The results of these analyses showed that the effects of thinking about death got significantly larger with longer delays between the manipulation and the dependent variable. This was not true of the other threats. Thus, by leveraging the power of the many studies conducted in this area, Martens and colleagues (2011) were able to make an empirically based inference that the processes involved in each of these different kinds of threats may differ. That inference would have remained conjecture without the meta-analytic results.

Interim Summary

To summarize up to this point, researchers in psychological science utilize empirical methods to test hypotheses about the relationships between variables. They have many kinds of designs at their disposal, ranging from basic survey methodologies, to neuroscience techniques, to qualitative inquiries that can be transformed into meaningful numeric indices. Across all of these approaches, researchers need to be aware of the strengths and limitations that are inherent in the methods they choose and would be advised to avoid overinterpreting the findings of any one single study. Meta-analyses that assess effects/relationships across a research literature, though not without their own limitations (e.g., publication biases), can provide evidence for the robustness of particular findings and inform the overall utility of the theoretical frameworks meant to explain them.

JUDGMENT CALLS AND BEST PRACTICES

Existential psychological science, as the section above attests, is not unidimensional in terms of the kinds of psychological studies that it features. Scholars in this area utilize all of the kinds of studies that researchers have at their disposal, including cross-sectional correlation designs, laboratory experiments, field experiments, longitudinal diary methods, and neuroscience techniques. These studies are carried out in diverse contexts, ranging from the traditional psychology laboratory to online, virtual, and "real-world" settings. The diversity of methods employed is a strength of this area and is a credit to the many innovative social scientists who seek to answer questions about the psychological processes tethered to existential concerns. It also brings into focus the assortment of options and design choices that researchers must wrestle with when they are designing an empirical study. Where does one start? Is it best to start with a correlational study or proceed directly to an experiment? Does a 10-week diary study make sense? Answers to these kinds of questions are not always clear-cut and require a consideration of multiple factors (e.g., available resources, access to data).

I'm not going to pretend that there is one established way for selecting among the many options that a researcher has when starting a program of inquiry. In fact, what I'm going to lay out below contains thoughts and plans that I don't always follow in my own research, depending on competing demands like resource availability and anticipated timelines (e.g., the need for a student to complete a dissertation). Nevertheless, I hope to sketch out a few things to potentially consider when selecting among possible designs.

BUILDING UPON EXISTING MATERIALS VERSUS CREATING SOMETHING NEW

First, I think it's useful to think about whether you are trying to detect an effect that has never been detected before, or whether you're looking to build upon and extend research that is already established in the literature. The optimal approach to the latter case may be to simply start with the type of study that is most robust in the existing literature and build upon that kind of design. That may be especially true for many pockets of existential psychological science, where effective approaches to testing core hypotheses are already established. TMT, for example, has well-established experimental methods that are central to research in that area (Cox et al., 2019). Cross-sectional correlation designs are less optimal for testing TMT hypotheses and researchers looking to build upon and/or extend a question informed by TMT would be well advised to leverage existing TMT methodologies. In the former case, when looking to detect an effect that has never been detected, I think it reasonable to consider the design that has the most potential power to detect the effect of interest. This might be especially advisable in light of contemporary psychological science's justifiable emphasis on power and reproducibility (e.g., Nosek et al., 2022; Shrout & Rodgers, 2018; Tackett et al., 2019).

What this means for a particular research project can vary. Sometimes it might mean conducting a straightforward cross-sectional correlation study using reliable and valid measures (if they exist) of the key constructs. Detecting a simple correlation might have limited inferential value for causal processes, but it could provide important "proof-of-concept" evidence before moving to a study that requires the creation of an entirely new manipulation or a sizable commitment of resources. In other situations, starting with an experiment might make sense if manipulations and procedures can successfully be developed. I guess the message, here, is to be thoughtful about how you plan to start and to err on the side of seeking maximal power, not just in terms of sample size but also in terms of the measures employed, to detect a relationship in the early stages of a research design.

THE SUITABILITY OF ONLINE DATA COLLECTION

A second consideration that may be relevant in contemporary psychological science is a decision about whether or not to carry out the study online or in the laboratory. The particular research question and kind of design needed for that research question (e.g., diary vs. experiment) is obviously going to significantly impact this decision process. However, it is not uncommon for researchers to face legitimate choices about how to collect their data. As with the type of design, I would encourage researchers to think carefully about how the data collection method might relate to the relative power of their study to detect a reliable association or effect. This might be most important in the early stages of a research project, when simply determining whether an effect of interest can be reliably detected is essential. It's possible, for example, that an online environment might introduce enough random variation to weaken the overall impact of manipulation or to obscure associations that might be relatively small to begin with. Data-quality concerns (e.g., inattentiveness) in online environments are well documented (Newman et al., 2021) and the lack of environmental control might "wash out" the impact of an otherwise well-designed manipulation or valid effect. Given this, it may be prudent to choose the testing environment that will enable researchers to eliminate the most "noise" and to most powerfully test the hypothesized effect. A controlled laboratory environment may be ideal.

At the same time, however, there are factors that can attenuate some of the concerns that online studies might introduce and make an online study appropriate for a particular research application. For example, it's possible that paradigms that have been validated for online use already exist in a certain area of scholarship. A thorough literature review and assessment of research practices in a specific research area might highlight these paradigms and give researchers more confidence in opting for an online study if their planned study involves the same methodological features. It is also sometimes the case that a researcher might need to opt for an online study even when empirical justification for doing so is lacking. In these situations, the researcher should be mindful of the validity threats that online studies introduce and take preventative steps to reduce them. Scholars should consult the many excellent resources on these issues that exist (Chmielewski & Kucker, 2020; Gosling & Mason, 2015; Newman et al., 2021), but here are few important highlights.

For studies sampling from popular crowdsourcing platforms (e.g., Amazon Mechanical Turk, CloudResearch, Prolific), steps should be taken to protect against data-quality threats that might easily emerge in those kinds of venues (though these steps may be applicable to all online research). This includes bot detection procedures (see Irish & Saba, 2023; Simone et al., 2023), the use of participants vetted for good data quality (see Hauser et al., 2023), and appropriate incentivization for participation (Newman et al., 2021).

Researchers should also specifically consider options for identifying inattentive participants in their collected data sets. Attention checks can include items that ask participants to ignore the question and "click" a certain spot on the screen, items that have a clear right or wrong answer, and items that instruct participants to select a specific response option if they are paying attention (see Gummer et al., 2021). The idea is that these items will identify inattentive responders based on an incorrect response to the attention check. It is important to note that there is debate about the effectiveness of these kinds of checks (Roth & Yakobi, 2024), as well as evidence showing that including them can systematically change attention instead of assessing it (Hauser & Schwarz, 2015). Existential psychology researchers would be well advised to consider these issues. For example, because the inclusion of attention checks can bias people to be more systematic in their thinking (Hauser & Schwarz, 2015), including them could effectively eliminate effects that are grounded in less systematic and more intuitive ways of processing information. TMT effects (Simon et al., 1997) and perceptions of meaning in life (Heintzelman & King, 2016; Hicks et al., 2010) are two types of existential phenomena that could be affected. A "seriousness" check that asks participants to directly report on whether they tried to provide serious and valid responses at the end of the study (Aust et al., 2013) may be a better option in many situations. Using participants vetted for providing quality data (Hauser et al., 2023) is also advisable. The main point is that confidence in the attentiveness of participants is important for the validity of a study, and researchers should consider ways to enhance and detect attentiveness that do not introduce further validity concerns.

In sum, researchers face a number of broad decisions before drilling down to the operational measures critical to their research question. At minimum, they must decide on a study type (e.g., experimental vs. nonexperimental) and whether to conduct the study in a controlled environment (e.g., laboratory) or via the convenience of an online study platform. It would be impossible to outline all the factors that might influence these decisions, and researchers need to think carefully about what approach is most appropriate and feasible for their specific situation. Regardless, transparent reporting of why a particular approach was adopted and an honest appraisal of its strengths and weaknesses should be made available.

BEST PRACTICES AND A COMMENT ON SAMPLE-SIZE ESTIMATION

One of the biggest shifts in psychological science that has occurred during my career, which began around 2005, is the field's enhanced scrutiny on statistical power, reproducibility, and replicability. I suspect that anyone reading this chapter and handbook will have had some exposure to the many recommendations and commentaries on the importance of utilizing robust and transparent methodologies. Many excellent resources exist that cover the "replication crisis" in psychology (Maxwell et al., 2015; Nosek et al., 2022; Shrout & Rodgers, 2018), transparency in psychological science (Hales et al., 2019; Hardwicke & Vazire, 2023; Klein et al., 2018), preregistration (Simmons et al., 2021), and statistical power and sample-size justification (Lakens, 2022). Optimal existential psychological science will follow current "best-practice" recommendations and should include procedures that enhance confidence in the robustness and validity of any findings that emerge.

One area in this space that, at least in my experience, creates a lot of confusion at the study design phase is the determination of sample size. Although formal a priori power analyses using programs like G*Power (Faul et al., 2009) are ideal, the determination of an anticipated effect size for those power analyses can be ambiguous in a lot of situations. In addition, even when a documented average effect size exists in the literature, concerns about whether or not that effect size is accurate are reasonable. Publication bias and meta-analyses that include underpowered studies (Giner-Sorolla et al., 2024) can all lead to an inaccurate—and in many cases overestimated—effect size. For this reason, I find it more than reasonable to follow the clear recommendations of Giner-Sorolla and colleagues (2024). They (p. 18) note that a priori power analyses can be justified based on (1) estimates from an accurate and unbiased literature specific to the paradigm and question at hand; (2) estimates from biased literature that has been adequately corrected; (3) strong relevant theory; (4) if research addresses basic theoretical questions, basic practical effect size, usually based on the capacity of a typical lab to perform follow-up work to the question; and (5) if research is applied, practical effect size, usually based on the minimum change in raw units that would be cost-effective or otherwise seen as meaningful and useful. Regardless of how it is justified, transparency about the determination of sample size is essential.

CONCLUSION

I suspect that anyone willing to slog their way through a handbook chapter on existential psychology research methods is likely passionate about the empirical examination of existential concerns. I share that passion. For me, the opportunity to ask *and potentially answer* questions about the psychological processes involved in people's efforts to confront the "big questions" of their own lives is tremendously invigorating. That many of these concerns are also linked to important social outcomes like mental health (Iverach et al., 2014), suicide (Kleiman & Beaver, 2013), prejudice (Das et al., 2009), environmental concern (Vess & Arndt, 2008), and civic engagement (Maffly-Kipp et al., 2023) only affirms that there might be broader "meaning" in existentially oriented psychological science. Yet, to accurately understand existential processes and harness their practical significance, the science underlying existential inquiry must be sound. Adhering to core principles of psychological science methods and best-practice recommendations as they emerge is crucial for doing this work in the "right way."

REFERENCES

Abeyta, A. A., Juhl, J., & Routledge, C. (2014). Exploring the effects of self-esteem and mortality salience on proximal and distally measured death anxiety: A further test of the dual process model of terror management. *Motivation and Emotion, 38,* 523–528.

Abeyta, A. A., Routledge, C., Juhl, J., & Robinson, M. D. (2015). Finding meaning through emotional understanding: Emotional clarity predicts meaning in life and adjustment to existential threat. *Motivation and Emotion, 39,* 973–983.

Adler, J. M., Dunlop, W. L., Fivush, R., Lilgendahl, J. P., Lodi-Smith, J., McAdams, D. P., . . . Syed, M. (2017). Research methods for studying narrative identity: A primer. *Social Psychological and Personality Science, 8*(5), 519–527.

Adler, J. M., Lodi-Smith, J., Philippe, F. L., & Houle, I. (2016). The incremental validity of narrative identity in predicting well-being: A review of the field and recommendations for the future. *Personality and Social Psychology Review, 20*(2), 142–175.

Aust, F., Diedenhofen, B., Ullrich, S., & Musch, J. (2013). Seriousness checks are useful to improve data validity in online research. *Behavior Research Methods, 45,* 527–535.

Chmielewski, M., & Kucker, S. C. (2020). An MTurk crisis?: Shifts in data quality and the impact on study results. *Social Psychological and Personality Science, 11*(4), 464–473.

Cox, C. R., Darrell, A., & Arrowood, R. B. (2019). The method behind the science: A guide to conducting terror management theory research. In C. Routledge & M. Vess (Eds.), *Handbook of terror management theory* (pp. 85–132). Academic Press.

Cronbach, L. J., & Meehl, P. E. (1955). Construct validity in psychological tests. *Psychological Bulletin, 52*(4), 281.

Das, E., Bushman, B. J., Bezemer, M. D., Kerkhof, P., & Vermeulen, I. E. (2009). How terrorism news reports increase prejudice against outgroups: A terror management account. *Journal of Experimental Social Psychology, 45*(3), 453–459.

Faul, F., Erdfelder, E., Buchner, A., & Lang, A. G. (2009). Statistical power analyses using G*Power 3.1: Tests for correlation and regression analyses. *Behavior Research Methods, 41*(4), 1149–1160.

Ferguson, C. J., & Brannick, M. T. (2012). Publication bias in psychological science: Prevalence, methods for identifying and controlling, and implications for the use of meta-analyses. *Psychological methods, 17*(1), 120–128.

Giner-Sorolla, R., Montoya, A. K., Reifman, A., Carpenter, T., Lewis, N. A., Jr., Aberson, C. L., . . . Soderberg, C. (2024). Power to detect what?: Considerations for planning and evaluating sample size. *Personality and Social Psychology Review, 28,* 276–301.

Gosling, S. D., & Mason, W. (2015). Internet research in psychology. *Annual Review of Psychology, 66*(1), 877–902.

Gray, K. (2017). How to map theory: Reliable methods are fruitless without rigorous theory. *Perspectives on Psychological Science, 12*(5), 731–741.

Greenberg, J., Pyszczynski, T., & Solomon, S. (1986). The causes and consequences of a need for self-esteem: A terror management theory. In *Public self and private self* (pp. 189–212). Springer.

Greenberg, J., Pyszczynski, T., Solomon, S., Simon, L., & Breus, M. (1994). Role of consciousness and accessibility of death-related thoughts in mortality salience effects. *Journal of Personality and Social Psychology, 67*(4), 627.

Gummer, T., Roßmann, J., & Silber, H. (2021). Using instructed response items as attention checks in web surveys: Properties and implementation. *Sociological Methods and Research, 50*(1), 238–264.

Hales, A. H., Wesselmann, E. D., & Hilgard, J. (2019). Improving psychological science through transparency and openness: An overview. *Perspectives on Behavior Science, 42,* 13–31.

Hamaker, E. L., Kuiper, R. M., & Grasman, R. P. (2015). A critique of the cross-lagged panel model. *Psychological Methods, 20*(1), 102.

Hardwicke, T. E., & Vazire, S. (2023). Transparency is now the default at psychological science. *Psychological Science.*

Hauser, D. J., Moss, A. J., Rosenzweig, C., Jaffe, S. N., Robinson, J., & Litman, L. (2023). Evaluating CloudResearch's Approved Group as a solution for problematic data quality on MTurk. *Behavior Research Methods, 55*(8), 3953–3964.

Hauser, D. J., & Schwarz, N. (2015). It's a trap!: Instructional manipulation checks prompt systematic thinking on "tricky" tasks. *Sage Open, 5*(2).

Hayes, J., & Schimel, J. (2018). Unintended effects of measuring implicit processes: The case of death-thought accessibility in mortality salience studies. *Journal of Experimental Social Psychology, 74,* 257–269.

Hayes, J., Schimel, J., Arndt, J., & Faucher, E. H. (2010). A theoretical and empirical review of the death-thought accessibility concept in terror management research. *Psychological Bulletin, 136*(5), 699–739.

Heintzelman, S. J., & King, L. A. (2016). Meaning in life and intuition. *Journal of Personality and Social Psychology, 110*(3), 477–492.

Heintzelman, S. J., & King, L. A. (2019). Routines and meaning in life. *Personality and Social Psychology Bulletin, 45*(5), 688–699.

Hicks, J. A., Cicero, D. C., Trent, J., Burton, C. M., & King, L. A. (2010). Positive affect, intuition, and feelings of meaning. *Journal of Personality and Social Psychology, 98*(6), 967–979.

Hicks, J. A., Trent, J., Davis, W. E., & King, L. A. (2012). Positive affect, meaning in life, and future time perspective: an application of socioemotional selectivity theory. *Psychology and Aging, 27*(1), 181.

Hill, P. L., & Weston, S. J. (2019). Evaluating eight-year trajectories for sense of purpose in the health and retirement study. *Aging and Mental Health, 23*(2), 233–237.

Irish, K., & Saba, J. (2023). Bots are the new fraud: A post-hoc exploration of statistical methods to identify bot-generated responses in a corrupt data set. *Personality and Individual Differences, 213,* 112289.

Iverach, L., Menzies, R. G., & Menzies, R. E. (2014). Death anxiety and its role in psychopathology: Reviewing the status of a transdiagnostic construct. *Clinical Psychology Review, 34*(7), 580–593.

Kernis, M. H., & Goldman, B. M. (2006). A multicomponent conceptualization of authenticity: Theory and research. *Advances in Experimental Social Psychology, 38,* 283–357.

Klackl, J., Jonas, E., & Kronbichler, M. (2014). Existential neuroscience: Self-esteem moderates neuronal responses to mortality-related stimuli. *Social Cognitive and Affective Neuroscience, 9*(11), 1754–1761.

Kleiman, E. M., & Beaver, J. K. (2013). A meaningful life is worth living: Meaning in life as a suicide resiliency factor. *Psychiatry Research, 210*(3), 934–939.

Klein, O., Hardwicke, T. E., Aust, F., Breuer, J., Danielsson, H., Mohr, A. H., . . . Frank, M. C. (2018). A practical guide for transparency in psychological science. *Collabra: Psychology, 4*(1), 20.

Lakens, D. (2022). Sample size justification. *Collabra: Psychology, 8*(1), 33267.

Landa, I., & English, T. (2022). Variability in state authenticity predicts daily affect and emotion regulation. *Emotion, 22*(8), 1995.

Maffly-Kipp, J., Holte, P. N., Stichter, M., Hicks, J. A., Schlegel, R. J., & Vess, M. (2023). Civic hope and the perceived authenticity of democratic participation. *Social Psychological and Personality Science, 14*(4), 419–427.

Maffly-Kipp, J., & Vess, M. (2024). Meaning through fantasy?: Fantasy proneness positively predicts meaning for people high in depression. *Journal of Positive Psychology,* 1–12.

Martela, F., Laitinen, E., & Hakulinen, C. (2024). Which predicts longevity better: Satisfaction with life or purpose in life? *Psychology and Aging, 39*(6), 589–598.

Martens, A., Burke, B. L., Schimel, J., & Faucher, E. H. (2011). Same but different: Meta-analytically examining the uniqueness of mortality salience effects. *European Journal of Social Psychology, 41*(1), 6–10.

Maxwell, S. E., Lau, M. Y., & Howard, G. S. (2015). Is psychology suffering from a replication crisis? What does "failure to replicate" really mean? *American Psychologist, 70*(6), 487.

McAdams, D. P., & McLean, K. C. (2013). Narrative identity. *Current Directions in Psychological Science, 22*(3), 233–238.

McKenna-Plumley, P. E., Turner, R. N., Yang, K., & Groarke, J. M. (2023). "It's a feeling of complete disconnection": Experiences of existential loneliness from youth to older adulthood. *BMC Psychology, 11*(1), 408.

McKenna-Plumley, P. E., Turner, R. N., Yang, K., & Groarke, J. M. (2024). The Brief Scale of Existential Loneliness: Scale development and psychometric evaluation. *Current Psychology.*

Menzies, R. E., Sharpe, L., & Dar-Nimrod, I. (2019). The relationship between death anxiety and severity of mental illnesses. *British Journal of Clinical Psychology, 58*(4), 452–467.

Mohideen, F., & Heintzelman, S. J. (2023). Routines and meaning in life: Does activity content or context matter? *Personality and Social Psychology Bulletin, 49*(7), 987–999.

Moreau, D., & Gamble, B. (2022). Conducting a meta-analysis in the age of open science: Tools, tips, and practical recommendations. *Psychological Methods, 27*(3), 426–432.

Newman, A., Bavik, Y. L., Mount, M., & Shao, B. (2021). Data collection via online platforms: Challenges and recommendations for future research. *Applied Psychology, 70*(3), 1380–1402.

Newman, D. B., Nezlek, J. B., & Thrash, T. M. (2018). The dynamics of searching for meaning and presence of meaning in daily life. *Journal of Personality, 86*(3), 368–379.

Nosek, B. A., Hardwicke, T. E., Moshontz, H., Allard, A., Corker, K. S., Dreber, A., . . . Vazire, S. (2022). Replicability, robustness, and reproducibility in psychological science. *Annual Review of Psychology, 73*(1), 719–748.

Proulx, T., & Heine, S. J. (2006). Death and black diamonds: Meaning, mortality, and the meaning maintenance model. *Psychological Inquiry, 17*(4), 309–318.

Pyszczynski, T., Greenberg, J., & Solomon, S. (1999). A dual-process model of defense against conscious and unconscious death-related thoughts: An extension of terror management theory. *Psychological Review, 106*(4), 835–845.

Pyszczynski, T., Greenberg, J., Solomon, S., Arndt, J., & Schimel, J. (2004). Why do people need self-esteem? A theoretical and empirical review. *Psychological Bulletin, 130*(3), 435.

Quirin, M., Klackl, J., & Jonas, E. (2019). Existential neuroscience: A review and brain model of coping with death awareness. In C. Routledge & M. Vess (Eds.), *Handbook of terror management theory* (pp. 347–367). Elsevier.

Reis, H. T., & Judd, C. M. (Eds.). (2000). *Handbook of research methods in social and personality psychology.* Cambridge University Press.

Roth, Y., & Yakobi, O. (2024). Attention!: Do we really need attention checks? *Journal of Behavioral Decision Making, 37*(2), e2377.

Routledge, C., Arndt, J., Wildschut, T., Sedikides, C., Hart, C. M., Juhl, J., . . . Schlotz, W. (2011). The past makes the present meaningful: Nostalgia as an existential resource. *Journal of Personality and Social Psychology, 101*(3), 638.

Schnell, T., & Becker, P. (2006). Personality and meaning in life. *Personality and Individual Differences, 41*(1), 117–129.

Schmeichel, B. J., Gailliot, M. T., Filardo, E. A., McGregor, I., Gitter, S., & Baumeister, R. F. (2009). Terror management theory and self-esteem revisited: The roles of implicit and explicit self-esteem in mortality salience effects. *Journal of Personality and Social Psychology, 96*(5), 1077.

Schönbrodt, F. D., & Perugini, M. (2013). At what sample size do correlations stabilize? *Journal of Research in Personality, 47*(5), 609–612.

Seli, P., Beaty, R. E., Marty-Dugas, J., & Smilek, D. (2019). Depression, anxiety, and stress and the distinction between intentional and unintentional mind wandering. *Psychology of Consciousness: Theory, Research, and Practice, 6*(2), 163.

Shrout, P. E., & Rodgers, J. L. (2018). Psychology, science, and knowledge construction: Broadening perspectives from the replication crisis. *Annual Review of Psychology, 69*(1), 487–510.

Simmons, J., Nelson, L., & Simonsohn, U. (2021). Pre-registration: Why and how. *Journal of Consumer Psychology, 31*(1), 151–162.

Simon, L., Greenberg, J., Harmon-Jones, E., Solomon, S., Pyszczynski, T., Arndt, J., & Abend, T. (1997). Terror management and cognitive-experiential self-theory: Evidence that terror management occurs in the experiential system. *Journal of Personality and Social Psychology, 72*(5), 1132–1146.

Simone, M., Cascalheira, C. J., & Pierce, B. G. (2023). A quasi-experimental study examining the efficacy of multimodal bot screening tools and recommendations to preserve data integrity in online psychological research. *American Psychologist, 79*(7), 956–969.

Tackett, J. L., Brandes, C. M., King, K. M., & Markon, K. E. (2019). Psychology's replication crisis and clinical psychological science. *Annual Review of Clinical Psychology, 15*(1), 579–604.

Van den Bos, K. (2009). Making sense of life: The existential self trying to deal with personal uncertainty. *Psychological Inquiry, 20*(4), 197–217.

Vess, M., & Arndt, J. (2008). The nature of death and the death of nature: The impact of mortality salience on environmental concern. *Journal of Research in Personality, 42*(5), 1376–1380.

Vess, M., Brooker, R. J., Schlegel, R. J., & Hicks, J. A. (2019). Daily mental lapses and the subjective experience of true self-alienation. *Journal of Research in Personality, 78,* 148–152.

Vess, M., Leal, S. A., Hoeldtke, R. T., Schlegel, R. J., & Hicks, J. A. (2016). True self-alienation positively predicts reports of mindwandering. *Consciousness and Cognition, 45,* 89–99.

Vess, M., & Maffly-Kipp, J. (2022). Intentional mindwandering and unintentional mindwandering are differentially associated with the experience of self-alienation. *Personality and Individual Differences, 185,* 111289.

Waytz, A., Hershfield, H. E., & Tamir, D. I. (2015). Mental simulation and meaning in life. *Journal of Personality and Social Psychology, 108*(2), 336.

Williams, H., & Vess, M. (2016). Daydreams and the true self: Daydreaming styles are related to authenticity. *Imagination, Cognition and Personality, 36*(2), 128–149.

Wood, A. M., Linley, P. A., Maltby, J., Baliousis, M., & Joseph, S. (2008). The authentic personality: A theoretical and empirical conceptualization and the development of the Authenticity Scale. *Journal of Counseling Psychology, 55*(3), 385.

Yang, Y., Sedikides, C., Wang, Y., & Cai, H. (2024). Nature nurtures authenticity: Mechanisms and consequences. *Journal of Personality and Social Psychology, 126*(1), 79–104.

SECTION II

DEATH, AGING, AND TIME

CHAPTER 6

Back to the Future

Terror Management Theory—Review and Preview

Sheldon Solomon, Jeff Greenberg, *and* Tom Pyszczynski

Terror management theory (TMT) was inspired by cultural anthropologist Ernest Becker's (1962/1971, 1973, 1975) efforts to integrate and synthesize ideas from anthropology, biology, humanities, philosophy, psychoanalysis, religion, social psychology, and sociology in order to delineate the motivational underpinnings of human behavior. The central ideas were initially introduced in a chapter by Greenberg and colleagues (1986) that proposed that anxiety inherent in awareness of the inevitability of death is a driving force behind much human behavior, and that this potential for anxiety is managed by an anxiety-buffering system consisting of self-esteem and cultural worldviews. The present chapter marks 48 years of our collaboration, likely making us the longest lasting trio in the history of scientific inquiry. Here we review the development, empirical assessment, and conceptual refinements of TMT by highlighting three *Advances in Experimental Social Psychology* chapters, considering where TMT currently stands in contemporary psychological discourse, and noting various applications and current/future directions for TMT.

The authors share equal responsibility for this chapter.

A TMT OF SOCIAL BEHAVIOR: THE PSYCHOLOGICAL FUNCTIONS OF SELF-ESTEEM AND CULTURAL WORLDVIEWS

A more thorough presentation of TMT appeared in our first *Advances* chapter (Solomon et al., 1991). It described Becker's analysis of human behavior, and our attempt to systematize these ideas with TMT; basic TMT research hypotheses and initial research findings; our epistemological stance on the relationship between theory and research; and aspirations for future inquiry.

Our early research surrounded two questions central to social psychological discourse at the time. First, *What is the nature and function of self-esteem?* Although William James argued that self-esteem was as vital for human survival and well-being as basic emotions such as fear and anger, subsequent theory and research did little to clarify what self-esteem consisted of, how it was acquired and maintained, and what psychological functions it served. Second, *What are the psychological underpinnings of "Man's inhumanity to man"?* Why is human history rife with wars interwoven with persistent hostility toward others who do not share our religious or political beliefs? World War

II shifted the focus of social psychology toward understanding prejudice, totalitarianism, conformity, and obedience. Yet our graduate studies left us believing that some core aspects of these phenomena were still not being addressed.

After assuming academic positions in the early 1980s, we were delighted to encounter cultural anthropologist Ernest Becker's *The Birth and Death of Meaning* (1962/1971), *The Denial of Death* (1973), and *Escape from Evil* (1975). We were enthralled by Becker's interdisciplinary focus, motivational orientation, and commitment to the enlightenment view that knowledge and insight about human affairs can and should be utilized to foster psychological well-being and social progress.

Becker's analysis commences with the Darwinian assumption that humans share with all forms of life a basic biological predisposition toward self-preservation in the service of survival and reproduction, with the collateral recognition that human adaptation is heavily based on our sociability, culture, and cognitive abilities. We are social creatures who coordinate and cooperate with others to construct and maintain a host of elaborate institutions and meaning systems that facilitate our collective survival: cultures. Moreover, the capacity for abstract symbolic thought renders humans capable of conceiving things that do not yet exist and then transforming imagination into reality.

Such social and cognitive proclivities, which have enabled humankind to proliferate in a wide range of natural environments, also engender explicit self-awareness, resulting in awe and dread. Self-awareness is awesome, with the potential to yield a deep appreciation of and reverence for living. It is also, however, dreadful, yielding a poignant realization that humans are, like all living things, destined to die, and that one can be obliterated at any moment.

Awareness of the inevitability of death in an animal with diverse biological and psychological systems oriented toward survival creates the potential for debilitating existential terror that is both intolerably aversive and likely to undermine effective instrumental and social behavior. Humans manage existential terror by constructing and maintaining *cultural worldviews:* humanly constructed and socially validated beliefs that minimize death anxiety by embedding us in a symbolic conception of reality that allows us to view ourselves as beings of *value* in a world of *meaning* rather than mere material creatures fated to obliteration upon death.

Cultural worldviews account for the origin of the universe, prescribe what constitutes appropriate conduct, and provide hope of literal or symbolic immortality. *Literal immortality* can include ideas central to many of the world's great religions, such as heavens, souls, afterlives, and reincarnations. It can also include attempts to literally live forever, by pursuing fountains of youth, magical elixirs, and medical solutions to the problem of death. *Symbolic immortality* consists of the belief that remnants of one's existence will persist in perpetuity, by, for example, having children, amassing huge fortunes, being part of a great and enduring tribe or nation, producing great works of science or art, and performing noble acts of public service.

Self-esteem is the belief that one is a person of value in a world of meaning and is attained by believing that one is living up to the standards of value of one's cultural worldview. The primary function of self-esteem, as well as the cultural worldviews from which self-esteem is derived, is to minimize anxiety in general and death anxiety in particular. Self-esteem acquires its anxiety-buffering qualities over the course of the socialization process. Long before babies have the capacity to survive on their own or have any awareness of death, distress in response to unmet needs or physical danger instigates the formation of physical and psychological attachments to primary caretakers who nurture and protect their offspring. Self-esteem and cultural worldviews develop their anxiety-buffering capacity as an outgrowth of these attachment processes.

As they mature, children are incorporated into their social milieus by learning the language, beliefs, and customs of their culture. Parental affection becomes increasingly contingent on children behaving in accord with cultural dictates. Children are praised and rewarded when they behave appropriately, producing feelings of psychological security and well-being. Inappropriate behavior generates different parental reactions, ranging from punishment to rebuke to sullen indifference, all entailing a lack of affection, resulting in anxiety and insecurity. Children thus associate being "good" with being safe and being "bad" with being helpless and vulnerable; this is how stable high self-esteem becomes an anxiety buffer.

Then, as children become explicitly aware of the inevitability of their own death, as well as their parents' fallibility and mortality, the anxiety-buffering qualities of self-esteem ultimately depend on the promises of security and death transcendence afforded by the larger culture. Self-esteem is now obtained by meeting the culturally prescribed standards associated with specific social roles and values of the cultural worldview the child has internalized over the course of the socialization process.

In sum, TMT posits that the uniquely human awareness of death elicits potentially debilitating existential terror that is "managed" by embracing cultural worldviews and self-esteem striving by living up to the values of their worldview. People manage potential terror by construing themselves as persons of value in a world of meaning who are therefore eligible for literal and/or symbolic immortality. Because of the protection from the potential for terror these psychological structures afford, people are powerfully motivated to maintain faith in their cultural worldviews and satisfy the standards of value associated with them. Moreover, threats to one's cultural worldview or self-esteem instigate compensatory processes to bolster faith in their worldview and fortify confidence in their self-worth.

EMPIRICAL ASSESSMENTS OF TMT

Initial empirical assessments of the central tenets of TMT were focused on two central hypotheses: (1) the *anxiety-buffer hypothesis*—if self-esteem buffers anxiety, people with higher self-esteem should experience less anxiety and anxiety-related difficulties—and (2) the *mortality salience* hypothesis—if cultural worldviews serve to manage existential terror, making people aware of their own mortality (*mortality salience*; MS) should magnify their need for the protection afforded by their beliefs.

The Anxiety-Buffer Hypothesis

To move beyond a large body of correlational evidence consistent with the anxiety-buffer hypothesis, we assessed whether situationally elevated self-esteem would reduce anxiety in response to subsequent threats. Specifically, Greenberg and colleagues (1992b) gave participants positive or neutral personality feedback before having them view graphic depictions of death or a neutral film. Although neutral self-esteem participants showed a significant increase in self-reported anxiety in response to the death-related video, those who received a self-esteem boost showed no such increase. In a second study, after receiving positive feedback or no feedback on a supposed IQ test, participants anticipated either receiving painful electrical shocks or watching a series of colored lights while physiological responses were being assessed. Results indicated that while all participants were more aroused in anticipation of electrical shocks than colored lights, this effect was significantly diminished when self-esteem was increased. These studies provided convergent evidence that self-esteem buffers anxiety that is not confined to self-esteem-related threats.

The Mortality Salience Hypothesis

MS was posited to instigate efforts to bolster faith in the cultural worldview (*cultural worldview defense*), reflected by increased agreement with and affection for those who share their beliefs, and increased hostility and disdain for those who oppose their beliefs or merely harbor different beliefs. MS was originally induced by having people respond to two open-ended questions: "Please describe the emotions that the thought of your own death arouses in you" and "Write down as specifically as you can, what you think will happen to you physically as you die and once you are dead." Control participants responded to parallel questions about neutral activities such as eating or watching television, or aversive but not fatal experiences such as an upcoming exam, failure, extreme pain, having a limb amputated, or being socially excluded. Many other MS inductions have been used in subsequent studies, for example, being interviewed in front of a funeral parlor, or subliminal exposure to the word *dead* or *death*. These diverse operationalizations established the construct validity of the MS manipulation.

In the first MS experiment, Rosenblatt and colleagues (1989) predicted and found that following MS, Tucson municipal court judges, whose role it is to uphold the law, set substantially higher bonds for an alleged prostitute than judges in the control condition. Additional studies replicated this finding with student participants, but only those who believed that prostitution was morally reprehensible. This finding established that defensive reactions to MS are not indiscriminately negative, but rather, depend on the values of the individual's internalized worldview. Further studies found that this effect was not due to heightened self-awareness, general anxiety, negative affect, or physiological arousal. And an additional study showed that MS effects are not limited to negative reactions; in response to MS, participants recommended a higher monetary reward for a citizen who reputedly behaved in a heroic fashion by thwarting a bank robbery.

Taking Stock I

Based on this research, we concluded that TMT was conceptually and empirically sound pending the outcome of future inquiry. We acknowledged the importance of independent replications; studying individual and cross-cultural differences; and delineating the intrapsychic processes underlying mortality salience effects.

Additionally, following cultural anthropologist Marvin Harris's (1979) view that researchers should make their epistemological assumptions explicit, we presented our take on the scientific pursuit of knowledge based on Laudan's (1977) *Progress and Its Problems: Towards a Theory of Scientific Growth*. After arguing that theories cannot be unequivocally confirmed or disconfirmed, Laudan proposed that theories should be evaluated in terms of *problem-solving utility* in the context of an ongoing dialectic between theory, research, and specific historical factors. Laudan's pragmatic epistemic approach is compelling and consistent with the historical development of social psychology.

We ended the chapter with the hope that TMT might ultimately contribute to the development of "an applied theoretical social psychology"—a general account of human thoughts, feelings, and behavior that inspires empirical research and suggests actionable insights for enhancing psychological well-being and fostering social progress.

TMT OF SELF-ESTEEM AND CULTURAL WORLDVIEWS: EMPIRICAL ASSESSMENTS AND CONCEPTUAL REFINEMENTS

A decade after TMT's original inception, the second *Advances* chapter (Greenberg et al., 1997) summarized the standing of the anxiety-buffer and mortality salience hypotheses; described moderating and mediating variables of MS effects; and concluded with a discussion of lingering theoretical and empirical concerns.

The Anxiety-Buffer Hypothesis

Additional research in support of the causal role of self-esteem as an anxiety buffer was presented, and theoretical and methodological concerns regarding this line of inquiry were then addressed. Specifically, we explained:

1. Why alternative accounts of self-esteem, such as Leary and colleagues' (1995) sociometer theory positing that self-esteem is a barometer of social approval rather than as an existential anxiety buffer were problematic; for example, if self-esteem was a barometer of social approval, defensive distortions to protect and maximize self-esteem would be horribly maladaptive.
2. How the idea of self-esteem as an anxiety buffer is unique to Becker and TMT by noting that while other theories assume a relationship between self-esteem and anxiety, TMT is the only theory that provides an explicit account of how (and why) self-esteem and anxiety are related. Moreover, the finding that increased self-

esteem reduces anxiety and physiological arousal after watching a graphic death video and in anticipation of receiving electrical shocks is particularly compelling because it demonstrates the generality of self-esteem as an anxiety buffer beyond threats that directly undermine self-esteem.

3. How self-esteem could be differentiated from positive affect in the previously reported experiments. Specifically, some studies manipulated self-esteem without associated increases in positive affect, and the effects remained statistically significant after the effects of affect were eliminated by analysis of covariance.

The MS Hypothesis

We first cited successful efforts by independent researchers in the United States, Germany, and Israel to replicate basic MS effects (e.g., greater punishment for moral transgressors, increased bias toward one's own culture over others) and in some cases to extend them (e.g., physical distancing from an outgroup member). In addition to increasing confidence in the validity and robustness of MS effects, other scholars' research and commentary—both supportive and critical—of these findings were indicative of TMT becoming an increasingly influential topic of inquiry in social psychological discourse.

A theoretical account of prejudice and xenophobia was then presented. To the extent that cultural worldviews function to mitigate existential terror, the mere existence of different worldviews is often threatening because accepting the validity of alternative conceptions of reality undermines confidence in the veracity of one's own beliefs, and in so doing, may unleash the existential terror cultural worldviews are erected to forestall. To restore psychological equanimity, people denigrate others with different beliefs, simultaneously striving to convince and/or coerce them into disposing of their worldviews and adopting their own, or physically annihilating them to affirm the superiority of their own cultural worldview.

Consistent with this analysis, Greenberg and colleagues (1990) demonstrated that Christian participants had more favorable reactions to fellow Christians and less favorable reactions to Jewish targets in response to MS, and MS increased American participants' favorable reactions to an essay and its author expressing support for U.S. economic and foreign policies, and increased their negative reactions to an anti-U.S. essay and its author. These findings were then conceptually replicated with a behavioral measure of physical aggression. Specifically, following an MS or control induction, conservative and liberal American participants in a supposed study of food preferences allotted a variable amount of hot sauce to a liberal or conservative fellow participant who did not like spicy food, but would be required to consume (which served as a measure of aggression; McGregor et al., 1998). Hot sauce allotment did not differ in the control condition depending on whether the other person had the same or different political orientation as the participant, or in response to MS if the target shared the same political orientation as the participant. However, allocation increased substantially and significantly in response to MS if the target's political orientation was at odds with the participant's.

Next, we reviewed recent research to establish that intimations of mortality have a pervasive effect on human affairs. For example, in response to MS, people engage in greater prosocial behavior toward ingroup members; make higher estimates of social consensus for their beliefs; are reluctant to handle sacred cultural religious and political icons in a sacrilegious fashion; and avoid stimuli that increase self-awareness.

The Death-Thought Accessibility Hypothesis

Given that mortality salience increases worldview defense, presumably because bolstering confidence in one's beliefs buffers existential terror, we developed a complementary hypothesis: that threatening cherished aspects of cultural worldviews or self-esteem should make implicit death thoughts (*death-thought accessibility*; DTA) come more readily to mind and fortifying those resources should reduce DTA. DTA is generally measured by asking participants to complete word stems, including some that could be completed with neutral or death-related words; for example, C O F F _ _ could be COFFEE or COFFIN, and G R _ V E could be GROVE or GRAVE.

In accord with the DTA hypothesis, threats to the worldview, self-esteem, and close relationships increase DTA and worldview defense, and high self-esteem reduces DTA (for a review, see Hayes et al., 2010). For example, DTA increased when Christian fundamentalists were confronted with logical inconsistencies in the Bible (Friedman & Rholes, 2007); creationists read an article providing strong evidence for evolution, or Canadians read an article condemning their cultural values (Schimel et al., 2007); participants read an article claiming that progress is illusory (Rutjens et al., 2009); and atheists read an essay arguing that the theory of evolution cannot account for the origin of life and that was in favor of intelligent design (Hayes et al., 2015). Moreover, DTA increased after participants received negative feedback about their intelligence, were told their personality was incompatible with their career aspirations, or that they were ill-prepared to give an upcoming speech (Hayes et al., 2008), or when participants were asked to consider undesirable aspects of themselves (Ogilvie et al., 2008).

Moderation

Additional moderators of MS effects were also established, including self-esteem, depression, political orientation, and rational–experiential cognitive or emotional mindset.

Self-Esteem

To the extent that self-esteem serves as an effective bulwark against existential terror—a central tenet of TMT—high self-esteem was hypothesized and subsequently demonstrated to decrease cultural worldview defense in response to MS (Harmon-Jones et al., 1997). Specifically, participants with moderate self-esteem, or who did not receive a self-esteem boost, reported increased preference for a pro-U.S. author relative to an anti-U.S. author following an MS induction; however, this MS effect was not obtained for high self-esteem participants or for those who received favorable personality feedback that enhanced self-esteem.

Depression

A complementary hypothesis was that depression would have the opposite effect as self-esteem in moderating MS effects, based on Becker's assumption that depression is associated with difficulties gleaning an adequate sense of meaning and value. Accordingly, Simon and colleagues (1996) found that mildly depressed participants responded to an MS induction with stronger support for pro-U.S. students or (in a second study) students who shared their attitudes about domestic issues such as the legality of flag burning. Moreover, mildly depressed participants given an opportunity to engage in worldview defense after an MS induction subsequently reported a great sense of meaning in life, suggesting that affirming one's cultural worldview serves to confer meaning (Simon et al., 1998).

Political Orientation

Given that *liberal* means "tolerant and open-minded," and that conservatives are less prone to harbor such inclinations, Greenberg and colleagues (1992a) demonstrated that while conservatives reminded of death disparaged liberals more than usual, liberals reminded of death had more favorable impressions of conservatives. In a second study, participants primed with the value of tolerance in America did not disparage different others in response to MS.

Rational versus Experiential Mindset

Research also showed that MS effects emerge when people are in an experiential, but not a rational, mindset. This finding resulted from efforts to understand why some researchers, in ours and other labs, had difficulty replicating basic MS effects. Experimenters who produced MS effects tended to dress and act casually and delivered instructions to participants in a relaxed, natural manner, whereas MS effects were scarce when experimenters dressed and spoke more formally and awkwardly. This led to the idea, based on cognitive–experiential self theory (Kirkpatrick &

Epstein, 1992) distinction between rational and experiential cognitive systems, that differences in formality influenced participants' mindsets. The rational system is deliberative, effortful, abstract, and primarily linguistic; it operates actively and consciously based on logic and evidence, activated primarily when situational cues suggest the need for careful analysis. The experiential system, in contrast, is the default and dominant system in most circumstances, characterized by automatic and rapid preconscious information processing that seems self-evidently valid. This led us to suspect that for MS effects to emerge, participants must be in a relaxed intuitive mindset rather than a more structured analytic one.

Simon and colleagues (1997) tested this hypothesis by manipulating the appearance and demeanor of the experimenter (informal dress and expression vs. formal dress and expression) and found that MS increased worldview defense in the informal experimenter condition but not in the formal experimenter condition. Another study replicated this finding with a more direct manipulation of mindset, using written instructions to the participants to encourage either rational or experiential processing. As predicted, MS increased cultural worldview defense, but only in the experiential mindset condition.

Mediation

Trying to understand another failure to replicate MS effects led to the development of the dual-process model of responses to conscious and nonconscious death thoughts that mediate MS effects (Pyszczynski et al., 1999). Specifically, conscious death thoughts and nonconscious but highly accessible death thoughts instigate distinct defensive reactions. *Proximal* defenses suppress death-related thoughts or push the problem of death into the distant future by denying one's vulnerability. They are directly focused on the problem of death, (superficially) rational, and activated when death thoughts are in current focal attention. *Distal* defenses function to control the potential for anxiety engendered by the knowledge that death is inevitable by boosting self-esteem and fortifying faith in one's cultural worldview. Such defenses are experiential, not related to the problem of death in any semantic or logical way, and increasingly activated as DTA increases, up to the point when such thoughts become conscious, and proximal defenses are initiated.

Direct support for this model includes Greenberg and colleagues' (2000) demonstration that immediately after an MS induction, people engaged in proximal defense (i.e., vulnerability-denying defensive distortions) but showed no evidence of distal defense (i.e., exaggerated regard for similar others and disdain for dissimilar others); however, after a delay and distraction, distal defense was obtained but proximal defense was not.

Taking Stock II

TMT was now fortified by replications and extensions of basic research findings; support for a third core hypothesis (DTA); delineation of and support for theoretically relevant moderating variables; and the development and empirical assessment of the dual-process model of responses to conscious and nonconscious death thoughts that unfold in a predictable temporal pattern and underlie MS effects. Further research was suggested to extend the range of inquiry to include evolutionary considerations and to explore psychological disorders from a TMT perspective.

30 YEARS OF TMT: FROM GENESIS TO REVELATION

When the third *Advances* chapter was published (Pyszczynski et al., 2015), TMT was firmly embedded in experimental existential psychology, an established subdiscipline of experimental social psychology exploring universal human existential concerns—death, freedom and choice, identity, isolation, meaninglessness—with experimental methods (Greenberg et al., 2004). Moreover, there were now substantial bodies of evidence in support of the basic TMT hypotheses, including replications in over 20 different countries, summarized and evaluated in reviews and/or meta-analyses: anxiety buffer (Pyszczynski et al., 2004), mortality salience (Burke et al., 2010), and death-thought accessibility (Hayes et al., 2010). There were also reviews of TMT analyses of a wide variety of social psychological phenomena, including close relationships (Mikulincer et al., 2003), prejudice (Greenberg et al., 2009), terrorism (Pyszczynski et al., 2003), health-related behavior (Goldenberg & Arndt, 2008), prosocial behavior (Vail et al., 2012), and sexuality and animality (Goldenberg, 2012).

A brief recap of prior basic research and the dual-process model of reactions to conscious and nonconscious death thoughts was followed by TMT analyses of the evolution of the human mind and culture; how human beings relate to their bodies and the rest of the natural world; and the role that "mismanagement" of existential terror plays in psychological disorders. We then provided detailed responses to theoretical and empirical criticisms of TMT and concluded with recommendations for future inquiry.

Evolution, Body and Soul, and Terror Mismanagement

The Role of Death Awareness in the Evolution of Culture and Consciousness

Cultural worldviews likely serve multiple adaptive functions by enhancing survival through fostering social cohesion and cooperation, as well as facilitating transmission of cumulative cultural knowledge over generations. Indeed, our ancestors likely engaged in sophisticated abstract and symbolic thought perfused with supernatural beliefs prior to the emergence of the explicit awareness of death. Over time however, increasing cognitive complexity amplified self-awareness to the point of recognizing that one's own death is inevitable and could come at any time. Explicit awareness of personal mortality would be psychologically debilitating, likely rendering people fearful, timid, and passive, and disinclined to take risks.

Such psychological dis-ease in the wake of burgeoning awareness of death inspired early humans to develop cultural worldviews that offered hope of immortality; such worldviews, which in many cases eventually culminated in a single omniscient and omnipotent god, then became popular and were culturally selected for and transmitted successfully over generations. Concurrently, rituals developed that physically instantiated cultural belief systems with icons and ceremonies that served as a behavioral expression of the prevailing cultural narrative. Art, architecture, and music were invented and refined in this context in the broad service of assuaging existential apprehensions.

Archeological, anthropological, and historical evidence is consistent with this account (Solomon et al., 2015). Art, jewelry, and ritual burials with grave goods originated at roughly the same time as the cognitive capacities that made death awareness possible. Thereafter, humans throughout the world, regardless of culture, had one psychodynamic feature in common: a radical disinclination to die, resulting in ardent pursuit of immortality via searching for magical lands and elixirs of life; embracing sexual and nutritional habits to forestall aging; and constructing elaborate gateways to the afterlife such as pyramids and underground cities with terra-cotta armies.

Body and Soul

Becker argued that the human body is a source of anxiety and distress because it is the part of us that undeniably and quite visibly deteriorates, dies, and decays. A common human innovation to cope with this distress is a worldview that construes people as "more" than their physical bodies, with their "true essence" consisting of a soul, spirit, mind, or other nonmaterial entity that transcends the limitations of their bodies and will persist after their bodies have died. While the specific nature of souls varies considerably between cultures and throughout history, every soul construct renders the prospect of immortality possible because souls are detachable from the bodies in which they are embedded.

Denial of our creaturely nature also entails drawing a clear distinction between humans and other animals and distancing from the aspects of our bodies that remind us of our animality. Evidence for this analysis was provided by studies showing that reminders of death increase self-reported disgust in response to animals and bodily excretions, as well as increased belief that humans are distinct from animals (Goldenberg et al., 1999,

2001). Other research has shown that disgust-eliciting stimuli and reminders of similarities between humans and other animals increase DTA (Cox et al., 2007).

The connection between the human body and animality is particularly pronounced during sexual encounters, when one realizes that humans have much in common with fornicating animals at a farm or zoo. This is why sexuality is so heavily regulated and ritualized in all cultures. Research has shown that MS decreases the appeal of the physical (but not romantic) aspects of sex among those high in neuroticism; importantly, this effect occurs regardless of level of neuroticism when similarities between humans and other animals are made salient. Moreover, making the physical aspects of sex salient increases DTA, but this effect is eliminated when participants are first induced to think about romantic love. Aspects of these lines of research are reviewed in this volume by Lifshin and colleagues (Chapter 7), Courtney and colleagues (Chapter 10), and Goldenberg and colleagues (Chapter 38).

Psychological Disorders as Terror Mismanagement

In *The Denial of Death*, Becker (1973) argued that while "normal" people manage existential terror by perceiving themselves as valuable participants in a meaningful universe, some individuals are unable or unwilling to subscribe to the prevailing cultural worldview, perhaps because of biological predisposition, neuroanatomical abnormalities, traumatic experiences, or chronic stress. They instead adopt behavioral and psychological affectations in response to intimations of mortality that Yalom (1980) described as "clumsy modes of managing terror." Strachan and colleagues (2007) demonstrated that in response to MS, spider phobics decrease the amount of time they voluntarily view pictures of spiders; individuals with obsessive–compulsive disorder use more soap and water to wash their hands; and socially anxious individuals spend more time in voluntary isolation. Moreover, MS increases psychological dissociation and anxiety-sensitivity (being anxious about being anxious), a putative precursor of PTSD (Kosloff et al., 2006). Research has also shown that PTSD is associated with a disruption of normal anxiety-buffering processes (Pyszczynski & Kesebir, 2011). This work and subsequent research on the role of death anxiety in mental health problems is reviewed in this volume by Menzies (Chapter 9).

Criticisms of TMT

Serious engagement with critical scholars has been a vital element of the TMT enterprise, as it is for science in general, impelling us to clarify our thinking and design research to address empirical inconsistencies and unexpected findings. In this *Advances* chapter we discussed various criticisms of TMT and why we did not find them compelling.

Some scholars reject TMT on the grounds that, because they rarely think about dying, the theory is obviously wrong. In response, we noted that it is precisely because most people are comfortably ensconced in a cultural worldview that infuses their lives with meaning and value that death is not on their minds. Moreover, Greenberg and colleagues (1995) used a death-anxiety scale as an MS induction and found that participants who reported the least death-anxiety had the strongest worldview defense thereafter.

Another criticism is that TMT is fundamentally unfalsifiable because it claims that death has a pervasive effect on the totality of human experience, and by attempting to explain everything it ultimately explains nothing. Not true. While TMT, following Becker, does indeed posit that concerns about death are ubiquitous, there have always been theoretically relevant dispositional and situational factors that yield falsifiable hypotheses.

Objections to TMT from evolutionary psychologists include that TMT is wrong because it was originally framed in terms of a self-preservation instinct rather than genetic transmission, and that adaptation to death anxiety is incompatible with natural selection, which is limited to domain-specific selection pressures. In response, we pointed out that in the first *Advances* chapter we wrote that "Some have argued (e.g., Dawkins, 1976) that the need for self-preservation at the individual level is ultimately in the service of preserving our genes rather than ourselves per se. We have no quarrel with this assertion, and accepting it would not significantly alter our conceptual analysis." Thereafter, we provided extensive arguments that selection pressures can result from internal psychological conditions in support of the claim that TMT is quite compatible with contemporary evolutionary theorizing (Landau et al., 2007).

Perhaps the most common and enduring criticism of TMT regards the extent to which death is uniquely responsible for the phenomena that we were trying to explain. In response to this possibility, we included many aversive control conditions for comparison with MS, none of which produced the same effects as a MS induction. It has also been argued that death is a specific manifestation of broader superordinate psychological concerns, such as meaning, significance, or certainty. Of course, from a TMT perspective, certainty regarding the meanings provided by one's worldview and significance provided by self-esteem are essential components of the anxiety-buffering system. Awareness of death adds death denial as a powerful motivator that often usurps the pragmatic functions of meaning and certainty. People often prefer comforting illusions to more accurate beliefs. If uncertainty was really the major concern with death, then knowing that they were certain to die a painful death, that there is definitely no afterlife, and that they would be largely forgotten by most people a year or so after they die would be comforting; we're quite certain it is not. Moreover, history is replete with examples of people going to extraordinary lengths to avoid dying—for example, building pyramids, searching for the Fountain of Youth or the Elixir of Life—in spite of no rational basis for knowing whether the meaning systems that inspire such pursuits are valid.

We have conducted dozens of studies showing that threats to certainty and meaning do not produce effects parallel to MS. Others have found effects similar to MS for these threats (e.g., McGregor et al., 2001). Recent research suggests, however, that some manipulations of meaninglessness and uncertainty also increase DTA, supporting a TMT account that undermining meaning or certainty arouses implicit concerns about mortality because they undermine anxiety-buffering beliefs. Finally, alternative explanations for MS effects cannot explain or provide an alternative account of the dual-process model of proximal and distal defenses that underlie MS effects.

Taking Stock III

We concluded that TMT has been highly generative and many hypotheses that have been derived from the theory have been supported empirically, and further that the research programs have led to refinements regarding moderators and mediators of mortality salience effects and variables that affect levels of DTA and death anxiety. Furthermore, applications of TMT have been shown to be useful in understanding many domains of human concern and behavior. We also noted various remaining questions regarding potential clinical applications of TMT; determinants of various forms of terror management, for better (e.g., awe, gratitude, humility) and worse (e.g., mindless devotion to charismatic leaders, insatiable desire for money and stuff); the relationship between proximal and distal defenses; and the implications of cultural differences in how death is construed.

TMT AND THE REPLICATION CRISIS

TMT is currently a very active focus of theory and research in experimental existential psychology (e.g., *Handbook of Terror Management Theory*; Routledge & Vess, 2019) and continues to generate a considerable amount of debate and discussion within the field. Because there have been some failures to replicate some findings (e.g., Sætrevik & Sjåstad, 2022; Schindler et al., 2023), some have called the entire TMT literature into question.

Two broad problems that have not received adequate attention when assessing the replicability of mortality salience effects are that MS effects depend on the prevailing cultural worldviews of the participants, and there are times and places in which mortality is pervasively salient such that there is really no control condition to compare to an MS induction. For example, many studies reporting failure to replicate MS effects were conducted during the height of the deadly COVID-19 pandemic, when death thoughts were likely highly accessible for everyone.

One replication effort illustrating a lack of consideration of context and moderating variables was Klein and colleagues (2019, 2022), a collaboration of 17 labs attempting to replicate the effect of MS on evaluations of essays supportive and critical of the United States. They initially reported that they were unable to replicate previous findings that MS increases preference for essays favorable to one's country over unfavorable ones, even with procedural advice from the authors of the original study. This is, however, highly misleading, because they did not follow the most important advice given by the authors. Among other points, because the study was conducted very shortly after Donald Trump had won the 2016 U.S. presidential election, we suggested the essays needed modification, noting that the anti-American essay developed for use in 1992 focused on how the United States served the wealthy and was plagued by prejudice and actually supported the worldview of many Americans reeling from Trump's election.

Additionally, Chatard and colleagues (2020) reviewed the reported analyses and discovered that they (ironically) did not follow their own preregistered data-analysis plan, and that *none* of the groups that attempted to replicate the study without input from the original authors included a delay or distraction between the MS induction and dependent measures. When reanalyzing these data, Chatard and colleagues found MS effects under some but not all conditions, consistent with the moderators that had already been established.

Like virtually all findings in psychology, and many if not most areas of science, TMT effects sometimes do not replicate. Though some argue that this suggests the effect is not "real," we think it naive to think that research assessing complex, multidetermined attitudes and behavior conducted at one time and place will always yield the same findings when the study is done by different researchers in a different time and place.

Rather than viewing inconsistent findings across studies as evidence that an effect is suspect, we think it more useful to view them as a sign that additional conceptual analysis is in order. Additionally, theoretically derived TMT effects have been found in well over one thousand studies; concluding that these effects are suspect based on a much smaller set of failures to replicate does nothing to explain these findings, nor provide insight into the important real-world phenomena the theory was designed to explain. Indeed, MS effects have been obtained in a variety of recent studies that have taken context into account (e.g., Courtney et al., 2021; Fairlamb & Courtney, 2022; Qi, 2023; Vail et al., 2019a).

This is not to say that failures to replicate should be ignored. We have long viewed resolution of inconsistent findings as one of the highest priorities for theory development and refinement regarding TMT, and indeed, almost all domains of psychological research.

CURRENT AND FUTURE APPLICATIONS OF TMT

TMT remains robust and viable by Laudan's (1977) epistemological standard of problem-solving utility presented earlier: A sound theory engages scholars' interest to broach questions of current concern that yield assessable hypotheses that are subsequently confirmed (or if not confirmed, the theory is refined or ultimately abandoned).

We also would like to think that TMT has had a positive influence on psychological discourse, and other fields as well, including marketing, management and policy, robotics, political science, environmental studies, animal rights advocacy (see Lifshin et al., Chapter 7, this volume), hospice care, culture, religion, film, and gender studies, and the study of terrorism. For example, regarding terrorism, Kruglanski and colleagues' (2022) work on understanding terrorism as a quest for significance builds on our analysis and research (Pyszczynski et al., 2003, 2006, 2008), and a recent paper uses TMT to understand the ideology of ISIS and how it recruits new potential martyrs in refugee camps in Syria (Garshasbi & Karimi Maleh, 2024).

We next consider some directions TMT research has been going.

TMT and the Environment

Biologists and environmental scientists now recognize the connection between TMT and humankind's disinclination to respond effectively to climate change. People striving for self-esteem, who are embedded in cultural worldviews that are disassociated from nature, place value on wealth and material consumption, and are predicated on an overreliance on technology and assumptions of inevitable progress, will likely respond in a counterproductive fashion when intimations of mortality are aroused (e.g., Dickinson, 2009). Accordingly, environmental and sustainability scholars propose "that TMT insights and methods should be better integrated into research designs to guide climate communications and to generate the comprehensive cultural and behavioral changes needed to address societies' climate problems" (Smith et al., 2022).

TMT and Politics

TMT research has had political implications from very early on, when in 1990 we found that MS increased Americans' positive reactions to a pro-U.S. essay and negative reactions to an anti-U.S. essay (Greenberg et al., 1990), and that MS led politically conservative Americans to be more negative to a liberal critic, whereas liberals were less prone to react to MS with negativity toward a conservative critic (Greenberg et al., 1992a). Similarly, high authoritarians became more negative toward different others after MS, but low authoritarians did not (Greenberg et al., 1990), and sometimes have reacted to MS with more positivity, for example toward immigrants (e.g., Weise et al., 2012).

When the 9/11 attacks occurred, we, along with journalists and colleagues, realized that the effects we were finding in the lab were writ large across the United States. We then proposed a simple characterization of worldviews as providing either a "rock" or a "hard place" for coping with existential anxiety (Pyszczynski et al., 2003). "Rock" worldviews are generally rigid and absolute, depicting the world in black-and-white terms with explicit determinations of good and bad and specifications for transcending death. Such views foster existential security but are also typically intolerant of alternative conceptions of reality, demonizing the evil other. "Hard place" worldviews, in contrast, acknowledge that absolute truth is unattainable and that there are viable alternative conceptions of reality. Such views foster openness to different ideas and perspectives and tolerance of others, but increase existential apprehensions because they lack existential certainty, rendering adherents prone to self-medication and dedication to passing cultural fads.

Generally, extreme or fundamentalist worldviews of all types, whether right-wing or left-wing, religious or secular, capitalist or communist, are the kinds of rock-type worldviews promoted by demagogues and become increasing appealing to people when scary times bring death and vulnerability close to consciousness. Becker (1973) proposed that in times of massive upheaval that lead people to lose confidence in their prevailing worldview, fear of death will draw people toward passionate devotion to seemingly larger-than-life ideological demagogues who proclaim to be divinely ordained to rid the world of evil.

Supporting these ideas, MS increased support for hypothetical charismatic leaders (Cohen et al., 2004), for George W. Bush prior to his reelection in 2004 (Landau et al., 2004), and for Donald Trump prior to his election in 2016 (Cohen et al., 2017). More recently, Hinkley (2021) found that mortality rates in communities in the United States are positively correlated with right-wing authoritarian attitudes, and, in a large cross-cultural study of 69 countries, Kakkar and Sivanathan (2017) found that people prefer dominant leaders (like alpha males in a primate community who generally rule by fear) rather than prestige leaders (who are admired and respected by virtue of their wisdom and expertise) in times of economic uncertainty where citizens perceive a lack of personal control.

TMT and Health Psychology

The terror management health model (TMHM; Courtney et al., Chapter 10, this volume; Goldenberg & Arndt, 2008) extended TMT into health psychology by positing that health decisions result from proximal defenses that often involve commitment to engage in healthier behavior, followed by distal defenses to bolster a sense of meaning and value that often lead to unhealthy behavior. For example, immediately after MS, residents of South Florida who read about the dangers of too much exposure to the sun reported that they would use a more powerful sunscreen and spend less time at the beach (proximal defense). However, 5 minutes after MS, participants who based their self-esteem on their appearance reported that they would use a less powerful sunscreen and spend more time at the beach (distal defense; Routledge et al., 2004).

There is now a substantial body of research documenting how proximal and distal reactions to intimations of mortality influence fitness and exercise, eating behaviors, smoking behaviors, and health-related decision making in general; and TMHM is particularly relevant in the aftermath of COVID-19 pandemic when most people were saturated with explicit and implicit death thoughts. TMT (Pyszczynski et al., 2021) and TMHM (Courtney et al., 2020) theorists have provided explanatory frameworks of reactions to COVID-19 that have in turn yielded interesting and potentially important research.

TMT, Psychological Disorders, and Clinical Applications

TMT research demonstrating that MS amplifies symptoms of various psychological disorders led to the development of anxiety-buffer disruption theory (ABDT; Pyszczynski & Kesebir, 2011) to explain reactions to traumatic events and the onset and maintenance of posttraumatic stress disorder (PTSD). From this perspective, PTSD occurs when typical mechanisms that provide a sense that one is a person of value in a world of meaning are disrupted in response to traumatic events. Individuals with PTSD do not respond to MS with typical worldview defense and lack the capacity to manage anxiety effectively thereafter (see e.g., Vail et al., 2018, 2019b, 2019c, 2020).

Based on TMT, ABDT, and related research, death anxiety has subsequently been identified as a transdiagnostic construct (see Iverach et al., 2014; Menzies, this volume, Chapter 9): that is, death anxiety occurs across a range of psychological disorders across different diagnostic categories and increases vulnerability to the development and maintenance of those psychological disorders. Accordingly, designing effective therapeutic interventions to diminish death anxiety should be a high priority for clinicians, particularly at a historical moment where environmental, economic, political, and psychological instability have produced wholesale psychological dis-ease, and rendered traditional treatments relatively ineffective (Guthrie, 2023). Consistent with this notion, research suggests reduction of death anxiety is a common outcome of effective treatments for trauma, ranging from mindfulness (Park & Pyszczynski, 2019) to psychedelics (Moreton et al., 2020), and that reductions in death anxiety are reflected in alterations of neural activity (Dor-Ziderman et al., 2019).

Reducing death anxiety is also crucial for treatment of terminally ill people in palliative care settings, where interventions to enhance meaning (e.g., meaning-centered group psychotherapy; Breitbart et al., 2010) and value (e.g., dignity therapy; Chochinov et al., 2011) have proven demonstrably effective. More recently, clinicians have integrated the palliative care literature with TMT to develop the concept of *existential maturity* (Emanuel et al., 2021) as a generalizable state characterized by death acceptance, sense of meaning and purpose, and feelings of awe and transcendence. Assessing the efficacy of various strategies to foster death acceptance is an important goal for future research.

From an even broader perspective, some cultural worldviews may be better for quelling existential concerns and hence mental health than others (see e.g., Rowe, 2023). Based on Becker's arguments in *Escape from Evil* (1975), we have suggested that cultural worldviews should be judged in terms of the extent to which they serve the material needs of their members given current technology and natural resources; the extent to which they serve the psychological needs of their members by espousing standards of value that are realistically attainable for the average individual; and the extent to which these needs are addressed without undue harm to others (within and outside the culture).

TMT and Art

TMT is also seeping into popular culture. In 2018, Canadian painter Kim Dorland presented *Terror Management Theory* at The Delphian Gallery, noting that TMT "has been very much on my mind these days that the state we're in on so many different fronts (environment, politics) is pretty ominous." Shortly thereafter, Ahmed Khaled Tawfik examined the psychodynamics of cultural disruption and its defense mechanisms with explicit reference to TMT in the dystopian science fiction novel *Utopia* (2011). And there are now numerous songs called *Terror Management Theory* and two albums with the theory in their titles.

There is also a documentary about Becker and TMT, *Flight from Death: The Quest for Immortality* (Shen, 2003), and it seems that these ideas are seeping into streaming shows and movies. For example, the film *Barbie* is partly about what happens when Barbie learns about mortality; and one of the themes, elucidated by Roberts and Goldenberg (2024), is that humans cope with their mortality through imbuing life with meaning and with idealized fantasies that can live on beyond our physical deaths.

TAKING STOCK: BACK TO THE FUTURE

On the cusp of oblivion as scholars (and ultimately as humans!), we wrote this chapter looking at TMT backward and forward in part as an existential balm to garner a wisp of symbolic immortality for ourselves. More importantly, however, our hope is that current and future scholars and clinical practitioners will find the chapter inspirational and informative.

For 40 years we have insisted that a primary goal of TMT is to inspire others to partake of Ernest Becker's work directly. Becker remains in our estimation one of the most important and underappreciated thinkers of the last few millennia—integrating and synthesizing critical insights from science, religion, the humanities, and popular culture to provide a powerful and parsimonious account of human affairs.

When people read Becker—students, colleagues, and laypeople alike—it often gives them a useful new way of understanding themselves, others they know, history, and current events. We have been hopeful our TMT work would do the same and help this view of us humans become part of how we all understand each other and ourselves. Toward this goal, we are gratified that TikToks and YouTubes about the theory have garnered millions of viewers.

Meanwhile, our hope is that this chapter is informative in providing a reasonably accurate historical overview of the development and refinement of TMT. Although we, not surprisingly, still find TMT a vibrant theory with a promising future, this is ultimately not for us to determine. Perhaps TMT will eventually be replaced by a different depiction of coping with mortality. That is science. Regardless, TMT has contributed to the development of the burgeoning field of experimental existential psychology and has had an impact on many fields beyond psychology, and theory and research will continue toward understanding the role of death and other existential concerns in important domains of human behavior.

REFERENCES

Becker, E. (1971). *The birth and death of meaning: An interdisciplinary perspective on the problem of man.* Free Press. (Original work published 1962)

Becker, E. (1973). *The denial of death.* Free Press.

Becker, E. (1975). *Escape from evil.* Free Press.

Breitbart, W., Rosenfeld, B., Gibson, C., Pessin, H., Poppito, S., Nelson, C., . . . Olden, M. (2010). Meaning-centered group psychotherapy for patients with advanced cancer: A pilot randomized controlled trial. *Psycho-Oncology, 19*(1), 21–28.

Burke, B. L., Martens, A., & Faucher, E. H. (2010). Two decades of terror management theory: A meta-analysis of mortality salience research. *Personality and Social Psychology Review, 14*(2), 155–195.

Chatard, A., Hirschberger, G., & Pyszczynski, T. (2020). A word of caution about Many Labs 4: If you fail to follow your preregistered plan, you may fail to find a real effect. *Collabra: Psychology, 8*(1), 12345.

Chochinov, H. M., Kristjanson, L. J., Breitbart,

W., McClement, S., Hack, T. F., Hassard, T., & Harlos, M. (2011). Effect of dignity therapy on distress and end-of-life experience in terminally ill patients: A randomised controlled trial. *Lancet Oncology, 12*(8), 753–762.

Cohen, F., Solomon, S., & Kaplin, D. (2017). You're hired!: Mortality salience increases Americans' support for Donald Trump. *Analyses of Social Issues and Public Policy, 17*(1), 339–357.

Cohen, F., Solomon, S., Maxfield, M., Pyszczynski, T., & Greenberg, J. (2004). Fatal attraction: The effects of mortality salience on evaluations of charismatic, task-oriented, and relationship-oriented leaders. *Psychological Science, 15*(12), 846–851.

Courtney, E., Felig, R., & Goldenberg, J. (2021). Together we can stop the spread of COVID-19: The interactive effects of priming collectivism and mortality salience on virus-related health behaviour intentions. *British Journal of Social Psychology, 61,* 410–431.

Courtney, E. P., Goldenberg, J. L., & Boyd, P. (2020). The contagion of mortality: A terror management health model for pandemics. *British Journal of Social Psychology, 59*(3), 607–617.

Cox, C. R., Goldenberg, J. L., Pyszczynski, T., & Weise, D. (2007). Disgust, creatureliness and the accessibility of death-related thoughts. *European Journal of Social Psychology, 37*(3), 494–507.

Delphian Gallery. (n.d.). Kim Dorland—terror management theory. https://delphiangallery.com/kim-dorland/.

Dickinson, J. L. (2009). The people paradox: Self-esteem striving, immortality ideologies, and human response to climate change. *Ecology and Society, 14*(1), 34.

Dor-Ziderman, Y., Lutz, A., & Goldstein, A. (2019). Prediction-based neural mechanisms for shielding the self from existential threat. *NeuroImage, 202,* 116080.

Emanuel, L., Solomon, S., Fitchett, G., Chochinov, H., Handzo, G., Schoppee, T., & Wilkie, D. (2021). Fostering existential maturity to manage terror in a pandemic. *Journal of Palliative Medicine, 24*(2), 211–217.

Fairlamb, S., & Courtney, E. (2022). An existential perspective on interpersonal closeness and social distancing during the COVID-19 pandemic. *Psychology and Health, 39*(8), 1059–1076.

Friedman, M., & Rholes, W. S. (2007). Successfully challenging fundamentalist beliefs results in increased death awareness. *Journal of Experimental Social Psychology, 43*(5), 794–801.

Garshasbi, R., & Karimi Maleh, A. (2024). Fear of death: Al-Hawl's children and the security threat in the Middle East. *Behavioral Sciences of Terrorism and Political Aggression.*

Gerwig, G. (Director). (2023). *Barbie* [Film]. Warner Bros.

Goldenberg, J. L. (2012). A body of terror: Denial of death and the creaturely body. In P. R. Shaver & M. Mikulincer (Eds.), *Meaning, mortality, and choice: The social psychology of existential concerns* (pp. 93–110). American Psychological Association.

Goldenberg, J. L., & Arndt, J. (2008). The implications of death for health: A terror management health model for behavioral health promotion. *Psychological Review, 115*(4), 1032–1053.

Goldenberg, J. L., Pyszczynski, T., Greenberg, J., Solomon, S., Kluck, B., & Cornwell, R. (2001). I am not an animal: Mortality salience, disgust, and the denial of human creatureliness. *Journal of Experimental Psychology: General, 130*(3), 427–435.

Goldenberg, J. L., Pyszczynski, T., McCoy, S. K., Greenberg, J., & Solomon, S. (1999). Death, sex, love, and neuroticism: Why is sex such a problem? *Journal of Personality and Social Psychology, 77*(6), 1173–1187.

Greenberg, J., Arndt, J., Simon, L., Pyszczynski, T., & Solomon, S. (2000). Proximal and distal defenses in response to reminders of one's mortality: Evidence of a temporal sequence. *Personality and Social Psychology Bulletin, 26*(1), 91–99.

Greenberg, J., Koole, S. L., & Pyszczynski, T. (Eds.). (2004). *Handbook of experimental existential psychology.* Guilford Press.

Greenberg, J., Landau, M. J., Kosloff, S., & Solomon, S. (2009). How our dreams of death transcendence breed prejudice, stereotyping, and conflict. In T. Nelson (Ed.), *The handbook of prejudice, stereotyping, and discrimination* (pp. 309–332). Psychology Press.

Greenberg, J., Pyszczynski, T., & Solomon, S. (1986). The causes and consequences of a need for self-esteem: A terror management theory. In R. F. Baumeister (Ed.), *Public self and private self* (pp. 189–212). Springer-Verlag.

Greenberg, J., Pyszczynski, T., Solomon, S., Rosenblatt, A., Veeder, M., Kirkland, S., & Lyon, D. (1990). Evidence for terror management theory II: The effects of mortality salience on reactions to those who threaten or bolster the cultural worldview. *Journal of Personality and Social Psychology, 58*(2), 308–318.

Greenberg, J., Simon, L., Harmon-Jones, E., Solomon, S., Pyszczynski, T., & Lyon, D. (1995).

Testing alternative explanations for mortality salience effects: Terror management, value accessibility, or worrisome thoughts? *European Journal of Social Psychology, 12*(4), 417–433.
Greenberg, J., Simon, L., Pyszczynski, T., Solomon, S., & Chatel, D. (1992a). Terror management and tolerance: Does mortality salience always intensify negative reactions to others who threaten one's worldview? *Journal of Personality and Social Psychology, 63*(2), 212–220.
Greenberg, J., Solomon, S., & Pyszczynski, T. (1997). Terror management theory of self-esteem and cultural worldviews: Empirical assessments and conceptual refinements. In M. P. Zanna (Ed.), *Advances in experimental social psychology* (Vol. 29, pp. 61–139). Academic Press.
Greenberg, J., Solomon, S., Pyszczynski, T., Rosenblatt, A., Burling, J., Lyon, D., . . . Pinel, E. (1992b). Why do people need self-esteem?: Converging evidence that self-esteem serves an anxiety-buffering function. *Journal of Personality and Social Psychology, 63*(6), 913–922.
Guthrie, D. (2023). How I learned to stop worrying and love the eco-apocalypse: An existential approach to accepting eco-anxiety. *Perspectives on Psychological Science, 18*(1), 210–223.
Harmon-Jones, E., Simon, L., Greenberg, J., Pyszczynski, T., Solomon, S., & McGregor, H. (1997). Terror management theory and self-esteem: Evidence that increased self-esteem reduced mortality salience effects. *Journal of Personality and Social Psychology, 72*(1), 24–36.
Harris, M. (1979). *Cultural materialism: The struggle for a science of culture*. Random House.
Hayes, J., Schimel, J., Arndt, J., & Faucher, E. H. (2010). A theoretical and empirical review of the death-thought accessibility concept in terror management research. *Psychological Bulletin, 136*(5), 699–739.
Hayes, J., Schimel, J., Arndt, J., & Faucher, E. H. (2015). Delay and death-thought accessibility: A meta-analysis. *Personality and Social Psychology Bulletin, 41*(12), 1682–1696.
Hayes, J., Schimel, J., Faucher, E. H., & Williams, T. J. (2008). Evidence for the DTA hypothesis II: Threatening self-esteem increases death-thought accessibility. *Journal of Experimental Social Psychology, 44*(3), 600–613.
Hinckley, R. A. (2021). Local existential threat, authoritarianism, and support for right-wing populism. *Social Science Journal.*
Iverach, L., Menzies, R. G., & Menzies, R. E. (2014). Death anxiety and its role in psychopathology: Reviewing the status of a transdiagnostic construct. *Clinical Psychology Review, 34*(7), 580–593.
Kakkar, H., & Sivanathan, N. (2017). When the appeal of a dominant leader is greater than a prestige leader. *Proceedings of the National Academy of Sciences, 114*(26), 6734–6739.
Kirkpatrick, L. A., & Epstein, S. (1992). Cognitive-experiential self-theory and subjective probability: Further evidence for two conceptual systems. *Journal of Personality and Social Psychology, 63*(4), 534–544.
Klein, R. A., Cook, C. L., Ebersole, C. R., Vitiello, C. A., Nosek, B. A., Chartier, C. R., . . . Ratliff, K. A. (2019, December 11). *Many Labs 4: Failure to replicate mortality salience effect with and without original author involvement.* https://www.cos.io/blog/many-labs-4-failure-replicate-mortality-salience-effect-and-without-original-author-involvement.
Klein, R. A., Vianello, M., Hasselman, F., Adams, B. G., Adams, R. B., Alper, S., . . . Nosek, B. A. (2022). Many Labs 4: Failure to replicate mortality salience effect with and without original author involvement. *Collabra: Psychology, 8*(1), 35271.
Kosloff, S., Solomon, S., Greenberg, J., Cohen, F., Gershuny, B., Routledge, C., & Pyszczynski, T. (2006). Fatal distraction: The impact of mortality salience on dissociative responses to 9/11 and subsequent anxiety sensitivity. *Basic and Applied Social Psychology, 28*(4), 349–356.
Kruglanski, A. W., Molinario, E., Jasko, K., Webber, D., Leander, N. P., & Pierro, A. (2022). Significance-quest theory. *Perspectives on Psychological Science, 17*(4), 1050–1071.
Landau, M. J., Solomon, S., Greenberg, J., Cohen, F., Pyszczynski, T., Arndt, J., . . . Cook, A. (2004). Deliver us from evil: The effects of mortality salience and reminders of 9/11 on support for President George W. Bush. *Personality and Social Psychology Bulletin, 30*(9), 1136–1150.
Landau, M. J., Solomon, S., Pyszczynski, T., & Greenberg, J. (2007). On the compatibility of terror management theory and perspectives on human evolution. *Evolutionary Psychology, 5*(3), 476–519.
Laudan, L. (1977). *Progress and its problems: Towards a theory of scientific growth.* University of California Press.
Leary, M. R., Tambor, E. S., Terdal, S. K., & Downs, D. L. (1995). Self-esteem as an interpersonal monitor: The sociometer hypothesis. *Journal of Personality and Social Psychology, 68*(3), 518–530.
McGregor, H. A., Lieberman, J. D., Greenberg,

J., Solomon, S., Arndt, J., Simon, L., & Pyszczynski, T. (1998). Terror management and aggression: Evidence that mortality salience motivates aggression against worldview-threatening others. *Journal of Personality and Social Psychology, 74*(3), 590–605.

McGregor, I., Zanna, M. P., Holmes, J. G., & Spencer, S. J. (2001). Compensatory conviction in the face of personal uncertainty: Going to extremes and being oneself. *Journal of Personality and Social Psychology, 80*(3), 472–488.

Mikulincer, M., Florian, V., & Hirschberger, G. (2003). The existential function of close relationships: Introducing death into the science of love. *Personality and Social Psychology Review, 7*(1), 20–40.

Moreton, S. G., Szalla, L., Menzies, R. E., & Arena, A. F. (2020). Embedding existential psychology within psychedelic science: Reduced death anxiety as a mediator of the therapeutic effects of psychedelics. *Psychopharmacology, 237,* 21–32.

Ogilvie, D. M., Cohen, F., & Solomon, S. (2008). The undesired self: Deadly connotations. *Journal of Research in Personality, 42*(3), 564–576.

Park, Y. C., & Pyszczynski, T. (2019). Reducing defensive responses to thoughts of death: Meditation, mindfulness, and Buddhism. *Journal of Personality and Social Psychology, 116*(1), 101–118.

Pyszczynski, T., Greenberg, J., & Solomon, S. (1999). A dual-process model of defense against conscious and unconscious death-related thoughts: An extension of terror management theory. *Psychological Review, 106*(4), 835–845.

Pyszczynski, T. A., Greenberg, J., & Solomon, S. (2003). *In the wake of 9/11: The psychology of terror.* American Psychological Association.

Pyszczynski, T., Greenberg, J., Solomon, S., Arndt, J., & Schimel, J. (2004). Why do people need self-esteem?: A theoretical and empirical review. *Psychological Bulletin, 130*(3), 435–468.

Pyszczynski, T., Abdollahi, A., Solomon, S., Greenberg, J., Cohen, F., & Weise, D. (2006). Mortality salience, martyrdom, and military might: The Great Satan versus the axis of evil. *Personality and Social Psychology Bulletin, 32*(4), 525–537.

Pyszczynski, T., Rothschild, Z., & Abdollahi, A. (2008). Terrorism, violence, and hope for peace: A terror management perspective. *Current Directions in Psychological Science, 17*(5), 318–322.

Pyszczynski, T., & Kesebir, P. (2011). Anxiety buffer disruption theory: A terror management account of posttraumatic stress disorder. *Anxiety, Stress and Coping: An International Journal, 24*(1), 3–26.

Pyszczynski, T., Lockett, M., Greenberg, J., & Solomon, S. (2021). Terror management theory and the COVID-19 pandemic. *Journal of Humanistic Psychology, 61*(2), 173–189.

Pyszczynski, T., Solomon, S., & Greenberg, J. (2015). Thirty years of terror management theory: From genesis to revelation. In J. M. Olson & M. P. Zanna (Eds.), *Advances in experimental social psychology* (Vol. 52, pp. 1–70). Academic Press.

Qi, J. (2023). The terror management function of descendent continuity: Evidence that descendent continuity acts as a distal and proximal defense. *Personality and Social Psychology Bulletin, 49,*125–137.

Roberts, T. A., & Goldenberg, J. L. (2024, January 11). Barbie's existential crisis and the fight for reproductive justice. *Ms. Magazine.* https://msmagazine.com/2024/01/11/death-barbie-abortion-supreme-court/.

Rosenblatt, A., Greenberg, J., Solomon, S., Pyszczynski, T., & Lyon, D. (1989). Evidence for terror management theory 1: The effects of mortality salience on reactions to those who violate or uphold cultural values. *Journal of Personality and Social Psychology, 57*(4), 681–690.

Routledge, C., Arndt, J., & Goldenberg, J. L. (2004). A time to tan: Proximal and distal effects of mortality salience on sun exposure intentions. *Personality and Social Psychology Bulletin, 30*(10), 1347–1358.

Routledge, C., & Vess, M. (Eds.). (2019). *Handbook of terror management theory.* Elsevier Academic Press.

Rowe, J. K. (2023). *Radical mindfulness: Why transforming fear of death is politically vital.* Routledge.

Rutjens, B. T., van der Pligt, J., & van Harreveld, F. (2009). Things will get better: The anxiety-buffering qualities of progressive hope. *Personality and Social Psychology Bulletin, 35*(5), 535–543.

Sætrevik, B., & Sjåstad, H. (2022). Failure to replicate terror management theory: Evidence from a multi-lab study. *Collabra: Psychology, 8*(1), 35271.

Schimel, J., Hayes, J., Williams, T., & Jahrig, J. (2007). Is death really the worm at the core?: Converging evidence that worldview threat increases death-thought accessibility. *Journal of Personality and Social Psych*ology, *92*(5), 789–803.

Schindler, M., Treger, S., & Benau, E. M. (2023).

Not so terrifying after all?: A set of failed replications of the mortality salience effects of terror management theory. *PLOS One, 18*(5), e0285267.

Shen, P. (Director). (2003). *Flight from death: The quest for immortality* [Film]. Koch Entertainment.

Simon, L., Arndt, J., Greenberg, J., Pyszczynski, T., & Solomon, S. (1998). Terror management and meaning: Evidence that the opportunity to defend the worldview in response to mortality salience increases the meaningfulness of life in the mildly depressed. *Journal of Personality, 66*(3), 359–382.

Simon, L., Greenberg, J., Harmon-Jones, E., Solomon, S., & Pyszczynski, T. (1996). Mild depression, mortality salience, and defense of the worldview: Evidence of intensified terror management in the mildly depressed. *Personality and Social Psychology Bulletin, 22*(1), 81–90.

Simon, L., Greenberg, J., Harmon-Jones, E., Solomon, S., Pyszczynski, T., Arndt, J., & Abend, T. (1997). Terror management and cognitive-experiential self-theory: Evidence that terror management occurs in the experiential system. *Journal of Personality and Social Psychology, 72*(5), 1132–1146.

Smith, L. K. M., Ross, H. C., Shouldice, S. A., & Wolfe, S. E. (2022). Mortality management and climate action: A review and reference for using terror management theory methods in interdisciplinary environmental research. *WIREs Climate Change, 13(4).*

Solomon, S., Greenberg, J., & Pyszczynski, T. (1991). A terror management theory of social behavior: The psychological functions of self-esteem and cultural worldviews. In M. P. Zanna (Ed.), *Advances in experimental social psychology* (pp. 91–159). Academic Press.

Solomon, S., Greenberg, J., & Pyszczynski, T. (2015). *The worm at the core: On the role of life in death.* Random House.

Strachan, E., Schimel, J., Arndt, J., Williams, T., Solomon, S., Pyszczynski, T., & Greenberg, J. (2007). Terror mismanagement: Evidence that mortality salience exacerbates phobic and compulsive behaviors. *Personality and Social Psychology Bulletin, 33*(8), 1137–1151.

Tawfik, A. K. (2011). *Utopia* (C. Rossetti, Trans.). Bloomsbury Qatar Foundation Publishing. (Original work published 2008)

Vail, K., Arndt, J., Vess, M., Routledge, C., & Rutjens, B. T. (2012). When death is good for life: Considering the positive trajectory of terror management. *Personality and Social Psychology Review, 16*(4), 303–329.

Vail, K. E., Courtney, E., & Arndt, J. (2019a). The influence of existential threat and tolerance salience on anti-Islamic attitudes in American politics. *Political Psychology, 40*(6), 1143–1162.

Vail, K. E., Courtney, E., Goncy, E., Cornelius, T., & Edmondson, D. (2019b). Anxiety buffer disruption: Relationship threat, death-anxiety, and coping appraisals among low and high posttraumatic stress symptom samples. *Journal of Social and Clinical Psychology, 38*(6), 501–511.

Vail, K. E., Goncy, E., & Edmondson, D. (2019c). Anxiety buffer disruption: Worldview threat, death thought accessibility, and worldview defense among low and high posttraumatic stress symptom samples. *Psychological Trauma: Theory, Research, Practice, and Policy, 11*(6), 647–655.

Vail, K. E., Morgan, A., & Kahle, L. (2018). Self-affirmation attenuates death-thought accessibility after mortality salience, but not among a high-posttraumatic stress sample. *Psychological Trauma: Theory, Research, Practice, and Policy, 10*(1), 112–120.

Vail, K. E., Reed, D., Goncy, E., Cornelius, T., & Edmondson, D. (2020). Anxiety buffer disruption: Self-evaluation, death anxiety, and stressor appraisals among low and high posttraumatic stress symptom samples. *Journal of Social and Clinical Psychology, 39*(4), 353–382.

Weise, D., Arciszewski, T., Verlhiac, J., Pyszczynski, T., & Greenberg, J. (2012). Terror management and attitudes toward immigrants: Differential effects of mortality salience for low and high right-wing authoritarians. *European Psychologist, 17*(1), 63–72.

Yalom, I. D. (1980). *Existential psychotherapy.* Basic Books.

CHAPTER 7

The Nature Problem

Wilderness, Animals, and the Human Body

Uri Lifshin, Sarah E. Wolfe, Lauren K. M. Smith, Stylianos Syropoulos, Immo Fritsche, *and* Fabian M. Hess

What is a human being? What is an animal, a plant, or the planet? Beliefs about our relationships with other animals and nature relate to historical, evolutionary, biological, religious, scientific, economic, geographic, and psychological factors (e.g., Herzog, 2010; Lifshin, 2023; Rowan et al., 2021). They affect crucial aspects of our lives, relationships, and decisions about how we exist within nature (Dhont et al., 2019; Fritsche & Hoppe, 2019; Wolfe & Tubi, 2019). From an existential psychological perspective, nature is two faced. It is the source of all life, goodness, plenty, awe, meaning, and inspiration; but it also poses a problem for humans: It reminds us of what small, mortal, uncertain, vulnerable, and potentially insignificant creatures we are. This "nature problem" can increase our need for psychological security and defensive responses and influence our attitudes and behaviors toward nature, ourselves, and each other (Becker, 1975; Dhont et al., 2019; Fritsche & Hoppe, 2019; Smith et al., 2022). In this chapter, we review existential theory and research, particularly in the framework of terror management theory (TMT; Greenberg et al., 1986; Goldenberg et al., 2000; Solomon et al., Chapter 6, this volume), pertaining to human ambivalence toward the body, nonhuman animals, and nature more broadly. In each section, we briefly highlight directions for future research.

THE BODY PROBLEM

> Mortality is connected to the natural animal side of his existence; and so man reaches beyond and away from that side. So much so that he tries to deny it completely.
>
> —Becker (1975, p. 92)

Building on the interdisciplinary thinkers such as Kierkegaard, Freud, Rank, Kafka, Tillich, Brown, Reich, Lifton, and others, Ernest Becker (1971, 1973, 1975) illuminated the fundamental human need to "deny death." Becker noted that "we are gods with anuses" (1973, p. 51); as Gods we have the capacity to govern life on this planet, but as all other defecating animals, we end up as food for worms and plants. His insights on existential absurdity illustrate how corporal self-awareness contains a problem—a potential for overwhelming anxiety. To prevent this anxiety from manifesting, we humans create death-transcending cultures that provide us with worldviews and symbolic identities. Our cultural beliefs allow us to think of ourselves as more than merely biological mortal creatures—as valuable persons in a meaningful world who may somehow overcome our bodies' limitations. Cultural worldviews provide beliefs in immortal souls (Greenberg et al., 2020) and symbolic routes for death transcendence through national identification, art, science, professional achievements, consumption, and in the memories of future generations (Florian & Mikulincer, 1998; Greenberg et al., 1986; Lifton, 1979; Sani et al., 2009). The more people live up to the cultural standards of value and maintain self-esteem, the more they may enjoy a protective sense of immortality (Florian & Mikulincer, 1998; Greenberg et al., 1992; Lifshin et al., 2021).

Human solutions to the problem of death are not without a cost. Becker pointed out that "the irony of man's condition is that the deepest need is to be free of the anxiety of death and annihilation; but it is life itself which awakens it, and so we must shrink from being fully alive" (1973, p. 66). The realization that we *are* essentially mortal animals, juxtaposed with the basic motivation to avoid death anxiety, requires us to repress our own time-limited-y bodies. In *Life against Death*, Brown wrote that "The incapacity to die, ironically but invisibly, throws mankind out of the actuality of living. . . . the result is the denial of life (repression)" (1959, p. 284). Both Becker and Brown argued that this need to repress life—to deny death—is the core of human neurosis. This neo-Freudian-psychodynamic perspective suggests that sexual urges and desires ("id") must be regulated and controlled by cultural norms and morals ("superego") to avoid death anxiety. Hence Freud's Oedipus conflict is an effort not merely to overcome sexual attraction to the opposite sex parent, but to repress one's physical, fragile, and mortal reality by becoming a culturalized and socialized person who may enjoy literal/symbolic immortality.

Terror management theory (Goldenberg et al., 1986, 2000b; Solomon et al., Chapter 6, this volume) applied Becker's insights to generate empirical research on the existential psychological motivation to disassociate from the body and from animals; the need to deny our "human creatureliness"—our flesh-and-blood body with animalistic needs and desires. TMT researchers considered broad and foundational questions about the death-anxiety suppressing quality of human distancing from animals; disgust from biological aspects of human and animal bodies; the ambivalent nature of human sexuality; and the role of cultural worldviews in moderating these relationships (for reviews, see Cox et al., 2020; Goldenberg et al., 2019). Below, we delineate the main lines of research in these domains.

Findings

Goldenberg and colleagues (1999) theorized that sex poses a psychological threat due to its potential to expose our core animal (mortal) nature. They hypothesized that stripped from the veil of cultural sublimation, *physical* sex would be associated with creatureliness and death, and that mortality salience (MS) would render it as less appealing or even existentially threatening, especially among neurotic (anxious/emotionally unstable) individuals. Congruently, MS (vs. control condition) caused high-neuroticism participants to rate physical (vs. romantic) aspects of sex as less appealing (Study 1). Furthermore, thoughts of physical sex increased death-thought accessibility (DTA) to conscious awareness among high-neuroticism individuals (Studies 2–3), an effect that was mitigated by associating sex with meaningful love (Study 3). Goldenberg and colleagues (2002) went on to demonstrate that thinking about physical (vs. romantic) aspects of sex increased DTA when being reminded of human–animal similarities (vs. differences). They also found that MS led participants to feel less attracted to the physical aspects of sex when they were primed with thoughts of human–animal similarities, but not with human–animal differences.

Goldenberg and colleagues (2001) directly supported the TMT of disassociation from animals by showing that after MS (vs. control condition) participants rated an essay that described humans as unique and distinctly different from animals more preferably than an essay that portrayed humans as similar to other animals. MS also increased disgust about images related to human creatureliness (i.e., human body products) and animals (also see Bassett & Sonntag, 2010).

Relatedly, Tracy and colleagues (2011) found that after MS, participants were more rejective of Darwin's theory of animal origin of humans (vs. a creationist human origin).

Cox and colleagues (2007b) further hypothesized and found that thinking of "disgusting" human body products such as urine, feces, or vomit (vs. speaking in public) and reading a "humans are animals" essay (vs. "humans are unique") increased DTA. Trait-level individual differences in perceived similarity of the self to other animals (PSSA) also predict existential concerns. Lifshin and colleagues (2023) found that individuals who scored high on measures of PSSA also reported higher trait anxiety and DTA than those with low PSSA scores.

Being compared to an animal may be also especially upsetting. Feelings of metadehumanization of one's group or self-dehumanization are associated with increased anxiety, depression, and substance abuse (Fontesse et al., 2021) and can provoke people to reciprocate by aggressing against and counterdehumanizing the insulting outgroup (Kteily et al., 2016). El-Hout and Salomon (2022) demonstrated that immigrants witnessing an animal-based dehumanization (vs. criminalization) of other immigrants had increased threat-related cardiovascular reactivity. Motyl and colleagues (2010, 2013) hypothesized and found that because MS motivates people to disassociate from animals, making aggression seem more animalistic can reduce aggressive behaviors and attitudes as a defense strategy after MS priming.

Perhaps the best evidence for a terror management-based body disassociation comes from Goldenberg and colleagues' (2006) series of behavioral studies. They demonstrated that after MS (vs. aversive controls), participants who scored high on neuroticism spent less time experiencing physical sensations that were either unpleasant (submerging one's arm in icy water, Study 1) or pleasant (placing one's foot in a massager, Studies 2–3). Thus, death awareness can lead people, especially those high in neuroticism, to "flight" from physical sensations.

There is also evidence that death thoughts motivate avoidance from stimuli that increase body-related self-awareness. Arndt and colleagues (1998, Study 1) found that MS reduced the time participants spent in a cubicle containing a large mirror. Findings from existential neuroscience indicate that death-related stimuli caused a reduction of activity in the insular cortex, a brain region that governs bodily self-monitoring/awareness processes (Han et al., 2010; Shi & Han, 2013; for reviews, see Quirin et al., 2019; Quirin & Northoff, Chapter 12, this volume). Klackl and colleagues (2014) discovered that reduced insula activity after death reminders was more pronounced among individuals with high self-esteem. Presumably, individuals with high self-esteem (which are typically also low in neuroticism) were more successful in disassociating from their bodily self.

Yet not all people devalue their bodies when they are reminded of mortality. For some individuals, the body can serve as a self-esteem source when it is perceived to meet one's cultural standards. Goldenberg and colleagues (2000b) found that although MS reduced appearance monitoring for respondents with a more negative body esteem, it increased identification with one's body and made the physical aspects of sex more appealing for respondents with a more positive body esteem. Goldenberg and Shackleford (2005) showed that MS decreased self-reported feelings of body–self integration only for people with low body-esteem.

Existential concerns manifest in attitudes not only toward one's own body but also to judgments of others, especially of women. Menstruation, pregnancy, and breastfeeding—the "trio of terror" (Morris et al., 2014)—are undeniable similarities between (female) humans and other mammals. The social regulations of women's bodies and measuring their appearance against cultural standards may have evolved as a response (Fahs, 2017). Cox and colleagues (2007a) showed that MS provoked more negative reactions toward breastfeeding (but not bottle-feeding) women. Roberts and colleagues (2002) demonstrated that, after MS, men avoided and/or felt more negatively about a woman who dropped a tampon (vs. a hairclip). Morris and Goldenberg (2015) illustrated how following a mortality reminder, heterosexual men preferred images of literally objectified women—women melded with an object—to images of women and object presented together but as distinct entities. Concerningly, MS also led men to be more accepting of violence toward sexualized women (Landau et al., 2006).

There is also evidence that terror management underlines negativity toward transgender individuals. Higher disgust sensitivity and inductions of disgust can increase prejudice against transgender/sexual individuals, especially gay men (Kiss et al., 2020). Studies show that disbelief in human evolution from animals, low-PSSA, and "speciesism" beliefs predict disgust sensitivity (e.g., Lifshin et al., 2023) and negative attitudes and support for discriminatory behaviors against transgender/sexual individuals (Caviola et al., 2019; Syropoulos et al., 2022). Webster and Saucier (2011) found that MS increased negative attitudes toward gay men (but not toward lesbians), and that this effect was mediated by stereotypic gender role beliefs.

Body objectification has double-edged consequences: It provides a source of self-esteem for women who perceive themselves as aligned with cultural beauty standards, while deviance from these standards could make women particularly vulnerable to (self-)devaluation and existential concerns (Goldenberg et al., 2019). This premise was tested in experiments showing, for example, that for American female participants, MS increased liking of unhealthy tanning when paired with an advertisement showing an attractive tan woman (Routledge et al., 2004). Morris and colleagues (2014) showed that MS led women (but not men) to literally self-objectify in conditions where women's reproductive features were salient. Beyond self-objectification, MS increased female participants' restraint with breast self-examinations when primed with human–animal similarities, but not with human–animal differences (e.g., Goldenberg et al., 2008).

Future Directions

Research indicates that thinking of ourselves as animals relates to existential concerns (e.g., Cox et al., 2007b; Goldenberg et al., 1999; Lifshin et al., 2023). It may therefore be of value to examine if PSSA—as a contextual factor or an individual difference variable—might contribute to anxiety or other somatoform related disorders. According to anxiety-buffer disruption theory (e.g., Yetzer & Pyszczynski, 2019), psychological disorders might result from a disruption in death-anxiety-buffering mechanisms (e.g., cultural worldviews, self-esteem, close relationships). Thus, creatureliness-denial motivation (e.g., PSSA) may also relate to various health-related attitudes and behaviors (e.g., Arndt & Goldenberg, 2017).

Finally, future research may test ways by which people may reduce their distancing from the body as a response to MS. For example, findings show that practicing mindfulness meditation allows people to withstand high DTA without suppression and defensive responses (Niemiec et al., 2010; Park & Pyszczynski, 2019). This may also help moderate the negative effects of terror management needs on attitudes toward nature (Kashdan et al., 2011; Koller, 2021). However, there is also contradictory evidence suggesting that prolonged exposure to death might lead to deficiencies in psychological well-being (Mösler et al., 2022; Yetzer & Pyszczynski, 2019) or to chronic high levels of defensiveness (Fernandez et al., 2010).

ATTITUDES TOWARD ANIMALS

Are we better than Lizards or Potatoes?

There are many reasons for the psychological distance between humans and animals (e.g., Dhont et al., 2019; Lifshin, 2023; Rowan et al., 2021). Evolutionary anthropologists suggest that hunting animals for food was probably a key factor in human evolution and our differentiation from other prehistoric primates (e.g., Becker, 1971; Stanford, 1999; Wilkins et al., 2012). Humans have historically used animals for such purposes as food, farming, clothing, travel, scientific advancements, protection, comfort, and entertainment (e.g., Rowan et al., 2021). Animals can also harm humans, leading to genetic predispositions toward fearing and aggressing against certain animals (e.g., Öhman & Mineka, 2001). Animosity toward other animals may also arise from competition for limited resources (e.g., Basak et al., 2023; Becker, 1971). These factors contribute to a general social dominance orientation that motivates and justifies negative attitudes and behaviors toward animals (Dhont et al., 2019; Hoffarth et al., 2019).

From an existential psychology standpoint, terror management needs motivate people to feel different from and superior to other mortal animals (Becker, 1973, 1975; Goldenberg et al., 2000, 2001; Marino & Mountain, 2015). As reviewed above, initial findings by Goldenberg and colleagues (2001) regarding the motivation to disassociate from animals set the foundations for TMT research on attitudes toward animals. Studies then tested the hypothesis that thinking about death might not just make people disassociate from animals but also assert their superiority over them.

Findings

Beatson and Halloran (2007) conducted the first experiment testing how terror management motivation might affect attitudes toward animals. They exposed participants to an MS or a control condition, as well as to a creatureliness prime or control condition, and then measured positive and negative attitudes toward animals. Results showed that the effect of MS was moderated by self-esteem: Low-self-esteem participants reported more negative attitudes toward animals after MS, but those with high self-esteem did not. Presumably, high-self-esteem participants felt protected, and did not need to aggress against animals as a terror management strategy. Beatson and colleagues (2009) found that even pet owners responded to MS and reminders of human creatureliness with less positive attitudes toward pets regardless of self-esteem.

Soenke and colleagues (2018) hypothesized that after MS people would reject evidence for animal superiority over humans, and that undermining human superiority over animals would elevate existential concerns. In Study 1, MS (vs. control) increased negative reactions to an article describing dolphins as smarter than humans, but not to an article that did not compare dolphins to humans. In Study 2, reading that dolphins are smarter than humans increased DTA compared to reading about dolphin intelligence without a comparison to humans.

Lifshin and colleagues (2017) exposed participants to subliminal death primes (the word *dead*) or control primes (the word *pain* or *fail*) and then asked them to report their attitudes toward killing animals in different domains. Across five experiments, death primes increased support for killing animals, compared to the control conditions, beyond preexisting attitudes toward animals and demographic or individual differences variables. But, in line with TMT, the effect was moderated by a self-esteem enhancement manipulation (Study 4). Increased support for killing animals was also associated with feelings of power-based invulnerability (e.g., "I feel powerful," "I can escape dangerous situations"; Lifshin et al., 2017, Study 5).

Fairlamb and colleagues (2023) replicated this effect and demonstrated that it may be moderated by environmental-contingent self-worth (ECSW). From a TMT perspective, people who are highly invested in values related to animal protection should defend these values more vigorously after MS. They conducted a series of online experiments in which they first measured ECSW (unlike Lifshin et al., 2017, that measured preexisting attitudes several weeks before the experiment), then exposed participants to a subtle death prime (the word *death* on a T-shirt or a death-word completion task), and then measured motivation for killing and protecting animals. In contrast to Lifshin and colleagues (2017), although low-ECSW participants supported killing animals more after death primes compared to after control primes, high-ECSW participants supported killing animals less and wanted to protect animals more after the death prime. Fairlamb and colleagues (2023, Study 3) also replicated the indirect effect of death primes on feelings of power-based invulnerability. Here there was a moderated mediation effect: After death primes, for low-ECSW participants, increased support for killing animals predicted more feelings of power-based invulnerability, while for high-ECSW participants, decreased support for killing animals predicted a lower sense of power and invulnerability.

Another factor that relates to TMT and attitudes toward animals is religion. There are major differences between types of religions and beliefs, as some may sanctify animals and treat them with awe and respect, while others objectify them and justify their abuse (e.g., Cox et al., 2020; Gray & Young, 2011; Herzog, 2010; Preston & Baimel, 2021). There are also different variations in beliefs within a given religion, which may emphasize human dominion or nature stewardship (Eckberg & Blocker, 1996; Ng & Eom, 2023; Pasaribu et al., 2022; Shin & Preston, 2021), or on the level of religious fundamentalism (e.g., Cox et al., 2020; DeLeeuw et al., 2007; Eckberg & Blocker, 1996; Preston & Shin, 2022; Vess et al., 2012). Some worldviews may grant animals immortal souls and include them in the spiritual realm (e.g., in Hinduism, humans can be reincarnated into an animals). This may render PSSA as less threatening and reduce or defuse the need to disassociate from animals (Caruana, 2020; Gray & Young, 2011; Herzog, 2010; Lifshin & Greenberg, 2019; Serpell, 2009; Wrenn, 2020). However, in most industrialized countries, animals might be considered as soulless, inferior creatures that may be commodified and without fundamental rights (e.g., Cox et al., 2020; Goldenberg et al., 2000b; Lifshin, 2023). This view is crystalized in Descartes's (1649) classis mechanistic view: "One [argument] is that it is more probable that worms, flies, caterpillars and other animals move like machines than that they have immortal souls" (also see Rowan et al., 2021). If nonhuman animals are thought to be soulless, high PSSA might be especially threatening and increase existential concerns (e.g., Becker, 1973, 1975; Cox et al., 2020; Goldenberg et al., 2001; Lifshin, 2023; Wrenn, 2020).

Lifshin and colleagues (2018, in press-b) suggested that the relationship between religiosity and support for killing animals may be curvilinear, evidencing that students who were either very religious or not religious at all supported killing animals more than moderately religious ones. Importantly, belief in God was associated with less support for killing animals compared to disbelief. From a TMT standpoint, religion and beliefs in God may provide more protection against death anxiety (e.g., Greenberg et al., 2020) than disbelief and atheism and thereby reduce defensive aggression against animals. However, high religiosity (fundamentalism) might lead to more disassociation from and negative attitudes toward animals (e.g., Cox et al., 2020; DeLeeuw et al., 2007; Preston & Baimel, 2021; Preston & Shin, 2022; Rabinovitch & Parzuchowski, 2025), especially after MS (e.g., Vess et al., 2012).

Future Directions

Future studies may test how defensive negativity toward animals may be modified. One approach may be enhancing people's security-providing psychological structures (anxiety buffers). So far, studies have used self-esteem to this end (Beatson & Halloran, 2007; Lifshin et al., 2017, Study 4). One caveat is that in some cases self-esteem may depend upon feeling superior to other animals. Strengthening other anxiety buffers such as attachment security (e.g., Capozza et al., 2022; Mikulincer & Shaver, 2007) or immortality beliefs (e.g., Dechesne et al., 2003; Lifshin et al., 2021; Piotrowski et al., 2020; Sani et al., 2009) may also "do the trick." Researchers may also consider whether attachment to pets, as an individual trait and/or as a security prime, reduces negativity toward animals after MS (e.g., Zilcha-Mano et al., 2012).

Insights on the moderating effects of environmental values and ECSW (e.g., Fairlamb et al., 2023; Vess & Arndt, 2008) and of norm salience (Fritsche et al., 2010) may be further applied to improve the human–animal relationship. For instance, Lifshin and colleagues (2022b) found that even after MS, telling people about a new a pro-animal rights law increased support for animal rights, compared to a control condition that did not mention the new legislation.

Human–animal relations may also be improved by increasing solidarity with animals (Amiot & Bastian, 2017) and PSSA by humanizing animals (rather than "animalizing" humans; e.g., Bastian et al., 2012; Lifshin et al., 2024). However, there is still no evidence that these manipulations are effective in conjunction with existential threat (cf. Beatson & Halloran, 2007; Goldenberg et al., 2001). Perhaps relating animals to cultural immortality or other spiritual beliefs may render them as less threatening and more valued (e.g., Billet et al., 2023; Cox et al., 2020; Lifshin & Greenberg, 2019; Preston & Baimel, 2021; Wrenn, 2020).

Researchers could also examine how existential motivations influence social dominance orientations, political worldviews, or other beliefs and cognitions that justify animal exploitation and resistance to change (Caviola et al., 2019; Dhont et al., 2019;

Hoffarth et al., 2019). Evidence suggests that MS can increase sensitivity to cognitive dissonance (Jonas et al., 2003), and support for authoritative, system-justifying, or discriminating worldviews and ideologies (Bassett, 2010; Cohen et al., 2017). For example, MS may increase cognitive dissonance regarding past pro/anti-environmental behavior in decision-making contexts relating to animals. Factors that moderate MS responses, such as strengthen anxiety buffers, may reduce cognitive dissonance after MS. Other factors may reduce social dominance and speciesism. Pöllänen and colleagues (2022) found that classic psychedelic drug use was associated with reduced speciesism and "ego dissolution," which predicted more desire to help animals. Forstmann and Sagioglou (2017) found that psychedelics predicted higher self-identification with nature and engagement in pro-environmental behaviors (also see Nilsson & Stålhammar, 2024). Further experimental and longitudinal research may verify this possibility.

Finally, researchers should consider that animals are diverse, and that people may have different psychological reactions to different animals (e.g., Herzog, 2010; Patinadan & Dillon, 2022; Sevillano & Fiske, 2023). Existential concerns may also affect attitudes toward plant life, for example, the perception of plant sentience (Segundo-Ortin & Calvo, 2023).

DISASSOCIATION FROM ANIMALS AND CULTURAL WORLDVIEW DEFENSE

> "Away from the animal; away from sexuality!" are the guiding principles of the formation of all human ideology. This is the case whether it is disguised in the fascist form of racially pure "supermen," the communist form of proletarian class honour, the Christian form of man's "spiritual and ethical nature," or the liberal form of "higher human values." All these ideas harp on the same monotonous tune: "We are not animals."
>
> —Reich (1946, p. 339)

How do we convince ourselves that we are different from other animals? According to TMT (Goldenberg et al., 2000b), people mask their animality through culture and symbolic identities. Our cultures provide us with ways of separating ourselves from nature by creating sophisticated beliefs systems, languages, values, norms, costumes, institutions, and engaging in art and science. We clothe our bodies, adorn ourselves with precious jewelry, anoint ourselves with fragrance, and do it all via "unnatural" technologies that distinguish us from other animals.

Findings

Lifshin and colleagues (2022a) demonstrated that affirmations of cultural worldviews can reduce PSSA among people who attach high importance to their cultural identity and right-wingers. This effect was stronger after MS (Study 4), supporting its terror management function. However, findings were only replicated in some countries and important variations exist. In fact, opposite effects were observed in countries that worship animals, such as India and Nepal.

Lifshin and colleagues (in press-a) hypothesized that if cultural worldviews help reduce PSSA, then low-PSSA individuals should exhibit more (cultural/national) ingroup biases and outgroup negativity, especially after existential threat (e.g., Greenberg et al., 1990). In contrast, high-PSSA individuals may perceive similarity across humanity and a shared ingroup identity with outgroup members (Bastian et al., 2012; Costello & Hodson, 2010). Supporting these hypotheses, low-PSSA was associated with higher ingroup identification and glorification, political right-wing views, prejudice, outgroup negativity, and support for militarism (Studies 1a–1d). After death primes, low-PSSA individuals exhibited more cultural worldview defense and negative attitudes toward members of other cultures (Studies 2–5). Conversely, MS increased high-PSSA individuals' positive attitudes toward outgroups (Studies 4–5).

Syropoulos and colleagues (2022) generalized the link between PSSA and outgroup negativity in large, nationally representative samples. They hypothesized and found that disbelief in human evolution (an indication of low-PSSA) predicted prejudice, racism, support for discriminatory behaviors against minorities, and militaristic attitudes toward outgroups in the United States (Studies 1 and 5); and higher ingroup biases, outgroup prejudice, and lower support for conflict resolution in 45 different countries (Studies 2–4). Mediational analyses indicated that PSSA partially accounted for the link between belief in evolution and prejudice (Studies 7–8), beyond religiosity, political views, and demographics (also see Caviola et al., 2019).

Researchers have also examined high-PSSA individuals' terror management strategies. Lifshin and colleagues (2023) theorized that if high-PSSA individuals are less invested in ingroup identities and nationalistic worldviews, they may be more inclined to pursue personal creativity as a terror management strategy, but also more vulnerable to existential concerns. They found that PSSA correlated with investment in creativity, especially after death primes (Studies 3–4), and that high-PSSA individuals had heightened trait-anxiety and DTA (Studies 5–6), and increased state-anxiety following negative feedback about their creativity (Study 6).

Future Directions

Research is needed to better understand how to change PSSA, and how this may affect terror management. Bastian and colleagues (2012) demonstrated humanizing animals may have such effects but did not test it in conjunction with existential threat. Lifshin and colleagues (2024) found that brief text and video manipulations to humanize animals heightened cross-cultural similarity and lowered ingroup identification and glorification, thereby indirectly affecting attitudes toward war and peacemaking in the context of the Israeli–Palestinian and American–Iranian conflict. However, these effects were small, and the manipulations did not consistently change PSSA.

Future research could also test if on a broader level, cultures, nations, religions, and organizations differ in PSSA, and if it can account for variations in support for, and engagement in, intercultural violence or discriminatory policies and laws. Understanding this dynamic may advance endeavors to improve both human–animal and human-to-human intergroup relations (e.g., Gradidge et al., 2023; Lifshin et al., in press-a; Syropoulos et al., 2022).

HUMANS, WILDERNESS, AND THE CHANGING ENVIRONMENT

Humans' relationship with nature is characterized by deep ambivalence. In myths and fairy tales, nature as the place beyond rational civilization has been both magically appealing and horrifying. For thousands of years, humanity sought to control, cultivate, and dominate nature. We build large dams and irrigation systems to control water and use fire to increase soil fertility or reduce wildfires. We also dominate nature through culturally sanctioned aesthetics across scales: urban planners, landscape architects, and household gardeners all aspire to create and maintain "natural spaces" according to predetermined cultural standards, thereby bringing the wilderness predictably and visually under human control (Vitousek et al., 1997).

As a species, we've largely rejected the unknown and "untamed" wilderness lands that surround us. The wilderness just outside of civilizations' borders triggers peoples' fascination, discomfort, and terror (Fritsche & Hoppe, 2019; Koole & van den Berg, 2005). *Everyone* experiences some aspect of "wilderness" as a threat—whether that aspect is the unpredictability of a storm, a raging river, or a looming grizzly bear (van den Berg & ter Heijne, 2005). Wilderness confronts people with the invalidation of human morals, existential threat, and the realization of unpredictability and uncontrollability (Fritsche & Hoppe, 2019).

Meanwhile, our relationship with nature has become increasingly important as humanity faces significant climate and environmental threats. These threats pose major challenges for decisions about resource use policies and adaptation or mitigation programming (Wolfe & Tubi, 2019). Studies indicate that fears related to the natural environment could be crucial drivers of peoples' environmental and social responses (e.g., Fritsche et al., 2018). Fear is most widely employed in the public domain of environmental changes—but often with mixed results (O'Neill & Nicholson-Cole, 2009; Uhl et al., 2018). Researchers have suggested that climate-change skepticism is a psychological coping response to the fears generated by worrisome climate information (Feinberg

& Willer 2011; Haltinner & Sarathchandra, 2018; Lifshin et al., 2016). TMT scholars tested the role of existential concerns in environmental attitudes, and how these may affect other defensive compensatory responses (for reviews, see Fritsche & Hoppe, 2019; Lifshin & Greenberg, 2019; Smith et al., 2022; Wolfe & Tubi, 2019).

Findings

Koole and van den Berg (2005) conducted seminal studies on the existential psychology of wilderness. They demonstrated that although wilderness is generally perceived as more beautiful than cultivated nature, wilderness primes were associated with increased conscious thoughts about death (Study 1) and preconscious DTA (Study 4). They also showed that MS reduced aesthetic preference of wilderness over cultivated landscapes (Studies 2 and 5). Other studies extended this point by showing that death primes can increase willingness to excessively deplete natural resources from the forest in a simulated game (Kasser & Sheldon, 2000) and decrease concern about climate change (Dickinson, 2009; Valmori et al., 2024), ecological sustainability (e.g., Hu et al., 2018), or possible nuclear catastrophes (Selimbegović et al., 2016).

The effects of existential concerns on attitudes toward nature can depend on preexisting pro-environmental cultural values and self-esteem. Studies show that low-ECSW individuals reported more negative attitudes toward the natural environment after MS compared to after control primes, while for high-ECSW individuals, MS increased positive attitudes toward the environment (Valmori et al., 2024; Selimbegović et al., 2016; Vess & Arndt, 2008). Fritsche and Häfner (2012) showed that MS decreased people's motivation to protect the environment for its own sake ("biocentric"), but not their egoistic ("anthropocentric") pro-environmental motivation. Again, ECSW moderated this effect, highlighting the TMT dynamic.

Importantly, the moderating effects of preexisting attitudes on defensive responses after MS may depend on the cognitive salience of descriptive and injunctive cultural norms. Fritsche and colleagues (2010) demonstrated that when cultural pro-environmental norms—but not irrelevant norms—are in focal attention, death primes can increase pro-environmental attitudes and behaviors. Harrison and Mallett (2013) showed that MS increased collective ecoguilt when pro-environmental values were made salient.

Researchers also examined climate and extreme weather events as mortality reminders (for review, see Smith et al., 2022). Smith and Wolfe (2023) tested whether water crises serve as a potential mortality reminder, among Canadian and American online participants. In that study, drowning and drinking contaminated water crisis reminders—but not dehydration—increased DTA similarly to MS vs. a control.

Other studies examined how nature may elicit a sense of awe, which may also facilitate compensatory responses congruent with TMT (for review, see Jiang et al., 2024). Nature-related awe can result in diminished sense of self ("small self") and increased prosocial behaviors (e.g., Piff et al., 2015); decreased tolerance for uncertainty and increased supernatural belief and perception of intentionality (Valdesolo & Graham, 2014); and motivation for self-transcendence and authentic self-pursuit (Jiang & Sedikides, 2022). Hornsey and colleagues (2018) demonstrated the perceived psychological threat of awe primes—being reminded of the vastness of the universe—can be moderated by self-esteem.

Drawing attention to global climate catastrophes can increase people's sense of shared threat and reduce intergroup conflicts, especially among individuals with a strong sense of shared identity (Pyszczynski et al., 2012). But environmental threats can also increase defensive social responses aimed at restoring a subjective sense of control through the ingroup (Barth et al., 2021; Fritsche, 2022). Fritsche and colleagues (2012) demonstrated how salient climate change threat elevated German and U.K. participants' authoritarian attitudes and derogation of specific threatening groups in society (e.g., violent offenders). Barth and colleagues (2018) extended these findings, showing that salient climate change threat increased students' conformity with an apparent student majority norm of radical (vs. nonradical) left-wing action (i.e., attacking a sexist professor).

Smith and Wolfe (2025) found that water crisis reminders influenced environmental identity polarization similarly to mortality reminders (compared to control conditions). People's increased "groupiness" in response to threatening climate change also results in derogation of cultural minority groups, such as the Muslim and Pakistani communities in the United Kingdom (Shanaah et al., 2024). Interestingly, this effect was only observed among participants who considered the United Kingdom's collective capability to control climate change to be low. Thus, environmental threat may trigger intergroup hostility when ingroup agency cannot be expressed in terms of a project of collective agency, such as fighting climate change threats.

Existential concerns may also be channeled to promote climate sustainability-related actions. A large body of research suggests that an increased sense of personal legacy and of generativity relate to pro-environmental attitudes and behaviors and to concern about climate change (e.g., Lifshin et al., 2016; Syropoulos et al., 2023, 2024; Vlasceanu et al., 2024; Zaval et al., 2015). Researchers have also examined how religious messages related to nature stewardship may increase pro-environmentalism (Preston & Baimel, 2021; Shin & Preston, 2021). Finally, people's current health may also be used to promote pro-environmentalism. Cote and Wolfe (2017) observed that Canadian pro-bottled water ad campaigns leaned heavily on water's life-giving properties and incorporated health, safety, and aesthetics themes to bolster their audience's self-esteem—positioning *their* water as a product to help avoid death.

Future Directions

Research opportunities related to humans' relationships with nature are abundant. Many of the ways to improve attitudes toward animals mentioned in the previous sections (e.g., strengthening anxiety buffers; relating nature to norms, values, and beliefs; using psychedelic drugs) may apply to increasing environmental concerns and positive attitudes toward nature more broadly. Furthermore, research by Chen and colleagues (2024) suggests that attachment to one's environment ("place attachment") may afford a sense of psychological security that can mitigate death-related concerns. Future studies may examine how nature-related place attachment may moderate the effects of existential threats on environmental attitudes and behaviors.

In the context of climate change, Wolfe and Tubi (2019) highlighted four categories specific to adaptation and mitigation research: climate change communications, collective action, transformational responses, and related "hero projects." These inquires may help practitioners and policymakers avoid inducing defenses that could hamper mitigation and adaptation, and could instigate population-level action. Smith and colleagues (2022) proposed that TMT research could identify and evaluate the real and imagined nature scenarios that act as existential threats and trigger defensive responses (e.g., Fritsche et al., 2012; Smith & Wolfe, 2023). Fritsche (2024) highlighted ways in which threats may create a "momentum" for collective pro-ecological transformations.

Future research could also explore how disgust and creatureliness reminders prompt unconscious existential concerns and influence responses to environmental problems and solutions. One example may be being unwilling to adopt necessary sewage-water recycling practices (Rozin et al., 2015; Shouldice & Wolfe, 2024; Wester et al., 2016). This research may then extend to test how disgust can influence behaviors touching on all aspects of daily life—from support for climate policies, participation in car sharing (Hazée et al., 2019), to engaging in environmental education (Bixler & Floyd, 1999).

REFERENCES

Amiot, C. E., & Bastian, B. (2017). Solidarity with animals: Assessing a relevant dimension of social identification with animals. *PLOS One, 12,* e0168184.

Arndt, J., & Goldenberg, J. L. (2017). Where health and death intersect: Insights from a terror management health model. *Current Directions in Psychological Science, 26,* 126–131.

Arndt, J., Greenberg, J., Simon, L., Pyszczynski, T., & Solomon, S. (1998). Terror management and self-awareness: Evidence that mortality salience provokes avoidance of the self-focused state. *Personality and Social Psychology Bulletin, 24,* 1216–1227.

Barth, M., Masson, T., Fritsche, I., Fielding, K., & Smith, J. R. (2021). Collective responses to global challenges: The social psychology of pro-environmental action. *Journal of Environmental Psychology, 74,* 101562.

Barth, M., Masson, T., Fritsche, I., & Ziemer, C. T. (2018). Closing ranks: Ingroup norm conformity as a subtle response to threatening climate change. *Group Processes and Intergroup Relations, 21,* 497–512.

Basak, S. M., Rostovskaya, E., Birks, J., & Wierzbowska, I. A. (2023). Perceptions and attitudes to understand human-wildlife conflict in an urban landscape: A systematic review. *Ecological Indicators, 151,* 110319.

Bassett, J. F. (2010). The effects of mortality salience and social dominance orientation on attitudes toward illegal immigrants. *Social Psychology, 41.*

Bassett, J. F., & Sonntag, M. E. (2010). The effects of mortality salience on disgust sensitivity among university students, older adults, and mortuary students. *Open Psychology Journal, 3,* 1–8.

Bastian, B., Costello, K., Loughnan, S., & Hodson, G. (2012). When closing the human-animal divide expands moral concern: The importance of framing. *Social Psychological and Personality Science, 3,* 421–429.

Beatson, R. M., & Halloran, M. J. (2007). Humans rule!: The effects of creatureliness reminders, mortality salience and self-esteem on attitudes towards animals. *British Journal of Social Psychology, 46,* 619–632.

Beatson R. M., Loughnan S., Halloran M. J. (2009). Attitudes toward animals: The effect of priming thoughts of human-animal similarities and mortality salience on the evaluation of companion animals. *Society and Animals, 17,* 72–89.

Becker, E. (1971). *The birth and death of meaning* (2nd ed.). Free Press.

Becker, E. (1973). *The denial of death.* Free Press.

Becker, E. (1975). *Escape from evil.* Free Press.

Billet, M. I., Baimel, A., Sahakari, S. S., Schaller, M., & Norenzayan, A. (2023). Ecospirituality: The psychology of moral concern for nature. *Journal of Environmental Psychology, 87,* 102001.

Bixler, R. D., & Floyd, M. F. (1999). Hands on or hands off?: Disgust sensitivity and preference for environmental education activities. *Journal of Environmental Education, 30,* 4–11.

Brown, N. O. (1959). *Life against death: The psychoanalytic meaning of history.* Wesleyan University Press.

Capozza, D., Falvo, R., & Di Bernardo, G. A. (2022). Priming attachment security and outgroup humanization: The mediation role of intergroup emotions. *PLOS One, 17,* e0265714.

Caruana, L. S. J. (2020). Different religions, different animal ethics? *Animal Frontiers, 10,* 8–14.

Caviola, L., Everett, J. A. C., & Faber, N. S. (2019). The moral standing of animals: Towards a psychology of speciesism. *Journal of Personality and Social Psychology, 116,* 1011–1029.

Chen, R., Chen, Y., & Jiang, Z. (2024). Why humans form place attachment: A terror management perspective. *Journal of Environmental Psychology, 100,* 102489.

Cohen, F., Solomon, S., & Kaplin, D. (2017). You're hired!: Mortality salience increases Americans' support for Donald Trump. *Analyses of Social Issues and Public Policy, 17,* 339–357.

Costello, K., & Hodson, G. (2010). Exploring the roots of dehumanization: The role of animal–human similarity in promoting immigrant humanization. *Group Processes and Intergroup Relations, 13,* 3–22.

Cote, S. A. & Wolfe, S. E. (2017). Evidence of mortality salience and psychological defenses in bottled water campaigns. *Applied Environmental Education and Communication.*

Cox, C. R., Arrowood, R. B., & Swets, J. A. (2020). Of flesh and blood: Death, creatureliness, and incarnational ambivalence toward the Divine. In K. E. Vail III & C. Routledge (Eds.), *The science of religion, spirituality, and existentialism* (pp. 387–403). Academic Press.

Cox, C. R., Goldenberg, J. L., Arndt, J., & Pyszczynski, T. (2007a). Mother's milk: An existential perspective on negative reactions to breast-feeding. *Personality and Social Psychology Bulletin, 33,* 110–122.

Cox, C. R., Goldenberg, J. L., Pyszczynski, T., & Weise, D. (2007b). Disgust, creatureliness and the accessibility of death-related thoughts. *European Journal of Social Psychology, 37,* 494–507.

Dechesne, M., Pyszczynski, T., Arndt, J., Ransom, S., Sheldon, K. M., van Knippenberg, A., & Janssen, J. (2003). Literal and symbolic immortality: The effect of evidence of literal immortality on self-esteem striving in response to mortality salience. *Journal of Personality and Social Psychology, 84,* 722–737

DeLeeuw, J. L., Galen, L. W., Aebersold, C., & Stanton, V. (2007). Support for animal rights as a function of belief in evolution, religious fundamentalism, and religious denomination. *Society and Animals, 15,* 353–363.

Dhont, K., Hodson, G., Loughnan, S., & Amiot, C. E. (2019). Rethinking human–animal relations: The critical role of social psychology. *Group Processes and Intergroup Relations, 22,* 769–784.

Dickinson, J. L. (2009). The people paradox: Self-esteem striving, immortality ideologies, and human response to climate change. *Ecology and Society, 14,* 34.

Eckberg, D. L., & Blocker, T. J. (1996). Christianity, environmentalism, and the theoretical problem of fundamentalism. *Journal for the Scientific Study of Religion, 35,* 343–355.

El-Hout, M., & Salomon, K. (2022). Villains or vermin?: The differential effects of criminal and animal rhetoric on immigrant cardiovascular responses. *Group Processes and Intergroup Relations, 25,* 1939–1957.

Fahs, B. (2017). Mapping "gross" bodies: The regulatory politics of disgust. *Aesthetic Labour,* 83–99.

Fairlamb, S., Stan, A. E., & Lovas, K. (2023). To protect or to kill?: Environmental contingent self-worth moderates death prime effects on animal-based Attitudes. *Personality and Social Psychology Bulletin.*

Feinberg, M., & Willer, R. (2011). Apocalypse soon?: Dire messages reduce belief in global warming by contradicting just-world beliefs. *Psychological Science, 22,* 34–38.

Fernandez, S., Castano, E., & Singh, I. (2010). Managing death in the burning grounds of Varanasi, India: A terror management investigation. *Journal of Cross-Cultural Psychology, 41,* 182–194.

Florian, V., & Mikulincer, M. (1998). Symbolic immortality and the management of the terror of death: The moderating role of attachment style. *Journal of Personality and Social Psychology, 74,* 725–734.

Fontesse, S., Demoulin, S., Stinglhamber, F., de Timary, P., & Maurage, P. (2021). Metadehumanization and self-dehumanization are linked to reduced drinking refusal self-efficacy and increased anxiety and depression symptoms in patients with severe alcohol use disorder. *Psychologica Belgica, 61,* 238–247.

Forstmann, M., & Sagioglou, C. (2017). Lifetime experience with (classic) psychedelics predicts pro-environmental behavior through an increase in nature relatedness. *Journal of Psychopharmacology, 31,* 975–988.

Fritsche, I. (2022). Agency through the we: Group-based control theory. *Current Directions in Psychological Science, 31,* 194–201.

Fritsche, I. (2024). It's getting dark, but we will see: Gaining collective momentum in face of existential environmental threat. *Global Environmental Psychology, 2,* Article e12979.

Fritsche, I., Barth, M., Jugert, P., Masson, T., & Reese, G. (2018). A social identity model of pro-environmental action (SIMPEA). *Psychological Review, 125,* 245–269.

Fritsche, I., Cohrs, J. C., Kessler, T., & Bauer, J. (2012). Global warming is breeding social conflict: The subtle impact of climate change threat on authoritarian tendencies. *Journal of Environmental Psychology, 32,* 1–10.

Fritsche, I., & Häfner, K. (2012). The malicious effects of existential threat on motivation to protect the natural environment and the role of environmental identity as a moderator. *Environment and Behavior, 44,* 570–590.

Fritsche, I., & Hoppe, A. (2019). We supernaturals: Terror management and people's ambivalent relationship with nature. In C. Routledge & M. Vess (Eds.), *Handbook of terror management theory* (pp. 157–178). Elsevier Academic Press.

Fritsche, I., Jonas, E., Kayser, D. N., & Koranyi, N. (2010). Existential threat and compliance with pro-environmental norms. *Journal of Environmental Psychology, 30,* 67–79.

Goldenberg, J. L., Arndt, J., Hart, J., & Routledge, C. (2008). Uncovering an existential barrier to breast self-exam behavior. *Journal of Experimental Social Psychology, 44,* 260–274.

Goldenberg, J. L., Cox, C. R., Pyszczynski, T., Greenberg, J., & Solomon, S. (2002). Understanding human ambivalence about sex: The effects of stripping sex of meaning. *The Journal of Sex Research, 39,* 310–320.

Goldenberg, J. L., Hart, J., Pyszczynski, T., Warnica, G. M., Landau, M., & Thomas, L. (2006). Ambivalence toward the body: Death, neuroticism, and the flight from physical sensation. *Personality and Social Psychology Bulletin, 32,* 1264–1277.

Goldenberg, J. L., McCoy, S. K., Pyszczynski, T., Greenberg, J., & Solomon, S. (2000a). The body as a source of self-esteem: The effect of mortality salience on identification with one's body, interest in sex, and appearance monitoring. *Journal of Personality and Social Psychology, 79,* 118–130.

Goldenberg, J. L., Morris, K. L., & Boyd, P. (2019). Terror management is for the birds and the bees: An existential perspective on the threat associated with human corporeality. In C. Routledge & M. Vess (Eds.), *Handbook of terror management theory* (pp. 227–242). Elsevier Academic Press.

Goldenberg, J. L., Pyszczynski, T., Greenberg, J., & Solomon, S. (2000b). Fleeing the body: A terror management perspective on the problem of human corporeality. *Psychology and Social Psychology Review, 4,* 200–218.

Goldenberg, J. L., Pyszczynski, T., Greenberg, J., Solomon, S., Kluck, B., & Cornwell, R. (2001). I am not an animal: Mortality salience, disgust, and the denial of human creatureliness. *Journal of Experimental Psychology: General, 130,* 427–435.

Goldenberg, J. L., Pyszczynski, T., McCoy, S. K., Greenberg, J., & Solomon, S. (1999). Death, sex, love, and neuroticism: Why is sex such a problem? *Journal of Personality and Social Psychology, 77,* 1173–1187.

Goldenberg, J. L., & Shackelford, T. I. (2005). Is it me or is it mine?: Body-self integration as a function of self-esteem, body-esteem, and mortality salience. *Self and Identity, 4,* 227–241.

Gradidge, S., Alcañiz-Colomer, J., & Loughnan, S. (2023). Inhuman animals: Moving dehumanization into the domain of human-animal relations. *Current Opinion in Behavioral Sciences, 50,* 101249.

Gray, P. B., & Young, S. M. (2011). Human–pet dynamics in cross-cultural perspective. *Anthrozoös, 24,* 17–30.

Greenberg, J., Helm, P. J., Landau, M. J., & Solomon, S. (2020). Dwelling forever in the house of the lord: On the terror management function of religion. In K. E. Vail III & C. Routledge (Eds.), *The science of religion, spirituality, and existentialism* (pp. 3–20). Academic Press.

Greenberg, J., Pyszczynski, T., & Solomon, S. (1986). The causes and consequences of a need for self-esteem: A terror management theory. In R. F. Baumeister (Ed.), *Public self and private self* (pp. 189–212). Springer.

Greenberg, J., Pyszczynski, T., Solomon, S., Rosenblatt, A., Veeder, M., Kirkland, S., & Lyon, D. (1990). Evidence for terror management theory II: The effects of mortality salience on reactions to those who threaten or bolster the cultural worldview. *Journal of Personality and Social Psychology, 58,* 308–318.

Greenberg, J., Solomon, S., Pyszczynski, T., Rosenblatt, A., Burling, J., Lyon, D., . . . Pinel, E. (1992). Why do people need self-esteem?: Converging evidence that self-esteem serves an anxiety-buffering function. *Journal of Personality and Social Psychology, 63,* 913–922.

Haltinner, K., & Sarathchandra, D. (2018). Climate change skepticism as a psychological coping strategy. *Sociology Compass, 12,* e12586.

Han, S., Qin, J., & Ma, Y. (2010). Neurocognitive processes of linguistic cues related to death. *Neuropsychologia, 48,* 3436–3442.

Harrison, P. R., & Mallett, R. K. (2013). Mortality salience motivates the defense of environmental values and increases collective ecoguilt. *Ecopsychology, 5,* 36–43.

Hazée, S., Van Vaerenbergh, Y., Delcourt, C., & Warlop, L. (2019). Sharing goods? Yuck, no!: An investigation of consumers' contamination concerns about access-based services. *Journal of Service Research, 22,* 256–271.

Herzog, H. A. (2010). *Some we love, some we hate, some we eat: Why it's so hard to think straight about animals.* Harper.

Hoffarth, M. R., Azevedo, F., & Jost, J. T. (2019). Political conservatism and the exploitation of nonhuman animals: An application of system justification theory. *Group Processes and Intergroup Relations, 22,* 858–878.

Hornsey, M. J., Faulkner, C., Crimston, D., & Moreton, S. (2018). A microscopic dot on a microscopic dot: Self-esteem buffers the negative effects of exposure to the enormity of the universe. *Journal of Experimental Social Psychology, 76,* 198–207.

Hu, S., Zheng, X., Zhang, N., & Zhu, J. (2018). The impact of mortality salience on intergenerational altruism and the perceived importance of sustainable development goals. *Frontiers in Psychology, 9,* 1399.

Jiang, T., Hicks, J. A., Yuan, W., Yin, Y., Needy, L., & Vess. M. (2024). The unique nature and psychosocial implications of awe. *Nature Reviews Psychology, 3,* 475–488.

Jiang, T., & Sedikides, C. (2022). Awe motivates authentic-self pursuit via self-transcendence: Implications for prosociality. *Journal of Personality and Social Psychology, 123,* 576–596.

Jonas, E., Greenberg, J., & Frey, D. (2003). Connecting terror management and dissonance theory: Evidence that mortality salience increases the preference for supporting information after decisions. *Personality and Social Psychology Bulletin, 29,* 1181–1189.

Kashdan, T. B., Afram, A., Brown, K. W., Birnbeck, M., & Drvoshanov, M. (2011). Curiosity enhances the role of mindfulness in reducing defensive responses to existential threat. *Personality and Individual Differences, 50,* 1227–1232.

Kasser, T., & Sheldon, K. M. (2000). Of wealth and death: Materialism, mortality salience, and consumption behavior. *Psychological Science, 11,* 348–351.

Kiss, M. J., Morrison, M. A., & Morrison, T. G. (2020). A meta-analytic review of the association between disgust and prejudice toward gay men. *Journal of Homosexuality, 67,* 674–696.

Klackl, J., Jonas, E., & Kronbichler, M. (2014). Existential neuroscience: Self-esteem moderates neuronal responses to mortality-related stimuli. *Social Cognitive and Affective Neuroscience, 9,* 1754–1761.

Koller, S. (2021). Towards degrowth?: Making

peace with mortality to reconnect with (one's) nature: an ecopsychological proposition for a paradigm shift. *Environmental Values, 30,* 345–366.

Koole, S. L., & Van den Berg, A. E. (2005). Lost in the wilderness: Terror management, action orientation, and nature evaluation. *Journal of Personality and Social Psychology, 88,* 1014–1028.

Kteily, N., Hodson, G., & Bruneau, E. (2016). They see us as less than human: Metadehumanization predicts intergroup conflict via reciprocal dehumanization. *Journal of Personality and Social Psychology, 110,* 343–370.

Landau, M. J., Greenberg, J., Solomon, S., Martens, A., Goldenberg, J. L., Gillath, O., . . . Pyszczynski, T. (2006). The Siren's call: Terror management and the threat of men's sexual attraction to women. *Journal of Personality and Social Psychology, 90,* 129–146.

Lifshin, U. (2023). *Anxiety management and animal rights: Past, present and future.* Unpublished manuscript, The Hebrew University of Jerusalem.

Lifshin, U., & Greenberg, J. (2019). Relating Mary Midgley's insights to recent social psychological theory and research on humans' relationships with other animals. In C. Tandy (Ed.), *Death and anti-death: Vol. 17. One year after Mary Midgley, twenty years after Iris Murdoch* (pp. 131–162). Ria University Press.

Lifshin, U., Greenberg, J., & Sullivan, D. (2018). Religiosity and support for killing animals: Evidence of a curvilinear relationship. *Anthrozoös, 13,* 695–709.

Lifshin, U., Greenberg, J., Syropoulos, S., Helm, P. J., Leidner, B., Mikulincer, M., & Sullivan, D. (in press-a). I am not an animal—I am an American: Disassociation from animals and importance of cultural group identity. *Group Processes & Intergroup Relations.*

Lifshin, U., Greenberg, J., Syropoulos, S., Leidner, B., Helm, P. J., Sullivan, D., Horner, D., & Mikulincer, M. (2023). Perceived similarity of the self to animals, creativity, and anxiety: A terror management analysis. *Personality and Social Psychology Bulletin, 49,* 251–266.

Lifshin, U., Greenberg, J., Weise, D., & Soenke, M. (2016). It's the end of the world and I feel fine: Soul belief and perceptions of end-of-the-world scenarios. *Personality and Social Psychology Bulletin, 42,* 104–117.

Lifshin, U., Greenberg, J., & Zestcott, C. (in press-b). Religiosity and support for killing animals: A replication of the curvilinear relationship. *Society & Animals.*

Lifshin, U., Greenberg, J., Zestcott, C. A., & Sullivan, D. (2017). The evil animal: A terror management theory perspective on the human tendency to kill animals. *Personality and Social Psychology Bulletin, 43,* 743–757.

Lifshin, U., Helm, P. J., Mikulincer, M., Sullivan, D., & Greenberg, J. (2022a). *Cultural worldview affirmation and disassociation from animals: Evidence that affirmation of cultural worldviews can reduce perceived similarity of the self to animals.* Unpublished manuscript, Reichman University.

Lifshin, U., Horner, D., & Greenberg, J. (2022b). *The effect of pro-animal rights laws on attitudes towards killing animals.* Unpublished manuscript, Reichman University/University of Arizona.

Lifshin, U., Horner, D. E., Helm, P. J., Solomon, S., & Greenberg, J. (2021). Self-esteem and immortality: Evidence regarding the terror management hypothesis that high self-esteem is associated with a stronger sense of symbolic immortality. *Personality and Individual Differences, 175,* 110712.

Lifshin, U., McLamore, Q., Mikulincer, M., & Greenberg, J., & Leidner, B. (2024). *Increasing perceived similarity of the self to animals to reduce intergroup hostility and promote peace.* Unpublished manuscript, The Hebrew University of Jerusalem.

Lifton, R. J. (1979). *The broken connection: On death and the continuity of life.* Basic Books.

Marino, L., & Mountain, M. (2015). Denial of death and the relationship between humans and other animals. *Anthrozoös, 28,* 5–21.

Mikulincer, M., & Shaver, P. R. (2007). Boosting attachment security to promote mental health, prosocial values, and inter-group tolerance. *Psychological Inquiry, 18,* 139–156.

Morris, K. L., & Goldenberg, J. (2015). Objects become her: The role of mortality salience on men's attraction to literally objectified women. *Journal of Experimental Social Psychology, 56,* 69–72.

Morris, K. L., Goldenberg, J. L., & Heflick, N. A. (2014). Trio of terror (pregnancy, menstruation, and breastfeeding): An existential function of literal self-objectification among women. *Journal of Personality and Social Psychology, 107,* 181–198.

Mösler, T., Poppek, S., Leonhard, C., & Collet, W. (2022). Effects of a mortality salience exercise during mindfulness-based self-practice/self-reflection on physical and mental well-being among cognitive-behavior therapy trainees. *American Journal of Applied Psychology, 10,* 13–19.

Motyl, M., Hart, J., Cooper, D. P., Henick, N., Goldenberg, J., & Pyszczynski, T. (2013). Creatureliness priming reduces aggression and support for war. *British Journal of Social Psychology, 52,* 648–666.

Motyl, M., Hart, J., & Pyszczynski, T. (2010). When animals attack: The effects of mortality salience, infrahumanization of violence, and authoritarianism on support for war. *Journal of Experimental Social Psychology, 46,* 200–203.

Ng, S. T., & Eom, K. (2023). Religious stewardship and pro-environmental action: The mediating roles of environmental guilt and anger. *Psychology of Religion and Spirituality.*

Niemiec, C. P., Brown, K. W., Kashdan, T. B., Cozzolino, P. J., Breen, W. E., Levesque-Bristol, C., & Ryan, R. M. (2010). Being present in the face of existential threat: The role of trait mindfulness in reducing defensive responses to mortality salience. *Journal of Personality and Social Psychology, 99,* 344–365.

Nilsson, M., & Stålhammar, S. (2024). Psychedelics and inner dimensions of sustainability: A literature review. *European Journal of Ecopsychology, 9,* 4–47.

Öhman, A., & Mineka, S. (2001). Fears, phobias, and preparedness: Toward an evolved module of fear and fear learning. *Psychological Review, 108,* 483–522.

O'Neill, S., & Nicholson-Cole, S. (2009). "Fear won't do it": Promoting positive engagement with climate change through visual and iconic representations. *Science Communication, 30,* 355–379.

Park, Y. C., & Pyszczynski, T. (2019). Reducing defensive responses to thoughts of death: Meditation, mindfulness, and Buddhism. *Journal of Personality and Social Psychology, 116,* 101–118.

Pasaribu, D., Takwin, B., & Martens, P. (2022). The role of religious narratives and religious orientation towards concerns for the natural environment and animal welfare. *PLOS One, 17,* e0271515.

Patinadan, P. V., & Dillon, D. B. (2022). Friends, food or worth fighting for?: A proposed stereotype content model for nonhuman animals. *Human-Animal Interactions.*

Piff, P. K., Dietze, P., Feinberg, M., Stancato, D. M., & Keltner, D. (2015). Awe, the small self, and prosocial behavior. *Journal of Personality and Social Psychology, 108,* 883–899.

Piotrowski, J. P., Żemojtel-Piotrowska, M., & Clinton, A. (2020). Spiritual transcendence as a buffer against death anxiety. *Current Psychology, 39,* 994–1000.

Pöllänen, E., Osika, W., Stenfors, C. U., & Simonsson, O. (2022). Classic psychedelics and human–animal relations. *International Journal of Environmental Research and Public Health, 19,* 8114.

Preston, J. L., & Baimel, A. (2021). Towards a psychology of religion and the environment. *Current Opinion in Psychology, 40,* 145–149.

Preston, J. L., & Shin, F. (2022). Opposing effects of spirituality and religious fundamentalism on environmental attitudes. *Journal of Environmental Psychology, 80,* 101772.

Pyszczynski, T., Motyl, M., Vail, K. E. III, Hirschberger, G., Arndt, J., & Kesebir, P. (2012). Drawing attention to global climate change decreases support for war. *Peace and Conflict: Journal of Peace Psychology, 18,* 354–368.

Quirin, M., Klackl, J., & Jonas, E. (2019). Existential neuroscience: A review and brain model of coping with death awareness. In C. Routledge & M. Vess (Eds.), *Handbook of terror management theory* (pp. 347–367). Elsevier Academic Press.

Rabinovitch, A., & Parzuchowski, M. (2025). Egalitarian and continuity-based views mediate the link between nonreligiosity and concern for animals in a Judeo–Christian context. *Journal of Environmental Psychology,* 102780.

Reich, W. (1946). *The mass psychology of Fascism.* Orgone Institute Press.

Roberts, T. A., Goldenberg, J. L., Power, C., & Pyszczynski, T. (2002). "Feminine protection": The effects of menstruation on attitudes towards women. *Psychology of Women Quarterly, 26,* 131–139.

Routledge, C., Arndt, J., & Goldenberg, J. L. (2004). A time to tan: Proximal and distal effects of mortality salience on sun exposure intentions. *Personality and Social Psychology Bulletin, 30,* 1347–1358.

Rowan, A. N., D'Silva, J. M., Duncan, I. J. H. H., & Palmer, N. (2021). Animal sentience: History, science, and politics. *Animal Sentience, 31*(1).

Rozin, P., Haddat, B., Nemeroff, C., & Slovic, P. (2015). Psychological aspects of the rejection of recycled water: Contamination, purification and disgust. *Judgement and Decision Making, 10,* 50–63.

Sani, F., Herrera, M., & Bowe, M. (2009). Perceived collective continuity and ingroup identification as defence against death awareness. *Journal of Experimental Social Psychology, 45,* 242–245.

Segundo-Ortin, M. & Calvo, P. (2023). Plant sentience?: Between romanticism and denial: Science. *Animal Sentience, 33.*

Selimbegović, L., Chatard, A., Er-Rafiy, A., & Pyszczynski, T. (2016). Nuclear accident reminders and support for nuclear energy: Paradoxical effect. *Journal of Environmental Psychology, 48,* 87–100.

Serpell, J. A. (2009). Having our dogs and eating them too: Why animals are a social issue. *Journal of Social Issues, 65,* 633–644.

Sevillano, V., & Fiske, S. T. (2023). Animals are diverse: Distinct forms of animalized dehumanization. *Current Opinion in Behavioral Sciences, 51,* 101265.

Shanaah, S., Fritsche, I. & Osmundsen, M. (2024). The effect of climate change threat on public attitudes towards ethnic and religious minorities and climate refugees. *Group Processes and Intergroup Relations.*

Shi, Z., & Han, S. (2013). Transient and sustained neural responses to death-related linguistic cues. *Social Cognitive and Affective Neuroscience, 8,* 573–578.

Shin, F., & Preston, J. L. (2021). Green as the gospel: The power of stewardship messages to improve climate change attitudes. *Psychology of Religion and Spirituality, 13,* 437–447.

Shouldice, S. A., & Wolfe, S. E. (2024). *Death, disgust, and water reuse: The psychological impact of mortality fears on climate mitigation and adaptation efforts.* Unpublished manuscript, Royal Roads University.

Smith, L. K. M., Ross, H. C., Shouldice, S. A., & Wolfe, S. E. (2022). Mortality management and climate action: A review and reference for using terror management theory methods in interdisciplinary environmental research. *Wiley Interdisciplinary Reviews: Climate Change, 13,* e776.

Smith, L. K. M., & Wolfe, S. E. (2023). Dead in the water: Mortality messaging in water crisis communication and implications for pro-environmental outcomes. *People and Nature,* 1336–1352.

Smith, L. K. M., & Wolfe, S. E. (2025). Beyond the watery grave: Death and water reminders as (un)expected ways to increase environmental identity. *PsyEcology, 16.*

Soenke, M., Cohen, F., Greenberg, J., & Lifshin, U. (2018). Are you smarter than a cetacean?: Death reminders and concerns about human intelligence. *Society and Animals, 26,* 469–489.

Stanford, C. B. (1999). *The hunting apes: Meat eating and the origins of the human behaviour.* Princeton University Press.

Syropoulos, S., Law, K. F., Kraft-Todd, G. Mah, A., & Markowitz, E., & Young, L. (2024). Responsibility to future generations: A strategy for combatting climate change across political divides. *British Journal of Social Psychology.*

Syropoulos, S., Lifshin, U., Greenberg, J., Horner, D. E., & Leidner, B. (2022). Bigotry and the human-animal divide: (Dis)belief in human evolution and bigoted attitudes across different cultures. *Journal of Personality and Social Psychology, 123,* 1264–1292.

Syropoulos, S., Watkins, H., Goodwin, G. P., & Markowitz, E. (2023). Disentangling the effects of impact-oriented versus reputation-focused legacy motives on intergenerational concern and action. *Journal of Environmental Psychology, 90,* 102092.

Tracy, J. L., Hart, J., & Martens, J. P. (2011). Death and science: The existential underpinnings of belief in intelligent design and discomfort with evolution. *PLOS One, 6,* e17349.

Uhl, I., Klackl, J., Hansen, N., & Jonas, E. (2018). Undesirable effects of threatening climate change information: A cross-cultural study. *Group Processes and Intergroup Relations, 21,* 513–529.

Valdesolo, P., & Graham, J. (2014). Awe, uncertainty, and agency detection. *Psychological Science, 25,* 170–178.

Valmori, A., Carraro, L., Guidetti, M., Lenzi, M., & Castelli, L. (2024). The impact of mortality salience on environmental concerns and diet intentions: The moderating role of political orientation and RWA. *Current Psychology.*

van den Berg, A. E., & ter Heijne, M. (2005). Fear versus fascination: An exploration of emotional responses to natural threats. *Journal of Environmental Psychology, 25,* 261–272.

Vess, M., & Arndt, J. (2008). The nature of death and the death of nature: The impact of mortality salience on environmental concern. *Journal of Research in Personality, 42,* 1376–1380.

Vess, M., Arndt, J., & Cox, C. R. (2012). Faith and nature: The effect of death-relevant cognitions on the relationship between religious fundamentalism and connectedness to nature. *Social Psychological and Personality Science, 3,* 333–340.

Vitousek, P., Mooney, H., Lubchenco, J., & Melillo, J. (1997). Human domination of earth's ecosystems. *Science, 277.*

Vlasceanu, M., Doell, K. C., Bak-Coleman, J. B., Todorova, B., Berkebile-Weinberg, M. M., Grayson, S. J., . . . Van Bavel, J. J. (2024). Addressing climate change with behavioral science: A global intervention tournament in 63 countries. *Science Advances, 10,* 1–19.

Webster, R. J., & Saucier, D. A. (2011). The effects of death reminders on sex differences in prejudice toward gay men and lesbians. *Journal of Homosexuality, 58,* 402–426.

Wester, J., Timpano, K. R., Çek, D., & Broad, K. (2016). The psychology of recycled water: Factors predicting disgust and willingness to use. *Water Resources Research, 52,* 3212–3226.

Wilkins, J., Schoville, B. J., Brown, K. S., & Chazan, M. (2012). Evidence for early hafted hunting technology. *Science, 338,* 942–946.

Wolfe, S. E., & Tubi, A. (2019). Terror management theory and mortality awareness: A missing link in climate response studies? *Wiley Interdisciplinary Reviews: Climate Change, 10,* e566.

Wrenn, C. L. (2020). Discriminating spirits: Cultural source theory and the human–nonhuman boundary. *Mortality, 25,* 348–363.

Yetzer, A. M., & Pyszczynski, T. (2019). Terror management theory and psychological disorder: Ineffective anxiety-buffer functioning as a transdiagnostic vulnerability factor for psychopathology. In C. Routledge & M. Vess (Eds.), *Handbook of terror management theory* (pp. 417–447). Elsevier Academic Press.

Zaval, L., Markowitz, E. M., & Weber, E. U. (2015). How will I be remembered?: Conserving the environment for the sake of one's legacy. *Psychological Science, 26,* 231–236.

Zilcha-Mano, S., Mikulincer, M., & Shaver, P. R. (2012). Pets as safe havens and secure bases: The moderating role of pet attachment orientations. *Journal of Research in Personality, 46,* 571–580.

CHAPTER 8

Near-Death Experiences

An Overview and Implications for Mortality

Natasha A. Tassell-Matamua, Bruce Greyson,
and Philip J. Cozzolino

Near-death experiences (NDEs) are profound psychological phenomena often coinciding with near-death events. They comprise a consistent presentation of phenomenologically distinct features that transcend temporospatial perception (Tassell-Matamua & Holden, 2020) and contravene current understandings of conscious experience touted by Western scientific models of reality (Facco & Agrillo, 2012; Greyson, 2010a; van Lommel, 2010). They are believed to occur in approximately 10–20% of those who survive a life-threatening incident (Parnia et al., 2023; Zingrone & Alvarado, 2009). No one can categorically explain why they occur, when they will occur, where they will occur, or what causes them. Despite increased scholarly attention, much is still unknown about NDEs. What is certain, however, is these occurrences are existentially relevant. From their earliest known historical documentation, NDEs have been linked to the meaning, purpose, and value of human existence, and continue to effect important transformations in those who have them, as well as in those who learn about them. To contextualize their place in the science of existential psychology, we provide an overview of what is currently known about NDEs, before delving into their implications for better understanding and giving meaning to mortality.

A BRIEF HISTORY

NDEs are a long-standing and entrenched part of humanity's fabric. Representations of unusual death-related occurrences, like what we now call NDEs, extend back to ancient Sumeria and Egypt (Schroter-Kunhardt, 1993). The earliest known written account comes from ancient Greece in the *Myth of Er*, the concluding story in Plato's *Republic* authored around 380 B.C.E. NDEs are depicted in art from the 1500s (Martial et al., 2020). During the 1800s French philosophy and medical articles used the expression *experiences de morte imminente* (e.g., Egger, 1896) to denote occurrences that resemble contemporary NDE descriptions. Within the past 40 years interest in NDEs has blossomed, in part initiated by the publication of Moody's book *Life After Life* (1975), which enabled the general populace to access information about NDEs. More recently, the reach of social media and popular literature (e.g., Greyson, 2021a; Moorjani, 2012) has increased visibility of NDE narratives and arguably assisted in changing societal discourses from those that categorically rejected such unexplainable phenomena a century ago, to now accepting and actively pursuing information about NDEs and how they enhance understandings about the human experience.

Perhaps because of Moody's book, the scholarly field of near-death studies emerged. The International Association for Near-Death Studies was established in 1978, followed by the first academic journal dedicated to near-death studies (initially titled *Anabiosis,* now called the *Journal of Near-Death Studies [JNDS]*) in 1982. These helped consolidate efforts to methodically document NDEs within Western[1] scholarship. From an initial focus on case reports and descriptions of the structure and content of NDE features, studies transformed into those focused on verifying NDEs quantitatively and investigating their covariation with presumed antecedents and aftereffects. Due to such changes and on account of the perplexing questions NDEs raise for an increasing number of disciplines, the field of near-death studies is now multidisciplinary, with experts across various fields (e.g., neurology, psychiatry, religion, coma science, Indigeneity, parapsychology, among others) investing capabilities to understand NDEs more comprehensively. Once restricted to publication in bespoke journals such as JNDS, NDE studies are now found in numerous scholarly modalities, including highly cited journals (e.g., *Lancet*, *Trends in Cognitive Science*, *Frontiers*), international conference presentations, and online mediums (e.g., podcasts).

The term *near-death experience* is well popularized in Western societies, and NDEs are better understood than when the field of near-death studies first emerged in the English-speaking world 40 years ago. Yet much is still unknown about NDEs and their long history with humanity.

NDE PHENOMENOLOGY

Because their occurrence is unpredictable, their content highly subjective, and their causation unknown, what constitutes an NDE remains subject to debate. Moody (1975) proposed a prototypical NDE comprised 15 features that occurred in sequential order. Ring (1980) suggested NDEs unfold sequentially over five steps. Martial and colleagues (2018) recently noted an absence of prototypical sequences in their sample of NDE experiencers (NDErs). Yet, Greyson's (1983) four categories of quintessential features—cognitive, affective, transcendental, and paranormal—remain the most widely cited.

Cognitive features include changed perceptions of linear time as moving slower, moving faster, or being nonexistent, in comparison to everyday waking consciousness (Schwaninger et al., 2002). They can also include instantaneous and rapid recollection of long-forgotten memories. Known as *life reviews*, they are reported by 13–50% of NDErs (Cassol et al., 2018), are evident in literature as far back as 1795 (Noyes & Kletti, 1977), and are known in French and theosophical writings of the mid-1800s (Alvarado, 2011; Marjanen et al., 2022). An awareness of the impact of one's actions on others often occurs as part of memory recall (van Lommel, 2006).

Affective features include intense feelings of happiness, joy, peace, unconditional love, unity, and interconnectedness with the cosmos. Particularly common are feelings of peace (e.g., Schwaninger et al., 2002). Unpleasant, void, or distressing emotions, including fear, panic, terror, loneliness, and anxiety, have been less commonly documented, possibly due to underreporting (Cassol et al., 2019). The emotions felt during an NDE are typically inexplicable, meaning NDErs struggle to find terminology that sufficiently captures the magnitude, intensity, and accuracy of the feelings (Zingrone & Alvarado, 2009).

Transcendental features go beyond one's usual state of being. Most common is the encountering of others, usually deceased, with whom the person often (but not always) has a significant relationship with during life. Particularly intriguing are cases where the NDEr encountered someone they thought was alive, only to later find the person died during the period the NDE occurred (Greyson, 2010b); as well as cases where the being was unknown to the person during their NDE, but later discovered to be a person of significance (i.e., an unknown biological parent, deceased sibling; van Lommel, 2010). Other transcendental features include encountering benevolent and loving spiritual beings and apparent travel to another realm.

Paranormal features include extraordinary perceptual abilities beyond the five commonly cited sensory modalities and logical deduction. Most common are out-of-body experiences (OBEs), which involve the perception of events in real time, from a disembodied position. Particularly compelling are those OBE cases where the events observed are externally verified by others (Parnia et al., 2014; Rivas & Smit, 2013; Smit, 2008). Additional paranormal features include precognitive abilities, such as perceiving future events, and extrasensory perception, where accurate knowledge of others' thoughts, feelings, and location are often simultaneously obtained in the absence of any overt information exchange.

These four categories of features are the reference point for describing NDEs; yet limitations remain. There may exist other, yet to be acknowledged (in scholarly literature), NDE features not accounted for by these categorizations. NDE research overall is dominated by English-language accounts and research methodologies and methods emanating from the Global North[2] (Tassell-Matamua, 2025). A growing number of NDE studies from populations where English is not the primary language and categorized as Global South have been published (e.g., Ferrara Carunchio & de Oliveira Maraldi, 2020; Ghasemmianejad Jahromi & Long, 2021; Tassell-Matamua, 2013). However, cultural diversity in NDE research must be more thoroughly considered if NDE features are to be better understood.

Similarly, NDE literature remains dominated by adult accounts, despite concerns about the limited NDE accounts from children (e.g., Bush, 1983) and suggestions that more children may have NDEs than adults (Hashemi et al., 2023). Although Serdahely (1991) compared childhood NDEs reported by adults to those reported by children and showed only 2 out of 47 variables differed (adults described more time distortions and sense of timelessness), which suggests adults' recollections of their childhood NDEs are not embellished or diminished over time, most studies documenting children's NDEs have been of adults retrospectively recalling the NDEs they had as a child. While not problematic per se and notwithstanding Serdahely's work, such recollection is interpreted through the lens of the (now) adult (Thomas & O'Connor, 2023), with their subsequent layers of life experience and years of integration of the NDE. Children's reports are valuable for enhancing understandings about NDEs, yet children remain underinvolved in NDE research.

Finally, because the current categories of NDE features have been derived from quantitative approaches, Cassol and colleagues (2018) suggested qualitatively examining NDE narratives may provide additional, richer insights into their phenomenology. Their thematic analysis of 34 NDE accounts showed coherence with many of the NDE features described above, but without a plethora of case reports analyzed using a range of methods informed by diverse methodologies, definitive conclusions regarding NDE features cannot be assumed.

DEFINITIONAL DEBATES

Notwithstanding the concerns noted above, given the relatively consistent findings about NDE features and perhaps due to them typically being described as "more real than real" by NDErs (Thonnard et al., 2013), the psychological reality of NDEs is less in doubt, while their ontological reality remains subject to debate. Part of the challenge centers around two main definitional concerns.

The first relates to how and if NDEs can be objectively verified. Attempts to develop metrics to sufficiently measure NDEs began shortly after the inception of the field of near-death studies with Ring's (1980) Weighted Core Experience Index (WCEI), which lacked statistical reliability and validity due to not being based on psychometric analyses. Consequently, Greyson (1983) developed the NDE Scale to capture NDE "depth" according to the perceived intensity of features. This scale has served as *the* standardized means for measuring NDEs for the past 30 years, continues to be widely cited in NDE literature, and has been translated into 13 languages. More recently, Martial and colleagues (2020) developed the NDE-C scale, to "quantify NDEs in a more complete way" (p. 1), due to concerns the Greyson scale does not address all prototypical NDE features, the wording is not always clear, and it is not able to sufficiently differentiate NDEs from other types of mystical experiences that occur in non-life-threatening situations (e.g., Charland-Verville et al., 2014).

The second concern relates to the timing of NDEs, and more specifically whether they are the exclusive domain of clinical death or not. While NDEs often coincide with a life-threatening event, comparable experiences are also reported in situations where there was no known physiological threat of dying (e.g., Kelly et al., 2007; van Lommel, 2013). Introduction of the term *NDE-like* was only recently coined and based on concerns the term *near-death experience* may be a misnomer if used to represent experiences occurring in non-life-threatening situations (Facco & Agrillo, 2012). Recent calls to demarcate those NDEs where clinical death is verifiable from those NDEs where there is no verification of clinical death have echoed this concern. Parnia and colleagues (2022) suggest the term *recalled experiences of death* (RED) in lieu of the term *near-death experience.*

Combined, these definitional concerns ignite internal debates within the NDE research community and raise questions important to the ongoing advancement of the field.

EXPLANATORY MODELS

NDEs are a "biological paradox" (Xu et al., 2023, p. 1) because they are unanticipated, complex, organized, and comprehensive experiences of perception that occur often (although not always) while the experiencer is behaviorally nonresponsive to the external world. Thus, the question remains—what causes them? Even in the absence of a comprehensive and consensually agreed definition, attempts to answer this question have been extensive and focused on whether NDEs occur in some groups of people more than others, as well as attempts to explain their underlying mechanisms.

Regarding whether some groups of people might be more susceptible to an NDE, the answer appears to be an unequivocal "no." Studies have failed to produce conclusive and consistent evidence to suggest variables, such as age, sex, religious affiliation, among others, influence the occurrence of NDEs (Greyson, 2021b). It seems NDEs can happen to any person, anywhere, anytime.

Regarding mechanisms involved in manufacturing NDEs, the answer is less clear. Numerous studies and theories, most grounding their propositions in material reductionist philosophies, have linked NDE features with particular biological, psychological, and pathological causes. Although comprehensively addressed elsewhere (e.g., Greyson, 2009; Kelly et al., 2007), we briefly overview them here.

Biological Explanations

Biological explanations are the most consistently proposed and often the default of the uninformed or skeptical. Linking NDEs to biological causality ignites passionate debate among scholars (Kondziella & Martial, 2022) because most contemporary scientific theories, even in the absence of direct proof, propose consciousness is manufactured by the brain and has a physiological basis (Damasio, 2012; Grossberg, 2021; Klemm, 2014). The explanations generated to date imply NDEs can be accounted for biologically through blood gases, neurochemicals, and/or specific anatomic structures or processes of the brain.

Theories implicating blood gases propose a depletion or reduction of oxygen to the brain and/or elevated carbon dioxide (CO_2) levels in the blood trigger the unusual sensations described by NDErs. Yet it remains highly unlikely blood gases are responsible for the NDE in its entirety, as NDErs do not necessarily have higher levels of CO_2 in the brain compared to non-NDErs (Parnia et al., 2001). Equally, van Lommel and colleagues (2001) noted if anoxia is a necessary factor in *manufacturing* NDEs, cardiac arrest patients should have a much higher incidence of NDEs given anoxia is a typical feature of this medical condition.

The secretion of neurochemicals has also been proposed in NDE causality, such as endorphins (Carr, 1981, 1982; Guevara & Sotelo, 1997) or a ketamine-like endogenous agent being released during extreme stress situations (Corazza & Schifano, 2010; Jansen, 1997a). Associating NDEs with psychoactive chemicals need not negate the metaphysical reality of NDEs, as Jansen himself noted "ketamine is a door to a place we cannot normally get to; it is definitely not evidence that such a place does not exist" (1997b, pp. 94–95).

More recently, commonalities between psychedelic experiences and NDEs have been noted (Fritz et al., 2024; Michael et al., 2023; Timmerman et al., 2018), leading scholars to propose the same neural mechanisms may be involved in the production of both. What these findings mean for deepening understandings about NDE causality remains subject to further investigation, but overall the abovementioned neurochemical theories remain insufficient to account for the totality of NDE features.

Anesthesia has been proposed as accounting for some NDE features (Ghoneim & Block, 1992). While previous research revealed brain activity is completely deactivated during anesthesia, making usual perceptual processes inaccessible (e.g., Shulman et al., 2003; White & Alkire, 2003), cases of awareness were still known albeit considered rare (Cobcroft & Forsdick, 1993), ranging from between 0.2% and 1.5% of surgical patients and largely due to administration of an insufficient quantity of anesthesia (Ghoneim & Block, 1997). Most NDEs still notably occur in the absence of anesthesia, rendering it unlikely as a comprehensive explanation for how NDEs are manufactured.

Certain anatomic areas and processes of the brain have been hypothesized as playing a role in NDEs. Perhaps the most intriguing is the temporo-parieto-occipital junction, due to a recent study of four comatose patients showing gamma activity after mechanical ventilation was stopped (Xu et al., 2023). However, in two patients such activity occurred *before* their hearts stopped, but was not seen after their hearts stopped, and those same two patients showed no evidence of regaining consciousness during that period (van Lommel & Greyson, 2023). Other studies have shown increased alpha activity in frontal and posterior brain regions during NDE *recall* (e.g., Martial et al., 2019), although retrospective recollection of an event is not the same as in-the-moment subjective experience, so such brain regions cannot be assumed to constitute evidence of a *manufacturing* role in NDEs. Findings from other studies imply specific brain regions may be related to particular NDE features (e.g., Beauregard et al., 2009; Facco et al., 2019); yet it remains to be seen whether these same structures account for the totality of NDE features.

Psychological Explanations

Psychological explanations propose that NDEs are constructed entirely within the "mind" and are a consequence of defense mechanisms and/or cultural conditioning. Defense mechanisms are unconscious psychological processes (e.g., denial, dissociation, projection) that protect the individual from anxiety-provoking situations, often brought on by external stressors (e.g., Akhtar, 2018; Cramer, 2015; VandenBos, 2015). In relation to NDEs, features such as pleasant feelings and sensations, dissociation, and pleasant imagery (e.g., of deceased others or light) are proposed to distract the individual from the life-threatening situation and potential death, thus alleviating death anxiety. While such a theory speaks to the power of the human psyche to construct reality, many life-threatening events associated with NDEs occur so suddenly (e.g., car accident) the NDEr is not able to process they may die. Equally, not all NDEs happen under life-threatening situations (Charland-Verville et al., 2014) nor do all NDEs have the pleasant affect and sensations presumed to serve as defense mechanisms (Bush, 2009; Cassol et al., 2019; Greyson, 2023).

Another psychological explanation proposes NDEs are constructed from "cultural conditioning"; the idea expectations regarding what happens during the dying process and in the so-called afterlife influence the manifestation of NDEs. All cultures have narratives associated with death and dying that infiltrate the collective psyche of specific groups. Common examples are religious movements; Christians may believe they will see Christ and go to heaven when they die, while Muslims may believe they will enter Barzakh until the Day of Judgment, and these may indeed unfold in an NDE of someone who identifies as either Christian or Muslim. More subtle but no less powerful are social discourses that occur in secular societies where religious adherence may not be dominant (e.g., Aotearoa New Zealand), yet beliefs about death and dying are inherent in popular literature, social media, and through systems such as law and education, which shape and are shaped by collective ways of believing and thinking (i.e., worldviews). If cultural conditioning were strongly implicated in the manufacture of NDEs, NDE phenomenology should be highly relative to cultural context. Although the universality of NDEs is often implied in NDE literature (e.g., Peinkhofer et al., 2021), and NDE accounts in the United States were the same before and after Moody's 1975 book introduced the concept of NDEs (Athappilly et al., 2006), research to date has attempted to interpret NDEs almost exclusively through the lens of the Global North (Tassell-Matamua, 2025). This unintended bias excludes at least half of the world's population, making it difficult to determine the extent cultural context influences NDE phenomenology.

Others have argued that if cultural conditioning played a role in manufacturing NDEs, children would not adhere to such cultural ideas in their NDEs because they are too young to have been socialized about what death is and its implications for self and others (although recent literature implies children who experience terminal lucidity at the end of life do indeed have an understanding of what death entails; see Roehrs et al., 2023). Yet children report NDEs consistent with the religious/spiritual beliefs of their cultural context (e.g., Serdahely, 1991). Cultural conditioning has also been proposed to explain encounters with deceased others, in that the person having the NDE maintains an unconscious wish to connect with their dead significant other. Notably, this explanation would not apply in NDEs where the deceased person encountered was not yet known to have died, so-called Peak in Darien experiences (Greyson, 2010b, 2021a). Equally, Kelly (2001) found visions of deceased persons are more frequent with life-threatening conditions of sudden onset, such as accident or cardiac arrest, where the time to contemplate death is limited or nonexistent. Finally, the feature of seeing deceased others is but one aspect of NDEs among many others, so while this explanation may be a fitting (albeit nonverifiable) aspect of specific cases where an NDE occurred, it cannot be applied to all NDEs where a deceased other has been encountered.

Psychopathological Explanations

Psychopathological explanations involve speculative links between NDEs and a variety of psychological conditions. Greyson (2000, 2007) found heightened dissociative symptoms in NDErs compared to non-NDErs, although the level of symptoms was within the normal range and lower than would be expected in those on the pathological spectrum of depersonalization/derealization disorder (DDD) (DSM-5-TR; American Psychiatric Association, 2022). While once proposed as a potential precursor or explanation for NDE phenomenology, Greyson's and more recent findings showing no association between dissociative symptoms and NDEs or NDE-like experiences (Bicego et al., 2023), along with the typical symptoms of DDD (which can include sensory anesthesia, limited affect, and nonvolitional action and speech), suggest dissociation is highly unlikely to cause NDEs.

Fantasy proneness has been suggested as causal in NDEs (Martial et al., 2018), yet findings from separate studies are inconsistent. Martial and colleagues found individuals who had an NDE-like experience scored significantly higher on fantasy proneness than NDErs did, yet NDErs did not score significantly different from matched controls. More recently, Bicego and colleagues (2023) found fantasy proneness was associated with NDE *recollection*. While it may play a role in memory recollection for some, findings to date cannot reliably link the two.

Claims that NDEs are merely hallucinations remain insufficient as an explanation. Individuals who have experienced both an NDE and hallucinations (on separate occasions) indicate they are very different and can be differentiated from each other (Sartori et al., 2006), including pervasive differences in the context in which the two kinds of experience occur, the content of the experience, how it is remembered, and how it affects the individual (Greyson, 2014). Other studies indicate NDEs are often inherently meaningful and complex, while drug-induced hallucinations are not (Bates & Stanley, 1985), and most NDEs continue to occur outside the context of recreational drug use. When experiences that could be misinterpreted as hallucinations (i.e., hearing internal voices) occur post-NDE, these are positively accepted and responded to, which contrasts with the negative attitudes to such occurrences that are reported by psychiatric populations (Greyson & Liester, 2004).

Overall, explanations with psychopathology as a base cannot reliably or convincingly be implicated in or predict how NDEs are produced.

Nonmaterialist Explanations

Nonmaterialist explanations are a further way NDE causality can be understood. While causal mechanisms (i.e., biological, psychological, psychopathological) are often cited when reviewing NDEs, nonmaterialist suggestions for how NDEs occur have dominated much of the literature on NDEs over the past 40 years, until very recently when neurological explanations began to proliferate. Proponents of nonmaterialist explanations generally adopt a view that is nonmaterial, nonreductionistic, and sympathetic to the idea NDEs may be explained by adopting other understandings of reality. Synonymous with notions of transcendence, these understandings suggest that rather than being manufactured by the brain either physiologically or psychologically, NDEs occur because consciousness is primary in constructing reality and need not have a functioning human brain to have the experience of awareness. Rather, consciousness just simply is, and the minimization of brain function during NDEs (via life-threatening circumstances) more readily enables this awareness than when the brain is fully functioning and filtering awareness. Of course, such a seemingly radical explanation for NDEs requires extraordinary proof. Obtaining evidence that will be readily accepted as valid and legitimate when material reductionism is the privileged mode of understanding reality and wields so much power, remains challenging. Yet understanding nonmaterialist perspectives provides a useful foundation for discussing changes that occur after NDEs, as well as their existential relevance.

AFTEREFFECTS AND EXISTENTIAL IMPLICATIONS

Almost without exception, NDEs produce a metamorphosis in those who have them. Numerous studies attest to transformative and wide-ranging changes, known as aftereffects, that NDEs have on those who report them, as well as on those who have not had an NDE but learn about them (e.g., Ghasemiannejad Jahromi et al., 2023; Tassell-Matamua et al., 2017). Such changes raise interesting questions related to the science of existential psychology; some of those questions we address here.

Perhaps the most notable change after an NDE is how NDErs view mortality. It seems that nearly dying (NDE) or the thought that one might die (so-called NDE-like), catalyzes a reduced fear of dying in the future. A loss of the fear of death is the most consistent and widely reported change after an NDE. Studies indicate as many as 80–100% of NDErs report no longer fearing death, despite most claiming to fear death prior to their NDE (e.g., Bianco et al., 2019; Flynn, 1986; Greyson, 2003; Ring, 1984; Sabom, 1982; Sutherland, 1990). This loss of death fear is maintained over time (Sabom, 1982; Sutherland, 1990; van Lommel et al., 2001). Many NDErs endorse the idea of a recycled existence, where one lives in perpetuity in a "spiritual body" (Lindsay & Tassell-Matamua, 2021, p. 310). Indeed, an increase in afterlife beliefs and reincarnation has also been observed (Lindsay & Tassell-Matamua, 2021; Sutherland, 1990; van Lommel et al., 2001). Although the reincarnation finding was once criticized as due to biased samples (Sabom, 1998), it has remained relatively consistent over time (e.g., Lindsay & Tassell-Matamua, 2021; Sutherland, 1990).

In addition, spirituality is commonly endorsed post-NDE, while affiliation with and beliefs around religion may alter (Greyson & Khanna, 2014; Khanna & Greyson, 2014a, 2014b; Ring, 1980; Tassell-Matamua & Steadman, 2017). Spirituality becomes favored over religion, with NDErs often preferring the term *spiritual* to *religious* to describe their newfound understandings about the workings of the universe. Such are the spiritual changes evoked by NDEs, Shushan (2011, 2012) hypothesized many religious systems may have their origin in NDEs.

Alterations to life circumstances also often occur and can include termination of and isolation away from significant relationships, changes in employment, and reduced consumerism and materiality, among others (Corazza & Schifano, 2010; Ghasemiannejad Jahromi, 2021; Stout et al., 2006). Other notable effects include enhanced psychic abilities (Greyson, 1983; Sutherland, 1989), electromagnetic sensitivity (Greyson et al., 2015; Nouri & Holden, 2008), and subjective sleep alterations (Lindsay & Tassell-Matamua, 2020; Lindsay et al., 2023).

The worldview-related consequences observed in many individuals post-NDE, which are often enduring (Greyson, 2022), include modified values; an increased belief in an afterlife; greater concern or compassion for other people; an enhanced appreciation and subjective quality of life; positive attitude toward self; reduced negative affect and cognitions; a greater "thirst" for knowledge; and a sense of purpose and meaning in life, among others (Greyson, 2003; van Lommel et al., 2001).

Combined, such changes are among the most prevalent of the outcomes assessed by existential psychologists in people coping with knowledge of mortality. Studies have yet to reveal the underlying mechanisms catalyzing such changes (although some have tried; see Pehlivanova et al., 2022; Tassell-Matamua & Lindsay, 2016), yet research supporting terror management theory (TMT; Greenberg et al., 1986; Solomon, Greenberg, & Pyszczynski, Chapter 6, this volume) may provide some insights. TMT posits that a potentially overwhelming fear of death motivates individuals to behave in a manner that assuages that fear, leading humans to embrace specific social beliefs and standards imbued with value and that become abstract or symbolic representations of the self (e.g., being a good Christian or a highly regarded scientist) that offer the hope of existing beyond death either literally or symbolically. By conforming and adhering to such worldview-relevant expectations, individuals develop a sense of meaning, bolster their self-esteem, and sustain a sense of death transcendence by qualifying for spiritual or symbolic sense of continuance beyond death.

TMT's dual-process model describes the *proximal* and *distal* defenses that individuals employ to ward off death anxiety (Greenberg et al., 2000). Proximal defenses are activated once mortality is salient, and manifest as direct attempts to remove death-related thoughts from current focal attention (Arndt et al., 2005). These direct defenses are motivated by a "not me, not now" reaction (Chaplin, 2000) that serves the function of denying one's vulnerability to death. There is some evidence from TMT research that when death thought is close to focal attention, individuals may minimize the importance of culturally prescribed extrinsic goals such as wealth and fame (Kosloff & Greenberg, 2009), which could help reorient them toward intrinsic goals. When applied to NDEs, this may partially explain the often reported reorientation toward purpose and meaning and away from materialism and consumerism.

The bulk of TMT research, however, has explored the consequences of mortality awareness once thoughts of death are not in focal attention but are high in accessibility. The distal defenses typically observed in these studies show individuals with high death-thought accessibility become especially motivated to invest in and defend their worldview and strive for self-worth. This evidence shows subtle manipulations of death can generate in individuals increased stereotyping (Schimel et al., 1999), heightened levels of greed (Kasser & Sheldon, 2000), enhanced support for military interventions that would kill thousands of foreigners (Pyszczynski et al., 2006), and a move toward religious fundamentalism (Friedman, 2008). Such findings, of course, are in direct contrast to what is typically reported by those who have NDEs, but this may be either because NDErs' death cognitions remain in focal attention or because NDErs have quelled their death fears through afterlife beliefs, thus reducing their need to pursue symbolic bases for continuance beyond death (see, e.g., Dechesne et al., 2003).

That said, there have been efforts in experimental existential psychology to link the lessons learned from NDE research with the writings of Heidegger (1962) and Yalom (1980) to develop an extended model of mortality awareness (Cozzolino, 2006; Cozzolino et al., 2004). This work suggests that abstract/subtle reminders of mortality are more likely to activate psychological processes related to abstract representations of the self, such as worldviews. Conversely, this model suggests that concrete mortality awareness that individuates and specifies thoughts of death, has the potential to activate psychological processes tied to the person's intrinsic values while also reducing their desire to satisfy external demands and expectations. Put simply, there is nothing abstract about the concept of death for people who have experienced the cognitive, affective, transcendental, and paranormal features of an NDE. For these individuals, death often shifts from being an unknowable mystery to be feared (at least in Western societies) into being an experiential reality that becomes integrated into the self.

Thus, at a conceptual level the model assumes that individuals can think about death in one of two ways, either as an abstract concept (i.e., "What do I think about death?") or as a specific and individuated reality (i.e., "What do I think about *my* death?"). Based on this distinction, Cozzolino and colleagues (2004) validated a manipulation called "death reflection" in which participants imagine themselves dying in an apartment fire guided by vivid imagery, such as "It is getting very hard to breathe and the heat from the flames is almost unbearable." Participants also respond to four open-ended questions designed to individuate death further and to tap into two key elements of NDEs (i.e., life review and perspective taking; see Ring & Elsaesser-Valarino, 1998). Evidence shows that death-reflection processes can increase prosocial behavior (Blackie & Cozzolino, 2011), identity integration (Blackie et al., 2016), authentic and autonomous motivation (Arena et al., 2024), gratitude (Frias et al., 2011), and even higher body weight and shape satisfaction among young women (Alleva et al., 2020).

CONCLUSION

While there is much known about NDEs and the profound and enduring life changes they induce, particularly to notions of mortality, much is still unknown about these intriguing experiences. The thought of death seems to generate anxiety in many, at least in Western societies, notably because death is viewed as an exclusively physical process that ultimately results in annihilation of the self-concept (Carpentier & Van Brussel, 2012). Yet, when questioned about their changed attitude to death, many NDErs state it is because they have already died once, recognize it is neither terrible nor final, and understand it is merely a transition to another state of living. This of course does not mean *anxiety* about death is eliminated altogether. *How* one dies might still cause apprehension, as well as the death of significant others and the sorrowful pain that would cause. Yet it seems what happens at the time of death and after is no longer the subject of fear or denial. Death is no longer death (as we know it in Western societies), but rather a continuation of life, albeit in another form.

Research has yet to convincingly demonstrate how NDEs cause changes in engagement with death, the afterlife, spirituality, and life in general, although there is some existential psychology literature, such as TMT and its dual-process model (and extensions of that model; i.e., Cozzolino, 2006), that has potential for explaining some of the nuances of these changes. So it seems interest in NDEs will continue to grow, both among the general public as well as in Western scholarship. Consequently, NDE researchers must be cognizant of the implications continued delineation of NDEs will have in general, and for existential psychology in particular. For example, will the current definitional issues lead humanity to more enlightened existential understandings of themselves and others, or not? Will differentiating NDEs (actual death) and NDEs (no death) combined with a greater understanding of the neurological basis of NDEs (which has become so prominent over the past decade) ultimately matter to those who have NDEs? Would the implications of the experience change if people knew the neurological basis (if any) of NDEs? How might this influence their attempts to understand, integrate, and relate the experience to existential concerns of mortality?

While such questions are not likely easily answered, what is certain is that NDEs have had a long history with humanity and, given increases in reports of the past few decades, will continue to be ever present in our collective social discourses. The extent NDEs continue to influence and inform the science of existential psychology remains promising.

NOTES

1. We use the terms *Western* and *West* to refer to the social norms, values, customs, beliefs and rituals, political ideologies and systems, cultural artifacts, technologies, systems, and processes that are dominant within industrialized countries with a current population that largely comprises people from European descent who have a Judeo-Christian heritage.

2. We use Tassell-Matamua's (2025) descriptions. The *Global North* includes North America, Western Europe, and so-called developed parts of Australasia (including Japan, Australia, Singapore, and Aotearoa New Zealand) and the Middle East (including Dubai). The *Global South* includes those countries across Africa, South America, some parts of the Middle East, and so-called developing parts of Australasia, as well as Indigenous communities regardless of geographical locale.

REFERENCES

Akhtar, S. (2018). *Comprehensive dictionary of psychoanalysis*. Routledge.

Alleva J. M., Atkinson M. J., Schwarten S., Theden A., Waldén M. I., & Martijn C. (2020). The potential benefits of death reflection for improving women's body image. *Body Image, 35,* 192–200.

Alvarado, C. S. (2011). Panoramic memory, affect, and sensations of detachment in the dying: Discussions published in France, 1889–1903. *Journal of Near-Death Studies, 30*(2), 63–82.

American Psychiatric Association. (2022). *Diagnostic and statistical manual of mental disorders* (5th ed., text rev.). Author.

Arena, A. F. A., MacCann, C., Moreton, S. G., Menzies, R. E., & Tiliopoulos, N. (2024). Living authentically in the face of death: Predictors of autonomous motivation among individuals exposed to chronic mortality cues compared to a matched community sample. *Omega, 89,* 379–403.

Arndt, J., Routledge, C., Cox, C. R., & Goldenberg, J. L. (2005). The worm at the core: A terror management perspective on the roots of psychological dysfunction. *Applied and Preventative Psychology, 11,* 191–213.

Athappilly, G. K., Greyson, B., & Stevenson, I. (2006). Do prevailing societal models influence reports of near-death experiences?: Comparison of accounts reported before and after 1975. *Journal of Nervous and Mental Disease, 194,* 218–222.

Bates, B. C., & Stanley, A. (1985). The epidemiology and differential diagnosis of near-death experience. *American Journal of Orthopsychiatry, 55,* 542–549.

Beauregard, M., Courtemanche, J., & Paquette, V. (2009). Brain activity in near-death experiencers during a meditative state. *Resuscitation, 80,* 1006–1010.

Bianco, B., Testoni, I., Palmieri, A., Solomon, S., & Hart, J. (2019). The psychological correlates of decreased death anxiety after a near-death experience: The role of self-esteem, mindfulness, and death representations. *Journal of Humanistic Psychology, online.*

Bicego, A., Cassol, H., Simon, J., Fritz, P., Abagnale, S., Vanhaudenhuyse, A., . . . Martial, C. (2023). Personality traits and pattern of beliefs of near-death(-like) experiencers. *Frontiers in Human Neuroscience, 17,* 1124739.

Blackie, L. E. R., & Cozzolino, P. J. (2011). Of blood and death: A test of dual-existential systems in the context of prosocial intentions. *Psychological Science, 22,* 998–1000.

Blackie, L. E., Cozzolino, P. J., & Sedikides, C. (2016). Specific and individuated death reflection fosters identity integration. *PLOS One, 11*(5), e0154873.

Bush, N. E. (1983). The near-death experience in children: Shades of the prison-house reopening. *Anabiosis: Journal of Near-Death Studies, 3*(2), 177–193.

Bush, N. E. (2009). Distressing Western near-death experiences: Finding a way through the abyss. In J. M. Holden, B. Greyson, & D. James (Eds.), *The handbook of near-death experiences: Thirty years of investigation* (pp. 63–86). Praeger/ABC-CLIO.

Carr, D. B. (1981). Endorphins at the approach of death. *Lancet, 1,* 390.

Carr, D. B. (1982). Pathophysiology of stress-induced limbic lobe dysfunction: A hypothesis for NDEs. *Anabiosis: Journal of Near-Death Studies, 2,* 75–89.

Carpentier, N., & Van Brussel, L. (2012). On the contingency of death: A discourse-theoretical perspective on the construction of death. *Critical Discourse Studies, 9*(2), 99–115.

Cassol, H., Martial, C., Annen, J., Martens, G., Charland-Verville, V., Majerus, S., & Laureys, S. (2019). A systematic analysis of distressing near-death experience accounts. *Memory, 27,* 1122–1129.

Cassol, H., Petre, B., Degrange, S., Martial, C., Charland-Verville, V., Lallier, F., . . . Laureys, S. (2018). Qualitative thematic analysis of the phenomenology of near-death experiences. *PLOS One, 13*(2), e0193001.

Chaplin, S. (2000). *The psychology of time and death.* Sonnet Press.

Charland-Verville, V., Jourdain, J.-P., Thonnard, M., Ledoux, D., Donneau, A.-F., Quertemont, E., & Laureys, S. (2014). Near-death experi-

ences in non-life-threatening events and coma of different etiologies. *Frontiers in Human Neuroscience, 8*(203), 1–8.
Cobcroft, M. D., & Forsdick, C. (1993). Awareness under anesthesia: The patients' point of view. *Anaesthesia and Intensive Care, 21,* 837–843.
Corazza, O., & Schifano, F. (2010). Near-death states reported in a sample of 50 misusers. *Substance Use and Misuse, 45*(6), 916–924.
Cozzolino, P. J. (2006). Death contemplation, growth, and defense: Converging evidence of dual-existential systems? *Psychological Inquiry, 17,* 278–287.
Cozzolino, P. J., Staples, A. D., Meyers, L. S., & Samboceti, J. (2004). Greed, death, and values: From terror management to transcendence management theory. *Personality and Social Psychology Bulletin, 30,* 278–292.
Cramer P. (2015). Understanding defense mechanisms. *Psychodynamic Psychiatry, 43*(4), 523–552.
Damasio, A. (2012). *Self comes to mind: Constructing the conscious brain.* Vintage.
Dechesne, M., Pyszczynski, T., Arndt, J., Ransom, S., Sheldon, K. M., Van Knippenberg, A., & Janssen, J. (2003). Literal and symbolic immortality: The effect of evidence of literal immortality on self-esteem striving in response to mortality salience. *Journal of Personality and Social Psychology, 84*(4), 722.
Egger, V. (1896). Le moi des mourants. *Revue Philosophique de la France et de 'Étranger, 21,* 26–38.
Facco, E., & Agrillo, C. (2012). Near-death-like experiences without life-threatening conditions or brain disorders: A hypothesis from a case report. *Frontiers in Psychology, 3,* 490.
Facco, E., Casiglia, E., Al Khafaji, B. E., Finatti, F., Duma, G. M., Mento, G., . . . Tressoldi, P. (2019). The neurophenomenology of out-of-body experiences induced by hypnotic suggestions. *International Journal of Clinical and Experimental Hypnosis, 67*(1), 39–68.
Ferrara Carunchio, B., & de Oliveira Maraldi, E. (2020). A survey of near-death experiences in Brazil: Exploring socio-demographic characteristics and relationship to psychopathology and mystical experiences. *Études Sur la Mort, 153,* 89–103.
Flynn, C. P. (1986). *After the beyond: Human transformation and the near-death experience.* Prentice Hall Direct.
Frias, A., Watkins, P. C., Webber, A. C., & Froh, J. J. (2011). Death and gratitude: Death reflection enhances gratitude. *Journal of Positive Psychology, 6,* 154–162.
Friedman, M. (2008). Religious fundamentalism and responses to mortality salience: A quantitative text analysis. *International Journal for the Psychology of Religion, 18,* 216–237.
Fritz, P., Lejeune, N., Cardone, P., Gosseries, O., & Martial, C. (2024). Bridging the gap: (A) typical psychedelic and near-death experience insights. *Current Opinion in Behavioral Sciences, 55,* 101349.
Ghasemiannejad Jahromi, A. (2021). The aftereffects of near-death experiences on the lives of near-death experiencers: A qualitative study. *Journal of Qualitative Research in Health Sciences, 10*(2), 83–91.
Ghasemiannejad Jahromi, A., & Long, J. (2021). The phenomenology of Iranian near-death experiences. *Journal of Near-Death Studies, 38*(3), 180–200.
Ghasemiannejad Jahromi, A., Qaderi Bagajan, K., Jamshidi, B., & Zakiei, A. (2023). Effects of knowledge of near-death experiences (NDEs) on life changes in people without NDEs. *OMEGA: Journal of Death and Dying.*
Ghoneim, M. M., & Block, R. I. (1992). Learning and consciousness during general anesthesia. *Anesthesiology, 76,* 279–305.
Ghoneim, M. M., & Block, R. I. (1997). Learning and memory during general anesthesia: An update. *Anesthesiology, 87,* 387–410.
Greenberg, J., Arndt, J., Simon, L., Pyszczynski, T., & Solomon, S. (2000). Proximal and distal defenses in response to reminders of one's mortality: Evidence of a temporal sequence. *Personality and Social Psychology Bulletin, 26,* 91–99.
Greenberg, J., Pyszczynski, T. & Solomon, S. (1986). The causes and consequences of the need for self-esteem: A terror management theory. In R. F. Baumeister (Ed.), *Public self and private self* (pp. 189–212). Springer-Verlag.
Greyson, B. (1983). The Near-Death Experience scale: Construction, reliability, and validity. *Journal of Nervous and Mental Disease, 171,* 369–375.
Greyson, B. (2000). Dissociation in people who have near-death experiences: Out of their bodies or out of their minds? *Lancet, 355,* 460–463.
Greyson, B. (2003). Incidence and correlates of near-death experiences in a cardiac care unit. *General Hospital Psychiatry, 25,* 269–276.
Greyson, B. (2007). Near-death experiences: Clinical applications. *Revista de Psiqiatria Clínica, 34,* 49–57.
Greyson, B. (2009). Explanatory models for near-death experiences. In J. M. Holden, B. Greyson, & D. James (Eds.), *The handbook of near-death experiences: Thirty years of investigation* (pp. 213–234). Praeger/ABC-CLIO.

Greyson, B. (2010a). Implications of near-death experiences for a postmaterialist psychology. *Psychology of Religion and Spirituality, 2*, 37–45.

Greyson, B. (2010b). Seeing deceased persons not known to have died: "Peak in Darien" experiences. *Anthropology and Humanism, 35*(2), 159–171.

Greyson, B. (2014). Differentiating spiritual and psychotic experiences: Sometimes a cigar is just a cigar. *Journal of Near-Death Studies, 32*, 123–136.

Greyson, B. (2021a). *After: A doctor explores what near-death experiences reveal about life and beyond*. Macmillan.

Greyson, B. (2021b). Near-death experiences. In E. F. Kelly & P. Marshall (Eds.), *Consciousness unbound: Liberating mind from the tyranny of materialism* (pp. 17–56). Rowman & Littlefield.

Greyson, B. (2022). Persistence of attitude changes after near-death experiences: Do they fade over time? *Journal of Nervous and Mental Disease, 210*(9), 692–696.

Greyson, B. (2023). The darker side of near-death experiences. *Journal of Scientific Exploration, 37*(4), 683–698.

Greyson, B., & Khanna, S. (2014). Spiritual transformation after near-death experiences. *Spirituality in Clinical Practice, 1*(1), 43–55.

Greyson, B., & Liester, M. B. (2004). Internal voices following near-death experiences. *Journal of Humanistic Psychology, 44*, 320–336.

Greyson, B., Mitchell B., Liester, M., Monument, C., Kinsey, L., Alsum, S., & Fox, G. (2015). Electromagnetic phenomena reported by near-death experiencers. *Journal of Near-Death Studies, 33*, 213–243.

Grossberg, S. (2021). *Conscious mind, resonant brain: How each brain makes a mind*. Oxford University Press.

Guevara, P., & Sotelo, J. (1997). Could endorphins participate in the limbic pathways responsible for NDEs after acute cerebral hypoxia? *Journal of Near-Death Studies, 15*(3), 225–226.

Hashemi, A., Oroojan, A. A., Rassouli, M., & Ashrafizadeh, H. (2023). Explanation of near-death experiences: A systematic analysis of case reports and qualitative research. *Frontiers in Psychology, 14*, 1048929.

Heidegger, M. (1962). *Being and time*. Harper & Row.

Jansen, K. (1997a). The ketamine model of the near-death experience: A central role for the N-methyl-D-aspartate receptor. *Journal of Near-Death Studies, 16*, 5–26.

Jansen, K. (1997b). Response to commentaries on "The ketamine model of the near-death experience." *Journal of Near-Death Studies, 16*, 79–95.

Kasser, T., & Sheldon, K. M. (2000). Of wealth and death: Materialism, mortality salience, and consumption behavior. *Psychological Science, 11*, 348–351.

Kelly, E. W. (2001). Near-death experiences with reports of meeting deceased people. *Death Studies, 25*(3), 229–249.

Kelly, E. W., Greyson, B., & Kelly, E. F. (2007). Unusual experiences near death and related phenomena. In E. F. Kelly, E. W. Kelly, A. Crabtree, A. Gauld, M. Grosso, & B. Greyson (Eds.), *Irreducible mind: Toward a psychology for the 21st century* (pp. 367–422). Rowman & Littlefield.

Khanna, S., & Greyson, B. (2014a). Daily spiritual experiences before and after near-death experiences. *Psychology of Religion and Spirituality, 6*(4), 302–309.

Khanna, S., & Greyson, B. (2014b). Near-death experiences and spiritual well-being. *Journal of Religion and Health, 53*(6), 1605–1615.

Klemm, W. R. (2014). *Mental biology: The new science of how the brain and mind relate*. Prometheus.

Kondziella, D., & Martial, C. (2022). Response to: Near-death experiences and the importance of transparency in subjectivity, ontology and epistemology. *Brain Communications, 4*(1), fcab305.

Kosloff, S., & Greenberg, J. (2009). Pearls in the desert: Death reminders provoke immediate derogation of extrinsic goals, but delayed inflation. *Journal of Experimental Social Psychology, 45*, 197–203.

Lindsay, N., O'Sullivan, L., Gibson, R., Ladyman, C., & Tassell-Matamua, N. (2023). Near-death experiences and sleep disturbance: An exploratory study using wrist actigraphy. *Journal of Nervous and Mental Disease, 211*(11), 856–861.

Lindsay, N., & Tassell-Matamua, N. A. (2020). Subjective sleep quality after a near-death experience. *Journal of Near-Death Studies, 38*(2), 65–86.

Lindsay, N., & Tassell-Matamua, N. (2021). Near-death experiences and afterlife belief: A mixed-method analysis. *Psychology of Religion and Spirituality, 13*(3), 304–313.

Marjanen, J., Savinainen, A., & Jouko, S. (2022). *From death to rebirth. Teachings of the Finnish Sage Pekka Ervast*. Literary Society of the Finnish Rosy Cross.

Martial, C., Cassol, H., Charland-Verville, V., Merckelbach, H., & Laureys, S. (2018). Fantasy proneness correlates with the intensity of near-death experience. *Frontiers in Psychiatry, 9*, 190.

Martial, C., Mensen, A., Charland-Verville, V., Vanhaudenhuyse, A., Rentmeister, D., Bahri, M. A., . . . Faymonville, M.-E. (2019). Neurophenomenology of near-death experience memory in hypnotic recall: A within-subject EEG study. *Scientific Report, Fa,* 14047.

Martial, C., Simon, J., Puttaert, N., Gosseries, O., Charland-Verville, V., Nyssen, A. S., . . . Cassol, H. (2020). The Near-Death Experience Content (NDE-C) scale: Development and psychometric validation. *Consciousness and Cognition, 86,* 103049.

Michael, P., Luke, D., & Robinson, O. (2023). This is your brain on death: A comparative analysis of near-death experience and subsequent 5-methoxy-DMT experience. *Frontiers in Psychology, 14.*

Moody, R. A. (1975). *Life after life.* Mockingbird Books.

Moorjani, A. (2012). *Dying to be me.* Hay House.

Nouri, F. M., & Holden, J. M. (2008). Electromagnetic aftereffects of near-death experiences. *Journal of Near-Death Studies, 27,* 83–110.

Noyes, R., & Kletti, R. (1977). Depersonalization in response to life-threatening danger. *Comprehensive Psychiatry, 18*(4), 375–384.

Parnia, S., Waller, D. G., Yeates, R., & Fenwick, P. (2001). A qualitative and quantitative study of the incidence, features and aetiology of near death experiences in cardiac arrest survivors. *Resuscitation, 48,* 149–156.

Parnia, S., Keshavarz Shirazi, T., Patel, J., Tran, L., Sinha, N., O'Neill, C., . . . Deakin, C. D. (2023). AWAreness during Resuscitation—II: A multi-center study of consciousness and awareness in cardiac arrest. *Resuscitation, 191,* 109903.

Parnia, S., Post, S. G., Lee, M. T., Lyubomirsky, S., Aufderheide, T. P., Deakin, C. D., . . . Shirazi, T. K. (2022). Guidelines and standards for the study of death and recalled experiences of death—A multidisciplinary consensus statement and proposed future directions. *Annals of the New York Academy of Sciences, 1511*(1), 5–21.

Parnia, S., Spearpoint, K., de Vos, G., Fenwick, P., Goldberg, D., Yang, J., . . . Schoenfeld, E. R. (2014). AWARE—AWAreness during REsuscitation—A prospective study. *Resuscitation, 85(12),* 1799–1805.

Pehlivanova, M., Carroll, A., & Greyson, B. (2022). Which near-death experience features are associated with reduced fear of death? *Mortality.*

Peinkhofer, C., Martial, C., Cassol, H., Laureys, S., & Kondziella, D. (2021). The evolutionary origin of near-death experiences: A systematic investigation. *Brain Communications, 3*(3), fcab132.

Pyszczynski, T., Abdollahi, A., Solomon, S., Greenberg, J., Cohen, F., & Weise, D. (2006). Mortality salience, martyrdom, and military might: The great Satan versus the axis of evil. *Personality and Social Psychology Bulletin, 32,* 525–537.

Ring, K. (1980). *Life at death: A scientific investigation of the near-death experience.* Coward, McCann & Geohegan.

Ring, K. (1984). *Heading toward omega: In search of the meaning of the near-death experience.* William Morrow.

Ring, K., & Elsaesser-Valarino, E. (1998). *Lessons from the light: What we can learn from the near-death experience.* Moment Point Press.

Rivas, T., & Smit, R. H. (2013). A near-death experience with veridical perception described by a famous heart surgeon and confirmed by his assistant surgeon. *Journal of Near-Death Studies, 31*(3), 179–186.

Roehrs, P., Fenwick, P., Greyson, B., Kellehear, A., Kothe, K., Nahm, M., . . . Woollacott, M. (2023). Terminal lucidity in a pediatric oncology clinic. *Journal of Nervous and Mental Disease.*

Sabom, M. B. (1982). *Recollections of death: A medical investigation.* Harper & Row.

Sabom, M. B. (1998). *Light and death.* Zondervan.

Sartori, P., Badham, P., & Fenwick, P. (2006). A prospectively studied near-death experience with corroborated out-of-body perceptions and unexplained healing. *Journal of Near-Death Studies, 25*(2), 69–84.

Schimel, J., Simon, L., Greenberg, J., Pyszczynski, T., Solomon, S., Waxmonski, J., & Arndt, J. (1999). Support for a functional perspective on stereotypes: Evidence that mortality salience enhances stereotypic thinking and preferences. *Journal of Personality and Social Psychology, 77,* 905–926.

Schroter-Kunhardt, M. (1993). A review of near death experiences. *Journal of Scientific Exploration, 7,* 219–239.

Schwaninger, J., Eisenberg, P. R., Schechtman, K. B., & Weiss, A. N. (2002). A prospective analysis of near-death experiences in cardiac arrest patients. *Journal of Near-Death Studies, 20,* 215–232.

Serdehaly, W. J. (1991). A comparison of retrospective accounts of childhood near-death experiences with contemporary pediatric near-death experience accounts. *Journal of Near-Death Studies, 9*(4), 219–224.

Shulman, R. G., Hyder, F., & Rothman, D. L. (2003). Cerebral metabolism and consciousness. *Compets Rendus Biologies, 326,* 253–273.

Shushan, G. (2011). *Conceptions of the afterlife in early civilizations: Universalism, constructivism, and near-death experience.* Bloomsbury.

Shushan, G. (2012). *Near-death experience and the origins of afterlife beliefs.* YouTube. www.youtube.com/watch?v=QVeoV14J2dY.

Smit, R. H. (2008). Corroboration of the dentures anecdote involving veridical perception in a near-death experience. *Journal of Near-Death Studies, 27*(1), 47–61.

Stout, Y. M., Jacquin, L. A., & Atwater, P. M. H. (2006). Six major challenges faced by near-death experiencers. *Journal of Near-Death Studies, 25*(1), 49–62.

Sutherland, C. (1989). Psychic phenomena following near-death experiences: An Australian study. *Journal of Near Death Studies, 8*(2), 93–102.

Sutherland, C. (1990). Changes in religious beliefs, attitudes, and practices following near-death experiences: An Australian study. *Journal of Near-Death Studies, 9*(1), 21–31.

Tassell-Matamua, N. (2013). Phenomenology of near-death experiences: An analysis of a Māori case study. *Journal of Near-Death Studies, 32,* 107–117.

Tassell-Matamua, N. A. (2025). Power and privilege in the study of near-death experiences. In B. Flanagan & K. Clough (Eds.), *The Routledge handbook of research methods in spirituality and contemplative studies* (pp. 271–282). Routledge.

Tassell-Matamua, N. A., & Holden, J. M. (2020). Near-death experiences: The mystical–feeling of "crossing over" and its impact on faith and spirituality. In K. E. Vail, III & C. Routledge (Eds.), *The science of religion, spirituality and existentialism* (pp. 51–66). Elsevier.

Tassell-Matamua, N. A., & Lindsay, N. (2016). "I'm not afraid to die": The loss of the fear of death after a near-death experience. *Mortality, 21*(1), 71–87.

Tassell-Matamua, N. A., Lindsay, N., Bennett, S., Valentine, H., & Pahina, J. (2017). Does learning about near-death experiences promote psycho-spiritual benefits in those who have not had a near-death experience? *Journal of Spirituality in Mental Health, 19(2),* 95–115.

Tassell-Matamua, N. A., & Steadman, K. L. (2017). I feel more spiritual: Increased spirituality after a near-death experience. *Journal for the Study of Spirituality, 7*(1), 35–49.

Thomas, D., & O'Conner, G. (2023). Exploring near death experiences with children post-intensive care: A case series. *EXPLORE.*

Thonnard, M., Charland-Verville, V., Brédart, S., Dehon, H., Ledoux, D., Laureys, S., & Vanhaudenhuyse, A. (2013). Characteristics of near-death experiences memories as compared to real and imagined events memories. *PLOS One, 8*(3), e57620.

Timmermann, C., Roseman, L., Williams, L., Erritzoe, D., Martial, C., Cassol, H., . . . Carhart-Harris, R. (2018). DMT models the near-death experience. *Frontiers in Psychology, 9,* 1424.

VandenBos, G. (Ed.). (2015). *American Psychological Association dictionary of psychology* (2nd ed.). American Psychological Association.

van Lommel, P. (2006). Near-death experience, consciousness, and the brain: A new concept about the continuity of our consciousness based on recent scientific research on near-death experience in survivors of cardiac arrest. *World Futures, 62,* 134–151.

van Lommel, P. (2010). *Consciousness beyond life: The science of the near-death experience.* HarperCollins.

van Lommel, P. (2013). Non-local consciousness: A concept based on scientific research on near-death experiences during cardiac arrest. *Journal of Consciousness Studies, 20,* 7–48.

van Lommel, P., & Greyson, B. (2023). Invited commentary: Critique of recent report of electrical activity in the dying human brain. *Journal of Near-Death Studies, 41*(1), 3–8.

van Lommel, P., van Wees, R., Meyers, V., & Elferrich, I. (2001). Near death experience in survivors of cardiac arrest: A prospective study in the Netherlands. *Lancet, 358,* 2039–2045.

White, N. S., & Alkire, M. T. (2003). Impaired thalamocortical connectivity in humans during general-anesthetic-induced unconsciousness. *NeuroImage, 19,* 402–411.

Xu, G., Mihaylova, T., Li, D., & Borjigin, J. (2023). Surge of neurophysiological coupling of gamma oscillations in the dying human brain. *Proceedings of the National Academy of Sciences, 120*(19), e2216268120.

Yalom, I. D. (1980). *Existential psychotherapy.* Basic Books.

Zingrone, N. L., & Alvarado, C. S. (2009). Pleasurable Western adult near-death experiences: Features, circumstances, and incidence. In J. M. Holden, B. Greyson, & D. James (Eds.), *The handbook of near-death experiences: Thirty years of investigation* (pp. 17–40). Praeger/ABC-CLIO.

CHAPTER 9

Death Anxiety and Mental Health

Rachel E. Menzies

The awareness of death is a universal aspect of human existence (Yalom, 2008). By the end of the first decade of life, most children have developed a complete understanding of death's inevitability and irreversibility (Menzies & Menzies, 2018). Each of us must then continue into adulthood with the knowledge of our own eventual demise. The numerous ways in which humans attempt to grapple with this fear have been explained through theoretical frameworks such as terror management theory (TMT; see, e.g., Greenberg, 2012). TMT outlines the buffers with which humans are equipped (i.e., cultural worldviews and self-esteem), allowing us to function and thrive despite our awareness of our own mortality.

In line with this, many people may use adaptive strategies to cope with death anxiety (e.g., bolstering self-worth or pursuing activities that will offer a sense of meaning in life). However, some may instead rely on maladaptive behaviors, such as avoidance or excessive efforts to prevent death (Yalom, 2008). As a result, death anxiety has been argued to be a transdiagnostic construct, underlying the development of a range of mental health problems (Iverach et al., 2014). How might death anxiety underlie mental illnesses? According to TMT, ineffective anxiety buffers may lead a person to have a psychological vulnerability to the fear of death (Maxfield et al., 2014). Such buffers may be impacted by a variety of causes, including genetic predispositions, stressful life events, or insecure attachment styles. Psychopathology has similarly been viewed as a maladaptive attempt to cope with the fear of death, such as by distilling broad existential dread into specific feared objects (e.g., germs or spiders; Strachan et al., 2007).

Iverach and colleagues (2014) argued that death anxiety may therefore underlie the "revolving door" of mental illnesses. That is, it is a common clinical observation that an individual may experience various disorders across their lifespan. For example, a person may experience separation anxiety as a child, before developing obsessive–compulsive disorder (OCD) as an adolescent (for which they may receive successful treatment), before later returning to treatment in adulthood with health anxiety. This clinical observation has been supported by growing empirical data. A meta-analysis of 27 studies revealed that, on average, an individual will experience *twice* the number of disorders across their life as they have at present (Menzies et al., 2024b). For instance, a person who is currently suffering from two disorders will have previously experienced (and recovered from) an additional two different disorders earlier in their life. These findings highlight the importance of identifying key causal mechanisms that may underpin the development of these manifestly differently conditions, of which death anxiety is one promising candidate.

If death anxiety underpins psychopathology, one would expect the fear of death to be closely linked with symptoms of mental illnesses. A body of research has revealed relationships consistent with this. One meta-analysis of 99 studies demonstrated that, on average, there is a moderate correlation between death anxiety and symptoms of psychopathology (Menzies et al., 2024a). In addition, across 11 studies using experimental designs, death anxiety had a moderate impact on clinically relevant behaviors. This meta-analytic finding suggests that the fear of death is playing a *causal* role, by driving symptoms of certain disorders (Menzies et al., 2024a). Not only has death anxiety been implicated in one's current mental health concerns, so too has it been shown to predict mental health across the lifespan. For example, individuals with high levels of death anxiety have been shown to experience greater numbers of mental illnesses across the lifespan; a finding that remains significant after controlling for potential confounds such as neuroticism (Menzies et al., 2019).

Death anxiety has therefore been linked to broad psychological distress and high rates of disorders. To what extent does the fear of death contribute to individual mental health diagnoses? Is its impact universal across psychopathology, or do certain disorders appear uniquely relevant to the dread of death?

ANXIETY DISORDERS

Anxiety disorders have been linked to fears of death for close to a century (e.g., Kingman, 1928). While this notion remained largely speculative for most of the 20th century, growing research has revealed the role of death anxiety in driving and maintaining a range of anxiety disorders.

Specific Phobias

Specific phobias have long been theorized to stem from death anxiety (Kingman, 1928). The most common phobic objects (e.g., heights, spiders, snakes) all have the direct potential to cause death, contributing to evolutionary accounts of such phobias as serving a protective function across human history (Zuccala & Menzies, 2022). In addition to this evolutionary perspective, others have argued that phobias may be a result of channeling death anxiety into a more specific and manageable threat that is easier to avoid than death itself (Strachan et al., 2007).

Numerous studies have demonstrated significant relationships between death fears and phobic symptoms. Moderate to large correlations have been found between death anxiety and symptoms of claustrophobia (Menzies et al., 2019) and blood-injury phobia (de Jong & Merckelbach, 1998). Furthermore, symptoms of spider phobia and height phobia are predicted by the patient's estimated likelihood of a fatal bite or fall, respectively (Jones & Menzies, 2000; Menzies & Clarke, 1995). That is, patients who believed a spider bite was more likely to result in death showed greater avoidance of spiders in the laboratory. In one mortality salience study, Strachan and colleagues (2007) demonstrated that spider phobics who were primed with death showed greater avoidance of spider-related stimuli and greater estimates of threat (i.e., higher perceived likelihood of a fatal bite). Such findings offer strong support for the causal role of death anxiety in specific phobias, at least in relation to spider phobias and the fear of heights.

Agoraphobia and Separation Anxiety

Agoraphobia is characterized by fear and avoidance of places that might cause panic or in which escape might be difficult (American Psychiatric Association, 2022). Symptoms of agoraphobia typically include catastrophic beliefs about danger (e.g., that harm will befall the individual if they leave the home) in addition to hypochondriacal concerns, suggesting the potential relevance of death anxiety (Foa et al., 1984; Furer et al., 1997). Furthermore, the onset of this disorder is often preceded by an experience of loss or physical threat, such as illness or the death of a family member (Foa et al., 1984). Consistent with this, strong correlations have been found between death anxiety and agoraphobia (Menzies et al., 2019).

Separation anxiety has been similarly linked to death anxiety. This disorder is characterized by fear of being separated from attachment figures and caregivers, and persistent worry about losing them, including through death (American Psychiatric Association, 2022). Correlational studies have demonstrated significant links between death anxiety and separation anxiety both in student samples (Caras, 1995) and in samples of people with agoraphobia (Fleischer-Mann, 1995). In borderline and schizophrenic patients, Walser (1984) observed strong interrelationships between death anxiety and separation anxiety, concluding that the latter may in fact mask the former. However, at present, no experimental studies have been conducted to examine whether death anxiety may play a causal role in agoraphobia or separation anxiety disorder.

Social Anxiety

While social anxiety may not seem directly relevant to death anxiety, evolutionary perspectives may shed some light on their potential connection. Fear of negative evaluation, which characterizes social anxiety, has been argued to stem from mortality concerns (Zuccala & Abbott, 2021). In our species' early evolutionary history, being judged negatively by peers and consequently rejected by our tribe would have heightened the individual's risk of premature death. As a result, social anxiety may have served a protective function against death, similar to that of specific phobias.

Numerous studies have now supported the relationship between death anxiety and social anxiety, with strong positive correlations found between the two constructs (e.g., Lowe & Harris, 2019; Menzies et al., 2019; Zuccala et al., 2021). Death anxiety has also been shown to have a causal impact on social anxiety symptoms. For example, Strachan and colleagues (2007) demonstrated that mortality salience increases avoidance of a staged group discussion among students high in social anxiety. Finch and colleagues (2016) used an eye-tracking procedure to examine the role of death anxiety in attentional biases characterizing social anxiety. Among socially anxious participants, death reminders increased vigilance toward social threat, indicated by heightened initial bias toward angry facial expressions.

Taken together, these two studies suggest that death anxiety underlies two key maintaining factors in social anxiety: social avoidance and attentional biases to social threat. However, Zuccala and Abbott (2021) found somewhat conflicting findings. In a sample of participants diagnosed with social anxiety, mortality salience failed to produce differences in self-reported anxiety surrounding a public-speaking task. While the authors concluded that death anxiety may therefore not underlie social anxiety, the reliance on self-reported measures (in contrast to behavioral measures) may offer another explanation for these findings. Meta-analytic studies have suggested that the impact of mortality salience on clinically relevant symptoms may be greater for covertly measured behavioral symptoms (e.g., avoidance) rather than self-reported symptoms (Menzies et al., 2024b). This may explain the absence of findings concerning self-reported measures of social anxiety. In any case, given the more ambiguous theoretical relationship between death anxiety and social anxiety, this disorder warrants further investigation.

Panic Disorder

Panic disorder, characterized by hypervigilance to and catastrophic interpretations of bodily sensations, has been argued to stem from death anxiety (Furer et al., 1997). For example, patients with panic disorder commonly worry that their chest sensations may be a sign of a heart attack, requesting specialist appointments and medical investigation. Consistent with this, large correlations have been found between panic disorder symptoms and death anxiety (Menzies et al., 2019, 2021a). In one experimental study, Menzies and colleagues (2021a) utilized a sample of patients with a "scanning" disorder (i.e., a disorder in which patients typically "scan" their body for symptoms of illness). Nearly half of this group consisted of patients diagnosed with panic disorder. Among these patients, mortality salience increased behaviors relevant to panic disorder, including time spent checking one's body for symptoms, tendency to view symptoms as threatening, and intention to visit a doctor. Thus, death anxiety appears to play a causal role in panic disorder symptoms, supporting arguments in favor of targeting death fears directly in the treatment of this disorder (Randall, 2001).

SOMATIC SYMPTOM-RELATED DISORDERS

Many somatic symptom-related disorders have clear links to mortality concerns, with symptoms centering on anxiety around one's physical health (Furer et al., 1997). Similarly to panic disorder, patients with these conditions frequently monitor their body for signs of illness, seek reassurance from others as to their health, and interpret benign sensations as signs of imminent disease. Unsurprisingly, then, symptoms of hypochondriasis have been shown to be correlated with death anxiety (Noyes et al., 2002). Furthermore, patients with hypochondriasis report higher fears of death than healthy controls (Kellner et al., 1987). The condition once known as hypochondriasis was later recategorized into two different disorders: illness anxiety disorder and somatic symptom disorder (American Psychiatric Association, 2013). As one might expect, these more recent diagnoses remain related to death anxiety, showing a similar pattern of relationships between mortality concerns and disorder symptoms (Menzies et al., 2019).

The aforementioned study by Menzies and colleagues (2021a) explored the causal role of death anxiety in somatic symptom-related disorders, in addition to panic disorder. The "scanning disorder" group primarily consisted of patients with a somatic symptom-related disorder; specifically, 68% of this group had either somatic symptom disorder or illness anxiety disorder. As described above, mortality salience increased relevant clinical behavior in these conditions, including checking one's body for symptoms, perceiving benign symptoms as indicative of poorer health, and desire to visit a doctor in the near future (Menzies et al., 2021a). As a result, death anxiety appears to play a strong causal role in at least these two somatic symptom-related disorders, underscoring the need to consider this construct in treatment.

OBSESSIVE–COMPULSIVE AND RELATED DISORDERS

The diagnostic category of obsessive–compulsive disorder (OCD) and related disorders has attracted the most research regarding the role of death anxiety. Menzies and colleagues (2015) argued that death anxiety may underpin most presentations of OCD. For example, contamination concerns are typically dominated by compulsive attempts to prevent serious illnesses, such as HIV (Jones & Krochmalik, 2003). In patients with the checking subtype of OCD, the compulsive checking of power outlets, stoves, and locks are often attempts to prevent electrocution, fires, and home invasion (Vaccaro et al., 2010). In the aggressive obsessions, immense distress is caused by the belief that one may harm or kill oneself or another (see, e.g., Chawla et al., 2022). In other presentations, a person with OCD may carry out magical rituals and/or engage in counting or tapping compulsions in the belief that doing so will keep them or their loved ones safe from harm (Menzies et al., 2015).

A number of studies have supported the direct link between mortality concerns and OCD symptoms. In a treatment-seeking clinical sample, Menzies and colleagues (2020) revealed that death anxiety was significantly correlated with the severity of all six symptom domains of OCD, that is, contamination, checking, obsessions, hoarding, indecisiveness, and "just right" experiences. In addition, death anxiety has been shown to predict the trajectory toward OCD; specifically, patients with higher death anxiety were more likely to experience a higher number of disorders prior to developing OCD (Menzies et al., 2021c). By contrast, patients with lower death anxiety were more likely to develop OCD as their first disorder, leading authors to speculate whether certain OCD-specific concerns (e.g., sexual obsessions) may not be associated with death at all. This explanation was later bolstered by Chawla and colleagues (2022), who found that sexual obsessions in OCD were uniquely explained by other existential concerns (e.g., guilt, identity, and meaninglessness), but not death anxiety. On the other hand, death anxiety remained the sole existential concern to significantly predict aggressive obsessions, after controlling for relevant confounds.

Experimental findings have lent further support for the potentially causal role of death anxiety in OCD. First, Strachan and colleagues (2007) used a mortality salience design in students who scored high or low on a measure of handwashing frequency. They found that among the group high in washing, reminders of death led to a significant increase in handwashing behavior in the laboratory, highlighting the role of death anxiety in driving compulsive washing. This was later replicated and extended in a study involving treatment-seeking patients diagnosed with OCD (Menzies & Dar-Nimrod, 2017). In this study, a sample of OCD patients was categorized as either having the contamination subtype of OCD, or another subtype of this disorder (e.g., compulsive checking). Menzies and Dar-Nimrod (2017) found that mortality salience led those with contamination-based OCD to spend twice as long washing their hands, as well as using significantly more soap and paper towels. Notably, for the group who had other subtypes of OCD, no increase in washing behavior was observed following the death reminder. Thus, death anxiety has been repeatedly shown to play a causal role in the contamination subtype of OCD. However, it remains to be seen whether its role in compulsive washing generalizes to behaviors in other subtypes of OCD.

Body Dysmorphic Disorder

A handful of studies have explored death anxiety in other obsessive–compulsive and related disorders, such as body dysmorphic disorder (BDD). Death anxiety has been shown to be significantly correlated with BDD symptoms, both in clinical (Menzies et al., 2019) and community samples (Menzies et al., 2023). In a subsample of men who scored in the clinical range for muscle dysmorphia (a subtype of BDD), mortality salience increased relevant behaviors, including selecting larger food portions (consistent with trying to gain muscle mass) and reporting having exercised more (Menzies et al., 2023). These effects were not found in men who reported low levels of muscle dysmorphia symptoms.

Hoarding Disorder

Hoarding disorder is another related condition in which death anxiety has been explored. This condition is characterized by a strong emotional attachment to possessions and difficulty discarding them, leading to an accumulation of clutter in the home (American Psychiatric Association, 2022). Why might mortality concerns drive hoarding behaviors? Frost and Steketee (2011) noted that many people with hoarding disorder view their accumulated possessions as an "attempt to achieve immortality—to produce something that would outlive [them]" (p. 105), and "a legacy to pass on to their heirs or even the world" (p. 55). Hoarding has also been conceptualized as a direct response to loss. People who hoard are significantly more likely to have experienced either the death of a family member (Sanchez et al., 2023) and hospitalization or serious illness earlier in their life (Hartl et al., 2005), compared to healthy controls. In another study, a loss or death was the most common singular event identified to trigger the onset of hoarding behavior (Frost & Steketee, 2011).

Two studies demonstrated a significant correlation between death anxiety and hoarding severity, including one in a clinical treatment-seeking sample (Brown & Menzies, 2025; Menzies et al., 2020). Only one experimental study has been conducted thus far with an explicit focus on hoarding. Brown and Menzies (2025) examined this question in a community sample. Their findings indicated that mortality salience did not influence any of the hoarding-related symptoms in the overall sample (i.e., intent to acquire new items, intent to discard items, and attachment to objects; Brown & Menzies, 2025). This finding raises the question of whether death anxiety may not be as relevant to hoarding disorder as theorized. Given the body of qualitative and quantitative cross-sectional research suggesting a relationship between mortality concerns and hoarding behaviors, further research may be needed, using treatment-seeking samples with a formal diagnosis of hoarding disorder, to elucidate this relationship.

TRAUMA-RELATED DISORDERS

The fear of death has been argued to relate in various ways to the etiology and maintenance of trauma-related disorders, including posttraumatic stress disorder (PTSD). The first diagnostic criterion for PTSD centers on exposure to actual or perceived threat of death (American Psychiatric Association, 2022). That is, a person's perception that the traumatic event may have resulted in their own death or the death of another person is viewed as a fundamental cause of PTSD. In fact, it is this etiological event, revolving around confrontation with death, which distinguishes PTSD from other mental health conditions and their symptoms. Meta-analytic studies have shown that the degree to which one perceives a threat to their life is a significant predictor of PTSD symptoms (Karima et al., 2023), further highlighting the central role of death in this disorder.

Second, such life-threatening events have been argued to heighten fear of death, leading PTSD symptoms to emerge (Cheung et al., 2005). Third, building upon TMT, anxiety-buffer disruption theory (Pyszczynski & Kesebir, 2011) proposes that PTSD is the consequence of disrupted anxiety buffers (e.g., self-esteem and cultural worldviews), leaving the individual vulnerable to death anxiety (Kesebir et al., 2011; Maxfield et al., 2014). The theory also posits that fragile preexisting buffers (e.g., strength of one's meaning-providing worldview, self-esteem, and close relationships) predispose people to this disruption in response to traumatic events.

Consistent with this, death anxiety is strongly correlated with severity of PTSD symptoms in groups such as veterans (Martz, 2004) and earthquake survivors (Abdollahi et al., 2011). In addition, in a study of people exposed to military operations, death anxiety was found to explain an additional 40.4% of variance in PTSD symptoms (Ron, 2015). Showing support for the anxiety-buffer disruption theory, Chatard and colleagues (2012) investigated responses to mortality salience in individuals with PTSD following a civil war. They found that for participants with high levels of PTSD symptoms, death primes increased the accessibility of death thoughts. On the other hand, no such effect was found for participants with low levels of PTSD symptoms. These findings suggest that buffers among individuals with PTSD may be impaired, leaving them unable to effectively suppress thoughts of death following a life-threatening event. Similarly, Vail and colleagues (2018) demonstrated that among participants with low PTSD symptoms, engaging in buffers such as self-affirmation prevented death reminders from increasing death-thought accessibility. By contrast, for people with high PTSD symptoms, self-affirmation failed to prevent mortality salience from increasing the accessibility of death thoughts. Put simply, PTSD symptoms appear to be associated with ineffective anxiety buffers, which are unable to keep death thoughts at bay.

Despite these promising findings, more research is needed to elucidate the potential causal role of death anxiety in PTSD. Thus far, studies have focused on evaluating the anxiety-buffer disruption theory, relying primarily on death-thought accessibility as the outcome variable. That is, no studies have investigated whether mortality salience impacts relevant *behaviors* in PTSD (e.g., avoidance of trauma-related stimuli), leaving open the question of whether death anxiety does indeed play a causal role in driving symptoms of this disorder.

MOOD DISORDERS

While much of the research thus far has focused on anxiety-related disorders, existential issues have similarly been argued to drive symptoms of mood disorders. For example, the dread of death may contribute to feelings of hopelessness, meaninglessness, and amotivation that characterizes depressive disorders (Ghaemi, 2007; Simon et al., 1998). Consistent with this, depressive symptoms have been shown to be significantly correlated with death anxiety across various populations, including people with chronic physical illnesses (e.g., Miller et al.,

2012; Sharpe et al., 2024) and outpatients with a diagnosed mood disorder (Menzies et al., 2019; Öngider & Özışık Eyüboğlu, 2013).

One experimental study demonstrated that levels of death-thought accessibility (i.e., the degree to which a person is preoccupied with thoughts about death) predicted symptoms of depression (Fairlamb & Juhl, 2022). That is, among participants with low self-worth, completing more death-related words in a word fragment task was significantly associated with depressive symptoms. Such a finding is consistent with thoughts of death being listed as part of the diagnostic criteria for major depressive disorder (American Psychiatric Association, 2022).

Only a handful of experimental studies have been conducted examining mortality salience and depression. Simon and colleagues (1996, 1998) used this paradigm among participants with mild depression. This revealed that mortality salience led to greater worldview defense for this group compared to individuals without depression. Such findings suggest that depressive symptoms may be due to insufficient buffers in the face of death anxiety. In addition, when depressed participants had the opportunity to defend their cultural worldview, they reported increased sense of purpose in life compared to participants who were not given this opportunity. It is therefore possible that endorsing cultural worldviews may help increase meaning in life among people with mild depression.

Finally, Menzies and colleagues (2021) used a mortality salience design with a subsample of outpatients diagnosed with depression. This group demonstrated increased desire to visit a medical specialist following death reminders. This finding suggests that they may have had weaker buffers against death anxiety, therefore driving them to seek reassurance. However, reassurance seeking is not a core behavior characterizing depressive disorders, and it more typically features in anxiety disorders. Thus, the studies conducted so far have not explicitly measured differences in depressive behavior following mortality salience, instead measuring only defensive behaviors or behaviors relevant to other mental health conditions. As a result, further research is needed to examine the degree to which death anxiety drives symptoms of depression.

ADDICTIONS

Problematic substance use has long been argued to stem from death anxiety. Becker (1973) proposed that self-medicating with substances may be an attempt to distract from the knowledge of death, writing that "modern man is drinking and drugging himself out of awareness" (p. 284). In line with this, Wisman and colleagues (2015) proposed the *existential escape hypothesis*. That is, they argued that "escaping" from the self (such as through substance use) is one means of coping with death anxiety, particularly for individuals with lower levels of self-esteem.

A number of studies have explored this possibility in the area of substance use and addictions. For example, among outpatients diagnosed with alcohol use disorder, a large correlation has been found between death anxiety and severity of addiction (Menzies et al., 2019). A series of experimental studies have demonstrated the potential causal role of death anxiety in such substance use problems. Ein-Dor and colleagues (2014) found that participants in the mortality salience condition were three times more likely to purchase an alcoholic drink at a beverage stand. Similarly, reminders of death have been linked to increased willingness to binge drink (Jessop & Wade, 2010) as well as greater consumption of alcohol at a nightclub (Wisman et al., 2015) and of an ostensibly alcoholic beverage in the laboratory (McCabe & Bartholow, 2019). Another study demonstrated that mortality salience increased self-reported cravings for cannabis among frequent cannabis users (Nagar & Rabinovitz, 2015).

Unlike the behaviors that characterize many other mental health problems, such as the avoidance and hypervigilance featured in the anxiety-related conditions described above, behaviors in addictions often increase the individual's risk of death. How might a fear of death account for behaviors that actually increase one's risk of death, such as problematic substance use? Studies from TMT have indicated that when thoughts of death are within conscious awareness, people engage in proximal defenses; that is, suppressing thoughts of death, denying their vulnerability, or choosing to engage in protective health behaviors. However, when thoughts of death are no longer within conscious awareness, proximal defenses are instead engaged; people attempt to defend their cultural worldviews and bolster their self-esteem (Pyszczynski et al., 1999). Thus, if the use of an addictive substance offers a source of self-esteem, a reminder of death may drive an individual to use that substance *more,* after the thoughts of death have slipped out of conscious awareness.

In line with this finding, several studies have demonstrated that when an addictive behavior is a source of self-esteem, death reminders may fail to produce healthy changes in behavior. This has particularly been explored in the context of tobacco use. For example, among participants whose self-esteem is linked to smoking, an antismoking campaign focusing on health consequences had no significant impact on their intention to quit (Martin & Kamins, 2010). Instead, campaigns focusing on the social consequences of addiction (rather than focusing on the risk to one's life) appear to be more beneficial. For example, Arndt and colleagues (2009) found that among participants who sourced self-esteem from smoking, mortality salience increased susceptibility to an antismoking campaign that highlighted negative social impacts of smoking.

It also appears that the impact of death anxiety is not unique to substance addictions. In fact, Rockloff and colleagues (2014) found that among problem gamblers, mortality salience increased urges to gamble. Thus, death anxiety may be a driving force in a range of addictions, including behavioral addictions.

EATING DISORDERS

Eating disorders may initially appear unrelated to death anxiety. This class of disorders have among the highest mortality rates of all mental illnesses, as the severe food restriction that characterizes conditions like anorexia nervosa may lead to life-threatening complications and lifelong medical problems (Farber et al., 2007). For example, the rate of death among people with anorexia nervosa is more than five times that of the general population (Fichter & Quadflieg, 2016).

At first glance, this may suggest that eating disorders are characterized by a *lack* of anxiety about death. While women with eating disorders have been shown to have a preoccupation with death, with high levels of death-related ideation (Farber et al., 2007), one could argue that this is a natural consequence of the higher risk of mortality faced by such women. Similarly, the high levels of death anxiety experienced by women with anorexia nervosa compared to matched controls (Giles, 1996) could again be argued to be a consequence of the eating disorder, as opposed to this fear itself driving the disordered eating.

While not dismissing the potential bidirectional nature of the relationship, why might death anxiety play a causal role in eating disorders? From a TMT perspective, women who experience eating disorders may be striving for the thinness promoted by their cultural worldview. That is, given that the "thin ideal" is a key part of beauty standards for women, aspiring to this ideal may be one way that women can enhance their self-esteem and protect against death anxiety, even if their eating behaviors simultaneously heighten their risk of death (see, e.g., Goldenberg et al., 2005).

In line with this theoretical account, death anxiety has been shown to predict eating disorder symptoms in community samples (Le Marne & Harris, 2016). Most notably, this finding remains significant above and beyond other well-established transdiagnostic constructs in eating disorders, such as self-esteem and perfectionism (Le Marne & Harris, 2016). Exploring the direction of causality more clearly, using a mortality salience design, Goldenberg and colleagues (2005) found that reminders of death led women to select smaller food portions, and to rate themselves as farther from their ideal thinness. This finding was found only for women; the absence of this effect in men adds further weight to the explanation proffered by TMT (i.e., that women are striving for the thin ideal promoted by their culture, an ideal that is irrelevant for men). While this study by Goldenberg and colleagues was conducted in a student sample, the finding was later replicated in a clinically relevant sample of women, of which the majority had previously sought treatment for disordered eating (Forrester et al., 2024).

These experimental findings suggest that death anxiety may be a driver, rather than solely a consequence, of the body dissatisfaction and desire for thinness that characterizes eating disorders. It remains to be seen however if death anxiety may underpin eating disorders that are not characterized by food restriction (e.g., binge-eating disorder). However, given this set of findings and the poor treatment outcomes for this class of disorders, it is worth considering whether death anxiety may be a promising treatment target (van den Berg et al., 2019).

PSYCHOTIC DISORDERS

While psychotic disorders may similarly not appear related to death anxiety, a relationship between the two has been proposed since the 1960s. Searles (1961) argued that delusions of grandeur and omnipotent hallucinations may be one way of coping with one's own insignificance in the face of mortality. It is possible that persecutory delusions may serve an equivalent function. For example, while the belief that one is subject to targeted government surveillance may cause significant distress, it may also provide a sense that one is an important, special, or powerful person, in contrast to the reality of one's actual insignificance.

Only a handful of studies have examined death anxiety in the context of psychosis. Walser (1984) found that people with schizophrenia report significantly higher death anxiety than those without this disorder. Similarly, death anxiety has been shown to be positively correlated with both schizophrenia symptoms (Lonetto & Templer, 1986) and schizotypy (i.e., personality traits associated with the vulnerability for schizophrenia and psychotic-like experiences; Easden et al., 2023). However, more research is needed to elucidate this relationship. Experimental research is particularly needed given that the causal direction may be the reverse. That is, it is equally possible that psychotic symptoms may heighten one's level of death anxiety, rather than the reverse.

PERSONALITY DISORDERS

One domain that has received far less attention in relation to death anxiety is that of personality disorders. Among the studies that do exist, they thus far focus selectively on borderline personality disorder (BPD). In a review of existential issues in BPD, Liu and colleagues (2023) emphasized the lack of research on death anxiety in this condition, relative to other existential constructs such as identity concerns, meaninglessness, and isolation. However, given that many common deficits in BPD are known buffers against death anxiety (e.g., secure relationships, sense of meaning, stable self-worth, all of which are typically diminished in BPD), one could argue that people with BPD may be more vulnerable to mortality concerns.

The two studies that exist appear to support this notion. In a nonclinical community sample, Gershuny and colleagues (2004) reported that BPD symptoms increased alongside self-reported death anxiety. A later study by Menzies and colleagues (2025) examined existential issues among people with a self-reported diagnosis of BPD. They found that death anxiety was elevated among this sample compared to community norms. This finding was replicated in a sample of hospital outpatients who had a confirmed diagnosis of BPD. Furthermore, death anxiety was positively correlated with symptom severity in both of these BPD samples (Menzies et al., 2025). However, more research is needed to examine whether these findings generalize to personality disorders outside of BPD.

CLINICAL IMPLICATIONS

In light of the above research highlighting the central role of death anxiety in mental illness, there have been burgeoning calls to consider this construct in the conceptualization and treatment of psychopathology (Iverach et al., 2014). On the one hand, the recognition of the role of death anxiety in the etiology of certain disorders is not new (e.g., illness anxiety; see, e.g., Furer et al., 2007). However, there is a growing recognition of the need to both assess and directly treat death anxiety in clinical populations. This recognition is reflected in the recent development of self-report scales for specific use among clinical groups, including clinical cutoff thresholds and subscales measuring treatment targets (e.g., Menzies et al., 2022a).

Importantly, current standard treatments do not traditionally address death anxiety. Instead, they typically focus on disputing the patient's fears of particular *causes* of death, rather than death itself (Iverach et al., 2014). For example, in the case of contamination-based OCD, gold-standard treatments may seek to challenge the patient's beliefs about the likelihood of contracting a serious illness through contact with perceived contaminants, in addition to the severity of that illness if it were to occur (Krochmalik et al., 2001). Similarly, for a patient with a phobia of spiders, treatment would center on evaluating the likelihood and danger of being bitten, to reduce the patient's inflated estimate of threat (Choy et al., 2007). In both cases, the reduced estimate of threat could occur either through cognitive interventions (e.g., education about the immune system or nonfatality of spider bites) or through direct learning (e.g., exposure to perceived contaminants or spiders). Regardless of the exact methods used, both treatments would focus on the *proximal* cause of death (e.g., fatal illness or spider bite) rather than addressing the fear of death itself. As a result, while such treatments produce significant improvements in symptoms of the disorder (e.g., reductions in handwashing or spider avoidance), they are unlikely to produce any changes on attitudes to death. This notion is supported by preliminary data suggesting that standard treatments do not produce changes in existential issues, including death anxiety (Menzies et al., 2025).

If standard treatments are failing to address death anxiety, they may also be contributing to the revolving door of psychopathology described above (Menzies et al., 2024b). That is, if death anxiety continues to escape clinical attention, an individual may recover from OCD following disorder-specific treatment, only to later develop a different disorder in the future. Given this, it is vital to identify which treatments may be more effective at targeting death anxiety.

TREATING DEATH ANXIETY

Existential Therapy

A number of treatments have been proposed to ameliorate death anxiety. Since the 1980s, existential therapists have emphasized and sought to target this fear (Yalom, 1980). Yalom (1980) also argued that treating death anxiety should produce improvements in a person's symptoms, consistent with the transdiagnostic argument proposed by Iverach and colleagues (2014). To this end, Yalom (2008) proposed various cognitive strategies for beginning to address mortality concerns. For example, he discussed the concept of "rippling" (i.e., the notion that we continue to influence others after our own death, due to the subtle ways our beliefs, behaviors, or values have shaped those of the people around us during our life). Yalom used rippling as an antidote to fears of one's own transiency and the feelings of meaninglessness and insignificance that can stem from this. In addition, Yalom emphasized the use of various philosophical approaches in order to address fears of death. For example, to address fears of nothingness following death, Yalom discussed the use of the "symmetry" argument from Epicurean philosophy (i.e., the notion that the nonexistence after death will be the same nonexistence we experienced prior to our birth). Furthermore, to encourage a focus on making the most of one's life, rather than fixating on its end, he encouraged Nietzsche's thought experiment about the eternal return, in which an individual is asked to contemplate how they would feel upon discovering that they would be forced to relive each moment of their life over again for all eternity. Lastly, Yalom encouraged consideration of the potential benefits of mortality. Specifically, he argued that "the physicality of death destroys us, but the idea of death saves us." That is, consideration of death can motivate action and allow us to make more authentic and deliberate choices.

Thus, existential therapy offers a number of cognitive approaches for death anxiety, as introduced by Yalom (2008). In particular, it encourages direct examination of beliefs underpinning this fear (e.g., that nonexistence would be unpleasant), in addition to a refocusing on the quality, rather than length, of one's life. While such treatment approaches appear likely to alleviate fear of death, at present no randomized controlled trials (RCTs) have been conducted. Thus, the efficacy of existential therapy on death anxiety is currently unclear.

TMT and Relevant Treatment Components

While not commonly considered in the development and evaluation of clinical interventions, TMT can shed much light on potential treatment targets for ameliorating death anxiety. The past four decades of TMT research have demonstrated that building faith in one's cultural worldview and bolstering one's self-esteem can protect an individual from the dread of death (Pyzczsynski et al., 2015). That is, a sense that one is living a meaningful life, that one is recognized by and connected to others, and that one is a valuable contributor to the world, has been shown repeatedly to be protective against death anxiety. Given this vast body of research (e.g., Burke et al., 2010), it is logical to expect that treatments that deliberately target these buffers may alleviate fears of death.

Consistent with the TMT argument that weakened buffers may leave an individual vulnerable to psychopathology, low self-esteem has been implicated in the development of numerous mental health conditions, including depression, eating disorders, social anxiety, OCD, personality disorders, and more (for review, see Zeigler-Hill, 2011). Self-esteem has increasingly attracted attention as a potential treatment target. Previous studies have revealed the benefits of self-esteem interventions for a range of mental health outcomes, including body image (O'Dea & Abraham, 2000), depression (Waite et al., 2012), and suicidal behaviors (Dat et al., 2022). However, at present, no studies have examined whether interventions targeting self-esteem are beneficial in alleviating death anxiety. Further research is needed to address this question.

By contrast, more research has examined interventions that aim to build a sense of meaning in life. In relation to death anxiety, the majority of existing interventions have been evaluated among people imminently facing death. Interventions that focus on meaning have been purported to have the largest impact on death anxiety among patients with advanced cancer (Grossman et al., 2018). For example, RCTs have demonstrated that group logotherapy (an intervention based on creating meaning) leads to reduced death anxiety relative to a no-treatment control group, among a small sample of cancer patients (e.g., Emafti et al., 2019; Heidary et al., 2023). In particular, meaning-centered psychotherapy has been implemented as both an individual and group-based treatment at end of life (Breitbart, 2002). This treatment aims to build a meaningful interpretation of life, with experiential exercises highlighting one's historical and family legacy, and building connection with nature and art. This treatment has been shown in multiple RCTs to produce significant improvements in outcomes such as desire for hastened death, as well as anxiety, spiritual well-being, quality of life, and sense of meaning, among patients with advanced cancer (Breitbart et al., 2010, 2018).

Similarly, dignity therapy has also been shown to be an effective psychological intervention in end-of-life settings. Dignity therapy guides the individual to reflect on their life and leave behind a physical "life review document" with which to share their story with loved ones. This process enhances the individual's sense of personal significance, their ability to build a meaningful narrative of their life, and through sharing this with others, their connection with friends and family. Dignity therapy has been shown to produce significant improvements in quality of life, spiritual well-being, and depression among patients with a terminal prognosis (Chochinov et al., 2011). In addition, while no studies have yet examined death anxiety specifically, meta-analytic findings indicate the positive effects of dignity therapy on general anxiety (Zhang et al., 2022).

Thus, interventions such as dignity therapy and meaning-centered psychotherapy, which both center on building buffers identified in TMT, have shown promise in addressing existential distress at end of life. However, it remains to be seen whether the effects of such interventions are unique to end-of-life settings and groups without psychiatric diagnoses or whether they generalize to samples of individuals with mental illnesses. While this is currently unclear, the strategies and findings of these interventions are consistent with those found in experimental studies with the general population; that is, that meaning, self-esteem, and close relationships reduce defensive responses and anxious behaviors following reminders of death.

Acceptance and Commitment Therapy

Acceptance and commitment therapy (ACT) has also introduced tasks that may in theory help address death anxiety. For example, ACT encourages the visualization of one's funeral, the writing of one's own eulogy, in addition to one's tombstone inscription (Hayes & Smith, 2005). While such tasks are not explicitly designed to target death anxiety, these components could be beneficial at helping the individual confront this fear. The strong focus on building a meaningful life aligned with one's values could also be argued to help mitigate mortality concerns. Such techniques fit neatly alongside a TMT approach to psychopathology. That is, clarifying one's core values and committing to live by them may be one way of bolstering cultural worldviews, self-esteem, and one's sense of meaning. Thus, ACT interventions may theoretically have a twofold benefit for death anxiety: (1) habituation to (and normalization of) death-related stimuli through written exposure tasks and (2) bolstering of one's buffers through values-driven living, in accordance with TMT.

At present, only a small number of studies have evaluated ACT in relation to death anxiety. These have indeed suggested that ACT produces significant improvements in death anxiety among patients with cancer (Farahi & Khalatbari, 2019) and HIV (Mirzaeidoostan et al., 2019). However, RCTs are lacking, and existing studies have been limited by small sample sizes, and a lack of individuals diagnosed with mental illnesses.

Cognitive-Behavioral Therapy

Cognitive-behavioral therapy (CBT) has also been proposed as a suitable intervention for death anxiety. Such treatments involve (1) identifying and challenging maladaptive beliefs about death (e.g., the belief that dying will be painful or that one would not cope with the death of a loved one) and (2) targeting maladaptive behaviors that are argued to maintain death anxiety (e.g., avoidance; Furer et al., 2007). The majority of studies evaluating CBT treatments have centered on the latter, with a heavy focus on graded exposure therapy (Menzies et al., 2018). These interventions typically involve helping participants systematically face avoided death-related stimuli (e.g., cemeteries or mental images of dying). CBT is arguably the therapy modality that has garnered the most attention in relation to death anxiety, with a number of treatment manuals having been published (Furer et al., 2007; Menzies & Veale, 2022; Menzies et al., 2022b). At present, CBT is the only therapy that has been evaluated in a clinical sample of individuals with mental health diagnoses. Among a small group of participants with a mental disorder, an online self-guided CBT program (*Overcome Death Anxiety*; Menzies et al., 2021b) produced notable improvements in this fear; 90% of completers demonstrated a clinically reliable reduction in at least one facet of death anxiety (Menzies et al., 2023a). However, as of yet, no RCTs have been conducted.

Summary of Treatment Evidence

One meta-analysis has examined RCTs of psychological treatments for death anxiety (Menzies et al., 2018). This revealed that CBT produced significant improvements in this fear compared to control conditions and compared with other treatments. As a result, treatments focusing on CBT are likely to be most efficacious in alleviating death anxiety. However, there are several limitations that warrant attention (see, e.g., Menzies & Menzies, 2022). First, despite the promising findings from RCTs of CBT, none have been conducted among participants with diagnosed mental illnesses. Furthermore, no

RCTs have examined whether treating death anxiety does in fact produce direct improvements in broader mental health, either immediately posttreatment or longitudinally. If death anxiety underpins the "revolving door," as theorized, then one would expect that treatments targeting death anxiety should both (1) reduce the symptoms of an individual's current disorder (e.g., OCD) *and* (2) inoculate the individual against the development of a different disorder in the future. At present, this claim remains untested and largely theoretical. It also remains to be seen whether death anxiety treatments are contraindicated for particular clinical groups, such as those who are suicidal. This is a particularly important question given recent research that suggests that death anxiety may be protective against suicidal intent (Sims et al., 2024).

CONCLUSIONS

In sum, death anxiety appears to be a key transdiagnostic construct across a range of mental health problems, with numerous studies demonstrating its causal role in driving clinical symptoms. Fortunately, death anxiety can be effectively ameliorated through psychological treatments. CBT appears to be most effective (Menzies et al., 2018), although treatment components from other modalities (e.g., ACT, existential psychotherapy) warrant consideration and further evaluation.

Given the strong evidence of the role of death anxiety in driving psychopathology, one would expect that treatment that reduces death anxiety would lead to improvements in relevant mental illnesses. However, further research is sorely needed to examine this possibility. If this theoretical argument is indeed supported, it may offer promising new pathways to addressing the high comorbidity in mental health and reducing the global burden of psychopathology, which is vital given that psychological distress is on the rise in many populations (e.g., Bor et al., 2014; Jorm & Kitchener, 2021). Psychological treatment remains costly and often inaccessible, with a shortage of practitioners resulting in lengthy treatment wait lists, particularly in rural and remote areas (Zinchenko & Hyland, 2021). The development of online death anxiety treatments has ensured that interventions for this important construct will be scalable, cost-effective, and accessible worldwide (Menzies et al., 2023a). It remains to be seen whether such interventions do indeed produce long-term improvements above and beyond standard treatments, offering some hope at abating the revolving door of mental illness.

REFERENCES

Abdollahi, A., Pyszczynski, T., Maxfield, M., & Lusyszczynska, A. (2011). Posttraumatic stress reactions as a disruption in anxiety-buffer functioning: Dissociation and responses to mortality salience as predictors of severity of posttraumatic symptoms. *Psychological Trauma: Theory, Research and Practice, 3*(4), 329–341.

American Psychiatric Association. (2013). *Diagnostic and statistical manual of mental disorders* (5th ed). Author.

American Psychiatric Association. (2022). *Diagnostic and statistical manual of mental disorders* (5th ed., text rev.). Author.

Arndt, J., Cox., C. R., Goldenberg, J. L., Vess, M., Routledge, C., & Cohen, F. (2009). Blowing in the (social) wind: Implications of extrinsic esteem contingencies for terror management and health. *Journal of Personality and Social Psychology, 96,* 1191–1205.

Becker, E. (1973). *The denial of death.* Free Press.

Bor, W., Dean, A. J., Najman, J., & Hayatbakhsh, R. (2014). Are child and adolescent mental health problems increasing in the 21st century? A systematic review. *Australian and New Zealand Journal of Psychiatry, 48*(7), 606–616.

Breitbart, W. (2002). Spirituality and meaning in supportive care: Spirituality and meaning-centered group psychotherapy intervention in advanced cancer. *Support Cancer Care, 10,* 272–280.

Breitbart, W., Pessin, H., Rosenfeld, B., Applebaum, A. J., Lichtenthal, W. G., Li, Y., . . . Fenn, N. (2018). Individual meaning-centered psychotherapy for the treatment of psychological and existential distress: A randomized controlled trial in patients with advanced cancer. *Cancer, 124*(15), 3231–3239.

Breitbart, W., Rosenfeld, B., Gibson, C., Pessin, H., Poppito, S., Nelson, C., . . . Olden, M. (2010). Meaning-centered group psychotherapy for patients with advanced cancer: A pilot randomized controlled trial. *Psycho-Oncology, 19,* 21–28.

Brown, G., & Menzies, R. E. (2025). *Buried in belongings: Investigating the relationship between death anxiety and hoarding.* Manuscript in preparation.

Burke, B. L., Martens, A., & Faucher, E. H. (2010). Two decades of terror management theory: A meta-analysis of mortality salience research. *Personality and Social Psychology Review, 14*(2), 155–195.

Caras, G. W. (1995). The relationships among psychological separation, the quality of attachment, separation anxiety and death anxiety. *Dissertation Abstracts International, Section B: The Sciences and Engineering, 56,* 3436.

Chatard, A., Pyszczynski, T., Arndt, J., Selimbegovic, L., Konan, P. N., & Van der Linden, M. (2012). Extent of trauma exposure and PTSD symptom severity as predictors of anxiety-buffer functioning. *Psychological Trauma: Theory, Research, Practice, and Policy, 4,* 47–55.

Chawla, S., Menzies, R. E., & Menzies, R. G. (2022). Existential concerns in OCD with aggressive and sexual obsessions. *Journal of Obsessive-Compulsive and Related Disorders, 32,* 100710.

Cheung, M. C., Dennis, I., Easthope, Y., Werrett, J., & Farmer, S. (2005). A multiple-indicator multiple-cause model for posttraumatic stress reactions: Personality, coping, and maladjustment. *Psychosomatic Medicine, 67,* 251–259.

Chochinov, H. M., Kristjanson, L. J., Breitbart, W., McClement, S., Hack, T. F., Hassard, T., & Harlos, M. (2011). Effect of dignity therapy on distress and end-of-life experience in terminally ill patients: a randomised controlled trial. *Lancet Oncology, 12*(8), 753–762.

Choy, Y., Fyer, A. J., & Lipsitz, J. D. (2007). Treatment of specific phobia in adults. *Clinical Psychology Review, 27*(3), 266–286.

Dat, N. T., Mitsui, N., Asakura, S., Toyoshima, K., & Kusumi, I. (2022). The effectiveness of self-esteem-related interventions in reducing suicidal behaviors: A systematic review and meta-analysis. *Frontiers in Psychiatry, 13,* 925423.

de Jong, P. J., & Merckelbach, H. (1998). Blood-injection-injury phobia and fear of spiders: Domain specific individual differences in disgust sensitivity. *Personality and Individual Differences, 24*(2), 153–158.

Easden, D., Gurvich, C., Kaplan, R. A., & Rossell, S. L. (2023). Exploring fear of death and psychosis proneness: Positive schizotypy as a function of death anxiety and maladaptive coping. *Clinical Psychologist, 27*(1), 35–44.

Ein-Dor, T., Hirschberger, G., Perry, A., Levin, N., Cohen, R., Horesh, H., & Rothschild, E. (2014). Implicit death primes increase alcohol consumption. *Health Psychology, 33*(7), 748–751.

Emafti, M. F., Hedayatizadeh-Omran, A., Noroozi, A., Janbabai, G., Tatari, M., & Modanloo, M. (2019). The effect of group logotherapy on spirituality and death anxiety of patients with cancer: An open-label randomized clinical trial. *Iranian Journal of Psychiatry and Behavioral Sciences, 13*(3).

Fairlamb, S., & Juhl, J. (2022). Death thoughts predict increased depression for those with low self-worth. *Death Studies, 46*(4), 1021–1026.

Farahi, S., & Khalatbari, J. (2019). Effectiveness of acceptance and commitment therapy on the life expectancy, resilience and death anxiety in women with cancer. *International Journal of Applied Behavioral Sciences, 6*(3), 9–19.

Farber, S. K., Jackson, C. C., Tabin, J. K., & Bachar, E. (2007). Death and annihilation anxieties in anorexia nervosa, bulimia, and self-mutilation. *Psychoanalytic Psychology, 24*(2), 289–305.

Fichter, M. M., & Quadflieg, N. (2016). Mortality in eating disorders—Results of a large prospective clinical longitudinal study. *International Journal of Eating Disorders, 49*(4), 391–401.

Finch, E. C., Iverach, L., Menzies, R. G., & Jones, M. (2016). Terror mismanagement: Evidence that mortality salience exacerbates attentional bias in social anxiety. *Cognition and Emotion, 30*(7), 1370–1379.

Fleischer-Mann, J. (1995). Exploration of attachment-separation, fear of death and separation anxiety in agoraphobia. *Dissertation Abstracts International, Section B: The Sciences and Engineering, 56,* 2370.

Foa, E. B., Steketee, G., & Young, M. C. (1984). Agoraphobia: Phenomenological aspects, associated characteristics, and theoretical considerations. *Clinical Psychology Review, 4*(4), 431–457.

Forrester, M., Sharpe, L., & Menzies, R. E. (2024). Starving off death: Mortality salience impacts women's body image and disordered eating. *Death Studies.*

Frost, R. O., & Steketee, G. (2011). *Stuff: Compulsive hoarding and the meaning of things.* Mariner Books.

Furer, P., Walker, J. R., Chartier, M. J., & Stein, M. B. (1997). Hypochondriacal concerns and somatization in panic disorder. *Depression and Anxiety, 6*(2), 78–85.

Furer, P., Walker, J. R., & Stein, M. B. (2007). *Treating health anxiety and fear of death: A practitioner's guide*. Springer Science & Business Media.

Gershuny, B. S., Najavits, L. M., Wood, P. K., & Heppner, M. (2004). Relation between trauma and psychopathology: Mediating roles of dissociation and fears about death and control. *Journal of Trauma and Dissociation, 5*(3), 101–117.

Ghaemi, S. N. (2007). Feeling and time: The phenomenology of mood disorders, depressive realism, and existential psychotherapy. *Schizophrenia Bulletin, 33*(1), 122–130.

Giles, A. H. (1996). Death anxiety toward self and mother in clients with anorexia nervosa. *Dissertation Abstracts International, Section B: The Sciences and Engineering, 56*, 0522.

Goldenberg, J. L., Arndt, J., Hart, J., & Brown, M. (2005). Dying to be thin: The effects of mortality salience and body-mass-index on restricted eating among women. *Personality and Social Psychology Bulletin, 31*, 1400–1412.

Greenberg, J. (2012). Terror management theory: From genesis to revelations. In P. R. Shaver & M. Mikulincer (Eds.), *Meaning, mortality, and choice: The social psychology of existential concerns* (pp. 17–35). American Psychological Association.

Grossman, C. H., Brooker, J., Michael, N., & Kissane, D. (2018). Death anxiety interventions in patients with advanced cancer: A systematic review. *Palliative Medicine, 32*(1), 172–184.

Hartl, T. L., Duffany, S. R., Allen, G. J., Steketee, G., & Frost, R. O. (2005). Relationships among compulsive hoarding, trauma, and attention-deficit/hyperactivity disorder. *Behaviour Research and Therapy, 43*(2), 269–276.

Hayes, S. C., & Smith, S. (2005). *Get out of your mind and into your life: The new acceptance and commitment therapy*. New Harbinger.

Heidary, M., Heshmati, R., & Hayes, J. (2023). Effect of group logotherapy on anxiety about death and existential loneliness in patients with advanced cancer: A randomized controlled trial. *Cancer Nursing, 46*(1), E21–E30.

Iverach, L., Menzies, R. G., & Menzies, R. E. (2014). Death anxiety and its role in psychopathology: Reviewing the status of a transdiagnostic construct. *Clinical Psychology Review, 34*, 580–593.

Jessop, D. C., & Wade, J. (2010). Fear appeals and binge drinking: A terror management theory perspective. *British Journal of Health Psychology, 13*(4), 773–788.

Jones, M. K., & Krochmalik, A. (2003). Obsessive-compulsive washing. In R. G. Menzies & P. de Silva (Eds.), *Obsessive-compulsive disorder: Theory, research and treatment* (pp. 121–137). Wiley.

Jones, M. K., & Menzies, R. G. (2000). Danger expectancies, self-efficacy and insight in spider phobia. *Behaviour Research and Therapy, 38*(6), 585–600.

Jorm, A. F., & Kitchener, B. A. (2021). Increases in youth mental health services in Australia: Have they had an impact on youth population mental health? *Australian and New Zealand Journal of Psychiatry, 55*(5), 476–484.

Karima, F. H., Demartoto, A., & Murti, B. (2023). Effects of social support, perceived threat, and witnessing death on the risk of post-traumatic stress disorder: Meta-analysis. *Journal of Epidemiology and Public Health, 8*(3), 396–409.

Kellner, R., Abbott, P., Winslow, W. W., & Pathak, D. (1987). Fears, beliefs, and attitudes in DSM-III hypochondriasis. *Journal of Nervous and Mental Disease, 175*, 20–25.

Kesebir, P., Luszczynska, A., Pyszczynski, T., & Benight, C. (2011). Posttraumatic stress disorder involves disrupted anxiety-buffer mechanisms. *Journal of Social and Clinical Psychology, 30*, 819–841.

Kingman, R. (1928). Fears and phobias: Part II. *Welfare Mag, 19*, 303–308.

Krochmalik, A., Jones, M. K., & Menzies, R. G. (2001). Danger ideation reduction therapy (DIRT) for treatment-resistant compulsive washing. *Behaviour Research and Therapy, 39*(8), 897–912.

Le Marne, K. M., & Harris, L. M. (2016). Death anxiety, perfectionism and disordered eating. *Behaviour Change, 33*(4), 193–211.

Liu, C., Menzies, R. E., & Menzies, R. G. (2023). A systematic review of existential concerns in borderline personality disorder. *Journal of Humanistic Psychology*.

Lonetto, R., & Templer, D. I. (1986). *Death anxiety*. Hemisphere.

Lowe, J., & Harris, L. M. (2019). A comparison of death anxiety, intolerance of uncertainty and self-esteem as predictors of social anxiety symptoms. *Behaviour Change, 36*(3), 165–179.

Martin, I. M., & Kamins, M. A. (2010). An application of terror management theory in the design of social and health-related anti-smoking appeals. *Journal of Consumer Behaviour, 9*(3), 172–190.

Martz, E. (2004). Death anxiety as a predictor of posttraumatic stress levels among individuals with spinal cord injuries. *Death Studies, 28*(1), 1–17.

Maxfield, M., John, S., & Pyszczynski, T. (2014). A terror management perspective on the role of death-related anxiety in psychological dysfunction. *Humanistic Psychologist, 42*, 35–53.

McCabe, S., & Bartholow, B. D. (2019). Mortality salience leads to greater consumption of an ostensibly alcoholic beverage on Friday versus other weekdays. *British Journal of Health Psychology, 24*(4), 847–858.

Menzies, R. E., & Dar-Nimrod, I. (2017). Death anxiety and its relationship with obsessive-compulsive disorder. *Journal of Abnormal Psychology, 126,* 367–377.

Menzies, R. E., Julien, A., Sharpe, L., Menzies, R. G., Helgadóttir, F. D., & Dar-Nimrod, I. (2023a). Overcoming death anxiety: A phase I trial of an online CBT program in a clinical sample. *Behavioural and Cognitive Psychotherapy, 51*(4), 374–379.

Menzies, R. E., McMullen, K., Riotto, G. D., Iliescu, S., Petrovic, B., & Remfrey, M. (2024a). From dread to disorder: A meta-analysis of the impact of death anxiety on mental illness symptoms. *Clinical Psychology Review, 113,* 102490.

Menzies, R. E., & Menzies, R. G. (2022). Death anxiety and mental health: Requiem for a dreamer. *Journal of Behaviour Therapy and Experimental Psychiatry, 78,* 10187.

Menzies, R. E., Richmond, B., Sharpe, L., Skeggs, A., Liu, J., & Coutts-Bain, D. (2024b). The "revolving door" of mental illness: A meta-analysis and systematic review of current versus lifetime rates of psychological disorders. *British Journal of Clinical Psychology, 63*(2), 178–196.

Menzies, R. E., Sharpe, L., & Dar-Nimrod, I. (2019). The relationship between death anxiety and severity of mental illnesses. *British Journal of Clinical Psychology, 58,* 452–467.

Menzies, R. E., Sharpe, L., & Dar-Nimrod, I. (2021a). The effect of mortality salience on bodily scanning behaviors in anxiety-related disorders. *Journal of Abnormal Psychology, 130*(2), 141–151.

Menzies, R. E., Sharpe, L., & Dar-Nimrod, I. (2022a). The development and validation of the death anxiety beliefs and behaviours scale (DABBS). *British Journal of Clinical Psychology, 61*(4), 1169–1187.

Menzies, R. E., Sharpe, L., Favaloro, B., & Kearney, J. (2025). The role of existential concerns in borderline personality disorder and their responsiveness to dialectical behaviour therapy. *Clinical Psychologist, 29*(1), 29–42.

Menzies, R. E., Sharpe, L., Helgadóttir, F. D., & Dar-Nimrod, I. (2021b). Overcome death anxiety: The development of an online CBT program for fears of death. *Behaviour Change, 38*(4), 235–249.

Menzies, R. E., Sharpe, L., Richmond, B., & Cunningham, M. L. (2023b). "Life's too short to be small": An experimental exploration of the relationship between death anxiety and muscle dysmorphia symptoms. *Body Image, 44,* 43–52.

Menzies, R. E., & Veale, D. (2022). *Free yourself from death anxiety: A CBT self-help guide for a fear of death and dying.* Jessica Kingsley.

Menzies, R. E., Zuccala, M., Sharpe, L., & Dar-Nimrod, I. (2018). The effects of psychosocial interventions on death anxiety: A meta-analysis and systematic review of randomised controlled trials. *Journal of Anxiety Disorders, 59,* 64–73.

Menzies, R. E., Zuccala, M., Sharpe, L., & Dar-Nimrod, I. (2020). Subtypes of obsessive-compulsive disorder and their relationship to death anxiety. *Journal of Obsessive-Compulsive and Related Disorders, 27,* 100572.

Menzies, R. E., Zuccala, M., Sharpe, L., & Dar-Nimrod, I. (2021c). Are anxiety disorders a pathway to obsessive-compulsive disorder?: Different trajectories of OCD and the role of death anxiety. *Nordic Journal of Psychiatry, 75*(3), 170–175.

Menzies, R. G., & Clarke, J. C. (1995). Danger expectancies and insight in acrophobia. *Behaviour Research and Therapy, 33*(2), 215–221.

Menzies, R. G., & Menzies, R. E. (2018). Fear of death: Nature, development and moderating factors. In R. E. Menzies, R. G. Menzies, & L. Iverach (Eds.), *Curing the dread of death: Theory, research and practice* (pp. 21–40). Australian Academic Press.

Menzies, R. G., Menzies, R. E., & Dingle, G. (Eds.) (2022b). *Existential concerns and cognitive-behavioral procedures: An integrative approach to mental health.* Springer Nature.

Menzies, R. G., Menzies, R. E., & Iverach, L. (2015). The role of death fears in obsessive-compulsive disorder. *Australian Clinical Psychologist, 1,* 6–11.

Miller, A. K., Lee, B. L., & Henderson, C. E. (2012). Death anxiety in persons with HIV/AIDS: A systematic review and meta-analysis. *Death Studies, 36*(7), 640–663.

Mirzaeidoostan, Z., Zargar, Y., & Zandi Payam, A. (2019). The effectiveness of acceptance and commitment therapy on death anxiety and mental health in women with HIV in Abadan City, Iran. *Iranian Journal of Psychiatry and Clinical Psychology, 25*(1), 2–13.

Nagar, M., & Rabinovitz, S. (2015). Smoke your troubles away: Exploring the effects of death cognitions on cannabis craving and consumption. *Journal of Psychoactive Drugs, 47*(2), 91–99.

Noyes, R., Stuart, S., Longley, S. L., Langbehn, D. R., & Happel, R. L. (2002). Hypochondriasis and fear of death. *Journal of Nervous and Mental Disease, 190,* 503–509.

O'Dea, J. A., & Abraham, S. (2000). Improving the body image, eating attitudes, and behaviors of young male and female adolescents: A new educational approach that focuses on self-esteem. *International Journal of Eating Disorders, 28*(1), 43–57.

Öngider, N., & Özışık Eyüboğlu, S. (2013). Investigation of death anxiety among depressive patients. *Turkish Journal of Clinical Psychiatry, 16*(1), 34–46.

Pyszczynski, T., Greenberg, J., & Solomon, S. (1999). A dual-process model of defense against conscious and unconscious death-related thoughts: An extension of terror management theory. *Psychological Review, 106*(4), 835–845.

Pyszczynski, T., & Kesebir, P. (2011). Anxiety buffer disruption theory: A terror management account of posttraumatic stress disorder. *Anxiety, Stress, and Coping, 24*(1), 3–26.

Pyszczynski, T., Solomon, S., & Greenberg, J. (2015). Thirty years of terror management theory: From genesis to revelation. In M. P. Zanna & J. M. Olson (Eds.), *Advances in experimental social psychology* (Vol. 52, pp. 1–70). Academic Press.

Randall, E. (2001). Existential therapy of panic disorder: A single system study. *Clinical Social Work Journal, 29,* 259–267.

Rockloff, M. J., Browne, M., Li, E., & O'Shea, T. (2014). It's a sure bet you're going to die: Existential terror promotes gambling urges in problem players. *Gambling Research, 26*(1), 33–43.

Ron, P. (2015). It is not their war: The impact of military operations on Philippine migrant care workers for elderly people in Israel. *Clinical Interventions in Aging,* 1053–1061.

Sanchez, C., Linkovski, O., van Roessel, P., Steinberg, N. M., McCarthy, E., Muñoz Rodríguez, P. A., . . . Rodriguez, C. I. (2023). Early life stress in adults with hoarding disorder: A mixed methods study. *Journal of Obsessive-Compulsive and Related Disorders, 37,* 100785.

Searles, H. F. (1961). Schizophrenia and the inevitability of death. *Psychiatric Quarterly, 35*(4), 631–665.

Sharpe, L., Menzies, R. E., Richmond, B., Todd, J., & Shaw, J. (2024). The development and validation of the worries about recurrence or progression scale (WARPS). *British Journal of Health Psychology, 29*(2), 454–467.

Simon, L., Arndt, J., Greenberg, J., Pyszczynski, T., & Solomon, S. (1998). Terror management and meaning: Evidence that the opportunity to defend the worldview in response to mortality salience increases the meaningfulness of life in the mildly depressed. *Journal of Personality, 66*(3), 359–382.

Simon, L., Greenberg, J., Jones, E. H., Solomon, S., & Pyszczynski, T. (1996). Mild depression, mortality salience and defense of the worldview evidence of intensified terror management in the mildly depressed. *Personality and Social Psychology Bulletin, 22*(1), 81–90.

Sims, M. A., Menzies, R. E., & Menzies, R. G. (2024). A systematic review of the relationship between death anxiety, capability for suicide, and suicidality. *Death Studies, 48*(1), 16–26.

Strachan, E., Schimel, J., Arndt, J., Williams, T., Solomon, S., Pyszczynski, T., & Greenberg, J. (2007). Terror mismanagement: evidence that mortality salience exacerbates phobic and compulsive behaviors. *Personality and Social Psychology Bulletin, 33*(8), 1137–1151.

Vaccaro, L. D., Jones, M. K., Menzies, R. G., & Clare, T. S. (Eds.). (2010). *Danger ideation reduction therapy for obsessive-compulsive checkers: A comprehensive guide to treatment.* Australian Academic Press.

Vail, K. E., Morgan, A., & Kahle, L. (2018). Self-affirmation attenuates death-thought accessibility after mortality salience, but not among a high post-traumatic stress sample. *Psychological Trauma: Theory, Research, Practice, and Policy, 10*(1), 112–120.

van den Berg, E., Houtzager, L., de Vos, J., Daemen, I., Katsaragaki, G., Karyotaki, E., . . . Dekker, J. (2019). Meta-analysis on the efficacy of psychological treatments for anorexia nervosa. *European Eating Disorders Review, 27*(4), 331–351.

Waite, P., McManus, F., & Shafran, R. (2012). Cognitive behaviour therapy for low self-esteem: A preliminary randomized controlled trial in a primary care setting. *Journal of Behavior Therapy and Experimental Psychiatry, 43*(4), 1049–1057.

Walser, C. B. (1984). *Death anxiety and separation anxiety in borderline and schizophrenic patients.* Doctoral dissertation, California School of Professional Psychology, Berkeley.

Wisman, A., Heflick, N., & Goldenberg, J. L. (2015). The great escape: The role of self-esteem and self-related cognition in terror management. *Journal of Experimental Social Psychology, 60,* 121–132.

Yalom, I. D. (1980). *Existential psychotherapy.* Basic Books.

Yalom, I. D. (2008). *Staring at the sun: Overcoming the terror of death.* Jossey-Bass.

Zeigler-Hill, V. (2011). The connections between self-esteem and psychopathology. *Journal of Contemporary Psychotherapy, 41,* 157–164.

Zhang, Y., Li, J., & Hu, X. (2022). The effectiveness of dignity therapy on hope, quality of life, anxiety, and depression in cancer patients: a meta-analysis of randomized controlled trials. *International Journal of Nursing Studies, 132*, 104273.

Zinchenko, O., & Hyland, J. (2021). An audit of waiting times in the outpatient clinic in Inverness Sector A NHS Highland during the COVID-19 pandemic. *BJPsych Open*, 7(Suppl. 1), S113.

Zuccala, M., & Abbott, M. J. (2021). Social anxiety disorder and the fear of death: An empirical investigation of the terror management approach towards understanding clinical anxiety. *Cognitive Therapy and Research, 45*, 628–641.

Zuccala, M., & Menzies, R. E. (2022). Fears of death and their relationship to mental health. In R. G. Menzies, R. E. Menzies, & G. Dingle (Eds.), *Existential concerns and cognitive-behavioral procedures: An integrative approach to mental health*. Springer Nature.

Zuccala, M., Modini, M., & Abbott, M. J. (2021). The role of death fears and attachment processes in social anxiety: A novel hypothesis explored. *Australian Journal of Psychology, 73*(3).

CHAPTER 10

Health in the Spotlight and Shadow of Death

The Terror Management Health Model

Emily P. Courtney, Jamie L. Goldenberg, *and* Jamie Arndt

In 2020, people worldwide were reminded that life is precarious. Death tolls from COVID-19 flashed across television screens and newspaper headlines, and people barricaded themselves in their homes to flee the threat. During the peak of the pandemic, many people put health first, masking and washing and maintaining the recommended 6 feet of distance, whereas others used different tactics, from outright denial to excessive alcohol use. After some time of acclimating to the threat, some people adopted masks as their new uniform while others marched in the street to preserve what they saw as the values of individual freedom.

In short, in a rather condensed time period, worldwide human behaviors reflected some of the many variations of how people deal with health-relevant situations, and what we suggest is a key catalyst of these behaviors, deeply rooted existential concerns about mortality. The terror management health model (TMHM; Arndt & Goldenberg, 2017; Goldenberg & Arndt, 2008) is a model of behavioral health decisions that considers how human beings are motivated to manage psychological concerns associated with the awareness of their mortality, and that the processes of doing so have wide ranging implications for human health. In this chapter we present this model and its foundational research, the application and research on the COVID-19 pandemic, and some recent advances in the literature that highlight future directions and insight.

TERROR MANAGEMENT THEORY AND THE TMHM: A BRIEF OVERVIEW

Terror management theory (TMT; Greenberg et al., 1986) builds upon the writings of Ernest Becker (e.g., 1962, 1973) and other existential theorists to explain that the human experience comes with the burden of knowledge—including the knowledge of one's own finitude. For humans to function with a semblance of equanimity, terror instigated by the understanding that everyone (including oneself) dies must be managed. This terror management is accomplished through two primary mechanisms, what TMT dubs a dual-process model of defense against the awareness of mortality (Pyszczynski et al., 1999). First, individuals must do what they can to avoid being paralyzed with fear of death, and so they push the threat from the forefront of their mind. *Proximal defenses* constitute a first line of protection, occurring in response to conscious awareness of mortality. When proximal defenses effectively relegate thoughts of death to the back of the mind, or if a death reminder was subtler (i.e., subconscious/implicit) to begin with, a second line of defense is activated. *Distal defenses*, in contrast, are not directly related to the problem of death, but rather activate the constructed ideologies, the sense of meaning, the abstract and culturally contextual standards that make life feel worth living.

In much TMT literature, both proximal and distal defenses are studied experimentally using manipulations of *mortality salience* (MS), wherein individuals are reminded of their own eventual death and defense activation is measured (Burke et al., 2010). This methodological approach seeks to exaggerate and thus capture psychological processes that are presumed to otherwise operate throughout daily affairs. In terms of proximal defenses, which aim to remove death awareness from focal attention, death reminders lead to immediate attempts at threat reduction, such as through cognitive suppression (Arndt, Greenberg, Solomon, et al., 1997) or vulnerability denial (Greenberg et al., 2000). Once thoughts of death are no longer conscious but still accessible (either following proximal defense activation or via a subliminal or subtle mortality reminder; e.g., Arndt, Greenberg, Pyszczynski, et al., 1997), distal defenses come into play. This arm of the dual-process system aims to mitigate not an imminent sense of death threat but instead the threat associated with being mortal: People want to live on beyond the physical literally or symbolically, and so distal defenses manifest as attempts to adhere to and defend cultural worldviews and bolster self-esteem (Pyszczynski et al., 2015).

Much of human health behavior occurs amid the backdrop of mortality if not under the glare of the fatal spotlight. Indeed, this may be especially true with respect to cancer, which is so chronically and severely associated with a death sentence (Moser et al., 2014, 2021) that even the mere mention of cancer can serve to activate death-related cognitions and psychological efforts to manage that activation (e.g., suppression; Arndt et al., 2007). Given the inextricable link between life, death, and health behavior, the TMHM (Arndt & Goldenberg, 2017; Goldenberg & Arndt, 2008) applies TMT's dual-process model to investigate the role of conscious and nonconscious mortality awareness on health behaviors and intentions. In the TMHM, conscious mortality awareness and ensuing proximal defenses lead to immediate health-based responses focused on threat reduction; nonconscious mortality awareness and ensuing distal defenses lead to health-based responses focused on that which bolsters the self. Experimental evidence supports this dual-process perspective. In an initial study (Arndt et al., 2003), individuals who were reminded of death reported immediate intentions to engage in more exercise compared to those who were not thinking of death. But after a delay period during which death awareness faded from consciousness, only those who included exercise in their feelings of self-esteem reported more exercise intentions. These findings set the stage to elucidate when—and for whom—the awareness of mortality can lead to different health behaviors.

EVIDENCE OF THE TMHM

Proximal Health Behavior Defenses

A wide range of health decisions result from efforts to reduce perceptions of risk (Sheeran et al., 2014). TMHM posits that such efforts are partly driven by, and thus magnified in response to, conscious awareness of mortality where the operative goal is to reduce the perceived risks associated with conscious thoughts of death. Sometimes these proximal defenses help facilitate adaptive health intentions. For example, individuals reminded of mortality in the context of deadly melanoma (compared to a control topic) reported more immediate intentions to reduce sun exposure and wear sunscreen (Routledge et al., 2004). Similarly, as noted earlier, death reminders also facilitated immediate increases in intentions to exercise (Arndt et al., 2003). In other studies, however, participants seemed to go in a different direction, and denied the health threat (Cooper et al., 2010) or avoided cancer screenings (Arndt et al., 2006).

Moderating Factors

Because proximal defenses are aimed at removing death-related thought from focal attention, in a health context, these defenses are often moderated by factors more directly relevant to the risk perceptions that threaten to make death a conscious concern. Consider the findings of Taubman-Ben-Ari and Findler (2005) and Bozo and colleagues (2009). In these studies, a death reminder led younger and middle-aged adults to report higher intentions to engage in health-promoting behaviors, while older adults responded to MS with comparatively lower health intentions. Although speculative, age may have been functioning as a proxy for perceived risk or fatalistic perceptions.

More direct evidence comes from studies measuring individual differences in adaptive coping, health optimism, and response efficacy, all of which have a history of predicting beneficial responses to health threats and illness information. In Arndt and colleagues (2006), individuals higher in adaptive coping responded to MS with more interest in health behavior involvement, an effect that did not emerge among those with lower adaptive coping. Similarly, women higher in health optimism reported greater intentions to perform breast self-exams (BSEs) when reminded of death, while women lower in health optimism responded with comparatively lower BSE intentions. Further, health optimism and response efficacy interacted with conscious death awareness to predict safe sun behaviors (Cooper et al., 2010), a pattern that did not hold once death faded from conscious awareness. In short, when there is a sense that people can effectively deal with the health threat, conscious thought of mortality can engage proactive health protection efforts. However, because proximal defenses hinge more on the reduction of *perceived risk*, rather than reduction of *actual risk*, when individuals lacked health optimism, adaptive coping strategies, or response efficacy, they tended to respond with denial or avoidance-based strategies, potentially ushering one more quickly to the grave.

Distal Health Behavior Defenses

The TMHM informs not only the decisions people make when they are consciously thinking about death, or proximal defenses to mortality salience, but also how and why seemingly unrelated motivations impact health when thoughts of death are activated but not conscious—which is presumably very often in the context of health decisions. Under these conditions, people's "health" decisions are informed not just by health concerns, but also by an individual's broader system of meaning (i.e., cultural worldview) and the contingencies for self-esteem and social influence it prescribes.

Health-Risk Behavior

As with proximal defenses, people's reactions to nonconscious thoughts of death are not always adaptive. This is because people sometimes derive meaning and value from behaviors that can jeopardize their health. And therefore, seemingly sensible human beings respond to the awareness of their mortality by engaging in behaviors that are likely to bring it on more quickly.

Risky sex, drugs, smoking, drinking, and fast driving are some of the domains in which this idea has been studied in the context of terror management research. The overarching finding is that when mortality concerns are activated, but not conscious, health concerns take a back seat to the need for self-esteem. The first associated evidence came from research on reckless driving (Taubman Ben-Ari et al., 1999), finding that individuals who derived self-esteem from fast driving, reported behavior intentions to drive fast and even drove faster and more recklessly on a driving simulator after a traditional MS manipulation, where a delay followed an explicit reminder of mortality. Other research showed these effects were more common among men, who tended to derive self-esteem from taking risks (Hirschberger et al., 2002), and these findings extended to risky sexual behavior (Lam et al., 2009).

From this perspective we can make sense of some of the complexities associated with the effects of on-pack, graphic cigarette labels depicting blackened cancer-afflicted lungs, tracheotomy scars, rotten teeth, and the general threat of dying. Although generally effective at reducing smoking, they can elicit variable reactions (Cameron et al., 2015; Strong et al., 2021). Hansen and colleagues (2010) examined reactions to these fear-inducing cigarette pack labels and found that individuals high in smoking-based self-esteem responded with even more positive attitudes toward smoking; when the packages lacked graphic labels, those at all levels of smoking esteem reported more negative smoking attitudes. Similarly, those who derived esteem from regular cannabis use responded to reminders of their mortality (compared to a control topic) with more cravings and marijuana use intentions (Nagar & Rabinovitz, 2015).

Similar to smoking behaviors, alcohol use can also have implications for how some people derive esteem and identity (Lindgren et al., 2016).[1] In a field study, implicitly priming death (compared to pain) on a flyer led passerby college students to drink more alcoholic than nonalcoholic beverages (Ein-Dor et al., 2014). In another field study, individuals with low self-esteem actually consumed more alcohol in a nightclub than those with high self-esteem following MS (Wisman et al., 2015). Making matters worse, following MS, those who derived esteem from engaging in binge-drinking reported more intentions to binge drink (Jessop & Wade, 2008). Part of these reactions may reflect the cultural norms and value surrounding alcohol use. In McCabe and Bartholow (2019), MS led to more consumption of an ostensibly alcoholic beverage on a Friday than on a Monday, consistent with cultural scripts about alcohol use. These studies suggest a more nuanced approach to health behavior change: The threat of dying is not necessarily sufficient to change attitudes for those who derive esteem from risky behaviors.

Moderating Factors

In highlighting a critical role of self-esteem in distal defenses to mortality concerns, the TMHM offers guidelines for what may be important moderating factors in outcomes relevant to health. To illustrate, we return first to studies on suntanning. Whereas immediately after a mortality reminder, participants indicated greater interest in high-SPF products (Routledge et al., 2004) and safe sun behaviors (especially when those behaviors were presented as effective for reducing skin cancer risk; Cooper et al., 2010, 2014), when mortality priming was followed by a delay, interest in engaging in skin cancer risk reduction shifted depending on esteem-relevant factors. Specifically, a focus on appearance became a more critical moderating variable. Among women for whom having tan skin served as a source of self-esteem, a delay following MS led to less interest in high-SPF products (Routledge et al., 2004), a result that was expounded upon in studies where appearance standards were made salient. When (female) participants were presented with images of beautiful women with tan skin, MS followed by a delay instigated greater interest in tanning and other unsafe sun behaviors, compared to when participants were not reminded of death (Cox et al., 2009). However, when participants were presented with alternative appearance standards (e.g., "pale can be pretty" or a photo of UV damage to women's skin), salient mortality led to decreased tanning intentions, choosing high-SPF sunscreen products, and other sun protection responses (Cox et al., 2009; Morris, Cooper, et al., 2014).

These studies underscore the importance of societal forces in shaping how people derive self-esteem and thus influencing how reminders of mortality affect the decisions people make. Of course, as Carl Rogers and other humanistic perspectives have long taught us, people vary in the extent to which their sense of self-worth is contingent on such external validation. And among those who depend on such external validation, it can be used to productively direct decision making. Accordingly, women high in extrinsic self-esteem reported greater interest in tanning following MS, but importantly, reported lower interest in tanning if they were also presented with the notion that pale can be pretty (Arndt et al., 2009). Similarly, among those who had extrinsic motivation to smoke (Arndt et al., 2009), focusing on social consequences of smoking habits served as a more effective means of encouraging quitting intentions and negative attitudes toward smoking behaviors (Martin & Kamins, 2007, 2009, 2019; Wong et al., 2017) compared to focusing on actual physical death from smoking. In sum, the social forces that shape people's sense of self-value can be powerful factors in the health-relevant decisions that people make under the shadow of mortality.

Such susceptibility to the influence of social forces invites further consideration of how and when such standards, or social exemplars, might be useful in health-messaging campaigns. The prototype willingness model (Gerrard et al., 2008) has been useful in this respect. The model suggests that a person's construal of others who do or do not engage in certain behaviors affects an individual's willingness to emulate those behaviors. Integrating insights from the prototype willingness model with TMHM, protypes have been used to shift the relevance of health behavior, such as exercise (i.e., making it more a basis of self-worth, Arndt et al., 2009), as a distal defense. And these manipulations, such as visualizing a prototypically healthy eater or an unhealthy smoker, when paired with MS, have been shown to influence health behaviors. In a field experiment focused on food consumption, grocery shoppers who completed a packet of questionnaires that either did or did not contain a mortality reminder before entering the store purchased comparatively more healthy, nutritious foods (McCabe et al., 2015). Smokers' self-concepts were also affected by a prototype and MS manipulation, such that they endorsed a nonsmoker identity and heightened negative attitudes toward smokers (McCabe et al., 2014). This same pattern held longitudinally, where over the course of the 3 weeks, smokers reported a reduction in a sense of identity related to smoking behaviors, as well as reduced smoking frequency and more attempts at quitting (Morris et al., 2019).

Similar to research on prototypes, other societal exemplars, such as celebrity endorsement on products, can shift the appeal of certain behavior to one's sense of identity and its relevance as a distal defense. McCabe and colleagues (2014) compared the effects of conscious versus nonconscious MS on how individuals respond to health-based recommendations from different sources. In two studies, the researchers manipulated MS, the presence or absence of a delay, and the source of a health-based recommendation for a brand of bottled water: either a medical doctor or a celebrity. After these manipulations, participants indicated how much they would pay for a "healthy" water product and had the chance to actually consume as much of the "healthy" water product as they pleased. When death was conscious, participants reported willingness to pay more and consumed more of the "healthy" water when it was endorsed by a medical professional; when death was nonconscious, participants preferred the "healthy" water when it was endorsed by celebrity. In a final study, nonconscious mortality awareness led individuals to report safer alcohol consumption intentions when, in contrast to the endorsement of a medical professional, safe drinking was endorsed by the movie star Sandra Bullock.

Overall, considering the variety of moderating factors related to the health issues themselves, the aforementioned studies all indicate a critical consideration in trying to influence adaptive rather than maladaptive health-based responses to death awareness. Social and contextual factors like beauty standards, prototypes, and exemplars inform the impact of death awareness on distal defenses, and whether individuals engage in adaptive or maladaptive behaviors with respect to health.

The Body as an Existential Threat

In elucidating a critical impact of existential concerns on motivations related to health, the TMHM identifies a death-adjacent threat: the body. The physicality of the body, and its fallibility to health threats, stands to unravel the symbolic ways that people manage terror, making the body itself an existential threat (Goldenberg, 2005; Goldenberg et al., 2000). As a result, salient mortality leads to a literal and metaphorical distancing from the more creaturely aspects of the body like physical, tactile experiences and bodily functions (Goldenberg et al., 2001, 2006). In the context of health behavior, this means that people may avoid certain health behaviors because of an existential threat associated with the physicality of the body.

Goldenberg and colleagues (2008) investigated the relevance of concerns about the physicality of the body in the context of breast cancer screening. When women read an essay that highlighted the ways that humans are similar to other animals (i.e., human creatureliness), compared to an essay about human uniqueness, women decreased their intentions to conduct breast self-exams (BSEs) under conditions where mortality was salient. Priming creatureliness, compared to human uniqueness or a control topic, also led women to conduct shorter breast examinations on a realistic torso model (an experience that was found to increase the nonconscious accessibility of death). In both studies, thinking about the more creaturely aspects of the body undermined women's engagement with breast exams. Presumably this is because the salience of creatureliness increases anxiety when one has to confront the physical body and this anxiety inhibits the examination behavior. A third study tested this directly. Using a misattribution of arousal paradigm (Zanna & Cooper, 2000), women age 35 or older were primed with creatureliness and then told that they were going to be sampling a health-supplement beverage with either energizing or relaxing herbal additives, with side effects that might include mild anxiety or mild drowsiness. The women who were primed with creatureliness spent less time conducting their own BSEs after drinking the "calming" beverage, when they could not externalize the source of their anxiety; compared to when they were able to misattribute their anxiety as a side effect of the "energizing" beverage.

Anxiety, of course, abounds in any setting where health threats might be particularly salient, and certain people—such as those high in neuroticism—are especially prone to feelings of anxiety. If anxiety undermines bodily engagement when creatureliness is salient, then those high in neuroticism should be more restrained and uncomfortable with breast exams when reminded of human creatureliness. Goldenberg and colleagues (2009) examined the role of trait-level neuroticism among women faced with mammography. When mortality was salient, women high in neuroticism reported less willingness to undergo a mammogram. And when actually in the clinic situation that would likely arouse concerns about mortality, they reported more physical and psychological discomfort during a mammogram when they had been primed with creatureliness, compared to human uniqueness.

Given the inevitable confrontation with the body in various health behavior, it is critical to identify ways to mitigate the avoidance that can be aroused by concerns with human creatureliness. As with other distal defenses, creatureliness concerns may be ameliorated via the salience of social value in conjunction with a health behavior. BSEs, which involve an intimate interaction with an especially creaturely body part, can be encouraged through their framing. When BSEs were presented as an empowering practice rather than a practical one, death awareness in both a naturalistic (i.e., mammography clinic) and in-lab experimental paradigm led women to report greater intentions to engage in BSEs in the future (Cooper et al., 2011).

Empowering women to overcome the threat of their physical bodies presents an intuitive and positive direction for encouraging health engagement. But, and somewhat ironically, there is reasoning derived from TMT to suggest that the objectification of women's bodies can relieve the existential distress associated with its creatureliness (Goldenberg & Roberts, 2011; see Goldenberg et al., Chapter 38, this volume). Objectification, in which the body is viewed as an object that defines women's worth, is associated with a host of negative consequences for women (e.g., shame, disordered eating; Fredrickson & Roberts, 1997; Moradi & Huang, 2008) but, at the same time, functions to disconnect the body from its creatureliness and death. The body in a sense becomes a symbolic platform through which one can derive self-esteem, or at least try to obtain self-esteem. Therefore, when mortality concerns are heightened, women's appearance becomes a more pressing concern (Grabe et al., 2005), especially for individuals who are highly invested in appearance standards (Goldenberg & Roberts, 2011; Grabe et al., 2005), and especially when concerns about the body's creatureness are salient (Morris, Goldenberg, et al., 2014). Thus, from this perspective, objectification can function as a terror management mechanism.

Based on this reasoning, Morris and colleagues (2013) argued that self-objectification can serve as a form of self-affirmation to encourage breast cancer screening following reminders of breast cancer's deadliness. In this study, the researchers first measured women's trait-level tendency to self-objectify, and then primed either objectifying media (i.e., a *Sports Illustrated* Swimsuit Edition) or competence-based media (i.e., a *Sports Illustrated* cover featuring soccer phenom Mia Hamm, which produced no effects throughout the study). Subsequently, in lieu of a standard TMT death prime, women were given an instructional brochure on conducting a BSE, where the prime explicitly mentioned that breast cancer can lead to death in young women, while the control topic simply stated that BSEs are an important part of women's health. After priming death, only women high in self-objectification, relative to those low in self-objectification, who viewed the objectifying magazine image responded to the threat of breast cancer death with increased BSE intentions and more positive attitudes toward the magazine cover, indicating a healthy response despite the connection to an unhealthy trait (i.e., self-objectification).

Along similar lines, the theoretical framework of adaptive self-objectification (ASO; Courtney & Goldenberg, 2021) integrates existing breast cancer awareness campaigns, existential perspectives, and the potential for women to localize objectification to specific areas of the body in order to reduce the implication of creatureliness during difficult illnesses like breast cancer. Women are prone to conflating their own bodies with literal objects in the presence of both mortality and creatureliness reminders (Morris, Goldenberg, et al., 2014). As such, it follows that viewing the especially threatening parts of the body (like the breasts, which are afflicted by cancer in roughly 13% of women; National Cancer Institute, 2023) as inert and replaceable (Nussbaum, 1995), sick and medicalized (Langellier & Sullivan, 1998) objects, rather than a part of one's sense of self, could be a mechanism underlying difficult and painful treatment decisions like radiation and mastectomy; and even the death-thought activating process of conducing a self-exam (Courtney, 2024). This same theorizing extends to other organs rife with social meaning, such as the uterus, ovaries, and even testicles. Generally speaking, there is hope for self-objectification to be presented in such a way that it appeals to esteem while also encouraging potentially adaptive health outcomes.

Summary

The existing literature on the TMHM provides a breadth of evidence for the inextricable link between death and health—with explanations for why individuals may or may not engage in healthy behaviors. When death is consciously accessible, individuals engage in proximal strategies for perceived risk reduction, whether they're health-facilitating intentions to exercise more (Arndt et al., 2003) or willingness to wear stronger sunblock (Routledge et al., 2004); or health-defeating intentions to avoid screening (Arndt et al., 2006) or deny the health threat entirely (Cooper et al., 2010). Either way, the thought of death is relegated out of focal attention; at which point, distal defensiveness in the form of health behaviors' relationship to individual esteem and meaning take over. It is under these conditions that the model also recognizes that there is an existential threat associated with the physical body, and this further complicates people's decisions to engage in behaviors that have implications for health. From the perspective of the TMHM, it is critical to find or establish a connection between health behaviors and meaning and value to encourage individuals to defend against existential concerns with behaviors that stave off death rather than bring it on sooner.

APPLICATIONS OF THE TMHM: THE CASE OF COVID-19

As highlighted at the outset of this chapter, the COVID-19 pandemic was an opportunity to observe the TMHM in action and consider how best to apply its tenets to promote behavior to reduce the health threat. A majority of existing TMHM investigations up to 2020 were controlled lab studies designed to isolate the influence of existential threat (whether in the form of conscious or nonconscious MS, a relevant deadly health threat, or the body's creatureliness) and specific moderating factors on proximal and distal health intentions and behaviors. While controlled studies provide foundational support for the theoretical perspective, naturalistic settings can blur the salience of death and its conscious versus nonconsciously driven consequences. The pandemic allowed for a unique line of research buttressed by the TMHM's frameworks, while highlighting areas in which the framework can be further honed.

The TMHM as applied specifically to the pandemic (TMHM-[P]andemic; Courtney et al., 2020) integrated public health research with TMT's dual-process approach to predict both proximal and distal defensiveness in response to conscious and nonconscious death awareness aroused by near-constant visibility of COVID-19 (Pyszczynski et al., 2020). At the onset of the pandemic, individuals were bombarded with news reports of death tolls and refrigeration truck morgues, mortality was constantly consciously salient (Fairlamb, 2022) and death anxiety became a dominant topic in daily discourse (Barnes, 2021; Chew, 2022). With that death anxiety came spikes in psychological distress (Hossain et al., 2020; Menzies & Menzies, 2020) and a necessitation for activation of TMT defenses.

First, proximal defenses aimed at reducing perceived risk. For some, those actions looked like denial or suppression of the deadliness of COVID-19 (e.g., comparisons to the seasonal flu); for others, they looked like a focus on hand-washing, sanitizing grocery bags, and adherence to social distancing. However, as lockdowns persisted, COVID-19 death tolls took a backseat to social unrest due to damages associated with both pandemic-necessitated shutdowns and systemic injustice. From the perspective of the TMHM/TMHM-P, this uprising of ideological variables in the public eye despite quotidian death reminders represented the "push and pull between proximal and distal defenses": Yes, individuals wanted to stay safe and healthy, but sources of esteem combated the focus on health (Pyszczynski et al., 2020). In turn, and considering the chaotic overlap between the conscious and nonconscious death awareness instigated by COVID-19, identifying moderating factors was of critical importance.

Moderating Factors

The pandemic allowed for a case study of the TMHM literature, and the TMHM-P (Courtney et al., 2020) employed the model's primary principles as a first step to understanding responses to COVID-19. Following the methodological paradigms standard to TMT/TMHM investigations, researchers aimed to determine some of the social, contextual, and individual variables that informed responses to rampant naturalistic death reminders.

In the presence of MS, accompanying salience of cultural worldviews can differentially inform distal defenses. Courtney and colleagues (2021) found that, when COVID-19-related death was made salient, priming collectivism (compared to individualism) heightened intentions to comply with curve-flattening recommendations like social distancing and abiding by lockdowns. However, priming individualism (compared to collectivism) led to lower vaccination intentions (an arguably exclusively individual decision, despite the benefits for others) when death was nonconsciously accessible. Further exemplifying the role of worldviews, shoehorning cultural symbols into health-relevant actions can serve to improve attitudes as well as intentions to engage with those behaviors. When face masks were emblazoned with a cultural symbol important to the participant (e.g., a pride flag or symbol for the National Health Service compared to a plain surgical mask), MS served to heighten positive interpersonal perceptions and feelings of solidarity (Perach & Limbu, 2022). Additionally, while health optimism played a proximal role in heightening mask-wearing intentions when mortality was salient, those with self-esteem contingent on external appearance reported distal interest in wearing an aesthetically pleasing face mask (Fairlamb et al., 2022). As such, the simple act of wearing a mask became not only a health behavior, but one that could signal worldview investment and draw feelings of esteem.

Importantly, though, cultural worldviews are not universal: The aforementioned studies illustrate that patterns of responses to COVID-19 death reminders are contingent on values relevant to the study populations. For example, and highlighting the findings in Courtney and colleagues' studies on individualism and collectivism, Harvell-Bowman (2023) and Miller and Ma (2021) argued that the salience of ingroup-specific ideology (like individualism in the United States) in conjunction with a COVID-19 death reminder would be more likely to produce adaptive health outcomes and combat psychological reactance (Dimoff et al., 2021). As noted, though, the reality of death awareness is not as tidy as conscious or nonconscious, especially when an existential threat is as unfamiliar, confusing, and polarized as COVID-19 (Kim & Kreps, 2020). This noisiness was exemplified in big-data investigations using TMT as a framework: Google searches and tweets were not only about health behaviors, but the anxieties and death-related aspects of COVID-19 were also associated with search and tweets about racial division, religion, material objects/purchasing behaviors, methods of bolstering individual achievement, and attempts at social connection (Barnes, 2021; Chew, 2022; Kwon & Park, 2022; Liu et al., 2023; Wang, 2023). At a grand scale, distal defenses depending on relevant cultures were made evident: even in people's internet search histories and social media communications.

The role of macrolevel cultural worldviews on differential defensive responses to the existential threat of COVID-19 is clear; but individual differences also helped or hindered COVID-19 health intentions and engagement, even to the extent that health behaviors became worldviews in themselves. For example, existential anxiety predicted individual intentions to get vaccinated, but researchers also found a positive relationship between existential anxiety and adoption of conspiracy beliefs that in turn predicted lower vaccination intentions, reflecting individual internalization of ideological strife and mistrust (Scrima et al., 2022). However, internalization of health behaviors also showed promise. Fairlamb and Courtney (2022) found that COVID-19-based death reminders early in the pandemic led to proximal intentions to social distance; however, in a proceeding study, intentions to social distance arose in a distal context, as well. This result was moderated by attachment style, such that those with more secure attachments intended to social distance more, even despite a desire for interpersonal closeness. This, and much of the aforementioned work on COVID-19, shows evidence for the manner in which adaptive health behaviors (like social distancing or exercise) could become laden with an additional dimension of self-esteem and meaning, with positive downstream effects.

Summary

COVID-19 had overwhelmingly negative impact on the general populous: In the wake of a daily blitzkrieg of death reminders, prepandemic efforts to stay healthy were no longer sufficient, the worldviews that once provided meaning became tenuous, and a new way of life began to emerge—with a level of collective psychological distress not previously observed (Pyszczynski et al., 2020). However, COVID-19 allowed researchers to extend the TMHM outside the lab and consider more cultural and individual nuance than in previous studies, all in a setting in which death awareness organically oscillated between the conscious and nonconscious. Given the ecologically valid and methodologically diverse approaches to applying the TMHM to the pandemic, a new era of TMHM literature can continue to advance and refine the theoretical foundation with creativity, novelty, and generalizability.

BEYOND COVID-19: ADVANCES IN TMHM RESEARCH

The case of COVID-19 exemplified that the TMHM can be tested using a variety of new approaches, with attention paid to a variety of moderating factors. Advances in research methods and considerations for commonplace, naturalistic existential threats in the context of health can further not only TMHM research, but also the manner in which individuals approach their own health and health care. We know from previous research and highlighted by COVID-19 that the existential dynamics of engagement with health are dependent on the target of that engagement and their characteristics—their cultural worldviews, their sources of esteem, and ultimately, what is best for each individual as they navigate their health.

First, COVID-19 afforded a sustained death reminder for individuals of all backgrounds. Theoretically relevant, real-time empirical data guided lines of inquiry: incidence, prevalence, and mortality rates; vaccination uptake; internet search volumes; and more. As such, future research may consider other big-data approaches to investigating the TMHM. Further, longitudinal work employing methods like ecological momentary assessment and real-time data capture will serve to expand theory to the daily reality in which people live. Additionally, researchers may consider behavioral engagement, rather than behavioral intentions, as important outcomes of interest. Using the TMHM as a guide, advances in methodology can provide insight into existential dynamics underlying engagement with health.

The TMHM asserts that adoption of adaptive health behaviors is contingent on a person's individual level of knowledge, background, and desire to engage in those behaviors for the purposes of building esteem under the duress of nonconscious mortality awareness, which runs in parallel to the concept of patient-centered care (PCC; Robinson et al., 2008). PCC emphasizes a partnership between health care providers and patients based on the characteristics of the patient, wherein personal relevance and perception of health issues is a necessary starting point in both health engagement and health care seeking. PCC and the TMHM alike ask: Do people even see themselves as susceptible to health risk, especially one that could kill them, and do they feel as if they'd be able to make the right choices if they are?

PCC, as guided by the TMHM, could mean many things. For different people, different health issues may be more concerning, relevant, and thus worth addressing than others. Preliminary evidence from Courtney and Goldenberg (2024, 2025) indicates that health issues like COVID-19, breast cancer, and substance use disorders carry heavier existential weight than asthma or skin cancer. Family history and ensuing personal relevance also bear implications for existential threat and health engagement. Courtney and Goldenberg (2025) found that, among women with a family history of breast cancer (compared to those without a family history) who perceived themselves as vulnerable to a diagnosis of their own, breast cancer was perceived as significantly deadlier, which in turn predicted esteem contingent on engagement in risk reducing and early detection behaviors, which subsequently predicted intentions to do so. These studies show that individuals must feel at risk, and effective health behaviors must connect with esteem in order to facilitate adaptive engagement with individual health.

Imbuing health behaviors with meaning at both the individual and broader scales through the lens of the TMHM should also help facilitate adaptive health engagement. Framing healthy behaviors as a positive practice that one can autonomously opt into, rather than demands or requirements that could facilitate resistance to health (Bessarabova & Massey, 2020), may encourage individuals to do right by themselves, both in a practical health sense and by bolstering feelings of esteem and meaning. There are a multitude of ways in which people can be encouraged to draw both individual and cultural meaning from health: from public health campaigns (e.g., Breast Cancer Awareness Month, November for Men's Health; Courtney & Goldenberg, 2021, 2025) to PCC to prototypes. Public health experts, communications and marketing professionals, and health care providers alike may consider painting health behaviors as lifestyle-adjacent. The important thing is that people recognize the risk of different health problems, recognize their own risk of those health problems, and recognize that effective health management can contribute to individual esteem.

CONCLUSION

Foundational to TMT and the TMHM is the idea that death is the worm that eats at the collective core: We know we'll die, it's just a matter of how. Many health issues are deadly for a variety of reasons, and that connection between death and health-related attempts to stave off its threat (regardless of its reality) is a primary motivator for both adaptive and maladaptive health engagement. This engagement is contingent on a variety of individual difference factors that interplay with the awareness of death: from cultural values like freedom, to cultural or celebrity icons, to individual susceptibility, to family history and vicarious health experiences.

COVID-19 afforded TMHM researchers the opportunity to naturalistically examine health engagement with constant death awareness. We now have more information we can use to inform the way we communicate about health. We know that we must imbue health behaviors with meaning, especially for those at increased risk. It may also be important to refrain from sanitizing health information: Your health could kill you and you will die; wouldn't you like to do your best to live healthily in the meantime?

And yes, health is largely an individual decision: Reminding those at risk that they will die while also providing esteem-based health solutions may change individual behavior, but larger-scale, systems-level thinking (Carey et al., 2015; Leischow et al., 2008) is necessary for broad-scale change. Individual behaviors only go so far in facilitating health in living conditions rife with pollution and chronic exposure to environmental carcinogens. We must consider ways in which public health, health communications, health care, and our larger systemic framework consider health facilitation across social status and culture. Death is a universal problem, and so is our health: Macrolevel changes to the system and a macrolevel focus on the cultural value of health are needed to facilitate health above and beyond individual behaviors and individual differences. The TMHM is a cornerstone for a constantly shifting (and hopefully improving) way of understanding the ways in which we can help people help themselves build longer, healthier lives—despite an inevitable expiration date.

NOTE

1. These studies have focused on the social or cultural value of alcohol use and thus conceptualized alcohol use as a distal defense against mortality awareness. However, given alcohol's and alcohol expectancies' connection to (perceived) anxiety reduction (Boness et al., 2021), there may also be situations where alcohol and other drug use could function as an attempted proximal defense to mitigate conscious concerns with mortality.

REFERENCES

Arndt, J., Cook, A., Goldenberg, J. L., & Cox, C. R. (2007). Cancer and the threat of death: The cognitive dynamics of death-thought suppression and its impact on behavioral health intentions. *Journal of Personality and Social Psychology, 92*(1), 12–29.

Arndt, J., Cox, C. R., Goldenberg, J. L., Vess, M., Routledge, C., Cooper, D. P., & Cohen, F. (2009). Blowing in the (social) wind: Implications of extrinsic esteem contingencies for terror management and health. *Journal of Personality and Social Psychology, 96*(6), 1191–1205.

Arndt, J., & Goldenberg, J. L. (2017). Where health and death intersect: Insights from a terror management health model. *Current Directions in Psychological Science, 26*(2), 126–131.

Arndt, J., Greenberg, J., Pyszczynski, T., & Solomon, S. (1997). Subliminal exposure to death-related stimuli increases defense of the cultural worldview. *Psychological Science, 8*(5), 379–385.

Arndt, J., Greenberg, J., Solomon, S., Pyszczynski, T., & Simon, L. (1997). Suppression, accessibility of death-related thoughts, and cultural worldview defense: Exploring the psychodynamics of terror management. *Journal of Personality and Social Psychology, 73*(1), 5–18.

Arndt, J., Routledge, C., & Goldenberg, J. L. (2006). Predicting proximal health responses to reminders of death: The influence of coping style and health optimism. *Psychology and Health, 21*(5), 593–614.

Arndt, J., Schimel, J., & Goldenberg, J. L. (2003). Death can be good for your health: Fitness intentions as a proximal and distal defense against mortality salience. *Journal of Applied Social Psychology, 33*(8), 1726–1746.

Barnes, S. J. (2021). Understanding terror states of online users in the context of COVID-19: An application of terror management theory. *Computers in Human Behavior, 125,* 106967.

Becker, E. (1962). *The birth and death of meaning: A perspective in psychiatry and anthropology.* Free Press.

Becker, E. (1973). *The denial of death.* Free Press.

Bessarabova, E., & Massey, Z. B. (2020). Testing terror management health model and integrating its predictions with the theory of psychological reactance. *Communication Monographs, 87*(1), 25–46.

Boness, C. L., Watts, A. L., Moeller, K. N., & Sher, K. J. (2021). The etiologic, theory-based, ontogenetic hierarchical framework of alcohol use disorder: A translational systematic review of reviews. *Psychological Bulletin, 147*(10), 1075.

Bozo, Ö., Tunca, A., & Šimšek, Y. (2009). The effect of death anxiety and age on health-promoting behaviors: A terror-management theory perspective. *Journal of Psychology, 143*(4), 377–389.

Burke, B. L., Martens, A., & Faucher, E. H. (2010). Two decades of terror management theory: A meta-analysis of mortality salience research. *Personality and Social Psychology Review, 14*(2), 155–195.

Cameron, L. D., Pepper, J. K., & Brewer, N. T. (2015). Responses of young adults to graphic warning labels for cigarette packages. *Tobacco Control, 24*(e1), e14–e22.

Carey, G., Malbon, E., Carey, N., Joyce, A., Crammond, B., & Carey, A. (2015). Systems science and systems thinking for public health: A systematic review of the field. *BMJ Open, 5*(12), e009002.

Chew, P. K. H. (2022). Big data analysis of terror management theory's predictions in the COVID-19 pandemic. *OMEGA: Journal of Death and Dying.*

Cooper, D. P., Goldenberg, J. L., & Arndt, J. (2010). Examining the terror management health model: The interactive effect of conscious death thought and health-coping variables on decisions in potentially fatal health domains. *Personality and Social Psychology Bulletin, 36*(7), 937–946.

Cooper, D. P., Goldenberg, J. L., & Arndt, J. (2011). Empowering the self: Using the terror management health model to promote breast self-examination. *Self and Identity, 10*(3), 315–325.

Cooper, D. P., Goldenberg, J. L., & Arndt, J. (2014). Perceived efficacy, conscious fear of death and intentions to tan: Not all fear appeals are created equal. *British Journal of Health Psychology, 19*(1), 1–15.

Courtney, E. P. (2024). Adaptive self-objectification. *Open Science Framework. https://osf.io/tr862.*

Courtney, E. P., Felig, R. N., & Goldenberg, J. L. (2021). Together we can slow the spread of COVID-19: The interactive effects of priming collectivism and mortality salience on virus-related health behaviour intentions. *British Journal of Social Psychology.*

Courtney, E. P., & Goldenberg, J. L. (2021). Adaptive self-objectification in the context of breast cancer: A theoretical integration of the terror management health model and research on objectification. *Applied Psychology: Health and Well-Being.*

Courtney, E. P., & Goldenberg, J. L. (2024). *The terror management health model and death-based fear appeals: A systematic review.* Unpublished manuscript, Department of Psychology, University of South Florida.

Courtney, E. P., & Goldenberg, J. L. (2025, in press). Breast health esteem to motivate breast health behavioral intentions: An application of the terror management health model. *Current Oncology.*

Courtney, E. P., Goldenberg, J. L., & Boyd, P. (2020). The contagion of mortality: A terror management health model for pandemics. *British Journal of Social Psychology,* bjso.12392.

Cox, C. R., Cooper, D. P., Vess, M., Arndt, J., Goldenberg, J. L., & Routledge, C. (2009). Bronze is beautiful but pale can be pretty: The effects of appearance standards and mortality salience on sun-tanning outcomes. *Health Psychology, 28*(6), 746–752.

Dimoff, J. D., Dao, A. N., Mitchell, J., & Olson, A. (2021). Live free and die: Expanding the terror management health model for pandemics to account for psychological reactance. *Social and Personality Psychology Compass, 15*(3).

Ein-Dor, T., Hirschberger, G., Perry, A., Levin, N., Cohen, R., Horesh, H., & Rothschild, E. (2014). Implicit death primes increase alcohol consumption. *Health Psychology, 33*(7), 748–751.

Fairlamb, S. (2022). The relationship between COVID-19-induced death thoughts and depression during a national lockdown. *Journal of Health Psychology, 27*(12), 2770–2776.

Fairlamb, S., Cinnirella, M., & Iahr, I. (2022). The proximal and distal effects of mortality salience on COVID-19-related health perceptions and intentions. *Journal of Applied Social Psychology, 52*(10), 965–976.

Fairlamb, S., & Courtney, E. (2022). An existential perspective on interpersonal closeness and social distancing during the COVID-19 pandemic. *Psychology and Health.*

Fredrickson, B. L., & Roberts, T.-A. (1997). Objectification theory: Toward understanding women's lived experiences and mental health risks. *Psychology of Women Quarterly, 21*(1997), 1787–1791.

Gerrard, M., Gibbons, F. X., Houlihan, A. E., Stock, M. L., & Pomery, E. A. (2008). A dual-process approach to health risk decision making: The prototype willingness model. *Developmental Review, 28*(1), 29–61.

Goldenberg, J. L. (2005). The body stripped down. *Current Directions in Psychological Science, 14*(4), 224–228.

Goldenberg, J. L., & Arndt, J. (2008). The implications of death for health: A terror management health model for behavioral health promotion. *Psychological Review, 115*(4), 1032–1053.

Goldenberg, J. L., Arndt, J., Hart, J., & Routledge, C. (2008). Uncovering an existential barrier to breast self-exam behavior. *Journal of Experimental Social Psychology, 44*(2), 260–274.

Goldenberg, J. L., Hart, J., Pyszczynski, T., Warnica, G. M., Landau, M., & Thomas, L. (2006). Ambivalence toward the body: Death, neuroticism, and the flight from physical sensation. *Personality and Social Psychology Bulletin, 32*(9), 1264–1277.

Goldenberg, J. L., Pyszczynski, T., Greenberg, J., & Solomon, S. (2000). Fleeing the body: A terror management perspective on the problem of human corporeality. *Personality and Social Psychology Review, 4*(3), 200–218.

Goldenberg, J. L., Pyszczynski, T., Greenberg, J., Solomon, S., Kluck, B., & Cornwell, R. (2001). I am not an animal: Mortality salience, disgust, and the denial of human creatureliness. *Journal of Experimental Psychology: General, 130*(3), 427–435.

Goldenberg, J. L., & Roberts, T.-A. (2011). The Birthmark: An existential account of the objectification of women. In R. M. Calogero, S. Tantleff-Dunn, & J. K. Thompson (Eds.), *Self-objectification in women: Causes, consequences, and counteraction* (pp. 77–99). American Psychological Association.

Goldenberg, J. L., Routledge, C., & Arndt, J. (2009). Mammograms and the management of existential discomfort: Threats associated with the physicality of the body and neuroticism. *Psychology and Health, 24*(5), 563–581.

Grabe, S., Routledge, C., Cook, A., Andersen, C., & Arndt, J. (2005). In defense of the body: The effect of mortality salience on female body objectification. *Psychology of Women Quarterly, 29*(1), 33–37.

Greenberg, J., Arndt, J., Simon, L., Pyszczynski, T., & Solomon, S. (2000). Proximal and distal defenses in response to reminders of one's mortality: Evidence of a temporal sequence. *Personality and Social Psychology Bulletin, 26*(1), 91–99.

Greenberg, J., Pyszczynski, T., & Solomon, S. (1986). The causes and consequences of a need for self-esteem: A terror management theory. In R. F. Baumeister (Ed.), *Public self and private self* (pp. 189–212). Springer.

Hansen, J., Winzeler, S., & Topolinski, S. (2010). When the death makes you smoke: A terror management perspective on the effectiveness of cigarette on-pack warnings. *Journal of Experimental Social Psychology, 46*(1), 226–228.

Harvell-Bowman, L. A. (2023). Exploring the existential implications of COVID-19 in health communication. *American Behavioral Scientist.*

Hirschberger, G., Florian, V., Mikulincer, M., Goldenberg, J. L., & Pyszczynski, T. (2002). Gender differences in the willingness to engage in risky behavior: A terror management perspective. *Death Studies, 26*(2), 117–141.

Hossain, M. M., Tasnim, S., Sultana, A., Faizah, F., Mazumder, H., Zou, L., . . . Ma, P. (2020). Epidemiology of mental health problems in COVID-19: A review. *F1000Research, 9,* 636.

Jessop, D. C., & Wade, J. (2008). Fear appeals and binge drinking: A terror management theory perspective. *British Journal of Health Psychology, 13*(4), 773–788.

Kim, D. K. D., & Kreps, G. L. (2020). An analysis of government communication in the United States during the COVID-19 pandemic: Recommendations for effective government health risk communication. *World Medical and Health Policy, 12*(4), 398–412.

Kwon, S., & Park, A. (2022). Understanding user responses to the COVID-19 pandemic on Twitter from a terror management theory perspective: Cultural differences among the US, UK and India. *Computers in Human Behavior, 128,* 107087.

Lam, S. R., Rios Morrison, K., & Smeesters, D. (2009). Gender, intimacy, and risky sex: A terror management account. *Personality and Social Psychology Bulletin, 35*(8), 1046–1056.

Langellier, K. M., & Sullivan, C. F. (1998). Breast talk in breast cancer narratives. *Qualitative Health Research, 8*(1), 76–94.

Leischow, S. J., Best, A., Trochim, W. M., Clark, P. I., Gallagher, R. S., Marcus, S. E., & Matthews, E. (2008). Systems thinking to improve the public's health. *American Journal of Preventive Medicine, 35*(2), S196–S203.

Lindgren, K. P., Ramirez, J. J., Olin, C. C., & Neighbors, C. (2016). Not the same old thing: Establishing the unique contribution of drinking identity as a predictor of alcohol consumption and problems over time. *Psychology of Addictive Behaviors, 30*(6), 659–671.

Liu, Y., Cai, L., Ma, F., & Wang, X. (2023). Revenge buying after the lockdown: Based on the SOR framework and TPB model. *Journal of Retailing and Consumer Services, 72,* 103263.

Martin, I. M., & Kamins, M. (2007). Relationships can disappear in a puff of smoke: A test of TMT and risk perceptions on smoking behavior. *Advances in Consumer Research, 34*(2003), 312–313.

Martin, I. M., & Kamins, M. A. (2009). An application of terror management theory in the design of social and health-related anti-smoking appeals. *Journal of Consumer Behaviour, 9*(3), 172–190.

Martin, I. M., & Kamins, M. A. (2019). Effectively using death in health messages: Social loss versus physical mortality salience. *Journal of Consumer Behaviour, 18*(3), 205–218.

McCabe, S., Arndt, J., Goldenberg, J. L., Vess, M., Vail, K. E., Gibbons, F. X., & Rogers, R. (2015). The effect of visualizing healthy eaters and mortality reminders on nutritious grocery purchases: An integrative terror management and prototype willingness analysis. *Health Psychology, 34*(3), 279–282.

McCabe, S., & Bartholow, B. D. (2019). Mortality salience leads to greater consumption of an ostensibly alcoholic beverage on Friday versus other weekdays. *British Journal of Health Psychology, 24*(4), 847–858.

McCabe, S., Vail, K. E., Arndt, J., & Goldenberg, J. L. (2014). Hails from the crypt: A terror management health model investigation of the effectiveness of health-oriented versus celebrity-oriented endorsements. *Personality and Social Psychology Bulletin, 40*(3), 289–300.

Menzies, R. E., & Menzies, R. G. (2020). Death anxiety in the time of COVID-19: Theoretical explanations and clinical implications. *Cognitive Behaviour Therapist, 13,* e19.

Miller, C. H., & Ma, H. (2021). How existential anxiety shapes communication in coping with the coronavirus pandemic. In H. D. O'Hair & M. J. O'Hair (Eds.), *Communicating science in times of crisis* (pp. 54–80). Wiley.

Moradi, B., & Huang, Y. P. (2008). Objectification theory and psychology of women: A decade of advances and future directions. *Psychology of Women Quarterly, 32*(4), 377–398.

Morris, K. L., Cooper, D. P., Goldenberg, J. L., Arndt, J., & Gibbons, F. X. (2014). Improving the efficacy of appearance-based sun exposure interventions with the terror management health model. *Psychology and Health, 29*(11), 1245–1264.

Morris, K. L., Cooper, D. P., Goldenberg, J. L., Arndt, J., & Routledge, C. (2013). Objectification as self-affirmation in the context of a death-relevant health threat. *Self and Identity, 12*(6), 610–620.

Morris, K. L., Goldenberg, J. L., Arndt, J., & McCabe, S. (2019). The enduring influence of death on health: insights from the terror management health model. *Self and Identity, 18*(4), 378–404.

Morris, K. L., Goldenberg, J. L., & Heflick, N. A. (2014). Trio of terror (pregnancy, menstruation, and breastfeeding): An existential function of literal self-objectification among women. *Journal of Personality and Social Psychology, 107*(1), 181–198.

Moser, R. P., Arndt, J., Han, P. K., Waters, E. A., Amsellem, M., & Hesse, B. W. (2014). Perceptions of cancer as a death sentence: Prevalence and consequences. *Journal of Health Psychology, 19*(12), 1518–1524.

Moser, R. P., Arndt, J., Jimenez, T., Liu, B., & Hesse, B. W. (2021). Perceptions of cancer as a death sentence: Tracking trends in public perceptions from 2008 to 2017. *Psycho-Oncology, 30*(4), 511–519.

Nagar, M., & Rabinovitz, S. (2015). Smoke your troubles away: Exploring the effects of death cognitions on cannabis craving and consumption. *Journal of Psychoactive Drugs, 47*(2), 91–99.

National Cancer Institute. (2023). *Cancer stat facts: Female breast cancer.* Surveillance, Epidemiology, and End Results Program. https://seer.cancer.gov/statfacts/html/breast.html.

Nussbaum, M. C. (1995). Objectification. *Philosophy and Public Affairs, 24*(4), 249–291.

Perach, R., & Limbu, M. (2022). Can culture beat Covid-19?: Evidence that exposure to facemasks with cultural symbols increases solidarity. *British Journal of Social Psychology, 61*(3), 991–1010.

Pyszczynski, T., Lockett, M., Greenberg, J., & Solomon, S. (2020). Terror management theory and the COVID-19 pandemic. *Journal of Humanistic Psychology, 61*(2), 173–189.

Pyszczynski, T., Solomon, S., & Greenberg, J. (1999). A dual-process model of defense against conscious and unconscious death-related thoughts: An extension of terror management theory. *Psychological Review, 106*(4), 835–845.

Pyszczynski, T., Solomon, S., & Greenberg, J. (2015). Thirty years of terror management theory. In J. M. Olson & M. P. Zanna (Eds.), *Advances in experimental social psychology* (pp. 1–70). Academic Press.

Robinson, J. H., Callister, L. C., Berry, J. A., & Dearing, K. A. (2008). Patient-centered care and adherence: Definitions and applications to improve outcomes. *Journal of the American Academy of Nurse Practitioners, 20*(12), 600–607.

Routledge, C., Arndt, J., & Goldenberg, J. L. (2004). A time to tan: Proximal and distal effects of mortality salience on sun exposure intentions. *Personality and Social Psychology Bulletin, 30*(10), 1347–1358.

Scrima, F., Miceli, S., Caci, B., & Cardaci, M. (2022). The relationship between fear of COVID-19 and intention to get vaccinated.

The serial mediation roles of existential anxiety and conspiracy beliefs. *Personality and Individual Differences, 184,* 111188.

Sheeran, P., Harris, P. R., & Epton, T. (2014). Does heightening risk appraisals change people's intentions and behavior?: A meta-analysis of experimental studies. *Psychological Bulletin, 140*(2), 511–543.

Strong, D. R., Pierce, J. P., Pulvers, K., Stone, M. D., Villaseñor, A., Pu, M., . . . Messer, K. (2021). Effect of graphic warning labels on cigarette packs on US smokers' cognitions and smoking behavior after 3 months. *JAMA Network Open, 4*(8), e2121387.

Taubman-Ben-Ari, O., & Findler, L. (2005). Proximal and distal effects of mortality salience on willingness to engage in health promoting behavior along the life span. *Psychology and Health, 20*(3), 303–318.

Taubman Ben-Ari, O., Florian, V., & Mikulincer, M. (1999). The impact of mortality salience on reckless driving: A test of terror management mechanisms. *Journal of Personality and Social Psychology, 76*(1), 35–45.

Wang, T. H. (2023). The urge to search: A multinational model of prepurchase behavior during COVID-19. *Social Behavior and Personality: An International Journal, 51*(1), 1–18.

Wisman, A., Heflick, N., & Goldenberg, J. L. (2015). The great escape: The role of self-esteem and self-related cognition in terror management. *Journal of Experimental Social Psychology, 60,* 121–132.

Wong, N. C. H., Nisbett, G. S., & Harvell, L. A. (2017). Smoking is so ew!: College smokers' reactions to health- versus social-focused antismoking threat messages. *Health Communication, 32*(4), 451–460.

Zanna, M. P., & Cooper, J. (2000). Dissonance and the pill: An attribution approach to studying the arousal properties of dissonance. In E. T. Higgins & A. W. Kruglanski (Eds.), *Motivational science: Social and personality perspectives* (pp. 306–312). Psychology Press.

CHAPTER 11

Suicide

The Fatal Withdrawal from Life

Joseph Hayes *and* Robert W. G. Tupper

Why do people commit suicide? Given the evolutionary propensity to preserve one's life, the fact that people intentionally kill themselves seems absurd. As such, one would expect acts of suicide to be exceedingly rare. Yet according to the World Health Organization (WHO; 2021), suicide accounts for approximately 1% of all deaths, amounting to over 700,000 deaths per year worldwide. Moreover, given the stigma of mental illness and the amoral (or even illegal) status of suicidal acts in many countries, these figures are necessarily *under*estimates, not to mention the fact that they are only counting suicidal acts that end in death. Plus, all of this speaks only to suicidal *acts*. It says nothing of suicidal thoughts, which are far more pervasive (Klonsky et al., 2016). Thus, suicidality (including thoughts, attempts, and deaths) is far more common than one might expect at first blush.

The science of existential psychology has yet to offer a compelling theory of why people commit suicide. In fact, the dominant theoretical perspective in existential psychology (namely, terror management theory [TMT]; Greenberg et al., 1986) argues that nearly all our daily activity is influenced by the universal *fear* of death. How could so many people commit suicide if they are so afraid of dying? Indeed, the mere existence of suicide is often used as a critique of TMT (e.g., Muravan & Baumeister, 1997). In this chapter, we propose a theory of suicide that integrates TMT with goal regulation theory. In brief, we argue that suicide is the ultimate manifestation of *fatalistic withdrawal* (Hayes et al., 2016)—a goal-disengagement process initiated by the knowledge of inevitable death. Although death awareness will often invigorate life-affirming behavior, the fact that death is inevitable can also make living seem futile and can therefore lead people to give up on life and commit suicide.

GOAL REGULATION THEORY

The most basic premise of goal regulation theory is that intentional behavior is driven by a system of goals (see, e.g., Carver & Scheier, 1998). Goals are cognitive representations of the purpose (or intended outcome) of behavior that allow people to regulate their own actions toward desired ends—even over long periods of time. Goals are organized into a broad, hierarchical system where lower-order actions (e.g., tie my shoes) are guided by higher-order programs (e.g., go for a run) that are, in turn, guided by even higher-order principles (e.g., be fit). From this perspective, even the smallest of muscle movements can be cybernetically controlled by broader goal constructs (Carver & Scheier, 1998). Overall, the function of the goal system is to provide intentional self-regulation of behavior that is modulated by thoughts and values (i.e., top down) rather than driven by preprogramed instincts or reflexive learning processes (i.e., bottom up; cf., Davis & Panksepp, 2018).

According to Carver and Scheier (1998), goal processes involve setting standards by which current goal progress can be evaluated, and monitoring whether behavior is in line with these standards. Building upon objective self-awareness theory (Duval & Wickland, 1972), they argued that self-focused attention triggers a comparison of one's current state with a salient goal standard. If a discrepancy is detected, then the individual experiences negative affect and becomes motivated to engage efforts to bring the self in line with the standard. In other words, they increase effort toward achieving the goal until the standard is met, the goal is abandoned, or self-awareness is reduced (see Carver & Scheier, 1998, for detailed discussion).

Although bringing the self in line with standards to achieve personally important goals may seem relatively straightforward, successfully accomplishing goals is often fraught by setbacks and roadblocks. This is especially true for long-term goals that entail controlling behavior over long periods of time (e.g., get a PhD). When such goals are initially set, there is almost always a degree of uncertainty about whether they will be achieved. Situational constraints or personal shortcomings might impede or prevent goal progress and all efforts may ultimately end in failure. And in the case of broad-level goal principles (e.g., be a good friend), success can never be achieved once and for all. Such goals require sustained commitment to lower-order actions that are consistent with the broader principle or value standard. Missteps are always possible, and "success" is therefore often tenuous.

According to goal regulation theory, when people encounter prolonged difficulties in their goal pursuits, they may pause to reassess the likelihood of success (Carver & Scheier, 1998). Depending on how important the goal may be to one's overall self-concept, this pause may be characterized by high levels of anxiety and self-doubt. On a neurobiological level, this anxious state represents the affective component of a broader suite of processes performed by the behavioral inhibition system (BIS; Gray & McNaughton, 2000). The BIS is activated whenever a person experiences motivational conflict, and its primary function is to resolve these conflicts. In this case, the conflict is between the desire to continue goal activity to obtain a positive outcome (i.e., the goal) and to cease goal activity to avoid a negative outcome (i.e., frustrative nonreward). Obviously, one cannot simultaneously pursue a goal and give up on it. Thus, the purpose of the BIS is to regulate motivational conflicts so that one of these behavioral outputs takes precedence (McNaughton & Corr, 2004).

In many cases, goal impedances can be overcome with persistent effort. In general, if the individual remains confident in their abilities (cf. Bandura, 1977) or feels that there is still hope of success (Carver & Scheier, 1998), they will persist in goal-directed activity until the difficulties are overcome. In such cases, the anxious BIS-state effectively kicks behavior into a higher gear and promotes invigorated goal approach motivation (McGregor et al., 2010). In other cases, however, the individual may conclude that no action can be taken to overcome the goal impedance. One of the main functions of the BIS is to stop approach-oriented behavior that may lead to negative outcomes (e.g., wasted energy expenditure, unintended injury/death) rather than the desired positive outcome (McNaughton & Corr, 2004). The BIS will therefore tend to side with disengagement (or goal withdrawal) when no viable solution to the impedance can be found. In these cases, the goal will be abandoned, and all effort aimed at goal attainment, including the subroutines and specific actions that functionally service this goal, will be terminated.

From a goal regulation perspective, goal disengagement is never fully accomplished until an alternative goal is activated (Carver & Scheier, 1998). The alternative goal need not be connected to the disengaged goal, but oftentimes disengagement itself can facilitate efforts to attain the higher-level principle that the disengaged goal was intended to serve. For instance, if a student is not successful in their attempts to gain admission to a graduate program in clinical psychology, they may turn their attention to the broader purpose of this goal (e.g., to help people in need) and reallocate resources to achieving the broader purpose via alternate means (e.g., seek admission to a different educational or skills-based program aimed at helping people in need). Thus, goal withdrawal is often an adaptive means of flexibly adjusting to situational constraints (see Brandtstädter & Renner, 1990; Hubley & Scholer, 2022; Wrosch et al., 2003). Once again, this is a crucial function of the BIS—to prevent futile goal persistence so that energy can be redirected toward more fruitful goal pursuits.

In summary, goal regulation theory offers a top-down, systematic perspective on the self-regulation of behavior. Although there are many other interesting and important aspects to this theoretical perspective (see Carver & Scheier, 1998, for a fulsome review), we emphasize the goal dynamics of persistence and withdrawal in the interest of understanding suicide. Accordingly, we maintain that suicide can be understood by viewing life itself in goal-related terms and focusing on the basic goal regulation mechanisms of persistence and withdrawal.

A GOAL REGULATION PERSPECTIVE ON LIVING

In many ways, *living* is a goal just like any other. People generally want to live; they approach activities that sustain life and behave in ways that promote survival. What makes this goal somewhat unique (i.e., the goal to *be* alive, or to *continue* living from one moment to the next) is that it is a superordinate goal at the highest levels of the goal hierarchy that guides many subordinate activities (a system concept; see Carver & Scheier, 1998). In other words, the goal to continue living is underpinned by innumerable ongoing, daily tasks (e.g., earning money, buying food, eating), and therefore plays a central role in the overall self-regulation of behavior. Indeed, one may even conceive of the goal to continue living as the highest-level goal in the entire system (Hayes et al., 2016; Pyszczynski et al., 1990).

The Problem of Inevitable Death

The main threat to the ongoing viability of the goal to continue living is, of course, death. Death represents the end of life—the point at which the goal to continue living has failed. As such, thoughts of death activate feelings of anxiety by initiating BIS-processes (Jonas et al., 2014; Tritt et al., 2012). Hundreds of empirical studies on TMT have elucidated how people react to thoughts of death (for reviews, see Routledge & Vess, 2019; Solomon et al., Chapter 6, this volume).

Our perspective represents only a slight divergence from TMT. In our view, the crux of TMT is the conflict between the biological self-preservation instincts and the knowledge of inevitable death. This conflict is the driving force behind all terror management motivation, as this is what leads to the anxiety/terror that must be managed to maintain equanimity. We do not disagree with this perspective but, rather, add that living is a psychological goal in addition to a biological imperative. In other words, while humans are biologically programed to survive, we also tend to endorse survival as a goal that we *intentionally* strive to maintain. This distinction may appear trivial, but the idea that goals function independently of biological drives is an important function of self-regulation. Indeed, many of our goals run counter to biological drives, which gives us the flexibility to control our own actions (e.g., refraining from eating fatty foods in the service of the goal to maintain an idealized body image). In the case of living, however, our goal to continue living tends to be perfectly aligned with our survival instincts. But these are nevertheless separate motivational processes.

The main thrust of distinguishing between instinctual and goal-based motivations to live is that the awareness of death is at odds with both these survival tendencies. And importantly, we argue that death poses an even greater threat to the psychological goal to live than it does to the biological propensity to survive. Goals are more flexible than instincts (by design, they are meant to allow the organism to flexibly adapt to their environment rather than be rigidly driven by predetermined instincts; see Davis & Panksepp, 2018), and they are especially sensitive to cues of inevitable failure (Carver & Scheier, 1998). And while all goals have the *possibility* of failure, the trouble with the goal to continue living is that it is *guaranteed* to fail because death is inevitable. All people recognize this fact from a relatively early age (e.g., Speece & Brent, 1984). And from a goal regulation perspective, the fact that death is inevitable is highly problematic because, when a goal is certain to fail, the BIS will trigger an impulse to withdraw from that goal. In essence, the knowledge of inevitable death makes the goal to continue living seem futile.

Although goal withdrawal is typically adaptive—especially when it facilitates reallocation of energy/motivation toward alternative goals—withdrawal from the goal to continue living is highly maladaptive (Hayes & Hubley, 2017). Since living is a superordinate system concept, abandoning this goal entails simultaneously withdrawing from all subordinate goals that serve the purpose of sustaining life. This would constitute a system-wide collapse in the goal motivation system. We term this state *fatalistic* withdrawal, because it entails abandoning all intentional self-regulation and resigning oneself to fate (Hayes et al., 2016). And for the current purposes, we also maintain that fatalistic withdrawal can be *fatal* by promoting self-destructive behavior, including overt attempts to end life via suicide. As such, an organism that understands the inevitability of death must have a means of preventing fatalistic withdraw from life. Otherwise, all goal-directed intentions to preserve life are imperiled due to the realization that death is inescapable.

A Symbolic Solution

Drawing from the writings of Becker (1973) and TMT (Greenberg et al., 1986), we maintain that humans found a way around this dilemma by creating a symbolic world (i.e., a cultural drama) that offers the potential for continued existence beyond death. On a goal regulation level, this solution entails abstracting the goal to continue living to an even higher order system concept—namely, *to exist*. From this vantage, being physically alive is a means of existing in the world, but existence can also be attained symbolically by having an identity and playing character roles in an ongoing symbolic drama—aspects of existence that do not inevitably end with physical death (Becker, 1973).

Although the goal to remain physically alive is doomed to fail and therefore prone to withdrawal, the goal to exist symbolically is not similarly doomed because symbols transcend the physical body and can thus exist indefinitely. Figure 11.1 offers a simplified illustration of the hierarchical goal system as we conceptualize it. This figure combines elements of Carver and Scheier's (1998) classic

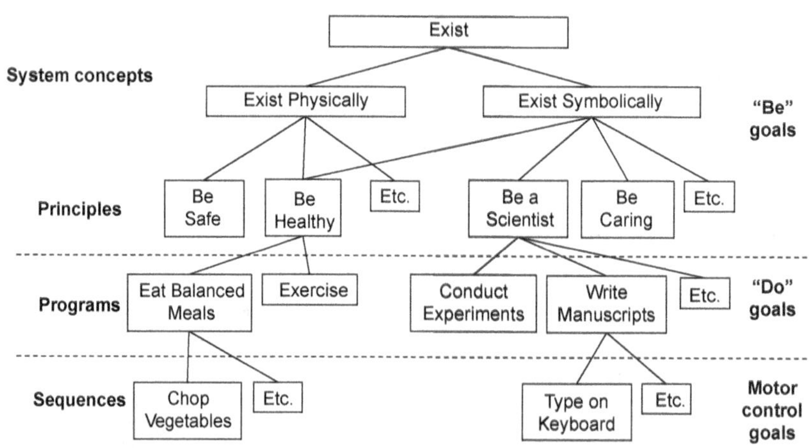

FIGURE 11.1. Simplified illustration of the hierarchical organization of the goal to continue living. Adapted from Carver and Scheier (1998) and Pyszczynski et al. (1990).

goal theory with similar conceptualizations of the goal system from a TMT perspective (e.g., Pyszczynski et al., 1990).

In this example, the goal to exist can be achieved physically or symbolically at the system concept level, and each of these system concepts has associated lower-order principles and programs. As previously mentioned, the physical side of existence is supported by the principle-level goals of being safe, being healthy, and so forth. Any goal that maximizes physical life and minimizes the potential for death is governed by this system concept.

The symbolic side of existence, on the other hand, is supported by measuring up to the cultural value standards necessary to achieve symbolic life continuity.[1] This side of existence is the typical purview of TMT research related to worldviews and self-esteem (see, e.g., Solomon et al., Chapter 6, this volume). Figure 11.1 depicts a person who aspires to live symbolically as a scientist, a caring person, and any number of other goal principles that offer a meaningful symbolic existence. At the program level, to exist symbolically as a scientist the individual must adhere to standards that convey this identity, such as conducting experiments and writing compelling manuscripts. Consistent with TMT, the extent to which this person feels successful in adhering to these value standards will determine their overall feeling of symbolic significance or self-esteem. In brief, symbolic goals offer meaning to life by providing purpose to our actions and suggesting that what we do matters in the grand scheme of things (cf., George & Park, 2016).

Preventing Fatalistic Withdrawal

According to our model, the main function of pursuing a symbolic form of existence is to satisfy the higher-order goal to exist, which cannot be accomplished through physical means because living (physically) is doomed to fail by the inevitability of death. On this matter, our perspective is identical to TMT and consistent with some of the earliest theoretical statements of the theory that specify the goal dynamics of pursuing direct (i.e., physical) and symbolic forms of self-preservation (Pyszczynski et al., 1990). However, whereas TMT focuses on the *anxiety-buffering* function of symbolic goal engagements following mortality reminders, we argue that symbolic existence goals also function to prevent fatalistic withdrawal from life. In fact, withdrawing from a conflicted goal can reduce anxiety by terminating BIS processes (McNaughton & Corr, 2004; see also Hayes et al., 2017). Recall that the BIS serves to regulate motivational conflict in a way that promotes either goal persistence or goal withdrawal. Regardless of which of these outcomes prevails, so long as the organism has regained a unidirectional motivational state, the BIS process and associated anxiety will be reduced. However, rather than being a healthy adaptation that reduces anxiety and promotes daily functioning, fatalistic withdrawal is a maladaptive means of reducing death anxiety and must therefore be prevented to ensure optimal functioning.

In essence, we view the goal to remain physically alive (depicted on the left side of Figure 11.1) as terminally prone to collapse considering that death is inevitable. In other words, the goal to remain physically alive cannot function on its own in an organism that is aware of the inescapability of death. People need a reason to maintain physical life, because staying alive for its own sake is futile. By supporting the broader goal to exist, symbolic existence goals (depicted on the right side of Figure 11.1) function to sustain the goal system and prevent collapse. Symbolic existence goals offer reasons to continue living despite the inevitability of death. Principle-level goals, such as being helpful to one's community, being a prolific scientific researcher, or being a loving caretaker of one's children, are all symbolic ways of being/existing that offer reason to remain alive. In brief, the symbolic side of the goal system functions to maintain the will to live physically, even though we fully understand that one day we will die.

A GOAL REGULATION PERSPECTIVE ON SUICIDE: THE PATH TOWARD SELF-DESTRUCTION

Our main argument in this chapter is that normally adaptive goal-withdrawal processes become maladaptive when applied to the goal to continue living. Withdrawal from life triggers a general collapse in the goals system and may ultimately lead a person to seek death by suicide. To be clear, we are not arguing that suicide is an inevitable outcome of fatalistic withdrawal. Rather, we maintain that suicide represents the ultimate manifestation of this more general withdrawal process—the final stop on an often much longer progression that is initiated by withdrawal from life. In this section, we draw upon existing theories of suicide to paint a general picture of the steps that may often be taken in this progression. It stands to reason that each step in the progression may not be necessary, and most people who start down this path do not proceed all the way to the end.

Failure to Maintain Symbolic Existence

According to our theory, the viability of symbolic existence is crucially important in preventing fatalistic withdrawal from life, especially when thoughts of death are salient. When a person feels that they have failed to create a symbolic self that is worthy of death transcendence, and there is no hope of remedying the situation, our theory suggests that they will begin to withdraw from life, setting the stage for suicide. Given the futility of living physically vis-à-vis the inevitability of death, without a viable means of existing symbolically, the highest goal in the hierarchy (the goal to exist) will be abandoned and the entire goal system will collapse. The precise circumstances that may lead a person to conclude that efforts to exist symbolically cannot be successful are likely many and varied. But all should entail significant damage to the perceived ability to live up to internalized standards associated with the possession of a critically important symbolic identity. Several lines of evidence are consistent with this reasoning.

Threats to the Symbolic Self

First, dozens of experimental studies in support of TMT show that threats to important sources of symbolic identity or self-esteem increase death-thought accessibility (DTA; Hayes et al., 2010). For example, thinking about undesirable aspects of oneself, failing to live up to important self-defining value standards, or being led to believe that one's personality is ill suited for one's desired career goals have all being shown to increased DTA (Hayes et al., 2008; Ogilvie et al., 2008). Moreover, failure to live up to important cultural definitions of success has been found to increase the cognitive accessibility of suicide-related thoughts (Chatard & Selimbegović, 2011). Thus, when people experience significant threats to their ability to achieve the goals that convey a desired symbolic identity, they have trouble managing death-related concerns and may begin to contemplate suicide.

Second, threats to important interpersonal relationships have also been linked to DTA and suicidality. Both the interpersonal theory of suicide (Joiner, 2005) and the three-step theory (Klonsky & May, 2015) identify thwarted belongingness or the failure to form meaningful interpersonal connections as a precipitating factor in suicidality. According to Baumeister and Leary (1995), belongingness is a fundamental human need, and close personal relationships are an important part of the means through which people buffer death-related anxiety (Mikulincer et al., 2003). Feeling loved and valued by significant others is pivotal in feeling that one's existence matters (George & Park, 2014), and being ostracized is akin to not existing at all on a symbolic level (Williams, 2007). In the words of Rosenberg and McCullough (1981), "existence loses its point and savor when one no longer makes a difference" (p. 180). This sentiment is consistent with the idea that people will lose the motivation to continue living when they fail to create and maintain a symbolic self that is worthy of continued existence.

Persistent Pain

Another consideration in understanding motivations for suicide is the subjective experience of life when people fail to meet symbolic value standards. According to Carver and Scheier (1998), progressing toward goals produces positive affect, whereas failure to achieve progress produces negative affect. When the goal in question is a self-defining feature of one's symbolic existence, and no alternatives for satisfying this goal exist, the negative affect will be persistent and may become a significant source of psychological suffering. According to Klonsky and May's (2015) three-step theory, persistent pain is the first step in the path toward suicide. Thus, significant failures can promote suicidality by creating persistent psychological pain that is difficult or impossible to eliminate by making progress toward self-defining existential goals.

Klonsky and May (2015) argued that the pain that promotes suicidality can be either psychological or physical. Consistent with our perspective, not only does the experience of chronic physical pain produce a negative subject experience of existence, but it can also impede one's ability to create and maintain the symbolic self. Research on the social effects of pain suggests that chronic pain interrupts important social roles (e.g., friendships, occupation, leisure, family), which can in turn lead to depression (Harris et al., 2003). Similarly, a qualitative analysis of the narratives expressed by chronic pain sufferers included reports of having lost important social or occupational roles, which ultimately led to a loss of self-esteem and hope for the future (Walker et al., 2006).

Failure to Mount Symbolic Defenses When Death Is Salient

Additional evidence for the role of symbolic existence goals in preventing fatalistic withdrawal from life can be gleaned from studies investigating how people respond to explicit reminders of death (i.e., mortality salience [MS]). For instance, Routledge and colleagues (2010) found that MS reduced self-reported vitality (i.e., energy for living) among people with low self-esteem. Since self-esteem is attained by feeling that one is living up to symbolic value standards and therefore qualifies for symbolic death transcendence (Lifshin et al., 2021), people with low self-esteem have greater difficulty preventing the impulse to withdraw from life when mortality is salient. Similarly, Mikulincer and Shaver (2012) found that when MS was followed by experimental manipulations that impeded symbolic existence goals, such as contemplating undesired aspects of oneself or separation from attachment figures, participants showed impaired performance on an effortful remote associates test and reported increased feelings of helplessness and despair.

The most direct evidence that death reminders can cause fatalistic withdrawal comes from a series of studies by Hayes and colleagues (2016) who found that MS and salient thoughts of failure at an important symbolic life goal (e.g., career goals, relationship goals) led participants who were dissatisfied with their life to report wanting to live shorter lives (12 years less, on average) than control participants. Hayes and Hubley (2023) replicated these results using a measure that assesses agreement with self-statements (e.g., "I want to continue living"). Results showed significantly reduced desire to live among low self-esteem participants who were reminded of death and failure.

Consistent with the notion that abandoning the desire to live triggers a general collapse in the goal system (as indicative of fatalistic withdrawal), Hayes and colleagues (2016) found that the same conditions that reduced the desire to live also reduced generalized goal approach motivation and the willingness to delay gratification (a hallmark of intentional self-regulation; e.g., Mischel et al., 1989). These conditions also increased self-reported fatalism (e.g., "It doesn't really matter what I do") and reduced future-oriented time perspective. Critically, these effects were found to be mediated by pessimism toward the future—a sense of hopelessness that things will ever get better. Consistent with Klonsky and May's (2015) three-step theory, the mere hope that things can improve is enough to maintain the will to live, even when life is full of abject suffering. But when hope is lost, the individual feels permanently and irreparably trapped in a state of symbolic failure (cf. entrapment; O'Connor & Kirtley, 2018). In essence, they may feel like they are already symbolically dead. And since the will to exist physically is predicated on the viability of continued symbolic existence, our model suggests that they will succumb to the impulse to withdraw from life and may consider suicide.

On an emotional level, Hayes and colleagues (2016) found that withdrawal from life was associated with *reduced* anxiety. This is consistent with our goal regulation perspective, because any resolution to the conflict between the desire to live and the knowledge of death (persistence or withdrawal) should deactivate the BIS (Hayes et al., 2017; Jonas et al., 2014). Thus, giving up on the goal to continue living may be emotionally appealing by providing relief from the BIS-mediated anxiety that would otherwise persist when efforts to exist symbolically fail. However, Hayes and colleagues also found that withdrawal from life led to significant increases in depression. Thus, giving in to the impulse to withdraw from life entailed trading one negative emotion (i.e., anxiety) for another (i.e., depression). From this perspective, suicide is connected to depression (Hawton et al., 2013) because both stem from a broader process of withdrawal from life.

In summary, several lines of evidence are consistent with the idea that symbolic existence goals function to prevent fatalistic withdrawal from life. When these symbolic goals are threatened or lost, and hope for the future appears lost, the impulse to withdraw grows stronger and people may be unable to remain engaged in life.

Mental Disengagement

Although we argue that the process of withdrawing from life is triggered by a failure or loss of symbolic existence, the process likely begins with mental disengagement. According to goal regulation theory, disengagement from goals at the highest level of the goal hierarchy is often not possible given that no alternative goals exist at the same level. Carver and Scheier (1998) maintained that goal disengagement can never be complete until another goal is identified, toward which approach-oriented activity can be redirected. But being alive is a precondition for all goal activity. One cannot abandon living in the interest of doing something else. Under these circumstances, the only option remaining is to disengage mentally by reducing self-awareness and thus circumventing the self-standard comparison process that is inherent in goal striving. This is the underlying logic of the escape theory of suicide (Baumeister, 1990), where people attempt to escape self-awareness to avoid the pain of failure.

Following the logic of escape theory, Wisman and colleagues (2015) proposed an *existential escape hypothesis* stating that people who are unable to mount symbolic defenses against the awareness of inevitable death (such as those with low self-esteem) will instead seek to reduce existential anxiety by deactivating the self and reducing self-awareness. This hypothesis is consistent with our perspective on fatalistic withdrawal and may represent the initial stages of the overall process of withdrawing from life. In support of this hypothesis, Wisman and colleagues found that MS led people with low self-esteem to avoid self-focused thought by choosing to write about someone else (instead of themselves) on a self-directed writing task or consuming higher amounts of alcohol during an evening at a nightclub. For people with low self-esteem, who may be otherwise unable to prevent fatalistic withdrawal by activating symbolic existence goals, reducing self-awareness may be the most viable means of escaping the anxious BIS process initiated by salient thoughts of inevitable death.

According to Baumeister (1990), escaping self-awareness can also be achieved through "cognitive deconstruction," which involves focusing away from higher-order meanings (e.g., be a good parent by caring for my children) in favor of lower-order goal construals (e.g., make a sandwich). By focusing on lower-order programs and motor-control sequences, the individual can avoid contemplation of the broader principle that may appear terminally conflicted or doomed to fail. In essence, the deconstructed state entails going through the motions without reflective attention to the purpose of these motions. Baumeister argued that focusing on lower-order goals through deconstruction reduces the pain of self-awareness following failure to live up to principle-level values. However, consistent with Carver and Scheier's (1998) perspective, this state of deconstruction is only a short-term fix, as awareness of the self can never be fully or permanently eliminated, except in suicide.

The Watershed of Withdrawing from Life

Carver and Scheier (1998) described the decision to persist versus withdraw as involving a watershed, akin to rainwater flowing in opposite directions at the top of a mountain ridge. Whereas the difference between persistence and withdrawal can be very small at first, once the process begins it may become difficult to reverse and can ultimately lead to behavior that is very far afield from where it began. We argue that fatalistic withdrawal from life follows precisely this trajectory. Although it likely starts small—a simple act of mental disengagement and the avoidance of self-awareness in the interest of reducing feelings of anxiety or depression stemming from failure—it can build over time and may eventually become entrenched, where the individual can see no way out other than to die by suicide.

Resistance to Reengaging in Life

One way in which fatalistic withdrawal can gain momentum and become entrenched is by leading a person to neglect the important goal principles that must be pursued to reestablish symbolic existence and thus revive the goal to live. Fatalism entails letting go of self-regulatory efforts and allowing oneself to drift, which will only consolidate failure and promote additional efforts to mentally disengage. Consistent with this idea, Hayes and Hubley (2017) found that depressed participants with low desire to live were reluctant to reengage life-affirming goals when asked to write about the reasons they have for living. Indeed, these participants showed markedly weak life affirmations. That said, when these participants *did* affirm life strongly, they reported feeling less depressed but more anxious thereafter. In effect, reviving the goal to continue living reversed the emotional consequences of fatalistic withdrawal (which entailed lower feelings of anxiety and heightened depression). We maintain that these anxious feelings can act as a barrier to reactivating the goal to continue living, thus explaining why fatalistically withdrawn participants were reluctant to do so in the first place. Indeed, depressed people often resist interventions aimed at improving their condition (see, e.g., Rothbaum et al., 2009) in part because they may feel hopeless, but also because having hope reactivates the motivational conflict between wanting to live and knowing that death is inevitable. Without viable symbolic goals that can offer meaning to life and keep the goal to continue living afloat, they will only remain anxious until they once again mentally disengage to escape self-awareness. Over time, they may develop a state of learned helplessness where they no longer try to revive the goal to continue living because such efforts only produced anxiety and renewed withdrawal when tried in the past.

Risk Taking and Deviance

Another way in which fatalistic withdrawal can gain momentum is by promoting risky or deviant behavior that would not normally be entertained by a person who is fully life-engaged. According to Baumeister (1990), attempts to reduce self-awareness through deconstruction often escalate over time, as behavior becomes increasingly detached (through deconstruction) from the higher-order principles that would normally inhibit problematic behavior (e.g., alcoholism, drug abuse). Similarly, fatalistic withdrawal might increase risky or deviant behavior by promoting a perception that one has little to lose in taking significant risks (Brezina et al., 2009). If a person has lost all reason to live, then the goal to preserve one's life no longer stands in the way of approaching dangerous situations. Moreover, if risky behavior has even the slightest hope of leading to positive outcomes, those dangerous situations may be seen as opportunities to rescue the goal to live from a state of hopeless despair.

In support of this reasoning, experimental studies suggest that under conditions of loss, people who are normally risk-averse can become motivated to engage in risky activity when it is seen as the only option available to return to the status quo (Scholer et al., 2010). Thus, risky behaviors such as high-stakes gambling or even crimes such as robbery and fraud, can appear justifiable from the vantage of someone who has already given up on life. Indeed, pathological gambling has consistently been linked to suicidality (Kristensen et al., 2023). And in the case of overtly dangerous acts (e.g., stunting, armed robbery), the person might even take solace in the idea that they will die if they are unsuccessful in their attempt. Such deaths would likely not be counted as "suicides" in official statistics but may well be driven by the same underlying fatalistic withdrawal process. In fact, similar arguments have been made to account for excess deaths associated with alcoholism and drug abuse among White, uneducated people in the United States (i.e., deaths of despair; Case & Deaton, 2020).

Overall, fatalistic withdrawal may build momentum over time by creating barriers to reengaging life-affirming goals and promoting maladaptive behaviors that only entrench the withdrawal process. Ultimately, hope of reviving the goal to live will be completely lost and suicide will become increasingly likely. We see this as akin to what O'Connor and Kirtley (2018) refer to as *entrapment*, where an initial defeat (i.e., failure to achieve an important symbolic existence goal) can progress toward suicidality when the person loses all hope of escaping that which defeats them. Similarly, both the interpersonal model of suicide (Joiner, 2005) and the three-step theory (Klonsky & May, 2015) argue that a loss of hope is necessary for suicide ideation to proceed to suicide plans and attempts.

Suicide as a Means of Preserving or Gaining Symbolic Existence

An additional consideration in the progression from fatalistic withdrawal to active attempts to die is that sometimes suicide can be seen as a means of preserving or gaining a sense of symbolic existence. Indeed, we can see several ways in which dying by suicide could function to provide the symbolic immortality or personal significance that is lacking.

First, in some cultures suicide is explicitly sanctioned (Pierre, 2015). In Japan, for instance, suicide can be an honorable way to die, especially when one has committed offenses that have brought shame upon oneself or one's family. From this perspective, suicide is a way to atone for transgressions and thus preserves the overall value of the symbolic self despite those transgressions. While suicide is not specifically valued in the West, public debate around physician-assisted suicide and the right to die is often centered around discussion of dying with dignity. This perspective maintains that continued life would only degrade the symbolic self, and that it is more dignified (i.e., heroic or worthy of honor and respect) to choose death over life.

Relatedly, the interpersonal model of suicide (Joiner, 2005) implicates feelings of burdensomeness in suicidality. A person who believes that they are a burden to significant others may see more value in dying than in living. More specifically, if they view the net value of their existence as negative, eliminating this value (i.e., bringing it to zero) can seem like a viable way of increasing their value. Plus, in the mind of the suicidal person who feels like a burden to their loved ones, it may appear courageous to commit suicide to spare them of this burden. Thus, suicide can be seen as an act of heroism, where the individual is willing to sacrifice themselves for the sake of their loved ones.

Another way in which suicide can be thought to contribute toward the greater good is in choosing to die as a martyr. Academic discussions of martyrdom often revolved around suicide terrorism, wherein people purposefully kill themselves to attack their enemies. According to TMT, suicide terrorism is motivated by the need for death transcendence and is perpetrated as a means of attaining symbolic significance or defending one's cultural worldview against detractors (Pyszczynski et al., 2003). Indeed, Pyszczynski and colleagues (2006) found that mortality salience increased Iranian participants' support for suicide martyrdom attacks against the United States and even increased their willingness to consider such attacks themselves. The suicide terrorist can thus be lauded as a cultural hero who will live forever as a martyr for a great cause. In many cases, they may also be lured by the promise of literal immortality and eternal rewards in paradise (i.e., heaven; see Pyszczynski et al., 2003). Similarly, Kruglanski and colleagues (2009) argued that acts of suicide terrorism are aimed are restoring a sense of significance that has been lost, gaining significance where it was previously lacking, or preventing a potential loss of significance that would result if they failed to act. Thus, suicide terrorists can be seen as cultural heroes who were ready to sacrifice themself for the group when it was needed.

From our perspective, suicide martyrdom may serve a double function that makes it particularly appealing for someone in a state of fatalistic withdrawal. More specifically, in addition to gaining symbolic existence, suicide martyrs also attain a means of ending their life. Although people who perpetrate these attacks are not always suicidal, several studies suggest they often wish to die and see suicide martyrdom as their chance to do so (Sheehan, 2014). A person in a state of fatalistic withdrawal may therefore see suicide martyrdom as a good opportunity to exist symbolically (or even eternally in Heaven) where they are unable to do so otherwise (McGregor et al., 2015), and to end their suffering by dying in the process.

Overcoming the Self-Preservation Instincts

Finally, even when all motivation to live has been lost and a person wants nothing more than to simply die, they must still contend with the biological instinct to survive. As previously discussed, we differentiate between the psychological goal to live and the biological instinct to preserve one's life. Whereas we argue that the psychological goal is fragile and prone to withdrawal, the biological instinct is hardwired and may not be so easily overridden. This distinction is an important feature of nearly all major theories of suicide (Joiner, 2005; Klonsky & May, 2015; O'Connor & Kirtley, 2018).

According to Joiner's (2005) interpersonal theory of suicide, the capacity to overcome the self-preservation instinct is an ability that can only be acquired through practice and habituation to physical or psychological pain. Joiner offered the example of military personnel who have become habituated to the potential danger and trauma of physical combat and are therefore more likely to die by suicide once they have acquired the desire to die. It is worth noting that Baumeister's (1990) proposed state of deconstruction, and the attendant reduction in inhibitions, would likely result in more opportunities to practice and habituate to pain, which is required according to Joiner's theory. Consistent with this idea, empirical studies suggest that acts of suicide often start small and escalate over time (Rudd et al., 1996). Furthermore, successive episodes of self-harm often become increasingly aggressive (O'Connor et al., 2000), and people who ultimately die by suicide are more likely to have had a history of deliberate self-harm than those who survive the attempt, even after controlling for the severity of disordered mood (Cavanaugh et al., 1999).

Interestingly, some evidence suggests that engaging in acts of self-harm may be self-reinforcing by virtue of reducing negative affect and increasing positive affect (Brain et al., 2002; Kemperman et al., 1997). Theoretically, for a person who wants to die, engaging in self-harm may leverage approach motivation, and thus temporarily relieve feelings of anxiety and depression (cf., McGregor et al., 2010). While these behaviors may ultimately lead a person to die by suicide, they may nevertheless offer relief from the psychological pain they are experiencing.

Joiner's (2005) theory also suggests those who die by suicide must acquire the practical means to do so. Whereas successive approximations through increasingly aggressive acts of self-harm may functionally accomplish this practical issue, having access to firearms, lethal drugs, or other means of ending life swiftly may circumvent (or at least minimize) the need for a lengthy process of learning to overcome the self-preservation instinct. Consistent with this idea, Swanson and colleagues (2003) reported that suicide rates are higher among anesthesiologists and other medical professionals (who have the practical means of ending their lives) than in the general population. Similarly, studies of population-level trends in death by suicide show that within the United States, rates of suicide are highest in states and cities where household gun ownership is more common (Miller et al., 2015). Consider also that joining a terrorist organization and committing to a suicide martyrdom attack will also provide the individual with a lethal means of ending life swiftly, which may offer additional motivation for suicide terrorism.

The Role of Impulsivity

Throughout this section, we have argued that suicide is the final step in an often long and drawn-out process. In some cases, however, a person may proceed to this final step more suddenly, acting impulsively and seemingly without much thought. Indeed, several studies have implicated impulsivity as a risk factor for suicidality (e.g., Beach et al., 2021; Rasmussen et al., 2024), and the integrated motivational–volitional model of suicide (O'Connor & Kirtley, 2018) suggests that impulsivity is a key volitional moderator of suicidal behavior. According to our model, suicide stems from a BIS-mediated motivational *impulse* to give up on the goal to continue living in the face of inevitable death. Thus, people who are high in trait impulsivity—especially those who lack perseverance (Whiteside & Lynam, 2001) or have a strong impulse to withdraw in the face of adversity (e.g., withdrawal aspect of neuroticism; DeYoung et al., 2007)—may be more likely to become fatalistically withdrawn because they are less able to override this impulse. Similarly, traits that predispose people to seek quick resolutions to motivational conflict that terminate the anxiety-ridden BIS process (e.g., anxiety sensitivity, intolerance of uncertainty; Allan et al., 2023) may also promote suicidality by hastening withdrawal from life. Consistent with this reasoning, recent research suggests that anxiety sensitivity (a fear of anxious affect) may promote suicide by increasing rumination and feelings of hopelessness (Jin et al., 2024). According to our model, the ability to linger in the anxious BIS-state when symbolic existence goals appear fraught should offer protection against fatalistic withdrawal by preventing a quick withdrawal resolution. Moreover, the ability to tolerate a potentially prolonged period of anxiety, without impulsively withdrawing as a means of reducing this anxiety, may be pivotal to regaining life-engagement among people already in a state of fatalistic withdrawal (Hayes & Hubley, 2017).

In addition to impulsive withdrawal, impulsive approach motivation may also promote suicidal behavior. Dozens of studies in the threat-defense literature suggest that reactively turning to approach-oriented action can mute threat-induced anxiety (see Jonas et al., 2014). Although reactive approach motivation is sometimes prosocial and magnanimous, it can also be belligerent, aggressive, and even self-destructive (e.g., McGregor et al., 2015). Thus, a person who feels trapped by failure in their symbolic life goals may see suicide or self-harm as an opportunity to gain symbolic value or to punish those deemed responsible for their failure (as discussed above), and they may impulsively approach this opportunity before fully thinking it through. The reduction of anxiety that accompanies the behavior can make it feel "right" to the individual. Plus, if they have already mentally disengaged from life, cognitive deconstruction may functionally impede their ability to connect the suicidal act with the broader implications of the action, thereby making the act of suicide more impulsive and apparently sudden. Alcohol intoxication may similarly promote impulsive death by suicide (Hufford, 2001). Whereas the self-preservation instinct is not so easily overcome, becoming intoxicated (to reduce self-awareness, anxiety, and/or blunt pain) coupled with a readily accessible means of dying (e.g., a firearm in the home) may facilitate impulsive acts of suicide that would not have occurred with a sober second thought.

With all of this noted, we nevertheless maintain that most suicides are likely not spur-of-the-moment impulsive acts (see Anestis et al., 2014). Furthermore, some personality traits that may promote impulsivity in one aspect of the withdrawal-from-life process may impede impulsivity in another aspect of the process. For instance, whereas neuroticism may predispose people to suicidality by promoting withdrawal in the face of adversity, it may also act as a barrier to suicidal behavior by increasing the fear of death (cf., Rappaport et al., 2017). Thus, the relationship between impulsivity and suicidality may be complex and often not straightforward. Our model nevertheless points toward aspects of the overall process that may be hastened or slowed by impulsive motivational withdrawal or approach.

Summary

To recap, we argue that suicide is the final step in a broader process of withdrawal from life. The process is likely not always straightforward, but we maintain that it begins with a significant failure in a person's efforts to create or maintain a symbolic self that is worthy of death transcendence. Without a symbolic sense of existence, the goal to live collapses due to the inevitability of death. Although the process can be quick and impulsive, it can also start small—with mental disengagement and cognitive deconstruction—and build over time due to lowered inhibitions and lack of attention to symbolic existence goals. Eventually, the individual may find themselves in a situation of no escape, where death seems imminent. At this point, they may seek personal significance and symbolic immortality via risky means that ultimately end in death or involve killing oneself in an act of suicidal martyrdom. Even still, the ability to intentionally inflict mortal harm to oneself is not an easy task, as it involves overcoming hardwired instincts to remain alive.

IMPLICATIONS FOR PRACTICE

The foregoing review combines TMT with goal regulation theory to suggest that suicidality stems from a broader tendency to withdraw from life when symbolic existence goals seem no longer viable. In this section, we draw from our proposed theory to briefly offer implications for preventing suicide. Many of these implications involve careful attention to the structure of an individual's goal system. According to our model, systemic features that facilitate ongoing efforts to exist symbolically should confer resilience in the face of adversity, which should in turn prevent fatalistic withdrawal from life, and consequently, suicidality.

One important feature of the goal system is the value standards by which "successful" goal achievement is judged. Feeling that one is living up to high standards of value may confer extra symbolic significance (Eidelman & Biernat, 2007), but if these standards are unrealistically high, they will be exceedingly difficult to achieve, which will promote self-standard discrepancies and increase the likelihood of goal withdrawal. Consistent with this reasoning, dozens of studies show a link between perfectionism and suicidality (Smith et al., 2018). Not surprisingly, high (vs. low) perfectionists are more likely to become suicidal following negative life events. Thus, supportive friends/family who convey that one's symbolic existence matters despite one's imperfections should mitigate suicides by preventing fatalistic withdrawal in the face of adversity.

Another important feature of the goal system is the number of principles that serve the broader goal of existing symbolically (e.g., be a scientist, be caring; see Figure 11.1). In general, having more principle-level goals should reduce the likelihood of fatalistic withdrawal by offering alternate means of existing symbolically when facing challenges in any specific goal (Pyszczynski et al., 1990). Moreover, turning to alternative goals can facilitate the abandonment of blocked goals without jeopardizing the higher-order goal to exist symbolically. While letting go of important self-defining goals can be difficult and painful, remaining committed to them often makes matters worse. Indeed, Pyszczynski and Greenberg's (1992) self-regulatory perseveration theory maintains that depression and suicide often stem from an inability to disengage from goals that have little chance of success. As previously mentioned, withdrawing from fraught goals is adaptive because it frees up resources that can be more usefully directed toward other goals that are more likely to be successful. This can only happen, however, if the person has other viable goals that serve the same higher-order function. A monolithic goal structure consisting of only a single means of symbolic existence is inherently fragile. In such cases, a person may perseverate on that goal, even with no chance of success, because letting go of it would entail abandoning the higher-order goal to exist symbolically. As such, perseveration may represent a desperate attempt to keep the higher-order goal afloat. If this goal is truly unachievable, however, perseveration only delays the inevitable collapse of the goal system. The only viable way out of the dilemma is to develop alternative principle-level goals that can support the higher-order goal to exist symbolically (see Pyszczynski & Greenberg, 1992).

Finally, our model suggests that people who are already fatalistically withdrawn must find a way to tolerate BIS-mediated anxiety if they are to prevent eventual suicide. Recall that Hayes and colleagues (2016) found that fatalistic withdrawal reduced anxiety (by terminating the BIS process) but increased depression (by causing the goal system to collapse). Furthermore, Hayes and Hubley (2017) were able to reverse these emotional effects (i.e., reduced depression but increased anxiety) by inducing depressed people to affirm goals that offered the hope of existing symbolically. These findings suggest that the way out of fatalistic withdrawal involves going through the BIS-mediated state of anxiety, and resisting the impulse to fall back into withdrawal, until real progress can be made toward principle-level goals that confer a meaningful symbolic existence. As previously discussed, however, people who are fatalistically withdrawn are often resistant to reactivating life-affirming goals because of the anxiety that is aroused in the process (Hayes & Hubley, 2017). Thus, our model suggests that fostering a tolerance of anxiety may be needed to lift a person out of fatalistic withdrawal and prevent them from proceeding down the path of self-destruction.

One method that may help people focus on principle-level goals while tolerating anxiety is acceptance and commitment therapy (ACT; Hayes et al., 2012). According to ACT, many psychological problems stem from the tendency to avoid negative emotions such as anxiety. Experiential avoidance is counterproductive, however, and ACT instead fosters a willingness to accept these negative emotions and to nevertheless move toward important self-defining goals and values. In the words of Blackledge and Hayes (2001), ACT encourages people to feel "feelings as feelings (e.g., experiencing emotions simply as constellations of physiological sensations, urges, and so on that have no intrinsic power to harm us or hold us back)." Within the present context, rather than impulsively withdrawing to reduce/avoid the anxiety that is experienced whenever one tries to achieve a valued goal, ACT would encourage people to mindfully notice these emotions, but to nevertheless align their behavior with their values. Clinical evidence suggests that when people follow the tenets of ACT, they do not necessarily experience less anxiety, but the anxiety seems less motivationally pertinent, and they are able to move toward the goals that matter to them despite the anxious affect (see Hayes et al., 2012). While many other clinical techniques may be equally effective in helping clients out of fatalistic withdrawal (and thus preventing suicide), ACT appears to be well-aligned with our goal regulation perspective. In brief, the goal of therapeutic efforts to prevent suicide among people in a depressive state of fatalistic withdrawal should be to encourage reactivation of the goal to live by fostering realistic progress in valued principle-level goals that offer a sense of meaningful symbolic existence.

NOTE

1. While we conceptualize the goal to exist symbolically as distinct from the goal to exist physically, these goals are not mutually exclusive, nor are they completely independent of one another. Consistent with any goal regulation theory, sometimes lower-order goals can serve multiple goals at higher-order levels. In Figure 11.1, we illustrate this with the goal principle of *being healthy*, which is typically a means of extending physical longevity, but can equally be an important aspect symbolic existence if one bases self-esteem on their physical appearance. By extension, the program-level goal of exercising can be a means of maintaining physical existence, while also maintaining the symbolic self.

REFERENCES

Allan, N. P., Gorka, S. M., Saulnier, K. G., & Bryan, C. J. (2023). Anxiety sensitivity and intolerance of uncertainty: Transdiagnostic risk factors for anxiety as targets to reduce risk of suicide. *Current Psychiatry Reports, 25,* 139–147.

Anestis, M. D., Soberay, K. A., Gutierrez, P. M., Hernandez, T. D., & Joiner, T. E. (2014). Reconsidering the link between impulsivity and suicidal behavior. *Personality and Social Psychology Review, 18,* 366–386.

Bandura, A. (1977). Self-efficacy: Toward a unifying theory of behavioral change. *Psychological Review, 84,* 191–215.

Baumeister, R. F. (1990). Suicide as escape from self. *Psychological Review, 97,* 90–113.

Baumeister, R. F., & Leary, M. R. (1995). The need to belong: Desire for interpersonal attachments as a fundamental human motivation. *Psychological Bulletin, 117,* 497–529.

Beach, V. L., Gissandaner, T. D., & Schmidt, A. T. (2021). The UPPS model of impulsivity and suicide: A systematic literature review. *Archives of Suicide Research, 26,* 985–1006.

Becker, E. (1973). *The denial of death.* Free Press.

Blackledge, J. T., & Hayes, S. C. (2001). Emotion regulation in acceptance and commitment therapy. *Journal of Clinical Psychology, 57,* 243–255.

Brain, K. L., Haines, J., & Williams, C. L. (2002). The psychopathology of repetitive self-mutilation. *Archives of Suicide Research, 6*, 199–210.

Brandtstädter, J., & Renner, G. (1990). Tenacious goal pursuit and flexible goal adjustment: Explication and age-related analysis of assimilative and accommodative strategies of coping. *Psychology and Aging, 5*, 58–67.

Brezina, T., Tekin, E., & Topalli, V. (2009). Might not be a tomorrow: A multimethods approach to anticipated early death and youth crime. *Criminology, 47*, 1091–1129.

Carver, C. S., & Scheier, M. F. (1998). *On the self-regulation of behavior*. Cambridge University Press.

Case, A., & Deaton, A. (2020). *Deaths of despair and the future of capitalism*. Princeton University Press.

Cavanaugh, J. T. O., Owens, D. G. C., & Johnstone, E. C. (1999). Suicide and undetermined death in southeast Scotland: A case-control study using the psychological autopsy method. *Psychological Medicine, 29*, 1141–1149.

Chatard, A., & Selimbegović, L. (2011). When self-destructive thoughts flash through the mind: Failure to meet standards affects the accessibility of suicide-related thoughts. *Journal of Personality and Social Psychology, 100*, 587–605.

Davis, K. L., & Panksepp, J. (2018). *The emotional foundations of personality: A neurobiological and evolutionary approach*. Norton.

DeYoung, C. G., Quilty, L. C., & Peterson, J. B. (2007). Between facets and domains: 10 aspects of the big five. *Journal of Personality and Social Psychology, 93*, 880–896.

Duval, S., & Wicklund, R. A. (1972). *A theory of objective self awareness*. Academic Press.

Eidelman, S., & Biernat, M. (2007). Getting more from success: Standard raising as esteem maintenance. *Journal of Personality and Social Psychology, 92*(5), 759–774.

George, L. S., & Park, C. L. (2014). Existential mattering: Bringing attention to a neglected by central aspect of meaning? In A. Batthyany & P. Russo-Netzer (Eds), *Meaning in positive and existential psychology* (pp. 39–51). Springer.

George, L. S., & Park, C. L. (2016). Meaning in life as comprehension, purpose, and mattering: Toward integration and new research questions. *Review of General Psychology, 20*, 205–220.

Gray, J. A., & McNaughton, N. (2000). *The neuropsychology of anxiety: An enquiry into the functions of the septo-hippocampal system* (2nd ed.). Oxford University Press.

Greenberg, J., Pyszczynski, T., & Solomon, S. (1986). The causes and consequences of a need for self-esteem: a terror management theory. In R. F. Baumeister (Ed.), *Public self and private self* (pp.189–212). Springer-Verlag.

Harris, S., Morley, S., & Barton, S. B. (2003). Role loss and emotional adjustment in chronic pain. *Pain, 105*, 363–370.

Hawton, K., Casanas i Comabella, C., Haw, C., & Saunders, K. (2013). Risk factors for suicide in individuals with depression: A systematic review. *Journal of Affective Disorders, 147*(1–3), 17–28.

Hayes, J., & Hubley, C. (2017). Between a rock and a hard place: When affirming life reduces depression, but increases anxiety. *Journal of Social and Clinical Psychology, 36*(10), 860–882.

Hayes, J., & Hubley, C. (2023). *The Desire to Live Scales (D2LS): A new tool for experimental existential research*. Poster presented at the International Convention of Psychological Science, Brussels, Belgium.

Hayes, J., Prentice, M., & McGregor, I. (2017). Giving in and giving up: Accommodation and fatalistic withdrawal as alternatives to primary control restoration. In M. Bukowski, I. Fritsche, A. Guinote, & M. Kofta (Eds.), *Coping with lack of control in a social world* (pp. 116–132). Routledge.

Hayes, J., Schimel, J., Arndt, J., & Faucher, E. H. (2010). A theoretical and empirical review of the death-thought accessibility concept in terror management research. *Psychological Bulletin, 136*, 699–739.

Hayes, J., Schimel, J., Faucher, E. H., & Williams, T. J. (2008). Evidence for the DTA hypothesis II: Threatening self-esteem increases death-thought accessibility. *Journal of Experimental Social Psychology, 44*, 600–613.

Hayes, J., Ward, C. L. P., & McGregor, I. (2016). Why bother?: Death, failure, and fatalistic withdrawal from life. *Journal of Personality and Social Psychology, 110*(1), 96–115.

Hayes, S. C., Strosahl, K. D., & Wilson, K. G. (2012). *Acceptance and commitment therapy: The process and practice of mindful change* (2nd ed). Guilford Press.

Hubley, C., & Scholer, A. A. (2022). Melting COVID-frozen goals: How goal disengagement supports well-being during the COVID-19 pandemic. *Motivation and Emotion, 46*, 752–768.

Hufford, M. R. (2001). Alcohol and suicidal behavior. *Clinical Psychology Review, 21*, 797–811.

Jin, Y., Woo, S., Kim, K., Kim, S. H., Roh, S., & Kim, S. (2024). The effect of anxiety sensitivity on repeated suicide attempts: The serial mediation effects of rumination and hopelessness and the moderated mediation effect of gender. *International Journal of Cognitive Therapy*.

Joiner, T. E. (2005). *Why people die by suicide.* Harvard University Press.
Jonas, E., McGregor, I., Klackl, J., Agroskin, D., Fritsche, I., Holbrook, C., . . . Quirin, M. (2014). Threat and defense: From anxiety to approach. In J. M. Olson & M. P. Zanna (Eds.), *Advances in experimental social psychology* (pp. 219–286). Academic Press.
Kemperman, I., Russ, M. J., & Shearin, E. (1997). Self-injurious behavior and mood regulation in borderline patients. *Journal of Personality Disorders, 11,* 146–157.
Klonsky, E. D., & May, A. M. (2015). The three-step theory (3ST): A new theory of suicide rooted in the "ideation to action" framework. *International Journal of Cognitive Therapy, 8*(2), 114–129.
Klonsky, E. D., May, A. M., & Saffer, B. Y. (2016). Suicide, suicide attempts, and suicide ideation. *Annual Review of Clinical Psychology, 12,* 307–330.
Kristensen, J., H., Pallesen, S., Bauer, J., Leino, T., Griffiths, M. D., & Erevik, E. K. (2023). Suicidality among individuals with gambling problems. *Psychological Bulletin, 150,* 82–106.
Kruglanski, A. W., Chen, X., Dechesne, M., Fishman, S., & Orehek, E. (2009). Fully committed: Suicide bombers; motivation and the quest for personal significance. *Political Psychology, 30,* 331–507.
Lifshin, U., Horner, D. E., Helm, P. J., Solomon, S., & Greenberg, J. (2021). Self-esteem and immortality: Evidence regarding the terror management hypothesis that high self-esteem is associated with a stronger sense of symbolic immortality. *Personality and Individual Differences, 175,* 110712.
McGregor, I., Hayes, J., & Prentice, M. (2015). Motivation for aggressive religious radicalization: Goal regulation theory and a personality × threat × affordance hypothesis. *Frontiers in Psychology, 6,* 1325.
McGregor, I., Nash, K., & Mann, N., & Phills, C. E. (2010). Anxious uncertainty and reactive approach motivation (RAM). *Journal of Personality and Social Psychology, 99,* 133–147.
McNaughton, N., & Corr, P. J. (2004). A two-dimensional neuropsychology of defense: Fear/anxiety and defensive distance. *Neuroscience and Biobehavioral Reviews, 28,* 285–305.
Mikulincer, M., Florian, V., & Hirschberger, G. (2003). The existential function of close relationships: Introducing death into the science of love. *Personality and Social Psychology Review, 7,* 20–40.
Mikulincer, M., & Shaver, P. R. (2012). Helplessness: A hidden liability associated with failed defenses against awareness of death. In P. R. Shaver & M. Mikulincer (Eds), *Meaning, mortality, and choice: The social psychology of existential concerns* (pp. 37–53). American Psychological Association.
Miller, M., Warren, M., Hemenway, D., & Azrael, D. (2015). Firearms and suicide in US cities. *Injury Prevention, 21,* 116–119.
Mischel, W., Shoda, Y., & Rodriquez, M. L. (1989). Delay of gratification in children. *Science, 244,* 933–938.
Muraven, M., & Baumeister, R. F. (1997). Suicide, sex, terror, paralysis, and other pitfalls of reductionist self-preservation theory. *Psychological Inquiry, 8,* 36–40.
O'Connor, R. C., & Kirtley, O. J. (2018). The integrated motivational-volitional model of suicidal behaviour. *Philosophical Transactions of the Royal Society B: Biological Sciences, 373,* 1754.
O'Connor, R. C., Sheehy, N. P., & O'Connor, D. B. (2000). Fifty cases of general hospital parasuicide. *British Journal of Health Psychology, 5,* 83–95.
Ogilvie, D. M., Cohen, F., & Solomon, S. (2008). The undesired self: Deadly connotations. *Journal of Research in Personality, 42,* 564–576.
Pierre, J. M. (2015). Culturally sanctioned suicide: Euthanasia, seppuku, and terrorist martyrdom. *World Journal of Psychiatry, 5,* 4–14.
Pyszczynski, T., Abdollahi, A., Solomon, S., Greenberg, J., Cohen, F., & Weise, D. (2006). Mortality salience, martyrdom, and military might: The Great Satan versus the Axis of Evil. *Personality and Social Psychology Bulletin, 32,* 525–537.
Pyszczynski, T., & Greenberg, J. (1992). *Hanging on and letting go: Understanding the onset, progression, and remission of depression.* Springer-Verlag.
Pyszczynski, T., Greenberg, J., Solomon, S., & Hamilton, J. (1990). A terror management analysis of self-awareness and anxiety: The hierarchy of terror. *Anxiety Research, 2,* 177–195.
Pyszczynski, T., Solomon, S., & Greenberg, J. (2003). *In the wake of 9/11: The psychology of terror.* American Psychological Association.
Rappaport, L. M., Flint, J., & Kendler, K. S. (2017). Clarifying the role of neuroticism in suicidal ideation and suicide attempt among women with major depressive disorder. *Psychological Medicine, 47,* 2334–2344.
Rasmussen, S., Martin, B., & Cramer, R. J. (2024). Multidimensional impulsivity and suicidal behaviour: A partial test of the integrated motivational-volitional (IMV) model of suicide. *Archives of Suicide Research.*
Rosenberg, M., & McCullough, B. C. (1981). Mattering: Inferred significance and mental

health among adolescents. *Research in Community & Mental Health, 2,* 163–182.
Rothbaum, F., Morling, B., & Rusk, N. (2009). How goals and beliefs lead people into and out of depression. *Review of General Psychology, 13,* 302–314.
Routledge, C., Ostafin, B., Juhl, J., Sedikides, C., Cathey, C., & Liao, J. (2010). Adjusting to death: The effects of mortality salience and self-esteem on psychological well-being, growth motivation, and maladaptive behavior. *Journal of Personality and Social Psychology, 99,* 897–916.
Routledge, C., & Vess, M. (2019). *Handbook of terror management theory.* Academic Press.
Rudd, M. D., Rajab, M. H., Orman, D. T., Stulman, D. A., Joiner, T. E. Jr., & Dixon, W. (1996). Effectiveness of an outpatient problem-solving intervention targeting suicidal young adults: Preliminary results. *Journal of Consulting and Clinical Psychology, 64,* 179–190.
Scholer, A. A., Zou, X., Fujita, K., Stroessner, S. J., & Higgins, E. T. (2010). When risk seeking becomes a motivational necessity. *Journal of Personality and Social Psychology, 99*(2), 215–231.
Sheehan, I. S. (2014). Are suicide terrorists suicidal?: A critical assessment of the evidence. *Innovations in Clinical Neuroscience, 11,* 81–92.
Smith, M. M., Sherry, S. B., Chen, S., Saklofske, D. H., Mushquash, C., Flett, G. L., & Hewitt, P. L. (2018). The perniciousness of perfectionism: A meta-analytic review of the perfectionism-suicide relationship. *Journal of Personality, 86,* 522–542.
Speece, M. W., & Brent, S. B. (1984). Children's understanding of death: A review of three components of a death concept. *Child Development, 55,* 1671–1686.
Swanson, S. P., Roberts, L. J., & Chapman, M. D. (2003). Are anaesthetists prone to suicide? A review of rates and risk factors. *Anaesthesia and Intensive Care, 31,* 434–445.
Tritt, S. M., Inzlicht, M., & Harmon-Jones, E. (2012). Toward a biological understanding of mortality salience (and other threat compensation processes). *Social Cognition, 30*(2012), 715–733.
Walker, J., Sofaer, B., & Holloway, I. (2006). The experience of chronic back pain: Accounts of loss in those seeking help from pain clinics. *European Journal of Pain, 10,* 199–207.
Whiteside, S. P., & Lynam, D. R. (2001). The five factor model and impulsivity: Using a structural model of personality to understand impulsivity. *Personality and Individual Differences, 30,* 669–689.
Williams, K. D. (2007). Ostracism: The kiss of social death. *Social and Personality Compass, 1,* 236–247.
Wisman, A., Heflick, N., & Goldenberg, J. L. (2015). The great escape: The role of self-esteem and self-related cognition in terror management. *Journal of Experimental Social Psychology, 60,* 121–132.
World Health Organization. (2021). *Suicide worldwide in 2019: Global health estimates.* www.who.int/publications/i/item/9789240026643.
Wrosch, C., Scheier, M. F., Carver, C. S., & Schultz, R. (2003). The importance of goal disengagement in adaptive self-regulation: When giving up is beneficial. *Self and Identity, 2,* 1–20.

CHAPTER 12

Existential Neuroscience

Bridging Philosophy, Psychology, and the Brain

Markus Quirin *and* Georg Northoff

After one of us (M. Q.) published an article titled "Existential Neuroscience" (Quirin et al., 2011), a colleague brought to my attention a philosophical internet blog criticizing the "hubristic" endeavor of investigating existentialist concerns using neuroscientific methods. Now, nearly a decade later, this field has firmly developed to become a recognized science, supported by a substantial body of research addressing diverse existential concerns (e.g., Caruso & Flanagan, 2017; Northoff, 2018; Quirin & Klackl, 2016; Quirin et al., 2019a; Schlosser, 2017). *Existential neuroscience* or *neuroexistentialism* has even been declared as the third wave of existentialism (Caruso & Flanagan, 2017). By intertwining philosophy, psychology, and neuroscience, existential neuroscience aims to untangle the neural underpinnings of existential concepts in order to find out how our brain processes concerns such as freedom, choice, or the quest for meaning. As such, this interdisciplinary fusion fuels the excitement of understanding ourselves at a deep level.

In the present chapter, we pass through the landscape where age-old philosophical inquiries into the nature of human existence converge with the innovative techniques and discoveries of modern neuroscience. We start by providing an overview of major existential concerns and their neural correlates. Next, we attempt to synthesize these findings into a brain model of existential concerns. Consequently, we apply this model to the topics of coping with mortality, uncertainty, and perceived absurdity, emphasizing the activation of the "integrative self" as a key neuropsychological network to restore autonomous regulation. We conclude with a discussion on relevant issues related to the present approach, including a monistic mind-brain perspective using the idea of spatiotemporal dynamics (Northoff, 2024; Northoff et al., 2020) and an outlook for future research.

EXISTENTIAL NEUROSCIENCE

Existential neuroscience is anchored in both existentialist philosophy and empirical existential psychology. *Existentialist philosophy* delves into the very essence of human existence, grappling with questions of freedom, choice, responsibility, and the search for meaning in an indifferent universe. Rooted in the works of thinkers like Jean-Paul Sartre, Martin Heidegger, Albert Camus, and Viktor Frankl, existentialism emphasizes individuality, authenticity, and the relentless exploration of our existence's fundamental truths. This philosophical perspective has made a significant impact on mainstream awareness and pop culture as, for example, reflected in Jim Morrison's words: "The most important kind of freedom is to be what you really are."

Existential psychology is grounded in philosophical existentialism and investigates the fundamental psychological mechanisms that underlie existential concerns through the application of empirical (including experimental) psychological methodologies (Greenberg et al., 2004). In addition, the applied side of existential psychology aims to assist individuals in dealing with major life issues (*existential psychotherapy*; Yalom, 1980).

Empirical research in existential psychology often focuses on understanding how individuals grapple with existential concerns, such as the inevitably of death (Burke et al., 2010; Greenberg et al., 1986; Routledge & Vess, 2018), and how these struggles impact mental well-being. For instance, Heidegger's notion of "existential anxiety" has spurred experimental research on how existential anxiety influences decision-making processes and emotional experiences (Greenberg et al., 2004). Moreover, Yalom (1980), founder of existential psychotherapy, emphasized the efficacy of existential approaches in addressing anxiety, depression, and meaninglessness (nihilism). Research in existential positive psychology, inspired by Frankl's emphasis on meaning, investigates how a sense of purpose and meaning contribute to life satisfaction and overall psychological health (Steger et al., 2008). These theoretical and empirical foundations collectively elucidate the intricate interplay between existential philosophy and psychology, enriching our understanding of the human experience and informing therapeutic interventions.

KEY EXISTENTIAL CONCERNS AND THEIR NEURAL CORRELATES

Table 12.1 presents a summary of critical brain regions that demonstrate activity detected by functional magnetic resonance imaging (fMRI) across various human concerns extensively discussed in existentialist literature. These findings are elaborated upon in the subsequent sections. Concerning the neural correlates of these existential concerns, it's crucial to acknowledge their multifaceted nature and their association with personalized experiences. Consequently, it is important to acknowledge that numerous other brain regions may contribute to their manifestation, and the comprehension of their neural mechanisms is an evolving process.

Uncertainty

Uncertainty, in a general sense, refers to a lack of sureness or confidence regarding a specific situation, outcome, or knowledge about the future. It involves a state of not being entirely clear, definite, or predictable, often accompanied by doubt, variability, or unpredictability (Merriam-Webster, n.d.). In his work *Being and Nothingness*, Jean-Paul Sartre (1943) argued that human beings are confronted with fundamental uncertainty and the burden of making choices without absolute knowledge or predetermined meanings.

Beings are constantly surrounded by uncertainties, and evolution has equipped them with neural strategies to address these challenges, such as learning and predicting. However, uncertainties vary in their magnitude and salience (content), which together determine the intensity of the uncertainty. While low levels of uncertainty can be stimulating (e.g., gambling, trying a new restaurant), high levels induce uneasiness and anxiety (Berlyne, 1960, 1966, 1973; Quirin et al., 2022b). Existential concerns, such as identity, worldview, and mortality threats, likely represent the highest intensities of uncertainty. However, it remains debated whether these existential threats differ from other types of threats solely in the quantity of uncertainty or also in quality. In fact, the certainty of human mortality presents a qualitative difference from many other threats, necessitating specific coping mechanisms (Pyszczynski et al., 2012).

Uncertainty processing involves a network of brain regions associated with decision making, risk assessment, and emotion regulation. Some key neural correlates of uncertainty include the anterior cingulate cortex (decision making, emotion regulation: Bot-

TABLE 12.1. Key Brain Structures Involved in Existential Concerns

Function	Region
Uncertainty, mortality salience, latent angst	**medial PFC** (prereflective evaluation and regulation of mortality salience, defensively or offensively); **anterior insula** (interoception, emotional responses to uncertainty, risk assessment and decision making); **amygdala** (fear and anxiety processing); **ventral striatum** ("nucleus accumbens": reward system, processes uncertainty related to potential rewards and punishments)
Love, attachment, connectedness	**ventral striatum** (infatuation, sexual striving), **medial PFC** (reward expectation, caring, unconditional love), **dorsomedial striatum** (social bonding, trust, attachment), **amygdala** (loss, fear of loss)
Self and identity, authenticity	**medial PFC, posterior cingulate cortex, precuneus** ("DMN": self-representations, sense of self, self-reflection, integration of goals, values, and preferences), **right anterior insula** (interoceptive awareness of emotions, preferences, and emotional resources), **ventral striatum** (reward processing), **ACC** (conflict resolution maintaining authenticity)
Absurdity versus meaning making	**superior temporal gyrus** (incongruity and violations of semantic or contextual expectations), **dorsolateral PFC** (reasoning, comprehension of incongruous or absurd situations), **amygdala** (affective aspects of absurdity), **medial PFC** (self-reflection, decision making, evaluating personal values and beliefs; reduced in depression), **ACC** (conflict monitoring and resolution, error detection, cognitive dissonance), **anterior insula** (interoceptive awareness of emotions contributing to meaning), **DMN** (self-reflection, introspection, contemplating one's life purpose)
Will	**medial PFC** (intuitive decision making, prereflective goals, effortless willpower/persistence, emotion regulation), **dorsolateral PFC** (cognitive control, working memory, analytical reflection, deliberate decision making and goals, effortful willpower/persistence).

Note. PFC, prefrontal cortex; ACC, anterior cingulate cortex; NA, nucleus accumbens; AI, anterior insula; DMN, default mode network.

vinick et al., 2004), the prefrontal cortex (PFC; decision making under uncertainty, cognitive control, and assessing potential outcomes: Ridderinkhof et al., 2004), the insula (interoception, emotional responses to uncertainty, risk assessment, and decision making: Preuschoff et al., 2008), the amygdala (fear and anxiety processing: Carlson et al., 2011), and the striatum (reward system, processes uncertainty related to potential rewards and punishments, influencing decision making and motivation: Preuschoff et al., 2006). Studies using methods other than fMRI report hemispheric asymmetries in the responses to uncertainty stimulated by societal threats (Prentice et al., 2020).

Mortality Salience and Latent Angst

Mortality salience pertains to an elevated state of consciousness characterized by a heightened awareness of one's own mortality or the inevitability of death. Given the inherent uncertainty surrounding the timing of one's demise and the unknowns regarding what may follow, death can be viewed as a profound and perhaps the most intense manifestation of uncertainty (Echebarria-Echabe, 2013; Van den Bos, 2009). This profound uncertainty likely explains why humans have developed spiritual and religious beliefs about the afterlife, envisioning possibilities beyond mere nothingness. Despite significant uncertainty regarding the exact timing and circumstances of death, the certainty of death itself is undeniable. Moreover, extensive evidence on the immediate psychological effects of heightened mortality awareness indicates that this phenomenon extends well beyond mere uncertainty (Greenberg et al., 1995; Landau et al., 2025).

Existentialist philosophers have offered various perspectives on death and existential threats, as well as on coping with the existential challenges they present. Yet nearly all of them emphasize the fundamental reality of death as an inherent part of human existence that finally gives life its meaning and urgency, for example, to live authentically. In his play *No Exit*, Jean-Paul Sartre posited that death gives life its value and meaning by imposing limits and defining choices. Friedrich Nietzsche influenced existentialist thought by discussing the concept of "eternal recurrence." For example, in *Thus Spoke Zarathustra* (1883) he encouraged individuals to embrace life and its challenges, including the inevitability of death, in order to live authentically. Søren Kierkegaard (2013), a precursor to existentialism, examined existential anxiety in his work *The Concept of Anxiety*. He argued that anxiety, often occurring nonconsciously ("latent angst"), arises from the human capacity for self-reflection and the realization of our own freedom and responsibility in the face of choices and uncertainties. Others, such as Albert Camus, emphasized absurdity of life resulting from the finality of life.

In the context of *terror management theory* (e.g., Greenberg et al., 1986, 1992; see also Burke et al., 2010), psychological studies have demonstrated that, when reminded of their mortality, individuals react with various psychological and emotional responses such as strengthened self-esteem or ingroup identity (e.g. Greenberg et al., 1986; see also Burke et al., 2010). Mortality awareness has also been shown to activate certain brain regions associated with processing fear, threat, and existential thoughts. When exposed to reminders of mortality, participants showed increased activation in the amygdala and anterior cingulate cortex (for reviews, see Quirin & Klackl, 2016; Quirin et al., 2019a). The PFC, particularly the ventromedial part, also plays a role in processing mortality salience, potentially in (defensively or offensively) modulating fear and emotional responses (Klackl et al., 2014; Yanagisawa et al., 2016). Additionally, several studies employing methods other than fMRI (i.e., not focusing on the activation of specific brain regions) have demonstrated direct and distinguishable effects of mortality salience on brain responses (Gyimes & Valentini, 2023), as well as how it moderates brain responses related to the avoidance of self-confrontation ("self-escape"; Chen et al., 2020; Luo et al., 2019) or reinforcement learning (Gao et al., 2020).

Latent Angst

Affective reactions to uncertainty and mortality salience, along with the mechanisms for coping with them, do not need to be conscious, a condition that alludes to the concept of *latent angst* (Kierkegaard, 2013). In fact, the neurobiological network that processes uncertainty is basic in a way that it involves evolutionarily older, deeper structures of the brain; that is, it is already a function of the animal brain. Accordingly, uncertainty processing and corresponding affective or behavioral reactions may escape the individual's awareness (Holbrook et al., 2011).

Indeed, many studies found automatic reactions, physiological or behavioral, to death reminders that largely occurred without conscious awareness of participants (e.g., Arndt et al., 2001; Quirin et al., 2021b). For example, death reminders engendered increases in striving for self-esteem and defense of one's worldview (Burke et al., 2010; Solomon et al., 1991), physiological arousal, subcortical rather than cortical brain activation (Quirin et al., 2011), or increases in negative affect as measured with an indirect rather than self-report test (Quirin et al., 2021b).

Kierkegaard's concept of latent angst corresponds with psychological research demonstrating that psychological phenomena such as affective processes, having been evolving early in evolution and already existing in (nonreflecting) mammals, can occur in a prereflective ("unconscious") way (e.g., Brosschot et al., 2010; Lane, 2008; Quirin et al., 2009, 2018; Winkielman & Berridge, 2004). Such prereflective forms of affect, when related to potential mortality threats, might be interpreted as latent angst (Heidegger, 1927) and have been measured using cognitive tests such as the Implicit Positive and Negative Affect Test (Quirin et al., 2009, 2018). A recently published study (Quirin et al., 2021b), for instance, revealed elevated scores in implicit but not explicit negative affect when asked to reflect about terror acts. Implicit negative affect also corresponded with activation in the amygdala but not in prefrontal areas, supporting the notion of latent (nonreflected) angst (Suslow et al., 2015).

Notably, processes generated by these areas, particularly the amygdala and related circuits, often operate below the level of conscious awareness. The amygdala plays a crucial role in rapid, automatic processing of emotional stimuli, especially fear and threat-related cues, even before conscious awareness (Whalen et al., 1998). Even the insular cortex, implicated in interoceptive awareness, may contribute to nonconscious anxiety by processing somatic sensations associated with anxiety responses (Critchley et al., 2002). Such evidence lends, at least partially, support to Kierkegaard's concept of latent angst.

Love, Attachment, Connectedness

Love is a multifaceted concept including diverse dimensions such as infatuation, romantic attachment, and broader social connectedness. *Infatuation*, experienced in the early stages of romance, is an intense emotional and cognitive state characterized by euphoria, desire, and a profound sense of bonding. In his novel *The Stranger* (1942b), Camus stressed the potential of love for alleviating the pain of inherent meaninglessness of life. In contrast, the later stages of romantic love, often termed *attachment*, encompass a deep, enduring emotional bond and an increased sense of security with a romantic partner.

Several existentialists discussed the role of love and attachment in autonomy, identity, and self-concept. Sartre (1943), for example, suggested that love can be seen as a struggle to balance the desire for personal autonomy with the need for connection and recognition (particularly, in states of emotional dependency). Similarly, in *The Second Sex*, de Beauvoir (1953) emphasized the importance of recognizing the autonomy and subjectivity of both partners in a relationship. Social connectedness in general, including friendship, encompasses feelings of belonging, companionship, and emotional support. Sartre delved into how our interactions with others mold our perception of self and consciousness, ultimately shaping and defining our identity. Heidegger (1927) similarly explored these ideas through his concept of *being-with-others* or "Mitsein."

Infatuation is strongly linked to the activation of pleasure centers in the brain, particularly regions associated with dopamine release such as the ventral tegmental area and the ventral striatum or "nucleus accumbens." Additionally, the release of "love hormones" like oxytocin and vasopressin, regulated by the hypothalamus, plays a pivotal role in fostering social bonding, trust, and attachment, and even attenuates defensive reactions to the major existential concern of mortality salience (Pfundmair et al., 2019). Research indicates that activity in the PFC undergoes alterations during infatuation, possibly due to changes in self-representation, including heightened self-esteem, and an overly positive perception of the other (e.g., Aron et al., 2005; Xu et al., 2011).

As romantic attachment progresses into later stages, oxytocin and vasopressin continue to play a significant role. Simultaneously, the activation of the amygdala, responsible for processing fear and pleasure, gains importance, reflecting the inherent association of attachment with the potential experience of loss. Additionally, the anterior cingulate cortex, implicated in emotion regulation and reward anticipation, becomes increasingly engaged in partner attachment. This can be interpreted as a manifestation of progressing social emotion regulation facilitated by the partner (Coan, 2010). Similarly, areas engaged in attachment and social connection, are also activated in the experience of their absence, that is, social isolation or "loneliness" (Cacioppo & Hawkley, 2009; Cacioppo et al., 2015; Eisenberger, 2012; Layden et al., 2017).

Self and Identity

Identity in terms of *personal identity* refers to an individual's distinct sense of self, encompassing their unique characteristics, beliefs, values, experiences, and memories. It represents an understanding of one's own continuity and distinctiveness over time, enabling a person to differentiate themselves from others (Erikson, 1959). One important aspect of (personal) identity is *social identity*, which refers to an individual's self-concept deriving from their membership or feeling of belonging to social groups referring to nationality, ethnicity, gender, profession, subcultural movements, or any other group. Social identity helps individuals define their self typically by adopting the characteristics, values, or norms associated with that group (Tajfel et al., 1979).

Heidegger (1927), for example, explored the concept of authenticity in relation to personal identity. He argued that individuals often live inauthentic lives, being absorbed by societal norms and expectations. Authenticity, according to Heidegger, involves confronting one's mortality and making choices that align with one's true self. This notion is compatible with psychological constructs of self-congruence, self-concordance, or self-determination. According to *self-determination theory* (e.g., Ryan & Deci, 2000), the strength of personal identification with societal values or goals can vary on a continuum from introjection to integration. Based on a neurocognitive approach, this continuum can be conceptualized as the strength of the connection between the value or goal in question and already existing self-aspects, that is, the integrative self (see also Quirin et al., 2021a).

The neural correlates of personal (including social) identity and the self are intricate and involve various brain regions associated with self-awareness, self-referential processing, memory, and social cognition. The medial PFC, particularly the ventromedial part (D'Argembeau et al., 2007), posterior cingulate cortex, and precuneus, that is, parts of the so- called default mode network, are often active during self-referential processing and the construction of one's sense of self (Amodio & Frith, 2006; Decety & Sommerville, 2003; Northoff et al., 2006). The anterior cingulate cortex is involved in integrating information related to self-representation and social cognition, contributing to self-awareness (Amodio & Frith, 2006). The adjacent anterior insula, particularly in the right cortex, performs similar integrative functions, plays a role in temporal continuity (Scalabrini et al., 2021), and contributes to emotional self-awareness (Craig, 2009). These brain regions and networks collectively contribute to the construction and representation of personal identity and the sense of self.

Authenticity

Authenticity refers to the congruence between an individual's actions, values, beliefs, and desires with their true self or core identity (Quirin & Kuhl, 2022), as described above. It involves being genuine, true to oneself, and behaving in ways that align with one's own beliefs and values, rather than succumbing to external pressures or societal expectations (Camus, 1942b; Sartre, 1943). From this perspective, self and identity, or the activation of underlying neural structures, do not inherently convey authenticity. This is because individuals may be aware of their personal goals and values but still fail to act in accordance with them. In "Existentialism Is a Humanism," Sartre (1946) argued that individuals are condemned to be free, and as such, they must take responsibility for creating their own essence through their actions and choices. Accordingly, in his opinion, authenticity involves embracing one's freedom and making choices that align with one's values and beliefs, which means to be true to oneself. Most existentialist thinkers consider living an authentic life, that is, in line with their "self," as a major source of meaning (Camus, 1942a; Frankl, 1963; Sartre, 1946). In fact, existentialists' claim for living authentic lives is in line with empirical results from psychological studies showing that authenticity, often investigated in terms of self-determination (e.g., Deci & Ryan, 2000) or self-concordance (Sheldon & Elliot, 1999), is associated with improved mental well-being, life satisfaction, and interpersonal relationships.

Authenticity (in terms of self-congruence or self-concordance with own preferences or values) was found to be associated with activity of the medial PFC adjacent to the anterior insula. The medial PFC is integral in self-reflection, decision making, and value processing (Euston et al., 2012; Hare et al., 2009), and reduced activity was found for individuals misconceiving others' expectations as self-chosen goals (Quirin et al., 2022a).

Less authentic (in terms of less intrinsically motivated) behaviors also go with reduced activity in the major reinforcement area, the ventral striatum ("nucleus accumbens") (Murayama et al., 2010). The anterior cingulate cortex is also relevant, aiding in conflict resolution that maintains authenticity (Botvinick, 2007). Interoceptive awareness, represented by the insular cortex, might contribute to authenticity by processing internal states and emotions (Craig, 2009).

Absurdity versus Meaning

Existentialists, Albert Camus in particular, have often emphasized that an individual's meaning in life derives from the inherent absurdity of existence and the absence of an objective or predetermined meaning to life. They have argued that individuals must confront this existential void and actively create their own meaning through authentic choices and actions. In his influential work *The Myth of Sisyphus*, Camus (1942a) explored the absurdity of existence and the human struggle to find meaning in an indifferent universe. He argued that individuals can find meaning and happiness through "rebellion" against the absurd, even in the face of existential threats (e.g., by embracing love). Absurdity, psychologically, refers to the inherent lack of meaning, coherence, or rationality in certain aspects of human existence or the universe (Corey, 2013). It embodies situations, beliefs, or experiences that leave individuals to grapple with the senselessness of life.

Absurdity perception involves various neural processes related to incongruity, surprise, and violations of logical or contextual expectations. Some key neural correlates of absurdity include the superior temporal gyrus, which is implicated in processing incongruity and violations of semantic or contextual expectations, fundamental to perceiving absurdity and attempting to make meaning out of it (Bottini et al., 1994). Moreover, it involves the anterior cingulate cortex, as it is associated with conflict monitoring, error detection, and processing cognitive dissonance (Van Veen & Carter, 2002), and the dorsolateral PFC, as it is involved in higher-order cognitive functions—including reasoning and comprehension of incongruous or absurd situations (Goel & Dolan, 2001). Not least, typically processing affective information (e.g., Phan et al., 2004), the amygdala may be engaged in the evaluation of the emotional or affective aspects of absurdity. However, it should be noted that the actual impression of absurdity arising from the detection of a logical conflict in working memory can be considered fleeting. It is plausible to assume that the motivational consequences of absurdity in terms of a lack of meaningful, higher-order life goals (i.e., frustration and dysthymia) are more strongly associated with reduced tonic activity in brain areas involved in meaning in life, or even with depression.

The neural correlates of meaning in life involve complex interplay among various brain regions associated with cognitive processing, emotional experiences, and self-reflection. The PFC, particularly its medial part, is associated with self-reflection, decision making, and evaluating personal values and beliefs, which are central to the perception of life's meaning (Kapogiannis et al., 2009). The anterior cingulate cortex is linked to emotional processing, particularly to emotional awareness, conflicts, appraisal, and regulation, contributing to the evaluation of life goals and values (Lane et al., 1998; Zhang & Peng, 2023). The anterior insula is involved in processing interoceptive awareness and emotions, which play a role in the subjective experience and assessment of life's meaning (Craig, 2009; Gu et al., 2013). The default mode network, including the medial PFC and posterior cingulate cortex, is active during self-reflection, introspection, and contemplating one's life purpose, contributing to the construction of meaning (Hassabis & Maguire, 2009).

Will

Will or "volition" encompasses the multifaceted processes inherent in decision making, the initiation of actions, and the steadfast commitment to sustaining them ("*willpower*") over the course of pursuing one's goals (Baumeister & Heatherton, 1996). According to existentialism, volition involves making choices that are authentic, aligning with one's values, beliefs, and personal essence, thereby creating meaning in one's life (Kierkegaard, 1843). Through authentic choices, individuals infuse their existence with purpose and significance, asserting their values and defining their own paths. However, individuals sometimes make nonauthentic choices that align more with social expectations than with their own preferences, life goals, or values. A general tendency toward adopting such "introjected" goals can lead to feelings of alienation, depression, or burnout (Deci & Ryan, 2000).

A BRAIN MODEL OF EXISTENTIAL CONCERNS

In the preceding sections, we examined concepts commonly explored in existentialist philosophy and relating to human needs, emotions, and cognitive worldviews. Also, we delved into the neural correlates associated with these concepts as applied in psychological research. In this section, we attempt to integrate these findings in a brain model of existential concerns against the background of major neuroscientific or neuroscientifically informed systems-dynamics theories of psychological functioning, such as the *theory of personality systems interactions* (Kuhl, 2000; Kuhl et al., 2021; Quirin & Kuhl, 2022; Quirin et al., 2019b), the *theory of predictive-and-reactive control systems* (Tops et al., 2010, 2014, 2017), *self-determination theory* (Deci & Ryan, 2000; Ryan & Deci, 2000), and the *theory of spatiotemporal dynamics* (Northoff, 2023, 2024; Northoff et al., 2020).

The *brain model of existential concerns* posits that two distinct brain networks are differentially involved in processing two clusters of existential concerns. One network becomes active in the presence of strong affect and arousal, typically elicited by objects, representations, and urgencies related to gaining reward or avoiding punishment (e.g., threats and uncertainty). In this case, the individual reacts to their environment attentionally or behaviorally, aiming to minimize losses and maximize gains. It can thus be termed a *reactive control system* (Tops et al., 2010, 2014, 2017). Reactive control narrows the individual's attention to uncertainties and potential dangers, prompting a focused and restricted type of information processing. Accordingly, the locus of control (determination) of experience and behavior predominantly lies in the external world ("external regulation"; Deci & Ryan, 2000).

The other network becomes active when the situation generally aligns with the individual's needs and goals, meaning there is an absence of strong emotion and arousal. This lack of urgency allows the individual to fulfill their self-extending needs and feel autonomous, having control over the situation. Accordingly, this network may be termed the *autonomous regulation system.* Since, in the absence of urgencies, the current situation is safe and relatively predictable, this network may also be called the *predictive control system* (Tops et al., 2010, 2014, 2017). The absence of urgencies facilitates broad information processing, enabling the simultaneous consideration of various representations and action alternatives, whether experienced directly or stored in memory. Such broad information processing is essential for the experience of intrinsic motivation and creativity (Kuhl, 2000; Kuhl et al., 2015; Quirin & Kuhl, 2022). The use of the distinct terms *control* and *regulation* is informed by the theory of personality systems interactions (Kuhl, 2000; Kuhl et al., 2021; see also Quirin & Kuhl, 2022). This theory leverages the different everyday-language connotations of the two terms, with *control* implying a sense of constraint or unfreedom, while *regulation* does not (Kuhl, 2000; Quirin et al., 2021).

Brain areas underlying reactive control refer to the mediodorsal thalamus, ventral pallidum, lateral limbic system structures (e.g., ventral striatum or "nucleus accumbens"), anterior hippocampal formation, amygdala, the dorsal anterior cingulate cortex, inferotemporal cortex, temporal pole, anterior insula, and areas of the inferior frontal gyrus. By contrast, autonomous regulation is supported mostly by dorsomedial structures, including the posterior cingulate cortex, precuneus, parahippocampal cortex, posterior hippocampal formation, anteroventral thalamus, dorsal striatum, medial prefrontal cortex, and dorsolateral prefrontal cortex (Tops et al., 2010, 2014, 2017). Figure 12.1 illustrates the locations of a selection of these brain regions.

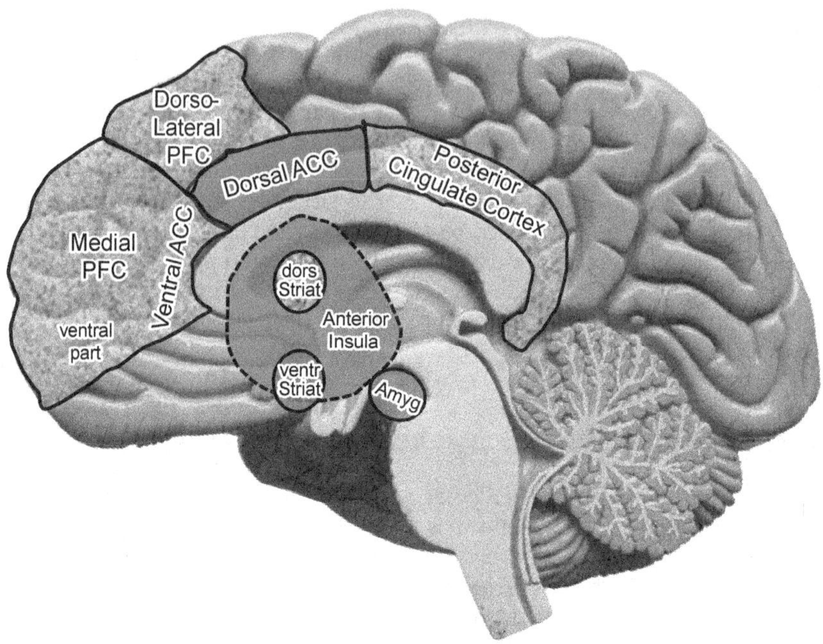

FIGURE 12.1. Major brain regions involved in autonomous regulation (textured/bright) versus reactive control (dark). The dashed line indicates a region located further behind. PFC, prefrontal cortex; ACC, anterior cingulate cortex; Amyg, amygdala; dors. Striat., dorsal striatum; ventr. Strat., ventral striatum ("nucleus accumbens").

As the functional properties of the two systems are inherently linked to aspects of existential concerns, the brain model of existential concerns posits that the activity of these brain networks and their respective cognitive-processing modes facilitate the generation and handling of specific existential concerns in everyday life (e.g., the absurdity of existence). Specifically, the reactive control system along with its narrow mode of cognitive processing facilitates thoughts and feelings associated with absurdity and uncertainty and related brain structures (e.g., Tops et al., 2010, 2014, 2017). For example, the perception of life as having no meaning reflects human dissatisfaction with the tendency to seek inherent value and purpose. This sense of absurdity can push an individual to either rebel against meaninglessness or abandon this search altogether, often leading to depression. In contrast, the autonomous regulation system, with its expansive mode of cognitive processing, is considered to facilitate authenticity, meaning making, and willpower (see Figure 12.1).

The Integrative Self

Autonomous regulation, like reactive control, is a mode of processing existing in mammals and birds already. However, the ability to process and integrate representations of preferences, goals, and values and utilize them for efficient goal pursuit constitutes a more recent, higher-level function of autonomous regulation. This advanced function can be attributed to the *integrative self*, which is considered the high-level variant of autonomous regulation consisting of interconnected representations encompassing personal memories, self-concepts, values, and preferences (Kuhl et al., 2015). According to self-determination theory and many other sociocultural theories, these self-aspects primarily, though not exclusively, originate from external values and opinions of parents and significant others, which have been integrated into the (integrative) self.

Conceptualized this way, this neuropsychological structure represents the entirety of genuine (authentic) self-aspects, which need not necessarily be consciously reflected upon, unlike the explicit self-concept (see also Northoff & Horvat, 2022). It is important to clarify that, diverging from certain psychological and philosophical conceptualizations of the self, the term *integrative self* specifically denotes a subsystem nested within the human psyche and brain, rather than encompassing the entirety of an individual's psyche (e.g., Quirin & Kuhl, 2022).

Because the integrative self deeply interconnects various self-aspects, it encompasses integrated goals rather than introjected ones—personal ideals rather than merely social expectations (Quirin et al., 2019b, 2021a, 2022a). Consequently, when the integrative self is activated, individuals are more likely to experience authenticity, find meaning, and resonate with their preferences. In other words, it is this high-level autonomous regulation system that is considered to be implicated in the processing of existential concerns such as authenticity, autonomy, and meaning making.

Additionally, intrinsic motivation stemming from basic (mammalian) needs and drives, such as hunger or sex, does not initially involve the self but rather engages low-level processes (Kuhl et al., 2021). In these instances, behavior is not regulated externally (i.e., under reactive control). Consequently, it can be described as autonomous or predictive, but not under the immediate regulation of the integrative self.

The examination of neural underpinnings of the integrative self and related existential concerns such as authenticity, personal identity, meaning making, and effortless will implies an overlapping network of regions implicated in these aspects, with a particular emphasis on the ventromedial PFC—an area that among others has been associated with self-referential processing (D'Argembeau et al., 2007; Northoff et al., 2006) and autonomous regulation (Tops et al., 2010, 2014, 2017).

As a preliminary conclusion, discernible patterns of brain activation associated with processing different existential concerns align with two primary control systems within the human brain: the reactive control system and the autonomous regulation system. The integrative self, as a higher-order autonomous regulation system, holds a distinct significance in addressing existential concerns typically linked to psychological well-being and personal growth. In the following sections, we delve into a detailed exploration of how reactive and autonomous modes, in conjunction with the integrative self, are intertwined with selected existential concerns.

NAVIGATING EXISTENTIAL CONCERNS: RESTORING AUTONOMOUS REGULATION THROUGH ENGAGEMENT OF THE INTEGRATIVE SELF

After having examined key existential concerns through the lens of the proposed brain model, we now address some neuropsychological mechanisms that may underlie transitions from reactive to autonomous regulation. This transition is crucial for coping with mortality salience and uncertainty by activating or strengthening personal identities and values, as well as coping with absurdity of life through meaning making, both of which are addressed below. Accordingly, the focus here is on the interaction and dynamics between the two brain systems, rather than on an examination of reactive and autonomous modes in relative isolation.

Personal Identities and Values: Coping with Mortality Salience and Uncertainty

Numerous investigations have delved into the neural underpinnings associated with coping mechanisms in response to mortality or uncertainty, as reviewed in previous work (Quirin & Klackl, 2016; Quirin et al., 2019a). These reviews conclude that both reminders of mortality and signals of uncertainty trigger activation in brain regions linked to salience and discrepancy detection and related negative affective states—central functions of the reactive control system and prominently involving the amygdala and the anterior cingulate cortex (see also Tritt et al., 2012).

Furthermore, mortality threats can activate areas of the PFC associated with autonomous regulation, including the integrative self. This activation might reflect a counteraction to downregulate reactive control. Specifically, activation of the left ventrolateral PFC plays a pivotal role in familiarity processing and semantic categorization, suggesting its involvement in upholding own worldviews and other schemata. In contrast, the left dorsolateral PFC emerges as a key player in amplifying signals related to appetitive goal pursuit and action orientation, and is thus involved in proactive coping associated with autonomous regulation (see also the concept of "reactive approach"; McGregor et al., 2010). Meanwhile, the ventromedial PFC is strongly engaged in processing self-representations encompassing self-chosen goals, preferences, values, and identity (Northoff et al., 2006) and has therefore been linked to the operating of the "integrative self" (Kuhl et al., 2015; Quirin et al., 2022a). This region is therefore considered to substantially contribute to the sustainable integration of adverse including death-related experiences (Quirin & Kuhl, 2022; Quirin et al., 2019b). Since this integration process necessitates a significant transformation of personal schemata from defensive and narrow to adaptive and broad worldviews, it can be termed *accommodative self-growth* (Quirin & Kuhl, 2022; Quirin et al., 2019b). A study using magnetoencephalography revealed that meditators exhibited brain responses to the combined presentation of death-related and self-related stimuli indicative of acceptance rather than denial, in contrast to nonmeditators. Furthermore, death acceptance was found to predict positive indicators of successful meditation (Dor-Ziderman et al., 2023).

Meaning Making: Coping with Absurdity

According to Camus (1942b), individuals need to rebel against the inherent absurdity of life by finding their subjective meanings. This key existentialist notion may be linked to a switch from reactive to autonomous regulation. From an epistemic standpoint, the perception of life's absurdity is inherently relative, stemming from an intentional construct that delineates an irreconcilable mismatch between perceived reality and one's worldview or goal schema. According to the present functional approach, a narrow, reactive processing mode may contribute to the perception of life's absurdity. This is because it narrows perception to the attainment of one's own goals (which appear absurd in the face of mortality), impeding the recognition and processing of benefits for others or society at large.

In conclusion, individuals naturally switch between the two control modes and their associated existential concerns and emotions as an adaptive way of coping with everyday challenges. Activating the integrative self, a specific predictive mode involving structures such as the ventromedial PFC, in response to adverse experiences broadens the scope of processing. This activation helps put problems and adverse experiences in perspective, facilitating their integration and consequently fostering wisdom.

DISCUSSION AND OUTLOOK

Albeit philosophical existentialism has long been captivating thinkers across disciplines, only throughout the last decade have researchers begun investigating the neural correlates of existential phenomena under the emerging field of existential neuroscience. The present work aimed to elucidate major neuropsychological mechanisms underlying existential concerns and integrate these findings with the ideas of prominent existentialist philosophers. The effort of combining philosophical insights with empirical rigor culminated in the development of a brain model of existential concerns.

As we tried to make clear, the interdisciplinary subject of existential neuroscience possesses promising avenues for integration with philosophical and psychological theories. This integrative attempt is useful as researchers can develop a more comprehensive understanding of human consciousness and behavior, and because it can finally offer practical implications for mental health interventions and existential well-being. However, every attempt to integrate different approaches or theories risks overlooking the nuanced distinctions within the subject matter. Consequently, the precise meanings of concepts used to describe existential concerns may vary between philosophical and psychological interpretations. While some of these variances might be relatively minor, others could represent significant points of contention. At this juncture, we leave it open for debate which of the drawn parallels pertain to minor differences and which to major divergences.

It may be important to mention that the neural correlates of existential concerns can be observed in neurotransmitter activity, though this was not the primary focus of the present work. For example, norepinephrine is strongly involved in the generation of arousal, anxiety, and uncertainty. In contrast, serotonin and gamma-aminobutyric acid help counteract these feelings by reducing activity in brain areas that contribute to their generation. Similarly, oxytocin and opioids have comparable effects, with oxytocin playing a crucial role in emotional bonding as well as both parental and romantic attachment (Feldman, 2012). Notably, these neurotransmitters do not operate independently; instead, they form complex neural circuits where they interact in intricate ways. Consequently, neurotransmitters may indirectly influence existential concerns through these interactions.

The final point of our discussion delves into the age-old philosophical question concerning the relationship between "body and soul," or more precisely, mind and brain (e.g., Fountoulakis, 2022). This question fundamentally underpins our model of existential neuroscience, which seeks to understand how existential concerns correlate with neural activity on an ontological level. Dualistic perspectives (e.g., Descartes, 1641/1951) posit that mind and brain are two distinct, causally interrelated entities. In contrast, monistic perspectives assert that matter and mind are ontologically identical, essentially "two sides of the same coin." Our model of existential concerns is based on a recently developed monistic theory, the *theory of spatiotemporal dynamics* (Northoff, 2023, 2024; Northoff et al., 2020). This theory posits that for monistic theories of mind and brain to hold, there must be a "common ground" or "common currency" shared by the two ontological domains of mind and (brain) matter, along with the network of entities interacting within each domain (i.e., cells versus representations). This common ground manifests in the spatiotemporal dynamics among these entities, highlighting how patterns of neural activity correspond with mental phenomena. This approach allows us to explore the integration of subjective experiences and objective brain functions, offering a comprehensive framework for understanding the mind-brain relationship in the context of existential neuroscience. According to Northoff (and his team), these spatiotemporal dynamics provide a framework for understanding how mental states emerge from brain states without reducing one to the other. The dynamic interactions within neural networks and the timing of neural oscillations create a coherent field in which mental processes can be mapped onto physical brain processes. This mapping facilitates the integration of subjective experiences and objective brain functions, thereby addressing the hard problem of consciousness by positing a unified basis for mental and neural phenomena. The unified basis consists here in the spatiotemporal dynamics that are shared by both neural and mental states. The shared spatiotemporal features then create the basic ontological existence and reality of both neural and mental features entailing monism. While the differentiation of neural and mental features is then more related to us and our employment of distinct viewpoints such as first- and third-person perspectives to conceive the shared spatiotemporal features in terms of neural and mental states.

Future research in existential neuroscience may focus on several key areas. First, the neural mechanisms, systems, and circuits underlying existential concerns and eventual cultural and contextual differences need further exploration. Second, future research may investigate how existential interventions, such as mindfulness practices or existential psychotherapy can influence brain function (e.g., shifts from reactive control to autonomous regulation) and structure (referring to neuroplasticity). Not least, exploring the ethical implications of neuroscientific findings on existential themes, including issues related to personal identity, will, decision making, and well-being, is of major importance.

SUMMARY AND CONCLUSION

The integration of philosophical existentialism with neuroscience, existential neuroscience, represents a promising frontier for advancing our knowledge of existential concerns such as authenticity, freedom, love, identity, search for meaning, and will. By embracing this interdisciplinary dialogue, researchers can pave the way for a more circumspect understanding of existential concerns and their neural substrates, ultimately enriching both philosophical discourse and scientific inquiry. Existential neuroscience can assist in the analysis and even substantiation of the causes, psychological components, and mechanisms underpinning existential concerns, and finally offer practical implications for mental health interventions and existential well-being.

ACKNOWLEDGMENTS

This research was made possible, in part, by the generous support of the John Templeton Foundation (Grant ID: JTF 62700) awarded to Markus Quirin.

REFERENCES

Amodio, D. M., & Frith, C. D. (2006). Meeting of minds: The medial frontal cortex and social cognition. *Nature Reviews Neuroscience, 7,* 268–277.

Arndt, J., Allen, J. J. B., & Greenberg, J. (2001). Traces of terror: Subliminal death primes and facial electromyographic indices of affect. *Motivation and Emotion, 25,* 253–277.

Aron, A., Fisher, H., Mashek, D. J., Strong, G., Li, H., & Brown, L. L. (2005). Reward, motivation, and emotion systems associated with early-stage intense romantic love. *Journal of Neurophysiology, 94,* 327–337.

Baumeister, R. F., & Heatherton, T. F. (1996). Self-regulation failure: An overview. *Psychological Inquiry, 7,* 1–15.

Berlyne, D. E. (1960). *Conflict, arousal, and curiosity.* McGraw-Hill.

Berlyne, D. E. (1966). Curiosity and exploration: Animals spend much of their time seeking stimuli whose significance raises problems for psychology. *Science, 153,* 25–33.

Berlyne, D. E. (1973). Aesthetics and psychobiology. *Journal of Aesthetics and Art Criticism, 31.*

Bottini, G., Corcoran, R., Sterzi, R., Paulesu, E., Schenone, P., Scarpa, P., . . . Frith, D. (1994). The role of the right hemisphere in the interpretation of figurative aspects of language A positron emission tomography activation study. *Brain, 117,* 1241–1253.

Botvinick, M. M. (2007). Conflict monitoring and decision making: Reconciling two perspectives on anterior cingulate function. *Cognitive, Affective, and Behavioral Neuroscience, 7,* 356–366.

Botvinick, M. M., Cohen, J. D., & Carter, C. S. (2004). Conflict monitoring and anterior cingulate cortex: An update. *Trends in Cognitive Sciences, 8,* 539–546.

Brosschot, J. F., Verkuil, B., & Thayer, J. F. (2010). Conscious and unconscious perseverative cognition: Is a large part of prolonged physiological activity due to unconscious stress? *Journal of Psychosomatic Research, 69,* 407–416.

Burke, B. L., Martens, A., & Faucher, E. H. (2010). Two decades of terror management theory: A meta-analysis of mortality salience research. *Personality and Social Psychology Review, 14,* 155–195.

Cacioppo, J. T., & Hawkley, L. C. (2009). Perceived social isolation and cognition. *Trends in Cognitive Sciences, 13,* 447–454.

Cacioppo, S., Grippo, A. J., London, S., Goossens, L., & Cacioppo, J. T. (2015). Loneliness: Clinical import and interventions. *Perspectives on Psychological Science, 10,* 238–249.

Camus, A. (1942a). *The myth of Sisyphus* [Le mythe de Sisyphe]. Éditions Gallimard.

Camus, A. (1942b). *The stranger* [L'Étranger]. Gallimard.

Carlson, J. M., Greenberg, T., Rubin, D., & Mujica-Parodi, L. R. (2011). Feeling anxious: Anticipatory amygdalo-insular response predicts the feeling of anxious anticipation. *Social Cognitive and Affective Neuroscience, 6,* 74–81.

Caruso, G., & Flanagan, O. (2017). *Neuroexistentialism: Meaning, morals, and purpose in the age of neuroscience.* Oxford University Press.

Chen, Y., Shen, Y., Shi, Z., Zhang, X., Li, H., Xu, X., . . . Yang, J. (2020). Mortality salience impairs self-referential processing: Neurophysiological and behavioral evidence. *Current Psychology, 39,* 782–792.

Coan, J. A. (2010). Adult attachment and the brain. *Journal of Social and Personal Relationships, 27,* 210–217.

Corey, G. (2013). *Theory and practice of counseling and psychotherapy.* Cengage Learning.

Craig, A. D. (2009). How do you feel—now?: The anterior insula and human awareness. *Nature Reviews Neuroscience, 10,* 59–70.

Critchley, H. D., Mathias, C. J., & Dolan, R. J. (2002). Fear conditioning in humans: The influence of awareness and autonomic arousal on functional neuroanatomy. *Neuron, 33,* 653–663.

D'Argembeau, A., Ruby, P., Collette, F., Degueldre, C., Balteau, E., Luxen, A., . . . Salmon, E. (2007). Distinct regions of the medial prefrontal cortex are associated with self-referential processing and perspective taking. *Journal of Cognitive Neuroscience, 19,* 935–944.

de Beauvoir, S. (1953). *The second sex* [Le deuxième sexe]. Knopf.

Decety, J., & Sommerville, J. A. (2003). Shared representations between self and other: A social cognitive neuroscience view. *Trends in Cognitive Sciences, 7,* 527–533.

Deci, E. L., & Ryan, R. M. (2000). The "what" and "why" of goal pursuits: Human needs and the self-determination of behavior. *Psychological Inquiry, 11,* 227–268.

Descartes, R. (1951). *Meditations on first philosophy.* Newcomb Livraria Press. (Original work published 1641)

Dor-Ziderman, Y., Schweitzer, Y., Nave, O., Trautwein, F.-M., Fulder, S., Lutz, A., . . . Berkovich-Ohana, A. (2023, August 21). Mindfulness meditators' brains show an acceptance of death which predicts positively-valenced meditative self-dissolution experiences. *Psychology Online Preprint Service.*

Echebarria-Echabe, A. (2013). Mortality salience and uncertainty: Similar effects but different processes? *European Journal of Social Psychology, 43,* 185–191.

Eisenberger, N. I. (2012). The pain of social disconnection: Examining the shared neural underpinnings of physical and social pain. *Nature Reviews Neuroscience, 13,* 421–434.

Erikson, E. H. (1959). Identity and the life cycle: Selected papers. *Psychological Issues, 1,* 1–171.

Euston, D. R., Gruber, A. J., & McNaughton, B. L. (2012). The role of medial prefrontal cortex in memory and decision making. *Neuron, 76,* 1057–1070.

Feldman, R. (2012). Oxytocin and social affiliation in humans. *Hormones and Behavior, 61,* 380–391.

Fountoulakis, K. N. (2022). *The human connectome.* Springer.

Frankl, V. E. (1963). *Man's search for meaning: An introduction to logotherapy.* Washington Square Press.

Gao, T., Zhou, Y., Li, W., Pfabigan, D. M., & Han, S. (2020). Neural mechanisms of reinforcement learning under mortality threat. *Social Neuroscience, 15,* 170–185.

Goel, V., & Dolan, R. J. (2001). The functional anatomy of humor: Segregating cognitive and affective components. *Nature Neuroscience, 4,* 237–238.

Greenberg, J., Koole, S. L., & Pyszczynski, T. (Eds.). (2004). *Handbook of experimental existential psychology.* Guilford Press.

Greenberg, J., Pyszczynski, T., & Solomon, S. (1986). The causes and consequences of the need for self-esteem: A terror management theory. In R. F. Baumeister (Ed.), *Public and private self* (pp. 189–212). Springer.

Greenberg, J., Pyszczynski, T., & Solomon, S. (1995). Toward a dual motive depth psychology of self and social behavior. In M. Kernis (Ed.), *Efficacy, agency, and self* (pp. 73–99). Plenum Press.

Greenberg, J., Simon, L., Pyszczynski, T., Solomon, S., & Chatel, D. (1992). Terror management and tolerance: Does mortality salience always intensify negative reactions to others who threaten one's worldview? *Journal of Personality and Social Psychology, 63,* 212–220.

Gu, X., Hof, P. R., Friston, K. J., & Fan, J. (2013). Anterior insular cortex and emotional awareness. *Journal of Comparative Neurology, 521,* 3371–3388.

Gyimes, I. L., & Valentini, E. (2023). Reminders of mortality: Investigating the effects of different mortality saliences on somatosensory neural activity. *Brain Sciences, 13.*

Hare, T. A., Camerer, C. F., & Rangel, A. (2009). Self-control in decision-making involves modulation of the vmPFC valuation system. *Science, 324,* 646–648.

Hassabis, D., & Maguire, E. A. (2009). The construction system of the brain. *Philosophical Transactions of the Royal Society B: Biological Sciences, 364,* 1263–1271.

Heidegger, M. (1927). *Sein und zeit.* State University of New York Press.

Holbrook, C., Sousa, P., & Hahn-Holbrook, J. (2011). Unconscious vigilance: Worldview defense without adaptations for terror, coalition, or uncertainty management. *Journal of Personality and Social Psychology, 101,* 451–466.

Kapogiannis, D., Barbey, A. K., Su, M., Zamboni, G., Krueger, F., & Grafman, J. (2009). Cognitive and neural foundations of religious belief. *Proceedings of the National Academy of Sciences, 106,* 4876–4881.

Kierkegaard, S. (1843). *Fear and trembling* [Frygt og bæven].

Kierkegaard, S. (2013). *Kierkegaard's writings, VIII, Volume 8: Concept of anxiety: A simple psychologically orienting deliberation on the dogmatic issue of hereditary sin* (Vol. 18). Princeton University Press.

Klackl, J., Jonas, E., & Kronbichler, M. (2014).

Existential neuroscience: Self-esteem moderates neuronal responses to mortality-related stimuli. *Social Cognitive and Affective Neuroscience, 9,* 1754–1761.

Kuhl, J. (2000). A functional-design approach to motivation and self-regulation: The dynamics of personality systems and interactions. In M. Boekaerts & P. R. Pintrich (Eds.), *Handbook of self-regulation* (pp. 111–169). Academic Press.

Kuhl, J., Quirin, M., & Koole, S. L. (2015). Being someone: The integrated self as a neuropsychological system. *Social and Personality Psychology Compass, 9,* 115–132.

Kuhl, J., Quirin, M., & Koole, S. L. (2021). The functional architecture of human motivation: Personality Systems Interactions Theory. In A. J. Elliot (Ed.), *Advances in motivation science* (Vol. 8, pp. 1–62). Elsevier.

Landau, M. J., Ryu, Y.-J., Greenberg, J., Chur, M., & Pyszczynski, T. (2025). Why is existential uncertainty distressing and persistent? A terror management perspective. In P. Carroll, K. Rios., & K. Oleson (Eds.), *Handbook of the uncertain self* (2nd ed., pp. 149–165). Routledge.

Lane, R. D. (2008). Neural substrates of implicit and explicit emotional processes: A unifying framework for psychosomatic medicine. *Psychosomatic Medicine, 70,* 214–231.

Lane, R. D., Reiman, E. M., Axelrod, B., Yun, L.-S., Holmes, A., & Schwartz, G. E. (1998). Neural correlates of levels of emotional awareness: Evidence of an interaction between emotion and attention in the anterior cingulate cortex. *Journal of Cognitive Neuroscience, 10,* 525–535.

Layden, E. A., Cacioppo, J. T., Cacioppo, S., Cappa, S. F., Dodich, A., Falini, A., & Canessa, N. (2017). Perceived social isolation is associated with altered functional connectivity in neural networks associated with tonic alertness and executive control. *Neuroimage, 145,* 58–73.

Luo, S., Wu, B., Fan, X., Zhu, Y., Wu, X., & Han, S. (2019). Thoughts of death affect reward learning by modulating salience network activity. *NeuroImage, 202.*

McGregor, I., Nash, K., Mann, N., & Phills, C. E. (2010). Anxious uncertainty and reactive approach motivation (RAM). *Journal of Personality and Social Psychology, 99,* 133–147.

Murayama, K., Matsumoto, M., Izuma, K., & Matsumoto, K. (2010). Neural basis of the undermining effect of monetary reward on intrinsic motivation. *Proceedings of the National Academy of Sciences, 107,* 20911–20916.

Nietzsche, F. (1883). *Thus spoke Zarathustra [Also sprach Zarathustra].* Verlag von Ernst Schmeitzner.

Northoff, G. (2018). *The spontaneous brain: From the mind-body to the world-brain problem.* MIT Press.

Northoff, G. (2023). *Neurowaves: Brain, time, and consciousness.* McGill-Queen's Press-MQUP.

Northoff, G. (2024). *From brain dynamics to the mind: Spatiotemporal neuroscience.* Elsevier Science.

Northoff, G., Heinzel, A., de Greck, M., Bermpohl, F., Dobrowolny, H., & Panksepp, J. (2006). Self-referential processing in our brain: A meta-analysis of imaging studies on the self. *Neuroimage, 31,* 440–457.

Northoff, G., & Horvat, S. (2022). The self and its time–A non-reductive neuro-phenomenological perspective on the brain's spontaneous activity. *Mind and Matter, 20,* 195–216.

Northoff, G., Wainio-Theberge, S., & Evers, K. (2020). Is temporo-spatial dynamics the "common currency" of brain and mind?: In quest of "spatiotemporal neuroscience." *Physics of Life Reviews, 33,* 34–54.

Pfundmair, M., Schindler, S., & Burgstaller, J. (2019). The role of oxytocin in terror management processes. *Psychoneuroendocrinology, 103,* 83–86.

Phan, K. L., Taylor, S. F., Welsh, R. C., Ho, S.-H., Britton, J. C., & Liberzon, I. (2004). Neural correlates of individual ratings of emotional salience: A trial-related fMRI study. *Neuroimage, 21,* 768–780.

Prentice, L., Klackl, J., Agroskin, D., Grossmann, I., Alexandrov, Y., Apanovich, V., . . . Jonas, E. (2020). Reaction to norm transgressions and Islamization threat in culturally tight and loose contexts: A cross-cultural comparison of Germany versus Russia. *Culture and Brain, 8,* 46–69.

Preuschoff, K., Bossaerts, P., & Quartz, S. R. (2006). Neural differentiation of expected reward and risk in human subcortical structures. *Neuron, 51,* 381–390.

Preuschoff, K., Quartz, S. R., & Bossaerts, P. (2008). Human insula activation reflects risk prediction errors as well as risk. *Journal of Neuroscience, 28,* 2745–2752.

Pyszczynski, T., Greenberg, J., & Arndt, J. (2012). Freedom versus fear revisited: An integrative analysis of the dynamics of the defense and growth of self. In M. R. Leary & J. P. Tangney (Eds.), *Handbook of self and identity* (2nd ed., pp. 378–404). Guilford Press.

Quirin, M., Jais, M., Di Domenico, S. I., Kuhl, J., & Ryan, R. M. (2021a). Effortless willpower?: The integrative self and self-determined goal pursuit. *Frontiers in Psychology, 12.*

Quirin, M., Kazén, M., & Kuhl, J. (2009). When nonsense sounds happy or helpless:

The Implicit Positive and Negative Affect Test (IPANAT). *Journal of Personality and Social Psychology, 97,* 500–516.

Quirin, M., Kerber, A., Küstermann, E., Radtke, E. L., Kazén, M., Konrad, C., . . . Kuhl, J. (2022a). Not the master of your volitional mind?: The roles of the right medial prefrontal cortex and personality traits in unconscious introjections versus self-chosen goals. *Frontiers in Psychology, 13.*

Quirin, M., & Klackl, J. (2016). Existential neuroscience: A review and outlook for the case of death awareness. In E. Harmon-Jones & M. Inzlicht (Eds.), *Social neuroscience: Biological approaches to social psychology* (pp. 124–142). Psychology Press.

Quirin, M., Klackl, J., & Jonas, E. (2019a). Existential neuroscience: A review and brain model of coping with death awareness. In C. Routledge & M. Vess (Eds.), *Handbook of terror management theory* (pp. 347–367). Elsevier.

Quirin, M., & Kuhl, J. (2022). The concert of personality: Explaining personality functioning and coherence by personality systems interactions. *European Journal of Personality, 36,* 274–292.

Quirin, M., Loktyushin, A., Arndt, J., Küstermann, E., Lo, Y.-Y., Kuhl, J., & Eggert, L. D. (2011). Existential neuroscience: A functional magnetic resonance imaging investigation of neural responses to reminders of one's mortality. *Social, Cognitive, and Affective Neuroscience, 25,* 559–570.

Quirin, M., Malekzad, F., Kazén, M., Luckey, U., & Kehr, H. M. (2021b). Existential threat: Uncovering implicit affect in response to terror reminders in soldiers. *Frontiers in Psychology, 12,* 1952.

Quirin, M., Malekzad, F., Paudel, D., Knoll, A. C., & Mirolli, M. (2022b). Dynamics of personality: The Zurich model of motivation revived, extended, and applied to personality. *Journal of Personality.*

Quirin, M., Tops, M., & Kuhl, J. (2019b). Autonomous motivation, internalization, and the integrative self: A self-regulation framework of interacting neuropsychological systems. In R. M. Ryan (Ed.), *The Oxford handbook of human motivation* (pp. 393–416). Oxford University Press.

Quirin, M., Wróbel, M., Pala, A. N., Stieger, S., Shanchuan, D., Hicks, J. A., . . . Padun, M. A. (2018). A cross-cultural validation of the Implicit Positive and Negative Affect Test (IPANAT): Results from ten nations across three continents. *European Journal of Psychological Assessment, 34,* 52–63.

Ridderinkhof, K. R., Ullsperger, M., Crone, E. A., & Nieuwenhuis, S. (2004). The role of the medial frontal cortex in cognitive control. *Science, 306,* 443–447.

Routledge, C., & Vess, M. (2018). *Handbook of terror management theory.* Academic Press.

Ryan, R. M., & Deci, E. L. (2000). Intrinsic and extrinsic motivations: Classic definitions and new directions. *Contemporary Educational Psychology, 25,* 54–67.

Sartre, J.-P. (1943). *Being and nothingness* [l'être et le néant]. Éditions Gallimard.

Sartre, J.-P. (1946). *Existentialism is a humanism* [L'existentialisme est un humanisme]. Les Editions Nagel.

Scalabrini, A., Wolman, A., & Northoff, G. (2021). The self and its right insula—Differential topography and dynamic of right vs. left insula. *Brain Sciences, 11,* 1312.

Schlosser, U. L. (2017). Experiences through the gradual expansion of consciousness, conscientiality and global ethics. In M. Masaeli (Ed.), *Spirituality and global ethics* (pp. 260–297). Cambridge Scholars.

Sheldon, K. M., & Elliot, A. J. (1999). Goal striving, need satisfaction, and longitudinal well-being: The self-concordance model. *Journal of Personality and Social Psychology, 76,* 482–497.

Solomon, S., Greenberg, J., & Pyszczynski, T. (1991). A terror management theory of social behavior: On the psychological functions of self-esteem and cultural worldviews. In M. P. Zanna (Ed.), *Advances in experimental social psychology* (Vol. 24, pp. 93–159). Academic Press.

Steger, M. F., Kashdan, T. B., Sullivan, B. A., & Lorentz, D. (2008). Understanding the search for meaning in life: Personality, cognitive style, and the dynamic between seeking and experiencing meaning. *Journal of Personality, 76,* 199–228.

Suslow, T., Ihme, K., Quirin, M., Lichev, V., Rosenberg, N., Bauer, J., . . . Lobsien, D. (2015). Implicit affectivity and rapid processing of affective body language: An fMRI study. *Scandinavian Journal of Psychology, 56,* 545–552.

Tajfel, H., Turner, J. C., Austin, W. G., & Worchel, S. (1979). An integrative theory of intergroup conflict. In M. J. Hatch & M. Schultz (Eds.), *Organizational identity: A reader* (pp. 56–66). Oxford University Press.

Tops, M., Boksem, M. A. S., Luu, P., & Tucker, D. M. (2010). Brain substrates of behavioral programs associated with self-regulation. *Frontiers in Cognition, 1.*

Tops, M., Boksem, M. A. S., Quirin, M., IJzerman, H., & Koole, S. L. (2014). Internally directed cognition and mindfulness: An integrative perspective derived from predictive and reactive control systems theory. *Frontiers in Psychology, 5.*

Tops, M., Quirin, M., Boksem, M. A. S., & Koole, S. L. (2017). Large-scale neural networks and the lateralization of motivation and emotion. *International Journal of Psychophysiology, 119,* 41–49.

Tritt, S. M., Inzlicht, M., & Harmon-Jones, E. (2012). Toward a biological understanding of mortality salience (and other threat compensation processes). *Social Cognition, 30,* 715–733.

Van den Bos, K. (2009). The social psychology of uncertainty management and system justification. In J. T. Jost, A. C. Kay, & H. Thorisdottir (Eds.), *Social and psychological bases of ideology and system justification* (pp. 185–209). Oxford University Press.

Van Veen, V., & Carter, C. S. (2002). The anterior cingulate as a conflict monitor: fMRI and ERP studies. *Physiology and Behavior, 77,* 477–482.

Whalen, P. J., Rauch, S. L., Etcoff, N. L., McInerney, S. C., Lee, M. B., & Jenike, M. A. (1998). Masked presentations of emotional facial expressions modulate amygdala activity without explicit knowledge. *Journal of Neuroscience, 18,* 411–418.

Winkielman, P., & Berridge, K. C. (2004). Unconscious emotion. *Current Directions in Psychological Science, 13,* 120–123.

Xu, X., Aron, A., Brown, L., Cao, G., Feng, T., & Weng, X. (2011). Reward and motivation systems: A brain mapping study of early-stage intense romantic love in Chinese participants. *Human Brain Mapping, 32,* 249–257.

Yalom, I. D. (1980). *Existential psychotherapy.* Basic Books.

Yanagisawa, K., Abe, N., Kashima, E. S., & Nomura, M. (2016). Self-esteem modulates amygdala-ventrolateral prefrontal cortex connectivity in response to mortality threats. *Journal of Experimental Psychology: General, 145,* 273–283.

Zhang, M., & Peng, Y. (2023). Anterior insula and dorsal anterior cingulate cortex as a hub of self-regulation: Combining activation likelihood estimation meta-analysis and meta-analytic connectivity modeling analysis. *Brain Structure and Function, 228,* 1329–1345.

CHAPTER 13

Time, Scarcity, and Savoring the Moment

Jaime L. Kurtz *and* Ryan Murphy

In 2021, 33-year-old Suleika Jaouad, author of the *New York Times* best-selling memoir *Between Two Kingdoms: A Memoir of a Life Interrupted* (2021), was diagnosed with leukemia. Despite her relative youth, this was not her first experience with a devastating, life-altering health crisis. Just a few years prior, she'd endured a lengthy treatment for the same disease. Yet, in her second experience with leukemia, she noticed a shift in perspective. In a social media post, she shared,

> This time, the experience is so different. I don't yearn for accomplishments, professional or otherwise. I don't think, "Oh, but I just want to write another book, meet more people, see more things." What I want is time. I want to look back on this year and remember all of the shapeless days, where I wasn't looking at my phone, wasn't working, where I was truly present with my friends and family. . . . Whatever it is I leave behind, I want it to reflect a respect for time.

While this quote reveals a complex interplay of thoughts, feelings, and motivations, it also demonstrates a simple truth: When one's perceived sense of time feels scarce, there is a natural emotional and motivational change, which can be life-altering. Busyness, novelty, and outward accomplishments take a backseat to quiet, simple pleasures, and a mindset of savoring becomes the desired goal.

In this chapter, we briefly define *savoring* and place it in the context of the emotion regulation and positive psychology literature. We then examine the role that scarcity plays in the savoring process. In short, when there is not much of a resource left, that resource increases in value (Cialdini, 1993). If one thinks of *time* as one such limited resource, an awareness of time's scarcity can increase the value of an experience, making it more likely to be fully enjoyed. Indeed, evidence suggests that when time in an experience is limited or running short, the experience in question—be it a vacation, a season, a college career, a romantic relationship, or even life itself—it is imbued with added value (Fredrickson & Carstensen, 1990; Garcia-Rada & Kim, T, 2021; Gregory et al., 2023; Kurtz, 2008; Shu & Gneezy, 2010). In short, experiences with an "expiration date" are more likely to be savored. However, cultivating a mindset of scarcity—where one is aware of the transience of an experience even in advance of an ending—can also foster savoring well in advance.

SAVORING DEFINED

Savoring is generally thought of as an internal process of emotion regulation in which people upregulate their positive feelings by directing attention to emotionally relevant events (Bryant, 1989, 2003; Bryant et al., 2011; Bryant & Veroff, 2007; Quoidbach et al., 2015b). Savoring can happen spontaneously (such as in a moment of awe), but it is more commonly thought of as an active process, requiring awareness and focus to reap its benefits. Among its many synonyms include basking, marveling, reveling, luxuriating, and reflecting (Bryant & Veroff, 2007). When people are able to fully attend to a positive experience, ascribe it with value, and amplify its enjoyment (perhaps by writing about it or sharing it with another person), they are likely to be savoring. On the other hand, when a person is distracted, unmotivated, or disinterested, even the most pleasurable things can slip by unnoticed.

In the positive psychology literature, savoring can be thought of as a key mechanism that helps explain why seemingly simple practices lead to significant changes in a person's happiness (Emmons & McCullough, 2003; Jose et al., 2012; Lyubomirsky & Layous, 2013; Toepfer & Walker, 2009). For example, consider the well-established connection between gratitude expression (e.g., counting one's blessings or writing down three good things that happened in a day) and happiness. What internal process drives this relationship? If a person is genuinely feeling gratitude, it is likely because their attention has been drawn to something positive that has been bestowed upon them. In short, they are savoring. When French writer François de la Rochefoucauld (1694/1930) stated that "happiness does not consist in things themselves but in the relish we have of them" (p. 51), he was actually describing the vitally important process of savoring. Put in the language of emotion regulation, the ability to strategically upregulate our positive emotions is a critical determinant of well-being (Bryant & Veroff, 2007; Quoidbach et al., 2015b).

The Challenge of Savoring

Although they did not describe it as savoring directly, in their model of positive emotion regulation, Quoidbach and colleagues (2015b) argued that people can simply choose to engage in activities that do not encourage emotion upregulation (such as staying indoors on a beautiful spring day). They can easily be distracted in the midst of a positive experience (imagine a person scrolling through their phone while in the presence of a sunset). Individual differences may also play a role. Although some people may be naturally better at savoring than others are (e.g., those with a high degree of mindfulness or dispositional gratefulness, Brown & Ryan, 2003; McCullough et al., 2002), others may lack the skills to emotionally capitalize on their positive experiences, or they may be unaware of savoring's rewards.

For all of its benefits, savoring often involves effort and concentration. It is generally thought of as a process that requires focused attention on the simple, quiet pleasantries that can easily go unnoticed. Perhaps these things are in a person's attentional background, not demanding much attention (imagine a driver passing a beautiful view while navigating a busy road). Or maybe these things have been subject to hedonic adaptation: Over time and through repeated exposure, a person just fails to notice and appreciate them (Lyubomirsky, 2011; Wilson & Gilbert, 2008). In cases like these, a sense of scarcity (Cialdini, 1993) is thought to be an effective trigger for the savoring process.

The Role of Scarcity in Savoring

While savoring might seem like a challenge—or, in today's busy, multitasking world, a luxury—a sense of scarcity seems to naturally encourage it. Again, when something is scarce, it is more valuable. Conversely, when a resource exists in abundance, it is easily taken for granted (Quoidbach et al., 2010, 2015a). Consider an ordinary pleasure: a large bowl of delicious chocolates. The first few might be enjoyable, but most people would be quickly satiated, and savoring the seemingly endless supply of chocolates would quickly become a challenge. But a simple reframing—one that creates a sense of scarcity—can change this. In one experiment, participants were asked to taste and rate a series of chocolates (O'Brien & Ellsworth, 2012). When they reached the fifth chocolate in the series, some participants were told "this is the last chocolate" while others were told it was "the next chocolate" (suggesting more were still to come). Those presented with the "last chocolate" rated it as more enjoyable than those told it was the "next chocolate." They were more likely to say it was their favorite and also rated the entire experiment as more pleasant.

Extending this over a longer period of time, Quoidbach and Dunn (2013) randomly assigned participants to one of three experimental conditions: Some were instructed to eat as much chocolate as they wanted over the course of the subsequent week, some were told to abstain from eating chocolate over the subsequent week, and some were given no instructions about chocolate consumption. Participants all returned 1 week later and taste-tested a piece of chocolate. Those who had been abstaining from eating chocolate savored this chocolate more (both in self-reported enjoyment and in blind coders' observations) and reported greater positive affect than the other two groups. These studies suggest that when something pleasant is scarce in number—whether it is the last in a sequence or when a person will be deprived of it for a period of time—it can be transformed into something worthy of savoring.

Scarcity of Time

While emphasizing the scarcity of number or quantity is certainly a useful way to promote savoring in everyday life, our primary focus here is the often powerful, poignant experience of time's scarcity, or temporal scarcity. Time is an innately limited resource, and it inevitably declines in abundance over the lifespan. In general, putting a priority on time (as compared to money) encourages happiness-enhancing strategies such as socializing (Mogilner, 2010). Adding in an element of scarcity might just make that difference in motivation even stronger.

Life's Scarcity

As time becomes more and more limited in various contexts, people tend to prioritize spending time in a meaningful way. Specifically, as Carstensen's socioemotional selectivity theory states, when life is nearing its end, people's goals tend to shift toward the things and the people that are most emotionally rewarding, and longer-term goals become less central (Carstensen et al., 1999; Fredrickson & Carstensen, 1990). Rather than focusing on activities that will benefit them in the future, people begin to place a greater emphasis on living in a way that is emotionally satisfying in the present.

Socioemotional selectivity theory (Carstensen et al., 1999) posits that by actively focusing on the present rather than deriving motivation from the past or future, people can become more motivated to emphasize emotion and meaning in their present lives. This theory links the ways in which we perceive time with the manner by which we prioritize social goals and relationship partners. Carstensen and her colleagues (1999) argued that this is because social interaction is fundamental to human survival and flourishing, and that people are "inherently agentic," behaving in a manner that facilitates eventual goal achievement. When one considers that people can often hold a variety of goals (including goals that stand in opposition to one another), it becomes quite necessary for them to optimize behavior according to how they prioritize these goals. Carstensen and colleagues argued that changing the way we view and value time influences the ways in which we go about the process of goal prioritization.

Their theory separates goals into two broad categories: goals based in knowledge acquisition and goals based in emotional regulation or satisfaction. Knowledge-acquisition goals motivate social behavior that allows for people to bolster their understanding of the social and physical world. These prepare people to thrive in the future. Networking at a professional conference or learning a language to facilitate future travels might qualify as knowledge acquisition goals—there is an investment of effort that will hopefully be rewarding in time. Emotion regulation goals motivate social behavior that facilitates the upregulation of positive emotions while helping people live meaningfully and build a sense of social belonging. These sorts of goals help people derive greater satisfaction in their present lives.

Examples might include inviting friends over for dinner or going to a favorite art museum: The emotional payoff is fairly immediate.

Social goals do not always fall squarely into one of these categories and have the capacity to overlap across dimensions, so this separation does not assume that knowledge-acquisition goals lack emotional content. Rather, Carstensen and colleagues believed they generally tend to serve one motivation over the other. When time is perceived as abundant, we tend to pursue more knowledge-acquisition goals, as we want to behave in a way that guides us toward a more optimal future. This does not mean that emotional rewards become unimportant—it simply means that it becomes easier to accept the delay of these rewards because the future seems expansive. However, when we perceive time as being scarce, the importance of an optimal future becomes diminished, and we become more oriented toward living in a meaningful and emotionally satisfying manner (Carstensen et al., 1999; Fredrickson & Carstensen, 1990). The combination of these two kinds of goals serves as the personal fuel source by which our social behavior is motivated. However, because the pursuit of information can often conflict with emotion regulation goals, we appraise the importance of our goals to decide on how to subsequently behave.

As this concept relates to lifespan development and aging, it seems that as people get older, they begin to place greater value on emotional satisfaction and the pursuit of meaning. This could be due to accrued wisdom and experience over one's life along with the understanding that their remaining time is beginning to run out. Research examined this possibility by comparing the cognitive appraisal of social partners in differing dimensions across different groups of people (Carstensen & Fredrickson, 1998). The first two studies examined a wide range of age groups and found that older age groups tended to place a greater level of value on the potential for emotional satisfaction from social partners than younger groups. The third study removed the confound of experience by studying participants who were similarly aged but separated into subgroups depending on whether they were HIV-negative, HIV-positive (but asymptomatic), or HIV-positive and actively experiencing AIDS symptoms. This study allowed for researchers to examine differences based on relative life expectancy, rather than on age. Researchers found the effect of temporal scarcity to be consistent in this study as well, as those who were HIV-positive and symptomatic prioritized social partners according to their affective value. The results of this study demonstrated how scarcity of time, rather than age, can be a powerful influence on the ways we choose to navigate our social world. In this scarcity mindset, time is precious, and it should not be wasted.

Scarcity in Phases of Life

The scarcity mindset need not apply to the ending of life as a whole; research suggests that it also applies to cherished *phases* of life. Consider the following passage from Sylvia Plath's diary (2000). She had been spending the summer with a family in a beach town. One day, as the end of summer was drawing near, she glanced at the calendar, and was struck by how quickly the time had passed her by:

> And so I leave the two streetlights at the end of Beach Bluff Avenue which shone in crosses of light through my door every night. And the crickets chirping on the wind. And the blue of Preston Beach water. Good-bye Castle Rock . . . and my quaint, crooked streets of Marblehead, with hollyhocks springing tall from the narrow dooryards. . . . I want to stay awake for the next three days and nights, drawing the threads of my summer cocoon neatly around me, to savor until dying of the last wave, the last dawn, this place, the leaving of which means leaving a great space of living. (pp. 178–179)

The passage highlights the cognitive and motivational components of this sort of mindset. Suddenly aware of time's scarcity, Plath was attending to her surroundings anew, expressing appreciation for pleasant subtleties that are very prone to hedonic adaptation. The crickets, the flowers, and the quaint, crooked streets suddenly shifted from the background to the forefront of her attention. She was deriving pleasure from these things in the same way she may have done when first arriving in the town. Moreover, she was motivated to make the most of the short amount of time she had left in Marblehead. She didn't want to squander any more time, but rather, she wanted to stay awake and make the most of every minute that remained. This demonstrates that, as we near the end of life's experiences, we are afforded the necessary clarity to savor them the best we can before time runs out.

To test this notion empirically, Kurtz (2008) recruited senior students (who were sad to be graduating) about 6 weeks before college graduation and asked them to write about their college experience. Some were reminded of the fact that graduation was very soon, while others were reminded that it was still somewhat far off. After 2 weeks of practicing these different mindsets, those asked to think that graduation was soon were significantly happier than they were at the start of the study. They were also more appreciative and more motivated to make the most of their remaining time. While counterintuitive, this suggests that thinking about the ending of a cherished life experience can motivate one to fully enjoy it while it lasts. The endings of positive life experiences are often still bittersweet or sad experiences (Ersner-Hershfield et al., 2008). However, if one were to spend their final time in these phases denying their approaching endings, they may be disappointed and regretful when the ending inevitably arrives. Alternatively, becoming presently aware of the limited time one has left in a phase of life can help them make the most of that time and amplify their overall experience. While the end result may not differ—the ending is still inevitable—awareness of time's scarcity impacts motivation and appreciation during these final windows of time.

While most of the research on scarcity and positive outcomes has examined it on an individual level, scarcity also has the potential to impact interpersonal relationships. Previous research suggests that people view spending quality time with their significant others as a vital strategy for relationship maintenance (Dindia & Baxter, 1987). This may be easily achievable for couples who live in close proximity, but opportunities for quality time in romantic relationships are significantly more limited for those whose partners do not live close to them. As a result, long-distance romantic relationships are characterized by a prevalent and often powerful sense of scarcity. One series of studies (Garcia-Rada & Kim, 2021) examined how time's scarcity—and couples' desiring more time together than they have—impacts long-distance relationships. In these relationships, couples tended to prioritize extraordinary shared experiences, particularly when maintaining the relationship was a strong goal. One reason for this is the desire to remain memorable to one another over time and distance—and extraordinary experiences foster this. But another motivator might be the simple fact that time spent together (in person) can be innately scarce for long-distance couples. Time is a precious resource and shouldn't be squandered on mundane activities.

Of course, time spent with a long-distance romantic partner and events like graduation day are fraught with immediate scarcity. In these instances, the endings are both imminent and rapidly approaching, which can create a natural and salient sense of temporal scarcity. But what about endings that are further out in time? After all, time is always running out—whether we are consciously aware of it or not. How temporally near must an ending be for a scarcity mindset to be possible? In other words, is it sufficiently powerful to know that college will end in a year? Two years? Someday? Or must the ending be closer in time in order to trigger savoring?

Curious as to whether savoring could be enhanced well in advance of an ending, a group of college freshmen and sophomores—who still had about 2–3 years left in college—were asked to imagine moving away from their college town in 30 days, to see if this would be enough to create a sense of scarcity and encourage savoring (Layous et al., 2017). Compared to a neutral control group who simply kept track of their daily activities, those living the month like it was their last showed a significant increase in happiness. Interestingly, this effect was driven by fulfillment of the core psychological needs—autonomy, competence, and interpersonal relatedness—that are related to well-being (Deci & Ryan, 2000). The students in the scarcity condition seemed to use their time in a more emotionally rewarding manner, prioritizing valued people and inherently meaningful activities. As one student in the scarcity condition said in her daily report,

> During this week I enjoyed the beautiful campus I live on by doing many different things. I walked around campus to classes instead of taking the bus. I sat on the quad and enjoyed the scenery. I also visited Skyline Drive off campus with my boyfriend to stargaze. . . . Focusing on others gives me a sense of purpose. I worked on homework and studied a lot. . . . I was productive but didn't spend too much time doing work without spending time with friends.

Perhaps the student felt like an active agent in her daily decision making, as time's scarcity helped clarify her priorities. She was choosing activities she felt skilled at and was also allowing herself to socialize with meaningful others. This study suggests that just imagining time running out may motivate people to mindfully attend, value, and savor. As explored below, the ability to induce a sense of temporal scarcity could have significant implications on our ability to design effective interventions to encourage savoring and happiness.

Vacations are another natural example of positive experiences that are characterized by time's scarcity. In one field study, visitors to popular tourist destinations, such as Chicago and London, were asked to indicate which attractions they had visited during their brief stay (Shu & Gneezy, 2010). (Imagine things like the Field Museum of Natural History and the Willis Tower in Chicago, and Westminster Abbey and the Tower Bridge in London.) A sample of residents of the same cities was also recruited and asked to complete the same task. Findings revealed that the tourists had visited a significantly larger number of popular attractions than the residents had, despite having had much less time to do so. (And it's not as if the residents of these cities were dispositionally less ambitious than the tourists—they reported visiting popular tourist attractions in other cities, just not in their own.) The brief timeline of travel comes with a sense of now-or-never. If one were to miss an attraction on a short trip, they may never have another opportunity to see it. Permanent residents do not feel the same pressure. Also, over time, they may have emotionally adapted toward these otherwise prominent fixtures (Lyubomirsky, 2011; Wilson & Gilbert, 2008). As a result, the residents may never seize opportunities to visit these attractions, despite their relative availability. Once again, time's scarcity is motivating. While we're unsure if the tourists actually savored the attractions they visited, they certainly set the stage for savoring by putting themselves in what many would consider a unique and pleasant experience.

Maximizing the Hedonic Value of Endings

Despite the emotional rewards associated with practicing savoring, it can still be difficult to reckon with the endings of positive life experiences once they arrive. A specific type of motivation that emerges in these moments is the desire to "end on a high note." The same way that television shows use their series finales to create satisfying endings to their stories, people want their final experiences within cherished life experiences to be memorable, or at least meaningful. Rituals such as graduation ceremonies and farewell dinners tap into this motivation. While this may be seen as an attempt to take advantage of remaining time, there are demonstrable benefits to this practice. The peak-end rule suggests that people are more likely to retroactively evaluate their experiences in a more positive light when they end in a positive manner (Fredrickson & Kahneman, 1993; Kahneman et al., 1993).

With this principle in mind, there are several ways a person can design an ending to maximize enjoyment. One way might be to focus on novelty—making farewell dinner reservations at a new and different hotspot. But another strategy would prioritize familiarity—going back to an old favorite. Even if it lacks excitement, it provides comfort and meaning. A recent series of studies (Winet & O'Brien, 2023) found that familiarity tends to win out in these moments, often because the familiar is more emotionally relevant. In explaining this effect, researchers referred to socioemotional selectivity theory: People tend to gravitate toward goals with greater emotional rewards attached as time becomes more limited (Carstensen et al., 1999). While novelty is exciting, it lacks the meaning and emotion often already associated with familiarity. As time begins to dwindle for people, it becomes preferable to capitalize on interactions with people, places, and things that they have already formed a meaningful connection with, because they now perceivably lack the time required to build new ones.

Interventions to Encourage Savoring via Scarcity

Drawing directly from previous research, we suggest that practicing a mindset of scarcity would encourage savoring and other positive outcomes. Surely, there are times when this mindset occurs spontaneously. For instance, college graduation day is naturally marked by an intense feeling of poignancy, a mixed affective state that has been shown to promote savoring behavior (Ersner-Hershfield et al., 2008). Across longer periods of time, previous research has also demonstrated that a general sense of uncertainty about the future can also motivate people to savor the present (Gregory et al., 2023).

Knowing we have the ability to induce a sense of scarcity rather than relying on an actual impending ending to promote savoring (Layous et al., 2017), it could be beneficial to acknowledge one's time as scarce across a variety of contexts and levels. Previously mentioned research offers the promising message that timelines are malleable, and this mindset of scarcity can be cultivated even in advance of an ending (Etkin et al., 2015; Kurtz, 2008; Layous et al., 2017). One practical suggestion, then, is to simply imagine that time in a cherished life experience is scarce. In doing so, people may feel an urgency to savor these life experiences, rather than taking them for granted.

Achieving this mindset requires a shift in one's perspective to better appreciate the full spectrum of possible experiences. In doing so, one can potentially learn to savor experiences across both ordinary and extraordinary contexts. Counterintuitively, this also means embracing negative life experiences. While experiencing adversity can have detrimental effects on well-being, experiencing negative events can help widen the range of experience one can draw from when evaluating their life (Croft et al., 2014). For example, if somebody were to only experience neutral or positive life experiences, their baseline evaluation of life would likely fall fairly close to their evaluation of positive experiences due to lack of alternative experiences for comparison. In this instance, their judgment would likely be clouded by a form of perceived abundance (Quoidbach et al., 2015a). After all, while many people often strive for positive or extraordinary life experiences, research suggests that a critical component of their value lies in their scarcity (Cialdini, 1993). Conversely, if one experiences a considerable range of positive and negative life events, it would likely be far easier for them to appreciate the more extraordinary experiences due to simple contrast. We are not suggesting that people actively seek out monotony or discomfort to help facilitate savoring. However, by mindfully considering their comprehensive life experience, they could experience greater capacity for savoring life's more ordinary pleasures (Bryant & Smith, 2015). This idea is well-encapsulated in the work of Viktor Frankl (1962), who wrote, "If there is a meaning in life at all, then there must be a meaning in suffering. Suffering is an ineradicable part of life, even as fate and death. Without suffering and death human life cannot be complete." In short, then, focusing on previous experiences of scarcity and struggle—while perhaps not enjoyable in the moment—may encourage savoring through sheer contrast. Similarly, thinking about time as short, even when an ending is not imminent, may help foster savoring as well.

Another promising intervention requires "mentally subtracting" a close other from one's life—essentially, imagining how life might have unfolded without this key person. To test the role of mental subtraction on positive outcomes, Koo and colleagues (2008) recruited a sample of married participants. Some were asked to imagine their life without their spouse; specifically, how they might not have met their spouse and what their present lives might be like without this person. Compared to a control group, these participants reported more happiness and more satisfaction with their marriages. Importantly, this finding was counter to what the participants had expected: They predicted that this mental subtraction would make them sad. Note that this study focused not on the imagined scarcity of time, but on the imagined scarcity (or absence) of a valuable person. However, we believe the underlying mechanism, whereby scarcity ascribes value, is similar.

Possible Mechanisms

Existing research suggests that the manner in which people behave is motivated, in part, by the perceived time they have to engage in particular experiences. This falls in line with previous research which has demonstrated how perceived scarcity can increase the value of resources (Cialdini, 1993). But what drives this effect? The available literature points toward several possible mechanisms. Understanding these can help explain the impact of scarcity on the capacity for savoring and recognition of savoring opportunities.

Motivation

Previous studies have established that people tend to respond with greater urgency (a "now or never" mentality) when faced with immediate endings rather than ones that are far off in time (Kurtz, 2008; Shu & Gneezy, 2010). This mentality is further demonstrated in a study examining people's preference of experience depending on the availability of time (Winet & O'Brien, 2023). Presented with choices between novel and familiar experiences, people tended to have a greater affinity for familiar experiences when time is limited. While people do actively seek out novelty, it can be easy to take familiar experiences for granted when they are perceived as readily available. Thus, it makes intuitive sense that when faced with the perceived ending of these experiences' availability, the veil becomes lifted and people experience clarity in their preferences and priorities.

Need Fulfillment

Another theory that attempts to explain the effect of scarcity on savoring can be found in a previously mentioned study, where college freshman and sophomores were asked to imagine having only 30 days left in their college town (Layous et al., 2017). These students reported an increase in subjective well-being compared to the control condition. Furthermore, they found that this effect was likely mediated by the satisfaction of core psychological needs (autonomy, competence, and connectedness; Deci & Ryan, 2000). While savoring may promote greater well-being in its own right, helping people feel as if they are in control of their lives, working effectively, and deriving meaning from their social relationships could certainly mediate this effect.

Meaning

Increased savoring behavior in the face of the upcoming end of one's time with cherished people, places, and experiences could also be attributed to the meaningfulness of endings. While endings can produce a variety of thoughts and emotions depending on individual differences, existing research posits that endings can produce a powerful sense of meaning in and of themselves. In the previously mentioned study on positivity bias for ending experiences, O'Brien and Ellsworth (2012) posed an interesting theory to explain the observed effect of salient temporal scarcity on savoring. They noted that "people might judge everyday 'last' events more positively because they generally signal an 'end' to the experience" (p. 2). While ending experiences can certainly be powerful or meaningful in their own right (e.g., graduation), the endings produced for the purpose of their study were rather insignificant on a personal level. They technically received their "last" piece of chocolate from the researchers, but what is to stop any of the participants from going to buy more chocolate after they leave the lab? Therefore, the overall significance of the results supports the idea that actively conceptualizing an upcoming loss motivates savoring behavior toward a perceived ending. It follows that a possible mechanism for the effect of scarcity on savoring could be the meaning often associated with the endings of life experiences.

Attention to the Positive

Another proposed mechanism for the effect of scarcity on savoring pertains to the relationship between affect and information processing (Ersner-Hershfield et al., 2008). In a study examining poignancy, an emotional state characterized by mixed feelings of happiness and sadness in the face of impending endings, researchers found that feeling poignancy can lead to an increased focus on positive stimuli, as opposed to negative stimuli. Participants were sorted into either the control condition or the experimental condition, where a sense of poignancy was induced, and then asked to view 30 emotionally charged images. Eye-tracking technology was used to analyze the participants' vision patterns to determine if there were differences in attentional tendencies between the groups. The study found that those in the experimental condition tended to focus more on positive images compared to negative ones, despite reporting a mixture of positive and negative emotions.

Based on previous research demonstrating how one's motivation often coincides with their visual patterns (Light & Isaacowitz, 2006), the researchers suggested that poignancy motivates a positive effect on information processing as a means of maximizing positive affective experiences. Given what we know about scarcity and how people respond to the approach of endings, this study suggests that people's capacity for savoring may be driven by a form of positivity bias. Poignancy is a bittersweet emotion often associated with endings, and the positive effect that it inspires could explain the increase of savoring activity in the face of temporal scarcity. People's attention becomes shifted from a neutral observation of their surroundings to being positively focused. This study suggests this could be an attempt to upregulate positive affect, which would fall in line with our previously established definition of savoring behavior. Therefore, it is quite possible that the focus of our attention could be a viable mechanism for the impact of scarcity on savoring.

FUTURE DIRECTIONS

In order to better understand the influence of scarcity on time perception, it is important to consider the wide range of contexts in which we experience scarcity. On a small scale, we might organize time into hours remaining in the day or the number of days remaining before a deadline. However, on a larger scale, we may think of time with regard to different multiyear chapters of our lives or even our entire lifespan. The various levels on which we perceive time could have significant implications for the influence of scarcity on behavior. For example, if somebody were unable to find time to practice a cherished hobby on a given day, they would most likely not shift their schedules to accommodate that activity—and why would they? They always have tomorrow to try again. However, if that same person were to be told they would permanently lose the ability to practice that hobby after 1 week, it stands to reason that their priorities would likely shift in order to better savor their remaining time with the activity. These varying reactions to different perceptions of temporal scarcity lend themselves to the idea that scarcity and its influence can be experienced in vastly different ways depending on context. While this theoretical scenario and explanation are intuitive, we know of little research that explores these nuances. Therefore, it is crucial to examine these differences across both small and large-scale periods of time.

Both small and large-scale sources of temporal scarcity impact our ability to savor across various contexts. One key difference between the two forms of scarcity lies in the balance between their salience and perceived permanence. Lower-level, daily scarcity is very salient, as it only requires you to consider the hours of a given day and how they can be spent. However, this time is often viewed as more inconsequential given the notion that time will "restart" the following day. Previous research supports this idea, as a series of studies on procrastination suggested that the tendency for people to put off unenjoyable tasks or activities extends to partaking in positive experiences as well (Shu & Gneezy, 2010). Their explanation for this phenomenon is that people falsely predict that they will have more time to participate in these experiences in the future and could end up missing out on them entirely as a result.

On the other hand, higher-level existential sources of scarcity often produce a powerful sense of permanence and irreversibility but can be difficult to actively focus on prior to their endings due to the overall experiences spanning much greater ranges of time. When people no longer have the ability to assume they will have more time down the line, it becomes much easier to recognize scarcity. Therefore, the challenge then becomes recognizing scarcity earlier and actively considering it when prioritizing goal-oriented behavior. Ultimately, the differences in how one considers time appear to coincide with differences in how scarcity can motivate savoring behavior.

Much of the savoring literature examines the process as it relates to more existential sources of temporal scarcity. Events like graduations, marriages, and funerals serve as the culmination and ending of larger-scale life processes like progressing through the education system, building a lifelong partnership, or even life itself. There is an element of permanence to these experiences and their endings; once the chapter is over, there is a perceivably irreversible transition from one state of being to another. For example, after someone graduates, they will conceivably never return to the same level of education as a student. However, while the effect that these experiences and transitions can have on our overall lives is immense, it is not wholly immediate. The experiences we have during these chapters of life are often spread out across long periods of time, and the changes we experience as a result occur gradually rather than all at once. Because of this, it can be difficult to notice change or perceive time as scarce depending on one's perspective.

Smaller-scale sources of scarcity tend to be more salient but lack the element of permanence ascribed to large-scale sources. On a daily level, one might experience temporal scarcity in feeling as if they lacked the proper time to complete a work task. However, the chances are likely that they would be able to finish it the next day, which may lessen the associated urgency.

While there is a substantial amount of information regarding savoring and how it is influenced by our perceptions of time, there are still many other complex questions that remain unanswered. Thinking about time's scarcity, particularly when it comes to valued people and life experiences, is not a mindset many people are pulled toward (it might be actively avoided!). Yet, this practice brings a surprising number of benefits. The extent to which people are willing to embrace a mindset of temporal scarcity, especially when thinking of cherished people, places, and experiences, is an interesting avenue for future research.

Also, what follows the ending? Could the ending of a positive experience create an unfortunate comparison with what is to follow, such as a restful vacation followed by a return to a high-stress workplace? It's easy to see how thinking about the ending of a cherished life experience might be a source of stress or worry (imagine a college student who has no clear plans following graduation). At what point does scarcity trigger genuine sadness or anxiety, rather than savoring?

Another interesting question relates to the nature of the ending. The research reviewed here focuses on positive life events with impending endings: college graduations, vacations, long-distance relationships, and so forth. But how does an impending ending affect hedonically neutral or even negative life events? Does the ending highlight the events' upsides? Or might the fact that they are soon ending make them even more intolerable, as it becomes more apparent that a brighter future lies just ahead?

An important avenue for future research regards differences in the experience and ability to savor among those with neurological or developmental disorders. For example, for those who struggle with executive dysfunction due to a condition like attention-deficit/hyperactivity disorder, time perception and attentional regulation may be experienced in vastly different ways. This could impact the ability to induce a state of salient scarcity, as well as whether the scarcity can produce the same positive effects on savoring and well-being. Those suffering from significant mental health disorders (e.g., depression, anxiety) could experience similar differences in these effects. These disorders can often contribute to a skewed perspective of reality due to the cognitive distortions they can incite or intensify. This could lead to an increased focus on a positive experience's ending having a potentially adverse effect rather than promoting savoring. While neurotypical individuals may be able to make the most of remaining time, those who are neurodivergent may find that perceived scarcity under these circumstances could serve as a deterrent to savoring.

Additionally, the effect of scarcity could also be impacted when several endings are impending at once. Rather than somebody feeling greater motivation to make the most of a particular experience or relationship, they may choose one or the other and feel disappointment in not being able to fully embrace both or all of them before they are gone. Previous studies indicate that perceived scarcity can provide clarity in the prioritization of goals (Layous et al., 2017), but what happens when decisions need to be made about prioritizing one positive experience or another? One study examined the impact of conflicting goals on people's well-being and how their perception of goal conflict appears to be related to their perceptions of time (Etkin et al., 2015). This research demonstrated a unique link between goal conflict and time perception, in that greater perceived conflict between goals leads to heightened stress and anxiety as well as a greater sense of temporal scarcity. This notion is a significant one, as the effect was found to be consistent across conflicts between goals competing for each other's time as well as goals that do not compete for time or other resources (e.g., money, health). Because of this, the impact cannot be explained away by increased time demands or the influence of scarcity on resource valuation on its own. People experience heightened time pressure, stress, and anxiety when experiencing goal conflicts—whether they are influenced by the available time to complete them or not.

Finally, to better assess the rich, complicated nature of how people experience endings—and mixed emotions in general—we would encourage future researchers to go beyond standard survey methodology. Qualitative or interview data would add important nuance to our understanding of these sorts of experiences. Imagine a person on the last day of a cherished vacation, or while spending time with a long-distance romantic partner. Survey data may indicate feelings of sadness as time is inevitably running out, but people might also experience happiness, as time's scarcity forces them to be fully present and grateful (Larsen et al., 2001). Do these emotions interact in an additive way, creating a sort of "upward spiral"? What other important elements are missing when looking only at numerical data? And how does the experience change as time is winding down?

BIG PICTURE

As life is filled with distractions and rigid social expectations for how one should be spending their time or working toward their ideal futures, it can be incredibly difficult to take in the present moment. The process of savoring is vital to our enjoyment of both ordinary and extraordinary moments and chapters, and to our overall well-being. Our experiences with savoring grow and evolve over the course of our lives as we gain age and experience—and more importantly, as our remaining time declines. The temporal scarcity we experience on a daily basis and over the course of our lives can bring about a myriad of different emotions but ultimately serves to help us enjoy the time that we have left.

In a world that has seemingly become disillusioned with the process of finding contentment with daily life while feeling the mounting weight of time pressure and loneliness (Gallup, 2023), one might argue the notion of increased temporal scarcity potentially serving as a tool to combat these pressures downplays or ignores reality. However, the ideas presented in this chapter outline the importance of pushing back against the feeling of helplessness that often accompanies endings. Rather than focusing on the imminent loss, people can find clarity of perspective and ideally sit for an extra second within life's small, simple pleasures. Rather than spending every waking moment searching for a path forward to the idealized lives we long for, we can better appreciate our actual lives and recognize the full magnitude of their significance.

In James Taylor's "Secret O' Life" (1977), he wrote that "the secret of life is enjoying the passage of time." While this may seem reductive to the greater components that influence the perceived quality of one's life, it rings true with the research presented in this chapter. To live meaningfully is to savor each moment—to grow throughout the process of one's lifespan and meet change with open arms, rather than with fear or regret. It is to live knowing perfection is unattainable, to learn from mistakes and not choose a lack of experience over the possibility of failure. Most importantly, it is to recognize the impermanence of life's moments and chapters, as well as the fleeting nature of life itself. By doing so actively, we begin to see life not as a series of chores and obligations en route to what we see as ideal, but to recognize just how lucky we are to be here at all. We only get to do this once; so we might as well find a way to enjoy it as best we can.

REFERENCES

Brown, K. W., & Ryan, R. M. (2003). The benefits of being present: Mindfulness and its role in psychological well-being. *Journal of Personality and Social Psychology, 84*(4), 822–848.

Bryant, F. B. (1989). A four-factor model of perceived control: Avoiding, coping, obtaining, and savoring. *Journal of Personality, 57,* 773–797.

Bryant, F. B. (2003). Savoring Beliefs Inventory (SBI): A scale for measuring beliefs about savouring. *Journal of Mental Health, 12,* 175–196.

Bryant, F. B., Chadwick, E. D., & Kluwe, K. (2011). Understanding the processes that regulate positive emotional experience: Unsolved problems and future directions for theory and research on savoring. *International Journal of Wellbeing, 1,* 107–126.

Bryant, F. B., & Smith, J. L. (2015). Appreciating life in the midst of adversity: Savoring in relation to mindfulness, reappraisal, and meaning. *Psychological Inquiry, 26*(4), 315–321.

Bryant, F. B., & Veroff, J. (2007). *Savoring: A new model of positive experience.* Erlbaum.

Carstensen, L. L., & Fredrickson, B. L. (1998). Influence of HIV status and age on cognitive representations of others. *Health Psychology, 17*(6), 494–503.

Carstensen, L. L., Isaacowitz, D. M., & Charles, S. T. (1999). Taking time seriously: A theory of socioemotional selectivity. *American Psychologist, 54*(3), 165–181.

Cialdini, R. B. (1993). *Influence: Science and practice.* HarperCollins.

Croft, A., Dunn, E. W., & Quoidbach, J. (2014). From tribulations to appreciation: Experiencing adversity in the past predicts greater savoring in the present. *Social Psychological and Personality Science, 5,* 511–516.

de la Rochefoucauld, F. (1930). *Moral maxims and reflections.* M. Gillyflower & J. Everingham. (Original work published 1694)

Deci, E. L., & Ryan, R. M. (2000). The "what" and "why" of goal pursuits: Human needs and the self-determination of behavior. *Psychological Inquiry, 11,* 227–268.

Dindia, K., & Baxter, L. A. (1987). Strategies for maintaining and repairing marital relationships. *Journal of Social and Personal Relationships, 4*(2), 143–158.

Emmons, R. A., & McCullough, M. E. (2003). Counting blessings versus burdens: An experimental investigation of gratitude and subjective well-being in daily life. *Journal of Personality and Social Psychology, 84,* 377–389.

Ersner-Hershfield, H., Mikels, J. A., Sullivan, S. J., & Carstensen, L. L. (2008). Poignancy: Mixed emotional experience in the face of meaningful endings. *Journal of Personality and Social Psychology, 94*(1), 158–167.

Etkin, J., Evangelidis, I., & Aaker, J. (2015). Pressed for time?: Goal conflict shapes how time is perceived, spent, and valued. *Journal of Marketing Research, 52*(3), 394–406.

Frankl, V. E. (1962). *Man's search for meaning: An introduction to logotherapy.* Beacon Press.

Fredrickson, B. L., & Carstensen, L. L. (1990). Choosing social partners: How old age and anticipated endings make people more selective. *Psychology and Aging, 5*(3), 335–347.

Fredrickson, B. L., & Kahneman, D. (1993). Duration neglect in retrospective evaluations of affective episodes. *Journal of Personality and Social Psychology, 65*(1), 45–55.

Gallup. (2023). *The global state of social connections.* www.gallup.com/analytics/509675/state-of-social-connections.aspx.

Garcia-Rada, X., & Kim, T. (2021). Shared time scarcity and the pursuit of extraordinary experiences. *Psychological Science, 32*(12), 1871–1883.

Gregory, A., Quoidbach, J., Haase, C. M., & Piff, P. (2023). Be here now: Perceptions of uncertainty enhance savoring. *Emotion, 23,* 30–40.

Jaouad, S. (2021). *Between two kingdoms: A memoir of a life interrupted.* Random House.

Jose, P. E., Lim, B. T., & Bryant, F. B. (2012). Does savoring increase happiness?: A daily diary study. *Journal of Positive Psychology, 7,* 176–187.

Kahneman, D., Fredrickson, B. L., Schreiber, C. A., & Redelmeier, D. A. (1993). When more pain is preferred to less: Adding a better end. *Psychological Science, 4*(6), 401–405.

Koo, M., Algoe, S. B., Wilson, T. D. & Gilbert, D. T. (2008). It's a wonderful life: Mentally subtracting positive events improves people's affective states, contrary to their affective forecasts. *Journal of Personality and Social Psychology, 95,* 1217–1224.

Kurtz, J. L. (2008). Looking to the future to appreciate the present: The benefits of perceived temporal scarcity. *Psychological Science, 19,* 1238–1241.

Larsen, J. T., McGraw, A. P., & Cacioppo, J. T. (2001). Can people feel happy and sad at the same time? *Journal of Personality and Social Psychology, 81*(4), 684–696.

Layous, K., Kurtz, J. L., Chancellor, J., & Lyubomirsky, S. (2017). Reframing the ordinary: Imagining time as scarce increases well-being. *Journal of Positive Psychology, 13,* 301–308.

Light, J. C., & Isaacowitz, D. M. (2006). The effect of developmental regulation on visual attention: The example of the "biological clock." *Cognition and Emotion, 20*(5), 623–645.

Lyubomirsky, S. (2011). Hedonic adaptation to positive and negative experiences. In S. Folkman (Ed.), *The Oxford handbook of stress, health, and coping* (pp. 200–224). Oxford University Press.

Lyubomirsky, S., & Layous, K. (2013). How do simple positive activities increase well-being? *Current Directions in Psychological Science, 22*(1), 57–62.

McCullough, M. E., Emmons, R. A., & Tsang, J. (2002). The grateful disposition: A conceptual and empirical topography. *Journal of Personality and Social Psychology, 82,* 112–127.

Mogilner, C. (2010). The pursuit of happiness: Time, money, and social connection. *Psychological Science, 21* (9), 1348–1354.

O'Brien, E., & Ellsworth, P. C. (2012). Saving the last for best: A positivity bias for end experiences. *Psychological science, 23*(2), 163–165.

Plath, S. (2000). *The unabridged journals of Sylvia Plath.* Anchor.

Quoidbach, J., & Dunn, E. W. (2013). Give it up: A strategy for combatting hedonic adaptation. *Social Psychological and Personality Science, 4,* 563–568.

Quoidbach, J. Dunn, E. W., Hansenne, M. & Bustin, G. (2015a). The price of abundance: How a wealth of experiences impoverishes savoring. *Personality and Social Psychology Bulletin, 41,* 393–404.

Quoidbach, J., Dunn, E. W., Petrides, K. V., & Mikolajczak, M. (2010). Money giveth, money taketh away: The dual effect of wealth on happiness. *Psychological Science, 21,* 759–763.

Quoidbach, J., Mikolajczak, M. & Gross, J. J. (2015b). Positive interventions: An emotion regulation perspective. *Psychological Bulletin, 141,* 655–693.

Shu, S. B., & Gneezy, A. (2010). Procrastination of enjoyable experiences. *Journal of Marketing Research, 47*(5), 933–944.

Taylor, J. (1977). Secret o' life [Recorded by James Taylor]. On *JT.* Columbia Records.

Toepfer, S. M., & Walker, K. (2009). Letters of gratitude: Improving well-being through expressive writing. *Journal of Writing Research, 1,* 181–198.

Wilson, T. D., & Gilbert, D. T. (2008). Explaining away: A model of affective adaptation. *Perspectives on Psychological Science, 3*(5), 370–386.

Winet, Y. K., & O'Brien, E. (2023). Ending on a familiar note: Perceived endings motivate repeat consumption. *Journal of Personality and Social Psychology, 124*(4), 707–734.

CHAPTER 14

Nostalgia

The Existential Value of Temporal Longing

Constantine Sedikides *and* Tim Wildschut

Nostalgia has ontological overtones. The emotion confers meaning in life and aids in existential coping. In this chapter we review literature showcasing nostalgia as an existential emotion.

DEFINITIONAL ISSUES

Nostalgia is "a sentimental longing or wistful affection for the past" (*New Oxford Dictionary of English*, 1998, p. 1266) or "an affectionate feeling you have for the past, especially for a particularly happy time" (*Collins English Dictionary*, 2023). Prototype analyses concur with dictionary definitions. A prototype is laypersons' comprehension of a construct "consisting of the most common features or properties of members of that category" (Horowitz et al., 1982, p. 183). The features can be central or peripheral to the construct. The former are more representative of the construct's essence than the latter (Rosch, 1975). Central features of nostalgia include "the past," "fond memories," "rose-tinted memory," "reliving," "feeling," "personal meaning," "childhood/youth," "social relationships," "memorabilia/keepsakes," "happiness," "missing," "longing/yearning," and "return to the past" (Hepper et al., 2012). Nostalgia, then, is an emotion that refers to a personally important and somewhat idealized past, often centered on one's childhood, close others, or momentous events (e.g., birthdays, weddings, graduations) involving the self as the protagonist or hero (Allison & Green, 2020; Wildschut et al., 2006). The emotion entails temporal retracing, fond reminiscing, tenderness, and joy, but also yearning for the irredeemably gone moments and a draw to return to them (Evans et al., 2021; Sedikides et al., 2015). Nostalgia is self-relevant, social, and ambivalent but mostly positive (Leunissen et al., 2021; Sedikides & Wildschut, 2019). It is experienced frequently (e.g., several times a week; Hepper et al., 2021; Wildschut et al., 2006), and across cultures (Hepper et al., 2014; Sedikides & Wildschut, 2022) or age groups (Hepper et al., 2021; Turner & Stanley, 2021).

Meaning in life is the subjective perception that one's existence has coherence (i.e., is consistent), purpose (i.e., is goal-oriented), and significance (i.e., matters; Igou et al., Chapter 48, this volume; King et al., 2016). Recent findings have accentuated the role of significance (Costin & Vignoles, 2020). Nevertheless, we focus here mostly on meaning in life as an inclusive construct. Only occasionally do we consider search for meaning in life, a quest likely to be instantiated when one endures meaning deficits (Steger et al., 2008).

Existential coping refers to ways in which individuals combat ontological threat, such as life meaninglessness or awareness of one's impermanence. It refers to struggles to regain meaning or pacify concerns about the inevitability of death (Galen, Chapter 55, this volume; Greenberg et al., 2004).

ON THE MEANINGFULNESS OF NOSTALGIA

Nostalgic reverie pertains to a personally important and meaningful past. Indeed, nostalgizing and meaningfulness have been typical motifs in novels and memoir (Batcho, 2023). More to the point, nostalgia is positively associated with meaning.

Evidence for this assertion comes from several studies. In Batcho and colleagues (2008), participants completed the Nostalgia Inventory (Batcho, 1995; e.g., "I miss . . .": "my family," "vacations I went on," "TV shows, movies") and reported how meaningful four sets of lyrics were to them. Nostalgia was positively related to lyric meaningfulness. In Routledge and colleagues (2011, Study 1), participants listened to popular songs and indicated whether they felt nostalgic and their lives were worth living. The more nostalgic they felt, the more meaningful they perceived their lives to be. In Routledge and colleagues, participants completed a nostalgia scale, the Southampton Nostalgia Scale (Sedikides et al., 2015; e.g., "How prone are you to feeling nostalgic?"; "How often do you experience nostalgia?"; "How important is it for you to bring to mind nostalgic experiences?") and two meaning scales, the Presence of Meaning in Life subscale of the Meaning in Life Questionnaire (Steger et al., 2006; "I understand my life's meaning") and the Purpose in Life Scale (McGregor & Little, 1998; e.g., "My personal existence is purposeful and meaningful"). Nostalgia was positively associated with meaning. The positive association between nostalgia and meaning has been found in additional studies using varying measures of the two constructs (Karagoz & Ramkissoon, 2023; Newman et al., 2020; Wu et al., 2020).

Nostalgia is linked to meaning in work settings as well (Leunissen et al., 2018, Study 1). Employees reported the level of nostalgia they felt for their organization in the prior month and the extent to which they found their work meaningful (Positive Meaning subscale of the Work and Meaning Inventory; Steger et al., 2012; e.g., "I have found a meaningful career"). Nostalgia for their organization was positively related to deriving meaning from their work.

ON THE PURVEYANCE OF MEANING IN LIFE: NOSTALGIA AS A MOTIVATIONAL FORCE

Nostalgia has the capacity to promote meaning in life. This principle relies on nostalgia's motivational potency (Sedikides & Wildschut, 2023). Indeed, nostalgia is construed as an approach-oriented emotion (Van Tilburg et al., 2018). Moreover, nostalgia incites an approach orientation (e.g., "I go out of my way to get things I want," "I will often do things for no other reason than that they might be fun;" Stephan et al., 2014). As sociologist Fred Davis (1979, p. 420) asserted:

> It [nostalgia] reassures us of past happiness and accomplishment; and, since these still remain on deposit, as it were, in the bank of our memory, it simultaneously bestows upon us a certain worth, irrespective of how present circumstances may seem to question or obscure this. And current worth, as our friendly bank loan officer assures us, is titled to at least some claim on the future as well.

Below we review literature showing that nostalgia builds meaning and has notable downstream consequences.

Nostalgia Fosters Meaning

Nostalgia is induced with a variety of techniques (Wildschut & Sedikides, 2024). The most common one is the Event Reflection Task (ERT; Sedikides et al., 2015; Wildschut et al., 2006), a vivid autobiographical writing exercise. Typically, in the experimental condition, participants read a definition of nostalgia (e.g., "a sentimental longing for one's past"), ponder an event in their lives that makes them feel nostalgic, immerse themselves in the experience, list keywords capturing the gist of it, and describe in writing the experience and how it makes them feel. In the control condition, participants follow the same protocol, but for an ordinary event in their lives. Finally, participants complete a manipulation check assessing level of felt nostalgia.

Nostalgia, induced by the ERT, increases meaning (Leunissen et al., 2018; Sedikides et al., 2018; Van Tilburg et al., 2019), measured with the meaning subscale of the Nostalgia Functions Scale (e.g., "life is meaningful," "life has a purpose"; Hepper et al., 2012). It does so even when the ERT involves a more stringent control condition, namely, a desired future event. Bringing to mind a desired future event (e.g., graduating, finding a good job, forming a close relationship) would likely infuse life with meaning (Feldman, 2013). Yet participants who reflect on a nostalgic event report higher meaning (measured with the Presence of Meaning in Life subscale of the Meaning in Life Questionnaire; Steger et al., 2006) than those who reflect on a desired future event (Routledge et al., 2012, Experiment 1). Moreover, nostalgia enhances meaning, not only among healthy adults, but also among vulnerable groups, such as Syrian refugees residing in Saudi Arabia (Wildschut et al., 2019) and dementia patients (Ismail et al., 2018). Nostalgia confers meaning regardless of participants' level of neuroticism (Frankenbach et al., 2021) or resilience (Wildschut et al., 2019), and can do so vicariously (i.e., by reading another person's nostalgic remembrances; Wildschut et al., 2018), and across cultures (Hepper et al., 2023).

Nostalgia fosters meaning when manipulated by asking participants to relay personal experiences that correspond to central (as opposed to peripheral) features of the nostalgia prototype (Hepper et al., 2012, Study 7). In addition, it instils meaning when induced through nonnarrative techniques such as music (Routledge et al., 2011, Study 1), song lyrics (Routledge et al., 2011, Study 2), scents (Reid et al., 2015), and foods (Reid et al., 2023). Characteristically, nostalgia elevates meaning independently of positive affect (Sedikides & Wildschut, 2018) and of reflection (i.e., a genuine interest in one's attitudes, feelings, or self) or brooding (i.e., a repetitive and persistent focus on one's self, typically dwelling on the consequences of one's negative affective states; Jiang et al., 2021).

Like future desired events, positive past events can also be a source of meaning in life (King et al., 2006). We address this issue later in the chapter (Routledge et al., 2012, Experiment 3). Here, we are concerned with the possibility that reflecting on the nostalgic past differs from reflecting on the positive past in search for meaning. People instigate a quest for meaning when they are short on it (Steger et al., 2008). As such, if they find meaning in nostalgizing, then they will terminate their quest. Indeed, participants are more likely to cease their quest for meaning (Search for Meaning subscale of the Meaning in Life Questionnaire; Steger et al., 2006; e.g., "I am looking for something that makes my life feel meaningful"), when contemplating a nostalgic event instead of a positive past event (Routledge et al., 2012, Experiment 2).

How Does Nostalgia Foster Meaning?

Nostalgia nurtures meaning in life through assorted mechanisms. One of them is mental transportation, that is, mental time travel to the relevant event and reexperiencing it as if one were there (Wheeler et al., 1997). Evans and colleagues (2021) manipulated nostalgia (ERT), assessed mental transportation (Green & Brock, 2000; e.g., "I could picture myself in the scene of the events that I wrote about"), and measured meaning in life (meaning subscale of the Nostalgia Functions Scale; Hepper et al., 2012). Mental transportation mediated the effect of nostalgia on meaning. Reliving intensely a nostalgic event suffused it with meaningfulness (see also Waytz et al., 2015).

Another mechanism is ritual engagement. Rituals (e.g., decorating the Christmas tree, exchanging wedding rings) are noninstrumental and symbolic activities geared toward achieving a desired outcome. In a longitudinal study, Yin and colleagues (2025, Study 4) assessed nostalgia (Southampton Nostalgia Scale; Sedikides et al., 2015), intentions to engage or actually engaging in common ritualistic behaviors (e.g., pasting couplets) during a traditional Chinese festival, and meaning in life (meaning in life subscale of the Nostalgia Functions Scale; Hepper et al., 2012). Nostalgia predicted ritualistic intentions and behaviors, which in turn predicted greater meaning in life. Ritualistic engagement renders life more coherent, purposeful, and significant.

An additional mechanism through which nostalgia relays meaning is social connectedness, a sense of acceptance and belongingness (Sedikides & Wildschut, 2019). In nostalgizing, "the mind is 'peopled'" (Hertz, 1990, p. 195). The nostalgizer reinstates symbolic bonds with close others, who are brought to life and join the present (Davis, 1979). Indeed, the content of nostalgic recollections is replete with social themes (e.g., interactions with close others; Abeyta et al., 2015; Wildschut et al., 2006). Social themes are key sources of meaningfulness (Lambert et al., 2010; Stillman et al., 2009), as is social connectedness (Stavrova & Luhmann, 2016). Nostalgia, induced via music (Routledge et al., 2011, Study 1), strengthens social connectedness (i.e., "feeling loved"), which, in turn, is associated with higher meaning in life (i.e., "life is worth living"). This mediational pattern was replicated in an experiment (Routledge et al., 2011, Study 2) where nostalgia was induced with the ERT, social connectedness was assessed with the Social Provisions Scale (Cutrona & Russell, 1987) comprising such provisions as secure attachment (e.g., "I have close relationships that provide me with a sense of security and emotional well-being") and social integration (e.g., "I feel part of a group of people who share my attitudes and beliefs"), and meaning was assessed with the Presence of Meaning in Life subscale of the Meaning in Life Questionnaire (Steger et al., 2006).

Nostalgia also transmits meaning through self-continuity, a sense of connection between one's past and current self (Sedikides et al., 2016). Self-continuity involves synthesizing personally relevant experiences (e.g., Thanksgiving dinners, family vacations) across time (Sedikides et al., 2023). That is, people construct narratives that bind their changing self. This process facilitates making sense of life events, perceiving the self as part of the broader culture (McLean et al., 2007), and understanding the present self in the context of the past self. Self-continuity, then, likely contributes to perceptions of one's life as coherent or predictable, and purposeful or significant. Consistent with this possibility, self-continuity is positively associated with meaning in life (Vignoles et al., 2006). More relevant, nostalgia, induced with the ERT, elevates self-continuity (Sedikides et al., 2016; e.g., "I feel connected with who I was in the past"), which conduces to greater meaning in life (van Tilburg et al., 2019).

Finally, nostalgia conveys meaning through a sequence of mechanisms. These are social connectedness and self-continuity. Nostalgia-elicited social connectedness augments self-continuity. The momentous occasions that are the fodder of nostalgic reverie often weave the narrative thread of relational bonds. For instance, nostalgic recollections of a family Christmas may incite recollections of other Christmases, culminating in a mental storyboard of one's bonds with family members over time, thus engendering self-continuity (Sedikides et al., 2016). These occasions, though, are also rich in social themes (Wildschut et al., 2006), resulting in greater meaning. Van Tilburg and colleagues (2019) documented this sequence (nostalgia → social connectedness → self-continuity → meaning) in two experiments. In Experiment 1, participants first listened to a nostalgic and then a control (i.e., happy) song. Subsequently, they reported their social connectedness (extent to which each song made them feel "connected to close others" and "loved"), self-continuity (extent to which each song made them feel "connected to your past" and "there is continuity in your life") and meaning (extent to which each song made them feel that "life is meaningful" and "life has a purpose"). Nostalgia-elicited social connectedness predicted self-continuity, which in turn predicted meaning in life. This serial mediational pattern was replicated in Experiment 2 that included the same measures but a between-subjects design (i.e., participants listened either to a nostalgic or nonnostalgic song).

Downstream Consequences of Nostalgia-Elicited Meaning

Nostalgia-elicited meaning in life has downstream consequences. One consequence is motivational. Sedikides and colleagues (2018, Experiments 1–2) induced nostalgia using the ERT, assessed meaning in life with the meaning subscale of the Nostalgia

Functions Scale (Hepper et al., 2012), and then assessed motivation to pursue one's more important (vs. less important) goals with a modified version of Milyavskaya and colleagues' (2012) task (e.g., "I want to put more time and effort into pursuing this goal"). Nostalgia increased meaning in life, which galvanized intentions to pursue one's most important goals, whether agentic (e.g., improving academic performance) or communal (e.g., having more friends).

Another downstream consequence of nostalgia-elicited meaning is behavioral. It refers to turnover intentions, a proxy of turnover (the two variables are correlated at 0.50; Tett & Meyer, 1993). Turnover entails human resource investment losses in training or expertise (Ton & Huckman, 2008), diminished job satisfaction (Krackhardt & Porter, 1985), lower productivity (Argote et al., 1995) among remaining employees, and reductions in company profits (Ton & Huckman, 2008). Nostalgia is an antidote to turnover intentions. Leunissen and colleagues (2018, Study 2) induced organizational nostalgia with a modified version of the ERT. Participants in the nostalgia condition were instructed to "bring to mind a nostalgic event that you have experienced in your organization. Specifically, try to think of a past event you experienced in your organization that makes you feel most nostalgic," whereas those in the control condition were instructed to "bring to mind an ordinary event that you have experienced in your organization. Specifically, try to think of a past event you experienced in your organization that is ordinary" (p. 47). Next, participants completed the Positive Meaning subscale of the Work and Meaning Inventory (Steger et al., 2012) and a turnover intentions scale (Van Dick et al., 2004; e.g., "I am thinking of quitting this job"). Nostalgia elevated meaning in one's work. Subsequently, work meaningfulness attenuated participants' turnover intentions.

A final consequence of nostalgia-elicited meaning is spirituality. Biskas and colleagues (2022, Study 3) manipulated nostalgia with the ERT, assessed meaning with the meaning in life subscale of the Nostalgia Functions Scale (Hepper et al., 2012), and measured spirituality with the Intrinsic Spirituality Scale (Hodge, 2003; e.g., "my spirituality answers my questions," "that growing spiritually is important in my life"). Nostalgia contributed to great spirituality through increases in meaning.

Summary

Nostalgia, no matter how it is induced, nourishes meaning in life through several mechanisms. These are mental transportation, ritual engagement, and—sequentially—social connectedness and self-continuity. Also, an infusion of nostalgia terminates the search for meaning. Furthermore, nostalgia affords, via rises in meaning, several benefits: galvanizing the resolve to pursue one's important goals, weakening employees' intentions to quit their job, and enhancing spirituality.

ON EXISTENTIAL COPING: NOSTALGIA AS A HOMEOSTATIC CORRECTIVE

Nostalgia has the capacity to counteract life meaninglessness and mortality awareness. This principle is based on the regulatory model of nostalgia (Wildschut & Sedikides, 2023). The model postulates that an adverse occasion (e.g., realizing the pointlessness or ephemerality of the daily routine) negatively influences one's current state (e.g., triggers loss of meaning in life, activates death cognitions), but also increases nostalgia. Subsequently, nostalgia positively impacts on one's current state (e.g., raises meaning in life, deactivates death cognitions). In this framework, nostalgia functions as a balancing feedback mechanism that sustains equilibrium. We are guided by the regulatory model in reviewing the pertinent literature, although the findings are fragmented, often testing isolated tenets rather than the full model.

Life Meaninglessness

Nostalgia counteracts threats to meaning in life and repairs meaning deficits. As Wallace, a character in Saul Bellow's *Mr. Sammler's Planet* (1970, p. 190) proclaimed, nostalgic memories "keep the wolf of insignificance from the door." We review pertinent evidence for this principle (see also Abeyta & Pillarisetty, 2023).

Nostalgia Counteracts Threats to Life's Meaning

Threats to life's meaningfulness elicit nostalgia. In an experiment by Routledge and colleagues (2011, Study 3), participants in the threat condition read an essay challenging the significance of life (p. 643): "There are approximately 7 billion people living on this planet. . . . The Earth is 5 billion years old and the average human life span across the globe is 68 years. What is 68 years of one person's rat-race compared to 5 billion years of history? We are no more significant than any other form of life in the universe." Participants in the control condition read a different essay, judged as equivalent on interest and originality, regarding limitations of computers (p. 643): "the computer never understood a word of this text. A computer does not comprehend what is stored in its 'memory' any more than a book in the library understands what it contains." Next, all participants reported their state nostalgia (e.g., "I feel nostalgic at the moment"; Wildschut et al., 2006). Participants in the meaning-threat condition felt more nostalgic than those in the control condition.

Further, nostalgia countervails threats to life's meaningfulness. In Routledge and colleagues (2011, Study 4), participants first underwent a nostalgia induction via the ERT. Then, they went through the same life meaninglessness versus computer limitations manipulation as above. Finally, they evaluated the essay (e.g., "is convincing in its points") and its author (e.g., "is a reliable source"). Derogating the threatening essay and its source would constitute defensive responding to threat (Greenberg et al., 1990). In the computer limitations condition, nostalgic participants' responses did not differ from those of controls. However, in the life meaninglessness condition, nostalgic participants disparaged the essay and its author *less* than controls; apparently, nostalgic participants did not feel the need to resort to defensive responding, as they were already fortified by the psychological resource of nostalgia.

The above results pattern was replicated with a different manipulation of life meaninglessness, surrealist art (Arndt et al., 2013). In contrast to representational art, surrealist art disrupts meaning, as objects defy regular or expected structures (Steger & Marsh, Chapter 51, this volume). In a relevant experiment by Routledge and colleagues (2012, Experiment 3), participants in the meaning-threat condition viewed René Magritte's *The Son of Man*, a surrealist painting portraying a man whose face is partially blocked by an apple, whereas participants in the control condition viewed John Constable's *Landscape with a Double Rainbow*, a representational painting portraying a rainbow (for details on this manipulation, see Proulx et al., 2010). Afterward, participants underwent a nostalgia induction via the ERT (although the control condition entailed a positive, as opposed to an ordinary, event). Lastly, they completed the Presence of Meaning subscale of the Meaning in Life Questionnaire (Steger et al., 2006). When exposed to representational art, nostalgic and control participants did not differ in their level of meaning. However, when exposed to surrealist art, nostalgic participants reported elevated meaning compared to controls. Nostalgic participants were better able to withstand the erosion of meaning instigated by the surrealist painting; nostalgia shielded them against meaning drops.

Boredom is "a state of low arousal and dissatisfaction, which is attributed to an inadequately stimulating situation" (Mikulas & Vodanovich, 1993, p. 3). In several experiments, Van Tilburg and colleagues (2013) manipulated boredom by having participants engage in repetitive activities, such as copying 10 (instead of two) references of journal articles about concrete mixtures. Boredom led to drops in meaning (Presence of Meaning subscale of the Meaning in Life Questionnaire; Steger et al., 2006), but gains in nostalgia (e.g., "Right now, I am feeling quite nostalgic"; Wildschut et al., 2006). Nostalgia, in turn, offset or suppressed loss of meaning. Stated otherwise, in the absence of nostalgia, drops in meaning would be more precipitous. This empirical sequence illustrates a test of the full regulatory model of nostalgia.

Nostalgia Repairs Meaning Deficits

Individuals with chronic meaning deficits are likely to have ill well-being, given that meaning is positively associated with well-being (Steger, 2014). Would these individuals benefit from nostalgia, assuming it raises well-being? An experiment addressed this question (Routledge et al., 2011, Study 5). First, participants completed the Purpose in Life scale, which was designed by Crumbaugh and Maholick (1964) to assess Frankl's (1959/1963) concept of noogenic neurosis, that is, existential frustration and emptiness. Participants, then, ranged from having meaning deficits to having meaning surfeits. Next, they underwent an ERT-based nostalgia induction. Lastly, they filled out Ryan and Frederick's (1997) subjective vitality scale (e.g., "At this moment, I feel alive and vital"; "I am looking forward to each new day"). In reflecting a heightened sense of alertness and energy for life, subjective vitality is an operationalization of eudaimonic well-being (Ryan & Deci, 2001). Nostalgia (vs. control) conferred no subjective vitality to participants with meaning surfeits but increased subjective vitality in participants with meaning deficits.

Individuals characterized by meaning deficits are also susceptible to stressful stimuli (Park & Folkman, 1997). Does nostalgia contribute to stress reduction? An experiment answered this question (Routledge et al., 2011, Study 6). First, participants responded to the item "My life has meaning" (embedded in several filler items), which helped the researchers form a continuum from meaning deficits to meaning surfeits. Then, participants were subjected to an ERT manipulation of nostalgia. Stress induction followed using the Trier Social Stress Test (Kirschbaum et al., 1993). It comprises both public speaking (i.e., persuading a hiring panel of one's suitability for a job) and mental arithmetic (i.e., subtracting serially, and as speedily and accurately as possible, 17 from 2,023). This protocol reliably intensifies stress responses (Schlotz et al., 2008). Immediately after the Trier Social Stress Test, participants reported their stress level (e.g., "I feel jittery). Nostalgia (vs. control) did not reduce stress in participants with meaning surfeits. However, nostalgia alleviated stress in participants with meaning deficits.

Loneliness is a risk factor for psychological ill-being or maladjustment (e.g., unhappiness, depression, anxiety; Brodeur et al., 2021; Erzen & Çikrikci, 2018). Persons high (vs. low) on loneliness are characterized by meaning deficits (Mwilambwe-Tshilobo et al., 2019; Stillman & Lambert, 2013). Does nostalgia conduce to life meaningfulness among lonely people? Abeyta and Juhl (2023, Study 1) assessed loneliness (UCLA Loneliness Questionnaire; Russell, 1996; "How often do you feel that you lack companionship?"), state nostalgia (Nostalgia Inventory; Batcho, 1995), and state meaning (Presence of Meaning subscale of the Meaning in Life Questionnaire; Steger et al., 2006). Nostalgia was related to greater meaning in life, especially among participants high (vs. low) on loneliness. Also, the negative association between loneliness and meaning in life was weaker among nostalgic participants than among non-nostalgic participants. In Study 2, Abeyta and Juhl assessed loneliness (as in Study 1), manipulated nostalgia (with the ERT), and measured meaning in life (via the meaning subscale of the Nostalgia Functions Scale; Hepper et al., 2012). Replicating the Study 1 findings, nostalgia raised meaning in life, especially among participants high (vs. low) on loneliness. Additionally, the negative association between loneliness and meaning in life was weaker in the nostalgia (than control) condition.

Disillusionment is a state of existential concern. It is accompanied by feeling confused, disconnected from one's social environment, hopeless, and lost. It occurs when a person's deeply held belief systems are discredited by life events or the state of the world (Janoff-Bulman & Berg, 1998; Maher et al., 2018). Maher and colleagues (2021, Study 3) manipulated disillusionment by presenting participants in the experimental condition with facts about global issues that challenged cherished justice and equality beliefs, and by asking participants in the control condition to work on a neutral (i.e., shape comparison; Gervey et al., 2005) task. Next, the researchers manipulated nostalgia with the ERT. Finally, the researchers assessed meaning in life with five items (e.g.,

"I feel a sense of meaningfulness"; Van Tilburg & Igou, 2011). In the absence of disillusionment, nostalgic and nonnostalgic participants reported equivalent levels of meaning. However, in the presence of disillusionment, nostalgic participants reported *reduced* meaning loss compared to nonnostalgic ones. Nostalgia prevented disillusioned participants from suffering drops in meaning; alternatively, nostalgia buffered disillusioned participants from meaninglessness.

Mortality Awareness

Nostalgia assuages the psychological consequences of mortality awareness. As Davis (1979, p. 41) remarked, nostalgia "quiet[s] our fears of the abyss." We report results from several studies that illustrate this principle.

Routledge and colleagues (2008, Experiment 1) tested whether dispositional nostalgia (Sedikides & Wildschut, 2024) has the potential to sustain meaning in the face of mortality awareness. First, they assessed nostalgia with the Time Perspective Inventory (Zimbardo & Boyd, 1999; e.g., "I get nostalgic about my childhood"). They proceeded with a mortality salience manipulation (Rosenblatt et al., 1989, p. 133). In the experimental (i.e., mortality salience) condition, participants were instructed to "Briefly describe the emotions that the thought of your own death arouses in you. Jot down, as specifically as you can, what you think will happen to you physically as you die and once you are physically dead." In the control (dental pain salience) condition, participants received similarly worded instructions, replacing "dental pain" with "death." After a 3-minute delay (intended to remove death reminders from focal attention; Arndt et al., 2004), participants completed the No Meaning Scale (Kunzendorf & Maguire, 1995; e.g., "My place in the universe is like that of an insignificant speck of dust," "Life is cruel joke"). In the control condition, participants high and low on nostalgia did not differ in meaning in life. However, in the experimental condition, participants high on nostalgia reported greater meaning than did those who were low on nostalgia. Alternatively, although reminders of one's finitude (compared to reminders of dental pain) decreased meaning among low nostalgia participants, they did not reduce meaning among high nostalgia participants. Nostalgia replenished meaning eroded by mortality cues.

Juhl and colleagues (2010, Study 1) examined whether dispositional nostalgia is associated with defensiveness to one's collective identity when confronted with harbingers of one's mortality. They started by assessing nostalgia with the Time Perspective Inventory (Zimbardo & Boyd, 1999). Afterward, they introduced the mortality salience manipulation mentioned above (Rosenblatt et al., 1989). Then, they presented participants with an essay, ostensibly written by a senior student, which demeaned their university or collective identity (e.g., "[this] just is not that great of a college to be honest. . . . I feel like I may have made a mistake by going to [this college]"; Dechesne et al., 2000). Participants lastly responded to questions that gauged defensiveness to the criticism. These questions pertained to attitudes toward the essay (e.g., "How much do you agree with this person's opinion?") and its author (e.g., "How much do you think you would like this person?"; Greenberg et al., 1990). Mortality salience led to more negative (i.e., more defensive) reactions than an aversive control condition among low nostalgia participants but did not do so among high nostalgia participants. Nostalgia served as a psychological or meaning resource that buffered participants from reacting negatively and with fear to a reminder of their mortality.

These findings were conceptually replicated in two other studies involving collective identity (Routledge et al., 2014). In Study 1, following completion of the Southampton Nostalgia Scale (Sedikides et al., 2015), participants underwent a mortality salience manipulation (control condition: extreme pain salience; Rosenblatt et al., 1989), and completed a nationalistic sacrifice measure (e.g., "I would die for my nation"). Mortality salience led to more willingness to die for one's country than an aversive control condition among low nostalgia participants but did not do so among high nostalgia participants. Individuals high on nostalgia were less defensive of their national identity. In Study 2, participants first engaged in a word-completion task (Greenberg et al., 1994) purported to quantify their level of death-thought accessibility. This task consists of 28 word fragments, six of which can be completed to create a death-related versus neutral word (e.g., COFF_ _ can be completed as COFFIN or COFFEE). The sum of completed death-related words constitutes the index of death-thought accessibility. Next, participants were subjected to nostalgia induction via the ERT. Lastly, they filled out a religious self-sacrifice measure (e.g., "I would die for my religion"). Mortality salience led to more death-thought accessibility (or death anxiety) than an aversive control condition among low nostalgia participants but did not do so among high nostalgia participants.

Routledge and colleagues (2008, Experiment 2) were concerned with the role of dispositional nostalgia in protecting against death ideation. They assessed nostalgia (Southampton Nostalgia Scale; Sedikides et al., 2015), manipulated mortality salience (Rosenblatt et al., 1989), and measured death-thought accessibility with the abovementioned word-completion task (Greenberg et al., 1994). In the pain salience condition, nostalgia was unrelated to death-thought accessibility. In the mortality salience condition, higher nostalgia was associated with reduced death-thought accessibility. Nostalgia sheltered against mortality awareness by combating death cognitions. These findings were replicated by manipulating nostalgia (Routledge et al., 2008, Experiment 3). The mortality salience manipulation (Rosenblatt et al., 1989) came first, followed by a nostalgia induction (ERT), and the abovementioned measure of death-thought accessibility (Greenberg et al., 1994). In the pain salience condition, the level of death-thought accessibility did not differ between participants high and low on nostalgia. In the mortality salience condition, however, nostalgia weakened death-thought accessibility relative to control. Taken together, nostalgia buffers against death ideation.

But does nostalgia buffer against fear of death (or death anxiety; Menzies, Chapter 9, this volume)? Juhl and colleagues (2010, Study 2) assessed nostalgia with the Southampton Nostalgia Scale (Sedikides et al., 2015), manipulated mortality salience (vs. pain salience; Rosenblatt et al., 1989), and measured fear of death with the Death of Self subscale of the Revised Collett-Lester Fear of Death Scale (Lester, 1990). This subscale consists of eight facets of death (e.g., "the shortness of life," "the total isolation of death"). In the extreme pain salience condition, nostalgic and nonnostalgic participants did not differ in their level of death fear. However, in the mortality salience condition, low nostalgics evinced more death fear than high nostalgics. Nostalgia buffered against fear of death.

SUMMARY

Nostalgia protects against loss of meaning in life. In particular, nostalgia is instigated by perceptions of life meaninglessness, reduces defensiveness to threats of meaninglessness, and helps individuals regain meaning in the presence of meaning-sapping boredom. Further, nostalgia restores lack of meaning. It increases subjective vitality and decreases stress in individuals with chronic meaning deficits, while boosting meaning among the lonely and the disillusioned. Moreover, nostalgia countervails the aversive consequences of mortality cues. Under the impact of such cues, it replenishes meaning, attenuates defensive responding, and palliates fear of death.

EPILOGUE

Although nostalgia has had a negative reputation since Johannes Hofer (1688/1934), a medical student at University of Basel, labeled it a brain disorder (Sedikides et al., 2004), empirical findings in the last two decades have rehabilitated its image. Our research program is part of the rehabilitation movement. We were concerned with the existential status of the emotion. Following a converging operations approach (Campbell & Fiske, 1959), we measured or manipulated the construct in multiple ways. Nostalgia enhances or sustains meaning and buttresses existential coping.

We reported mostly results of experiments, with the exception of a few cross-sectional studies and a longitudinal study. Is the existential relevance of nostalgia short-lived? An intervention (Layous et al., 2022) addressed this question. The intervention lasted for 6 weeks, with nostalgia reinstated (via the ERT) every week. Meaning in life (meaning subscale of the Nostalgia Functions scale; Hepper et al., 2012) was assessed at midintervention (Week 4) and postintervention (Weeks 7 and 8). Meaning was sustained throughout, especially among participants high on dispositional nostalgia. Nostalgia may also have long-term implications for well-being via the downstream consequences of its elicited meaning.

Several questions await empirical scrutiny. Does nostalgia impact on broader existential concerns (e.g., one's changing roles in developmental context, relevance to society, or legacy)? Assuming that the effect of nostalgia on meaning is mediated by social connectedness, is nostalgia more likely to impart meaning among low-avoidance than among high-avoidance individuals? (Heine & Mask, Chapter 34, this volume; Wildschut et al., 2010)? Can a person create and sustain meaning by engaging in anticipated nostalgia, "the foreseeing of looking back on life events and expecting to feel nostalgic about it in the future" (Cheung, 2023, p. 1)?

In conclusion, nostalgia is a wellspring of meaning in life, or, as the sociologist Janelle Wilson (2004) labeled it, a "sanctuary of meaning." It replenishes meaning, benefits psychologically persons with meaning deficits, and cushions against death cognitions or fear of death. Nostalgia is an existential emotion.

REFERENCES

Abeyta, A. A., & Juhl, J. (2023). Nostalgia restores meaning in life for lonely people. *Emotion, 23*(6), 1791–1795.

Abeyta, A. A., & Pillarisetty, S., (2023). Nostalgia supports a meaningful life. *Current Opinion in Psychology, 49,* Article 101520.

Abeyta, A. A., Routledge, C., Roylance, C., Wildschut, R. T., & Sedikides, C. (2015). Attachment-related avoidance and the social and agentic content of nostalgic memories. *Journal of Social and Personal Relationships, 32*(3), 406–413.

Allison, S. T., & Green, J. D. (2020). Nostalgia and heroism: Theoretical convergence of memory, motivation, and function. *Frontiers in Psychology, 11,* Article 577862.

Argote, L., Insko, C. A., Yovetich, N., & Romero, A. A. (1995). Group learning curves: The effects of turnover and task complexity on group performance. *Journal of Applied Social Psychology, 25*(6), 512–529.

Arndt, J., Cook, A., & Routledge, C. (2004). The blueprint of terror management: Understanding the cognitive architecture of psychological defense against the awareness of death. In J. Greenberg, S. L. Koole, & T. Pyszczynski (Eds.), *Handbook of experimental existential psychology* (pp. 35–53). Guilford Press.

Arndt, J., Landau, M. J., Vail, K. E., & Vess, M. (2013). An edifice for enduring personal value: A terror management perspective on the human quest for multilevel meaning. In K. D. Markman, T. Proulx, & M. J. Lindberg (Eds.), *The psychology of meaning* (pp. 49–69). American Psychological Association.

Batcho, K. I. (1995). Nostalgia: A psychological perspective. *Perceptual and Motor Skills, 80*(1), 131–143.

Batcho, K. I. (2023). Nostalgia in literature and memoir. *Current Opinion in Psychology, 50,* Article 101557.

Batcho, K. I., DaRin, M. L., Nave, A. M., & Yaworsky, R. R. (2008). Nostalgia and identity in song lyrics. *Psychology of Aesthetics, Creativity, and the Arts, 2*(4), 236–244.

Bellow, S. (1970). *Mr. Sammler's planet.* Viking Press.

Biskas, M., Juhl, J., Wildschut, T., Sedikides, C., & Saroglou, V. (2022). Nostalgia and spirituality: The roles of self-continuity and meaning in life. *Social Psychology, 53*(3), 152–162.

Brodeur, A., Clark, A. E., Fleche, S., & Powdthavee, N. (2021). COVID-19, lockdowns and well-being: Evidence from Google Trends. *Journal of Public Economics, 193,* 104346.

Campbell, D. T., & Fiske, D. W. (1959). Convergent and discriminant validation by the multitrait-multimethod matrix. *Psychological Bulletin, 56*(2), 81–105.

Cheung, W.-Y. (2023). Anticipated nostalgia. *Current Opinion in Psychology, 49,* Article 101521.

Collins English Dictionary. (2023). (14th ed.). Best Sellers Rank.

Costin, V., & Vignoles, V. L. (2020). Meaning is about mattering: Evaluating coherence, purpose, and existential mattering as precursors of meaning in life judgments. *Journal of Personality and Social Psychology, 118*(4), 864–884.

Crumbaugh, J. C., & Maholick, L. T. (1964). An experimental study in existentialism: The psychometric approach to Frankl's concept of noogenic neurosis. *Journal of Clinical Psychology, 20*(2), 200–207.

Cutrona, C. E., & Russell, D. (1987). The provisions of social relationships and adaptation to stress. In W. H. Jones & D. Perlman (Eds.), *Advances in personal relationships* (Vol. 1, pp. 37–67). JAI Press.

Davis, F. (1979). *Yearning for yesterday: A sociology of nostalgia.* Free Press.

Dechesne, M., Janssen, J., & van Knippenberg, A. (2000). Derogation and distancing as terror management strategies: The moderating role of need for closure and permeability of group boundaries. *Journal of Personality and Social Psychology, 79*(6), 923–932.

Erzen, E., & Çikrikci, Ö. (2018). The effect of loneliness on depression: A meta-analysis. *International Journal of Social Psychiatry, 64*(5), 427–435.

Evans, N. D., Reyes, J., Wildschut, T., Sedikides, C., & Fetterman, A. K. (2021). Mental transportation mediates nostalgia's psychological benefits. *Cognition and Emotion, 35*(1), 84–95.

Feldman, D. B. (2013). The meaning of hope and vice versa: Goal-directed thinking and the construction of a meaningful life. In J. A. Hicks & C. Routledge (Eds.), *The experience of meaning in life: Perspectives from the psychological sciences* (pp. 141–150). Springer.

Frankenbach, J., Wildschut, T., Juhl, J., & Sedikides, C. (2021). Does neuroticism disrupt the psychological benefits of nostalgia? A meta-analytic test. *European Journal of Personality, 35*(2), 249–266.

Frankl, V. E. (1963). *Man's search for meaning* (I. Lasch, Trans.). Beacon Press. (Original work published 1959)

Gervey, B., Igou, E. R., & Trope, Y. (2005). Positive mood and future-oriented self-evaluation. *Motivation and Emotion, 29*(4), 269–296.

Green, M. C., & Brock, T. C. (2000). The role of transportation in the persuasiveness of public narratives. *Journal of Personality and Social Psychology, 79*(5), 701–721.

Greenberg, J., Koole, S. L., & Pyszczynski, T. (Eds.). (2004). *Handbook of experimental existential psychology.* Guilford Press.

Greenberg, J., Pyszczynski, T., Solomon, S., Simon, L., & Breus, M. (1994). Role of consciousness and accessibility of death-related thoughts in mortality salience effects. *Journal of Personality and Social Psychology, 67*(4), 627–637.

Greenberg, J., Pyszczynski, T., Solomon, S., Rosenblatt, A., Veeder, M., Kirkland, S., & Lyon, D. (1990). Evidence for terror management theory II: The effects of mortality salience on reactions to those who threaten or bolster the cultural worldview. *Journal of Personality and Social Psychology, 58*(2), 308–318.

Hepper, E. G., Ritchie, T. D., Sedikides, C., & Wildschut, T. (2012). Odyssey's end: Lay conceptions of nostalgia reflect its original Homeric meaning. *Emotion, 12*(1), 102–119.

Hepper, E. G., Sedikides, C., Wildschut, T., Cheung, W.-Y., Abakoumkin, G., Arikan, G., . . . Zengel, B. (2023). Pancultural nostalgia in action: Prevalence, triggers, and psychological functions of nostalgia across cultures. *Journal of Experimental Psychology: General.*

Hepper, E. G., Wildschut, T., Sedikides, C., Ritchie, T. D., Yung, Y.-F., Hansen, N., . . . Zhou, X. (2014). Pancultural nostalgia: Prototypical conceptions across cultures. *Emotion, 14*(4), 733–747.

Hepper, E. G., Wildschut, T., Sedikides, C., Robertson, S., & Routledge, C. D. (2021). Time capsule: Nostalgia shields psychological wellbeing from limited time horizons. *Emotion, 21*(3), 644–664.

Hertz, D. G. (1990). Trauma and nostalgia: New aspects of the coping of aging holocaust survivors. *Israeli Journal of Psychiatry and Related Sciences, 27*(4), 189–198.

Hodge, D. R. (2003). The Intrinsic Spirituality Scale: A new six-item instrument for assessing the salience of spirituality as a motivational construct. *Journal of Social Service Research, 30*(1), 41–61.

Hofer, J. (1934). Medical dissertation on nostalgia. (C. K. Anspach, Trans.). *Bulletin of the History of Medicine, 2,* 376–391. (Original work published 1688)

Horowitz, L. M., French, R. P., & Anderson, C. A. (1982). The prototype of a lonely person. In L. A. Peplau & D. Perlman (Eds.), *Loneliness: A sourcebook of current theory, research and therapy* (pp. 183–205). Wiley.

Ismail, S., Christopher, G., Dodd, E., Wildschut, T., Sedikides, C., Ingram, T. A., . . . Cheston, R. (2018). Psychological and mnemonic benefits of nostalgia for people with dementia. *Journal of Alzheimer's Disease, 65*(4), 1327–1344.

Janoff-Bulman, R., & Berg, M. (1998). Disillusionment and the creation of value: From traumatic losses to existential gains. In J. Harvey (Ed.), *Perspectives on loss: A sourcebook* (pp. 35–44). Taylor & Francis.

Jiang, T., Cheung, W.-Y., Wildschut, T., & Sedikides, C. (2021). Nostalgia, reflection, brooding: Psychological benefits and autobiographical memory functions. *Consciousness and Cognition, 90,* Article 103107.

Juhl, J., Routledge, C., Arndt, J., Sedikides, C., & Wildschut, T. (2010). Fighting the future with the past: On the death-anxiety buffering function of nostalgia. *Journal of Research in Personality, 44*(3), 309–314.

Karagoz, D., & Ramkissoon, H. (2023). Nostalgic emotions, meaning in life, subjective well-being and revisit intentions. *Tourism Management Perspectives, 48,* Article 101159.

King, L. A., Heintzelman, S. J., & Ward, S. J. (2016). Beyond the search for meaning: A contemporary science of the experience of meaning in life. *Current Directions in Psychological Science, 25*(4), 211–216.

King, L. A., Hicks, J. A., Krull, J. L., & Del Gaiso, A. K. (2006). Positive affect and the experience of meaning in life. *Journal of Personality and Social Psychology, 90*(1), 179–196.

Kirschbaum, C., Pirke, K.-M., & Hellhammer, D. H. (1993). The "Trier Social Stress Test"—A tool for investigating psychobiological stress responses in a laboratory setting. *Neuropsychobiology, 28*(1–2), 76–81.

Krackhardt, D., & Porter, L. W. (1985). When friends leave: A structural analysis of the relationship between turnover and stayers' attitudes. *Administrative Science Quarterly, 30*(2), 242–261.

Kunzendorf, R. G., & Maguire, D. (1995). *Depression: the reality of "no meaning" versus the delusion of negative meaning.* Unpublished manuscript, University of Massachusetts.

Lambert, N. M., Stillman, T. F., Baumeister, R. F., Fincham, F. D., Hicks, J. A., & Graham, S. M. (2010). Family as a salient source of meaning in young adulthood. *Journal of Positive Psychology, 5*(5), 367–376.

Layous, K., Kurtz, J. L., Wildschut, T., & Sedikides, C. (2022). The effect of a multi-week nostalgia intervention on well-being: Mechanisms and moderation. *Emotion, 22*(8), 1952–1968.

Lester, D. (1990). The Collett-Lester fear of death scale: The original version and a revision. *Death Studies, 14*(5), 451–468.

Leunissen, J. M., Sedikides, C., Wildschut, T., & Cohen, T. R. (2018). Organizational nostalgia lowers turnover intentions by increasing work meaning: The moderating role of burnout. *Journal of Occupational Health Psychology, 23*(1), 44–57.

Leunissen, J. M., Wildschut, T., Sedikides, C., & Routledge, C. (2021). The hedonic character of nostalgia: An integrative data analysis. *Emotion Review, 13*(2), 139–156.

Maher, P. J., Igou, E. R., & van Tilburg, W. A. P. (2018). Brexit, Trump, and the polarizing effect of disillusionment. *Social Psychological and Personality Science, 9*(2), 205–213.

Maher, P. J., Igou, E. R., & van Tilburg, W. A. P. (2021). Nostalgia relieves the disillusioned mind. *Journal of Experimental Social Psychology, 92,* Article 104061.

McGregor, I., & Little, B. R. (1998). Personal projects, happiness, and meaning: On doing well and being yourself. *Journal of Personality and Social Psychology, 74*(2), 494–512.

McLean, K. C., Pasupathi, M., & Pals, J. L. (2007). Selves creating stories creating selves: A process model of self-development. *Personality and Social Psychology Review, 11*(3), 262–278.

Mikulas, W. L., & Vodanovich, S. V. (1993). The essence of boredom. *Psychological Record, 43,* 3–12.

Milyavskaya, M., Ianakieva, I., Foxen-Craft, E., Colantuoni, A., & Koestner, R. (2012). Inspired to get there: The effects of trait and goal inspiration on goal progress. *Personality and Individual Differences, 52*(1), 56–60.

Mwilambwe-Tshilobo, L., Ge, T., Chong, M., Ferguson, M. A., Misic, B., Burrow, A. L., . . . Spreng, R. N. (2019). Loneliness and meaning in life are reflected in the intrinsic network architecture of the brain. *Social Cognitive and Affective Neuroscience, 14*(4), 423–433.

New Oxford Dictionary of English. (1998). Nostalgia. Oxford University Press.

Newman, D. B., Sachs, M. E., Stone, A. A., & Schwarz, N. (2020). Nostalgia and well-being in daily life: An ecological validity perspective. *Journal of Personality and Social Psychology, 118*(2), 325–347.

Park, C. L., & Folkman, S. (1997). Meaning in the context of stress and coping. *Review of General Psychology, 1*(2), 115–144.

Proulx, T., Heine, S. J., & Vohs, K. D. (2010). When is the unfamiliar the uncanny?: Meaning affirmative after exposure to absurdist literature, humor, and art. *Personality and Social Psychology Bulletin, 36*(6), 817–829.

Reid, C. A., Green, J. D., Buchmaier, S., McSween, D. K, Wildschut, T., & Sedikides, C. (2023). Food-evoked nostalgia. *Cognition and Emotion, 37*(1), 34–48.

Reid, C. A., Green, J. D., Wildschut, T., & Sedikides, C. (2015). Scent-evoked nostalgia. *Memory, 23*(2), 157–166.

Rosch, E. (1975). Cognitive representations of semantic categories. *Journal of Experimental Psychology: General, 104*(3), 192–233.

Rosenblatt, A., Greenberg, J., Solomon, S., Pyszczynski, T., & Lyon, D. (1989). Evidence for terror management theory: I. The effects of mortality salience on reactions to those who violate or uphold cultural values. *Journal of Personality and Social Psychology, 57*(4), 681–690.

Routledge, C., Arndt, J., Sedikides, C., & Wildschut, T. (2008). A blast from the past: The terror management function of nostalgia. *Journal of Experimental Social Psychology, 44*(1), 132–140.

Routledge C., Arndt, J., Wildschut, T., Sedikides, C., Hart, C. M., Juhl, J., . . . Scholtz,

W. (2011). The past makes the present meaningful: Nostalgia as an existential resource. *Journal of Personality and Social Psychology, 101*(3), 638–652.

Routledge, C., Juhl, J., Abeyta, A., & Roylance, C. (2014). Using the past to promote a peaceful future: Nostalgia proneness mitigates existential threat induced nationalistic self-sacrifice. *Social Psychology, 45*(5), 339–346.

Routledge, C., Wildschut, T., Sedikides, C., Juhl, J., & Arndt, J. (2012). The power of the past: Nostalgia as a meaning-making resource. *Memory, 20*(5), 452–460.

Russell, D. W. (1996). UCLA Loneliness Scale (version 3): Reliability, validity, and factor structure. *Journal of Personality Assessment, 66*(1), 20–40.

Ryan, R. M., & Deci, E. L. (2001). On happiness and human potentials: A review of research on hedonic and eudaimonic well-being. *Annual Review of Psychology, 52,* 141–166.

Ryan, R. M., & Frederick, C. (1997). On energy, personality, and health: Subjective vitality as a dynamic reflection of well-being. *Journal of Personality, 65*(3), 529–565.

Schlotz, W., Kumsta, R., Layes, I., Entringer, S., Jones, A., & Wuest, S. (2008). Covariance between psychological and endocrine responses to pharmacological challenge and psychosocial stress: A question of timing. *Psychosomatic Medicine, 70*(7), 787–796.

Sedikides, C., Cheung, W. Y., Wildschut, T., Hepper, E. G., Baldursson, E., & Pedersen, B. (2018). Nostalgia motivates pursuit of important goals by increasing meaning in life. *European Journal of Social Psychology, 48*(2), 209–216.

Sedikides, C., Hong, E., & Wildschut, T. (2023). Self-continuity. *Annual Review of Psychology, 74,* 333–361.

Sedikides, C., & Wildschut, T. (2018). Finding meaning in nostalgia. *Review of General Psychology, 22*(1), 48–61.

Sedikides, C., & Wildschut, T. (2019). The sociality of personal and collective nostalgia. *European Review of Social Psychology, 30*(1), 123–173.

Sedikides, C., & Wildschut, T. (2022). Nostalgia across cultures. *Journal of Pacific Rim Psychology, 16,* 1–16.

Sedikides, C., & Wildschut, T. (2023). Nostalgia as motivation. *Current Opinion in Psychology, 49,* Article 101537.

Sedikides, C., & Wildschut, T. (2024). Trait nostalgia. *Personality and Individual Differences, 221,* 1–7.

Sedikides, C., Wildschut, T., & Baden, D. (2004). Nostalgia: Conceptual issues and existential functions. In J. Greenberg, S. L. Koole, & T. Pyszczynski (Eds.), *Handbook of experimental existential psychology* (pp. 200–214). Guilford Press.

Sedikides, C., Wildschut, T., Cheung, W.-Y., Routledge, C., Hepper, E. G., Arndt, J., . . . Vingerhoets, A. J. J. M. (2016). Nostalgia fosters self-continuity: Uncovering the mechanism (social connectedness) and the consequence (eudaimonic well-being). *Emotion, 16*(4), 524–539.

Sedikides, C., Wildschut, T., Routledge, C., Arndt, J., Hepper, E. G., & Zhou, X. (2015). To nostalgize: Mixing memory with affect and desire. *Advances in Experimental Social Psychology, 51,* 189–273.

Stavrova, O., & Luhmann, M. (2016). Social connectedness as a source and consequence of meaning in life. *Journal of Positive Psychology, 11*(5), 470–479.

Steger, M. F. (2014). Experiencing meaning in life: optimal functioning at the nexus of well-being, psychopathology, and spirituality. In P. T. P. Wong (Ed.), *The human quest for meaning: Theories, research, and applications* (2nd ed., pp. 165–184). Routledge.

Steger, M. F., Dik, B. J., & Duffy, R. D. (2012). Measuring meaningful work: The Work and Meaning Inventory (WAMI). *Journal of Career Assessment, 20*(3), 322–337.

Steger, M. F., Frazier, P., Oishi, S., & Kaler, M. (2006). The meaning in life questionnaire: Assessing the presence of and search for meaning in life. *Journal of Counseling Psychology, 53*(1), 80–93.

Steger, M. F., Kashdan, T. B., Sullivan, B. A., & Lorentz, D. (2008). Understanding the search for meaning in life: Personality, cognitive style, and the dynamic between seeking and experiencing meaning. *Journal of Personality, 76*(2), 199–228.

Stephan, E., Wildschut, T., Sedikides, C., Zhou, X., He, W., Routledge, C. D, . . . Vingerhoets, A. J. J. M. (2014). The mnemonic mover: Nostalgia regulates avoidance and approach motivation. *Emotion, 14*(3), 545–561.

Stillman, T. F., Baumeister, R. F., Lambert, N. M., Crescioni, A., DeWall, C., & Fincham, F. D. (2009). Alone and without purpose: Life loses meaning following social exclusion. *Journal of Experimental Social Psychology, 45*(4), 686–694.

Stillman, T. F., & Lambert, N. M. (2013). The bidirectional relationship of meaning and belonging. In J. Hicks & C. D. Routledge (Eds.), The experience of meaning in life (pp. 305–315). Springer.

Tett, R. P., & Meyer, J. P. (1993). Job satisfaction, organizational commitment, turnover intention, and turnover: Path analyses based on meta-analytic findings. *Personnel Psychology, 46*(2), 259–293.

Ton, Z., & Huckman, R. S. (2008). Managing the impact of employee turnover on performance: The role of process conformance. *Organization Science, 19*(1), 56–68.

Turner, J. R., & Stanley, J. T. (2021). Holding on to pieces of the past: Daily reports of nostalgia in a life-span sample. *Emotion, 21*(5), 951–961.

Van Dick, R., Christ, O., Stellmacher, J., Wagner, U., Ahlswede, O., Grubba, C., . . . Tissington, P. A. (2004). Should I stay or should I go? Explaining turnover intentions with organizational identification and job satisfaction. *British Journal of Management, 15*(4), 351–360.

Van Tilburg, W. A. P., & Igou, E. R. (2011). On boredom and social identity: A pragmatic meaning-regulation approach. *Personality and Social Psychology Bulletin, 37*(12), 1679–1691.

Van Tilburg, W. A. P., Igou, E. R., & Sedikides, C. (2013). In search of meaningfulness: Nostalgia as an antidote to boredom. *Emotion, 13*(3), 450–461.

Van Tilburg, W. A. P., Sedikides, C., Wildschut, T., & Vingerhoets, A. J. J. M. (2019). How nostalgia infuses life with meaning: from social connectedness to self-continuity. *European Journal of Social Psychology, 49*(3), 521–532.

Van Tilburg, W. A. P., Wildschut, T., & Sedikides, C. (2018). Nostalgia's place among self-conscious emotions. *Cognition and Emotion, 32*(4), 742–759.

Vignoles, V. L., Regalia, C., Manzi, C., Golledge, J., & Scabini, E. (2006). Beyond self-esteem: Influence of multiple motives on identity construction. *Journal of Personality and Social Psychology, 90*(2), 308–333.

Waytz, A., Hershfield, H. E., & Tamir, D. I. (2015). Mental simulation and meaning in life. *Journal of Personality and Social Psychology, 108*(2), 336–355.

Wheeler, M. A., Stuss, D. T., & Tulving, E. (1997). Toward a theory of episodic memory: The frontal lobes and autonoetic consciousness. *Psychological Bulletin, 121*(3), 331–354.

Wildschut, T., & Sedikides, C. (2023). Water from the lake of memory: The regulatory model of nostalgia. *Current Directions in Psychological Science, 32*(1), 57–64.

Wildschut, T., & Sedikides, C. (2024). Experimental nostalgia inductions: A primer. In T. Becker & D. Trigg (Eds.), *The Routledge handbook of nostalgia*. Routledge.

Wildschut, T., Sedikides, C., & Alowidy, D. (2019). *Hanin*: Nostalgia among Syrian refugees. *European Journal of Social Psychology, 49*(7), 1368–1384.

Wildschut, T., Sedikides, C., Arndt, J., & Routledge, C. D. (2006). Nostalgia: Content, triggers, functions. *Journal of Personality and Social Psychology, 91*(5), 975–993.

Wildschut, T., Sedikides, C., & Robertson, S. (2018). Sociality and intergenerational transfer of older adults' nostalgia. *Memory, 26*(8), 1030–1041.

Wildschut, T., Sedikides, C., Routledge, C., Arndt, J., & Cordaro, P. (2010). Nostalgia as a repository of social connectedness: The role of attachment-related avoidance. *Journal of Personality and Social Psychology, 98*(4), 573–586.

Wilson, J. L. (2004). *Nostalgia: Sanctuary of meaning*. University of Minnesota Publishing.

Wu, Z., Chen, Y., Geng, L., Zhou, L., & Zhou, K. (2020). Greening in nostalgia?: How nostalgic traveling enhances tourists' proenvironmental behaviour. *Sustainable Development, 28*(4), 634–645.

Yin, Y., Jiang, T., Wildschut, T., & Sedikides, C. (2025). Nostalgia, ritual engagement, and meaning in life. *Personality and Social Psychology Bulletin, 51*(10), 1884–1896.

Zimbardo, P. G., & Boyd, J. N. (1999). Putting time in perspective: A valid, reliable individual-differences metric. *Journal of Personality and Social Psychology, 77*(6), 1271–1288.

CHAPTER 15

An Existential Perspective on Aging into Older Adulthood

Molly Maxfield

Within the life cycle, age holds different meanings. Reminders of time's passing, such as birthdays, are signifiers of the increasing freedom and opportunities of youth and young adulthood one often revels in, such as "being old enough" to get one's driver's license or buy a beer, and they shift at some point to signifiers of change one may dread reaching, such as "being old enough" to retire or "too old" to drive. Yalom stated that at some point, "we apprehend that the path no longer ascends but slopes downward toward decline and diminishment" (2008, p. 5). When that shift toward decline occurs may be variable. Certainly, in later life, each passing year may bring increased awareness of losses, including the deaths of friends and family, as well as irrevocable changes in one's self, including health, housing, and care. Lifespan models of development suggest that personal growth is a constant endeavor, yet the many changes associated with older adulthood may feel like assaults on core aspects of one's identity in ways that create the impression of deterioration rather than development. Aging thus presents a series of challenges with existential themes, including death-related anxiety and its effects on relationships, meaning, identity, and freedom. In this existential perspective on aging, I review (1) the ways in which aging and older adulthood present an existential challenge, thereby influencing perceptions of aging and older adults, (2) the nature of older adults' perceptions of and responses to reminders of death, (3) the shifts in existential concerns that occur in later life, and (4) the ways in which an existential perspective has been, or could be, used to consider end-of-life planning and care. With what appears to be a long list of losses and decline, I also consider the resilience of older adults and suggestion that the limits on the human lifespan make life all the more cherished.

TERROR MANAGEMENT THEORY: A BRIEF OVERVIEW

Many findings covered in the present chapter are tests of, or are interpreted within the context of, terror management theory (TMT). Given the theory's prominence in the field of existential psychology and this handbook (see Solomon et al., Chapter 6), only a brief overview is provided here. Developed to explain death's relationship to human behavior and beliefs, TMT (Greenberg et al., 1986; Solomon et al., 2015) suggests that humans' unique cognitive abilities allow for projection into infinite imagined future outcomes but also that death is an unavoidable future outcome for all living beings. This awareness is particularly problematic because living beings also are biologically predisposed to strive for survival. The conflict between the desire for continued life and awareness of eventual death, its unpredictability and inevitability, creates the potential for debilitating death-related anxiety. Fortunately, humans have also developed the means for managing death-related anxiety. According to TMT, self-esteem, meaning and value derived from belonging to and meeting the standards of one's cultural worldview, and close interpersonal relationships comprise the three-part anxiety-buffering system, which is central to managing existential terror and meaningfully engaging in daily life.

To test the basic tents of TMT, three primary hypotheses were developed and tested. The anxiety-buffer hypothesis suggests that faith in one's cultural worldviews, close relationships, and self-esteem provide a buffer against anxiety and reduce defensive reactions to reminders of death, or mortality salience. The mortality salience hypothesis suggests that to the extent this three-part anxiety buffer provides protection from death-related anxiety, reminders of mortality will intensify justification and defense of components of the anxiety-buffering system. Finally, absent a reminder of mortality, threats to any portion(s) of the anxiety-buffering system, which protects people from mortality salience, lead to increased death-thought accessibility. (See Solomon et al., Chapter 6, this volume for full descriptions of TMT hypotheses and associated empirical support.)

For the purposes of the present chapter, familiarity with a few additional concepts/methodological points is essential. Specifically, in addition to hypotheses previously noted, mortality salience and death-thought accessibility are important methodologically, in that *mortality salience* refers to reminders of mortality, which lead to increased *death-thought accessibility*. In TMT research, mortality is made salient with a variety of experimental inductions: responding to open-ended questions about one's thoughts and feelings about death or to true/false questions about perceptions on death, study participation near a funeral home, or exposure to death-related words (e.g., *funeral*, *dead*, *skull*) embedded in a word search puzzle or quickly presented on a computer screen. To ensure that responses are specific to mortality salience and not simply a negative reaction following negative stimuli, researchers refer to the usage of "aversive control conditions" to convey that participants completed similar questions and inductions regarding negative topics unrelated to death (e.g., uncertainty, experiencing pain, dental pain, social isolation, failing an important test, paralysis). Death-thought accessibility refers to the availability of death-related concepts. A common measure of death-thought accessibility includes a word-stem completion task, with greater proportions of death-related word responses indicating greater death-thought accessibility (e.g., responding to DE_ _ with DEAD versus DEED or COFF_ _ with COFFIN versus COFFEE). It is also important to note the different types of defenses used when confronted with mortality salience. Proximal defenses are logically and clearly related to denying (e.g., suppression of death-related thoughts) or distancing from death (e.g., increase in healthy intentions); these tend to occur when death is in focal attention. Distal defenses are not obviously related to management of death-related anxiety and are focused on the defense and maintenance of the anxiety-buffering system (e.g., validation of sources of self-esteem, relationships, or cultural worldviews); distal defenses tend to occur when mortality is salient but not in focal attention. With this brief TMT overview in mind, I next consider the existential nature of aging.

AGING AS AN EXISTENTIAL CHALLENGE

The aging process is rife with signals of decline. Common age-related changes include declining eyesight and hearing, increasing aches and pains, decreasing stamina and mobility, slower processing speed, and declining memory abilities. In most cases, these changes start out small, even escaping attention initially, but the accumulation of age-related changes eventually becomes clear and leads to adjustments in behavior and functioning. Changes may range from fairly minimal to more significant. For example, declining vision may lead to avoidance of driving at night, which is fairly easy to accommodate. More drastically, declining mobility may require the use of an assistive device, such as a walker or wheelchair, which is not only an outward sign of aging but is also associated with increased need for support in activities of daily living (e.g., bathing, dressing, getting in and out of bed). In this sense, one's own body and its age-related changes are not only reminders of the constraints on remaining lifespan but also contribute to increasing limitations on one's previous level of functioning and independence. These reminders of decline and pending dependence are particularly problematic in cultures emphasizing the importance of youth, beauty, and vitality.

Perhaps then the many examples of age-associated loss are why older people may be resistant to identify as "older adults," particularly after reminders of negative stereotypes about aging (Weiss & Lang, 2012). The threshold of how one defines "older adult" varies but appears to increase with age (Chopik et al., 2018), with one sample defining "old age" as starting at approximately 10 years beyond their current age (Molden & Maxfield, 2017). Starting in middle age and continuing into late life, people consistently report younger subjective age, or the feeling that they are younger than their chronological age (Pinquart & Wahl, 2021). Refusing to identify as an older adult and reporting the feeling of being younger than one's age are ways of distancing one's self from older adulthood and have been associated with a variety of beneficial outcomes, including lower depressive symptoms as well as greater cognitive performance and perceived well-being (for a review and meta-analysis, see Alonso Debreczeni & Bailey, 2020). However, avoidance of appearing "old" can be problematic. For example, some people cite concerns about looking old as a reason to not use assistive devices and technology that are associated with disability and age (Astell et al., 2020). Poignantly then, people may place their health and well-being at risk in an attempt to maintain a more youthful appearance.

It is understandable that older adults would want to distance themselves from the identity of "older," given prevalent examples of ageism, particularly in Western cultures, with examples surfacing in the minimal representation of older adults in children's cartoons (Aydogmus & Gunbas, 2024) as well as negative portrayals in film (Ng et al., 2023), birthday cards (Lin & Walden, 2023, though interestingly highest for cards specifically directed at 30–60 years of age compared to younger and older groups), and social media (Levy et al., 2014), particularly during COVID-19 (Lichtenstein, 2021), though some of the ageism was benevolent in nature (Vervaecke & Meisner, 2021). Perhaps related to growing proportions of older adults, there is some evidence of rising incidents of positive media depictions of older adults in recent years; however, these depictions typically focus on people who are healthy, active, and in many ways defying aging processes and representations of the oldest-old are still relatively rare (Loos & Ivan, 2018).

Ageism is unique in that people presumably hope to have the opportunity to become an older adult via ongoing avoidance of death. Age-based attitudes change with age, with ageism appearing to peak in midlife (Bodner et al., 2012; Kite et al., 2005), perhaps related to hesitation about one's looming entrance into this less desirable group (Kite et al., 2005). Even older adults hold negative views of aging and older adults (Bodner et al., 2012) and are one of the few groups to lack an own-group bias (Kite et al., 2005). Within an older sample, individuals ages 81–98 viewed older adults in more stereotypical terms and indicated greater desire to avoid the company of same-aged individuals, compared to individuals ages 68–73 (Bodner et al., 2012). Examples of hostile ageism are evident in common stereotypes of older adults as frail, lacking competence, and having poor memory or generally compromised cognition. In the more benevolent vein, older individuals may be stereotyped as wise, kind individuals in need of assistance or support. Indeed, young adults generally view older adults as being high in warmth and low in competence (Cuddy et al., 2005; O'Connor & McFadden, 2012), which can inadvertently encourage dependent behavior among older adults (Baltes & Wahl, 1996). In this sense, older people are generally viewed as less competitive for resources and are met with pity (Cuddy et al., 2005)—a reaction most frequently directed downward in the social pecking order. Of course, positive attitudes about aging and older adulthood can exist in the absence of benevolent ageism. However, positive stereotypes about and attributions toward older adults are far less common, and negative stereotypes about aging have increased over time (Ng et al., 2015) and are more impactful than positive age-related stereotypes (Meisner, 2012).

Aside from culturally embedded negative perceptions of aging, there is evidence for the interconnectedness of mortality salience and older individuals. Young adult participants had greater death-thought accessibility after viewing photographs of older adults compared to participants who viewed photographs of young adults, suggesting that older adults act as a reminder of mortality for young adults. Furthermore, young adults rated older adults less favorably and rated themselves as being less similar to older adults only after mortality salience but not after an aversive control topic unrelated to death; this pattern was not observed in similarity ratings when the comparison group included teenagers (Martens et al., 2004). Greater death-related anxiety among college students has also been associated with greater fear about looking older (Chonody & Teater, 2016). And young adults had the highest levels of death-thought accessibility after reading about an older adult diagnosed with dementia compared to young and older adults with any other health condition (O'Connor & McFadden, 2012). Taken together, these results point to the existential component of aging and ageism as well as the unique position of dementia in existential concerns, as I discuss later in this chapter.

DEATH ANXIETY IN LATER LIFE

In spite of the changes and losses occurring in late life and the many examples of ageism and association of older adults with mortality, older adulthood is not without its advantages. The accumulation of life experience and wisdom are benefits of the aging process and appear to be reflected in the general tendency for older adults to have greater positive affect and lower negative affect (Carstensen et al., 2011; Mroczek & Kolarz, 1998), greater satisfaction (Carstensen, 1992) and less stress associated with interpersonal relationships (Birditt et al., 2005), and more stable self-esteem (Meier et al., 2011) compared to young adults. According to TMT, the maintenance of self-esteem, meaningful interpersonal connections, and sources of meaning support psychological well-being and provide a buffer to help manage the anxiety, particularly death-related anxiety, suggesting that older adults may be well-equipped to manage this existential concern.

Age-Related Differences in Self-Reported Death Anxiety

In terms of straightforward self-reports, the relationship between death-related anxiety and age is somewhat unclear but generally suggests there are age-related shifts. In a study spanning the adult lifespan, death anxiety was highest among people in their 20s and declined in successive decades, leveling out by age 60. Women in their early 50s were an exception, as they exhibited a "secondary spike" of death anxiety though levels were still lower than individuals in their 20s (Russac et al., 2007). Of note, women generally reported higher death-related anxiety than men, in this study and others. Various explanations have been offered as to why, including women's tendency to acknowledge and discuss fears more openly than men, greater likelihood of serving in a caregiver role of an older adult compared to men (Kastenbaum, 2000), and greater external locus of control, which has been associated with greater death-related anxiety (Sadowski et al., 1979). A review of studies investigating death anxiety specifically among older adults suggests that death anxiety peaks in midlife, then declines into older adulthood before stabilizing in very old age (Fortner & Neimeyer, 1999). Importantly though, most studies of death-related anxiety among older adults include community-dwelling samples in relatively good health, and results may be less representative of the experience of feelings about mortality when very close to life's end. Limited studies with residents of nursing homes and individuals with more physi cal problems seem to report greater death-related anxiety (for a review, see Fortner et al., 2000), highlighting both the heterogeneity of older adults and the many variables influencing death-related anxiety.

An additional limitation is the predominant cross-sectional approach to examining death-related anxiety, thus providing insight into what may be cohort effects. However, longitudinal work with adults ages 50–90 years old seems supportive of the existing literature, with death-related anxiety declining over a span of 4 years, even after controlling for self-perceived health, chronic illnesses, and gender (Chopik, 2017). In support of TMT's supposition that close interpersonal relationships provide protection from death-related anxiety, individuals with greater social support reported lower fear of death over time (Chopik, 2017). Notably, this study used a single item to measure frequency of death fear over the past week, thus providing a limited, more simplistic assessment compared to the majority of investigations of self-reported death anxiety. Nevertheless, its consistency with other studies supports the general pattern of decline in death-related anxiety with age.

Death-related anxiety may change according to developmental stage. Per Erikson's (1950) theory of psychosocial development, older adulthood is generally characterized by the challenge of achieving ego integrity, or acceptance of and satisfaction with one's life, as opposed to despair, or the sense of failure and regret about the past. Greater levels of ego integrity are associated with lesser death-related anxiety (Haroon et al., 2018), even more so among older adults in independent living situations compared to those residing in a nursing home (Goebel & Boeck, 1987). Among older adults, pessimism is associated with greater death anxiety, though optimism is not (Barnett et al., 2018), and older adults' religiosity, specifically intrinsic beliefs, also predicts greater ego integrity, which is associated with lower death anxiety (Hui & Coleman, 2013).

Aside from ego integrity and religious beliefs, beliefs about aging are also associated with death-related anxiety. Among older adults, more anxiety about one's own aging process and negative views and stereotypes of older adults were both associated with greater death-related anxiety (DePaola et al., 2003). Among a sample of adults (29–100 years old), aging anxiety and death anxiety were positively associated (Bodner et al., 2015). Self-reported death anxiety is not necessarily predictive of responses to reminders of mortality (e.g., Greenberg et al., 1995). A series of studies using TMT methods presents additional insight into age-related differences in behavioral responses to increased awareness of death.

Age-Related Differences in Responses to Mortality Salience

Initial hypotheses about older adults' responses to mortality salience were tentative. Being closer to life's end and experiencing more frequent and personal reminders of mortality, such as the deaths of similarly aged individuals and changes in their own health status, may lead older adults to display greater defensiveness in response to mortality salience. It is also possible that increased exposure to death-related reminders could create a level of immunity, such that older adults have no noticeable response to increased awareness of mortality. Lastly, the literature on emotional well-being in late life may point to greater acceptance of death, surfacing in decreased defensiveness among older adults.

Empirical studies of older adults' reactions to mortality affirmed each of these possible outcomes, highlighting the importance of moderating variables and study methods. My colleagues and I (2007) initially observed that older adults did not respond to a mortality salience induction with increased defensiveness (Study 1); we therefore considered the possibility that older adults were no longer affected by mortality salience. However, older adults displayed lower levels of defensiveness after exposure to a subtle reminder of death (e.g., death-related words embedded in a word search puzzle) compared to a control condition (Study 2), suggesting that older adults still respond to mortality salience but in less defensive, more positively oriented ways that may indicate a level of acceptance of death. A follow-up study revealed that executive functioning (a complex set of cognitive skills associated with decision making, reasoning, and managing multiple sources of information, among other things) moderated older, but not younger adults' responses to death (Maxfield et al., 2012). Greater executive functioning among older adults predicted less punitive responses toward moral transgressors after a mortality reminder, whereas lesser executive functioning among older adults was associated with greater punitiveness following a mortality reminder. In this sense, we learned that some older adults, specifically those with lesser executive functioning, maintained the defensiveness of traditional cultural worldviews observed among young adults. The moderating effect of executive functioning was specific to older adults though. Among young adults, mortality salience led to greater defensiveness compared to an aversive control, regardless of their executive-functioning status. Interestingly, memory functioning did not moderate mortality salience effects for older or young participants, suggesting that it is the specific combination of complex executive functioning and the experience of age that is critical to positively managing responses to mortality salience.

It appeared, then, that older adults were responsive to mortality salience, but that responses may be more positively oriented in this age range. Perhaps the changes in humans' social, physical, and cognitive functioning that occur with age require changes in approaches to defending against death. Based on Erikson's (1950) work suggesting that increasing age is accompanied by increased concern for future generations, my colleagues and I considered the possibility that reminders of mortality would lead to greater generative concern among older, but not young adults. In fact, older adults report greater generative concern after contemplating mortality compared to those in a control condition. The same pattern was not observed among young adults, as their generative concern did not vary according to experimental condition (Maxfield et al., 2014). Further, older adults' greater generative concern after a reminder of death remains, even after controlling for preexisting levels of generativity (Major et al., 2016). This pattern extends to generative behavior in the form of charitable giving, too. Older adults in a mortality salience condition made larger donations compared to older adults in a control condition, whereas young adults made smaller donations in a mortality salience condition compared to a control condition, and middle-aged adults' donations did not differ according to condition (Roberts & Maxfield, 2019). This set of results suggests that greater awareness of death among older adults prompts concern for future generations and others in need, and the findings also affirm that the anxiety-buffering system changes over time, allowing for adjustments to accommodate one's ability to bolster self-esteem, cultural worldviews, and relationships.

Examples of findings in which older and young adults respond similarly emerged when examining proximal defenses aimed at distancing one's self from death via health-promoting intentions. Immediately following a reminder of death, both young and older adults report greater intentions to engage in health-promoting behaviors compared to those in the control condition (Bevan et al., 2014). Interestingly, when midlife adults (ages 51–65) were included in a similar study, they reported lower health-related intentions after a mortality salience prime (Taubman-Ben-Ari & Findler, 2005). It thus appears that the desire to delay death via intentions to be healthy remains intact in young and older adulthood, but not midlife, thus highlighting the importance of including middle-aged participants in terror management studies. Midlife adults not only report the highest levels of explicit death-related anxiety (Fortner et al., 2000) but also respond to mortality salience with the counterintuitive approach of lower intentions for health-promoting behavior to delay death (Taubman-Ben-Ari & Findler, 2005). Middle-aged participants have been largely absent in terror management research, and their inclusion in future studies is important to understand strategies for managing death-related across the adult lifespan.

That older adults are able to manage their responses to mortality salience in arguably healthy ways is particularly impressive in the context of diminishing future time perspective (Brothers et al., 2014), raising the question: How do they do it? Several theories of aging put these findings into context and illuminate the ways older adults manage existential anxiety. The selection, optimization, and compensation (SOC) model suggests that age-related physical and/or cognitive declines are addressed by selectively engaging in fewer activities to focus on and optimize one's performance, perhaps using compensatory strategies when needed (Baltes & Baltes, 1990). In a similar vein, the lifespan theory of control proposes that the ways people manage a situation change over time. Typically, with age, people shift from focusing on primary control, in which people aim to control external environment and factors to create favorable situations, to secondary control, in which people adjust their internal reactions to the external environment (Heckhausen & Schulz, 1995). In reference to both the SOC model and lifespan theory of control, it may be that older adults are letting go of former sources of self-esteem that are no longer available to them and focusing on interests, relationships, and activities that are available, in combination with adjustment of internal expectations and reactions to their current level of functioning. In this way, as one's ability to maintain self-esteem and close relationships and meet the standards of the cultural worldview change over the lifespan, one must identify alternative sources of validation and self-esteem in order to develop an effective anxiety-buffering system. Yet cognitive functioning appears key to making these adjustments. Dynamic integration theory posits that the maintenance of cognitive resources provides the foundation upon which older adults can integrate, learn, and grow from their life experience to effectively regulate their emotions (Labouvie-Vief, 2009), as may be needed when confronted with reminders of mortality. And socioemotional selectivity theory suggests that the dwindling future time perspective associated with aging leads older adults to prioritize relationships and experiences known to boost positive emotions (Carstensen et al., 1999). That this orientation toward positivity is more pronounced among older adults with greater cognitive functioning (e.g., Knight et al., 2007; Mather & Knight, 2005) aligns with TMT findings that preservation of complex cognitive abilities is necessary for managing responses to mortality reminders (Maxfield et al., 2012). Importantly, the majority of the findings reviewed here include community-dwelling older adults who are able to participate in such research and exhibit intact or above average cognitive functioning. Therefore, positive adaptations to the challenges of aging may be more accessible to older adults in good health.

PRIMARY EXISTENTIAL CONCERNS IN LATER LIFE

Certainly, health is associated with quality of life (Michalos et al., 2000, 2001), creating a challenge for many older adults, as physical changes accumulate with age (National Council on Aging, 2022) and may result in declines in functioning or independence (Barile et al., 2013). And while advances in medical treatments delay death, some diagnoses and treatments may result in significant diminishments in daily life, as will be discussed in the next section. Here, I note that people anticipate that living with some diagnoses may be so threatening to their sense of self and meaning that they prefer death rather than continuing to live in a compromised state. Specifically, older adults are increasingly concerned about Alzheimer's disease and related dementias (ADRD), and they have identified Alzheimer's diseases as one of the most feared diagnoses (MetLife Foundation, 2011; Pitts, 2023). ADRD are prevalent (approximately 6.7 million Americans are living with Alzheimer's disease; Alzheimer's Association, 2023), are without cures, and are technically terminal, though they are not always thought of or treated as terminal diseases (Harrison et al., 2019). Dementias' symptom profiles affect cognitive functions, such as memory, language receptivity and expressivity, decision making, and reasoning, which contribute to declining functional independence. Dementias are associated with fluctuations in mood and changes in relationships related to increasing need for support and changing social engagement. Taken together, the symptoms of ADRD are uniquely terrifying in their ubiquity. Particularly in the earlier stages of dementia, people maintain awareness of the changes they are experiencing and may therefore be acutely aware of the secondary consequences of ADRD, which include negative effects on self-esteem, close relationships, and sources of meaning—the components of the anxiety-buffering system.

In early terror management study debriefings, several older participants reported that death would be preferable to living with Alzheimer's disease, leading researchers to examine dementia as an existential threat, one that might even be greater than death. Everyone experiences some degree of age-related cognitive decline (Salthouse, 2019), and most people know or have known someone with dementia. People therefore have some degree of familiarity with these diagnoses, yet their causes and means for reducing risk are complex, creating opportunities for confusion and worry among cognitively healthy individuals. The concept of *dementia-related anxiety* (also referred to as *dementia worry* or *anticipatory dementia*) is the fear of currently or eventually having a diagnosis of Alzheimer's disease or another type of dementia (Kessler et al., 2012).

The idea of dementia as a source of worry has been examined within the context of middle-aged adults, who have witnessed the deterioration of a parent with ADRD. They may fear experiencing a similar downward trajectory, often interpreting everyday forgetfulness as signs of an oncoming dementia process, often referred to as anticipatory dementia (Cutler & Hodgson, 1996). In longitudinal studies, individuals without objective cognitive impairment who report the subjective sense of cognitive decline that is worrisome are at greater risk for ADRD, suggesting that subjective decline when combined with worry may be an early indicator of ADRD (Jessen et al., 2014). Dementia-related anxiety can therefore be difficult to categorize—is the fear an unnecessary reaction to normal age-related decline? Or are the concerns an early indicator of a looming, dreaded disease?

Given dementia's ability to destabilize so many aspects of daily life, my colleagues and I anticipated that multiple factors could contribute to dementia-related anxiety, at least some of which would be existential in nature. A mixed-methods study, designed to assess what makes dementia so anxiety provoking, revealed clear existential themes in the causes of dementia-related anxiety, ways of coping with it, and its potential consequences. Middle-aged and older adults without dementia diagnoses were asked a series of open-ended questions concerning their thoughts and feelings about dementia, including their anticipated response to an imagined diagnosis of dementia (Maxfield et al., 2024). An inductive thematic analysis revealed several contributing factors, and themes with the most obviously existential undertones included fear of becoming a burden to others, fear of losing one's sense of self, and loss of independence and control. Similarly, a follow-up analysis of methods for managing dementia-related anxiety also uncovered parallels with the anxiety-buffering system (Maxfield et al., 2025). For example, a number of respondents cited interpersonal relationships as a source of comfort, noting close others could provide emotional and instrumental support and could be trusted to make the right decisions for their care if they themselves no longer had decisional capacity. Others sought comfort in the process of preparing and planning for the future, thereby allowing for end-of-life preparation in line with their personal values (affirmation of the cultural worldview) and as a way to minimize burden on close others (maintenance of relationships). Participants expressed personal responsibility to minimize their dementia risk via health-promoting behaviors, which grants a sense of control to avoid a disease process that is often viewed as uncontrollable, thus boosting self-esteem (Maxfield et al., 2025). Originally developed to understand death-related anxiety, the components of TMT's anxiety-buffering system appear to apply to dementia-related anxiety as well.

For some, a future dementia diagnosis represents a type of social death or death of the self. Among the same middle-aged and older adults interviewed about their thoughts and feelings about dementia, 42% of respondents anticipated that they would wish for hastened death (n = 14, 28%) or anticipated a more active desire to end their lives (n = 7, 14%) *if* they were diagnosed with ADRD (Maxfield et al., 2023). Merely imagining a dementia diagnosis prompts a sizable number of cognitively healthy middle-aged and older adults to anticipate a preference for death rather than life with compromised cognitive ability. Within the comments about the anticipated desire to limit life with dementia, three existentially charged themes emerged: concern about burdening others with one's care, devaluation of life and self with dementia, and desire for control. This sample was a predominantly White, highly educated population, and the findings likely reflect the strong emphasis certain groups place on cognitive status, for the reasons listed above—cognitive functioning is linked to maintaining the freedoms associated with living independently and avoiding burdening close others (Maxfield et al., 2024).

Of course, these are *anticipated* reactions to an imagined dementia diagnosis and may therefore be prone to affective forecasting errors often observed when considering future events believed to be highly impactful (Wilson & Gilbert, 2005). Although there are some findings documenting a lack of psychological distress in research settings after receiving a diagnosis (Carpenter et al., 2008) or test results documenting genetic risk for dementia (Galluzzi et al., 2022), there are also clear risk factors for suicide completion related to a dementia diagnosis: early onset cases (before age 65; Alothman et al., 2022), psychiatric diagnoses predating the dementia diagnosis (Choi et al., 2021), and soon after diagnosis (first 90 days; Alothman et al., 2022; Schmutte et al., 2022). It appears, then, that many people view a life with dementia as less valuable or tolerable based on dementia's anticipated ability to undermine key elements of self, meaning, freedom, and connectedness. Of course, the devaluation of life with dementia raises important and challenging questions about end-of-life decision making within the context of a disease process with the capacity to negatively affect complex decision making.

THE ROLE OF DEATH-RELATED ANXIETY IN END-OF-LIFE PLANNING AND CARE

Numerous medical advances over the past century have helped in the ongoing quest to push death into the future via longer lifespans. However, the medical advances that allow for longer lives inevitably lead to longer deaths. There is great variability in aging processes, particularly in terms of physical and cognitive health. Nevertheless, the medical side of aging is evident in that 94.9% of adults age 60 and older have at least one chronic health condition and 78.7% have two or more chronic health conditions (National Council on Aging, 2022). Furthermore, living with chronic health conditions creates challenges for quality of life, especially if one has multiple conditions (Barile et al., 2013). For better or worse, the combination of medical advances with high rates of chronic health conditions has led to a phenomenon frequently referred to as "medicalized" mortality—an approach to treat conditions and diseases to avoid death without consideration of patients' daily life. And this medicalization of mortality is particularly relevant for older adults, who may begin to feel defined by the age-related changes for which they are receiving treatment.

Diagnoses with more severe symptoms may lead to chronic pain and/or significant declines in functioning and independence that undermine quality of life to the extent some may question the meaning and value in living. The Death with Dignity movement focuses on providing the right to die a "good death" via a range of options, such as refusing or stopping life-sustaining treatments and even seeking medical aid in dying, also referred to as physician-assisted death, physician-assisted suicide, or euthanasia. Currently, 10 states and Washington, D.C., allow physician-assisted suicide. There are limited studies investigating *how* access to medical aid in dying influences the dying process, but research shows that individuals who seek out and use medical aid in dying are more likely to be male, older, well educated, and White, and cancer is by far the most common diagnosis (Kozlov et al., 2022). In a study limited to Oregon residents with advanced disease processes, those who sought out physician-assisted death had more years of education, were more likely to be unmarried, and reported higher levels of depression, hopelessness, and dismissive attachment styles, along with lower levels of spirituality compared to those who did not seek assistance with ending their lives (Smith et al., 2015). Physician-assisted death is a relatively recent option with minimal associated literature but the available research suggests that maintaining quality of life is central to the desire for continued life.

Aside from the desire to actively seek life's end, there are also medical decisions to manage care toward the end of life, often referred to as end-of-life care planning or advance care planning. This type of planning creates opportunities to express preferences for care, alleviates the need for decision making during stressful situations, and relieves family members of the burden of guessing how the individual would like to be treated. From the perspective of TMT, advance care planning should be appealing in that it provides opportunities to make decisions in line with personal values; however, TMT would also predict that people who are prone to avoid active focus on death-related topics would find the process of end-of-life planning to be a particular challenge. In fact, individuals who report avoidance of death-related thoughts are less likely to have completed health care and financial planning (Carr, 2012; Carr & Khodyakov, 2007). However, older age, experiencing the death of a loved one, poorer health, and recent hospitalizations predict greater likelihood of discussing one's end-of-life preferences (Carr, 2012; Carr & Khodyakov, 2007; Moorman & Inoue, 2013), providing more evidence that older adults' responses to mortality salience are different. Still though, only 28.8% of adults ages 65 and older have completed all components of advance care planning (Block et al., 2020), with many people delaying or avoiding the process, viewing it as unnecessary or aversive (Schickedanz et al., 2009). Further complicating a hard situation, providers also identify conversations about advance care plans as aversive and report difficulty knowing how or when to approach the topic (Tilburgs et al., 2018), highlighting the fact that avoidance of death-related conversations in medical settings may come from multiple sources. Among chronically ill older adults, those who were more religious and reported lower fear of death were more likely to broach the topic of end-of-life care with a provider (Dobbs et al., 2012). However, it is important to note that providers' professional orientations toward avoiding literal mortality, particularly if associated with their own personal preferences to avoid the topic of mortality, may create yet another hurdle for managing quality of life and care at the end of life.

CONCLUSIONS

The physical and cognitive changes of older adulthood signify approaching existential threats, such as declining independence, loss of loved ones, and approaching mortality, yet the experience and emotional changes that occur with age grant a level of control and perspective that facilitate management of these existential threats. It is this perspective that allows older adults to experience less fear of death, respond to death-related reminders with more positive responses, support future generations, and maintain emotional equanimity well into late life. In considering *how* some older adults manage their death-related fear when life's literal end is approaching, I look to the work of several existentially oriented theorists emphasizing the importance of symbolic immortality. For example, Becker (1973), Rank (see Menaker, 1982), and Erikson (1950), among others, highlighted the ways people strive to continue on after their death—perhaps genetically via children and grandchildren; financially via donations to valued causes and named scholarships or buildings; professionally via awards and recognition; artistically via creation of cherished music, paintings, or sculptures; and so on. Inspired by these theorists, TMT suggests that the troublesome awareness of literal mortality is combatted with sources of symbolic immortality. With age then, symbolic immortality becomes increasingly crucial for managing existential anxiety.

Importantly though, older adulthood is not without anxieties. As Atul Gawande (2014) wrote of his older patients: "It is not death that the very old tell me they fear. It is what happens short of death—losing their hearing, their memory, their best friends, their way of life." In this sense, viewing life and time as finite resources is not necessarily problematic regarding fear of one's own death, but fears of the many changes that could affect integrity of the self and identity, relevance of an increasingly outdated cultural worldview, sense of control and independence, and connections to close others remain. The apparent contrast between accumulation of loss and functioning with emotional well-being is often referred to as the "paradox of aging." It is important to remember, though, that the majority of experimental existential studies have focused on death-related anxiety and included community-dwelling older adults who maintain a level of independence and health that permits participation in these types of studies. Additional work investigating the anxiety-buffering systems of healthy older adult samples will advance our understanding of existential anxiety in late life. Furthermore, inquiries addressing shifting sources of fear and meaning in later life and studies including older adults with a greater range of physical and cognitive changes would be valuable additions to the literature addressing the questions of existence in the final stages of life.

REFERENCES

Alonso Debreczeni, F., & Bailey, P. E. (2020). A systematic review and meta-analysis of subjective age and the association with cognition, subjective well-being, and depression. *The Journals of Gerontology: Psychological and Social Sciences, 76*(3), 471–482.

Alothman, D., Card, T., Lewis, S., Tyrrell, E., Fogarty, A. W., & Marshall, C. R. (2022). Risk of suicide after dementia diagnosis. *JAMA Neurology, 79*(11), 1148–1154.

Alzheimer's Association. (2023). 2023 Alzheimer's disease facts and figures. *Alzheimer's and Dementia, 19*(4), 1598–1695.

Astell, A. J., McGrath, C., & Dove, E. (2020). "That's for old so and so's!": Does identity influence older adults' technology adoption decisions? *Ageing and Society, 40,* 1550–1576.

Aydogmus, M. E., & Gunbas, N. (2024). Psychological and demographic characteristics of older adults in cartoons on Netflix. *Journal of the American Geriatrics Society.*

Baltes, M. M., & Wahl, H. W. (1996). Patterns of communication in old age: The dependence-support and independence-ignore script. *Health Communication, 8*(3), 217–231.

Baltes, P. B., & Baltes, M. M. (1990). Psychological perspectives on successful aging: The model of selective optimization and compensation. In P. B. Baltes & M. M. Baltes (Eds.), *Successful aging: Perspectives from behavioral sciences* (pp. 1–34). Cambridge University Press.

Barile, J. P., Thompson, W. W., Zack, M. M., Krahn, G. L., Horner-Johnson, W., & Bowen, S. E. (2013). Multiple chronic medical conditions and health-related quality of life in older adults, 2004–2006. *Preventing Chronic Disease, 10,* 120282.

Barnett, M. D., Anderson, E. A., & Marsden, D. A. III. (2018). Is death anxiety more closely linked with optimism or pessimism among older adults? *Archives of Gerontology and Geriatrics, 77,* 169–173.

Becker, E. (1973). *The denial of death.* Free Press.

Bevan, A. L., Maxfield, M., & Bultmann, M. N. (2014). The effects of age and death awareness on intentions for health behaviours. *Psychology and Health, 29,* 409–421.

Birditt, K. S., Fingerman, K. L., & Almeida, D. M. (2005). Age differences in exposure and reactions to interpersonal tensions: A daily diary study. *Psychology and Aging, 20*(2), 330–340.

Block, B. L., Jeon, S. Y., Sudore, R. L., Matthay, M. A., Boscardin, W. J., & Smith, A. K. (2020). Patterns and trends in advance care planning among older adults who received intensive care at the end of life. *JAMA Internal Medicine, 180*(5), 786–789.

Bodner, E., Bergman, Y. S., & Cohen-Fridel, S. (2012). Different dimensions of ageist attitudes among men and women: A multigenerational perspective. *International Psychogeriatrics, 24*(6), 895–901.

Bodner, E., Shrira, A., Bergman, Y. S., & Cohen-Fridel, S. (2015). Anxieties about aging and death and psychological distress: The protective role of emotional complexity. *Personality and Individual Differences, 86,* 15–19.

Brothers, A., Chui, H., & Diehl, M. (2014). Measuring future time perspective across adulthood: Development and evaluation of a brief multidimensional questionnaire. *The Gerontologist, 54,* 1075–1088.

Carpenter, B. D., Xiong, C., Porensky, E. K., Lee, M. M., Brown, P. J., Coats, M., Johnson, D., & Morris, J. C. (2008). Reaction to a dementia diagnosis in individuals with Alzheimer's disease and mild cognitive impairment. *Journal of the American Geriatrics Society, 56*(3), 405–412.

Carr, D. (2012). The social stratification of older adults' preparations for end-of-life care. *Journal of Health and Social Behavior, 53,* 297–312.

Carr, D., & Khodyakov, D. (2007). End-of-life health care planning among young-old adults: An assessment of psychosocial influences.

Journals of Gerontology: Psychological and Social Sciences, 62B, S135–S141.

Carstensen, L. L. (1992). Social and emotional patterns in adulthood: Support for socioemotional selectivity theory. *Psychology and Aging, 7,* 331–338.

Carstensen, L. L., Isaacowitz, D. M., & Charles, S. T. (1999). Taking time seriously: A theory of socioemotional selectivity. *American Psychologist, 54,* 165–181.

Carstensen, L. L., Turan, B., Scheibe, S., Ram, N., Ersner-Hershfield, H., Samanez-Larkin, G. R., Brooks, K. P., & Nesselroade, J. R. (2011). Emotional experience improves with age: Evidence based on over 10 years of experience sampling. *Psychology and Aging, 26*(1), 21–33.

Choi, J. W., Lee, K. S., & Han, E. (2021). Suicide risk within 1 year of dementia diagnosis in older adults: A nationwide retrospective cohort study. *Journal of Psychiatry and Neuroscience, 46*(1), E119–E127.

Chonody, J. M., & Teater, B. (2016) Why do I dread looking old?: A test of social identity theory, terror management theory, and the double standard of aging. *Journal of Women and Aging, 28*(2), 112–126.

Chopik, W. J. (2017). Death across the lifespan: Age differences in death-related thoughts and anxiety. *Death Studies, 41*(2) 69–77.

Chopik, W. J., Bremner, R. H., Johnson, D. J., & Giasson, H. L. (2018). Age differences in age perceptions and developmental transitions. *Frontiers in Psychology, 9,* 67.

Cuddy, A. J. C., Norton, M. I., & Fiske, S. T. (2005). This old stereotype: The pervasiveness and persistence of the elderly stereotype. *Journal of Social Issues, 61,* 267–285.

Cutler, S. J., & Hodgson, L. G. (1996). Anticipatory dementia: A link between memory appraisals and concerns about developing Alzheimer's disease. *The Gerontologist, 36*(5), 657–664.

DePaola, S. J., Griffin, M., Young, J. R., & Neimeyer, R. A. (2003). Death anxiety and attitudes toward the elderly among older adults: The role of gender and ethnicity. *Death Studies 27*(4), 335–354.

Dobbs, D., Emmett, C. P., Hammarth, A., & Daaleman, T. P. (2012). Religiosity and death attitudes and engagement of advance care planning among chronically ill older adults. *Research on Aging, 34*(2), 113–130.

Erikson, E. (1950). *Childhood and society.* Norton.

Fortner, B. V., & Neimeyer, R. A. (1999). Death anxiety in older adults: A quantitative review. *Death Studies, 23*(5), 387–411.

Fortner, B. V., Neimeyer, R. A., & Rybarczyk, B. (2000). Correlates of death anxiety in older adults: A comprehensive review. In A. Tomer (Ed.), *Death attitudes and the older adult: Theories, concepts, and applications* (pp. 95–108). Brunner-Routledge.

Galluzzi, S., Mega, A., Di Fede, G., Muscio, C., Fascendini, S., Benussi, L., . . . Di Maria, E. (2022). Psychological impact of predictive genetic testing for inherited Alzheimer disease and frontotemporal dementia: The IT-DIAfN Protocol. *Alzheimer's Disease and Associated Disorders, 36*(2), 118–124.

Gawande, A. (2014). *Being mortal: Medicine and what matters in the end.* Metropolitan Books.

Goebel, B. L., & Boeck, B. E. (1987). Ego integrity and fear of death: A comparisons or institutionalized and independently living older adults. *Death Studies, 11*(3), 193–204.

Greenberg, J., Pyszczynski, T., & Solomon, S. (1986). The causes and consequences of a need for self-esteem: A terror management theory. In R. F. Baumeister (Ed.), *Public self and private self* (pp. 189–212). Springer.

Greenberg, J., Simon, L., Harmon-Jones, E., Solomon, S., Pyszczynski, T., & Lyon, D. (1995). Testing alternative explanations for mortality salience effects: Terror management, value accessibility, or worrisome thoughts. *European Journal of Social Psychology, 12,* 417–433.

Haroon, W., Khawaja, A. O., & Ghayas, S. (2018). Ego integrity, physical health status and death anxiety in older adults. *Journal of Behavioural Sciences, 28*(1), 18–32.

Harrison, K. L., Hunt, L. J., Ritchie, C. S., & Yaffe, K. (2019). Dying with dementia: Underrecognized and stigmatized. *Journal of American Geriatrics Society, 67*(8), 1548–1551.

Heckhausen, J., & Schulz, R. (1995). A lifespan theory of control. *Psychological Review, 102*(2), 284–304.

Hui, V. K. Y., & Coleman, P. G. (2013). Afterlife beliefs and ego integrity as two mediators of the relationship between intrinsic religiosity and personal death anxiety among older adult British Christians. *Research on Aging, 35*(2), 144–162.

Jessen, F., Amariglio, R. E., Boxtel, M., Breteler, M., Ceccaldi, M., Chételat, G., . . . Subjective Cognitive Decline Initiative (SCD-I) Working Group. (2014). A conceptual framework for research on subjective cognitive decline in preclinical Alzheimer's disease. *Alzheimer's and Dementia, 10*(6), 844–852.

Kastenbaum, R. (2000). *The psychology of death* (3rd ed.). Springer.

Kessler, E. M., Bowen, C. E., Baer, M., Froelich, L., & Wahl, H. W. (2012) Dementia worry: A psychological examination of an unexplored

phenomenon. *European Journal of Ageing, 9*(4), 275–284.
Kite, M. E., Stockdale, G. D., Whitley, B. E., Jr., & Johnson, B. T. (2005). Attitudes toward younger and older adults: An updated meta-analytic review. *Journal of Social Issues, 61*(2), 241–266.
Knight, M., Seymour, T. L., Gaunt, J. T., Baker, C., Nesmith, L., & Mather, M. (2007). Aging and goal-directed emotional attention: Distraction reverses emotional biases. *Emotion, 7,* 705–714.
Kozlov, E., Nowels, M., Gusmano, M., Habib, M., & Duberstein, P. (2022). Aggregating 23 years of data on medical aid in dying in the United States. *Journal of the American Geriatrics Society, 70*(10), 3040–3044.
Labouvie-Vief, G. (2009). Dynamic integration theory: Emotion, cognition, and equilibrium in later life. In V. L. Bengston, D. Gans, N. M. Pulney, & M. Silverstein (Eds.), *Handbook of theories of aging* (2nd ed., pp. 277–293). Springer.
Levy, B. R., Chung, P. H., Bedford, T., & Navrazhina, K. (2014). Facebook as a site for negative age stereotypes. *The Gerontologist, 54*(2), 172–176.
Lichtenstein, B. (2021). From "coffin dodger" to "boomer remover": Outbreaks of ageism in three countries with divergent approaches to Coronavirus control. *Journals of Gerontology: Psychological and Social Sciences, 76*(4), e206–e212.
Lin, S. S. H., & Walden, A. (2023). Ageism in birthday cards: A mixed-method content analysis. *The Gerontologist.*
Loos, E., & Ivan, L. (2018). Visual ageism in the media. In L. Ayalon & C. Tesch-Römer (Eds.), *Contemporary perspectives on ageism* (pp. 163–176). Springer.
Major, R. J., Whelton, W. J., Schimel, J., & Sharpe, D. (2016). Older adults and the fear of death: The protective function of generativity. *Canadian Journal on Aging, 35,* 261–272.
Martens, A., Greenberg, J., Schimel, J., & Landau, M. J. (2004). Ageism and death: Effects of mortality salience and perceived similarity to elders on reactions to elderly people. *Personality and Social Psychology Bulletin, 30,* 1524–1536.
Mather, M., & Knight, M. (2005). Goal-directed memory: The role of cognitive control in older adults' emotional memory. *Psychology and Aging, 20,* 554–570.
Maxfield, M., Greenberg, J., Pyszczynski, T., Weise, D., Kosloff, S., Soenke, M., . . . Blatter, J. (2014). Increases in generative concern among older adults following reminders of mortality. *International Journal of Aging and Human Development, 79,* 1–21.
Maxfield, M., Peckham, A., & James, D. L. (2024). "Terror is a better word": A qualitative analysis of dementia-related anxiety. *The Gerontologist.*
Maxfield, M., Peckham, A., James, D. L., & Koffer, R. E. (2025). "Why miss today worrying about tomorrow?": A qualitative investigation of ways to manage dementia-related anxiety. *Anxiety, Stress, and Coping, 38*(2), 219–233.
Maxfield, M., Peckham, A., James, D. L., Lathrop, L., & Fiske, A. (2023). Anticipated suicidal and death ideation in response to an imagined dementia diagnosis: A qualitative study. *Dementia, 22*(5), 1077–1096.
Maxfield, M., Pyszczynski, T., Cox, C., Kluck, B., Greenberg, J., Solomon, S., & Weise, D. (2007). Age related differences in responses to thoughts of one's own death: Mortality salience and judgments of moral transgressions. *Psychology and Aging, 22*(2), 341–353.
Maxfield, M., Pyszczynski, T., Greenberg, J., Pepin, R., & Davis, H. P. (2012). The moderating role of executive functioning in older adults' responses to a reminder of mortality. *Psychology and Aging, 27*(1), 256–263.
Meier, L. L., Orth, U., Denissen, J. A., & Kühnel, A. (2011). Age differences in instability, contingency, and level of self-esteem across the life span. *Journal of Research in Personality, 45,* 604–612.
Meisner, B. A. (2012). A meta-analysis of positive and negative age stereotype priming effects on behavior among older adults. *Journals of Gerontology: Psychological Sciences and Social Sciences, 67*(1), 13–17.
Menaker, E. (1982). *Otto Rank: A rediscovered legacy.* Columbia University Press.
MetLife Foundation. (2011). *What America thinks: MetLife Foundation Alzheimer's survey.* Harris Interactive.
Michalos, A. C., Hubley, A. M., Zumbo, B. D., & Hemingway, D. (2001). Health and other aspects of the quality of life of older people. *Social Indicators Research, 54*(3), 239–274.
Michalos, A. C., Zumbo, B. D., & Hubley, A. (2000). Health and the quality of life. *Social Indicators Research, 51,* 245–286.
Molden, J., & Maxfield, M. (2017). The impact of aging stereotypes on dementia worry. *European Journal of Ageing, 14*(1), 29–37.
Moorman, S. M., & Inoue, M. (2013). Persistent problems in end-of-life planning among young- and middle-aged American couples. *Journals of Gerontology: Psychological Sciences and Social Sciences, 68*(1), 97–106.
Mroczek, D. K., & Kolarz, C. M. (1998). The

effect of age on positive and negative affect: A developmental perspective on happiness. *Journal of Personality and Social Psychology,75,* 1333–1349.

National Council on Aging. (2022, April). *Chronic inequities: Measuring disease cost burden among older adults in the U.S.: A Health and Retirement Study analysis.* https://ncoa.org/article/the-inequities-in-the-cost-of-chronic-disease-why-it-matters-for-older-adults.

Ng, R., Allore, H. G., Trentalange, M., Monin, J. K., & Levy, B. R. (2015). Increasing negativity of age stereotypes across 200 years: Evidence from a database of 400 million words. *PLOS One, 10*(2), e0117086.

Ng, R., Indran, N., Yang, W. (2023). Portrayals of older adults in over 3000 films around the world. *Journal of the American Geriatrics Society, 71,* 2726–2735.

O'Connor, M. L., & McFadden, S. H. (2012). A terror management perspective on young adults' ageism and attitudes toward dementia. *Educational Gerontology, 38,* 627–643.

Pinquart, M., & Wahl, H.-W. (2021). Subjective age from childhood to advanced old age: A meta-analysis. *Psychology and Aging, 36*(3), 394–406.

Pitts, E. (2023, May 29). What diseases do Americans fear the most? *Deseret News.* www.deseret.com/2023/5/29/23721435/what-diseases-do-americans-fear-most-how-to-prevent-illness.

Roberts, J. R., & Maxfield, M. (2019). Mortality salience and age effects on charitable donations. *American Behavioral Scientist, 63*(14), 1863–1884.

Russac, R. J., Gatliff, C., Reece, M., & Spottswood, D. (2007). Death anxiety across the adult years: An examination of age and gender effects. *Death Studies, 31,* 549–561.

Sadowski, C. J., Davis, S. F., & Loftus-Vergari, M. C. (1979). Locus of control and death anxiety: A reexamination. *Omega, 10,* 203–210.

Salthouse, T. A. (2019). Trajectories of normal cognitive aging. *Psychology and Aging, 34*(1), 17–24.

Schickedanz, A. D., Schillinger, D., Landefeld, C. S., Knight, S. J., Williams, B. A., & Sudore, R. L. (2009). A clinical framework for improving the advance care planning process: Start with patients' self-identified barriers. *Journal of the American Geriatrics Society, 57*(1), 31–39.

Schmutte, T., Olfson, M., Maust, D. T., Xie, M., & Marcus, S. C. (2022). Suicide risk in first year after dementia diagnosis in older adults. *Alzheimer's and Dementia, 18*(2), 262–271.

Smith, K. A., Harvath, T. A., Goy, E. R., & Ganzini, L. (2015). Predictors of pursuit of physician-assisted death. *Journal of Pain and Symptom Management, 49*(3), 555–561.

Solomon S., Greenberg J., & Pyszczynski T. (2015). *The worm at the core: On the role of death in life.* Random House.

Taubman-Ben-Ari, O., & Findler, L. (2005). Proximal and distal effects of mortality salience on willingness to engage in health promoting behavior along the life span. *Psychology and Health, 20,* 303–318.

Tilburgs, B., Vernooij-Dassen, M., Koopmans, R., van Gennip, H., Engels, Y., & Perry, M. (2018). Barriers and facilitators for GPs in dementia advance care planning: a systematic integrative review. *PLOS One, 13*(6), e0198535.

Vervaecke, D., & Meisner, B. A. (2021). Caremongering and assumptions of need: The spread of compassionate ageism during COVID-19. *The Gerontologist, 61*(2), 159–165.

Weiss, D., & Lang, F. R. (2012). "They" are old but "I" feel younger: Age-group dissociation as a self-protective strategy in old age. *Psychology and Aging, 27*(1), 153–163.

Wilson, T. D., & Gilbert, D. T. (2005). Affective forecasting: Knowing what to want. *Current Directions in Psychological Science, 14*(3), 131–134.

Yalom, I. D. (2008). *Staring at the sun: Overcoming the terror of death.* Josey-Bass.

SECTION III

FREEDOM, AUTHENTICITY, AND MORAL RESPONSIBILITY

CHAPTER 16

Developmental Research on Children's Understanding of Choice and Constraints

Xin Zhao

"I have no choice."
"You do have a choice. And you've made it."

This conversation in *Game of Thrones* happened between Ned Stark and his wife, Catelyn Stark, right before Ned left Catelyn in Winterfell to start his position as Hand of the King in King's Landing. The exchange illustrates how we constantly consider, contemplate, and evaluate our own and others' choices. As human beings, we make choices all the time, ranging from important life-determining choices, such as which university to attend or which job offer to accept, to less significant everyday choices, such as what to eat for breakfast or what to wear to work.

Although choices are not always explicitly conscious, a critical aspect of one's life is identifying and reasoning about the choices one has, as well as the constraints on those choices. One's understanding of choice and constraints, including what one considers to be "choices" and what constitutes constraints in certain contexts, are usually influenced by multiple factors, some originating from the external world (e.g., physical laws, sociomoral norms) and some from the internal world (e.g., desires, goals, motivations). For instance, when deciding whether to travel to King's Landing to take the position of Hand of the King, Ned Stark must consider the physical situation (the long distance he needs to travel from Winterfell to King's Landing) as well as the sociomoral situation (requests from his best friend, King Robert Baratheon, and his obligation to his wife, who apparently does not want him to leave). His reasoning about choice is certainly also influenced by his own mental state (his goal and motivation to contribute to the development of the country).

While everyone may share some intuitions about choice and a desire for autonomous choice (Leotti et al., 2010; Ryan & Deci, 2000b), there can be individual variation in what people perceive as choices and the factors they believe constrain their choices. Importantly, these considerations of choice and constraints often guide people's goal-pursuing actions: Individuals who believe themself able to *choose* to perform a certain action are more likely to act on that choice; while those who believe that they do not have the ability to choose a certain action are less likely to exert any effort toward it. Moreover, considerations of choice also influence how one judges others' actions; people tend to assess whether actors acted freely or were constrained, and what alternative actions were available to them. Thus, one's beliefs in choice and free will play crucial roles in grappling with existential questions concerning our freedom, control, and responsibility for one's actions, as well as one's identity developing and pursuit of goals in life.

The topic of people's views of choice has received much attention in social psychology. Adults consider various factors, including physical situations, sociomoral factors, and individual mental states when reasoning about their choices (Baumeister et al., 2007; Baumeister & Monroe, 2014; Iyengar & De Voe, 2003; Miller et al., 2011; Nadelhoffer et al., 2014; Paulhus & Carey, 2011; Savani et al., 2008). Furthermore, adults value the freedom to choose in both important life-determining choices and less important everyday choices (Botti & Iyengar, 2004; Cordova & Lepper, 1996; Leotti et al., 2010; Ryan & Deci, 2000a). Yet beyond this baseline commonality, research has shown individual and cultural variation in adults' perceptions of choices, especially regarding what they perceive as choices and what factors they prioritize in decision making (Iyengar & DeVoe, 2003; Iyengar & Lepper, 1999; Kitayama et al., 2004; Miller et al., 1990, 2011; Savani et al., 2010). Importantly, people's beliefs in free will and choice have implications for their self-control behaviors, academic and job performance, and moral behaviors and judgments (Baumeister et al., 2009; Feldman et al., 2016; Job et al., 2010; MacKenzie et al., 2014; Rigoni et al., 2012; Shariff et al., 2014; Stillman et al., 2010; Vohs & Schooler, 2008).

With these findings, questions arise as to the developmental origins of these understandings of choice. What do children perceive as choices? What factors do children consider constraining their choices? How do individual and cultural variation emerge in childhood? Do children value the freedom to choose? How may children's understanding of choice relate to their own actions and interpretations of others' actions? Recent developmental research has started to answer these questions. In this chapter, I first lay out the theoretical accounts and then review recent empirical evidence on the development of understanding of choice and constraints, and the implications of these understandings on children's own self-regulatory behaviors, as well as on their judgments of others' actions. I also examine research on children's recognition of the social value of choice. At the end, I outline fruitful directions for future research.

THEORETICAL FRAMEWORK

Decades of theory and research in developmental psychology have shown that children gradually develop increasingly mature "theories" and knowledge in the physical, psychological and sociomoral domains (e.g., Gopnik & Wellman, 2012; Schult & Wellman, 1997; Wellman & Gelman, 1992). They gradually understand the physical laws of space and time (e.g., Baillargeon, 2004; Spelke, 1994); reason about others' desires, preferences, beliefs, and emotions (e.g., Wellman, 2014); and acquire social and moral norms (e.g., Rakoczy et al., 2008; Smetana, 2006). By preschool age, children readily develop a causal framework for explaining events and actions with reference to knowledge in the appropriate domains (e.g., Hickling & Wellman, 2001; Schult & Wellman, 1997). I think these domain-specific theories and knowledge lay the foundation for children to understand choices and constraints. As children understand the causes and motives of actions (e.g., someone eating ice cream because that person likes ice cream), they also come to understand that these causes and motives can sometimes become constraints for alternative actions (e.g., one may not be able to resist eating something one likes; see Kushnir, 2018, 2022). Importantly, I argue (and show later in this chapter) that, in preschool years, children begin to gradually understand that these causes (whether psychological, sociomoral, or other) do not necessarily lead to actions but are mediated by one's choices: One can choose to act according to these causes, but can also choose to act otherwise. For example, children gradually understand that one can choose to eat ice cream because one likes it, but also that one can choose not to eat ice cream; and they gradually understand that one can choose to eat soup because one's mom asks one to do so, but also that that same person can choose not to eat soup.

These understandings operate based on domain-specific knowledge, such that children understand some factors may create stronger constraints on actions than others; for example, physical laws may create stronger constraints than psychological desires. See Figure 16.1 for the theoretical model.

Children may also understand that many factors can influence choice. Sometimes these factors are consistent with each other; for example, a child wants to play outside, and their mom also encourages them to do so. However, conflicts between motives can also arise. A typical case involves conflicts between psychological desires and sociomoral obligations. For instance, a child may want to play outside, but at the same time, their mom needs their help to clean up dishes. As children consider conflicting motives, they may also gradually recognize that choosing an alternative usually incurs a cost and can be challenging. This could lead to the understanding of the praiseworthiness of making a costly choice to do the right thing, such as giving up the opportunity to play outside in order to help one's mom. Additionally, an understanding of choice also involves recognizing that people desire the opportunity to choose, and thus that respecting others' freedom to choose, rather than depriving them of it, is socially desirable. I propose (and demonstrate) that these understandings manifest in children's understanding and regulations of their own behaviors, as well as in their interpretations and evaluations of others' behaviors.

Cultural and social contexts can shape the emphasis children and adults place on different factors or constraints. For example, different motives may carry varying weights in different cultures, thus constraining actions in different ways. Considering cultural differences in emphasis on independent mental states versus interdependent norms and obligations (e.g., Markus & Kitayama, 1991), there may be particular cultural differences in how much psychological versus sociomoral motives matter in choice. Also, these culture-specific emphases may also shape how children interpret their own behaviors, and thus further shape how beliefs in choice are linked to behaviors.

In summary, I believe that children gradually develop a model of choice to understand their own and others' actions. This process relies on a general understanding of choice and domain-specific knowledge of causes and constraints in various domains (physical, psychological, sociomoral). These understandings include recognition of what constitutes choices and constraints, consideration of multiple motives for choice,

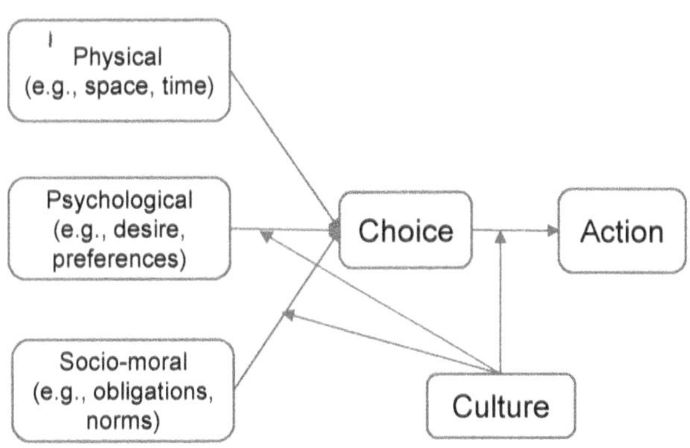

FIGURE 16.1. A theoretical model of children's understanding of choice. I propose that (1) children gradually understand that causes (e.g., physical, psychological, sociomoral) do not necessarily directly lead to actions but are mediated by one's choices: One can choose to act according to these causes, but they can also choose to act otherwise; (2) children gradually understand that multiple factors can influence choice and become increasingly able to consider conflicting motives and costly choice; and (3) culture can shape the emphasis children and adults place on different factors, particularly the relative importance of psychological versus sociomoral motives in influencing choice.

and the desire for choice. While explicit beliefs about choice and constraints may not emerge before preschool, previous work has suggested that some rudimentary sense of choice and constraints may already be in place in infancy and toddlerhood and may be evident in children's inferences of actions. Therefore, I briefly examine this work before presenting evidence on children's explicit beliefs about choice and constraints.

INFANCY AND TODDLERHOOD: CHOICES, CONSTRAINTS, AND INFERENCES OF HUMAN ACTIONS

When making inferences about human actions, even infants and toddlers not only care about the actual actions but also are sensitive to contextual information regarding whether the agent is "free to do otherwise" or is constrained. For example, in a classic study (Gergely et al., 2002), 14-month-olds saw an adult turn on a light box by leaning forward and touching its top with her forehead either freely (i.e., hands were free and were placed on the table) or with physical constraints (i.e., hands were occupied and constrained, as she was using her hands to wrap a blanket around herself). Infants were then asked to light up the box themselves. The rationale is that, in the constrained condition, the adult's hands were occupied; if she had had her hands free, she could have used her hands to light up the box. However, in the free condition, the adult could have used her hands to light up the box, but she didn't, and thus there must be some special meaning or function of using her head to touch the box. Therefore, if Gergely and colleagues' (2002) 14-month-olds understand this differentiation between constrained and freely chosen action, one would expect them to be more likely to imitate the exact action (using head to touch the box) in the free condition than in the constrained condition. This is exactly what Gergely and colleagues found. This differentiation between free versus constrained contexts has also been demonstrated in infants' inferences of preferences (Luo & Baillargeon, 2007; Ma & Xu, 2011), imitation (Gergely et al., 2002), predictions of future behaviors (Brandone & Wellman, 2009), and social learning (Behne et al., 2005).

There is also some indirect evidence suggesting that infants may have a desire for choice and an aversion to loss of control. In Sullivan and Lewis (2003), 4-month-old infants' actions of pulling initially led to slides and music; when these actions later became noncontingent and unpredictable, infants exhibited negative emotions, such as anger. Additionally, in another study, once infants acquired a skill, such as feeding or clothing themselves, they became resistant to parental attempts to control this ability (Kochanska & Aksan, 2004). These findings suggest that preference for choice and control may already be present in infancy.

In summary, some rudimentary intuition of choice and constraints seems to emerge as early as the first and second years of life. Infants and toddlers make inferences about agents' actions in a manner that is sensitive to whether the actions are free or constrained. Children also exhibit a desire for choice and control over their actions and environment. These reflections indicate children's early intuition of choice and constraints, which might serve as antecedents to a more explicit understanding of choice and constraints later in development.

EARLY AND MIDDLE CHILDHOOD: DEVELOPING BELIEFS ABOUT FREE WILL

Language development in childhood provides the opportunity to investigate children's explicit views about choice. A growing body of work on free will beliefs investigates how children across cultures explicitly reason about what they themselves and other people can choose to do and cannot choose to do (Chernyak et al., 2013; Kushnir, 2018; Kushnir et al., 2015). These studies show that some basic understanding of what are choices and what are not is already in place very early in development and shows little cultural variation: Children as young as 4 years old across cultures (United States, China, Singapore) say that one can freely choose to perform simple actions (e.g., getting off a stool), but cannot perform actions that are physically or epistemically constrained (e.g., floating in the air or copying a picture that cannot be seen, respectively; see Chernyak et al., 2013, 2019; Kushnir et al., 2015; Nichols, 2004; Wente et al., 2016; Zhao et al., 2021a).

In addition to physical or epistemic constraints, researchers have also investigated other more sophisticated motives and constraints that can shift children's reasoning about what are choices and what are not. One important type of constraint comes from internal desires. As adults, we think that even though one might really desire something, one can choose to act differently from one's desires. To investigate whether children hold such beliefs, a series of studies (Kushnir et al., 2015; Wente et al., 2016; Zhao et al., 2021a) asked children whether they thought someone could choose to refrain from a desired action (e.g., "Can Sally just choose to not eat a yummy cookie?") and whether someone could choose to engage in an undesired action (e.g., "Can Sally just choose to eat a bowl of yucky soup?"). The results showed that 4-year-olds seem to think one *has to* act according to their desires. It was not until age 6 or later that children across cultures (United States, China, Singapore, Peru) started to believe that one can *choose to* act against or inhibit their desires (Kushnir et al., 2015; Wente et al., 2016; Zhao et al., 2021a). There was also some cultural variation in that Singaporean and Peruvian children appeared to develop these free will beliefs about acting against desires later than U.S. and Chinese children did (Zhao et al., 2021a).

Another type of constraint comes from sociomoral norms. Using similar methods, studies have asked children in preschool and middle childhood to reason about whether one can choose to act against social or moral norms if one wants to. For example, in one story, children were asked if one can choose to wear pajamas to school even though it is not OK. They found that preschoolers across cultures typically did not believe one can choose to act against social or moral norms (Chernyak et al., 2013, 2019). Intriguingly, in middle childhood, children from Western and Eastern cultural contexts diverged in these beliefs (Chenrnyak et al., 2013; Kushnir, 2018). Around ages 7 and 8, U.S. children began to believe that one can choose to act contrary to social norms and conventions (Chernyak et al., 2013), whereas Singaporean and Nepalese children continued to believe that one cannot choose to do so and has to follow norms (Chernyak et al., 2013, 2019). Similarly, using more naturalistic and narrative measures, my colleague and I explored how U.S. and Chinese children talked about different types of choices—personal (toy preference), moral (sharing vs. stealing), and conventional (artifact use)—and found the most cultural differences in their stories about conventional choices: U.S. children were more likely to reference an agent's mental states (i.e., want, like), while Chinese children were more likely to use evaluative language (e.g., "It's weird/wrong") when talking about conventional choices (Zhao & Kushnir, 2019).

In short, during early and middle childhood, children across cultures begin to articulate beliefs about free will and choice with considerations of physical, internal, and sociomoral constraints. The developments of beliefs in free will and choice seem to differ by the types of constraints. Researchers observe more cultural similarities in consideration of physical and epistemic constraints but greater cultural variation in considerations of psychological and sociomoral constraints. Notably, these developing beliefs about free will and choice largely align with recent research revealing the development of imagination (Lane et al., 2016), counterfactual reasoning (Sobel, 2004), understanding of possibilities (Shtulman, 2009; Shtulman & Carey, 2007), and future thinking (Atance, 2008).

FREE WILL BELIEFS, CHOICE FREEDOM, AND BEHAVIORS: THE INFLUENCE OF CULTURE

As children gradually develop abstract beliefs in free will and choice, these beliefs can further shape how they perceive, interpret, and regulate their own behaviors, particularly in situations requiring difficult choices, such as self-control or prosocial behaviors. Recent research explores the relationship between children's beliefs in free will and self-control behaviors. In one study (Zhao et al., 2021a), my colleagues and I not only measured 4- to 8-year-olds' beliefs in free will to overcome desires using the items mentioned above (e.g., "Can Sally just choose to not eat a yummy cookie?"), but also administered a series of self-control tasks. For example, we conducted a toy-sort task where children were asked to sort a collection of attractive toys into baskets without playing with them. We found a positive relationship between children's belief in free will and their actual self-control behaviors among U.S. children. Those who were more likely to believe in free will to overcome desires were also more likely to perform better in self-control tasks. Along similar lines, recent theoretical arguments also suggest the possibility that choice may play an important role in executive functioning and self-regulation (Carlson, 2023).

Interestingly, my colleagues and I also found that the relationship between free will beliefs and self-control behaviors was moderated by culture; the correlation was only observed in the United States but not in the non-WEIRD (Western, educated, industrialized, rich, and democratic) cultures we sampled (China, Singapore, Peru; Zhao et al., 2021a). The culture-moderated relationship suggests that self-control may be experienced and interpreted differently across cultures. Previous research in cultural psychology indicated that individuals in U.S. and East Asian cultures differ in their views on the relationship between self and other, and on causal explanations of actions (e.g., Markus & Kityama, 1991; 2003; Morris & Peng, 1994). People in the United States tend to have an independent conception of self, and view intentional actions as stemming from individual desires, preferences, and subjective mental states, while people in East Asian cultures tend to have an interdependent conception of self, viewing agents as responding to situations, to social roles, and to expectations of other individuals. Consistent with this idea, children are socialized in quite different ways across cultures. When having conversations with their children, U.S. parents tend to emphasize individual mental states (e.g., preference, desires), while Asian parents tend to emphasize social norms and rules, and others' expectations (Wang, 2006). These cultural messages may shape how children interpret their self-control experience. U.S. children may interpret self-control as internally driven (e.g., by desires) and see their ability for self-control as evidence that they can choose to overcome desires, while children growing up in Asian cultures (where interdependence is emphasized) may view and interpret self-control as externally driven (for example by social norms or others' expectations). These different ways in experiencing and interpreting self-control may further lead to the culturally moderated relationships seen here. This is largely consistent with research showing culture-specific modes of self-regulation (e.g., Lamm et al., 2018). As Asian children's cultural worldviews may center around interdependence, social norms, and relatedness with others, their self-control behaviors may be correlated with their beliefs about choice to follow norms or social expectations.

Consistent with this possibility, another line of research examining the role of freedom of choice in children's prosocial behaviors has found similar cultural variation. In a study with U.S. preschoolers, Chernyak and Kushnir (2013) manipulated whether children were given a choice and how costly the choice was when engaging in prosocial behaviors (i.e., giving a sticker to a puppet). Children were assigned to one of three conditions: a *no choice* condition, where they were instructed to share a sticker with a puppet; a *non-cost-choice* condition, where they were offered a choice between giving the sticker to a puppet or putting the sticker away (i.e., they would not receive the sticker anyway); and a *costly choice* condition, where they were offered a choice between giving the sticker to a puppet or keeping the sticker for themselves. Although almost all children in all three conditions ended up giving the sticker to the puppet, in a subsequent context facing a new puppet, those children who had experienced a costly choice were more likely to share compared to those in the two other conditions. Similarly, Rapp and colleagues (2017) also found that 5-year-olds in Germany were more likely to engage in helping behaviors when they were given free choices than when were not given a choice (i.e., simply instructed to help). This research suggests that, for children in Western cultures, the experience of making a costly choice themselves may help them feel more internally motivated to act prosocially, which can facilitate their prosocial behaviors. This evidence aligns with recent research that parental autonomy support—of which providing choices for children is an important component—can promote children's self-control behaviors and executive functioning (Carlson, 2023; Castelo et al., 2022; Valcan et al., 2018). The evidence is also largely consistent with self-determination theory (SDT), which posits that autonomy is a basic need for human psychological well-being (Deci & Ryan, 2000), and that being able to act with a sense of choice and agency promotes motivation and performance.

While these studies suggest that freedom of choice enhances children's prosocial motivation and behaviors, recent research indicates that the impact of choice on behaviors may vary across cultures (Bao & Lam, 2008; Iyengar & Lepper, 1999). In recent work, Chinese children ages 4–5 were assigned to either a *self-choice* condition (the child could decide for themself whether to share with a puppet or not) or a *mother-choice* condition (the child's mother instructed the child to share). My colleagues and I measured prosocial motivation via children's feelings during the sharing task and their sharing behaviors toward a novel partner. Mothers also completed a questionnaire measuring the quality of mother–child relationship. We found that the mother–child relationship significantly moderated the effect of choice condition on children's sharing feelings. Children who had positive relationships with their mothers demonstrated positive feelings when their mothers made the choice for them, similar to when they made the choice themselves. However, those who had neutral or negative relationships with their mothers demonstrated worse feelings when their mothers made the choice for them compared to when they made the choice themselves. In a subsequent study, we also found that providing a reasonable explanation (e.g., "You should share a sticker with Mr. Monkey so that he can feel better") when making choices for the children can enhance children's prosocial motivation more than simply instructing them to share, and even more than asking them to make choices for themselves (Wu et al., 2023). These findings suggest that Chinese children's prosocial motivations do not necessarily decrease when others make choices for them; instead, they also feel motivated when they have a positive relationship with the person who made choice for them, or when the person who made the choice for them provided an explanation.

These findings together suggest that freedom of choice plays an important role in behaviors requiring self-regulation, but the specific effect may vary by culture. In cultures emphasizing independence (e.g., Western cultures), having the freedom to choose and believing one can control personal desires seems to be essential for behavioral regulation. However, in cultures emphasizing interdependence (e.g., East Asian cultures), identifying with choices made by others who are significant to the actor may be equally, if not more, motivating. This aligns with later arguments of self-determination theory, indicating that the achievement of autonomy isn't mutually exclusive from external influences (Deci & Ryan, 2000; Ryan & Deci, 2006). In other words, there can be different pathways to motivated self-regulation across cultures: Individuals may achieve it by exercising free will or personal choice, *or* by choosing to follow social expectations they identify with.

CHOICE AND SOCIAL AND MORAL JUDGMENT

Children's developing beliefs about free will and choice not only influence their own behaviors but also shape their social and moral judgments of others' behaviors, with important implications for existential questions concerning moral responsibility and praiseworthiness. Increasing evidence suggests that children consider agents' choices and constraints when evaluating their actions. For example, when observing agents violating moral norms, children as young as 4 years old protested more when the agent had freedom of choice than when they were constrained (Josephs et al., 2016). Similarly, research with Australian children revealed that, by age 6, moral judgments were influenced by the counterfactual choices available to the characters (Gautam et al., 2023). Children evaluated story characters more favorably if they *made a choice* to do something good than if they did something good but *did not* have a choice, and they evaluated the characters more negatively if they *made a choice* to do something bad than if they did something bad but *did not* have a choice. This research suggests that children are more likely to attribute intentionality and moral responsibility to actions when agents have the freedom to choose rather than when they are constrained. This understanding is increasingly incorporated into children's social and moral judgments during preschool years.

As children understand that one can choose to do otherwise, they may also understand that there can be multiple motives for choice, and that these motives can conflict with each other. For instance, one's personal desires may conflict with obligations, and thus choosing to overcome personal desires in order to act on obligations can be costly and difficult. As children increasingly make costly choices themselves, they may also gradually understand that making such a costly choice to do the "right" thing is particularly praiseworthy. In recent work (Zhao & Kushnir, 2023), my colleague and I investigated how children make social evaluations of actions that involve making a costly (versus noncostly) choice to act prosocially toward others. Children and adults were asked to compare a character who made a costly choice to perform a moral action (e.g., giving up playing outside to help her brother find a ball) versus a character who acted morally without making a costly choice (e.g., not liking playing outside and simply helping her brother). We found that older children (8- and 9-year-olds) and adults recognized the praiseworthiness of making a costly choice, while younger children (4- and 5-year-olds) did not. We also investigated costs originating from different domains; in some cases, the costs were psychological (e.g., forgoing a personal desire),while in others the costs were physical (e.g., traveling a long distance). We found that children first recognize physical cost at around 6–7 years old and then recognize psychological cost at around 8–9 years old. These findings suggest that as children understand that one can choose to do otherwise, these beliefs may further facilitate their understanding that making a costly choice to do the right thing is praiseworthy. In fact, in recent studies (Yang et al., 2023; Zhao & Yang, 2023), we found positive correlations between beliefs in choice and more favorable evaluations of the individuals making costly choices.

Along similar lines, this consideration of choice and constraints is also shown in children's inferences of others' preferences (Jara-Ettinger et al., 2015; Pesowski et al., 2016). Typically, children infer that one's choosing actions reflect one's personal preferences. For example, they believe that choosing toy A from a selection of toy A and toy B indicates a preference for toy A over toy B. Recent work suggests that, in these inferences, children also take into account the choices and constraints faced by the agent. For instance, in Pesowski and colleagues (2016), children heard a story about a girl choosing between two toy castles, one of which was obviously more attractive than the other. In the free choice condition, both options were accessible, while in the constrained condition, the better castle was out of reach for the girl. Interestingly, in both conditions, the girl chose the less interesting castle. When asked to infer the girl's preference, 5-year-olds (but not 3-year-olds) differentiated between these two conditions. They inferred that the girl preferred the less interesting toy castle in the free choice condition but did not make such an inference in the constrained condition.

In addition to physical constraints, children are also sensitive to sociomoral constraints when inferring others' preferences. In the same study, 5- to 6-year-olds were less likely to infer preferences from one's choosing actions when the unchosen item belonged to others (Pesowski et al., 2016). In a more complex scenario my colleagues and I examined recently, when observing someone choosing an apple from a set of two apples and one banana, 7-year-olds were also less likely to infer that the actor prefers an apple if there is someone waiting behind the actor, as they considered that the actor may intentionally be leaving a choice for the next person (Zang et al., 2023).

In summary, during early and middle childhood, as children develop a more sophisticated understanding of what one can and cannot choose to do, and as they accumulate more experience of making choices themselves, they incorporate this information into their inferences and judgments of others' actions. This is particularly evident in children's recognition of the praiseworthiness of making a costly choice to do the right thing. Children's consideration of different types of constraints (physical, psychological, etc.) also varies by age, suggesting the domain-specificity of these understandings. Additionally, recent evidence suggests that children's reasoning about various types of constraints may have important implications for their reasoning about stereotypes (Amemiya et al., 2022). It is a fruitful area to further examine how children construe the real world in terms of choice and constraints, and the consequences of these reasonings.

RECOGNIZING THE SOCIAL VALUE OF CHOICE

Another important aspect of understanding choice is to recognize that most people desire the freedom to choose for themselves (Deci & Ryan, 2011). People value the freedom to choose so much that they may also make social evaluations depending on whether one grants others the opportunity to choose or deprives others of such opportunity (Van Doesum et al., 2013; Van Lange & Van Doesum, 2015). Actions that are considerate and mindful of other people's freedom of choice have been termed *socially mindful actions* (Van Doesum et al., 2013). Recent research has shown that adults often behave in a way that leaves a choice for others and evaluate someone leaving a choice as nicer than someone leaving no choice (Van Doesum et al., 2013).

My colleagues and I recently conducted a series of studies to investigate whether children understand socially mindful actions—that is, whether they evaluate someone leaving a choice for others as prosocial. We developed a paradigm where preschoolers were told a story where children take turns to choose a snack during snack time. Children were asked to compare two characters, each of whom was asked to choose from a set of three fruits containing two common fruits and one unique fruit (e.g., two apples and one banana) with another person waiting behind. One character took one of the common fruits and left a choice between two different kinds of fruits for others, while the other took the unique fruit and did not leave a choice for others (e.g., choosing an apple from one apple and two bananas). See Figure 16.2 for an example of the stimuli. By age 6, both U.S. and Chinese children evaluated a character leaving a choice for others as nicer than a character leaving no choice (Zhao et al., 2021b). Also see Sierksma and colleagues (2022) for similar findings with children in the Netherlands. Children's ability to make these evaluations also correlated with theory-of-mind abilities (Zhao et al., 2022). Importantly, consistent with what I discussed in the previous section, children only make these evaluations when the agent had alternative choices (i.e., could have chosen to do otherwise), but not when they did not (e.g., there were only bananas available to begin with) (Zhao et al., 2021b).

This research shows that children recognize the social value of choice, but raises a follow-up question: Do children value choice no matter what, or do they flexibly consider

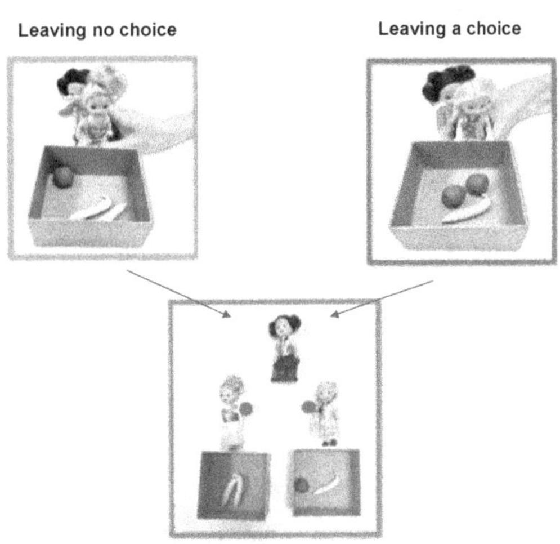

FIGURE 16.2. Example of the story setup in study examining children's evaluations of socially mindful actions.

other factors in their evaluations of the act of leaving a choice? My recent work has shown increasing evidence that children do not value choice blindly but instead take into account a range of factors. One thing children consider is the beneficiary's preference: When the beneficiary prefers the unique item, children as young as 4 years of age understand that it is nicer not to take away the only thing others prefer; however, when the beneficiary clearly prefers the item of which there are two, with age, children increasingly think that it is nicer to leave two identical but preferred items than to leave a diverse choice. These findings reveal that children increasingly develop a flexible appreciation of both others' preference and freedom of choice (Zang et al., 2023). Another factor children consider is whether the options available to choose from are desirable or aversive (Li & Zhao, 2024). For example, when the apples and bananas are damaged, do children and adults still consider leaving a choice as praiseworthy? My colleague and I found that adults' and 6-year-olds' evaluation of socially mindful actions was moderated by desirability of the options. Although they evaluated the act of leaving a choice for others as nicer than the act of leaving no choice even when the choosing options were undesirable, the effect was significantly smaller when the options were undesirable than when they were desirable. Along similar lines, there are other factors that have been shown to influence adults' values of choice, including the difficulty of choice, the burden of choice, the cognitive load of choice, and so on (Anderson, 2003; Greifeneder et al., 2010; Iyengar & Lepper, 2000; Schwartz, 2000, 2004; Steffel & Williams, 2018). Future research can delve further into how children balance the value of choice and the potential downsides of it.

Do children themselves behave in a way that leaves others with a choice? In an ongoing study, children ages 4 to 7 were asked to choose between two items of the same type and one unique item (e.g., two apples and one banana) in a line with another child (presented via video) waiting behind (Zhao & Li, 2024). See Figure 16.3 for an example of the procedure. My colleagues and I found that when asked spontaneously, children did not leave a choice for others; their choices aligned with their preferences and did not vary by age. However, when prompted to think about the next person's interest, children ages 6 and above (but not 4-year-olds) reliably left a choice for others. Children's choices were also significantly positively correlated with their theory-of-mind abilities.

In summary, these findings indicate that by age 6, children not only understand that one has the free will to choose for oneself but also understand that granting others the same choice is valuable and socially desirable. Their appreciation of the value of choice is flexible, taking into account vari-

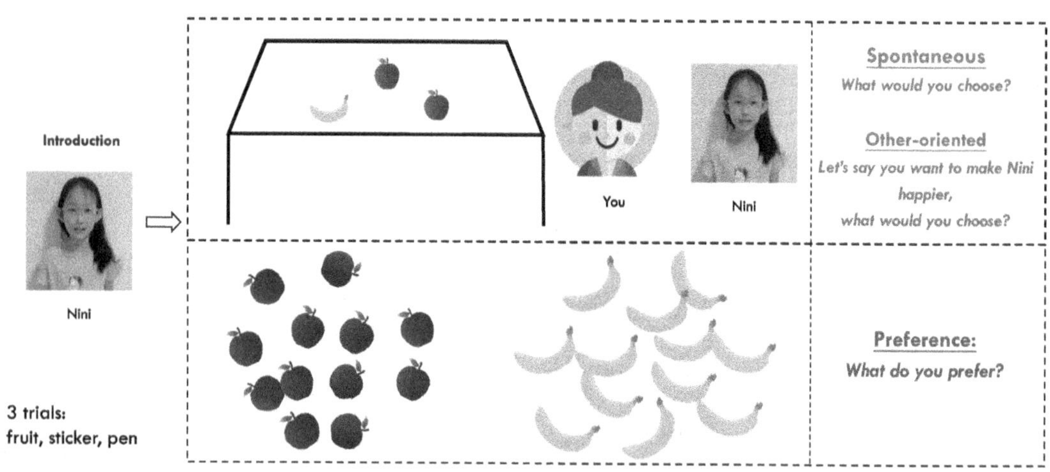

FIGURE 16.3. Procedure of study examining children's own socially mindful behaviors.

ous factors such as preference and desirability of options. By age 6, children also exhibit behaviors that leave a choice for others when prompted to consider others' perspectives. Moreover, these understandings and behaviors correlate with the development of theory-of-mind abilities.

CONCLUSIONS AND FUTURE DIRECTIONS

Taken together, the evidence I present in this chapter makes it clear that throughout early and middle childhood, children gradually develop a more explicit and sophisticated belief in choice and constraints, integrating their theories of the physical, psychological, and sociomoral domains into these beliefs. These developing beliefs have important implications for children's self-regulatory behaviors, prosocial behaviors, and social and moral judgments. Moreover, the ambiguity and complexity of choice allow cultural influences to play a role: As children are increasingly exposed to culture-specific influences, cultural differences emerge in their understanding of choice and constraints, as well as in how choice shapes their interpretation and regulation of behaviors. Culture seems to notably shape how self-control and prosocial behaviors are influenced by children's own beliefs about choice and whether they are given freedom of choice. These findings together suggest that even young children begin to understand the significance of choice and constraints in existential matters, including making sense and regulating one's actions, appreciating the value of agency and choice, and recognizing the moral responsibility and praiseworthiness of actions.

The findings in this chapter point to several important areas for future research. First, I have observed developmental changes and cultural variations in children's developing understanding of choice and constraints. What factors contribute to these developments and variations? Why are some individuals more likely to believe one can choose to overcome constraints than others? As children grow up, they may accumulate evidence that one can choose to overcome constraints. Children may get such evidence from their own experiences of making hard choices. As mentioned above, reflecting on experiences of making difficult choices may help children form more positive views about choice. Culture can shape how these experiences are interpreted and what views are formed (Zhao et al., 2021a). Children may also get this evidence via observations of others' actions; for example, seeing others wanting to do one thing but instead choosing to do otherwise may help children recognize the possibility of choice. There is suggestive evidence that, via observing other individuals persist or perform self-control behaviors, children can learn and generalize the value of persistence to a novel difficult task (Corriveau et al., 2016; Leonard et al., 2017). Future research can more directly test whether observing others' actions of making hard choices may help children better realize the possibility and the value of making such choices.

Another aspect that may contribute to the development and individual variation of choice beliefs may be adults' socialization input around the value of choice, such as parents' daily conversations with children and parental practices. Previous research on parental practices has shown that autonomy support promotes positive behavioral and emotional developmental outcomes in both Western and Eastern cultures, though the effect may be stronger in Western contexts (Pomerantz & Wang, 2009; Wang et al., 2007). However, less is known about the specific mechanisms underlying these effects. Examining the role of these parental practices on children's beliefs and views about choice, and their further relation to children's behaviors, may be an important future direction.

Second, children's beliefs about choice and free will may have important implications for their academic achievement. In recent work, my colleagues and I have begun to investigate children's views about choices in relation to various types of constraints in the academic domain, ranging from external environments (e.g., educational resources) to internal factors (e.g., talent), and their role in children's persistence. In a series of studies (Yang et al., 2023; Zhao & Yang, 2023), we have observed developmental changes, where children increasingly believe one can choose to overcome constraints to achieve academic success in early and middle childhood. They also increasingly recognize the value of overcoming constraints to succeed, evaluating those who do so more favorably than those who do not have constraints. Additionally, we found that these beliefs positively correlate with children's persistence challenge-seeking behaviors.

Finally, as I have shown, culture moderates the relationship between choice and children's behaviors. Although children across cultures behave similarly in self-control and prosocial behaviors, the pathways they take seem to differ across cultures. This is consistent with prior work showing that different interventions work for theory of mind development in U.S. versus Chinese children (Lu et al., 2008). These findings could have important practical implications on how to promote behavioral performance through different mindsets in different cultures.

REFERENCES

Amemiya, J., Mortenson, E., Ahn, S., Walker, C. M., & Heyman, G. D. (2022). Children acknowledge physical constraints less when actors behave stereotypically: Gender stereotypes as a case study. *Child Development, 93*(1), 72–83.

Anderson, C. J. (2003). The psychology of doing nothing: Forms of decision avoidance result from reason and emotion. *Psychological Bulletin, 129*(1), 139–167.

Atance, C. M. (2008). Future thinking in young children. *Current Directions in Psychological Science, 17*(4), 295–298.

Baillargeon, R. (2004). Infants' physical world. *Current Directions in Psychological Science, 13*(3), 89–94.

Bao, X., & Lam, S. (2008). Who makes the choice?: Rethinking the role of autonomy and relatedness in Chinese children's motivation. *Child Development, 79*(2), 269–283.

Baumeister, R. F., Masicampo, E. J., & DeWall, C. N. (2009). Prosocial benefits of feeling free: Disbelief in free will increases aggression and reduces helpfulness. *Personality and Social Psychology Bulletin, 35*(2), 260–268.

Baumeister, R. F., & Monroe, A. E. (2014). Recent research on free will: Conceptualizations, beliefs, and processes. *Advances in Experimental Social Psychology, 50,* 1–52.

Baumeister, R. F., Vohs, K. D., & Tice, D. M. (2007). The strength model of self-control. *Current Directions in Psychological Science, 16*(6), 351–355.

Behne, T., Carpenter, M., Call, J., & Tomasello, M. (2005). Unwilling versus unable: Infants' understanding of intentional action. *Developmental Psychology, 41,* 328–337.

Botti, S., & Iyengar, S. S. (2004). The psychological pleasure and pain of choosing: When people prefer choosing at the cost of subsequent outcome satisfaction. *Journal of Personality and Social Psychology, 87*(3), 312–326.

Brandone, A. C., & Wellman, H. M. (2009). You can't always get what you want infants understand failed goal-directed actions. *Psychological Science, 20,* 85–91.

Carlson, S. M. (2023). Let me choose: The role of choice in the development of executive function skills. *Current Directions in Psychological Science, 32*(3), 220–227.

Castelo, R. J., Meuwissen, A. S., Distefano, R., McClelland, M. M., Galinsky, E., Zelazo, P. D., & Carlson, S. M. (2022). Parent provision of choice is a key component of autonomy support in predicting child executive function skills. *Frontiers in Psychology.*

Chernyak, N., Kang, C., & Kushnir, T. (2019). The cultural roots of free will beliefs: How Singaporean and US Children judge and explain possibilities for action in interpersonal contexts. *Developmental Psychology, 55*(4), 866.

Chernyak, N., & Kushnir, T. (2013). Giving preschoolers choice increases sharing behavior. *Psychological Science, 24,* 1971–1979.

Chernyak, N., Kushnir, T., Sullivan, K. M., & Wang, Q. (2013). A comparison of American and Nepalese children's concepts of freedom of choice and social constraint. *Cognitive Science, 37,* 1343–1355.

Cordova, D. I., & Lepper, M. R. (1996). Intrinsic motivation and the process of learning: Beneficial effects of contextualization, personalization, and choice. *Journal of Educational Psychology, 88,* 715–730.

Corriveau, K. H., Min, G., Chin, J., & Doan, S. (2016). Do as I do, not as I say: Actions speak louder than words in preschoolers learning from others. *Journal of Experimental Child Psychology, 143,* 179–187.

Deci, E. L., & Ryan, R. M. (2000). The "what" and "why" of goal pursuits: Human needs and the self-determination of behavior. *Psychological Inquiry, 11*(4), 227–268.

Deci, E. L., & Ryan, R. M. (2011). Levels of analysis, regnant causes of behavior and well-being: The role of psychological needs. *Psychological Inquiry, 22*(1), 17–22.

Feldman, G., Chandrashekar, S. P., & Wong,

K. F. E. (2016). The freedom to excel: Belief in free will predicts better academic performance. *Personality and Individual Differences, 90,* 377–383.

Gautam, S., Owen Hall, R., Suddendorf, T., & Redshaw, J. (2023). Counterfactual choices and moral judgments in children. *Child Development, 94*(5), e296–e307.

Gergely, G., Bekkering, H., & Király, I. (2002). Rational imitation in preverbal infants. *Nature, 415,* 755.

Gopnik, A., & Wellman, H. M. (2012). Reconstructing constructivism: Causal models, Bayesian learning mechanisms, and the theory theory. *Psychological Bulletin, 138*(6), 1085.

Greifeneder, R., Scheibehenne, B., & Kleber, N. (2010). Less may be more when choosing is difficult: Choice complexity and too much choice. *Acta Psychologica, 133*(1), 45–50.

Hickling, A. K., & Wellman, H. M. (2001). The emergence of children's causal explanations and theories: Evidence from everyday conversation. *Developmental Psychology, 37*(5), 668.

Iyengar, S. S., & DeVoe, S. E. (2003, January). Rethinking the value of choice: Considering cultural mediators of intrinsic motivation. In *Nebraska Symposium on Motivation* (Vol. 49, pp. 129–174). University of Nebraska.

Iyengar, S. S., & Lepper, M. R. (1999). Rethinking the value of choice: A cultural perspective on intrinsic motivation. *Journal of Personality and Social Psychology, 76*(3), 349.

Iyengar, S. S., & Lepper, M. R. (2000). When choice is demotivating: Can one desire too much of a good thing? *Journal of Personality and Social Psychology, 79*(6), 995–1006.

Jara-Ettinger, J., Gweon, H., Tenenbaum, J. B., & Schulz, L. E. (2015). Children's understanding of the costs and rewards underlying rational action. *Cognition, 140,* 14–23.

Job, V., Dweck, C. S., & Walton, G. M. (2010). Ego depletion—Is it all in your head?: Implicit theories about willpower affect self-regulation. *Psychological Science, 21*(11), 1686–1693.

Josephs, M., Kushnir, T., Gräfenhain, M., & Rakoczy, H. (2016). Children protest moral and conventional violations more when they believe actions are freely chosen. *Journal of Experimental Child Psychology, 141,* 247–255.

Kitayama, S., Snibbe, A. C., Markus, H. R., & Suzuki, T. (2004). Is there any "free" choice?: Self and dissonance in two cultures. *Psychological Science, 15*(8), 527–533.

Kochanska, G., & Aksan, N. (2004). Development of mutual responsiveness between parents and their young children. *Child Development, 75*(6), 1657–1676.

Kushnir, T. (2018). The developmental and cultural psychology of free will. *Philosophy Compass, 13*(11), e12529.

Kushnir, T. (2022). Imagination and social cognition in childhood. *Wiley Interdisciplinary Reviews: Cognitive Science, 13*(4), e1603.

Kushnir, T., Gopnik, A., Chernyak, N., Seiver, E., & Wellman, H. M. (2015). Developing intuitions about free will between ages four and six. *Cognition, 138,* 79–101.

Lamm, B., Keller, H., Teiser, J., Gudi, H., Yovsi, R. D., Freitag, C., . . . Lohaus, A. (2018). Waiting for the second treat: Developing culture-specific modes of self-regulation. *Child Development, 89*(3), e261–e277.

Lane, J. D., Ronfard, S., Francioli, S. P., & Harris, P. L. (2016). Children's imagination and belief: Prone to flights of fancy or grounded in reality? *Cognition, 152,* 127–140.

Leonard, J. A., Lee, Y., & Schulz, L. E. (2017). Infants make more attempts to achieve a goal when they see adults persist. *Science, 357,* 1290–1294.

Leotti, L. A., Iyengar, S. S., & Ochsner, K. N. (2010). Born to choose: The origins and value of the need for control. *Trends in Cognitive Sciences, 14*(10), 457–463.

Li, S., & Zhao, X. (2024). Choosing among undesirable options: Children consider desirability of available choices in evaluation of socially mindful actions. *Cognitive Science, 48*(4), e13441.

Lu, H., Su, Y., & Wang, Q. (2008). Talking about others facilitates theory of mind in Chinese preschoolers. *Developmental Psychology, 44*(6), 1726.

Luo, Y., & Baillargeon, R. (2007). Do 12.5-month-old infants consider what objects others can see when interpreting their actions? *Cognition, 105,* 489–512.

Ma, L., & Xu, F. (2011). Young children's use of statistical sampling evidence to infer the subjectivity of preferences. *Cognition, 120,* 403–411.

MacKenzie, M. J., Vohs, K. D., & Baumeister, R. F. (2014). You didn't have to do that: Belief in free will promotes gratitude. *Personality and Social Psychology Bulletin, 40*(11), 1423–1434.

Markus, H. R., & Kitayama, S. (1991). Cultural variation in the self-concept. In *The self: Interdisciplinary approaches* (pp. 18–48). Springer.

Markus, H. R., & Kitayama, S. (2003, January). Models of agency: Sociocultural diversity in the construction of action. In *Nebraska Symposium on Motivation* (Vol. 49, pp. 1–58). University of Nebraska.

Miller, J. G., Bersoff, D. M., & Harwood, R. L. (1990). Perceptions of social responsibilities in India and in the United States: Moral imperatives or personal decisions? *Journal of Personality and Social Psychology, 58*(1), 33.

Miller, J. G., Das, R., & Chakravarthy, S. (2011). Culture and the role of choice in agency. *Journal of Personality and Social Psychology, 101*(1), 46–61.

Morris, M. W., & Peng, K. (1994). Culture and cause: American and Chinese attributions for social and physical events. *Journal of Personality and Social Psychology, 67*(6), 949.

Nadelhoffer, T., Shepard, J., Nahmias, E., Sripada, C., & Ross, L. T. (2014). The free will inventory: Measuring beliefs about agency and responsibility. *Consciousness and Cognition, 25*, 27–41.

Nichols, S. (2004). The folk psychology of free will: Fits and starts. *Mind and Language, 19*, 473–502.

Paulhus, D. L., & Carey, J. M. (2011). The FAD-Plus: Measuring lay beliefs regarding free will and related constructs. *Journal of Personality Assessment, 93*(1), 96–104.

Pesowski, M. L., Denison, S., & Friedman, O. (2016). Young children infer preferences from a single action, but not if it is constrained. *Cognition, 155*, 168–175.

Pomerantz, E. M., & Wang, Q. (2009). The role of parental control in children's development in Western and East Asian countries. *Current Directions in Psychological Science, 18*(5), 285–289.

Rakoczy, H., Warneken, F., & Tomasello, M. (2008). The sources of normativity: Young children's awareness of the normative structure of games. *Developmental Psychology, 44*(3), 875.

Rapp, D. J., Engelmann, J. M., Herrmann, E., & Tomasello, M. (2017). The impact of choice on young children's prosocial motivation. *Journal of Experimental Child Psychology, 158*, 112–121.

Rigoni, D., Kühn, S., Gaudino, G., Sartori, G., & Brass, M. (2012). Reducing self-control by weakening belief in free will. *Consciousness and Cognition, 21*(3), 1482–1490.

Ryan, R. M., & Deci, E. L. (2000a). Intrinsic and extrinsic motivations: Classic definitions and new directions. *Contemporary Educational Psychology, 25*(1), 54–67.

Ryan, R. M., & Deci, E. L. (2000b). Self-determination theory and the facilitation of intrinsic motivation, social development, and well-being. *American Psychologist, 55*(1), 68–78.

Ryan, R. M., & Deci, E. L. (2006). Self-regulation and the problem of human autonomy: Does psychology need choice, self-determination, and will? *Journal of Personality, 74*(6), 1557–1586.

Savani, K., Markus, H. R., & Conner, A. L. (2008). Let your preference be your guide?: Preferences and choices are more tightly linked for North Americans than for Indians. *Journal of Personality and Social Psychology, 95*(4), 861.

Savani, K., Markus, H. R., Naidu, N. V. R., Kumar, S., & Berlia, N. (2010). What counts as a choice?: US Americans are more likely than Indians to construe actions as choices. *Psychological Science, 21*(3), 391–398.

Schult, C. A., & Wellman, H. M. (1997). Explaining human movements and actions: Children's understanding of the limits of psychological explanation. *Cognition, 62*(3), 291–324.

Schwartz, B. (2000). Self-determination: The tyranny of freedom. *American Psychologist, 55*(1), 79.

Schwartz, B. (2004). The tyranny of choice. *Scientific American, 290*(4), 70–75.

Shariff, A. F., Greene, J. D., Karremans, J. C., Luguri, J. B., Clark, C. J., Schooler, J. W., . . . Vohs, K. D. (2014). Free will and punishment: A mechanistic view of human nature reduces retribution. *Psychological Science, 25*(8), 1563–1570.

Shtulman, A. (2009). The development of possibility judgment within and across domains. *Cognitive Development, 24*, 293–309.

Shtulman, A., & Carey, S. (2007). Improbable or impossible?: How children reason about the possibility of extraordinary events. *Child Development, 78*, 1015–1032.

Sierksma, J., Klootwijk, C. L. T., & Lee, N. C. (2022). Prosocial choices: How do young children evaluate considerate and inconsiderate behavior? *Developmental Psychology, 58*, 2013–2021.

Smetana, J. G. (2006). Social–cognitive domain theory: Consistencies and variations in children's moral and social judgments. In M. Killen & J. G. Smetana (Ed.), *Handbook of moral development* (pp. 137–172). Psychology Press.

Sobel, D. M. (2004). Exploring the coherence of young children's explanatory abilities: Evidence from generating counterfactuals. *British Journal of Developmental Psychology, 22*(1), 37–58.

Spelke, E. (1994). Initial knowledge: Six suggestions. *Cognition, 50*(1–3), 431–445.

Steffel, M., & Williams, E. F. (2018). Delegating decisions: Recruiting others to make choices we might regret. *Journal of Consumer Research, 44*(5), 1015–1032.

Stillman, T. F., Baumeister, R. F., Vohs, K. D., Lambert, N. M., Fincham, F. D., & Brewer, L. E. (2010). Personal philosophy and personnel achievement: Belief in free will predicts better job performance. *Social Psychological and Personality Science, 1*(1), 43–50.

Sullivan, M. W., & Lewis, M. (2003). Contextual determinants of anger and other negative expressions in young infants. *Developmental Psychology, 39*(4), 693–705.

Valcan, D. S., Davis, H., & Pino-Pasternak, D. (2018). Parental behaviours predicting early childhood executive functions: A meta-analysis. *Educational Psychology Review, 30,* 607–649.

Van Doesum, N. J., Van Lange, D. A., & Van Lange, P. A. (2013). Social mindfulness: Skill and will to navigate the social world. *Journal of Personality and Social Psychology, 105*(1), 86.

Van Lange, P. A., & Van Doesum, N. J. (2015). Social mindfulness and social hostility. *Current Opinion in Behavioral Sciences, 3,* 18–24.

Vohs, K. D., & Schooler, J. W. (2008). The value of believing in free will: Encouraging a belief in determinism increases cheating. *Psychological Science, 19*(1), 49–54.

Wang, Q. (2006). Culture and the development of self-knowledge. *Current Directions in Psychological Science, 15,* 182–187.

Wang, Q., Pomerantz, E. M., & Chen, H. (2007). The role of parents' control in early adolescents' psychological functioning: A longitudinal investigation in the United States and China. *Child Development, 78*(5), 1592–1610.

Wellman, H. M. (2014). *Making minds: How theory of mind develops.* Oxford University Press.

Wellman, H. M., & Gelman, S. A. (1992). Cognitive development: Foundational theories of core domains. *Annual Review of Psychology, 43*(1), 337–375.

Wente, A. O., Bridgers, S., Zhao, X., Seiver, E., Zhu, L., & Gopnik, A. (2016). How universal are free will beliefs? Cultural differences in Chinese and US 4- and 6-year-olds. *Child Development, 87,* 666–676.

Wu, W., Zhang, Q., & Zhao, X. (2023). Who makes the choice?: The influence of choice on preschoolers' sharing behaviors and feelings. *Acta Psychologica Sinica, 55*(11), 1815.

Yang, X., Zhao, X., Dunham, Y., & Bian, L. (2023). The development and predictors of a preference for strivers over naturals in the United States and China. *Child Development.*

Zang, L., Li, D., & Zhao, X. (2023). Preference matters: Knowledge of beneficiary's preference influences children's evaluations of the act of leaving a choice for others. *Journal of Experimental Child Psychology, 228,* 105605.

Zhao, X., & Kushnir, T. (2019). How U.S. and Chinese children talk about personal, moral and conventional choices. *Cognitive Development, 52,* 100804.

Zhao, X., & Kushnir, T. (2023). When it's not easy to do the right thing: Developmental changes in understanding cost drive evaluations of moral praiseworthiness. *Developmental Science, 26*(1), e13257.

Zhao, X., Li, D., & Yang, X. (2022). The relationship between preschoolers' understanding of considerate socially-mindful actions and theory of mind. *Acta Psychologica Sinica, 54*(8), 892.

Zhao, X., & Li, Z. (2024, March). *The development of socially mindful behaviors in early childhood.* Paper presented at the biennial meeting of the Cognitive Development Society, Pasadena, CA.

Zhao, X., Wente, A., Flecha, M. F., Galvan, D. S., Gopnik, A., & Kushnir, T. (2021a). Culture moderates the relationship between self-control ability and free will beliefs in childhood. *Cognition, 210,* 104609.

Zhao, X., & Yang, X. (2023). She succeeded despite lack of ability or resources: Children's consideration of constraint in beliefs and reasoning about academic achievement. *Developmental Psychology, 59*(3), 594.

Zhao, X., Zhao, X., Gweon, H., & Kushnir, T. (2021b). Leaving a choice for others: Children's evaluations of considerate, socially-mindful actions. *Child Development, 92*(4), 1238–1253.

CHAPTER 17

How the Existential Agent Functions

Free Will and Self-Regulation

Roy F. Baumeister

The capacity for autonomous, self-directed action is a vital part of the human mind and its psychology. This capacity has been explored and debated for centuries, especially under the rubric of free will. It has been of central importance to existentialist and phenomenological thinking as well. Indeed, Sartre's (1943/1956) *Being and Nothingness* devoted considerable effort to understanding the nature of consciousness (an important aspect of free will, given that experts and laypersons alike view consciousness as integral to free will; e.g., Shepherd, 2012). Heidegger's (1927) *Being and Time* had extended analyses of agency, as in how action can happen either authentically or automatically.

Self-control is a central part of free will, as evidenced by how frequently modern philosophical works on free will invoke examples of self-control (alongside rational choice) (e.g., Dennett & Caruso, 2021; Mele, 2006, 2022). This chapter covers how my research program on self-control led me into the topic of free will, including helping formulate a novel approach to the problem.

Specifically, I have come to think that free will can be studied scientifically—but that it requires reformulating the problem. Philosophical discussions of free will in recent decades have focused heavily on whether it is compatible with determinism (see below). Determinism holds that the future is already determined and so everything that happens is inevitable. Intuitively, that seems to contradict the notion that a person is free to choose among different ways of acting, because the eventual outcome has already been inevitable since the dawn of time.

I cannot imagine a scientific experiment proving that someone could or could not have acted differently in a particular situation, which is the crux of the philosophical debate. What psychological science can do is elaborate causal processes in the mind and environment that produce behaviors. The brain consists of neurons that manage to fire in coordinated patterns that ultimately produce action, by sending signals to the muscles on how to move. Insofar as there is free will, it will be found in the input into that motor control system: what happens in the mind just before it tells the muscles what to do. Psychology can illuminate how those processes work. Rather than debating whether free will could possibly exist, as philosophers do, psychologists can debate how the mental systems operate (see Baumeister, 2024).

Nevertheless, I do not dodge the question, if only so that readers can anticipate any possible biases or preferences on my part. Having spoken over recent decades with many scientists who reject free will, and many others who accept it, I find I largely agree with both. They are using wildly different definitions of what free will is. The next section explains the definitions. To me, however, the most striking thing about all those conversations is that the free will skeptics and the free will accepters largely agree about how behavior is caused. You might think they would be wildly different, but it is hard to find any specific differences. They both recognize the functioning of attitudes, numerical calculations, motivation, interpersonal concerns, and interpersonal influence, and the rest. Even more remarkably, both sides agree that the mental system by which human action is caused is drastically, even qualitatively different from anything else in nature.

Their disagreement is mainly focused on whether this extremely extraordinary form of action control deserves to be called "free will." But to me, the scientific problem is to understand how this system works, not to debate the term.

If pressed, I would say this. If this mental system were first discovered today, we would name it something other than "free will." But the term is close enough and, given that it has been in use for centuries, we should retain it. The more skeptically inclined may wish to use it ironically.

For me, the *free* part is less a problem than the *will* part. As I explain in the theory section of this chapter, there is a strong case for freedom, especially as considered in terms of degrees along a continuum and as features of the situation structure. (Less freedom when the situation is holding a gun to your head, for example.) But the *will* is not a recognized phenomenon in most modern psychology. Introductory textbooks do not contain chapters on the will. For me, the will in *free will* is purely metaphor (whereas the freedom is genuine), as in expressions such as "against his will."

DEFINITIONS

Free Will

Much of the seemingly endless debate about free will can be dismissed for scientific purposes as semantic squabbling over definitions. Scholars who argue against free will generally regard it as an exemption from causality or as something that operates outside of biological processes. Writing in the prestigious journal *Current Biology*, Montague (2008) explained that free will is closely related to belief in souls and that it means "your choices are not caused by physical events but instead emerge wholly formed from somewhere indescribable and outside the purview of physical descriptions," cannot have evolved by natural selection, and is "not even in principle within reach of scientific description" (p. R584). In similar fashion, Sapolsky (2023, 2024) described free will as actions that occur independent of all causality.

As I said earlier, I agree with these skeptics who reject the notion of free will if it is defined in such a fashion. My theory does not invoke souls causing behavior or exemptions from causality. Free will is just another kind of cause (or, more plausibly, a set of causes). This is not an extravagant hypothesis. Science has identified thousands of different kinds of causes, from electromagnetism to economic supply and demand, not to mention all the experiments in social psychology. Proposing that the human mental system for controlling action is a powerful development of a new set of causal processes, including greater flexibility of action, is just adding one more (albeit a fascinating one) to the giant heap.

In contrast to the scientifically dubious theories of souls causing action, free will proponents define it in a much more viable fashion. A useful definition was created by an interdisciplinary team of scientists and philosophers for a research grants competition. The team seems to have shared my skepticism about the will, for rather than putting the meaty substance into the definition of *free will* and therefore reifying it, it defined *free will* simply as the capacity for free action—and *free action* was defined as the capability to act differently in the same situation (Haggard et al., 2010).

The capacity to act differently in the same situation is an important and highly adaptive form of action control. It is closely related to the notion not of souls but of behavioral flexibility, which clearly has a long and fruitful evolutionary history. Even simple animals can improve their chances at survival and reproduction by varying their behavior. Learning itself depends on some degree of flexibility, so that the creature can alter its behavior based on previous outcomes. To be sure, action control processes in simple animals are a long way from human free will, but presumably the latter evolved from and builds on them.

Ordinary people also understand free will, and several researchers have explored those views, even while assuming that these cannot be expected to approach the sophistication and subtlety of expert philosophers. Monroe and Malle (2010, 2015) asked people how they understand free will. Their answers converged on making choices, doing what one wants, possibly after conscious deliberation, being unencumbered by external pressures and forces, and considering the future. Stillman and colleagues (2011) asked people to describe life experiences when they did versus did not act of their free will. The differences between the two sets of stories linked free will to reaching goals, advancing one's self-interest, conscious deliberation, doing what is morally right, and resisting external influence.

Self-Control

Self-control is a less contentious term than *free will.* Human mental systems exert control over themselves to change themselves. They alter how they think, how they act, how they feel, what they say, how they perform tasks and duties, and so on. Some writers distinguish self-control from self-regulation. For them, self-regulation is the broader term; all self-control is self-regulation. But they reserve self-control for deliberate, conscious actions, while self-regulation can be unconscious. Indeed, homeostasis can be counted as self-regulation: The body maintains a constant temperature, an average of 98.6 degrees Fahrenheit (or perhaps slightly less), sometimes producing fevers but then bringing the body temperature back to baseline, all occurring outside of conscious awareness but clearly a form in which the body regulates itself. As these patterns are not relevant to free will, I will not be discussing them, and so *self-control* and *self-regulation* function in this chapter as synonyms.

Other Relevant Terms

Culture is a system that organizes human interactions, large and small, based on shared information and shared understandings that include beliefs about the world, how things should be done, and behavior guidelines such as norms. Culture is learned, although it may organize and inform behaviors that have innate basis (e.g., sex, eating). The shared information is transmitted to the next generation. Culture is an advanced and improved way of being social. There are many social animals (including humankind), and a few dozen species may have small bits of culture (de Waal, 2001), but only humans are truly cultural animals in the sense that the majority of their actions involve culture.

Society is the culture plus the people living in it. A society is a group of individuals who interact and share the common identity. It normally has strict boundaries as to who belongs to the society and who does not (Moffett, 2019). Many cultures treat their members quite differently from outsiders, extending even to whether the same moral rules apply. For example, it may be entirely morally acceptable to rob, rape, enslave, and even kill outsiders, whereas it would be strongly immoral to do those things to other members of one's society.

THEORETICAL BASIS: HUMANS AS CULTURAL ANIMALS

Grand questions about human nature and behavior patterns are generally explained by invoking either nature or culture (the latter including socialization and environmental influences on upbringing, also called *nurture*). Free will and self-control are no different. The relative influence of nature and cultural nurture continues to be debated. My sense is that most thinkers acknowledge some role to each but debate what the mixture is.

My own approach treats nature and culture not as competing explanations but as complementary ones. Indeed, the basis of my thinking is that the human mind was shaped by natural selection—but with cultural participation as the main basis for that selection. Put another way, culture is humankind's strategy for solving the universal problems of survival and reproduction. Humans are essentially cultural animals, with culture as an advanced form of social life (Baumeister, 2005). The distinctively human traits are thus the result of biological adaptations to enable individual humans to flourish in a complex social environment organized with culture. These traits include the advanced human powers of self-control and any specifically human forms of free will.

This approach builds on the influential theory of cultural materialism (Harris, 1980), which asserts that whatever else a culture does, it must enable human beings to survive and reproduce, which means furnishing them with the necessary resources. In particular, using culture to organize society enables people to create more resources than they could if operating as lone individuals, such as by cooperative group hunting, and proceeding to farming and eventually to the modern global economic marketplace.

THEORY: SELF-CONTROL

Free will is a grander, more broadly encompassing (and more controversial) notion than self-control, so I begin by explicating self-control. This exposition will follow the path my own research and thinking took. I spent years studying self-control before the findings moved me on to the bigger questions of free will.

Early decades of scientific psychology focused on rats, and self-control (let alone free will) was not a popular topic of investigation. Self-control was left to the clinicians. Freud (1930, 1933/1965) posited that the psyche includes a *superego*, understood as the repository of cultural learning, including morals and ideals. In his view, the ego, as the system that dictates action, serves two masters, the virtuous superego prescribing culturally valued actions, and the id comprising basic innate drives that are often selfish and destructive.

Self-Awareness and Feedback Loops

Self-regulation theory and research took a big step forward with Carver and Scheier's (1981) adaptation of the feedback loop from cybernetic theory (originally developed to help steer long-range missiles toward military targets). These researchers had begun their careers studying self-awareness, a topic introduced to social psychology by Duval and Wicklund (1972). Carver and Scheier proposed that the very purpose of human self-awareness was to facilitate self-regulation. That is, the human self evolved to be able to direct attention toward itself so as to be able to alter its responses to bring them into line with personal and social standards. This assumption was stimulated in part by the recurrent finding that self-awareness nearly always involved comparison to standards (e.g., Wicklund, 1975). In plain terms, self-awareness was more than the basic "Oh, there I am" and instead more typically involved "How am I doing compared to goals and expectations?" The then-popular laboratory procedure of stimulating self-awareness by seating research participants in front of a mirror evoked not just recognition of one's own image as a familiar stimulus but also evaluative concerns. Typically, research participants who were made self-aware were motivated by that to perform better, to work harder, to be more honest and consistent, and in other respects to live up to positive norms (Carver & Scheier, 1981; Wicklund, 1975).

Carver and Scheier (1981, 1982) linked self-awareness to self-regulation with a feedback loop. The acronym TOTE captured the essential steps of the loop. TOTE stands for test, operate, test, exist. The simple but profound idea is that when people become self-aware, they perform a test of whether the self measures up to the relevant standard. Standards are ideas of how one should or should not be broadly understood. They include personal goals, moral virtue, social norms, parental expectations, professional ethics, laws, past performance, and social comparisons. If the test reveals that one falls short of these standards, then the system triggers the "operate" step, which means changing the self. At various points self-awareness performs another test to see whether the problem or discrepancy has been resolved. When a test finally indicates that the self does measure up to the standard, then the "exit" phase is triggered. The system exits the loop with no further testing or operating. Eventually, of course, self-awareness may perform another test and perhaps initiate further operations.

Emotions are relevant. A test that reveals some deficiency in the self will evoke negative emotions, which help the person realize the need to operate. When the standard is being met, positive emotions may be felt (especially when one first reaches the standard). In an important further refinement of the theory, Carver and Scheier (1990) noted that positive emotions do not necessarily wait until one reaches the goal. A positive emotion may occur simply by recognizing that one is making suitable progress toward the goal. Thus, a student or worker may feel good while performing an assignment long before it is completed, simply by recognizing that they have made sufficient progress to sustain the expectation that it will be completed on schedule. Conversely, negative emotions arise long before failure, based on recognizing that the task will not be completed on time or otherwise satisfactorily.

As an example of the feedback loop operation, someone may weigh themselves and decide they are overweight (the test). They might then operate by losing some weight, resulting in a more favorable test outcome, whereupon they can exit the loop. This is indeed what happens, though the operation of losing weight is often not straightforward. Hence further research on self-regulation focused on the "operate" phase.

Thus, individuals seeking help with self-regulation might profit from using the feedback loop. For example, someone worried about their weight might be advised to weigh themselves, compare this weight with their ideal weight by computing the difference. If they weigh too much, they should move to the "operate" phase and lose weight. They can test themselves periodically, and when their measured weight is equal to or better than their ideal weight, they can exit the loop. This is all valid, but some readers may wish for more details about how to succeed with the operation phase (losing weight). The next section builds on Carver and Scheier's work by seeking to explicate the operate phase.

Willpower and Ego Depletion

When first reading and summarizing the research literature on self-regulation, my colleagues and I noticed a surprising pattern (Baumeister et al., 1994): Performance at self-control seemed to deteriorate over time or when there were multiple demands on it. It seemed as if self-control depended on some energy supply (akin to the folk notion of willpower) that could become partly or severely depleted.

At the time, energy was an implausible and foreign notion to psychology. Research and theory were all besotted with information processing models, likening the brain to a computer. (This was back around 1990, when personal computers were first spreading through society.) But the computer analogy would predict the opposite result. If self-control operates like a computer program, then when it is already up and running, performance on the next self-control task should be facilitated. In contrast, an energy model suggests that it could be impaired.

Hence the initial studies based on the 1994 book compared participants who performed an initial self-control task with others who were assigned a neutral task—and then measured performance on a second, unrelated self-control task. Results consistently found that performance on the second task was worse for those who had already exerted self-control, contrary to the information processing model but consistent with the energy model (Baumeister et al., 1998; Muraven et al., 1998). This was true not only in my laboratory but in abundant other sources, reviewed by Muraven and Baumeister (2000). For example, vigilance researchers frequently observed that vigilance (which relies on attention regulation to maintain high performance) deteriorated over time.

We searched for previous theorists who had included energy as part of the self and had to go all the way back to Freud (1923/1961, 1933/1965) to find one. Freud had been rather vague about how the energy functioned and where it came from but, given that he had said the self involves energy, we borrowed his term (*ego*) and hence dubbed the pattern *ego depletion*. It was defined as a state of reduced willpower, reflected in impairments in self-regulatory functioning.

Three decades have now elapsed since the original publication of the energy model of self-control (Baumeister et al., 1994; Baumeister & Heatherton, 1996). Here I briefly summarize the major refinements, advances, and other developments.

The initial assumption was that the brain had temporarily run out of energy. This is implausible based on how the brain operates: Brain energy waxes and wanes but it is careful that it never runs out, which would probably bring death. Moreover, work by Muraven and colleagues (2006; Muraven & Slessareva, 2003) showed that participants in the depleted state can indeed still perform at a high level if sufficiently motivated (though they then show signs of even more severe depletion). Hence, a first shift was to understand ego depletion as conservation of diminished energy, rather than lacking sufficient energy to function. As with physical muscles, the human body naturally seeks to conserve energy, and it tries with increasing earnestness to conserve when it has already expended some.

The analogy between self-control and physical muscles was further extended by showing that self-control could be improved with training (Muraven et al., 1998; for a recent meta-analysis, see Friese et al., 2017). Thus, the state of ego depletion is akin to muscle tiredness right after exercise, whereas long-term improvement following frequent acts of self-control resembles how a muscle becomes stronger from exercise (after recovering from the initial tiredness, of course).

The finding that self-control can be improved by regular exercise has potentially important implications. The history of psychology has turned up mainly just two traits that produce benefits almost everywhere, with hardly any downside: intelligence and self-control. And despite decades' worth of evidence, there seems to be little prospect of interventions to produce lasting changes in intelligence. Self-control can be strengthened, however, even in early adulthood. Self-control may therefore be one of psychology's best hopes for contributing to improving life.

Our initial theory had used an energy model, but the energy was largely a metaphorical notion. A big change came with linking it to the body's actual energy system, as reflected by glucose in the bloodstream. A major investigation by Gailliot and colleagues (2007) reported three patterns consistent with the idea that glucose is a biological substrate to willpower. The first, which unfortunately has not replicated reliably and may have benefited in the initial difference from a rogue control condition, was that levels of blood glucose decrease from before to after self-control. There may be something to this notion, but on present evidence I do not endorse it.

The other two have fared much better, however. The second link to glucose was that people whose blood glucose is low exhibit relatively poor self-control. This finding in our lab turns out to have substantial additional evidence in nutrition research, which has shown in multiple ways that low blood glucose accompanies poor self-control (reviewed by Gailliot & Baumeister, 2007). Diverse evidence, ranging from diabetic hypoglycemia to laboratory manipulation of "glucose clamps," measurement of glucose levels among recently arrested juvenile delinquents, and randomized control studies of whether school pupils have breakfast, has confirmed the causally detrimental impact of low glucose on self-control.

The third pattern is that receiving a glucose dose counteracts effects of ego depletion. In the typical procedure, participants are given a glass of lemonade upon arriving at the experiment. Neither the participant nor the experimenter knows whether the lemonade was sweetened with sugar (big dose of glucose) or diet sweetener (no glucose), but studies have found very consistently that depletion manipulations fail to affect participants who got the sugar but remain strong and clear among those whose lemonade was artificially sweetened (e.g., Gailliot et al., 2007; Masicampo & Baumeister, 2008).

The next big advance was particularly relevant to existential concerns. While researching diverse findings for a large handbook chapter on the self (Baumeister, 1998), I came to realize that the executive aspect of the self was implicated in both self-control and decision making. Might choosing also cause ego depletion? An early single study found that agreeing to record a counterattitudinal speech (favoring large tuition increase) caused ego depletion, as measured by giving up quickly on a difficult task (Baumeister et al., 1998). Thus, the decision process seemingly created a depleted state. But it took a series of studies with multiple measures and procedures to establish that decision making did indeed deplete one's willpower and impair self-regulation (Vohs et al., 2008). Further studies showed that the effect goes in the other direction too: After exerting self-control, people simplify their decision process, often leading to poorer or less rational decisions (Pocheptsova et al., 2009).

Another big change to the research program and to the theory emerged by shifting focus from the state of ego depletion to chronic levels of self-control. Some people have better self-control than others. Trait measures for this were, however, antiquated and not highly reliable, so Tangney and colleagues (2004) developed a new questionnaire measure of the trait, including a popular short version. The original work included an effort to develop subscales that might reveal different aspects of self-control. But the factor structure did not replicate, and moreover the factors all seemed to predict the same outcomes about equally well, which renders them useless. The implication may be that self-control is a fairly monolithic trait. This has existential implications. The person acts as a unity, despite inner qualms or ambivalence, and despite conflicting desires. Being good or bad at self-control may be a general trait that can be applied in different domains (though given the limits to willpower, using it in some spheres may restrict its use in others). Habits may make some actions easier to perform than others, but the individual person's ability to form and break habits is the same central ability.

The measure of trait self-control proved very popular, and only a few years later de Ridder and colleagues (2012) published a meta-analysis with over a hundred studies. It confirmed that good self-control is associated with a wide range of positive outcomes, and no negative outcomes or downsides were found.

The most important point to emerge from the de Ridder meta-analysis, however, was the link to habits (see also Wood & Neal, 2007). Habits are automatic behaviors and therefore do not require much willpower or agency. De Ridder and colleagues (2012) had initially assumed that habits would be irrelevant to trait self-control, but they found the opposite. The implication is that people with good self-control use their self-control to break bad habits and form good ones. With that, they can coast through life rather easily. In contrast, people with low self-control are often struggling with problems and stresses they have brought on themselves (Baumeister et al., 2019).

Ego depletion and limited willpower provide a valuable reason for the importance of habits. Performing all one's actions with deliberate, conscious choice and control may be a compelling meditative exercise, but it will rapidly deplete one's willpower. Hence the human mind has evolved to automatize rapidly and easily, thereby moving the execution of desired behaviors from the realm of conscious and deliberate control to the automatic system.

Ego depletion theory came under fire in the 2010–2020 decade, from two directions. One proposed alternate explanations so as to jettison the limited-energy aspect. The other argued that the effect was not real. Obviously, at least one of these critiques must be completely wrong, because there cannot be a correct (alternate) explanation of a nonexistent effect. The alternate explanations typically focused only on a friendly corner of the data and generally did not extend to all the findings. The most forceful of them argued that no energy was depleted, but rather people simply lost motivation to exert themselves on the second task (Inzlicht & Schmeichel, 2012). There was no evidence that this happens, but it was plausible, and the paper received several awards. However, subsequent work, including my own, has failed to find any sign of reduced motivation on the second task.

The argument that ego depletion does not exist was fueled by the replication crisis, a widespread malaise spreading through social psychology during the second decade of the 21st century. A multisite replication by Hagger and colleagues (2016) reported null results. (Technically it was not a replication at all; their procedure had never been used before.) But it also was seriously confounded, given that manipulation checks showed that their peculiar manipulation had created frustration but not fatigue (the reverse of what should have been found). Thus, it failed to test the hypothesis. (Indeed, when the data were finally made public, one researcher reanalyzed them to control for the fatigue manipulation check and found that, to the very limited effect that the manipulation worked, the results significantly supported ego depletion; Dang, 2016.). As is typical in such cases, there was a lot of fanfare and hoopla about the ostensible failure, glossing over the deficiencies in the design—but the accumulating evidence in favor of ego depletion received less attention. A subsequent multisite replication found a significant result supporting ego depletion, both with the full sample and after excluding participants whose data might be questionable (Dang et al., 2021), and another found significant support with one analysis but not with the other (Vohs et al., 2021).

At present, a strong case can be made that ego depletion is the best replicated finding in all of social psychology (see Baumeister & Tice, 2022). A survey of all multisite replications in the field found only 4 clearly successful ones, out of 36 (Baumeister et al., 2023), one of which was for ego depletion. If successful multilab replication is a criterion, then ego depletion is one of only four, though there are a few ministudies that also do well, most notably the one-item anchoring adjustment effect. Added to that are more than 600 published findings in the literature, nearly all of which are consistent with ego depletion (Friese et al., 2017). None of them go in the opposite direction, which renders implausible the possibility of capitalizing on chance. There are multiple preregistered successful replications (Garrison et al., 2019), as well as multiple supportive findings outside the laboratory (some reviewed in Baumeister & Tice, 2022; see also Baumeister & Vohs, 2016). It is hard to identify any other finding in social psychology with a comparable record. My colleagues and I had supposed that cognitive dissonance would take over the top spot if its multisite replication succeeded, but it appears that it was not successful, or at best supporting only the minimal (consistency) part of the theory while failing to replicate the importance of personal choice and responsibility (Vaidis et al., 2024). Regardless of whether ego depletion has the single strongest case, it is clearly among social psychology's most widely replicated findings.

Transition from Self-Control to Free Will

Stumbling onto the willpower resource as a key to self-regulation was an intriguing challenge that took up a large part of my career for a long time. Crucially, self-control is a huge predictor of success in life (Mischel et al., 1988; Moffitt et al., 2011). If the willpower resource did nothing but fuel self-regulation, it would already be a hugely important feature of the psyche.

The turning point for me was finding that the willpower resource was also active in rational choice and decision making. That meant it was much bigger. What combines both self-control and rational choice? That is when I realized I had stumbled into the free will arena. Philosophical works on self-control are replete with examples of self-control and rational choice, but philosophers had no way of proving that both were forms of free will. But now my colleagues and I had found that they drew on the same resource and thus had an underlying common psychological phenomenon. If free will exists, this must be it. (It seems wildly implausible that human beings have free will but it has nothing to do with self-control and rational choice, as in these laboratory studies.) If free will does not exist, this is what is mistaken for it.

FREE WILL

This section lays out the main features of a scientific theory of this newly evolved (for humankind) mental system of action control. Again, that's what free will is in practice, or that's what is commonly mistaken for it.

Free Will Is (Mostly) Not for Random Action

Before laying out a scientific theory of free will, it is useful to address a common and misleading theme in scientific discussions of free will. Often scientists think free will should show up in data as random action. In their data it would appear as error variance. After all, error variance is what deviates from the causal process that one's study is seeking to establish. Scientists assume that free will would be exemption from their particular cause.

The link to randomness takes other forms. Some have speculated that quantum indeterminacy could contribute to randomness and hence be a foundation for free will.

However, as I have argued at length elsewhere (Baumeister, 2024), free will should not be confused with random action. The purpose of human free will is decidedly not to increase randomness in human behavior. This should be obvious based on the idea that humans are cultural animals, and their traits are adaptations to use and benefit from culture. Culture does not have much use for random action. Would you want a surgeon who did random things while operating on you or your loved ones? Would you want your teacher or boss to evaluate your work randomly? Au contraire, you want someone who exactly follows the proper procedures for best results.

As a useful trait for cultural animals, free will is more likely used for following rules than for acting randomly. Cultures flourish by producing and sharing resources, and this works best when people obey the rules and perform their duties properly. The example of following rules surprises people, because many intuitively assume that freedom would mean doing whatever one wants, with no rules. But no advanced mental powers are needed in order to do what one wants without rules. In contrast, to pursue one's enlightened self-interest within the framework of a complex society with abundant rules requires a rather sophisticated action control system.

Randomness may not be completely irrelevant to free will (Baumeister, 2024). In fact, Brembs (2011) proposed an evolutionary theory of free will based on the idea that some randomness might have been favored by natural selection. Simple animals who behaved somewhat randomly, thereby diverging from the most common patterns, would be able to avoid predators who wanted to eat them. Exploratory behavior might also benefit from randomness, since by definition exploration does not know in advance what will be found. Still, such advantages would have occurred early in evolution and are not specific to human free will. Human beings must occasionally make a random choice, such as when lacking information about the options. Mostly, however, randomness is irrelevant to human behavior and unhelpful for functioning in culture.

Freedom and Situational Structure

As noted earlier, some skeptics of free will like to insist that freedom must include complete exemption from all external and prior causes (e.g., Montague, 2008; Sapolsky, 2023, 2024). While being able to overcome a specific cause of action is the essence of self-control and undoubtedly an increment in freedom, does complete freedom require exemption from all causes?

I agree with Sapolsky and others that complete exemption from causality is a dubious notion. Moreover, why would that even evolve? Participating in culture for best results requires sophisticated understanding of rules, opportunities, and contingencies, so that one's action can be informed by them. This is the opposite of being untouched by them.

All-or-nothing debates may be theoretically elegant, but their value for psychological science is limited. Nearly all psychological phenomena lie along one continuum or another. It is common to speak of high and low self-esteem, for example, but as any researcher knows, data show that self-esteem levels are spread along a continuum of scores. Moreover, no one has completely high or low self-esteem.

Hence a central point in my theory is that freedom should be understood as a matter of degree. Some actions are freer than others. Nearly everyone can furnish memories of actions that were relatively free and others that were not so free. Indeed, Stillman and colleagues (2011) asked participants to do precisely that, and nobody was unable to comply with the request. Free actions included important personal decisions and pursuing one's goals. Unfree actions often meant being required by external rules or authority figures to do something one would not have chosen oneself. The difference between free and unfree action is apparently familiar to most people.

Furthermore, the continuum of relative freedom may exist without the endpoints being needed. There may be no complete freedom and no complete unfreedom. Regardless, most of human action lies along a continuum, with the agent having various degrees of liberty to choose what they want to do.

Another stumbling block for free will skeptics is how the mind could create freedom, possibly by taking the stream of causality in multiple different directions. But that is not a problem if we recognize the multiple possibilities as out there—as inherent in the situation structure rather than being created by the mind. The evolved role of the mind is thus simpler and more plausible. All the human mind has to do is recognize the alternate possibilities in the situation (and act on them), not create them as some metaphysical innovation.

My training as a social psychologist is relevant here. Social psychologists like to think of their discipline as elucidating the causal power of situations. We are trained to be alert to variations in situation structure, and human behavior is how the individual reacts to the press of the situation, including its threats, constraints, and opportunities. An early attempt to construct a theory of situation structure by scrutinizing and categorizing all the independent variables in social psychology experiments settled on five megadimensions, one of which was the matrix of possibilities (Baumeister & Tice, 1985). Many situations are defined by offering multiple alternative possibilities, such as threat, opportunity, contingencies, escape options, and many more. All these entail something that might happen but also might not. The human mind discerns these possibilities and acts so as to steer events toward some outcomes and away from others, such as success and failure. In the same situation, a mind that could not recognize the multiple possibilities would be less free to make the most advantageous decisions.

Free will thus evolved to make behavior more flexible and thereby more adaptive. It did not evolve to create new alternative possibilities in the world. Rather, it evolved to recognize them, so as to make better behavioral choices. (Better in the sense of improving one's prospects, ultimately in terms of more survival and reproduction.)

Distinctive and Cultural Features of Human (Free) Action

In order for human beings to function in a society with culture, indeed to function in ways that help the culture itself succeed, multiple advances over the simpler ape mentality have been useful. In general, the human agent needs to understand the social system and its informational basis in shared beliefs and values. The human agent needs to base their actions on what the culture offers, what it permits versus forbids, and what it values, as well as the agent's own wants and needs.

By way of putting vivid flesh on abstract bones, my research (2024) pointed to three common and influential forms of the human agent. These show free will in action, in practice. First, humans are moral agents, who share collective understanding about moral rights and wrongs, and who use that understanding to influence their actions—how their brains tell their muscles to move. Second, humans are economic agents, who exchange resources in a marketplace, and in the modern world regularly use money, with vary degrees of carefulness. Third, humans are information agents, who participate in building the shared body of knowledge, by acquiring, sharing, discussing and disputing information with other people (Baumeister et al., 2018). All of these are qualitatively far beyond what even our closest animal relatives do, and hence they are part of the human essence.

Almost everyone, including outspoken skeptics of free will, acknowledges that the human mental system for causing action is vastly different from what other animals do. Evolution created a remarkably new mental system for controlling behavior. If free will exists, this is it. If it does not exist, this is what is routinely mistaken for it.

Invoking the Future

One clear advantage of human thinking is extension through time. Most animals live almost entirely in the present. They react to their immediate environment. Their responses may be shaped by learning that occurred in previous situations, but it is not even clear that they can mentally replay those earlier experiences. (There may simply be an affective response to the current options based on whether similar actions had been rewarded or punished on previous occasions.) Evidence for the ability to imagine the future beyond a few minutes is scant. In contrast, human action often invokes events in the distant past or future.

In particular, human beings seem better able than other animals to mentally simulate multiple, alternative futures—clearly a powerful boost to freedom of choice. Redshaw and Suddendorf (2016) showed that human children past the age of 3 could reliably prepare for two different possible outcomes, whereas even adult chimpanzees and other apes could not learn to do this. (Human 2-year-olds could not master this and thus were more similar to the apes.) Being able to understand that there are multiple, alternative future possibilities, and to use that understanding to dictate one's present actions, renders one's actions freer as compared to creatures who cannot do this.

Another important impact of time consciousness on free will is that people can understand their lives as actions as part of ongoing stories. This is sometimes called the "narrative self" (e.g., McAdams, 2001, 2013, 2019). The animal mind is designed to react optimally to the immediate situation. The human mind can see the immediate situation as part of an ongoing saga rooted in the past but aiming toward a particular future, usually with a happy ending. This helps one make choices that may lead to happy endings even if they are not the most immediately appealing options. So compared to the average ape, human beings choose actions that are less immediately gratifying but that make them better off in the long run. Humans can also work toward long-term goals, resuming work after interruptions, sometimes finding alternate pathways and strategies when one approach is blocked, and in other ways benefiting from behavioral flexibility in the context of a time-extended pursuit of some goal.

Consciousness

Conscious thought presents a potent challenge for free will theory. Shepherd (2012) showed that ordinary people overwhelmingly assume that free will is the result of conscious thinking (see also Stillman et al., 2011). But some influential thinkers have disputed that conscious thoughts have any causal impact on behavior (Dijksterhuis & Nordgren, 2006; Huxley, 1874; Wilson, 2002). Many scientists were persuaded by Libet's (2004) research that conscious thoughts do not have any causal impact (presumably because they occur after brain activity, though others object that brain activity has to precede conscious experience because it creates it). Culture is also about linking conscious experiences, thoughts, and feelings of many individuals in cooperative fashion.

How does science establish causality? Experiments manipulate one variable with random assignment and measure outcomes on another variable. If the manipulated variable is a conscious thought or feeling, and the outcome variable is behavior, that would confirm that conscious thoughts cause behavior. With two talented colleagues I embarked on an ambitious though skeptical survey of the research literature to see whether such findings existed.

As it turned out, there were abundant and diverse findings indicating that conscious thoughts have a causal impact on behavior (Baumeister et al., 2011). Here are some examples, culled from the extensive literature review (see original review for references and specific findings). Thinking about doing something makes people more likely to actually do it. Mental practice improves eventual performance outcomes, above and beyond physical practice (for which it is not a substitute but an auxiliary boost). Anticipating, planning, and intending increase and improve eventual execution and goal attainment. Rethinking the past (reinterpreting what happened or doing counterfactual replays) improves learning and subsequent outcomes. Logical reasoning requires conscious thought to get correct answers reliably (though the unconscious seeks to fake it effectively). Considering other people's perspectives improves many interpersonal strategies and outcomes, such as in negotiation. Engaging in deliberate self-affirmation alters and improves behavioral outcomes, indeed manipulations of conscious self-regard in either direction can alter behavior. There are many more.

There should therefore be no doubt about the causal impact of conscious thoughts and feelings. Among other implications, this should validate an existential approach to understanding human beings, in both psychology and philosophy.

Scientifically, the fact that conscious thoughts cause behavior raises the further question of how that happens. What is the process? My colleagues and I went back through all the findings in studies experimentally establishing that conscious thoughts and feelings cause behaviors (Baumeister et al., 2011). Several key themes emerged.

First, the effects of conscious thoughts were indirect. The conscious thoughts were several steps removed from controlling the muscles. Often conscious thoughts involved mentally simulating events away from the immediate stimulus environment, such as recalling past promises or thinking about what someone else might be doing or intending.

Second, there was no proof that the active process of choice or agency was itself conscious. Conscious thinking clearly has plenty of causal impact on choice, but it remains possible that the unconscious uses consciousness to think through the options, and then it makes the choice outside of consciousness. Usually, of course, it then announces the choice in the conscious portion of the mind, which is helpful for coordinating input from other parts of the brain. In that model, conscious thought would precede and follow from choice, but the choosing itself might be made unconsciously. This is possible but not proven.

Third, impulses to act typically originate outside of consciousness. Motivational processes may originate in the older and unconscious parts of the brain, even though they will soon pass into consciousness and may be modified there. For example, thirst is not created by consciousness, originating more likely in the body's gradual drying out, or stimulated by a subliminal cue. Once thirst shows up in consciousness, the person may consciously ponder where and how to get something to drink.

Conscious thoughts also trigger other mental processes, and indeed some have argued that that is a central function of consciousness (Baars, 1988, 1997; Humphrey, 1986). Information is scattered through memory and around the brain, and a conscious thought about one thing enables associations to bring other relevant information to mind.

Limited Energy

Agentic processes consume energy. Indeed, it was my work on limited willpower that led me into discussions of free will. The ego depletion work was covered in the preceding section of this chapter. Nevertheless, the point is that evolution found a way to use the body's energy supply to support advanced psychological processes, thereby improving the control of action and enabling more adaptive behavioral outcomes.

Meaning and Ideas

Another major aspect of human free will is its ability to incorporate ideas, including quite abstract ones, into the causation of behavior.

The question of whether ideas move molecules is not just a metaphysical puzzle but also central to existential psychology and philosophy, given the emphasis on choice. Anyone who has taken college-level physics courses knows that the physical processes governing molecular activity have no place for ideas as causes, and this fact encourages simpleminded people to dismiss the possibility of free will. However, as Anderson (1972) argued in his classic statement of emergence (titled "More Is Different"), the sciences can be understood as existing in a hierarchy, of which physics is only the most fundamental, rather than being all-encompassing. The hierarchy proceeds from physics into chemistry, biology, physiology, psychology, and then on to sociology and economics. No processes can violate the more fundamental ones, but they do add new causes that are not reducible. For example, biological processes cannot violate the laws of chemistry—but they add new dimensions that are not fully explained by chemistry.

Ideas cannot be found at the molecular level or even in terms of brain chemistry. But brain processes represent ideas and use them to guide action. In that way, ideas enter into the causal stream of physical reality. Indeed, the causal power of ideas is a basic and probably indispensable assumption in most human sciences, from history to sociology.

Acknowledging the causal power of ideas takes human behavior beyond the realm of purely physical causation. This is true even insofar as the causation by ideas is mediated by physical processes, such as brain cell activity. Meaning is not fundamentally a physical reality (e.g., Baumeister, 1991; Baumeister & Landau, 2018). Among other indicators, meaning has none of the usual physical properties, such as mass, velocity, or chemical composition.

The importance of meaning is evident in the three sample agents mentioned earlier. The moral agent considers moral principles and may even debate them with others before acting. The economic agent understands the abstract value of money and uses it to guide trade. The information agent gives and takes information from others, relating it also to shared understandings.

CONCLUSION

The term *free will* is contentious and perhaps infelicitous. But the human mind took huge evolutionary steps forward in how it controls action, and no scientific theory about the mind can be complete without acknowledging this important reality. Multiple advances make the human mind freer in its actions than the minds of other animals who cannot plan for the future, incorporate abstract ideas into behavioral decisions, and the like. Self-control, rational choice, planning, and initiative are common, important, and highly adaptive forms of human action.

REFERENCES

Anderson, P. (1972). More is different. *Science, 177,* 393–396.

Baars, B. J. (1988). *A cognitive theory of consciousness.* Cambridge University Press.

Baars, B. J. (1997). *In the theater of consciousness: The workspace of the mind.* Oxford University Press.

Baumeister, R. F. (1991). *Meanings of life.* Guilford Press.

Baumeister, R. F. (1998). The self. In D. T. Gilbert, S. T. Fiske, & G. Lindzey (Eds.), *Handbook of social psychology* (4th ed., pp. 680–740). McGraw-Hill.

Baumeister, R. F. (2005). *The cultural animal: Human nature, meaning, and social life.* Oxford University Press.

Baumeister, R. F. (2024). *The science of free will.* Oxford University Press.

Baumeister, R. F., Bratslavsky, E., Muraven, M., & Tice, D. M. (1998). Ego depletion: Is the active self a limited resource? *Journal of Personality and Social Psychology, 74,* 1252–1265.

Baumeister, R. F., & Heatherton, T. F. (1996). Self-regulation failure: An overview. *Psychological Inquiry, 7,* 1–15.

Baumeister, R. F., Heatherton, T. F., & Tice, D. M. (1994). *Losing control: How and why people fail at self-regulation.* Academic Press.

Baumeister, R. F., & Landau, M. J. (2018). Finding the meaning of meaning: Emerging insights on four grand questions. *Review of General Psychology, 22,* 1–10.

Baumeister, R. F., Maranges, H. M., & Vohs, K. D. (2018). Human self as information agent: Functioning in a social environment based on shared meanings. *Review of General Psychology, 22,* 36–47.

Baumeister, R. F., Masicampo, E. J., & Vohs, K. D. (2011). Do conscious thoughts cause behavior? *Annual Review of Psychology, 62,* 331–361.

Baumeister, R. F., & Tice, D. M. (1985). Toward a theory of situational structure. *Environment and Behavior, 17,* 147–192.

Baumeister, R. F., & Tice, D. M. (2022). Ego depletion is the best replicated finding in all of social psychology. *Scholarly Journal of Psychology and Behavioral Sciences, 6.*

Baumeister, R. F., Tice, D. M., & Bushman, B. J. (2023). A review of multi-site replication projects in social psychology: Is it viable to sustain any confidence in social psychology's knowledge base? *Perspectives on Psychological Science, 18,* 912–935.

Baumeister, R. F., & Vohs, K. D. (2016). Strength model of self-regulation as limited resource: Assessment, controversies, update. *Advances in Experimental Social Psychology, 54,* 67–127.

Baumeister, R. F., Wright, B. R. E., & Carreon, D. (2019). Self-control "in the wild": Experience sampling study of trait and state self-regulation. *Self and Identity, 18,* 494–528.

Brembs, B. (2011). Towards a scientific concept of free will as a biological trait: Spontaneous actions and decision-making in invertebrates. *Proceedings of the Royal Society B: Biological Sciences, 278*(1707), 930–939.

Carver, C. S., & Scheier, M. F. (1981). *Attention and self-regulation: A control theory approach to human behavior.* Springer-Verlag.

Carver, C. S., & Scheier, M. F. (1982). Control theory: A useful conceptual framework for personality-social, clinical and health psychology. *Psychological Bulletin, 92,* 111–135.

Carver, C. S., & Scheier, M. E. (1990). Origins and functions of positive and negative affect: A control-process view. *Psychological Review, 97,* 19–35.

Dang, J. (2016). Commentary: A multilab preregistered replication of the ego depletion effect. *Frontiers in Psychology, 7,* 1155.

Dang, J., Barker, P., Baumert, A., Bentvelzen, M., Berkman, E., Buchholz, N., . . . Zinkernagel, A. (2021). A multilab replication of the ego depletion effect. *Social Psychological and Personality Science, 12*(1), 14–24.

de Ridder, D., Lensvelt-Mulders, G., Finkenauer, C., Stok, F. M., & Baumeister, R. F. (2012). Taking stock of self-control: A meta-analysis of how trait self-control relates to a wide range of behaviors. *Personality and Social Psychology Review, 16,* 76–99.

de Waal, F. (2001). *The ape and the sushi master: Cultural reflections of a primatologist.* Basic Books.

Dennett, D. C., & Caruso, G. D. (2021). *Just deserts: Debating free will.* Polity Press.

Dijksterhuis, A., & Nordgren, L. F. (2006). A theory of unconscious thought. *Perspectives on Psychological Science, 1,* 95–109.

Duval, S., & Wicklund, R. A. (1972). *A theory of objective self-awareness.* Academic Press.

Freud, S. (1930). Civilization and its discontents (J. Riviere, trans.). Hogarth Press.

Freud, S. (1965). *New introductory lectures on psychoanalysis* (J. Strachey, Trans.). Norton. (Original work published 1933)

Freud, S. (1961). The ego and the id. In J. Strachey (Ed. & Trans.), *The standard edition of the complete psychological works of Sigmund Freud* (Vol. 19, pp. 12–66). Hogarth Press. (Original work published 1923)

Friese, M., Frankenbach, J., Job, V., & Loschelder, D. D. (2017). Does self-control training improve self-control?: A meta-analysis. *Perspectives on Psychological Science, 12*(6), 1077–1099.

Gailliot, M. T., & Baumeister, R. F. (2007). The physiology of willpower: Linking blood glucose to self-control. *Personality and Social Psychology Review, 11,* 303–327.

Gailliot, M. T., Baumeister, R. F., DeWall, C. N., Maner, J. K., Plant, E. A., Tice, D. M., . . . Schmeichel, B. J. (2007). Self-control relies on glucose as a limited energy source: Willpower is more than a metaphor. *Journal of Personality and Social Psychology, 92,* 325–336.

Garrison, K. E., Finley, A. J., & Schmeichel, B. J. (2019). Ego depletion reduces attention control: Evidence from two high-powered preregistered experiments. *Personality and Social Psychology Bulletin, 45,* 728–739.

Haggard, P., Mele, A., O'Connor, T., & Vohs, K. D. (2010). *Lexicon of key terms.* www.freewillandscience.com/FW_Lexicon.doc.

Hagger, M. S., Chatzisarantis, N. L. D., Alberts, H., Octavianus Anggono, C., Batailler, C. Birt, A. R., . . . Zwienenberg, M. (2016). A multi-lab pre-registered replication of the ego-depletion effect. *Perspectives on Psychological Science, 11,* 546–573.

Harris, M. (1980). *Cultural materialism: The struggle for a science of culture.* Random House/Vintage.

Heidegger, M. (1927). *Sein und zeit* [Being and time]. Max Niemeyer Verlag.

Humphrey, N. (1986). *The inner eye.* Faber & Faber.

Huxley, T. (1874). On the hypothesis that animals are automata, and its history. *Nature, 10,* 362–366.

Inzlicht, M., & Schmeichel, B. J. (2012). What is ego depletion? Toward a mechanistic revision of the resource model of self-control. *Perspectives on Psychological Science, 7,* 450–463.

Libet, B. (2004). *Mind time: The temporal factor in consciousness.* Harvard University Press.

Masicampo, E. J., & Baumeister, R. F. (2008). Toward a physiology of dual-process reasoning and judgment: Lemonade, willpower, and expensive rule-based analysis. *Psychological Science, 19,* 255–260.

McAdams, D. P. (2001). The psychology of life stories. *Review of General Psychology, 5,* 100–122.

McAdams, D. P. (2013). The psychological self as actor, agent, and author. *Perspectives on Psychological Science, 8,* 272–295.

McAdams, D. P. (2019). "First we invented stories, then they changed us": The evolution of narrative identity. *Evolutionary Studies in Imaginative Culture, 3,* 1–18.

Mele, A. R. (2006). *Free will and luck.* Oxford University Press.

Mele, A. R. (2022). *Free will: An opinionated guide.* Oxford University Press.

Mischel, W., Shoda, Y., & Peake, P. K. (1988). The nature of adolescent competencies predicted by preschool delay of gratification. *Journal of Personality and Social Psychology, 54,* 687–696.

Moffett, M. (2019). *The human swarm: How our societies arise, thrive, and fall.* Basic Books.

Moffitt, T. E., Arseneault, L., Belsky, D., Dickson, N., Hancox, R. J., Harrington, H., . . . Caspi, A. (2011). A gradient of childhood self-control predicts health, wealth, and public safety. *Proceedings of the National Academy of Sciences, 108,* 2693–2698.

Monroe, A. E., & Malle, B. F. (2010). From uncaused will to conscious choice: The need to study, not speculate about people's folk concept of free will. *Review of Philosophy and Psychology, 1,* 211–224.

Monroe, A. E., & Malle, B. F. (2015). Free will without metaphysics. In A. Mele (Ed.), *Surrounding free will.* Oxford University Press.

Montague, R. P. (2008). Free will. *Current Biology, 18,* R584–R585.

Muraven, M., & Baumeister, R. F. (2000). Self-regulation and depletion of limited resources: Does self-control resemble a muscle? *Psychological Bulletin, 126,* 247–259.

Muraven, M., Shmueli, D., & Burkley, E. (2006). Conserving self-control strength. *Journal of Personality and Social Psychology, 91,* 524–537.

Muraven, M., & Slessareva, E. (2003). Mechanism of self-control failure: Motivation and limited resources. *Personality and Social Psychology Bulletin, 29,* 894–906.

Muraven, M., Tice, D. M., & Baumeister, R. F. (1998). Self-control as a limited resource: Regulatory depletion patterns. *Journal of Personality and Social Psychology, 74,* 774–789.

Pocheptsova, A., Amir, O., Dhar, R., & Baumeister, R. F. (2009). Deciding without resources: Resource depletion and choice in context. *Journal of Marketing Research, 46,* 344–355.

Redshaw, J., & Suddendorf, T. (2016). Children's and apes' preparatory responses to two mutually exclusive possibilities. *Current Biology, 26,* 1758–1762.

Sapolsky, R. (2023). *Determined.* Penguin.

Sapolsky, R. (2024). Life without free will: Does it preclude possibilities? *Possibility Studies and Society,* 2(3), 272–281.

Sartre, J.-P. (1956). *Being and nothingness* (H. E. Barnes, Trans.). Citadel Press. (Original work published 1943)

Shepherd, J. (2012). Free will and consciousness: Experimental studies. *Consciousness and Cognition, 21,* 915–927.

Stillman, T. F., Baumeister, R. F., & Mele, A. R. (2011). Free will in everyday life: Autobiographical accounts of free and unfree actions. *Philosophical Psychology, 24,* 381–394.

Tangney, J. P., Baumeister, R. F., & Boone, A. L. (2004). High self-control predicts good adjustment, less pathology, better grades, and interpersonal success. *Journal of Personality, 72,* 271–322.

Vaidis, D. C., Sleegers, W. W. A., van Leeuwen, F., DeMarree, K. G., Saetrevik, B., Ross, R. M., . . . Priolo, D. (2024). A multilab replication of the induced-compliance paradigm of cognitive dissonance. *Advances in Methods and Practices in Psychological Science, 7,* 1–26.

Vohs, K., Schmeichel, B., Lohmann, S., Gronau, Q. F., Finley, A. J., Ainsworth, S. E., . . . Albarracín, D. (2021). A multi-site preregistered paradigmatic test of the ego depletion effect. *Psychological Science, 32*(10), 1566–1581.

Vohs, K. D., Baumeister, R. F., Schmeichel, B. J., Twenge, J. M., Nelson, N. M., & Tice, D. M. (2008). Making choices impairs subsequent self-control: A limited-resource account of decision making, self-regulation, and active initiative. *Journal of Personality and Social Psychology, 94,* 883–898.

Wicklund, R. A. (1975). Objective self-awareness. In L. Berkowitz (Ed.), *Advances in experimental social psychology* (Vol. 8, pp. 233–275). Academic Press.

Wilson, T. D. (2002). *Strangers to ourselves: Discovering the adaptive unconscious.* Harvard University Press.

Wood, W., & Neal, D. T. (2007). A new look at habits and the habit-goal interface. *Psychological Review, 114*(4), 843–863.

CHAPTER 18

From Authenticity to I–Thou Relationships

Self-Determination Theory as a Framework for the Study of Existential–Phenomenological Psychology

Richard M. Ryan *and* William S. Ryan

Existentialism is often described as both a literary and a philosophical tradition focused on the issues of human freedom, authenticity, and meaning (Warnock, 2008). Fundamental to this tradition is the assumption that people can take responsibility for their actions and act in ways that are congruent with their values and interests, and in so doing be authentic. Existential authors also vividly describe the ways in which people can avoid that freedom and responsibility, acting with "double mindedness" (Kierkegaard, 1956), fallenness (Heidegger, 1927/1962), bad faith (Sartre, 1956), and other forms of being that are either intra- or interpersonally defensive and inauthentic.

Among contemporary theories in empirical psychology, *self-determination theory* (SDT; Ryan & Deci, 2017) is particularly relevant to these themes. A broad theory of motivation and wellness, SDT places central importance on human experience, and how interpretations of one's world shape behaviors. This in part reflects the influence of phenomenological traditions stemming from Brentano and Husserl on the development of "naive psychology" by Heider (1958) (see Spiegelberg, 1972) and later de Charms (1968), perspectives that were, in turn, foundational to SDT (Deci & Ryan, 1985). Even more relevant, SDT alone among modern empirically based theories emphasizes issues of autonomy and integration, which are deeply implicated in the major existentialists' conceptions of authenticity, freedom, and responsibility.

In this chapter, we discuss the relations between existential phenomenology and SDT, drawing conceptual parallels and reviewing what SDT research has shown concerning existentialism's more empirical claims. Beyond identifying parallels we also draw contrasts between SDT and some existential arguments, such as Sartre's (1956) famed claim that "existence precedes essence." Specifically, SDT holds that human existence is characterized by inherent integrative tendencies (a nature) that can be either supported or thwarted by social environments and embraced or defended against by the individual. At the same time, SDT provides an account of how human freedom can be exercised, and how the realization of our essential human needs and capacities facilitates living well or *eudaimonia* (Ryan et al., 2013).

We begin with a very brief overview of SDT, to set the stage for reviewing how the theory connects with key ideas within the existential–phenomenological tradition. These ideas include the topics of authenticity, freedom, and "I–Thou" interpersonal relationships, death anxiety, and other themes and concepts salient within both SDT and existential–phenomenological thought. We also discuss SDT's views on people's life aspirations as they relate to basic psychological needs and eudaimonia. Finally, we address the theory's departure from some existentialist assumptions insofar as SDT posits a specific human nature characterized by both basic psychological needs and inherent integrative tendencies. Throughout, our claim is that many tenets of existentialist thinking are consonant with SDT's analysis of motivation and human autonomy. Further, we suggest that SDT provides a framework for empirical research on many of these themes of existential import, from authenticity to death anxiety.

SELF-DETERMINATION THEORY

SDT, after more than four decades of development, has become a broad and empirically well-supported approach to human motivation and well-being (see Ryan et al., 2022). Because both the theory and its evidence base are extensively reviewed in other publications, herein we focus primarily on conceptual aspects of SDT that are directly relevant to existential themes. Most important in this regard, and unlike other empirically based theories, SDT places the issue of human autonomy at the center of its research and theorizing.

Types of Motivation and the Autonomy Continuum

SDT posits that all intentional behaviors vary in their relative autonomy, or the degree to which they are endorsed by the self and willingly engaged. The theory therefore specifies an array of motivations ranging from external regulation, in which others control one's actions via rewards and punishments, to fully autonomously motivated behavior, such as actions expressing one's most integrated values or abiding interests (Howard et al., 2017; Ryan & Connell, 1989). In Figure 18.1 we provide a general schematic of the continuum of autonomy, which entails a taxonomy of types of motivation for everyday activities. These include the following.

External Regulation

In the process of negotiating life one can be pushed and prodded along. Indeed, for many people what determines their day-to-day actions is too often a conspiracy of external pressures and seductions to which they succumb, without feeling much volition or choice. When externally regulated, people feel "I have to do this." Being externally regulated is not simply a personal fault but also is frequently the product of truly controlling or oppressive circumstances within families, schools, workplaces, and other proximal social contexts, as well as of more pervasive cultural, political, and economic conditions (Ryan & DeHaan, 2023). To the extent external regulation is predominant, one finds a person conforming to external demands and regulations without a sense of authorship or volition, with a loss of vitality and lowered satisfaction.

Introjection

Even without direct outward oppression, some people push and prod themselves along, living up to demands or images they have taken in, perhaps from parents, peers, or media. Meeting these internalized standards involves compliance with "shoulds" and "musts," lest one experience anxiety or blows to self-esteem. These standards lead many to focus on appearance, image, and other external, approval-based sources of self-esteem. Such living is researched within SDT as introjection, ego-involvement, contingent self-esteem, and other "internally controlling" motives (Ryan et al., 2016).

Identification and Intrinsic Motivation

People can also engage life with high autonomy and a sense of both valuing and fully standing behind their actions and interests. That is, actions can be self-determined in the sense that they are congruent and self-endorsed. Classically, SDT has highlighted intrinsic motivation, which pertains to activities that are inherently satisfying, as highly autonomous. Yet within SDT extrinsic and instrumental motives can also be autonomous. Specifically, *identification* represents motivation in which one has identified with the value of and rationale for an activity, such that even if it is not enjoyable, it is done willingly. As we elaborate below, when one's life activities are motivated by intrinsic motivation and identification they are also experienced as *authentic*—the person sees themselves as the author of their existence. Indeed, in a truly authentic life one must do some active authoring—make specific choices in the direction of goals and pursuits that are truly endorsed by the self.

Amotivation

All of the above types of regulation represent motivation. Even being externally controlled involves intentional action and effort. Yet SDT also considers amotivation as a common state. *Amotivation* describes an absence of motivation and energy to act. The two main sources of amotivation are lack of value (one sees no worth, meaning, or merit in the behavior) or lack of perceived competence (one feels helpless or too ineffective).

The Continuum of Autonomy

These varied types of motivation often co-occur within activities and life domains, as people can have mixed motives in their pursuits. Yet, although each of these types of motivation has its own unique characteristics, they also vary systematically in their relative autonomy, allowing them to be ordered along a continuum of motivation that has strong empirical support (e.g., see Howard et al., 2017). When amotivated, people fully lack either autonomy and/or competence for acting. Proceeding from external, to introjected, to identified, to integrated, one finds a greater degree of autonomy, reflecting increasing internalization of the value of an action. Finally, like integrated motivations, intrinsic motivation is typically a highly autonomous form of behavior. That these motivations reflect systematic differences in autonomy has been supported in many investigations using different methods, including meta-analytic evidence for the continuum (see Ryan et al., 2022).

Basic Psychological Needs

SDT addresses all these states of motivation, both alienated and autonomous, and

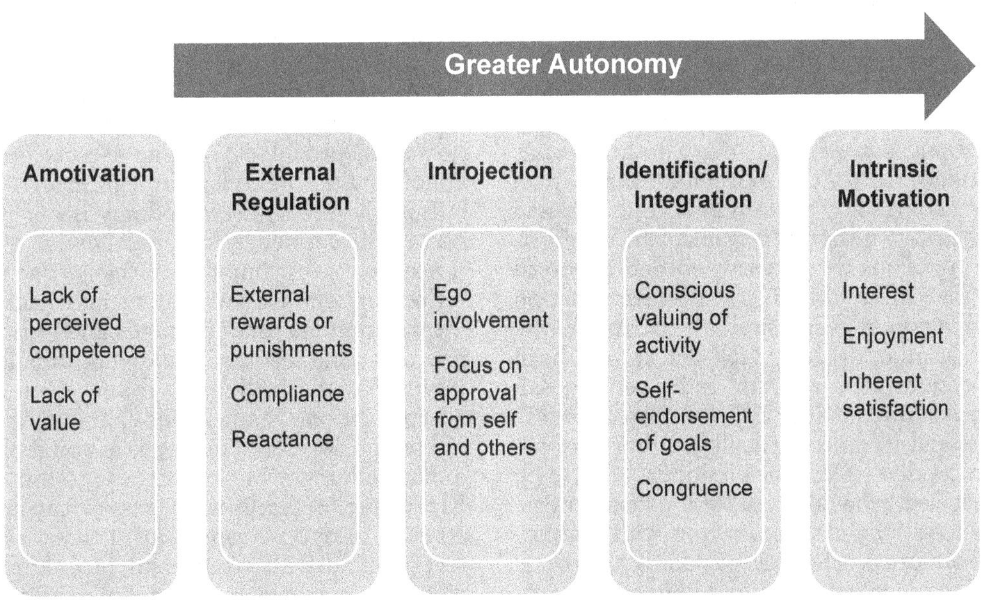

FIGURE 18.1. Continuum of autonomy: A taxonomy of types of motivation for everyday activities.

their variations and combinations in everyday social dynamics. Key to understanding these dynamics are satisfactions and frustrations of what SDT calls *basic psychological needs*. These are needs for autonomy (a sense of volition and "will"), competence (a sense of growth and effectiveness), and relatedness (connection and belonging). When these needs are met, people experience more vitality and empowerment, are energized by more autonomous forms of motivation, and experience greater integration. Specifically, they tend to be characterized by either more identified regulation or intrinsic motivation. Moreover, in contexts where these needs are supported, people experience greater psychological wellness. In fact, SDT argues that what makes these need-satisfactions *basic* is that they are essential to psychological growth, integrity, and wellness across development and cultures. Oppositely, frustration of these basic psychological needs is associated with diminished thriving and ill-being. For example, children of parents who tend to be very controlling or very cold or rejecting are more vulnerable to a variety of psychopathologies and forms of ill-being (see Ryan et al., 2016).

AUTONOMY, AUTHENTICITY, AND THE EXPERIENCE OF FREEDOM

We now further delve into the connections between SDT's conception of autonomy and the prominent existentialist themes of freedom and authenticity. It is a rich topic, as thinkers within the existentialist and phenomenological traditions have long depicted self-determination as possible, and as reflected in actions that are owned and endorsed by the self. Within SDT, self-determination and autonomy are similarly defined. One can be autonomous or self-determined both to actions that are fun and easily chosen (e.g., many intrinsically motivated behaviors) and to more difficult and burdensome choices that reflect one's abiding values (e.g., identified behaviors). Indeed, as existentialists have long claimed, acting with autonomy can often be difficult to do.

These conceptualizations of human autonomy can be traced to the Kantian assumption (Kant, 2017) that humans have a seemingly unique capacity for self-consciousness and reflection. This capacity allows one to take a "transcendent" perspective on one's own life, including the ability to evaluate one's own activities, values, and goals, and thus to potentially alter or reprioritize them (Korsgaard, 2009). This Kantian analysis was later extended by Husserl (1980), who provided a foundational methodology for existentialist philosophies by introducing phenomenological methods in which varied types of experience could be explored.

Applying Husserl's methodology, Pfander (1967) specifically researched the phenomenology of *self-determined* acts. He found that such acts appear "precisely not as an occurrence caused by a different agent but as an initial act of the ego-center itself" (p. 20). In Pfander's analysis, behaviors are truly self-determined only to the extent that they are (or would be) reflectively endorsed by the self or "ego center." Oppositely, non-self-determined acts are those people experience as being compelled by pressures from outside the self (such as external controls or introjections) that one does not fully or reflectively endorse or accept.

Phenomenologist Paul Ricoeur (1966) further elaborated this perspective in his classic work *Freedom and Nature*, clarifying that self-determination does not necessitate that an act be initiated by the self or occur in the absence of any external prompts. On the contrary, one can willingly join in with another's spontaneous idea, or even autonomously obey externally mandated rules or demands, provided that one ascents to, or concurs with, their merit or legitimacy.

Equally important, autonomy is not phenomenally defined by simply following one's inner feelings or impulses. Because one can reflect on one's own valuing and engagement with these inner demands and urgings, one can make choices as to what impulses, intuitions, and feelings to follow. One can accept that one is angry, for example, while autonomously choosing not to act on it. One might be hungry but still choose to fast. As Ricoeur (1966) argued, a person can even attempt to oppose aspects of their own nature (e.g., drives, traits, and inclinations), which he described as the "possibility of refusal," in which one willingly rejects or inhibits one's proclivities, temperament, or other impulses as they arise. Similarly, Sartre (1946/2007) stated, "the existentialist does not believe in the power of passion. . . . He thinks that man is responsible for his passion" (p. 5). In short, this means that part of being fully human entails selectively accepting and endorsing (or rejecting/inhibiting) not only prompts from the external world, but also those that arise from within.

These phenomenological findings are embedded in SDT's framework (see Ryan & Deci, 2017). In SDT, self-determination or autonomy applies not only to spontaneously motivated actions, but also to willingly complying with obligations, mandates, and pressures, the value of which one has fully internalized. And as we review below, listening to one's emotions and inner feeling is seen as important in SDT, and essential to integrative processes, but emotional signals are viewed as information rather than any infallible "organismic" wisdom.

SDT thus explicitly accepts, as do existential thinkers, that humans have capacities to selectively support some aspects of their natures and to oppose others. Our emotions, appetites, and traits make many ongoing demands on us, each of which we can reflectively consider and regulate. Some of these regulations (whether involving engagement or inhibition) will be the product of integrated value internalizations, others of internalized heteronomy and introjections. Indeed, in a SDT perspective, introjected motivation is often characterized by a kind of *willpower* in which one part of the person is overpowering another. Such "self-controlling" regulation should not be mistaken as autonomy, in which one is whole heartedly behind one's actions. Findings from SDT indeed suggest it is by working in accordance with one's needs, rather than opposing them, that typically represents the more congruent and autonomous forms of living (Vansteenkiste et al., 2023).

Freedom and Its Relations with Autonomy

SDT explicitly distinguishes between freedom and autonomy. Whereas freedom is defined within SDT as the absence of constraints, autonomy is rather the experience of endorsement and willingness to engage in particular actions. *Autonomy* concerns the self-governance or regulation by the self. Oppositely, *heteronomy* concerns being controlled or regulated by forces experienced as "outside" of oneself, whether these be other-controlled contingencies or self-controlling introjects. When autonomous, the individual stands behind or endorses their behavior, doing it willingly. When more heteronomous, the person is either divided in their motives or pressured to act in a self-controlling way.

One could, for example, have complete freedom (no constraints) and yet have no idea what to do with that freedom and therefore lack autonomy. Autonomy involves having aims and projects that are self-endorsed and volitionally undertaken, and thus entails a sense of direction, purpose, or goals. Although freedom from constraints can sometimes facilitate autonomy, it by no means guarantees it. In the context of freedom, one still needs valued goals or authentic interests to pursue, as well as a sense of competence to pursue them. That is, SDT argues that proactive agency requires more than freedom from constraints—it entails both autonomy and perceived competence.

Within existentialism the idea that we are "condemned" to freedom (Sartre, 1946/2007) expresses a somewhat different idea. It is that in every moment and in every situation one can always exercise choice and act with autonomy. In fact, whether one actively makes choices or lets circumstances push one around, for Sartre, one is enacting one's freedom. As Warnock (2008) reviewed, existentialist thinkers are not merely trying to logically prove that humans have such radical freedom, they are *evangelical*; they want to convince their readers and bring them the "good news" that they can choose their lives ahead.

Yet even in this tradition, this absolute freedom is bounded by the reality of one's circumstances and capacities. Sartre (1956) described such circumstance as one's *facticity*, the real conditions of one's life. Heidegger (1927/1962) similarly described *thrownness* as the place, time, culture, and context in which one finds oneself. These concepts of facticity and thrownness acknowledge that there is always a context within which one must exercise one's freedom, or alternatively within which one can shrink into inauthenticity, controlled motivation, and bad faith. Authentic autonomous actions are those that reconcile one's capacity for freedom with one's awareness of facticity.

Authenticity and Autonomy

The connections between SDT and existential conceptions of will and authenticity have been described in several previous articles (e.g., Ryan & Deci, 2004b, 2006; Ryan et al., 2012; Ryan & Ryan, 2019). These multiple reviews and discussions reflect the fact that existential thought is occupied by issues of autonomy, responsibility, and connection, all topics squarely within the frame of SDT.

The term *authentic* as used in the existential tradition has two primary meanings (Wild, 1965). First, it means something "proceeding from its reputed source or author." Second, *authentic* means "genuine or real." Both definitions of *authenticity* are relevant to our analysis and are embedded within SDT's viewpoint on autonomous functioning. In acting autonomously, a person "owns" their actions, identifies with them, and takes responsibility for them. They act willingly and sincerely. These are characteristics of the authorship aspect of authenticity. As for the genuineness or "real" aspect, autonomous actions take stock of what is actually occurring and what is truly possible (they do not ignore one's facticity). Actions are thus lacking in autonomy to the extent that they either (1) are experienced as not truly reflecting or emanating from the self or (2) are defensively out of touch with what is taking place either in the real world or within oneself. Living with illusions or in denial of one's circumstances and possibilities reflects a lack of authenticity and autonomy.

Self-Endorsement Requires Integration

In SDT it is argued that the self-endorsement of actions is typically a matter of degree. The more fully a person has integrated the value of an action, and the more it is fitting with basic needs and with the circumstances, the more autonomous and congruent it feels; one is "wholehearted." To the degree a goal or value is held defensively, such as in compartmentalization or biased reframing, then autonomy is compromised. Thus, in SDT, autonomy requires integration and active self-endorsement, a process that is seen as an ongoing and continual aspect of self-regulation.

As Ryan and Deci (2017) argued, the self is in essence a synthetic function, reflecting "an inherent tendency toward organization and integration" (p. 44), an assumption underlying all organismic theories (Ryan, 1995). However, this inevitably comes with the recognition that not all aspects of the personality (one's motives, values, and propensities) are well integrated; some will be merely introjected, or otherwise inauthentically espoused or compartmentalized. Acting with autonomy thus requires the ongoing process of synthesis and of determining, all things considered, the best courses of action.

Kierkegaard's view of authenticity is similarly connected to the issue of *self* as an integrative function. Indeed for him, the self was the continual activity of synthesis or integration. As he famously stated, the "self is a relation which relates itself to its own self . . . in short it is a synthesis" (1987, p. 146). Yet Kierkegaard strongly emphasized that this synthetic activity is neither automatic nor inevitable but instead is a continuous challenge. He argued that meeting this challenge requires ongoing self-questioning and reflection. To achieve a self is thus to be courageously engaged in "relating the self to the self" and taking responsibility for what one believes. In this view, an authentic person is "infinitely interested in his existence," and tries to act in congruence with what they truly believe, know, and feel. To fail at this task of selfhood (e.g., to be self-deceptive or defended) is to be inauthentic or in *despair*. As Taylor (1991) similarly described in his accounts of authenticity, it involves being "intrinsically open to challenge" (p. 222) and necessitates continual reevaluations of how one should act in order that "we can be called responsible for ourselves" (p. 224).

Heidegger (1927/1962) also distinguished authentic from inauthentic ways of being, even suggesting that most persons are typically not living authentically. Too often caught up in day-to-day pressures, fads, and events, they have little awareness of how or why they are doing what they are doing, existing instead in a "fallen" state. Yet individuals can engage their existence authentically. They can move toward a resolute, value-driven, way of being in the world. As Moran (2000, p. 240) suggested, for Heidegger such authenticity represented a movement toward wholeness: "humans have the urge to get their lives together, one wants to make it whole, to unify it." In later works, Heidegger made the connection between *whole* and *healthy*.

This viewpoint in which people have capacities for authenticity, and, by engaging them, feel more together and integrated relates directly to the SDT framework. SDT is fundamentally a theory of *self*, seeing its central function as that of integrating, to the degree one can, life experiences and events and using that information in the regulation of behavior. The self is responsible for creating and maintaining a coherent, organized personality in the face of a continuous stream of affordances, challenges, and threats impacting psychological thriving.

Thus, both SDT and existential psychology highlight the importance of autonomy and authenticity in human flourishing (DeRobertis & Bland, 2018). In the existential tradition, the awareness of one's freedom is often accompanied by the recognition of the responsibility to make authentic choices. In SDT, autonomy reflects the extent to which a person has engaged in this responsibility to act in ways that are congruent and true to oneself. Both traditions highlight the self as actively engaged in shaping its own identity and trajectories, and the importance of choice and responsibility in this ongoing process of self-creation. Further, in both traditions, experiencing autonomy and living authentically are seen as integral to a meaningful and fulfilling life (Ryan et al., 2008).

LISTENING TO ONESELF: SDT's CONNECTIONS OF AWARENESS AND AUTONOMY

SDT has been particularly focused on the conditions, both within the individual and in their social contexts, that are conducive to acting with autonomy. However, there are also intrapersonal actions associated with acting with autonomy. Most centrally, SDT argues that *awareness* is central to autonomy and healthy self-regulation. Especially critical to exercising autonomy and realizing authenticity is open, receptive awareness—a nondefensive observing and listening to oneself. SDT researchers have been studying two processes that facilitate such open and receptive awareness, namely mindfulness (Brown & Ryan, 2003) and integrative emotion regulation (Roth et al., 2019).

Mindfulness and Autonomy

Mindfulness is defined as open and receptive awareness of what is occurring (Brown et al., 2025). SDT specifically proposes that mindfulness conduces to more autonomous forms of motivation, those characterized by a sense of authenticity and self-endorsement. Mindfulness allows more awareness of internal phenomena, such as urges, emotions, impulses, and needs, as well as external conditions, such as temptations, conflicts, and pressures to act. And although mindfulness does not "cause" subsequent motivation, a more open, nondefensive awareness puts individuals in a better position to engage in meaningful choices and to better identify self-congruent actions (Ryan et al., 2021). For example, a person might mindfully observe inner discomfort as their friends try to pressure them to behave against certain personal values. That observation and awareness of inner conflict can then inform and hopefully facilitate more integrated choices concerning whether to "go along" or not.

Mindfulness is thus thought to support more autonomous forms of motivation. Yet greater awareness and openness may actually be associated with less motivation. SDT specifically suggests that controlled forms of motivation are in fact less likely to be enhanced by mindfulness or are even diminished. In this case a person becomes aware of the external source of motivation and its lack of "self"-support. Related to this, research shows that individuals higher in mindfulness are less easily influenced by extrinsic rewards (e.g., Brown et al., 2013). They are also less likely to be influenced by automatic responses and nonconscious defenses, conducing to more authentic actions (Levesque & Brown, 2007).

A recent meta-analysis by Donald and colleagues (2021) tested some of these overarching SDT formulations regarding how mindfulness relates to greater autonomy and more integrated forms of motivation. They located 89 studies, comprised of more than 25,000 participants, in which measures of motivation related to SDT's taxonomy and measures of mindfulness were both examined. Results revealed strong support for the positive association of mindfulness with autonomous forms of motivation, specifically intrinsic motivation and identified regulation. In contrast, mindfulness was negatively related to introjection, external regulation, and amotivation. In fact, associations with the SDT's autonomy continuum were graded in an expected way—the more autonomous the motive type, the stronger its association with mindfulness. As part of their review, Donald and colleagues also examined evidence across 21 experimental studies, finding that, here too, mindfulness enhancing interventions predicted more autonomous motivations.

Integrative Emotion Regulation

The organismic metatheory of SDT posits a general organizational tendency toward coherent self-regulation. That is, people are assumed to have an inherent propensity toward growth and integration, even though that general tendency can be obstructed or frustrated. As part of that organismic, integrative process, emotions are seen as of great value. Emotions, ideally, serve as *informational inputs* to self-regulation, rather than as direct activators or drivers of behavior. Whereas most other theories of coping and emotion regulation focus on the down-regulation of emotion, as if emotion was an interference with behavior, in SDT the emphasis is on acceptance of emotions and taking interest in what they are telling us. This process is described as *integrative emotion regulation* (IER; Roth et al., 2019; Ryan et al., 2016). It stands in contrast to suppressive regulation, or cognitive manipulations such as reframing that are aimed mostly at diminishing emotional impact, instead moving toward (rather than away from) one's emotional experience. IER is particularly relevant to the processes by which individuals can act authentically or in congruence with themselves.

In sum, the study of awareness via research on mindfulness and on IER suggests, in line with existential perspectives, that by engaging in our human capacities for mindfulness and reflective awareness we have the opportunity to guide life in a way that is choiceful, congruent, and authentic. In turn, the empirical evidence from SDT shows that such a way of living is predictive of higher-quality behavior, more persistence, and greater wellness.

THE INTERPERSONAL CONDITIONS FOR AUTONOMOUS, AUTHENTIC FUNCTIONING

A mainstay of SDT research has been social psychological—investigating how supports for basic psychological needs facilitate integrity and full functioning (Ryan & Ryan, 2019). Accordingly SDT claims that environments supporting autonomy, competence, and relatedness foster more autonomous and authentic forms of motivation, allowing people to live the freedom that existential philosophers so vividly celebrate.

Such influence can begin in early development. SDT research shows that controlling versus autonomy-supportive parenting styles foster very different outcomes. Controlling parenting not only interferes with healthy self-development (see meta-analysis by Bradshaw et al., 2025) it even disrupts the development of capacities to exert self-control and autonomy (e.g., Bindman et al., 2015). Research in education shows how controlling teaching styles inhibit autonomous motivations to learn and to integrate new knowledge (Reeve et al., 2022). Similarly, in people's work lives, controlling management styles lead to more disengaged, halfhearted workers, mediated by frustration of people's sense of autonomy (Slemp et al., 2018). Even in old age, controlling caregiver environments suppress autonomy and lead to less vitality (Bradshaw et al., 2024). Again, we cannot comprehensively review this social–interpersonal psychology of autonomy, but the evidence shows that across the lifespan and varied domains of activity, social conditions that support versus thwart autonomy, competence, and relatedness conduce to both more autonomous motivations to act and greater well-being.

Interpersonal supports for autonomy loom large within the SDT framework. It is argued that our relationships vary in terms of being autonomy supportive or controlling, leading people to be more or less authentic within them. Lynch and colleagues (2009), for example, did a cross-cultural study of Russian, American, and Chinese participants' experience of autonomy support within their close interpersonal relationships (e.g., to mother, father, romantic partners, friends, and roommates). They also measured the participants' "Big-Five" personality traits within each of these dyads, as well as their actual and ideal trait profiles in order to test the prediction first forwarded by humanistic psychologist Carl Rogers (1961) that discrepancies between ideal and actual self-characteristics would be negatively related to well-being, and to test the SDT prediction that partners' autonomy support would be associated with smaller discrepancies. As expected, discrepancies were negatively associated with wellness in all samples, and people's actual self-concept was closer to their ideal when they were with more autonomy-supportive partners. In short, participants were more able to be their ideal selves when with autonomy-supportive others. In a related cross-cultural study, Lynch and Sheldon (2020) found that the experience of *conditional regard* in one's relationships similarly predicted larger discrepancies between ideal and actual self-concept. They also reported that these discrepancies were associated with lower feelings of authenticity.

More recently within SDT, scholars have been studying not only such immediate contexts as school and work, but also the more pervasive conditions in societies that support versus thwart autonomy (Ryan & DeHaan, 2023). As an example, data show that when people perceive they have access to freedoms and resources within a culture, they have higher well-being, a result mediated by greater fulfillment of psychological needs for autonomy, competence, and relatedness (e.g., Bradshaw, DeHaan, et al. 2023; Martela et al., 2023). Thus, although SDT acknowledges the possibility of choice through reflective awareness, it also looks at social conditions that leave people without a sense of autonomy and documents the costs of that alienation.

INTERPERSONAL AUTHENTICITY: I AND THOU IN SDT

Another layer of authenticity that is of concern in both existentialism and in SDT is *interpersonal authenticity*. This means integration not only within oneself but also in interaction with others. This is not simply transparency, but rather a match between what one communicates and what one actually feels and intends (Ryan & Ryan, 2019).

Authentic relationships involve a respect for the person-ness of both parties. Here we enter into a deeper aspect of existential phenomenology, namely *social ontology* (see Ryan, 1989). From Husserl's *Cartesian Meditations* (1973) to Buber's influential *I and Thou* (1970), thinkers in the existential–phenomenological tradition have been concerned with both the ontology of others (how we know there are other minds) and what constitutes authentic relationships with others befitting their humanness. This literature reveals that we can be with and relate to others in distinct ways.

Sartre, for example, often portrayed human relations as a threat to freedom. In a famous passage in his *Being and Nothingness* (Sartre, 1956), he described "the look" phenomena, in which awareness of being observed by others undermines our freedom and autonomy. Testing this idea, Plant and Ryan (1985) indeed showed how observation by others can generate internally controlling states of ego involvement that undermine intrinsic motivation via diminished autonomy. But such interactions describe only some types of interaction, as within SDT people can also be with others in caring and autonomy supportive ways (e.g., Bradshaw et al., 2025).

In his dialogical approach, Buber (1970) specifically discussed the nature of authentic interactions, emphasizing the I–Thou relationship, where individuals engage with one another in a fully present and mutual manner that takes interest in and respects their perspective and viewpoint. This stands in contrast to the I–It relationship, where others are objectified, evaluated, or seen as a means to an end. Buber's relational philosophy is deeply rooted in the idea that meaningful existence is found in genuine encounters and connections with others.

Within SDT, *relationship motivation theory* (RMT; Ryan & Deci, 2017) is a relatively recent minitheory, which aims to specify the nature of interpersonal interactions that truly satisfy the need for relatedness. RMT argues that high-quality relationships are not "exchanges" between entities but rather interactions in which there is reciprocal respect for the selves of the individuals involved, and support of each other's basic psychological needs. Especially important is autonomy support, as it entails appreciation and consideration of the subjectivity and perspective of the other. Oppositely, *objectification* of the other denies their humanness. It represents a denial of their autonomy and their freedom to create themselves.

The concept of *mutuality of autonomy* within SDT further emphasizes not only the individual's autonomy but also the recognition and support of autonomy in others. This aligns with the idea that autonomy isn't solely an individualistic pursuit but is interconnected with social dynamics. Mutuality of autonomy represents the highest quality relationships, in which both relatedness and autonomy needs are satisfied. These concepts align with Buber's emphasis on the I–Thou relationship (Ryan & Deci, 2017), describing a relational stance where individuals acknowledge and engage with each other in a way that honors each person's autonomy. In the context of Buber's philosophy, this means approaching others not as objects or instruments for personal gain or exchange, but as unique individuals with their own autonomy and subjective experiences. In contrast, within I–It relationships one controls or treats others as objects.

Objectification takes many forms, but stereotypes and prejudices are a prime example (Legate & Ryan, 2014; Ryan et al., 2017). In prejudice one is predefining the other's character, without allowing that person to be other than the mold in which they are cast. As argued in RMT, stigma and prejudice present a denial of autonomy and relatedness, both delimiting the freedom of others by objectifying them, and also representing a form of ostracism and exclusion. Similar to positions taken in Sartre's (1948/1965) *Anti-Semite and Jew* and Fanon's (1967) *Black Skins, White Masks*, SDT argues that these ways of "relating" to others thwart autonomy and thereby dehumanize. This reflects, in Buber's terminology, an I–It relationship within which the freedom and experience of the other is ignored or oppressed.

Both SDT's mutuality of autonomy and Buber's social ontology highlight the importance of interpersonal authenticity (see Kaplan & Assor, 2012). Genuine connections, whether in the context of autonomy support in SDT or the I–Thou relationship in Buber's philosophy, involve an authentic recognition of the other's autonomy and a willingness to engage in a meaningful, reciprocal manner. This understanding of mutuality of autonomy has ethical implications. It suggests that ethical behavior involves not only respecting the autonomy of individuals but also fostering relationships that honor the autonomy of all parties involved (Ryan & Ryan, 2019). Indeed, recent work within SDT shows specifically how autonomy support is reflected in topics such as the quality of listening (Weinstein et al., 2021) and the acceptance of people's differences without stigmatizing them (e.g., Legate et al., 2019).

In sum, SDT's RMT and the social ontologies found in existential traditions like Buber's dialogical perspective converge in highlighting the significance of genuine, reciprocal relationships. Both perspectives emphasize the ethical and existential importance of recognizing and respecting the autonomy of individuals within the context of social interactions. This interconnected view reinforces the idea that autonomy is not only an individual pursuit but is intricately woven into the fabric of authentic, meaningful relationships.

TO HAVE OR TO BE?: INTRINSIC AND EXTRINSIC GOALS AND EUDAIMONIA IN SDT

Authenticity alone is no guarantee of wellness. Indeed, history is replete with examples of authentic but suffering individuals including, famously, both Kierkegaard and Nietzsche. Thus, a key question in existential thought has concerned what is entailed in a good life. In this regard, SDT distinguishes between hedonic well-being and eudaimonia. The former reflects a person's positive experience—having positive affect and avoiding negative affect. The latter, eudaimonia, concerns not affective outcomes, per se, but rather living well and pursuing what is valued and intrinsically worth doing. SDT, following the Aristotelian hypothesis, specifically suggests that living a eudaimonic life fosters outcomes such as vitality and meaning, and even if it is not focused on the attainment of pleasure, often yields positive emotions (Ryan et al., 2013). In contrast, SDT argues and shows that pursuit of selfish ends such as materialism, dominance, image, and fame often fail to yield the positive outcomes they promise, often because they fail to satisfy, or they even frustrate, autonomy and relatedness needs.

These ideas are formally laid out in SDT's *goal contents theory* (GCT; Bradshaw, 2023; Ryan & Deci, 2017). GCT posits that intrinsic life goals (i.e., pursuing goals such as personal growth, loving relationships, community, and health) enhance wellness, in large part because they satisfy basic psychological needs. They are typically pursued with autonomy, connect people with others, and foster a sense growth and competence. Success at intrinsic life goals has accordingly been associated with not only greater happiness but also lower ill-being (Kasser & Ryan, 1996, 2001).

GCT research contrasts intrinsic life goals with extrinsic life goals (e.g., pursuit of wealth, fame, power, and image). An emphasis on extrinsic aspirations is expected to, at best, only indirectly satisfy basic psychological needs, and the pursuit of these goals can also directly frustrate needs especially for autonomy and relatedness. For example, pursuit of money often compels people to give up time with family, outside interests, or other valued goals and activities. Pursuits of power or fame can lead to losses in relationships, even if one can feel competent and successful, as power often involves objectification of others, and fame, by contrast, the objectification of oneself by others.

Testing these ideas, Bradshaw, Conigrave, and colleagues (2023) conducted a systematic review and used multilevel structural equation modeling to meta-analytically evaluate the relations between intrinsic and extrinsic life goals and well-being and ill-being outcomes. Synthesizing 88 studies involving over 50,000 participants, they found that intrinsic aspirations were moderately and positively associated with well-being and moderately and negatively with ill-being. Results also supported the GCT hypothesis that to the extent that extrinsic aspirations predominate over intrinsic aspirations, the effects on well-being are negative and moderately sized. Such findings are important because they show how the aspirations we choose to follow shape happiness, with the irony that the more people are selfless in their pursuits, the more they seem to be self-fulfilled.

Similar ideas pervade existential humanistic thought. For example, humanistic psychologist Fromm (1981) raised what has been a recurring question in existential thought: What makes for a meaningful and good existence? Given our condition of freedom, what should we do with our lives? Fromm saw the connections here between the Aristotelian conception of eudaimonia and the fulfillment of true human needs. As he put it, optimal well-being involves distinguishing "between those needs (desires) that are only subjectively felt and whose satisfaction leads to momentary pleasure, and those needs that are rooted on human nature and whose realization is conducive to human growth and produces eudaimonia" (p. 4).

GCT argues that the reasons that a focus on intrinsic pursuits predicts wellness, whereas a focus on extrinsic pursuits (even when successful) does not, concerns the relations of these goals and aspirations with basic psychological needs. Intrinsic goals are more likely to fulfill these inherent human needs for autonomy, competence, and relatedness. Extrinsic goal pursuits, although sometimes competence confirming, are more likely to frustrate needs for autonomy and relatedness leading to lower wellness.

LIFE, DEATH, AND MEANING

Another common existentialist theme touched on by SDT research is that of death anxiety. Research has, for example, demonstrated that in older adults intrinsic goal attainment is associated with greater acceptance of one's own death and less death anxiety, whereas extrinsic goal attainment is negatively associated with death acceptance (Van Heil & Vansteenkiste, 2009). More generally, research shows that older adults who have experienced greater satisfactions of autonomy, relatedness, and competence in life show more adaptive death-related attitudes and death acceptance (Van der Kaap-Deeder et al., 2020) as well as greater meaning in life (see Tang et al., 2020). Greater autonomy is also associated with greater symbolic immortality, as well as sense of meaning in life, suggesting its contribution to this existential concern (Horner et al., 2021).

From the SDT point of view it is not avoidance of death but rather awareness of our finitude that can improve our ways of living (Ryan & Deci, 2004a). Illustrating this wisdom was a series of seven experiments by Niemiec and colleagues (2010). They drew on research from *terror management theory* (TMT; Greenberg et al., 1997), which has shown that presenting people with stimuli that make them aware of death, so-called *mortality salience* (MS) conditions, evokes defensive responses in which people tend to protect their worldviews and self-esteem. Niemiec and colleagues showed that under MS conditions, individuals low in mindfulness evidenced higher worldview defense and self-esteem striving, just as predicted by TMT. Yet this effect was not present in those higher in mindfulness. Those higher in mindfulness showed less suppression of death thoughts following MS exposure. Indeed, the experimental evidence indicated that more mindful individuals were more receptive to the death-related stimuli, attending to them more deeply, which in turn, partially mediated the inverse association between trait mindfulness and worldview defenses. These results suggest that mindful awareness helps people be more in touch with, and more fully emotionally integrate, potentially threatening stimuli, including mortality, and to react less defensively to them.

More recently Vail and Horner (2023) presented a series of seven studies investigating how a more self-determined orientation might help individuals deal with death-related anxieties and potentially ameliorate the impact of death awareness on wellness. First, they showed that MS stimuli (vs. non-death-related primes) increased death-thought accessibility, but not if participants had high need-satisfaction or were prompted to recall self-determined experiences. Next, they showed that higher need-satisfaction was associated with reduced death anxiety. Indeed, priming concepts of autonomy and self-determination eliminated the effect of MS on death anxiety. Another finding was that, although higher death-thought accessibility was related to lower life satisfaction, this effect was not significant for those high in need-satisfaction. They concluded that these findings suggest a self-determined orientation can be a buffer for existential concerns, including awareness of death.

HUMAN NATURE: ITS FREEDOM AND FACTICITY

The specification of inherent propensities toward integration and of basic psychological needs goes beyond the assumptions of many existentialists, who were either reluctant or opposed to characterizing what human nature entails. SDT instead puts forth a model of an authentic human nature grounded in the three basic psychological needs shared by all humans, and an active, integrative propensity.

Sartre (1956) famously declared that "existence precedes essence," highlighting that we humans are always free to define or redefine ourselves. Although SDT agrees that people can reflectively judge and choose to value or devalue what they are doing, what makes an activity valuable concerns what is intrinsically valued by humans. Thus, in contrast to Sartre, SDT posits that we humans have an *existence with an essence* that needs to be authentically realized. In this view there are inner guidelines for the self-realization that fit humanity better than others, namely basic psychological needs, and there are social conditions that can support or thwart that nature. We also have the freedom to allow that human capacity to guide us toward realization or to be led away from it. The goal of SDT is to both study and promote those social conditions and those forms of reflective and integrative awareness that allow us to be more authentic, more fulfilled, and more humane.

REFERENCES

Bindman, S. W., Pomerantz, E. M., & Roisman, G. I. (2015). Do children's executive functions account for associations between early autonomy-supportive parenting and achievement through high school? *Journal of Educational Psychology, 107*(3), 756–770.

Bradshaw, E. L. (2023). Causes, costs, and caveats: Reflections, and future directions for goal contents theory. In R. M. Ryan (Ed.), *The Oxford handbook of self-determination theory* (pp 139–159). Oxford University Press.

Bradshaw, E. L., Anderson, J., Banday, M., Basarkod, G., Daliri-Ngametua, R., Ferber, K., . . . Ryan, R. M. (2024). A quantitative meta-analysis and qualitative meta-synthesis of aged care residents' experiences of autonomy, being controlled, and optimal functioning. *The Gerontologist, 64*(5), gnad135.

Bradshaw, E. L., Conigrave, J. H., Steward, B. A., Ferber, K. A., Parker, P. D., & Ryan, R. M. (2023). A meta-analysis of the dark side of the American dream: Evidence for the universal wellness costs of prioritizing extrinsic over intrinsic goals. *Journal of Personality and Social Psychology, 124*(4), 873–899.

Bradshaw, E. L., DeHaan, C., Parker, P. D., Curren, R., Duineveld, J. J., Di Domenico, S. I., & Ryan, R. M. (2023). The perceived conditions for living well: Positive perceptions of primary goods linked with basic psychological needs and wellness. *Journal of Positive Psychology, 18*(1), 44–60.

Bradshaw, E. L., Duineveld, J. J., Conigrave, J. H., Steward, B. A., Ferber, K. A., Joussemet, M., Parker, P. D., & Ryan, R. M. (2025). Disentangling autonomy-supportive and psychologically controlling parenting: A meta-analysis of self-determination theory's dual process model across cultures. *American Psychologist, 80*(6), 879–895.

Brown, K. W., Goodman, R. J., & Inzlicht, M. (2013). Dispositional mindfulness and the attenuation of neural responses to emotional stimuli. *Social Cognitive and Affective Neuroscience, 8*(1), 93–99.

Brown, K. W., & Ryan, R. M. (2003). The benefits of being present: Mindfulness and its role in psychological well-being. *Journal of Personality and Social Psychology, 84*(4), 822–848.

Brown, K. W., Ryan, R. M., & Creswell, J. D. (Eds.). (2025). *Handbook of mindfulness* (2nd ed.). Guilford Press.

Buber, M. (1970). *I and thou* (R. G. Smith, Trans.; 2nd ed.). Scribner.

de Charms, R. (1968). *Personal causation: The internal affective determinants of behavior.* Academic Press.

Deci, E. L., & Ryan, R. M. (1985). *Intrinsic motivation and self-determination in human behavior.* Plenum Press.

DeRobertis, E. M., & Bland, A. M. (2018). Tapping the humanistic potential of self-determination theory: Awakening to paradox. *The Humanistic Psychologist, 46*(2), 105–128.

Donald, J. N., Bradshaw, E. L., Conigrave, J. H., Parker, P. D, Byatt, L., Noetel, M., & Ryan, R. M. (2021). Paths to the light and dark sides of human nature: A meta-analysis of the prosocial benefits of autonomy and the antisocial costs of control. *Psychological Bulletin, 147*(9), 921–946.

Fanon, F. (1967). *Black skins, white masks.* Grove.

Fromm, E. (1981). *To have or to be?* Bantam.

Greenberg, J., Solomon, S., & Pyszczynski, T. (1997). Terror management theory of self-esteem and cultural worldviews: Empirical assessments and conceptual refinements. In M. P. Zanna (Ed.), *Advances in experimental social psychology* (Vol. 29, pp. 61–139). Academic Press.

Heidegger, M. (1962). *Being and time.* HarperCollins. (Original work published 1927)

Heider, F. (1958). *The psychology of interpersonal relations.* Wiley.

Horner, D. E., Sielaff, A. R., & Greenberg, J. (2021). Autonomy, meaning, and the mediating role of symbolic immortality. *Journal of Humanistic Psychology.*

Howard, J. L., Gagné, M., & Bureau, J. S. (2017). Testing a continuum structure of self-determined motivation: A meta-analysis. *Psychological Bulletin, 143*(12), 1346–1377.

Husserl, E. (1973). *Cartesian meditations: An introduction to phenomenology* (D. Cairns, Trans.). Martinus Nijhoff. (Original work published 1931)

Husserl, E. (1980). *Phenomenology and the foundations of the sciences.* Springer.

Kant, I. (2017). *Kant: The metaphysics of morals.* Cambridge University Press.

Kaplan, H., & Assor, A. (2012). Enhancing autonomy-supportive I–Thou dialogue in schools: Conceptualization and socio-emotional effects of an intervention program. *Social Psychology of Education, 15,* 251–269.

Kasser, T., & Ryan, R. M. (1996). Further examining the American dream: Differential correlates of intrinsic and extrinsic goals. *Personality and Social Psychology Bulletin,* 22(3), 280–287.

Kasser, T., & Ryan, R. M. (2001). Be careful what you wish for: Optimal functioning and the relative attainment of intrinsic and extrinsic goals. In P. Schmuck & K. M. Sheldon (Eds.), *Life goals and well-being: Towards a positive psychology of human striving* (pp. 115–129). Hogrefe & Huber.

Kierkegaard, S. (1956) *Purity of heart is to will one thing*. Harper & Row.

Kierkegaard, S. (1987). *Fear and trembling, and the sickness unto death* (R. L. Perkins, Trans.). Mercer University Press.

Korsgaard, C. (2009). *Self-constitution: Agency, identity, and integrity*. Oxford University Press.

Legate, N., & Ryan, W. S. (2014). Autonomy support as acceptance for disclosing and developing a healthy lesbian, gay, bisexual or transgendered identity. In N. Weinstein (Ed.), *Human motivation and interpersonal relationships*. Springer Science + Business Media.

Legate, N., Weinstein, N., Ryan, W. S., DeHaan, C. R., & Ryan, R. M. (2019). Parental autonomy support predicts lower internalized homophobia and better psychological health indirectly through lower shame in lesbian, gay and bisexual adults. *Stigma and Health, 4*(4), 367–376.

Levesque, C., & Brown, K. W. (2007). Mindfulness as a moderator of the effect of implicit motivational self-concept on day-to-day behavioral motivation. *Motivation and Emotion, 31*(4), 284–299.

Lynch, M. F., La Guardia, J. G., & Ryan, R. M. (2009). On being yourself in different cultures: Ideal and actual self-concept, autonomy support, and well-being in China, Russia, and the United States. *Journal of Positive Psychology, 4*(4), 290–304.

Lynch, M. F., & Sheldon, K. M. (2020). Conditional regard, self-concept, and relational authenticity: Revisiting some key Rogerian concepts cross-culturally, through multilevel modeling. *Journal of Humanistic Psychology, 60*(2), 168–186.

Martela, F., Lehmus-Sun, A., Parker, P. D., Pessi, A. B., & Ryan, R. M. (2023). Needs and well-being across Europe: Basic psychological needs are closely connected with well-being, meaning, and symptoms of depression in 27 European countries. *Social Psychological and Personality Science, 14*(5), 501–514.

Moran, D. (2000). *Introduction to phenomenology*. Routledge.

Niemiec, C. P., Brown, K. W., Kashdan, T. B., Cozzolino, P. J., Breen, W. E., Levesque-Bristol, C., & Ryan, R. M. (2010). Being present in the face of existential threat: The role of trait mindfulness in reducing defensive responses to mortality salience. *Journal of Personality and Social Psychology, 99*(2), 344–365.

Pfander, A. (1967). Motives and motivation (H. Spiegelberg, Trans.). In A. Pfander (Ed.), *Munchener philosophische abhandlungen (festschrift fur Theodor Lipps)* [Phenomenology of willing and motivation: And other phaenomenlogica] (pp. 163–195). Northwestern University Press.

Plant, R. W., & Ryan, R. M. (1985). Intrinsic motivation and the effects of self-consciousness, self-awareness, and ego-involvement: An investigation of internally-controlling styles. *Journal of Personality, 53,* 435–449.

Reeve, J., Ryan, R. M., Cheon, S. H., Matos, L., & Kaplan, H. (2022). *Supporting students' motivation*. Taylor & Francis.

Ricoeur, P. (1966). *Freedom and nature: The voluntary and the involuntary*. Northwestern University Press.

Rogers, C. R. (1961). *On becoming a person: A therapist's view of psychotherapy*. Mariner Books.

Roth, G., Vansteenkiste, M., & Ryan, R. M. (2019). Integrative emotion regulation: Process and development from a self-determination theory perspective. *Development and Psychopathology, 31*(3), 945–956.

Ryan, R. M. (1989). Social ontology and its relevance for psychological theory. *New Ideas in Psychology, 7,* 115–124.

Ryan, R. M. (1995). Psychological needs and the facilitation of integrative processes. *Journal of Personality, 63*(3), 397–427.

Ryan, R. M., & Connell, J. P. (1989). Perceived locus of causality and internalization: Examining reasons for acting in two domains. *Journal of Personality and Social Psychology, 57*(5), 749–761.

Ryan, R. M., Curren, R. R., & Deci, E. L. (2013). What humans need: Flourishing in Aristotelian philosophy and self-determination theory. In A. S. Waterman (Ed.), *The best within us: Positive psychology perspectives on eudaimonic functioning* (pp. 57–75). American Psychological Association Books.

Ryan, R. M., & Deci, E. L. (2004a). Autonomy is no illusion: Self-determination theory and the empirical study of authenticity, awareness, and will. In J. Greenberg, S. L. Koole, & T. Pyszczynski (Eds.), *Handbook of experimental existential psychology* (pp. 449–479). Guilford Press.

Ryan, R. M., & Deci, E. L. (2004b). Avoiding death and engaging life as accounts of meaning and culture: A Comment on Pyszczynski, Greenberg, Solomon, Arndt, and Schimel (2004). *Psychological Bulletin, 130*(3), 473–477.

Ryan, R. M., & Deci, E. L. (2006). Self-regulation and the problem of human autonomy: Does psychology need choice, self-determination, and will? *Journal of Personality, 74*(6), 1557–1585.

Ryan, R. M., & Deci, E. L. (2017). *Self-determination theory: Basic psychological needs in motivation, development, and wellness.* Guilford Press.

Ryan, R. M., Deci, E. L., & Vansteenkiste, M. (2016). Autonomy and autonomy disturbances in self-development and psychopathology: Research on motivation, attachment, and clinical process. In D. Cicchetti (Ed.), *Developmental psychopathology: Vol. 1. Theory and method* (3rd ed., pp. 385–438). Wiley.

Ryan, R. M., & DeHaan, C. R. (2023). The social conditions for human flourishing: Economic and political influences on basic psychological needs. In R. M. Ryan (Ed.), *The Oxford handbook of self-determination theory* (pp. 1149–1172). Oxford University Press.

Ryan, R. M., Donald, J. N., & Bradshaw, E. L. (2021). Mindfulness and motivation: A process view using self-determination theory. *Current Directions in Psychological Science, 30*(4), 300–306.

Ryan, R. M., Duineveld, J. J., Di Domenico, S. I., Ryan, W. S., Steward, B., & Bradshaw, E. L. (2022). We know this much is (meta-analytically) true: A meta-review of meta-analytic findings evaluating self-determination theory. *Psychological Bulletin, 148*(11–12), 813–842.

Ryan, R. M., Huta, V., & Deci, E. L. (2008). Living well: A self-determination theory perspective on eudaimonia. *Journal of Happiness Studies, 9*(1), 139–170.

Ryan, R. M., Legate, N., Niemiec, C. P., & Deci, E. L. (2012). Beyond illusions and defense: Exploring the possibilities and limits of human autonomy and responsibility through self-determination theory. In P. R. Shaver & M. Mikulincer (Eds.), *Meaning, mortality, and choice: The social psychology of existential concerns* (pp. 215–233). American Psychological Association.

Ryan, W. S., Legate, N., Weinstein, N., & Rahman, Q. (2017). Autonomy support fosters lesbian, gay, and bisexual identity disclosure and wellness, especially for those with internalized homophobia. *Journal of Social Issues, 73*(2), 289–306.

Ryan, W. S., & Ryan, R. M. (2019). Toward a social psychology of authenticity: Exploring within-person variation in autonomy, congruence, and genuineness using self-determination theory. *Review of General Psychology, 23*(1), 99–112.

Sartre, J.-P. (2007). *Existentialism is a humanism.* Yale University Press. (Original work published 1946)

Sartre, J.-P. (1965). *Anti-semite and Jew.* Schocken Books. (Original work published 1948)

Sartre, J.-P. (1956). *Being and nothingness.* Philosophical Library.

Slemp, G. R., Kern, M. L., Patrick, K. J., & Ryan, R. M. (2018). Leader autonomy support in the workplace: A meta-analytic review. *Motivation and Emotion, 42*(5), 706–724.

Spiegelberg, H. (1972). *Phenomenology in psychology and psychiatry: A historical introduction.* Northwestern University Press.

Tang, M., Wang, D., & Guerrien, A. (2020). A systematic review and meta-analysis on basic psychological need satisfaction, motivation, and well-being in later life: Contributions of self-determination theory. *Psych Journal, 9,* 5–33.

Taylor, C. (1991). Responsibility for self. In P. French (Ed.), *The spectrum of responsibility* (pp. 214–224). St. Martin's Press.

Vail, K. E. III, & Horner, D. E. (2023). The captain of my soul: Self-determination and need-satisfaction help manage death-related cognition, anxiety, and well-being. *Journal of Personality and Social Psychology, 125*(6), 1308–1331.

Van der Kaap-Deeder, J., Soenens, B., Van Petegem, S., Neyrinck, B., De Pauw, S., Raemdonck, E., & Vansteenkiste, M. (2020). Live well and die with inner peace: The importance of retrospective need-based experiences, ego integrity and despair for late adults' death attitudes. *Archives of Gerontology and Geriatrics, 91,* 104184.

Van Hiel, A., & Vansteenkiste, M. (2009). Ambitions fulfilled?: The effects of intrinsic and extrinsic goal attainment on older adults' ego-integrity and death attitudes. *International Journal of Aging and Human Development, 68,* 27–51.

Vansteenkiste, M., Soenens, B., & Ryan, R. M. (2023). Basic psychological needs theory: A conceptual and empirical review of key criteria. In R. M. Ryan (Ed.), *The Oxford handbook of self-determination theory* (pp. 84–123). Oxford University Press.

Warnock, M. (2008). *Existentialism.* Oxford University Press.

Weinstein, N., Huo, A., & Itzchakov, G. (2021). Parental listening when adolescents self-disclose: A preregistered experimental study. *Journal of Experimental Child Psychology, 209,* 105178.

Wild, J. (1965). Authentic existence: A new approach to "value theory." In J. M. Edie (Ed.), *An invitation to phenomenology: Studies in the philosophy of experience* (pp. 59–78). Quadrangle.

CHAPTER 19

Solving the Existential Problem of Choice

Sartre, Free Will, Goal Breakthroughs, Courage, Autonomy, and Self-Concordance

Kennon M. Sheldon

Existential psychology addresses the most basic dilemmas and concerns of human existence—such as the problem of finding meaning given the world's seemingly inherent meaninglessness; the problem of affirming life despite the inevitability of death; the problem of being an authentic instead of a false self; and the problem of connecting with others despite our fundamental isolation from them (Pyszczynski et al., 2010). Arguably the most central problem of all, however, is *the problem of choice*—of somehow deciding what to do next, from among all the possibilities. Choice (i.e., behavioral selection) is perhaps most critical because it embodies our concrete response to all the other existential dilemmas, providing our means of dealing with them. Choice is where the "rubber meets the road" as we navigate our lives, turning mere deliberations into irrevocable actions.

Accordingly, the problem of choice (and its seeming absence, sometimes) has been addressed by nearly all existentially oriented writers and philosophers, including Søren Kierkegaard, Rollo May, Martin Heidegger, Friedrich Nietzsche, and Jean-Paul Sartre. In this chapter I specifically adopt Sartre's (1946, 1980) position on choice, attempting to derive a fresh perspective upon several relevant constructs from research psychology. Sartre argued that we humans are "condemned" to freedom, meaning that we have no choice but to create ourselves via our choices. Even when we make no explicit decision, or let others decide for us, this is still a choice that we have made, whether we recognize it or not. Of course, we always choose within situations and contexts, which can sometimes feel very pressuring or pose great difficulties. Still, we always have the final say over our behavior, like it or not (Libet, 1999). How could it be otherwise?

Sartre's position implies that the feeling of being compelled to make certain choices is an illusion—a sign of immaturity and/or an attempt to evade responsibility and emotional consequences for one's choices. Such misattributions involve mistaking mere difficulties (the situation is very difficult or pressuring) for the literal absence of choice ("I have zero degrees of freedom"), which, according to Sartre, is never the case. Similarly, Frankl (1946) insisted, with reference to his dehumanizing experiences in a Nazi prison camp, that one always has the freedom "to choose one's attitude in any given set of circumstances, to choose one's own way. And there are always choices to make." Since we cannot help but choose, the goal, for Sartre, Frankl, and many other existentially and humanistically oriented psychologists, is to learn to choose in a more authentic and responsible way—a way that is consistent with our deeply held values and our ideals concerning how humans should be (Rogers, 1964).

THE FREE WILL QUESTION

Sartre's "radical freedom" position relies on the assumption of human *free will*, a long-controversial claim in science and philosophy (Baumeister, 2008; Dennett, 2003; Harris, 2012; Sheldon, 2022). Here, it is worth briefly unpacking the concept of free will (versus determinism), because of the light it can shed on the existential problem of choice.

Free will, according to *Wikipedia*, is "the capacity or ability to choose between different courses of action unimpeded." Agents with free will deliberate about what to do, then make and enact decisions. Again, Sartre (1946) insisted that free will is inescapable, and that we are thus responsible for using it as wisely as we can.

The contrasting position is that all human behavior is *determined* by factors over which we have no knowledge and no control, such that the feeling of exercising free will is an illusion. According to determinism, Sartre's position on choice is nonsense. Instead of *always* choosing, we *never* choose—behavioral selection is instead determined by precognitive and automatic physical mechanisms. Determinism is a grounding assumption of most scientific inquiry and is prevalent even in psychology, as expressed in the scientist's desire to identify the simplest and most parsimonious mechanisms accounting for complex phenomena, including the most complex phenomenon of all, human behavior. Even today, a common ethos in psychology is to keep digging down to uncover the underlying physical or brain causes of behavior, with a corresponding reluctance to ascribe causality to "merely subjective" factors. In this view, supposed subjective causes are always reducible to physical causes and mechanisms, beneath or beyond the person's awareness and control. Accordingly, free will is impossible, and we cannot be held responsible for our actions (Harris, 2012; Sapolsky, 2023).

The dogma of determinism is far from universally accepted, however. For example, the "compatibilist" philosophical perspective insists that free will is conceptually consistent with brute physicality—that subjective agency has a solid place in the material universe and is not just an illusion. In this view, the choices made by human minds are legitimate potential causes of their bodies' behavior, which cannot be directly reduced to physical and nonpsychological causes. This is because choice is affected by the deliberations of a conscious person, making decisions in the present moment—an emergent process which is "more than" the neuronal events and brain systems that constitute it, although that deliberative process couldn't happen without the support of those events and systems. Indeed, human agency may have evolved within the physical universe as a radical new adaptive strategy, going beyond other animals and primates (Sheldon, 2024b). This adaptation allows humans to keep visualizing alternative possible futures and then deciding between them, moment by moment, within their often complex and shifting social and temporal worlds. If we couldn't decide "on the fly" as a temporally extended agent (or at least, as an agent-simulation, as will be discussed below), we couldn't function within ordinary human life. Brain diseases such as Alzheimer's disease and dementia illustrate what happens when people lose the brain capacity to exert temporally extended agency.

The compatibilist position seems intuitively plausible to most, and indeed, it is the norm among professional philosophers, with 59% subscribing to compatibilism and only 9% subscribing to hard determinism (Chalmers, 2014; Weinberg, 2020). Still, it remains possible that compatibilist intuitions merely reflect wishful or even magical thinking, problems to which even philosophers may fall prey (Harris, 2012). Also, it remains conceivable that more basic physical causes will be found that can fully account for behavioral selection, which would reduce subjective agency to a mere epiphenomenal illusion and invalidate Sartre's position. Because there are strong feelings on both sides, the free will versus determinism question remains unresolved and, to many, appears unsolvable.

To advance understanding of the possibility of free will (and hence, understanding of the existential problem of choice), a proper conceptual definition is needed, as well as a proper scientific model for testing that definition (Sheldon, 2022). As a goal researcher, I adopt the compatibilist definition proposed by philosopher Christian List in his book *Why Free Will Is Real* (2019). According to List's highly psychological approach, free will requires three related mental capabilities: the ability to generate alternative possibilities to consider, the ability to make a choice among them, and the ability to control action in service of that choice. Any system (natural or perhaps artificial) with these three capabilities has free will, by this definition. List showed that these abilities exist at a level of organization in the material universe (i.e., within the operations of the evolved human mind) that is of course constituted by, yet can also be downwardly regulating of, lower-level processes occurring in the brain and body. In a similar vein, Sperry's (1993) "monist-interactionist" position acknowledged that there is only one world yet insisted that mental processes can have a somewhat independent status in that world, which allows them to affect subsequent physical conditions in ways that mere knowledge of prior physical conditions could not have predicted. Given a fully functional human brain, agentic processes unfold by a logic of their own that is often determinative of the person's behavior, despite being influenced and sometimes biased by underlying physical or somatic conditions.

An analogy may be helpful. The behaviors of computers are determined by the programmed algorithms that run them. Of course, those behaviors could not occur without the support of the bits and bytes, the registers, and the cables—the physical machinery of the computer. But it is *the intentions of the programmer* that determine what the computer does, just as the *intentions of the driver* determine where a car goes. Similarly, by exerting our free will capacity, we program ourselves, imagining and selecting the intentions that drive our own machinery (will I turn the car right, toward the gym, or left, toward the ice cream store?). Of course, the computer programmer and the automobile driver are physically separate from the programmed computer and the driven car, whereas the "internal programmer," supposedly helping run its own mind, is not. Still, as I argue below, we internal agents have considerable independence from our constitutive machinery, because we are partially "cut off" from our implicit sources. Thus, we are free to make poor and even terrible choices, as well as brilliant and creative ones.

THE GOAL BREAKTHROUGH MODEL OF FREE WILL

If free will exists, how does it work? The recently proffered goal breakthrough model (GBM) offers a tangible and testable perspective on the goal selection process, one that is consistent with List's (2014, 2019) conception of the operation of free will (Sheldon et al., 2023b). It also offers a powerful lens for understanding the existential activity of making choices, including optimal choices. The GBM is presented and explicated below.

The GBM is designed to explain how people get new ideas for action. It is based on creative process models of cognitive discovery, generalized to the case of new goal or action discovery. The basic sequence leading from dissatisfaction to preparation to incubation to illumination and elaboration was first proposed by Wallas (1926). In that model, the would-be creator starts out trying to solve a problem (dissatisfaction). They exert conscious effort collecting information and looking for answers, often failing at first (preparation). Then their attention moves elsewhere, but the "gears keep churning"—activity continues beneath the surface (incubation). At some fortuitous moment, perhaps prompted by a momentary perception or event, a potential solution to the cognitive problem pops into mind (illumination). Then, the creator tests and applies the new idea (elaboration).

Many anecdotal examples of such a process exist, the most famous being Archimedes' realization, as he stepped into the bathtub, that the volume of the King's golden

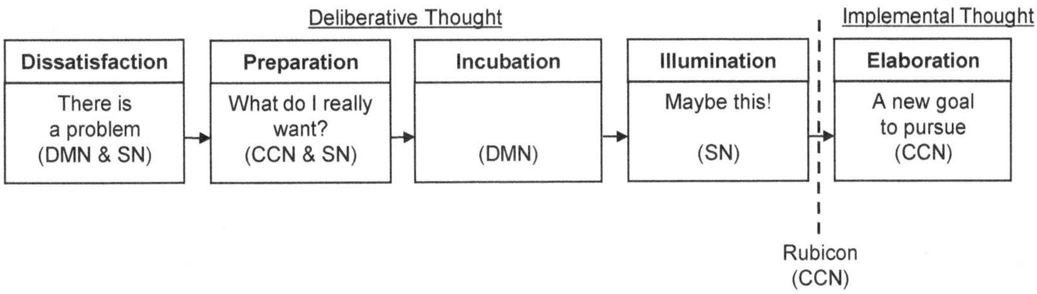

FIGURE 19.1. The goal breakthrough model.

crown could be measured by its water displacement. This allowed him to evaluate the purity of the gold that was used (given the crown's known weight). Hélie and Sun (2010) provided a modern update to the Wallas model, describing the interplay between explicit and implicit cognition, occurring over time, and leading to creative new ideas. Explicit cognition primes and "sets the stage" for the implicit mind, which operates much more holistically and can therefore provide fortuitous new connections and associations, although it may take time. Often, the iterative process continues in reciprocal fashion through a series of minibreakthroughs, until the final breakthrough is achieved (Hélie & Sun, 2010).

Translated to the case of new goal selection (as in Figure 19.1), a person may feel "stuck" in what they are doing, dissatisfied with the status quo. For example, a hedge fund manager might feel a sense of emptiness, even as they accumulate enormous piles of money. Or, a corporate lawyer might feel that their life has taken a wrong turn somewhere, away from the communitarian ideals that led them to law school in the first place (Sheldon & Krieger, 2004). At some point the sense of dissatisfaction may become too great to ignore, leading them to ask themselves new questions like "Is this all there is?" or "What was I really meant to do?" (preparation). Answers may take a long time to come; nevertheless, the fact that the person has begun posing explicit questions to themselves sets the implicit mind to work—priming it to identify possible answers (incubation). At some point, a creative new action possibility may emerge into consciousness (illumination), pointing a new way forward ("I could use my skills to work for this organization whose mission I actually believe in!"). Then the person might embark on a new career, hopefully improving their life and condition (elaboration).

Notably, the GBM is consistent with the well-known action phases or Rubicon model of goal-driven behavior proffered by Gollwitzer (2012) and others. In that model, the person first deliberates about what to do, a mindset in which they are objectively evaluating information and weighing possibilities. Then they "cross the Rubicon" to state a particular goal (as shown in Figure 19.1), leading to the three "implemental" phases of planning, acting, and evaluating the results of action. Within the latter three phases, the person is protecting their chosen intention and trying to make it come true, as an envisioned future state of the world and/or self. Notably, most action phases research has focused on the implementational phases of action rather than the deliberation phase. This may reflect Gollwitzer's (2012) assumption that options are plentiful, and that choosing among them merely involves applying a utility-based (expectancy-value) algorithm.

The GBM expands the initial deliberation phase of the action phases model, by identifying four potential subphases within that first phase, namely, dissatisfaction, preparation, incubation, and illumination. This is based on the observation that in some cases, attractive choice options may not be as plentiful as Gollwitzer suggests. In these cases, new or creative cognition may be required, to expand the decision space. The GBM also contracts the three implemental phases into a single phase called "elaboration," based on the creativity model from which it draws.

However, Gollwitzer's three implemental phases could be fit into the elaboration phase if desired, for a complete picture of the goal-striving process containing a total of seven boxes.

Figure 19.1 also depicts the high-level brain networks that support the GBM process. My colleagues and I (2024) reviewed neuroscience evidence concerning the GBM-relevant functioning of the default mode network (DMN; our mental "sketch pads" and the source of implicit cognition), the salience network (SN; in charge of recognizing the personal and emotional significance of material emerging from the DMN), and the cognitive control network (CCN; in charge of regulating cognition, making choices, and implementing planned behaviors; see Andrews-Hannah, 2012). Specifically, Sheldon and colleagues (2024) showed that dissatisfaction often arises from spontaneous musing in the DMN, which, when combined with SN activity, arises to awareness as a desire to do or change something. In cases where that "something" is not clear, the CCN can begin asking questions (like "What should I do here?"; "What might feel better?"), initiating the preparation phase of the process. Eventually answers may emerge, as enabled by the wide-ranging DMN functioning that has been primed by the CCN, and by the SN activity that signals when intriguing new possibilities emerge (the "aha!" moment). At this point it is incumbent on the CCN to "cross the Rubicon" to verbalize a choice ("I'll do that!"), and then to follow through in enacting that goal, by regulating the implemental phases of activity.

To complete explication of the figure, the GBM also contains two backward-pointing arrows representing additional ways the person can arrive at dissatisfaction, beyond unguided musing. First, a moment of illumination may be evaluated and found yet wanting, leading the person back to the drawing board of dissatisfaction. This represents the iterative process described by Hélie and Sun (2010), in which multiple moments of insight build toward a final, most complete insight. Second, the pursuit of a goal may be found wanting, in that it is too difficult or costly to achieve. This strategic evaluation process may cause the person to disengage from that goal, returning to the beginning to seek a new goal to pursue (Brandstätter & Berrmann, 2022). Third, a goal, once attained, may not yield the satisfaction and benefits that were expected (Sheldon, 2014). This emotional evaluation process can also return the person "back to the drawing board," to perhaps find something more fruitful to do.

Sheldon and colleagues (2023b) tested the basic GBM (excluding the backward-pointing arrows) in both a retrospective and a short-term longitudinal study. Participants described a past goal breakthrough (in Study 1) or desired new goal breakthrough (in Study 2) and then rated the various phases of the GBM sequence (either retrospectively, or over the subsequent few minutes). In both studies the rated intensity of initial question asking predicted the intensity of nonconscious thought during an incubation period, which predicted the brilliance of the illumination that resulted. Illumination in turn predicted increased felt integration and increased psychological need-satisfaction (Ryan & Deci, 2017) from before to after the breakthrough, as well as increased subjective well-being. The intensity of illumination also predicted greater past effort (in Study 1) and intended future effort (in Study 2) regarding the breakthrough goal that was identified.

In sum, the GBM of free will provides a novel way to conceptualize the choice process, which is the most self-defining existential activity according to Sartre and many other existential psychologists. It also provides a way to conceptualize the *optimal* choice process—namely, as one that is sensitive to internal signals, willing to pose new questions, and receptive and responsive to the possible answers provided by the implicit mind. Thus, the GBM shows how the conscious person can best interface with their own depths and sources, in service of optimal functioning (Sheldon, 2004). In particular, the GBM suggests that the two moments of (1) beginning to ask new questions and of (2) making a new choice based on the answers received, are where we psychological selves may have the most influence over our personal destinies.

Selves: Symbolic, True, and False

Most centrally, the free will question concerns the veracity of this common experience of deciding, as conscious selves, what to do in our lives—as in, "I've put on a couple of pounds lately, so I'll go to the gym, not the ice cream store." Is the experience of being a choosing self ("What do *I* want? *This*!") just an illusion, as the determinists insist, or is it somehow part of the determinative process? The GBM views it as potentially determinative. But who *are* we psychological selves who feel ourselves to be making such determinations, and what (if any) reality do we have? Obviously there is no objective homunculus (or "little man") inside of us, running the show (Metzner, 2009). What is it, then, that at least *feels* like a homunculus (i.e., a stable and tangible entity in the world), and even *acts* like one?

To address these questions, we need a functional definition of the self that is adequate to the task. In my recent book (Sheldon, 2022) I adopted the concept of the "symbolic self" (SS) proposed by Sedikides and Skowronski (1997, 2019). The SS is a complex and shifting neurofunctional aggregate that loosely integrates autobiographical information with current self-concepts, activated goals, perceived desires, and more. As argued by Sedikides and Skowronski, the SS is a "third-order" form of awareness, that goes beyond "first-order" awareness possessed by all animals (awareness of oneself in the world) and the "second-order" awareness possessed by brainy social species (awareness of oneself as an object seen from an external perspective). Phenomenologically, the SS is the feeling of being *us*, making decisions and living our lives, as best we can—the temporally extended agent, who is (ultimately) trying to pursue happiness. Of course, this agent is merely a flickering simulation, morphing over time as a function of countless factors. Still, it may have real effects on the world, as considered below.

According to Sedikides and Skowronski (1997), the SS evolved to enact three primary functions. The first function is to serve as an action executive, by selecting and regulating goals and behaviors. As "the person in charge," the SS is enjoined to make decisions (or to defer making them, which again, is still a decision). The second function is to create a "face" to interface with other people, as a social actor within the world. Hopefully we can connect effectively with others in the process, convincing them of our likeability and trustworthiness. The third is to defend the current structure of the SS, so that the person is never left without a guiding sense of identity. This function is important, because we shouldn't abandon our current sense of self based on small problems or inconsistencies; we'd quickly become helpless. But as we'll see below, the defensive functioning of the SS can impede the person's ability to make the most satisfying and fulfilling choices, in the long run.

How does the SS relate to the GBM? As the activated autobiographical agent, the SS likely influences all parts of the GBM sequence, but perhaps most so the parts requiring executive functioning—specifically, the task of asking oneself new questions about what to do, and the task of naming and enacting the new goal ideas that may result from those questions. The dissatisfied hedge fund manager feels themselves to be the character and agent in charge of their life, and based on their recurring feelings of dissatisfaction, they might begin asking themself what they can change—until promising new possibilities arrive; then hopefully, they have the courage to enact those possibilities.

To summarize, the SS is a high-level agent simulation whose functioning requires input and support from multiple regions and networks within the brain, even as it downwardly organizes the interactions between those regions and networks. It is the current or "actual self" in charge of interfacing both with the internal signals emerging "from below" and the external realities found "out in the world"—regulating (as needed) what is happening, both within and without.

But the next question is—how *well* does it regulate? That is, how effectively does the SS fulfill its functions? Obviously, peoples' goals and social performances are never perfect, and thus more learning is always required. In the case of action selection and regulation, one source of such learning doubtless comes in *learning more about oneself*—that is, about one's true or deeper preferences, desires, and inclinations, so that one's choices may be made based on the most accurate information possible, rather than based on the self-misunderstandings or even self-delusions that currently occupy one.

Based on this reasoning, I (2004, 2022) proposed that the SS also has a "fourth function"—namely, to accurately represent the totality from which it emerges, so that the person's true or deeper inclinations are expressed and given voice within their behavior. The need for such a function becomes clear when one considers dual-process models of cognition and motivation (Sheldon, 2014). Such models postulate a disjunction between nonconscious versus conscious processes, also called implicit versus explicit processes or system 1 versus system 2 processes (Kahneman, 2011). For example, motive disposition research finds that measures of implicit motivation (e.g., projective measures of the need for achievement) are barely correlated with explicit measures of the same construct (i.e., self-report measures of the need for achievement). People often do not know what they want, and when they are particularly "out of touch" with themselves, they may pay a price in health and well-being (McClelland et al., 1989).

To illustrate, a young woman who selects a career based mainly on her parents' wishes may choose very badly—for example, to become a doctor even though deep down, she has no love of science and quails at the sight of gore. In this case, her "actual" self (i.e., her current SS as an aspiring doctor) may be lodged in an inaccurate self-representation, a "false" or "introjected" self, which does not allow propensities in her implicit organism (her "true" self) to be expressed (such as her artistic or managerial talents). Fortunately, all people have an organismic valuing process that can help them overcome such disjunctions (Rogers, 1964; Sheldon et al., 2003)—growth-related information is always potentially available. But as viewed from the lens of the GBM, unleashing this valuing process may require the person to first recognize their unhappiness, then begin asking themselves questions about how to fix it. Again, conscious self-questioning may be key.

The Role of Existential Courage

It is important to emphasize how much courage such self-questioning can require! The SS defends itself (its third function; Sedikides & Skowronski, 1997) and may thus be resistant to improvements that threaten its current structure. In other words, the person's current self may in fact be a false self that fears recognizing their true self, because then the current introjected self may have to change (a kind of ego death). Thus, I (2024b) have argued that *existential courage* should be added to the Kernis and Goldman (2006) fourfold model of authentic functioning, in addition to awareness, unbiased processing, relational orientation, and authentic behavior. *Existential courage* is defined as the desire to understand the truth about ourselves, even if it leads to discomfort (Kramer, 2017; Woodard, 2010). Existential courage is what Sartre enjoined us to have, as we seek to use our free will more wisely. This truth-seeking desire can help people push through their own internal resistance to adduce fresh self-insights and action possibilities.

Stated in terms of the GBM: It likely takes considerable courage to recognize one's growing dissatisfaction with the status quo. If one doesn't acknowledge it, maybe one doesn't have to deal with it? Then it takes courage to begin asking oneself new questions (preparation). If one doesn't think about what to do, maybe the problem will solve itself? After illumination, it likely takes even more courage to cross the Rubicon to new action, committing one's time and resources to a perhaps irrevocable change in one's behavior (elaboration). It also takes courage to persist in the face of difficulties with one's new self-defining goal—there are doubtless temptations to try to retreat to the former status quo.

To summarize the argument thus far, people are condemned to choose. However, they often lack the information to make optimal choices or have identity commitments that encumber their choice-making. I have suggested that the "existential problem of choice" may be best solved when a person courageously seeks the truth about themselves and their deeper experiences, specifically, by asking themselves new questions. This helps activate the goal breakthrough process, engaging their nonconscious minds to provide them with new and better options to consider—options more concordant with the preferences of their "true" self (i.e., their implicit preferences, interests, motives, and growth impulses; Sheldon, 2014). A person who uses their free will in this way will gradually integrate their true self (or implicit) preferences into their current self (i.e., the activated SS), enabling them to make even better choices in the future. To a greater and greater extent, they use their whole brains in their decision making.

Autonomy, Self-Concordance, and the Possibility of Illusory Autonomy

Many of the issues discussed above can be profitably viewed from the lens of self-determination theory (SDT; Deci & Ryan, 1985; Ryan & Deci, 2017). According to SDT, humans have evolved a *need for autonomy*, that is, a need to feel like they cause, or at least own and agree with, their own behavior. In other words, we need to feel that we act with free will (Sheldon, 2024c). When people feel autonomous, they function more creatively and effectively, and benefit more from their actions, in terms of their felt need-satisfaction and well-being. In contrast, when people feel "controlled" in what they are doing, they fail to thrive in many ways (although notably, feeling controlled is still better than feeling helpless).

SDT postulates that people's need for autonomy is importantly affected by the social surround—do authorities in the person's life support the person's free choice, or do they try to control and constrain the person's choices? This postulate reflects SDT's early status as a social psychological theory of motivation. However, more recent research has focused on internal processes that affect a person's sense of autonomy, including self-concordance research (Sheldon & Elliot, 1999), mindfulness research (Brown & Ryan, 2003), and integrative emotion regulation research (Roth et al., 2019).

Self-concordance research is particularly relevant for this chapter on existential choice (Sheldon, 2014; Sheldon & Elliot, 1999). The self-concordance model focuses on peoples' spontaneous personal goal-setting process, postulating that when selecting goals, people may fail to pick goals that fully represent their true or implicit selves (as in the young woman mentioned above who is following her parent's wishes that she become a doctor, rather than divining her own wishes and talents). Longitudinal research shows that initial goal self-concordance predicts later need-satisfaction and hence boosted subjective well-being (Sheldon & Elliot, 1999), consistent with many other findings on the positive downstream effects of initiating activity with a sense of autonomous volition (summarized in Ryan & Deci, 2017). Self-concordance research builds on such research, showing an important internally generated means by which people can affect their own condition despite a negative social context—namely, by setting and pursuing personal goals that fully express and energize them. This can provide a direct channel for people's implicit preferences to affect the world.

Still, there are conundrums here. Self-concordance is typically operationalized via a relative autonomy index (Ryan & Deci, 2017; Sheldon et al., 2017), as the extent the person reports more autonomous than controlled motivation for pursuing their self-stated personal goals. Conversely, nonconcordance is operationalized as feeling more controlled than autonomous in pursuing one's goals. But recall the earlier discussion of Sartre's (1980) position on existential freedom—that we are *always* free, whether we recognize it or not, and thus that the feeling of being controlled in one's choices is an illusion, a misattribution that may help one evade responsibility and the emotional consequences of one's choices. In Sartrean terms, to be nonconcordant is to fail to recognize one's actual freedom in choosing the goals that one has stated.

Still, this failure may not "just" be a failure to face reality—it may also be diagnostic, as a kind of signal from one's deeper self. That is, the feeling of being controlled in one's goals may be a symptom, that one has not yet chosen well in one's goal selections—there is internal resistance to them. This symptom, though ultimately illusory, ontologically may serve as the "dissatisfaction" that can initiate the GBM process, if the person has the courage to return to the drawing board to reconsider their goals. For example: Imagine that the young woman described earlier finally becomes an unhappy doctor, having followed her parent's wishes. She feels it wasn't really her choice, but she is stuck with it now. According to Sartre it *was* her choice (obviously, it was a bad one), and she is always free to make a change—yet she remains in a psychological trap of her own making. But if she can find the courage to finally acknowledge and question her dissatisfaction, then she may yet extricate herself from that trap.

If there is such a condition as "illusory controlledness" (i.e., the feeling that one did not choose one's own goals when in fact, one did), is there also a condition of "*illusory autonomy*" (i.e., the feeling that one fully endorses one's goals, when in fact one does not really enjoy and value them)? In our lab my colleagues and I recently explored this possibility, with very interesting results. Again, self-concordance is typically measured via a relative autonomy index, the (very reasonable) assumption being that felt goal autonomy symptomizes "good fit" between the goal and the person's deeper preferences, a condition we called "objective self-concordance" (Sheldon et al., 2023a). This assumption has been validated in multiple experimental studies showing that people are higher in measured self-concordance (relative autonomy) when they are randomly assigned to a goal-type (i.e., an affiliative goal, an intrinsic goal, or a communal goal) that concretely matches their personality preferences (i.e., their high need for affiliation, high intrinsic values, or high communal orientation; Sheldon, 2014; Sheldon & Cooper, 2008; Sheldon & Schuler, 2011).

In our 2023 research my colleagues and I also tested a second type of self-concordance, exemplified when a person reports much autonomy in pursuing misfitting (objectively nonconcordant) goals. Specifically, participants were assigned to pursue either achievement goals or affiliation goals, after their achievement and affiliative motive dispositions were measured. As in the past experimental studies, objective self-concordance was defined as existing when the assigned goal matched the participants' prior measured dispositions and was reflected in higher self-concordance ratings in those cases. In contrast, subjective (and perhaps illusory) self-concordance was defined as existing when reported autonomy was still high, even when the assigned goal did not match. The person reports more ownership of the goal than would be expected. For example, a person more oriented toward affiliation than achievement, according to implicit or dispositional measures, may still claim autonomous ownership of an assigned (misfitting) achievement goal. Is this an illusion, or an adaptive process? Perhaps both.

To show how it may be adaptive, we need to consider an important principle of SDT—namely, that people have an organismic integration propensity that prompts them to internalize the doing of activities that they may not enjoy (Ryan & Deci, 2017). An example is a person who has come to pay their taxes willingly and even cheerfully, even though it is still not pleasant, because they value the system of taxation and the benefits it provides society (Sheldon et al., 2005). They have accepted being taxed, rather than feeling resistant to it. Such internalization is viewed as a mature response to the inevitability of having to do "non intrinsically motivated things" sometimes—by identifying with those things, the person may yet feel autonomous even though enjoyment is missing (Ryan & Stiller, 1991).

From this point of view, subjective self-concordance (claiming to enjoy and identify with goals that are not a good fit for one) may provide people with some benefits, helping them get on with what (seemingly) must be done. And indeed, Sheldon and colleagues (2023a) found independent main effects on intended effort and later attainment for both objective self-concordance (based on actual matching) and subjective self-concordance (based on asserting ownership despite not matching). My colleagues and I interpreted the latter effect as an SDT internalization effect, which can influence outcomes independently of objective self-concordance (matching).

Existential Overreach

"Getting on with one's chosen goals" sounds like an admirable existential attitude, involving the implementation phase of action. Once a choice has been made and the Rubicon has been crossed, it is time to start planning and acting, rather than continually questioning one's decisions, like Hamlet (Gollwitzer, 2012). Sartre believed that people should be "men of action." However, the possibility that the chosen goals, in some cases, may not well represent one's deeper or truer self, suggests a conundrum: that a person may keep pushing no matter what, rather than coming to realize that it is time to take note of their dissatisfaction and reconsider their choices. Sometimes one must disengage from one's former commitments (Brandstätter & Berrmann, 2022), to seek something new. In such cases, the existential fortitude to keep pressing onward in pursuit of one's verbalized goals may work *against* one's own best interests in the long run, by entrenching one ever more deeply into a suboptimal course of action. Suppose the young doctor presses on despite her unhappiness, even managing to become somewhat prominent within her field. How can she turn back?

In such cases, ideally, the most core meaning of existential courage—the desire to seek out the truth of oneself and one's experience (Kramer, 2017)—will hopefully reassert itself, to return the person from the goal implementation phases back to the goal deliberation phase (the second backward-pointing arrow in the GBM model; see Figure 19.1). Optimally, when one recognizes that a false self has been making one's choices, one would seek to overthrow that false self, in favor of greater truth in one's experience and living.

CONCLUSION

In this chapter I have considered the existential problem of choice, and its optimal resolution, from several novel angles. After adopting Sartre's idea that humans are radically free to make choices, whether they recognize (or like) it or not, I outlined a model of the optimal choice process based on creative cognition theory, a model that directly addresses the operation of free will. I showed that our identities (i.e., our activated symbolic selves) are intimately involved in our choice making, sometimes in defensive ways that impede wise choice. Still, even in these cases where the "problem of choice" has become especially pressing, we always have the capacity to become unstuck by recognizing our own dissatisfaction and beginning to ask ourselves new questions—if we can muster sufficient courage. In the process we may better integrate our deeper, implicit selves with our conscious choice-making selves, to forward our own growth and happiness.

REFERENCES

Andrews-Hanna, J. (2012). The brain's default network and its adaptive role in internal mentation. *Neuroscientist, 18(3)*, 251–270.

Baumeister, R. F. (2008). Free will in scientific psychology. *Perspectives on Psychological Science, 3*(1), 14–19.

Brandstätter, V., & Berrmann, K. (2022). Persistence and disengagement in personal goal pursuit. *Annual Review of Psychology, 73*, 271–299.

Brown, K. W., & Ryan, R. M. (2003). The benefits of being present: Mindfulness and its role in psychological well-being. *Journal of Personality and Social Psychology, 84*(4), 822–848.

Chalmers, D. (2014). What do philosophers believe? *Philosophical Studies, 170(3)*, 465–500.

Deci, E. L., & Ryan, R. M. (1985). *Intrinsic motivation and self-determination in human behavior.* Plenum Press.

Dennett, D. (2003). *Freedom evolves.* Penguin.

Frankl, V. (1946). *Man's search for meaning.* Beacon Press.

Gollwitzer, P. M. (2012). Mindset theory of action phases. In P. A. M. Van Lange, A. W. Kruglanski, & E. T. Higgins (Eds.), *Handbook of theories of social psychology* (Vol. 1, pp. 526–545). Sage.

Harris, S. (2012). *Free will.* Free Press.

Hélie, S., & Sun, R. (2010). Incubation, insight, and creative problem solving: A unified theory and a connectionist model. *Psychological Review, 117*(3), 994–1024.

Kahneman, D. (2011). *Thinking, fast and slow.* Farrar, Straus & Giroux.

Kernis, M. H., & Goldman, B. M. (2006). A multicomponent conceptualization of authenticity: Theory and research. In M. P. Zanna (Ed.), *Advances in experimental social psychology* (Vol. 38, pp. 283–357). Elsevier/Academic Press.

Kramer, R. M. (2017). To become or not to become?: Existential courage and the quest for identity. In S. T. Allison, G. R. Goethals, & R. M. Kramer (Eds.), *Handbook of heroism and heroic leadership* (pp. 262–282). Routledge/Taylor & Francis Group.

Libet, B. (1999). Do we have free will? *Journal of Consciousness Studies, 6(8–9)*, 47–57.

List, C. (2014). Free will, determinism, and the possibility of doing otherwise. *Noûs, 48*(1), 156–178.

List, C. (2019). *Why free will is real.* Harvard University Press.

McClelland, D. C., Koestner, R., & Weinberger, J. (1989). How do self-attributed and implicit motives differ? *Psychological Review, 96*(4), 690–702.

Metzner, T. (2009). *The ego tunnel: The science of the mind and the myth of the self.* Basic Books.

Pyszczynski, T., Greenberg, J., Koole, S., & Solomon, S. (2010). Experimental existential psychology: Coping with the facts of life. In S. T. Fiske, D. T. Gilbert, & G. Lindzey (Eds.), *Handbook of social psychology* (Vol. 1, 5th ed., pp. 724–757). Wiley.

Rogers, C. R. (1964). Toward a modern approach to values: The valuing process in the mature person. *Journal of Abnormal and Social Psychology, 68*(2), 160–167.

Roth, G., Vansteenkiste, M., & Ryan, R. M. (2019). Integrative emotion regulation: Process and development from a self-determination theory. *Developmental Psychopathology, 31*(3), 945–956.

Ryan, R. M., & Deci, E. L. (2017). *Self-determination theory: Basic psychological needs in motivation, development, and wellness.* Guilford Press.

Ryan, R. M., & Stiller, J. (1991). The social content of internalization: Parent and teacher influence on autonomy, motivation and learning. In P. R. Pintrich & M. L. Maehr (Eds), *Advances in motivation and achievement: Vol. 7. Goals and self-regulatory processes* (pp. 115–149). JAI Press.

Sapolsky, R. M. (2023). *Determined: A science of life without free will.* Penguin.

Sartre, J.-P. (1946). *L'existentialisme est un humanisme* (Collection Pensées). Nagel. (Translated as *Existentialism is a humanism*, J. Kulka & C. Macomber (Trans.), Yale University Press, 2007.)

Sartre, J.-P. (1980). *Being and nothingness: A phenomenological essay on ontology* (H. E. Barnes, Trans.). Washington Square Press. (Original work published 1943)

Sedikides, C., & Skowronski, J. J. (1997). The symbolic self in evolutionary context. *Personality and Social Psychology Review, 1*(1), 80–102.

Sheldon, K. M. (2004). *Optimal human being: An integrated multi-level perspective.* Erlbaum.

Sheldon, K. M. (2014). Becoming oneself: The central role of self-concordant goal selection. *Personality and Social Psychology Review, 18,* 349–365.

Sheldon, K. M. (2022). *Freely determined: What the new psychology of the self tells us about how to live.* Basic Books.

Sheldon, K. M. (2024a). *Beyond autonomy support: The importance of free will support.* Unpublished manuscript.

Sheldon, K. M. (2024b). Free will, authenticity, autonomy, self-concordance, and courage: Connecting the dots. In *Oxford handbook of authenticity.* Oxford University Press.

Sheldon, K. M. (2024c). The free will capacity: A uniquely human adaptation. *American Psychologist, 79*(7), 928–941.

Sheldon, K. M., Arndt, J., & Houser-Marko, L. (2003). In search of the organismic valuing process: The human tendency to move towards beneficial goal choices. *Journal of Personality, 71,* 835–869.

Sheldon, K. M., & Cooper, M. L. (2008). Goal striving within agentic and communal roles: Functionally independent pathways to enhanced well-being. *Journal of Personality, 76,* 415–447.

Sheldon, K. M., & Elliot, A. J. (1999). Goal striving, need satisfaction, and longitudinal well-being: the self-concordance model. *Journal of Personality and Social Psychology, 76*(3), 482–497.

Sheldon, K. M., Goffredi, R., & Schlegel, R. (2023a). Self-concordant goal-striving as internalized motivation: Benefits beyond person-goal fit. *Motivation Science, 9*(1), 53–61.

Sheldon, K. M., Goffredi, R., & Titova, L. (2023b). The goal breakthrough model: Explicit questions drive implicit processes. *Journal of Research in Personality, 104.*

Sheldon, K. M., Kasser, T., Houser-Marko, L., Jones, T., & Turban, D. (2005). Doing one's duty: Chronological age, felt autonomy, and subjective well-being. *European Journal of Personality, 19,* 97–115.

Sheldon, K. M., & Krieger, L. (2004). Does law school undermine law students?: Examining changes in goals, values, and well-being. *Behavioral Sciences and the Law, 22,* 261–286.

Sheldon, K. M., Lee, W., & Reeve, J. (2024). *Deciding the future: How psychological control processes regulate the brain to select goals.* Manuscript under review.

Sheldon, K. M., Osin, E. N., Gordeeva, T. O., & Suchkov, D. (2017). Evaluating the dimensionality of Self-determination theory's relative autonomy continuum. *Personality and Social Psychology Bulletin, 43,* 1215–1238.

Sheldon, K. M., & Schuler, J. (2011). Needing, wanting, and having: Integrating motive disposition theory and self-determination theory. *Journal of Personality and Social Psychology, 101,* 1106–1123.

Skowronski, J. J., & Sedikides, C. (2019). On the evolution of the human self: A data-driven review and reconsideration. *Self and Identity, 18*(1), 4–21.

Sperry, R. W. (1993). The impact and promise of the cognitive revolution. *American Psychologist, 48*(8), 878–885.

Wallas, G. (1926). *The art of thought.* Cape.

Weinberg, J. (2020). What philosophers believe: Results from the 2020 PhilPapers Survey. *Daily Nous*. https://dailynous.com/2021/11/01/what-philosophers-believe-results-from-the-2020-philpapers-survey/.

Woodard, C. R. (2010). The courage to be authentic: Empirical and existential perspectives. In C. L. S. Pury & S. J. Lopez (Eds.), *The psychology of courage: Modern research on an ancient virtue* (pp. 109–123). American Psychological Association.

CHAPTER 20

Authenticity and True Selves

Rebecca J. Schlegel *and* Grace N. Rivera

One of the fundamental questions people confront in their lives is "Who am I?" From an existential perspective, we are "thrown" into existence when we're born and we must make sense of that existence ourselves. We have to figure out who we are and how we fit into the world. For existential philosophers, the answer to the question "Who am I?" is determined by our choices. The self is not something we are born with, but something that we create through our choices (i.e., "existence precedes essence"; Aho, 2023). However, this doesn't seem to be how most people think about the self. Rather, work from our labs and others demonstrates that people tend to believe they have a set of immutable core attributes that makes them who they are (Christy et al., 2019; De Freitas, Cikara, et al., 2017; Dulaney et al., 2019; Kim et al., 2024; Lakoff & Johnson, 1999), and that this essence should set the path for their existence rather than vice versa (Kim et al., 2022). This self-perceived essence is what people commonly refer to as the "true self" (e.g., Christy et al., 2019).

In this chapter, we review a growing body of research that has examined the ways the lay idea of a true self informs how people approach questions surrounding selfhood and identity. In particular, we examine what people believe true selves to be and the downstream consequences these beliefs have on behavior and well-being, particularly the pursuit of meaning. Finally, we examine the closely related issue of authenticity, which is often used to refer to the idea of living a life consistent with one's true self. Specifically, we review what makes people feel authentic and whether the empirical evidence suggests the experience of authenticity actually requires a true self at all.

WHAT DO PEOPLE BELIEVE ABOUT TRUE SELVES?

For the purposes of this chapter, we set the question of whether true selves literally exist to the side. While we personally tend to agree with existential philosophers and other psychological theorists that it seems doubtful that true selves literally exist in an ontological sense (Baumeister, 1995; Jongman-Sereno & Leary, 2019; Strohminger et al., 2017), we contend that there are a lot of other interesting questions we can ask as existential psychologists about how people's beliefs surrounding the true self inform the way people think about themselves, their behavior, and what's meaningful in their lives. In that spirit, what do we know about what lay people think the true self is?

Lakoff and Johnson (1999) described the true self as a "complex metaphor" rooted in the visual image of a core-like entity within an external casing. The core-like entity represents who a person really is, whereas the external casing represents the observable/public-facing aspects of a person. These public-facing elements can be imbued to varying degrees with one's true self or false selves (e.g., versions of the self that feel as if they block or hide one's true self; much like a cover or mask around this casing; see Figure 20.1). This imagery is consistent with how humanistic theorists such as Carl Rogers (1961) described the experience of personhood and continues to be found in current theories rooted in the humanistic tradition such as the self-concordance model (Sheldon, 2014). This imagery is also consistent with the way lay people have described the true self as something that is discovered within one's self (Schlegel et al., 2012). People also have explicitly reported that they visualize the true self as a single solid entity (Landau et al., 2011).

People often also draw on this metaphor to describe behavior that is consistent (or not) with the true self (Lakoff & Johnson, 1999). For example, Rogers (1961) characterized the true self as something that can either expand to express itself in the right conditions or can be defensively hidden within the external casing when someone is faced with social threats. Consistent with this idea, Landau and colleagues (2011) found that priming people with expanding core-like entities led them to behave in ways that were consistent with self-expression, such as conforming less to other people's opinions.

Lakoff and Johnson (1999) also suggested that the true self metaphor is scaffolded by the prevalent folk theory that entities have "essences" that make them what they are, which is commonly referred to as psychological essentialism (Gelman, 2003). The link between psychological essentialism and true self beliefs can be found in a variety of studies that indirectly point to the similarities between how people reason about true selves and essentialist reasoning in other domains. For example, people typically locate essences as residing "deep within" the entity in question (Gelman & Wellman, 1991), which is consistent with the core-like entity metaphors described above. People also judge internal states (e.g., thoughts and feel-

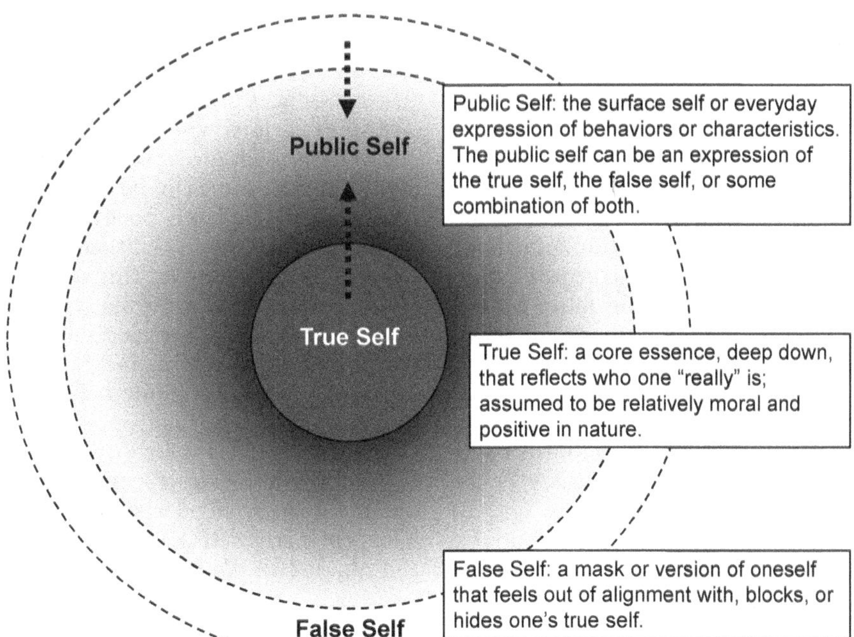

FIGURE 20.1. The true self as essentialist metaphor.

ings) as more diagnostic of a person's true self than their observable behavior (Andersen & Ross, 1984; Johnson et al., 2004), which only makes sense if people see the true self as the *internal* essence of a person.

In direct support for the idea that true self beliefs are linked to psychological essentialism, people explicitly believe that true selves have the same properties (e.g., immutability, informativeness, inherence) as other essences (Christy et al., 2019). For example, people were asked to rate a variety of personality characteristics on their relevance to the true self. They were then asked to imagine how likely it was that 30 years from now they'd have exactly the same amount of the characteristic as they do now. Results revealed the more closely linked a personal trait (e.g., empathy for others, enjoyment of blues music) was to the perceived true self, the more likely people believed it would not change at all over the next 30 years. Similarly, when asked to imagine what they would be like if they were born in a different historical era, the more closely linked a personality characteristic was to the perceived true self, the more likely people believed they would have the exact same amount of that trait even if they were born in a different era. Such results are precisely how people reason about other essences. Essences are believed to remain the same even across fairly radical changes in context. Individual differences in psychological essentialism also predict individual differences in belief in the true self and experimental manipulations of psychological essentialism affect participants' belief in true selves, thus providing fairly direct evidence that belief in a true self can be explained by people applying more general tendencies to essentialize to the self (Christy et al., 2019). Interestingly, self-essentialism predicts psychological well-being (Dulaney et al., 2019; Kim et al., 2024), perhaps because these beliefs promote feelings of self-knowledge and self-esteem (Christy et al., 2024).

Another interesting feature of essentialist reasoning is that people believe that essences are good. This pattern has been observed in a variety of domains; De Freitas, Tobia, Newman, and Knobe (2017) found that people perceive the essences of scientific papers, universities, conferences, nations, and bands to be normatively good. For example, when a nation is perceived to change for the worse, people think it is no longer the same nation because it is getting further from its perceived good essence. People make similar judgments about themselves and others, perceiving positive changes as bringing someone closer to their true self and negative changes as moving someone further away from their true self (Bench et al., 2015). As such, psychological essentialism also seems to drive a strong intuition that true selves are morally good (De Freitas, Tobia, et al., 2017), a belief referred to as the "good true self bias." This bias has been observed in multiple cultures and even among self-identified misanthropes who otherwise have pessimistic views of humanity (De Freitas et al., 2018; Newman et al., 2014; Strohminger et al., 2017). While numerous studies speak to the pervasiveness of the good true self bias, there are some limitations to it. Individuals high in the Dark Triad are less likely to see their own true selves as good (Maffly-Kipp et al., 2023), and people are willing to see a negative true self in someone else when motivated to punish someone for criminal acts (Maffly-Kipp et al., 2022).

This brings us to another key feature of essentialist reasoning, that people believe essences are causally powerful (Dar-Nimrod & Heine, 2011; Gelman, 2003). People believe essences give rise to the observable features of various types of entities (e.g., a lion's essence is what gives rise to its fierce hunting ability). The same can be said for true selves. In particular, people believe that true selves are what give rise to authentic behavior. In the case of true selves, this seems to be both a descriptive and a normative belief. People not only describe the true self as the source of authentic behavior, but they believe that true selves *should* guide behavior. We have referred to this normative belief as the "true-self-as-guide" lay theory of decision making. This lay theory suggests that if people want to make satisfying decisions, they should follow their true self (Kim et al., 2022; Schlegel et al., 2013). We have found the people rate following the true self at least as important as (and usually more important than) other commonly accepted decision-making strategies, such as considering who you ideally want to be, thinking carefully about the decision, or relying on intuition. Furthermore, people endorse the "true-self-as-guide" lay theory at relatively high levels in the United States, China, India, Singapore, and South Korea, suggesting this is not a uniquely American or individualist idea (Kim et al., 2022). Indeed, "true-self-as-guide" lay theory endorsement was positively associated with endorsement of the strategy "considering the effect of one's decisions on others" across samples, and this association was strongest in China, India, and South Korea. Thus, for those in countries with more collective cultural orientations, considering how a decision affects others is not viewed as at odds with following the true self. These two strategies may become increasingly intertwined for those higher in collectivism, possibly because others are seen as a part of the true self. These patterns are consistent with the idea that psychological essentialism is widespread across many nations and cultural traditions (Atran et al., 2002; Errington, 1989; Gil-White, 2001; Henrich et al., 2010).

In sum, people believe true selves are hidden within the person, stable over time, causally powerful, and morally good. Next, we ask why true self beliefs matter, with a particular eye toward meaning making.

WHY DO TRUE SELF BELIEFS MATTER?

Thinking about the self as an essence that is hidden within one's self has a number of downstream consequences. For example, the idea that you have an internal essence makes it possible that your beliefs about who you are could be wrong (e.g., Baumeister, 1987; Waterman, 1984; Waterman & Schwartz, 2013). Indeed, Baumeister (1987, p. 166) suggested that "the difficulty and the desirability of self-knowledge were well established cultural attitudes by the beginning of the 20th century." These cultural attitudes continue today. People commonly believe that self-discovery is a key ingredient to a life well-lived (Kierkegaard, 1989; G. N. Rivera et al., 2018; Ryan & Deci, 2004; Schlegel et al., 2013).

One reason self-discovery is highly valued is because the self exports meaning and value to other aspects of our lives (Baumeister, 1991; Schlegel et al., 2013; Waterman, 1993). For example, people often derive meaning from their careers. How does someone decide if their career is meaningful? While one person may find being an academic meaningful, others may see it as a frustratingly disconnected from the real world. There is no objective answer to whether any particular career is meaningful or not. Each person must decide for themselves which careers are meaningful to them. How are people supposed to approach such a question? On our view, people use the self (and the true self, in particular) to export personal meaning to these career options, as well as other major decisions in their lives (see Figure 20.2). Careers that are seen as consistent with one's perceived true self are deemed meaningful and valuable for that very reason. For example, being an academic may feel meaningful to someone because it allows them to express their deeply held values and explore interests that they believe emanate from their causally powerful essence. Because everyone has a unique true self-concept, this can explain why people find such a wide variety of careers meaningful versus not. The idea that people use their true self-concepts in this way is supported by the research asking people to defend various life decisions. Bellah and colleagues (1996, p. 76) found that most people could not answer this question without making reference to the self, leading them to conclude that "each self constitutes its own moral universe."

Consistent with such propositions, research has shown that a variety of true self relevant variables predict meaning in life and decision satisfaction. In the first set of studies on this topic, Schlegel and colleagues (2009) hypothesized that because people repeatedly use the true self to export meaning and value to other aspects of their life, feelings of meaningfulness and the true self-concept should be linked in people's minds such that the cognitive accessibility of the true self should relate to meaning in life judgments even in the absence of any explicit subjective experience of expressing the true self. Consistent with this hypothesis, both measured and manipulated cognitive accessibility of the true self positively predicted meaning in life judgments, a pattern not

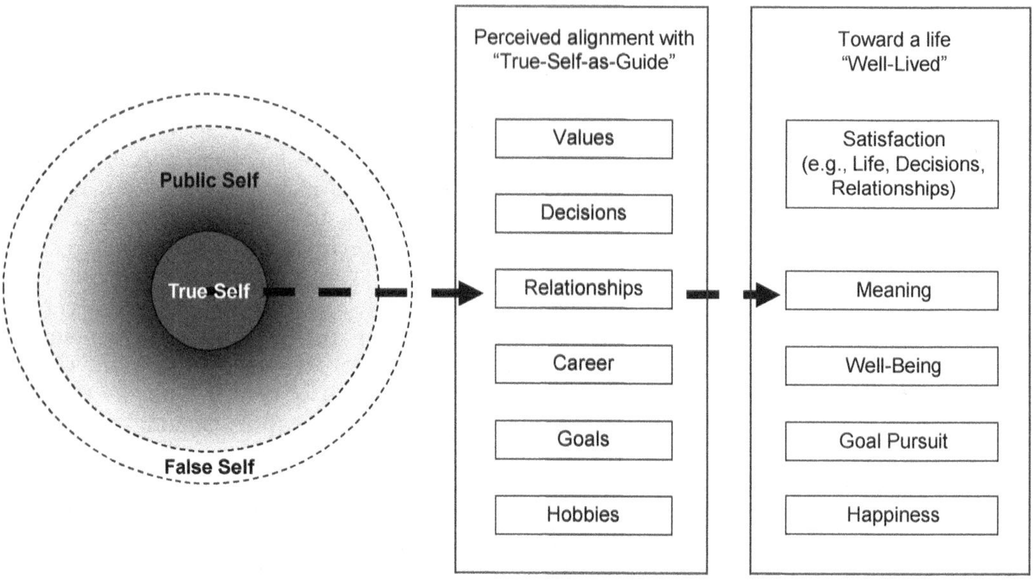

FIGURE 20.2. A true-self-as-guide lay theory approach.

observed for the actual self-concept (or the more public, everyday self-concept that reflects the "outer core" in the true self metaphor; Figure 20.1). These results suggest that it's the true self in particular that serves as a wellspring of meaning as opposed to the self in its entirety (see Figure 20.2).

A closely related line of work showed that the subjective feeling of knowing who you are also predicts higher meaning in life judgments (Schlegel et al., 2011). Critically, this work aimed to develop a novel method of assessing this feeling that did not rely on self-reported judgments of self-knowledge, instead relying on the metacognitive experience of ease (Schwarz, 1998; Schwarz & Clore, 1996) in a self-description task as a means of both measuring and manipulating feelings of true self-knowledge. Essentially, people use the ease with which they can describe something as a cue to how much they know about that thing. For example, if you were asked to describe the rules of baseball, the experience of ease or difficulty in recalling relevant rules would serve as a cue to how much you know about that topic. Thus, if true self-description tasks feel easy, it would serve as a cue to how much a person knows about their own true self. In contrast, the meta-cognitive experience of difficulty would suggest the person's true self-knowledge is lacking. Across three studies, both measured and manipulated meta-cognitive ease predicted higher meaning in life judgments. If the true self is being used to export meaning to other domains in our life, it makes sense that it's important to feel "in touch" with that true self. Replicating past work, similar effects were not observed for the actual/public self, again suggesting that it's the true self in particular that people use to make sense of their lives.

The effects observed on overall meaning in life judgments have also been observed in more specific domains as well. In one set of studies, Schlegel and colleagues (2013) found that perceived true self-knowledge predicted how satisfied people are with their decisions. For example, in one study my (R. J. S.) colleagues and I measured participants' feelings of true self-knowledge every day for 5 days and tracked how fluctuations in feelings of self-knowledge on the daily level predicted fluctuations in satisfaction with the same three decisions over that same period of time. This study used college students, so we assessed satisfaction with three decisions relevant to college student life (which university to attend, current major, whether or not to join certain student organizations on campus). We found that, at the within-person level, daily fluctuations in perceived true self-knowledge significantly predicted daily fluctuations in satisfaction with these college-relevant decisions. Consistent with previous studies, perceived knowledge of the actual/public self had no relationship with decision satisfaction. Additionally, the relationship between perceived true self-knowledge and decision satisfaction remained significant even after accounting for other relevant predictors, such as self-esteem and mood.

While these studies focused on the link between perceived *knowledge* of the true self and decision satisfaction, other work has demonstrated that perceptions of *following* the true self also predict decision satisfaction (Chen et al., 2022; Kim et al., 2021). In Chen and colleagues' (2022) work, participants were asked to complete moral dilemmas, such as the infamous "Trolley Problem," in which a person must decide if they would push a single stranger in front of a moving trolley to save the life of five other strangers (e.g., Koenigs et al., 2007). Participants who were instructed to use their true self as a guide were more satisfied with their decisions in these tough dilemmas than were those with no instructions or those who used alternate strategies such as logic or intuition. Such patterns are again consistent with the idea that people use their true self-concept to export meaning, value, and satisfaction to other aspects of their life. Kim and colleagues (2021) found similar patterns for major life decisions (e.g., choosing a major, choosing a romantic partner, moving). After generating a major decision, participants were asked to consider how they either used their true self or an alternative highly valued decision-making strategy, such as logic and rational thinking, to make that decision. Participants who were asked to consider how they used their true self to make the decision reported greater decision satisfaction than did those who were asked to consider how they used alternate strategies. This difference was explained by heightened perceptions that one had used their true self as a guide when making the decision. Importantly, in this work the shift in decision satisfaction was revealed even when there was no way that the experimental manipulation could lead to different decisions because participants were reflecting on previously made decisions. Simply *framing* a decision as guided by the true self can be powerful enough to boost one's satisfaction with a decision, even when one can't change anything about the decision itself. Thus, the true self may be an important feature of creating a satisfying narrative around a decision (and perhaps life more generally).

Taken together, there is plenty of evidence that true self beliefs matter for how people approach the existential questions that surround who they are and how the fit into the world. People experience more meaning in their lives to the extent that the believe they know who they are and live a life consistent with who they are. The perceived true self seems very effective at exporting meaning and value to the specific aspects of our life that contribute to a life that is experienced as satisfying.

TRUE SELVES AND AUTHENTICITY

The degree to which the public/actual self matches the underlying true self is often referred to as authenticity. Feeling authentic and appearing authentic to others are both important for a slew of intra- and interpersonal outcomes such as happiness, life satisfaction, affective well-being, liking, and trust (e.g., Goldman & Kernis, 2002; Liu & Perrewe, 2006; Sariçam, 2015; Wood et al., 2008). For example, in a meta-analysis of 65 samples (N = 18,637), authenticity shared a moderately strong positive relationship with well-being (r = .40; Sutton, 2020). This relationship may start as early as adolescence, with perceived authenticity predicting well-being in adolescent samples (Thomaes et al., 2017). Indeed, neither age nor gender changed the relationship between authenticity and well-being in the large meta-analysis, suggesting the relationship between authenticity and well-being is robust through the lifespan and similarly important for both men and women (Sutton, 2020). Regarding interpersonal outcomes, we tend to like and trust others who we deem to be more authentic (Liu & Perrewe, 2006). In the romantic domain, we are more satisfied with our relationships when we feel like we know our partner's true self (Wickam, 2013; Wickham et al., 2016), and when we feel our partner knows our own true self (G. R. Rivera et al., 2018).

Despite the fact that concerns about authenticity seem to be driven by concerns that behavior may not match what's inside ourselves (or others' selves), the emerging research suggests that the relationship between self-consistency and authenticity isn't as straightforward as it might seem. Below we review the existing evidence on what makes people feel authentic and what makes people appear authentic to others. We consider, as well, whether a true self is even necessary to explain the patterns observed in the literature despite the fact that people usually define it as consistency with the true self (e.g., Kernis & Goldman, 2006).

What Makes People Feel Authentic?

A quintessential study by Fleeson and Wilt (2010) raised the question of how important self-consistency is to the experience of authenticity. Specifically, Fleeson and Wilt asked people to report on their state levels of the Big Five and state authenticity in a variety of contexts. They consistently found that the social desirability of the state behavior (e.g., higher extraversion, lower neuroticism) was more predictive of authenticity than the congruence of that state behavior with people's traits. For example, highly extraverted behavior predicted authenticity for everyone, regardless of their self-reported level of trait extraversion, suggesting that even self-identified introverts report feeling more authentic when behaving in a more extraverted manner (see also Sheldon et al., 1997, for a similar pattern). Similarly, a meta-analysis on the relationship between authenticity and well-being found that this relationship was strongest when authenticity was measured using the Authenticity Inventory (Kernis & Goldman, 2006), which is less conceptually tied to the need to be consistent than are other widely used measures (Sutton, 2020). These findings go against most people's lay intuitions about what makes people feel authentic, with more people endorsing strict construals of authenticity that position authentic people as consistent across situations, compared to flexible construals (Jongman-Sereno & Leary, 2020). What is less clear is *why* self-consistency didn't appear to matter in the experience of authenticity.

One possible explanation is that the valence of behavior matters more for authenticity than the consistency of that behavior with the self-concept. On this view, authenticity judgments may be used in a self-enhancing manner to embellish one's strengths and downplay one's weaknesses (Guenther et al., 2023). From this perspective, positive self-attributes and positive behaviors will consistently feel more authentic because they are self-enhancing. Consistent with this perspective, authenticity and self-esteem are strongly linked (Heppner et al., 2008; Lenton, Bruder, et al., 2013). Furthermore, trait self-enactment and daily self-enhancement have been shown to predict reports of authenticity (Guenther et al., 2023), and multiple studies show that people are more likely to feel authentic when positive aspects of the self are salient (Bailey & Iyengar, 2023; Gan & Chen, 2017). In a particularly potent demonstration of this valence bias, Jongman-Sereno and Leary (2016) demonstrated that reflecting on (or even imagining) positive behavior made people feel more authentic than reflecting on (or imagining) negative behavior, even when both types of behavior were consistent with the self-concept. This connection between valence and authenticity is so strong that even experimental manipulations of positive affect make people feel more authentic, even when that positive affect is induced through something like a movie clip that has nothing to do with self-relevance (Chen et al., 2023; Lenton, Slabu, et al., 2013). Taken together, this evidence suggests that authenticity may be more about valence than consistency, leading some theorists to argue that authenticity reports are too contaminated by valence to be meaningful (Jongman-Sereno & Leary, 2019).

That said, another possible interpretation of this body of work is that we've been looking in the wrong place for consistency effects on authenticity. Indeed, Fleeson and Wilt (2010) argued that the valence effects they observed are also consistent with a humanistic perspective on authenticity. Humanistic perspectives suggest that engaging in positive behaviors should feel more authentic because the organismic valuing process guides people toward psychological growth and psychologically healthy choices (Rogers, 1961; Sheldon, 2014; Sheldon & Houser-Marko, 2001). This process should lead people to feel most authentic when they are engaged in behaviors that align with ideals and help them reach their unique potential (Heidegger, 2010; Medlock, 2012; Ryan & Deci, 2004; Sheldon, 2002, 2014; Zimmerman, 1986). Consistent with this perspective, Kim and colleagues (2019) demonstrated that promotion focus (or the tendency to approach goals in a way that emphasizes the achievements of personal ideals) predicts authenticity at the trait level and causally impacts authenticity at the state level when experimentally manipulated.

A humanistic understanding of authenticity also emphasizes the importance of self-ownership in authenticity (Ryan & Ryan, 2019; Vess, 2019). A variety of studies have established the importance of feelings of self-ownership to authenticity. For example, mind wandering predicts decreased authenticity when it is unintentional, but increased authenticity when intentional (Vess & Maffly-Kipp, 2022). Similarly, feelings of academic amotivation (i.e., not knowing *why* you are pursuing an academic goal) predict feelings of authenticity (Kim et al., 2017). Additionally, experimental manipulations that reduce belief in free will reduce people's feelings of true self-knowledge and the perceived authenticity of their actions, presumably because personal agency and self-ownership have been undermined (Seto & Hicks, 2016).

Interestingly (and perhaps counterintuitively given what we have just covered on self-ownership) a humanistic understanding of authenticity can also consider the role of self-transcendence in understanding authenticity (e.g., Jiang & Sedikides, 2022). For example, awe experiences elicit greater pursuit of one's authentic self (Yuan et al., 2024), a relationship that may be explained by the self-transcendent nature of awe experiences (Jiang & Sedikides, 2022; Keltner & Haidt, 2003). In our lab, we found that awe experiences positively predicted true self-knowledge to the extent that they increased perceptions of happiness (Cavallaro et al., 2025). Taken together, this work suggests that experiences that allow one to diminish focus on one's individual self and connect with the larger context may also promote authenticity.

What is challenging in teasing self-enhancement and humanistic perspectives apart is that most of the evidence for either perspective is consistent with the other perspective as well. As an example, let us also consider the body of work that suggests that people report feeling more authentic when they are reminded of their previous moral behaviors (Christy et al., 2016; Zhang et al., 2019) and when they are randomly assigned to argue in favor of values they hold relative to values they do not (Smallenbroek et al., 2017). From a self-enhancement perspective, this work could be interpreted as evidence that people are motivated to see their morally good behavior as more authentic than their morally questionable behavior in a self-distorting/defensive manner. From a humanistic perspective, these behaviors should feel more authentic because they are helping people get closer to their ideals. We suspect that both approaches have merit and that future work should continue to examine both and work to integrate these perspectives.

Another important question is what each perspective has to say about whether a true self is necessary for authentic experiences. A self-enhancement perspective does not require the existence of a true self at all. Rather, a self-enhancement perspective on authenticity simply suggests that people have overly positive true self-concepts (Bailey & Iyengar, 2023). A humanistic perspective does suggest a certain type of true self, but that true self does not perfectly align with the lay theories people have that link the true self to distinct essences for different people. Rather a humanistic perspective suggests that there is some common content across all "true selves" that guides people toward the nurturance of basic psychological needs. While this idea isn't necessarily inconsistent with the idea of a core encased in a larger casing, it certainly seems more nuanced than a simple set of unchanging essential traits. Future work should continue to explore the content people ascribe to their true self-concepts to further explore whether lay theories may be more linked to humanistic approaches than they might appear at first blush.

What Makes People Appear Authentic?

Far less research has examined what makes people appear authentic to others. However, a recent study found almost no correlation between self- and other-rated authenticity (Bailey & Levy, 2022), suggesting that people's judgments of whether someone else is being authentic are driven by something other than whether the target believes they are being authentic. In that study, the best predictor of rating others as authentic was one's own (self-rated) authenticity, suggesting that people who believe they are authentic think other people are too.

Other research points to the idea that we think people are authentic to the extent that they engage in behavior we see as morally good, likable, or otherwise positive and culturally desirable. Perhaps the most striking demonstration of this bias comes from work in which people were presented with vignettes describing a target that underwent some kind of change, either for the better or the worse (e.g., a caring father becomes a neglectful dad or vice versa; Newman et al., 2014). Across a variety of vignettes, participants consistently judged the positive behavior as a better reflection of the true self (i.e., more authentic). These studies also demonstrated that this effect depended on participants' own moral views. Vignettes varied such that perceived valence of the behavior would depend on the participant's political orientation (e.g., someone who previously denied global warming begins to support the environment). The perceived authenticity of the behavior in these vignettes depended on the participant's own political orientation. Liberals saw the more typically liberal behavior as more authentic than the alternative whereas conservative participants saw the more typically conservative behavior as more authentic.

The link between positivity and perceived authenticity is demonstrated across various social targets. For example, when participants were asked to consider changes people they knew had undergone, people were more likely to see positive changes (as opposed to negative changes) of close others as cases of true self-discovery (i.e., the person becoming more like their true self; Bench et al., 2015). Similarly, candidate preference strongly affects how authentic people view that behavior. For preferred candidates, people were motivated to see their preferred candidate as authentic in general and then interpret specific behaviors (e.g., honest talk) as evidence of that authenticity (Pillow et al., 2018). Finally, White and Crandall (2023) demonstrated a darker instantiation of these tendencies such that someone's own prejudice predicted how authentic they perceived someone else's prejudiced statements to be, further suggesting that people's own beliefs predict what they see to be authentic. We seem to find people who agree with us, are close to us, or conform to our own standards to be the most authentic.

Along similar lines, recent research (Rivera et al., 2024) tested multiple potential predictors of other-reported authenticity in a set of group interaction studies. The studies examined whether affect, Big Five personality states, and/or liking predicted judgments of others' authenticity. The most consistent and strongest predictor of perceiving someone else as authentic was whether the perceiver liked that target. One study probed the potential causal effect of liking on perceived authenticity by having participants interact with a research assistant who was trained to act in a likeable or dislikable manner (Rivera et al., 2024, Study 3). Results showed that experimentally manipulated likability enhanced perceived authenticity. In another study that used vignettes (Garrison et al., 2023), participants considered hypothetical targets who were faced with self-control conflicts (e.g., wanting to watch Netflix when you need to study) and made a decision to either act on the impulse (watch Netflix) or engage in self-control (study). While people showed some tendency to see other people's impulses as authentic, there was a large effect of valence such that people saw positive actions as authentic.

Taken together, this work, much like research on self-authenticity, suggests large valence effects on what makes other people seem authentic. Why might this be the case? We see at least a few potential explanations. First, because authenticity is viewed positively, authenticity judgments may be susceptible to halo effects (Lachman & Bass, 1985; Nisbett & Wilson, 1977) such that a general positive evaluation of a person leads to more specific positive judgments of that person. Another possibility is that people project their own perceived authenticity onto people they like. Given that most people perceive themselves as authentic (Bailey & Levy, 2022) and people project their own features onto people they like more than people they dislike (e.g., Davis, 2017), this would explain why liked targets are seen as more authentic than disliked targets. Finally, such patterns could again be explained by the good true self bias (De Freitas & Cikara, 2018; De Freitas, Cikara, et al., 2017; De Freitas et al., 2018; Newman et al., 2014) leading people to see behaviors they deem as good as more expressive of the presumed good true self of others. Notably, none of these explanations require the literal existence of a true self.

CONCLUSIONS

We began this chapter with the simple question "Who am I?" and explored what we know about how people approach this question, particularly as it relates to the consideration of a true self. While we leave the debate of whether there really is a true self to philosophers, we can confidently say that people's lay beliefs surrounding true selves matter and shape a whole host of individual and interpersonal well-being outcomes. It may be helpful to think of true selves like a secular soul belief—no one can prove that true selves (or souls) exist, yet the presence of belief in them surely guides human thoughts and behaviors in meaningful and interesting ways, ripe for ongoing scientific investigation. Belief in true selves likely stems from more general tendencies toward psychological essentialism, where people believe the true self functions like an essence deep inside us that gives rise to authentic behavior. Following from this essentialist thinking is a corresponding "true-self-as-guide" lay theory, which offers the wisdom that if one wants to live a meaningful and satisfying life, one should follow one's true self. The wisdom of such advice seemingly hinges on the general assumption that true selves are morally good (i.e., if true selves were generally assumed to be morally bad, then one wouldn't expect following them to lead to wholly meaningful and satisfying outcomes). In line with this, positivity and morality bias our judgments of the authenticity of both our own and others' behavior, though the conclusion of whether authenticity judgments are better explained by self-enhancement or humanistic perspectives is still debated. The study of true selves and authenticity is a multifaceted and growing field, which we expect will continue to give insight into how people navigate the question "Who am I?"

REFERENCES

Aho, K. (2023). Existentialism. In E. N. Zalta & U. Nodelman (Eds.), *The Stanford encyclopedia of philosophy*. Metaphysics Research Lab, Stanford University. https://plato.stanford.edu/archives/sum2023/entries/existentialism/.

Andersen, S. M., & Ross, L. (1984). Self-knowledge and social inference: I. The impact of cognitive/affective and behavioral data. *Journal of Personality and Social Psychology, 46*(2), 280–293.

Atran, S., Medin, D., & Sousa, P. (2002). Essentialism and folkbiology: Evidence from Brazil. *Journal of Cognition and Culture, 2*(3), 195–223.

Bailey, E. R., & Iyengar, S. S. (2023). Positive—more than unbiased—self-perceptions increase subjective authenticity. *Journal of Personality and Social Psychology, 125*(6), 1351–1372.

Bailey, E. R., & Levy, A. (2022). Are you for real?: Perceptions of authenticity are systematically biased and not accurate. *Psychological Science, 33*(5), 798–815.

Baumeister, R. F. (1987). How the self became a problem: A psychological review of historical research. *Journal of Personality and Social Psychology, 52*(1), 163–176.

Baumeister, R. F. (1991). *Meanings of life*. Guilford Press.

Baumeister, R. F. (1995). Self and identity. In *Advanced social psychology* (pp. 51–99). McGraw-Hill.

Bellah, R. N., Madsen, R., Sullivan, W. M., Swidler, A., & Tipton, S. M. (1996). *Habits of the heart: Individualism and commitment in American life* (Updated, Subsequent ed.). University of California Press.

Bench, S. W., Schlegel, R. J., Davis, W. E., & Vess, M. (2015). Thinking about change in the self and others: The role of self-discovery metaphors and the true self. *Social Cognition, 33*(3), 169–185.

Cavallaro, R. M., Church, M. H., Giddens, B.

J., & Rivera, G. N. (2025). Complex effects of awe on meaning in life and true self-knowledge. *Self and Identity, 24*(3), 189–216.

Chen, K., Zhang, H., Friedman, M., & Schlegel, R. J. (2022). The authentic catch-22: Following the true self promotes decision satisfaction in moral dilemmas. *Journal of Experimental Social Psychology, 102,* 104376.

Chen, K., Zhang, H., & Schlegel, R. J. (2023). Does being angry feel authentic?: A test of how affective valence and motivational direction differentially influence state authenticity. *Motivation and Emotion, 47*(5), 828–841.

Christy, A. G., Maffly-Kipp, J., Friedman, M., Cimpian, A., & Schlegel, R. J. (2024). Essentialist beliefs about the self predict psychological well-being. *Self and Identity, 23*(1–2), 127–174.

Christy, A. G., Schlegel, R. J., & Cimpian, A. (2019). Why do people believe in a "true self"?: The role of essentialist reasoning about personal identity and the self. *Journal of Personality and Social Psychology, 117*(2), 386–416.

Christy, A. G., Seto, E., Schlegel, R. J., Vess, M., & Hicks, J. A. (2016). Straying from the righteous path and from ourselves: The interplay between perceptions of morality and self-knowledge. *Personality and Social Psychology Bulletin, 42*(11), 1538–1550.

Dar-Nimrod, I., & Heine, S. J. (2011). Genetic essentialism: On the deceptive determinism of DNA. *Psychological Bulletin, 137*(5), 800–818.

Davis, M. H. (2017). Social projection to liked and disliked targets: The role of perceived similarity. *Journal of Experimental Social Psychology, 70,* 286–293.

De Freitas, J., & Cikara, M. (2018). Deep down my enemy is good: Thinking about the true self reduces intergroup bias. *Journal of Experimental Social Psychology, 74,* 307–316.

De Freitas, J., Cikara, M., Grossmann, I., & Schlegel, R. (2017). Origins of the belief in good true selves. *Trends in Cognitive Sciences, 21*(9), 634–636.

De Freitas, J., Sarkissian, H., Newman, G. E., Grossmann, I., De Brigard, F., Luco, A., & Knobe, J. (2018). Consistent belief in a good true self in misanthropes and three interdependent cultures. *Cognitive Science, 42,* 134–160.

De Freitas, J., Tobia, K. P., Newman, G. E., & Knobe, J. (2017). Normative judgments and individual essence. *Cognitive Science, 41*(Suppl. 3), 382–402.

Dulaney, E. S., Graupmann, V., & Quinn, K. A. (2019). Who am I and how often?: Variation in self-essentialism beliefs, cognitive style, and well-being. *Personality and Individual Differences, 136,* 148–159.

Errington, S. (1989). Fragile traditions and contested meanings. *Public Culture, 1*(2), 49–59.

Fleeson, W., & Wilt, J. (2010). The relevance of Big Five Trait content in behavior to subjective authenticity: Do high levels of within-person behavioral variability undermine or enable authenticity achievement? *Journal of Personality, 78*(4), 1353–1382.

Gan, M., & Chen, S. (2017). Being your actual or ideal self?: What it means to feel authentic in a relationship. *Personality and Social Psychology Bulletin, 43*(4), 465–478.

Garrison, K. E., Rivera, G. N., Schlegel, R. J., Hicks, J. A., & Schmeichel, B. J. (2023). Authentic for thee but not for me: Perceived authenticity in self-control conflicts. *Personality and Social Psychology Bulletin, 49*(12), 1646–1662.

Gelman, S. A. (2003). *The essential child: Origins of essentialism in everyday thought.* Oxford University Press.

Gelman, S. A., & Wellman, H. M. (1991). Insides and essences: Early understandings of the non-obvious. *Cognition, 38*(3), 213–244.

Gil-White, F. (2001). Sorting is not categorization: A critique of the claim that Brazilians have fuzzy racial categories. *Journal of Cognition and Culture, 1*(3), 219–249.

Goldman, B. M., & Kernis, M. H. (2002). The role of authenticity in healthy psychological functioning and subjective well-being. *Annals of the American Psychotherapy Association, 5*(6), 18–20.

Guenther, C. L., Zhang, Y., & Sedikides, C. (2023). The authentic self is the self-enhancing self: A self-enhancement framework of authenticity. *Personality and Social Psychology Bulletin.*

Heidegger, M. (2010). *Being and time.* State University of New York Press.

Henrich, J., Heine, S. J., & Norenzayan, A. (2010). The weirdest people in the world? *Behavioral and Brain Sciences, 33*(2–3), 61.

Heppner, W. L., Kernis, M. H., Nezlek, J. B., Foster, J., Lakey, C. E., & Goldman, B. M. (2008). Within-person relationships among daily self-esteem, need satisfaction, and authenticity. *Psychological Science, 19*(11), 1140–1145.

Jiang, T., & Sedikides, C. (2022). Awe motivates authentic-self pursuit via self-transcendence: Implications for prosociality. *Journal of Personality and Social Psychology, 123*(3), 576–596.

Johnson, J. T., Robinson, M. D., & Mitchell, E. B. (2004). Inferences about the authentic self:

When do actions say more than mental states? *Journal of Personality and Social Psychology, 87*(5), 615–630.

Jongman-Sereno, K. P., & Leary, M. R. (2016). Self-perceived authenticity is contaminated by the valence of one's behavior. *Self and Identity, 15*(3), 283–301.

Jongman-Sereno, K. P., & Leary, M. R. (2019). The enigma of being yourself: A critical examination of the concept of authenticity. *Review of General Psychology, 23*(1), 133–142.

Jongman-Sereno, K. P., & Leary, M. R. (2020). Self-judgments of authenticity. *Self and Identity, 19*(1), 32–63.

Keltner, D., & Haidt, J. (2003). Approaching awe, a moral, spiritual, and aesthetic emotion. *Cognition and Emotion, 17*(2), 297–314.

Kernis, M. H., & Goldman, B. M. (2006). A multicomponent conceptualization of authenticity: Theory and research. *Advances in Experimental Social Psychology, 38,* 283–357.

Kierkegaard, S. (1989). *The sickness unto death: A Christian psychological exposition of edification and awakening by anti-Climacus* (A. Hannay, Trans.). Penguin Classics.

Kim, J., Chen, K., Davis, W. E., Hicks, J. A., & Schlegel, R. J. (2019). Approaching the true self: Promotion focus predicts the experience of authenticity. *Journal of Research in Personality, 78,* 165–176.

Kim, J., Chen, K., Rivera, G. N., Hong, E. K., Kamble, S., Scollon, C. N., Sheldon, K. M., Zhang, H., & Schlegel, R. J. (2022). True-self-as-guide lay theory endorsement across five countries. *Self and Identity, 21*(8), 939–962.

Kim, J., Christy, A. G., Rivera, G. N., Hicks, J. A., & Schlegel, R. J. (2021). Is the illusion of authenticity beneficial?: Merely perceiving decisions as guided by the true self enhances decision satisfaction. *Social Psychological and Personality Science, 12*(1), 80–90.

Kim, J., Christy, A. G., Schlegel, R. J., Donnellan, M. B., & Hicks, J. A. (2017). Existential ennui: Examining the reciprocal relationship between self-alienation and academic amotivation. *Social Psychological and Personality Science, 10.*

Kim, Y., Dulaney, E., Wangchuk, G., Kim, K., & Graupmann, V. (2024). Self or non-self?: Self-essentialism and well-being in Tibetan Buddhist monks. *Journal of Cross-Cultural Psychology.*

Koenigs, M., Young, L., Adolphs, R., Tranel, D., Cushman, F., Hauser, M., & Damasio, A. (2007). Damage to the prefrontal cortex increases utilitarian moral judgements. *Nature, 446,* 908–911.

Kokkoris, M. D., & Kühnen, U. (2014). "Express the real you": Cultural differences in the perception of self-expression as authenticity. *Journal of Cross-Cultural Psychology, 45*(8), 1221–1228.

Lachman, S. J., & Bass, A. R. (1985). A direct study of halo effect. *Journal of Psychology, 119*(6), 535–540.

Lakoff, G., & Johnson, M. (1999). *Philosophy in the flesh: The embodied mind and its challenge to Western thought.* Basic Books.

Landau, M. J., Vess, M., Arndt, J., Rothschild, Z. K., Sullivan, D., & Atchley, R. A. (2011). Embodied metaphor and the "true" self: Priming entity expansion and protection influences intrinsic self-expressions in self-perceptions and interpersonal behavior. *Journal of Experimental Social Psychology, 47*(1), 79–87.

Lenton, A. P., Bruder, M., Slabu, L., & Sedikides, C. (2013). How does "being real" feel?: The experience of state authenticity. *Journal of Personality, 81*(3), 276–289.

Lenton, A. P., Slabu, L., Sedikides, C., & Power, K. (2013). I feel good, therefore I am real: Testing the causal influence of mood on state authenticity. *Cognition and Emotion, 27*(7), 1202–1224.

Liu, Y., & Perrewe, P. L. (2006). Are they for real?: The interpersonal and intrapersonal outcomes of perceived authenticity. *International Journal of Work Organisation and Emotion, 1*(3), 204–214.

Maffly-Kipp, J., Rivera, G. N., Schlegel, R. J., & Vess, M. (2022). The effect of true self-attributions on the endorsement of retributive and restorative justice. *Personality and Social Psychology Bulletin, 48*(8), 1284–1297.

Maffly-Kipp, J., Truong, T. N., Edens, J. F., & Vess, M. (2023). Dark triad traits are associated with a weaker morally-good true self bias in self-perceptions. *Self and Identity, 22*(5), 832–848.

Medlock, G. (2012). The evolving ethic of authenticity: From humanistic to positive psychology. *The Humanistic Psychologist, 40*(1), 38–57.

Newman, G. E., Bloom, P., & Knobe, J. (2014). Value judgments and the true self. *Personality and Social Psychology Bulletin, 40*(2), 203–216.

Nisbett, R. E., & Wilson, T. D. (1977). The halo effect: Evidence for unconscious alteration of judgments. *Journal of Personality and Social Psychology, 35*(4), 250–256.

Pillow, D. R., Crabtree, M. A., Galvan, M. J., & Hale, W. J. (2018). Not simply in the eye of the beholder: Authenticity as a product of candidate preference and unfettered speech. *Political Psychology, 39*(4), 849–868.

Rivera, G. N., Christy, A. G., Kim, J., Vess, M., Hicks, J. A., & Schlegel, R. J. (2018). Understanding the relationship between perceived authenticity and well-being. *Review of General Psychology.*

Rivera, G. N., Kim, J., Kelley, N. J., Hicks, J., & Schlegel, R. J. (2024). Liking predicts judgments of authenticity in real-time interactions more robustly than personality states or affect. *Personality and Social Psychology Bulletin.*

Rivera, G. R., Smith, C. M., & Schlegel, R. J. (2018). A window to the true self: The importance of I-sharing in romantic relationships. *Journal of Social and Personal Relationships.*

Rogers, C. R. (1961). *On becoming a person.* Houghton Mifflin.

Ryan, R. M., & Deci, E. L. (2004). Autonomy is no illusion: Self-determination theory and the empirical study of authenticity, awareness, and will. In J. Greenberg, S. L. Koole, & T. Pyszczynski (Eds.), *Handbook of experimental existential psychology* (pp. 449–479). Guilford Press.

Ryan, W. S., & Ryan, R. M. (2019). Toward a social psychology of authenticity: Exploring within-person variation in autonomy, congruence, and genuineness using self-determination theory. *Review of General Psychology, 23*(1), 99–112.

Sariçam, H. (2015). Life satisfaction: Testing a structural equation model based on authenticity and subjective happiness. *Polish Psychological Bulletin.*

Schlegel, R. J., Hicks, J. A., Arndt, J., & King, L. A. (2009). Thine own self: True self-concept accessibility and meaning in life. *Journal of Personality and Social Psychology, 96*(2), 473–490.

Schlegel, R. J., Hicks, J. A., Davis, W. E., Hirsch, K. A., & Smith, C. M. (2013). The dynamic interplay between perceived true self-knowledge and decision satisfaction. *Journal of Personality and Social Psychology, 104*(3), 542–558.

Schlegel, R. J., Hicks, J. A., King, L. A., & Arndt, J. (2011). Feeling like you know who you are: Perceived true self-knowledge and meaning in life. *Personality and Social Psychology Bulletin, 37*(6), 745–756.

Schlegel, R. J., Vess, M., & Arndt, J. (2012). To discover or to create: Metaphors and the true self. *Journal of Personality, 80*(4), 969–993.

Schwarz, N. (1998). Accessible content and accessibility experiences: The interplay of declarative and experiential information in judgment. *Personality and Social Psychology Review, 2*(2), 87–99.

Schwarz, N., & Clore, G. L. (1996). Feelings and phenomenal experiences. In E. T. Higgins & A. W. Kruglanski (Eds.), *Social psychology: Handbook of basic principles* (pp. 385–407. Guilford Press.

Seto, E., & Hicks, J. A. (2016). Disassociating the agent from the self: Undermining belief in free will diminishes true self-knowledge. *Social Psychological and Personality Science, 7,* 726–734.

Sheldon, K. M. (2002). The self-concordance model of healthy goal striving: When personal goals correctly represent the person. In E. L. Deci & R. M. Ryan (Eds.), *Handbook of self-determination research* (pp. 65–86). University of Rochester Press.

Sheldon, K. M. (2014). Becoming oneself: The central role of self-concordant goal selection. *Personality and Social Psychology Review, 18*(4), 349–365.

Sheldon, K. M., & Houser-Marko, L. (2001). Self-concordance, goal attainment, and the pursuit of happiness: Can there be an upward spiral? *Journal of Personality and Social Psychology, 80*(1), 152–165.

Sheldon, K. M., Ryan, R. M., Rawsthorne, L. J., & Ilardi, B. (1997). Trait self and true self: Cross-role variation in the Big-Five personality traits and its relations with psychological authenticity and subjective well-being. *Journal of Personality and Social Psychology, 73*(6), 1380–1393.

Smallenbroek, O., Zelenski, J. M., & Whelan, D. C. (2017). Authenticity as a eudaimonic construct: The relationships among authenticity, values, and valence. *Journal of Positive Psychology, 12*(2), 197–209.

Strohminger, N., Knobe, J., & Newman, G. (2017). The true self: A psychological concept distinct from the self. *Perspectives on Psychological Science, 12*(4), 551–560.

Sutton, A. (2020). Living the good life: A meta-analysis of authenticity, well-being and engagement. *Personality and Individual Differences, 153,* 109645.

Thomaes, S., Sedikides, C., van den Bos, N., Hutteman, R., & Reijntjes, A. (2017). Happy to be "me"?: Authenticity, psychological need satisfaction, and subjective well-being in adolescence. *Child Development, 88*(4), 1045–1056.

Vess, M. (2019). Varieties of conscious experience and the subjective awareness of one's "true" self. *Review of General Psychology, 23*(1), 89–98.

Vess, M., & Maffly-Kipp, J. (2022). Intentional mindwandering and unintentional mindwandering are differentially associated with the experience of self-alienation. *Personality and Individual Differences, 185,* 111289.

Waterman, A. S. (1984). Identity formation: Discovery or creation? *Journal of Early Adolescence, 4*(4), 329–341.
Waterman, A. S. (1993). Two conceptions of happiness: Contrasts of personal expressiveness (eudaimonia) and hedonic enjoyment. *Journal of Personality and Social Psychology, 64*(4), 678–691.
Waterman, A. S., & Schwartz, S. J. (2013). Eudaimonic identity theory. In A. S. Waterman (Ed.), *The best within us: Positive psychology perspectives on eudaimonia* (pp. 99–118). American Psychological Association.
White, M. H., & Crandall, C. S. (2023). Perceived authenticity as a vicarious justification for prejudice. *Group Processes & Intergroup Relations, 26*(3), 534–554.
Wickham, R. E. (2013). Perceived authenticity in romantic partners. *Journal of Experimental Social Psychology, 49*(5), 878–887.
Wickham, R. E., Williamson, R. E., Beard, C. L., Kobayashi, C. L. B., & Hirst, T. W. (2016). Authenticity attenuates the negative effects of interpersonal conflict on daily well-being. *Journal of Research in Personality, 60*, 56–62.
Wood, A. M., Linley, P. A., Maltby, J., Baliousis, M., & Joseph, S. (2008). The authentic personality: A theoretical and empirical conceptualization and the development of the Authenticity Scale. *Journal of counseling psychology, 55*(3), 385.
Yuan, W., Du, Y., & Jiang, T. (2024). How and when awe improves meaning in life: The role of authentic-self pursuit and trait authenticity. *Emotion, 24*(2), 412–430.
Zhang, H., Chen, K., Schlegel, R., Hicks, J., & Chen, C. (2019). The authentic moral self: Dynamic interplay between perceived authenticity and moral behaviors in the workplace. *Collabra: Psychology, 5*(1), 48.
Zimmerman, M. E. (1986). *Eclipse of self: The development of Heidegger's concept of authenticity* (2nd ed.). Ohio University Press.

CHAPTER 21

Don't Tread on Me

Freedom and Reactance to Autonomy Threat

Benjamin D. Rosenberg, Thomas B. Coulson II,
Christopher M. Falco, *and* Jason T. Siegel

Derived from cognitive dissonance theory (Festinger, 1957) and other cognitive inconsistency theories (for review, see Proulx et al., 2012), psychological reactance theory (PRT; Brehm, 1966) posits that people experience psychological reactance—a motivational state aimed at restoring freedom—when their freedom of behavior or belief is threatened or eliminated. Brehm's (1966) emphasis on the existential importance of freedom and its loss places PRT alongside the ideas of philosophers such as Kant (1797/1967), Sartre (1943/1956), Merleau-Ponty (1964), and Fromm (1941), who debated the existence and importance of free will. Viewpoints among these scholars varied widely; for instance, Sartre (1943/1956) suggested that freedom is absolute, equating free will with being human. Summarizing the range of ideas about freedom, Feldman (2017) noted, "Choice is important, as it is a fundamental factor in the understanding of the human psyche and is considered by thinkers to be a defining feature of human existence (Heidegger, 1927/1962; Sartre, 1943/1956) and sense of freedom (Kant, 1967)" (p. 5).

For many years, this debate about the existence and importance of freedom, free choice, and free will was largely the provenance of philosophers, with few empirical investigations informing their viewpoints (for review, see Feldman, 2017). More recently, psychologists and neuroscientists have made strides in defining and empirically studying the concept of free will as it relates to human behavior and cognition (for reviews, see Brass et al., 2019; Feldman, 2017). An important advancement is the acknowledgment that, as Brehm (1966) suggested, freedom of choice may be rooted in evolution, as it is likely adaptive for people to weigh their options and select appropriate actions (Vohs & Baumeister, 2004).

With these existential concerns in mind, this chapter briefly outlines the research and application of PRT, which have continued since its introduction over 50 years ago. In line with Rosenberg and Siegel's (2018) review of PRT, this chapter outlines and summarizes research that comprises five overlapping waves of PRT literature: 1) theory proposal and testing, 2) contributions from clinical psychology, 3) contributions from communication research, 4) measuring reactance, and 5) return to motivation. After covering these five waves, we discuss how principles from PRT could be applied when developing persuasive messages.

WAVE 1: THEORY PROPOSAL AND TESTING

Assumptions of PRT

Brehm (1966) developed PRT based on two main assumptions. First, people believe they can engage in a set of free behaviors (or *freedoms*). Second, when these freedoms are threatened or eliminated, people are often motivated to restore them. This motivational arousal, known as *reactance,* occurs even though freedom may not always be desired. These foundational assumptions led to predictions concerning the characteristics of freedoms, the nature of freedom threats, and the resultant effects of reactance (for review, see Brehm & Brehm, 1981).

Components of PRT

For clarity, researchers (e.g., Dillard & Shen, 2005) have segmented PRT into four sequential components: (1) the presence of freedom, (2) the threat or elimination of freedom, (3) reactance arousal, and (4) the restoration of freedom.

Freedoms

People believe they have a set of free behaviors—*freedoms*—they have engaged in before, can currently engage in, or could engage in in the future (Brehm, 1966). For a behavior to be perceived as a freedom, people must (1) be aware of the freedom and (2) feel capable of engaging in it (Wicklund & Brehm, 1968).

Elimination and Threats to Freedom

The *elimination* of freedom (Brehm, 1966) is anything that completely prevents people from engaging in a behavior or holding a particular position (e.g., outright bans; Avishai et al., 2023; Mazis et al., 1973). A *threat* to freedom is anything that limits but does not eliminate a behavior (e.g., attempted social influence; Brehm, 1966). Beneficial events can also act as threats and thus arouse reactance, such as when feeling pressured to return a favor (e.g., Krishnan & Carmen, 1979).

Reactance Arousal

Characteristics of the freedom itself influence reactance arousal. Brehm and Brehm (1981) proposed that more reactance is elicited when a greater proportion of freedoms are threatened. One study showed initial support for this relationship (Wicklund et al., 1970), though subsequent research is sparse (for an unsupportive exception, see Grabitz-Gniech et al., 1975). Additionally, Brehm (1966) noted that freedoms unique in fulfilling specific needs, when threatened, trigger more intense reactance than when other freedoms can fulfill the same need (e.g., removing a desired food from people who lack vs. have other foods to quell their hunger). However, this aspect has yet to be extensively studied (for an exception, see Goldman & Wallis, 1979).

Another factor that can determine how much reactance is aroused is the threat's characteristics, including threat severity, perceived intent to persuade, and vicarious threat (Brehm, 1966). Empirical studies have demonstrated that more severe threats induce stronger reactance (e.g., Rains & Turner, 2007). When people perceive high persuasive intent, their opposition to the advocated position tends to increase due to elicited reactance (Benoit, 1998; Jones & Brehm, 1970). Furthermore, vicarious experiences of threat, such as observing or learning about others having their freedoms threatened, can also evoke reactance (i.e., vicarious reactance; Sittenthaler et al., 2015b). However, direct threats to freedoms prompt an immediate physiological response, whereas vicarious threats lead to a delayed response (Sittenthaler et al., 2016; Steindl et al., 2015).

Restoration of Freedom

When freedoms are threatened or eliminated, reactance typically manifests in two primary ways (Brehm & Brehm, 1981). People may *directly* engage in the restricted behavior, known as the boomerang effect (Brehm, 1966), such as when underage college students drank more alcohol following an increase in the drinking age from 18 to 21 (Engs & Hanson, 1989). People may also express reactance *indirectly*, such as by observing or encouraging others to enact similar behaviors (Brehm & Brehm, 1981). For instance, if those newly underage college students were unable to drink as a method of freedom restoration, they might watch their friends do so instead. Additionally, people can alleviate the discomfort associated with reactance by showing hostility toward or derogating the source of a threat (Nezlek & Brehm, 1975; Rains, 2013). Alongside these behavioral responses, the attractiveness and desirability of restricted behaviors often increase (Brehm & Rozen, 1971; Brehm et al., 1966).

When Reactance Reduction Fails

When efforts to reduce reactance fail, people may stop feeling reactance and experience a sense of defeat or lost control (Brehm & Brehm, 1981; Wortman & Brehm, 1975); this resembles learned helplessness, where people accept their inability to restore freedoms after acknowledging that the threat exists (Seligman, 1975). We discuss learned helplessness further in Wave 5.

Additionally, personality traits (e.g., locus of control; Rotter, 1966) can affect reactance. For instance, people who are Type A (i.e., competitive, urgent, aggressive) exhibit higher reactance under threat than those who are Type B (i.e., relaxed, patient, easygoing; Rhodewalt & Marcroft, 1988). These results suggest that ability to cope with threats moderates reactance arousal (Brehm & Brehm, 1981), which aligns with findings that people assess situations through primary and secondary appraisal processes to determine if they are threatening (potentially harmful or loss-inducing) or challenging (leading to mastery or benefits; Brehm & Self, 1989; Folkman et al., 2000; Lazarus & Folkman, 1984).

WAVE 2: CONTRIBUTIONS FROM CLINICAL PSYCHOLOGY

PRT was identified as having substantial potential in clinical psychology (Brehm, 1976; Brehm & Brehm, 1981), with scholars reconceptualizing reactance as a trait (stable and enduring; Shoham et al., 2004) and a state (momentary and context-dependent; Brehm, 1966). Trait reactance is the "consistent tendency to perceive and react to situations as if one's freedoms were being threatened" (Kelly & Nauta, 1997, p. 1124); people with differing levels of trait reactance will perceive the same stimulus as more or less threatening to their freedom. For example, when participants were exposed to a message indicating a COVID-19 vaccination was mandatory (i.e., freedom-threatening) as opposed to voluntary, greater state reactance was reported—but only among those with higher levels of trait reactance (Soveri et al., 2024).

Perspectives on Reactance in Clinical Psychology

To better understand reactance among clients receiving psychotherapy, clinicians have described three approaches to examining trait reactance: reactance as a moderator, overcoming reactance in therapy, and reactance as a tailoring variable (for reviews, see Beutler et al., 2002; Shoham et al., 2004).

Reactance as a Moderator

Trait reactance moderates therapeutic success (for review, see Shoham et al., 2004); patients with higher trait reactance have shown less satisfaction and less expectation of change in therapy (Dowd et al., 1988). This decrease in therapeutic effectiveness can be attributed to patients perceiving their therapists' recommendations as freedom threatening (e.g., Tracey et al., 1989). Indeed, those high in trait reactance who experience bipolar disorder or depression adhere less to psychotropic medication (Lazary et al., 2023); people who exhibit high trait reactance may respond more positively to therapeutic styles that avoid confrontation (Gaume et al., 2023). Clients with higher trait reactance generally receive poorer prognoses than those with lower trait reactance (Beutler et al., 2002; Cautilli et al., 2005).

Overcoming Reactance in Therapy

Offering clients free choice in therapy is one method to prevent the adverse outcomes of reactance (Devine & Fernald, 1973). For example, students who were given a choice in treatments reported greater value and treatment effectiveness compared to those whose treatment was chosen for them (Gordon, 1976). Another method to address reactance in therapy is to encourage its arousal (for discussion, see Tennen et al., 1981) via paradoxical interventions (i.e., those that encourage symptomatic behavior; Dowd & Swoboda, 1984). However, research has indicated inconsistencies with using paradoxical interventions on client outcomes (e.g., Debord, 1989; Shoham-Salomon & Rosenthal, 1987; Swoboda et al., 1990).

Reactance as a Tailoring Variable

Research addressing the moderating effect of trait reactance and methods to overcome reactance in therapy suggests that therapists should tailor their therapy to patients' trait reactance levels (e.g., Beutler et al., 2018). Patients who are higher in trait reactance tend to respond better to therapy (e.g., using more pro-recovery language) when their therapists use a less structured approach that is more flexible and adaptive; conversely, patients low in trait reactance benefit more when therapy has a clear framework that encourages autonomy and shared decision making (Arnold & Vakhrusheva, 2016; Dowd & Siebel, 1990; Karno et al., 2010).

Debate over Trait Reactance

Although the previously mentioned research supports the conceptualization of reactance as a trait, other researchers have questioned its use and construct validity as a personality trait, suggesting that reactance is more effectively applied as a motivational state (Miron & Brehm, 2006; Shoham et al., 2004). Silvia (2006) highlighted the uneven nature of the evidence supporting trait reactance, noting inconsistencies in responses to reactance-inducing messages on the Hong Psychological Reactance Scale, a measure of trait reactance (Hong & Page, 1989). Further critiques focus on the low explanatory power of trait scales, suggesting they might only measure affect (Miron & Brehm, 2006).

WAVE 3: CONTRIBUTIONS FROM COMMUNICATION RESEARCH

In addition to the settings mentioned in Wave 2, researchers also started utilizing principles of PRT in communication research (for reviews, see Quick et al., 2013; Reynolds-Tylus, 2019). Branching from communication research examining low- and high-threat antidrinking messages (Bensley & Wu, 1991), scholars began investigating how messages can increase (e.g., controlling language; Buller et al., 1998) and decrease (e.g., narrative; Moyer-Gusé, 2008) reactance arousal.

High- and Low-Controlling Language

Building on Brehm's (1966) scholarship, researchers have explored how controlling language can cause reactance (Grandpre et al., 2003; Quick & Kim, 2009). These studies often compare high-controlling messages (high threat; "must," "ought," "should") with low-controlling ones (low threat; "perhaps," "possibly," "maybe"; Miller et al., 2007, p. 223). For example, Bensley and Wu (1991) found that high-threat messages increased college students' alcohol consumption more than low-threat messages did, demonstrating a boomerang effect (Brehm, 1966). This high- and low-threat message communication paradigm is the standard in PRT communication research (Burgoon et al., 2002). With this approach, results similar to the aforementioned alcohol consumption messages have been found repeatedly in various contexts, including health (e.g., Crano et al., 2017; Li & Shen, 2024; Richards et al., 2022) and consumer behavior (e.g., Zemack-Rugar et al., 2017).

Other Message Features Affecting Reactance Arousal

After establishing that strongly-worded messages consistently arouse reactance, researchers explored features that could instead reduce reactance (Quick et al., 2013). These are discussed in the "Practical Implications of PRT" section after Wave 5.

WAVE 4: MEASURING REACTANCE

Although *trait* reactance was considered to be measurable using observational (Shoham-Salomon et al., 1989) and self-report methods (Hong & Page, 1989; Merz, 1983), early research on PRT did not directly measure *state* reactance. Instead, outcomes like boomerang effects (Worchel & Brehm, 1970) and increased attractiveness of the eliminated freedom (Brehm & Rozen, 1971) were assessed. Despite early assertions that state reactance is immeasurable (Brehm, 1966; Brehm & Brehm, 1981), scholars have spent the last 20 years developing measures for directly measuring state reactance (Dillard & Shen, 2005; Lindsey, 2005; Sittenthaler et al., 2015a).

Measures of Trait Reactance

Questionnaire for Measuring Psychological Reactance

Merz (1983) developed the Questionnaire for Measuring Psychological Reactance (QMPR), an 18-item scale (e.g., "I react strongly to duties and regulations"), as an initial measure of trait reactance. While the QMPR initially showed some face and content validity (for review, see Shen & Dillard, 2007), subsequent evaluations indicated psychometric weaknesses, partly due to translation issues from its original German (Hong & Ostini, 1989; Tucker & Byers, 1987).

Therapeutic Reactance Scale

To address limitations of the QPMR (Merzs, 1983), Dowd and colleagues (1991) developed the 28-item Therapeutic Reactance Scale (TRS) to measure trait reactance. Initially, 112 items were developed from Brehm's (1966) description of reactance, which were subsequently refined to a final set of 28 items (e.g., "I am relatively opinionated"). Although the TRS demonstrated correlations with the K scale of the Minnesota Multiphasic Personality Inventory and measures of locus of control, its unidimensional nature prompted caution in its use, considering reactance's multidimensional aspects (Buboltz et al., 2002).

Hong Psychological Reactance Scale

Hong and Page (1989) developed the Hong Psychological Reaction Scale (HPRS) to address the deficits of the QMPR (Merz, 1983). The 14-item scale (e.g., "I find contradicting others stimulating") had four factors: emotional response to restricted choice, reactance to compliance, resisting influence from others, and reactance to advice and recommendations (Hong, 1992; Hong & Faedda, 1996). Despite evidence of validity in the form of correlations with trait anger and depression (while not correlating with self-esteem; Hong & Faedda, 1996), a confirmatory factor analysis (Thomas et al., 2001) suggested the HPRS needed major revisions like the TRS (Dowd et al., 1991). Recent research has indicated a single-factor solution to the HPRS, but this factor explained little variance in the scale (Waris et al., 2020); research has also indicated a bifactor structure (Moreira et al., 2020).

Observational Measure

Shoham-Salomon and colleagues (1989) developed an observational measure of trait reactance by coding patients' tone of voice. Patients were considered highly reactant if their tone was coded as spiteful, uninhibited, and active. Though initially demonstrating construct validity, later research found mixed evidence (Shoham et al., 1996). While seldom used (e.g., Levesque et al., 2008), this measure advanced direct reactance assessments beyond self-reports (e.g., Sittenthaler et al., 2015a).

Measures of State Reactance

Intertwined Model

Dillard and Shen (2005) were the first to create an in-depth state reactance measurement. After empirically testing four models based on previous literature (Dillard & Meijnders, 2002; Dillard & Peck, 2000; Kelly & Nauta, 1997), results supported the intertwined model (i.e., a combination of anger and negative cognitions). Researchers typically measure anger using a four-item scale (Dillard & Shen, 2005). However, there is more debate over how to measure negative cognitions (e.g., coders' ratings vs. a meta-cognitive scale; Reynolds-Tylus et al., 2021). The intertwined model was supported by a comparison of measures (Quick, 2012) and a meta-analysis (Rains, 2013). Notably, in line with PRT (Brehm, 1966), a serial mediation model is recommended, with perceived freedom threat predicting the intertwined construct (Rains, 2013).

Salzburg State Reactance Scale

Despite its widespread use (e.g., Kim et al., 2013), Sittenthaler and colleagues (2015c) noted limitations in Dillard and Shen's (2005) reactance measure, particularly its untested applicability beyond persuasion studies and nonstudent samples. In response, the Salzburg State Reactance Scale (Sittenthaler et al., 2015c) was developed, guided by earlier research (e.g., Jonas et al., 2009), using 10 items to assess emotional response, negative attitudes, and aggressive intentions across varied scenarios. Results indicated high internal consistency and correlations with other measures of state reactance (e.g., Lindsey, 2005).

Reactance to Health Warnings Scale

Based on Dillard and Shen's (2005) intertwined model, Hall and colleagues (2016, 2017) developed the Reactance to Health Warnings Scale (RHWS), to measure reactance to health messages across three dimensions: anger, perceived threat, and counterarguing the warning. Initially comprising 27 items, the RHWS was condensed to a three-item Brief RHWS with demonstrated reliability and validity (Hall et al., 2017).

Physiological Measurement of Reactance

Although Brehm (1966) associated psychological reactance with physiological arousal, few measured motivational states this way (e.g., Baum et al., 1986). Inspired by Wright's (2008) work on cardiovascular effort markers, Sittenthaler (2015a) tested a physiological reactance measure by assessing heart rate changes under illegitimate versus legitimate freedom threats. Results indicated that reactance involves both immediate physiological responses and slower cognitive responses. There has also been a recent movement to examine neurological correlates of psychological reactance (e.g., Mühlberger et al., 2020, 2024).

WAVE 5: RETURN TO MOTIVATION

Brehm (1966) initially defined reactance in PRT as a motivation to regain lost freedom. However, the construct's motivational focus was relatively deemphasized until Miron and Brehm (2006) connected it to other motivational theories (e.g., Brehm & Self, 1989). This reemphasis on reactance's motivational properties spurred the integration of PRT into broader motivational frameworks (e.g., Deci & Ryan, 2000; Leander et al., 2016; Schumpe & Leander, 2025; Steindl et al., 2015; Wright et al., 2015). Keeping this motivational aspect of PRT in mind, Wave 5 presents four avenues PRT has the potential to continue expanding: (1) factors affecting perceptions of freedom threats and freedom restoration, (2) catalysts of reactance beyond freedom threats, (3) outcomes of reactance beyond anger, negative cognitions, and boomerang effects, and (4) sequential reactance effects.

Factors Affecting Perceptions of Freedom Threats and Freedom Restoration

Though individual differences have long influenced reactance scholarship (Brehm & Brehm, 1981), recent research examines the impact of psychological states on responses to freedom threats, such as empathy (Shen, 2010) and self-affirmation (Schüz et al., 2013). Guided by Fromm's (1941) theorizing, Rosenberg and Siegel (2021) studied how uncertainty affects reactions to controlling and supportive scenarios. The authors found that reactance was greatest when participants felt safe and certain prior to exposure to a controlling message; when they felt uncertain, no differences in reactance emerged among those exposed to a controlling or supportive message. Therefore, uncertainty reduced people's negative perceptions of a freedom threat. Integrating prior literature, scholars have since posited that inducing uncertainty at different stages of the reactance process could reduce reactance toward persuasive communication, such as reducing the certainty of one's prior attitudes and reducing the certainty of one's metacognitive evaluations of messages (Adam-Troian & Bélanger, 2025).

Expanding Catalysts of Reactance

Experiences beyond direct threats or loss of freedoms, such as group categorization, can arouse reactance (Miron & Brehm, 2006). Even positive labels (e.g., "mother," p. 9) may induce reactance if they feel stereotypically limiting or discriminatory (Wicklund, 1974). Supporting this notion, Kray and colleagues (2001) suggested that explicitly activating gender stereotypes in negotiations led people to act contrary to stereotypical expectations. Although the primary paradigm for testing PRT involves using explicit verbal or written threats (e.g., Dillard & Shen, 2005), early studies testing implicit freedom threats, such as making a decision (e.g., Sullivan & Pallak, 1976) and publicly committing to a position (e.g., Andreoli et al., 1974), also demonstrated reactance arousal. Similarly, Graupmann and colleagues (2012) showed that group categorization (i.e., ingroup vs. outgroup) can affect reactance arousal, demonstrating that talking about other social groups or being in the presence of an outgroup member (e.g., police) can cause people to feel immediately threatened.

Expanding Outcomes of Reactance

PRT broadly affects behaviors and cognitions—reactance, as a negative motivational state, triggers various goal-directed outcomes (Hart, 2014; Proulx, 2012). Building on the theories of Lewin (1959) and Tolman (1932), more recent research suggests that reactance is related to outcomes associated with negative motivational states (i.e., changes in abilities, disposition, resource allocation, and perception; Rosenberg & Siegel, 2016). Although researchers have expressed interest in observing the relationship between reactance and other negative emotions (e.g., fear; Steindl et al., 2015), positive feelings (e.g., humor, determination) should also be explored. Additionally, Steindl and Jonas (2015) reported that interpersonal freedom threats aroused reactance, which biased subsequent cognitions and evaluations; future research could, therefore, examine how reactance-induced anger influences optimistic appraisals (e.g., Dunn & Schweitzer, 2005), riskier decision making (e.g., Baumann & DeSteno, 2012), and willingness to punish wrongdoers (e.g., Ask & Pina, 2011). Reactance also increases attention toward words related to the threatened object (Sprengholz et al., 2023) and affects subjective norm perceptions (Li & Shen, 2024).

Sequential Reactance Effects

Classic (i.e., learned helplessness; Wortman & Brehm, 1975) and contemporary (i.e., reactance decoy effect; Schumpe et al., 2020) scholarship have examined what happens when two freedom threats occur in such a way that the amount of reactance experienced is reduced. Additionally, recent work has examined a third phenomenon—the reactive spiral (Siegel & Rosenberg, 2025)—to address the circumstances when consecutive threats increase reactance.

Learned Helplessness

Learned helplessness occurs when people acknowledge a threat to their freedom but eventually accept their inability to overcome it and restore freedom (Wortman & Brehm, 1975), which can occur when people try but fail to reduce reactance (Brehm & Brehm, 1981). This can then lead to feelings of diminished control (Seligman, 1975). Perceived difficulty in freedom restoration appears to affect motivation to restore freedoms; motivation tends to be higher if freedom restoration is perceived as moderately difficult but lower when perceived as impossible (Mikulincer, 1988).

Reactance Decoy

A decoy can reduce reactance toward a persuasion attempt (Schumpe et al., 2020). The reactance decoy effect occurs when a persuasive message is preceded by another message that arouses reactance; this decoy message allows the recipient to vent their reactance toward the decoy object, thus reducing the ability of subsequent threats from the following message to cause reactance. This concept stems from previous research suggesting that preceding a target message with a message with a weaker argument or a less credible source can increase the target message's persuasiveness (Tormala & Clarkson, 2007). The reactance decoy can increase persuasiveness by reducing people's reactance and decreasing their need to reassert themselves when evaluating the proceeding message (Schumpe et al., 2020).

Reactive Spiral

Similar to Coyne's (1976) depressive spiral, whereby negative behaviors caused by depression lead to peer withdrawal, increasing isolation, and worsening depression (e.g., Joiner & Metalsky, 2001), a *reactive spiral* describes how being in a state of reactance can result in increased sensitivity to future freedom threats (Siegel & Rosenberg, 20242025). Based on work by Brehm and Brehm (1981) and Wicklund (1974), Siegel and Rosenberg (2025) proposed that two consecutive threats cause changes in processing and general hypersensitivity to subsequent threats. In this conceptualization, any two threats received in relatively close succession can result in the reactive spiral, so long as the first threat is sufficient to arouse reactance and the reactance does not dissipate. In line with numerous theories of affect and information processing (e.g., Forgas, 1995; Lerner et al., 2015), the reactive spiral occurs because the anger and negative cognitions resulting from an initial freedom threat influence subsequent information processing, thus affecting reactions to a second freedom threat (Siegel & Rosenberg, 2025).

PRACTICAL IMPLICATIONS OF PRT

One of PRT's greatest assets is its vast applied utility in various domains, a fact that was apparent early on in Brehm and Brehm's (1981) review and restatement of the theory; they included chapters on reactance in interpersonal relationships, clinical psychology, and social influence, among other topics. As summarized earlier, in the past four decades, scholars have explored the utility of PRT in explaining thought and behavior in a variety of domains, such as health communication and behavior (for reviews, see Quick et al., 2013; Reynolds-Tylus, 2019) and treatment of mental disorders (for review, see Beutler et al., 2002).

In line with this work, we examine how PRT's advances can enhance the effectiveness of persuasive communications—primarily by reducing reactance arousal, but in one instance, capitalizing on it. As an illustration of these possibilities, the following section examines 11 strategies for tailoring messages to influence parents' reactions to childhood vaccination requirements. We first explore one strategy already discussed in Wave 5 (uncertainty), then introduce 10 new strategies.

Uncertainty

As noted, participants who feel certain and safe have shown greater reactance to controlling messages than those who feel uncertain and vulnerable (Rosenberg & Siegel, 2021). Uncertainty could thus be vital in determining reactance elicited by a persuasive message. For example, parents who feel uncertain (e.g., about their lives) should be less likely to become reactant to a persuasive message about childhood vaccination compared to those feeling more certain. Reduced reactance to the message, in turn, could allow the message to more effectively persuade them to vaccinate their child.

Message Sensation Value

Novel messages have decreased reactance and enhanced message effectiveness (e.g., Kang et al., 2006). Palmgreen and colleagues (1991) defined one such novel approach, message sensation value, as the ability of a message's audiovisual features to evoke sensory and emotional responses. The high sensation value (HSV) of these messages helps shift focus away from the controlling elements of the messages, thus reducing perceived threats to freedom (Morgan et al., 2003; Quick, 2013). HSV messages have been shown to capture the attention of adolescents and lower their intentions to use drugs (Morgan et al., 2003).

An HSV message for childhood vaccination could use rapid, uplifting visuals of healthy, vaccinated children paired with dynamic music and bright colors. The narrative could show real-life stories of parents and children experiencing the benefits of vaccination, ending with a hopeful message emphasizing health and protection. Although the message would advocate for parents vaccinating their children, the HSV elements of the message could lessen the impact of its controlling elements.

Narrative

Narratives in messaging can reduce reactance and enhance persuasiveness (Quick et al., 2013). Moyer-Gusé and Nabi (2010) found that story-driven messages—such as those in TV dramas about teen pregnancy—decrease perceived persuasion, thereby reducing reactance and increasing intentions for safe sex among women compared to straightforward news broadcasts. Using a narrative approach, a message for childhood vaccination could tell the heartwarming story of a community coming together to protect its children, highlighting personal testimonials from parents about their positive experiences with vaccination. This story-driven message could create emotional engagement, reduce perceived persuasion, lower reactance, and increase vaccination acceptance.

Empathy

Making characters more relatable can increase feelings of empathy, which in turn reduces reactance and enhances persuasiveness by decreasing perceived threats (Shen, 2010, 2011). Shen (2010) demonstrated that empathy-inducing antismoking and antidrinking messages lowered reactance and indirectly improved ad effectiveness. This was achieved by participants empathizing with the characters, perceiving their messages as less threatening due to the connection with the characters.

Empathy might reduce reactance to childhood vaccination messages by featuring relatable stories of parents and children who have benefited from vaccines. This approach could make the characters' experiences and emotions more identifiable. By fostering a sense of connection and understanding, these messages could decrease perceived threats and resistance, enhancing the overall persuasiveness of the message.

Inoculation and Reactance

Inoculating (e.g., forewarning; McGuire, 1961) people about potential threats can increase or decrease reactance (Richards et al., 2017). Miller and colleagues (2013) found that preexposing participants to a reactance-*inducing* message increased resistance to later persuasive messages, like those promoting marijuana legalization. Conversely, forewarning participants about possible reactance reduced it, enhancing the persuasiveness of anti-binge-drinking campaigns (Richards & Banas, 2015; Richards et al., 2017). These inoculation effects are inconsistent (e.g., Karlsson et al., 2024) and may depend on other message factors (Bessarabova et al., 2013; Quick et al., 2015).

Messages aiming to increase childhood vaccinations could benefit from warning parents about the possible reactance-arousing aspects of the ad. For example, a message might state, "After listening to the following information, you might feel your freedom to choose to vaccinate your child is being threatened. However, the benefits of vaccines are powerful, and the recommendations for immunizing children make much sense given what is known about preventing disease." This message acknowledges the potential freedom threat, which could reduce reactance arousal while still advocating for the cause.

Low-Controlling Language

Autonomy-supportive messages can help reduce reactance (e.g., alcohol consumption; Bensley & Wu, 1991). Messages using low-controlling language (LCL; Staunton et al., 2022), which emphasize autonomy and use polite and implicit suggestions, support this approach, in contrast to messages using high-controlling language (HCL), which tend to be overtly persuasive and more likely to trigger reactance due to perceived freedom threats (for review, see Rains, 2013). This difference highlights the practical applications of using LCL in health communication strategies.

For example, LCL antismoking ads (e.g., "It's your health, your body, your brain") have led to adolescents reporting lower intentions to use cannabis compared to HCL ads (e.g., "Only complete idiots would do drugs"; Crano et al., 2017). Similarly, an ad targeting childhood vaccination could benefit from LCL, such as, "The choice to get your child vaccinated is yours," to reduce reactance arousal. There are times when HCL messages can be beneficial in enhancing message clarity and efficiency (for review, see Staunton et al., 2022), but they carry more risk of inducing reactance than LCL messages.

Restoration Postscripts

Reminding recipients at the end of a persuasive message of their freedom of choice to comply with the message (i.e., using a restoration postscript; Brehm & Brehm, 1981) can help lower reactance (Richards et al., 2022). For instance, phrases like "The choice is yours; you're free to decide for yourself" (Bessarabova et al., 2013) clearly emphasize the recipients' autonomy, reducing perceived threats to their freedom (Miller et al., 2007). This approach can also increase desired behavioral intentions (Reynolds-Tylus et al., 2022). Additionally, adding a brief statement such as "but you are free to refuse" to the end of a request can enhance compliance and reduce reactance (Carpenter & Pascual, 2016). Miller and colleagues (2007) found that adding a short postscript (i.e., reminding recipients that the choice was theirs) following a promotional health appeal made the message less threatening.

Returning to our example, it could be beneficial to add restoration postscripts after messages targeting childhood vaccination, such as, "Ultimately, the decision to vaccinate your child is yours. You know what is best for your child's health and well-being." However, it should be noted that postscripts can be ineffective or even counterproductive when used with messages employing LCL (Bessarabova et al., 2013) or if they are too short (Quick et al., 2015).

Providing Compliance Options

When offered only one way to comply with a directive, participants were more likely to comply with messages promising rewards rather than punishment; however, this difference diminished when they could pick from four options instead (Heilman & Garner, 1975). This finding demonstrates that offering multiple ways to comply with a persuasive message can minimize the reactance aroused by the message.

Campaigns aiming to persuade people could benefit from this approach. For instance, persuasive messages targeting cancer-preventive behaviors have aroused less reactance when offering two options (wearing sunscreen or protective clothing) instead of one (Shen, 2015). A childhood vaccination campaign could also reduce reactance by offering parents the choice to vaccinate their children at school clinics, local health fairs, or home visits by health care professionals. This multiple-option approach could minimize reactance by giving parents control over their compliance with the vaccination guidelines.

Source Characteristics

The source of a persuasive message can affect how one perceives the threat level of the message. Sources are more likely seen as freedom-threatening if seen as having power over the individual or being expert or authoritative (Brehm, 1966; Brehm & Brehm, 1981). This increased threat can lead to increased source derogation, thus increasing reactance to the message (Miller et al., 2007). However, sources seen as highly similar, such as peers, can minimize reactance and the detrimental effects of the threatening message (Song et al., 2018).

Although this research on source characteristics has been shown to work with persuasive messages such as those targeting wildlife disease policies (Song et al., 2018), childhood vaccination messages could also benefit from having more similar sources. Instead of doctors, who can sometimes be evaluated more negatively than peers (Crano et al., 2007), parents not identified as having expert or authoritative roles could advocate for childhood vaccination. The source having characteristics similar to the recipients could thus lessen the threatening impact of the requests made by the ad to vaccinate their child.

Mistargeting

Communication perceived as unintentionally overheard can be more effective in changing people's opinions than if the message targets them directly, but only if they believe the people they are overhearing are unaware of being overheard (Walster & Festinger, 1962). This has been demonstrated by smokers agreeing more with a message downplaying the link between smoking and lung cancer when they believed the speaker was unaware of their presence. With these findings in mind, Crano and colleagues (2007) developed the mistargeting strategy using persuasive messages indirectly—that is, directing the message to a person or group other than the true target. Mistargeting has notably been used to increase help-seeking intentions among people experiencing depression (e.g., "Do you know someone who fights depression?"; Lienemann & Siegel, 2016).

Persuasive messages about vaccination would likely benefit from using the mistargeting strategy. For example, instead of directly addressing parents regarding their children, ads could instead mistarget and state, "Thank you to all the parents who have vaccinated their children. You clearly understand the many benefits of doing so." In this instance, if a parent with unvaccinated children hears this message, the message will not be targeting them directly, thus potentially minimizing reactance arousal.

Reactance as a Persuasive Strategy

An alternative to reducing reactance is effectively inducing reactance to enhance persuasion (Turner, 2007). A "Truth" antitobacco campaign in Florida depicted cigarettes as manipulative, turning nonsmoking into a desirable outcome (Zucker et al., 2000). Positive campaign evaluations support this strategy's utility (Farrelly et al., 2002; Sly et al., 2001), with anger toward secondhand smoke associated with trait reactance and greater support for clean air policies (Quick et al., 2009). Similarly, a message targeting childhood vaccination could depict the consequences of people who refuse to vaccinate their children, highlighting the adverse effects it would have on their children (i.e., their child is more likely to get sick if other children are not vaccinated). This ad could trigger reactance by making people believe that their freedom to protect their child is threatened, thus leading them to favor childhood vaccination.

Interactions

Although incorporating any of the 11 proposed strategies would likely enhance persuasive effectiveness by reducing reactance, utilizing multiple strategies could maximize their effectiveness (e.g., Miller et al., 2007). An advertisement simultaneously using principles of LCL (Staunton et al., 2022), multiple compliance options (Shen, 2015), source characteristics (Song et al., 2018), and restoration postscripts (Miller et al., 2007) could be more effective in reducing reactance than only one strategy. With these strategies, a persuasive message targeting childhood vaccination could say, "Please consider vaccinating your child" instead of, "You must vaccinate your child," provide multiple avenues by which the child could be vaccinated, utilize other parents as similar peers, and remind parents of their autonomy at the end of the message by saying, "The choice is yours."

We are confident that using more than one strategy in one message could be effective; however, further research is needed to determine which strategies interact successfully, as combined strategies may not always produce anticipated effects (e.g., Bessarobova et al., 2013). However, persuasive messages aiming to minimize reactance arousal could benefit more from using multiple strategies simultaneously rather than using just one.

CONCLUSION

From Brehm's (1966) initial proposal, PRT remains a vital framework for understanding and addressing human responses to perceived threats to freedom. In this chapter, we have shown how, through five overlapping waves (Rosenberg & Siegel, 2018), PRT has evolved and expanded its relevance across various fields, particularly in clinical psychology and communication research. Practical strategies such as using empathy (Shen, 2010, 2011), inoculation (Richards et al., 2017), and low-controlling language (Staunton et al., 2022) have been identified as effective in reducing reactance, and they show promise in working better when together rather than separate (Miller et al., 2007). Additionally, concepts like the reactive spiral (Siegel & Rosenberg, 2025) further illuminate the complex interplay between sequential threats and reactance. Overall, PRT's integration with broader motivational frameworks (e.g., Schumpe & Leander, 2025) highlights its enduring relevance and provides a foundation for developing interventions to mitigate reactance and promote positive behavioral change.

REFERENCES

Adam-Troian, J., & Bélanger, J. J. (2025). The uncertainty-dissuasion model of reactance inhibition. *Motivation Science, 11*, 192–200.

Andreoli, V. A., Worchel, S., & Folger, R. (1974). Implied threat to behavioral freedom. *Journal of Personality and Social Psychology, 30*, 765–771.

Arnold, K. A., & Vakhrusheva, J. (2016). Resist the negation reflex: Minimizing reactance in psychotherapy of delusions. *Psychosis, 8*, 166–175.

Ask, K., & Pina, A. (2011). On being angry and punitive: How anger alters perception of criminal intent. *Social Psychological and Personality Science, 2*, 494–499.

Avishai, A., Ribisl, K. M., & Sheeran, P. (2023). Realizing the tobacco endgame: Understanding and mobilizing public support for banning combustible cigarette sales in the United States. *Social Science and Medicine, 327*, Article 115939.

Baum, A., Fleming, R., & Reddy, D. M. (1986). Unemployment stress: Loss of control, reactance and learned helplessness. *Social Science and Medicine, 22*, 509–516.

Baumann, J., & DeSteno, D. (2012). Context explains divergent effects of anger on risk taking. *Emotion, 12*, 1196–1199.

Benoit, W. L. (1998). Forewarning and persuasion. In M. Allen & R. W. Preiss (Eds.), *Persuasion: Advances through Meta-Analysis* (pp. 139–154). Hampton Press.

Bensley, L. S., & Wu, R. (1991). The role of psychological reactance in drinking following alcohol prevention messages. *Journal of Applied Social Psychology, 21*, 1111–1124.

Bessarabova, E., Fink, E. L., & Turner, M. (2013). Reactance, restoration, and cognitive structure: Comparative statics. *Human Communication Research, 39*, 339–364.

Beutler, L. E., Edwards, C., & Someah, K. (2018). Adapting psychotherapy to patient reactance level: A meta-analytic review. *Journal of Clinical Psychology, 74*(11), 1952–1963.

Beutler, L. E., Moleiro, C., & Talebi, H. (2002). Resistance in psychotherapy: What conclusions are supported by research. *Journal of Clinical Psychology, 58*, 207–217.

Brass, M., Furstenberg, A., & Mele, A. R. (2019). Why neuroscience does not disprove free will. *Neuroscience and Biobehavioral Reviews, 102*, 251–263.

Brehm, J. W. (1966). *A theory of psychological reactance*. Academic Press.

Brehm, J. W., & Rozen, E. (1971). Attractiveness of old alternatives when a new attractive alternative is introduced. *Journal of Personality and Social Psychology, 20*, 261–266.

Brehm, J. W., & Self, E. A. (1989). The intensity of motivation. *Annual Review of Psychology, 40*, 109–131.

Brehm, J. W., Stires, L. K., Sensenig, J., & Shaban, J. (1966). The attractiveness of an eliminated choice alternative. *Journal of Experimental Social Psychology, 2*, 301–313.

Brehm, S. S. (1976). *The application of social psychology to clinical practice*. Hemisphere.

Brehm, S. S., & Brehm, J. W. (1981). *Psychological reactance: A theory of freedom and control*. Academic Press.

Buboltz, W. C., Jr., Thomas, A., & Donnell, A. J. (2002). Evaluating the factor structure and internal consistency reliability of the Therapeutic Reactance Scale. *Journal of Counseling and Development, 80*, 120–125.

Buller, D. B., Borland, R., & Burgoon, M. (1998). Impact of behavioral intention on effectiveness of message features: Evidence from the Family Sun Safety Project. *Human Communication Research, 24*, 433–453.

Burgoon, M., Alvaro, E., Grandpre, J., & Voulodakis, M. (2002). Revisiting the theory of psychological reactance: Communicating threats to attitudinal freedom. In J. P. Dillard & M. Pfau (Eds.), *The persuasion handbook: Developments in theory and practice* (pp. 213–232). Sage.

Carpenter, C. J., & Pascual, A. (2016). Testing the reactance vs. the reciprocity of politeness explanations for the effectiveness of the "but you are free" compliance-gaining technique. *Social Influence, 11*(2), 101–110.

Cautilli, J., Riley-Tillman, T. C., Axelrod, S., & Hineline, P. (2005). Current behavioral models of client and consultee resistance: A critical review. *International Journal of Behavioral and Consultation Therapy, 1,* 147–164.

Coyne, J. C. (1976). Toward an interactional description of depression. *Psychiatry, 39,* 28–40.

Crano, W. D., Alvaro, E. M., Tan, C. N., & Siegel, J. T. (2017). Social mediation of persuasive media in adolescent substance prevention. *Psychology of Addictive Behaviors, 31,* 479–487.

Crano, W. D., Siegel, J. T., Alvaro, E. M., & Patel, N. M. (2007). Overcoming adolescents' resistance to anti-inhalant appeals. *Psychology of Addictive Behaviors, 21*(4), 516–524.

DeBord, J. B. (1989). Paradoxical interventions: A review of the recent literature. *Journal of Counseling and Development, 67,* 394–398.

Deci, E. L., & Ryan, R. M. (2000). The "what" and "why" of goal pursuits: Human needs and the self-determination of behavior. *Psychological Inquiry, 11,* 227–268.

Devine, D. A., & Fernald, P. S. (1973). Outcome effects of receiving a preferred, randomly assigned, or nonpreferred therapy. *Journal of Consulting and Clinical Psychology, 41,* 104–107.

Dillard, J. P., & Meijnders, A. (2002). Persuasion and the structure of affect. In J. P. Dillard & M. Pfau (Eds.), *The persuasion handbook: Developments in theory and research* (pp. 309–328). Sage.

Dillard, J. P., & Peck, E. (2000). Affect and persuasion: Emotional responses to public service announcements. *Communication Research, 27,* 461–495.

Dillard, J. P., & Shen, L. (2005). On the nature of reactance and its role in persuasive health communication. *Communication Monographs, 72,* 144–168.

Dowd, E. T., Hughes, S. L., Brockbank, L., Halpain, D., Seibel, C., & Seibel, P. (1988). Compliance-based and defiance-based intervention strategies and psychological reactance in the treatment of free and unfree behavior. *Journal of Counseling Psychology, 35,* 370–376.

Dowd, E. T., Milne, C. R., & Wise, S. L. (1991). The Therapeutic Reactance Scale: A measure of psychological reactance. *Journal of Counseling and Development, 69,* 541–545.

Dowd, E. T., & Seibel, C. A. (1990). A cognitive theory of resistance and reactance: Implications for treatment. *Journal of Mental Health Counseling, 12,* 458–469.

Dowd, E. T., & Swoboda, J. S. (1984). Paradoxical interventions in behavior therapy. *Journal of Behavior Therapy and Experimental Psychiatry, 15,* 229–234.

Dunn, J. R., & Schweitzer, M. E. (2005). Feeling and believing: The influence of emotion on trust. *Journal of Personality and Social Psychology, 88,* 736–748.

Engs, R., & Hanson, D. J. (1989). Reactance theory: A test with collegiate drinking. *Psychological Reports, 64,* 1083–1086.

Farrelly, M. C., Healton, C. G., Davis, K. C., Messeri, P., Hersey, J. C., & Haviland, M. L. (2002). Getting to the truth: Evaluating national tobacco countermarketing campaigns. *American Journal of Public Health, 92,* 901–907.

Feldman, G. (2017). Making sense of agency: Belief in free will as a unique and important construct. *Social and Personality Psychology Compass, 11,* e12293.

Festinger, L. (1957). *A theory of cognitive dissonance.* Stanford University Press.

Folkman, S., Lazarus, R. S., Dunkel-Schetter, C., DeLongis, A., & Gruen, R. J. (2000). The dynamics of a stressful encounter. In E. T. Higgins, & A. W. Kruglanski (Eds.), *Motivational science: Social and personality perspectives* (pp. 111–127). Psychology Press.

Forgas, J. P. (1995). Mood and judgment: The affect infusion model (AIM). *Psychological Bulletin, 117*(1), 39–66.

Fromm, E. (1941). *Escape from freedom.* Farrar & Rinehart.

Gaume, J., Blanc, S., Magill, M., McCambridge, J., Bertholet, N., Hugli, O., & Daeppen, J. B. (2023). Who benefits from brief motivational intervention among young adults presenting to the emergency department with alcohol intoxication: A latent-class moderation analysis. *Alcohol: Clinical and Experimental Research, 47(8),* 1614–1623.

Goldman, M., & Wallis, D. (1979). Restoring freedom when pressured not to select alternatives. *Psychological Reports, 44,* 563–566.

Gordon, R. M. (1976). Effects of volunteering and responsibility on the perceived value and effectiveness of a clinical treatment. *Journal of Consulting and Clinical Psychology, 44,* 799–801.

Grabitz-Gniech, G., Auslitz, K., & Grabitz, H. (1975). The strength of the reactance effect as a function of the absolute size and the relative reduction of freedom space. *Zeitschrift für Sozialpsychologie, 6,* 122–128.

Grandpre, J., Alvaro, E. M., Burgoon, M., Miller, C. H., & Hall, J. R. (2003). Adolescent reactance and anti-smoking campaigns: A theoretical approach. *Health Communication, 15,* 349–366.

Graupmann, V., Jonas, E., Meier, E., Hawelka, S., & Aichhorn, M. (2012). Reactance, the self, and its group: When threats to freedom come from the ingroup versus the outgroup. *European Journal of Social Psychology, 42,* 164–173.

Green, M. C., & Brock, T. C. (2000). The role of transportation in the persuasiveness of public narratives. *Journal of Personality and Social Psychology, 79,* 701–721.

Hall, M. G., Sheeran, P., Noar, S. M., Ribisl, K. M., Bach, L. E., & Brewer, N. T. (2016). Reactance to health warnings scale: Development and validation. *Annals of Behavioral Medicine, 50,* 736–750.

Hall, M. G., Sheeran, P., Noar, S. M., Ribisl, K. M., Boynton, M. H., & Brewer, N. T. (2017). A brief measure of reactance to health warnings. *Journal of Behavioral Medicine, 40,* 520–529.

Hart, J. (2014). Toward an integrative theory of psychological defense. *Perspectives on Psychological Science, 9,* 19–39.

Heidegger, M. (1962). *Being and time* (J. Macquarrie & E. Robinson, Trans.). Blackwell. (Original work published 1927)

Heilman, M. E., & Garner, K. A. (1975). Counteracting the boomerang: The effects of choice on compliance to threats and promises. *Journal of Personality and Social Psychology, 31(5),* 911–917.

Hong, S. (1992). Hong's Psychological Reactance Scale: A further factor analytic validation. *Psychological Reports, 70,* 512–514.

Hong, S., & Faedda, S. (1996). Refinement of the Hong Psychological Reactance Scale. *Educational and Psychological Measurement, 56,* 173–182.

Hong, S., & Ostini, R. (1989). Further evaluation of Merz's Psychological Reactance Scale. *Psychological Reports, 64,* 707–710.

Hong, S., & Page, S. (1989). A psychological reactance scale: Development, factor structure and reliability. *Psychological Reports, 64,* 1323–1326.

Joiner, T. E., Jr., & Metalsky, G. I. (2001). Excessive reassurance seeking: Delineating a risk factor involved in the development of depressive symptoms. *Psychological Science, 12,* 371–378.

Jonas, E., Graupmann, V., Kayser, D. N., Zanna, M., Traut-Mattausch, E., & Frey, D. (2009). Culture, self, and the emergence of reactance: Is there a "universal" freedom? *Journal of Experimental Social Psychology, 45,* 1068–1080.

Jones, R. A., & Brehm, J. W. (1970). Persuasiveness of one- and two-sided communications as a function of awareness there are two sides. *Journal of Experimental Social Psychology, 6,* 47–56.

Kang, Y., Cappella, J., & Fishbein, M. (2006). The attentional mechanism of message sensation value: Interaction between message sensation value and argument quality on message effectiveness. *Communication Monographs, 73,* 351–378.

Kant, I. (1967). *Kritik der praktischen Vernunft* [Critique of practical reason]. Felix Meiner Verlag. (Original work published 1797)

Karlsson, L. C., Mäki, K. O., Holford, D., Fasce, A., Schmid, P., Lewandowsky, S., & Soveri, A. (2024). Testing psychological inoculation to reduce reactance to vaccine-related communication. *Health Communication.*

Karno, M. P., Longabaugh, R., & Herbeck, D. (2010). What explains the relationship between the therapist structure patient reactance interaction and drinking outcome?: An examination of potential mediators. *Psychology of Addictive Behaviors, 24,* 600–607.

Kelly, A. E., & Nauta, M. M. (1997). Reactance and thought suppression. *Personality and Social Psychology Bulletin, 23,* 1123–1132.

Kim, S. Y., Levine, T., & Allen, M. (2013). Comparing separate process and intertwined models for reactance. *Communication Studies, 64,* 273–295.

Kray, L. J., Thompson, L., & Galinsky, A. (2001). Battle of the sexes: Gender stereotype confirmation and reactance in negotiations. *Journal of Personality and Social Psychology, 80,* 942–958.

Krishnan, L., & Carment, D. W. (1979). Reactions to help: Reciprocity, responsibility and reactance. *European Journal of Social Psychology, 9,* 435–439.

Lazary, J., Pogany, L., De las Cuevas, C., Tezanos, A. G., & de Leon, J. (2021). Adherence to psychiatric medications: Comparing patients with schizophrenia, bipolar disorder and major depression. *Neuropsychopharmacologia Hungarica, 23*(4), 363–373.

Lazarus, R. S., & Folkman, S. (1984). *Stress, appraisal, and coping.* Springer.

Leander, N. P., vanDellen, M. R., Rachl-Willberger, J., Shah, J. Y., Fitzsimons, G. J., & Chartrand, T. L. (2016). Is freedom contagious?: A self-regulatory model of reactance and sensitivity to deviant peers. *Motivation Science, 2,* 256–267.

Lerner, J. S., Li, Y., Valdesolo, P., & Kassam, K. S. (2015). Emotion and decision making. *Annual review of psychology, 66,* 799–823.

Levesque, D. A., Velicer, W. F., Castle, P. H., & Greene, R. N. (2008). Resistance among domestic violence offenders: Measurement development and initial validation. *Violence Against Women, 14,* 158–184.

Lewin, K. (1959). *Field theory in social science.* Harper & Brothers.

Li, R., & Shen, L. (2024). The role of subjective norm in persuasion through the restoration of personal freedom. *Health Communication.*

Lienemann, B. A., & Siegel, J. T. (2016). State psychological reactance to depression public service announcements among people with varying levels of depressive symptomatology. *Health Communication, 31,* 102–116.

Lindsey, L. M. (2005). Anticipated guilt as behavioral motivation an examination of appeals to help unknown others through bone marrow donation. *Human Communication Research, 31,* 453–481.

Mazis, M. B., Settle, R. B., & Leslie, D. C. (1973). Elimination of phosphate detergents and psychological reactance. *Journal of Marketing Research, 10,* 390–395.

McGuire, W. J. (1961). The effectiveness of supportive and refutational defenses in immunizing and restoring beliefs against persuasion. *Sociometry, 24,* 184–197.

Merleau-Ponty, M. (1964). *The primacy of perception.* Northwestern University Press.

Merz, J. (1983). A questionnaire for the measurement of psychological reactance. *Diagnostica, 29,* 75–82.

Mikulincer, M. (1988). The relationship of probability of success and performance following unsolvable problems: Reactance and helplessness effects. *Motivation and Emotion, 12,* 139–153.

Miller, C. H., Ivanov, B., Sims, J., Compton, J., Harrison, K. J., Parker, K. A., . . . Averbeck, J. M. (2013). Boosting the potency of resistance: Combining the motivational forces of inoculation and psychological reactance. *Human Communication Research, 39,* 127–155.

Miller, C. H., Lane, L. T., Deatrick, L. M., Young, A. M., & Potts, K. A. (2007). Psychological reactance and promotional health messages: The effects of controlling language, lexical concreteness, and the restoration of freedom. *Human Communication Research, 33,* 219–240.

Miron, A. M., & Brehm, J. W. (2006). Reactance theory—40 years later. *Zeitschrift für Sozialpsychologie, 37,* 9–18.

Moreira, P., Cunha, D., & Inman, R. A. (2020). Addressing a need for valid measures of trait reactance in adolescents: A further test of the Hong Psychological Reactance Scale. *Journal of Personality Assessment, 102(3),* 357–369.

Morgan, S. E., Palmgreen, P., Stephenson, M. T., Hoyle, R. H., & Lorch, E. P. (2003). Associations between message features and subjective evaluations of the sensation value of antidrug public service announcements. *Journal of Communication, 53,* 512–526.

Moyer-Gusé, E. (2008). Toward a theory of entertainment persuasion: Explaining the persuasive effects of entertainment-education messages. *Communication Theory, 18,* 407–425.

Moyer-Gusé, E., & Nabi, R. L. (2010). Explaining the effects of narrative in an entertainment television program: Overcoming resistance to persuasion. *Human Communication Research, 36,* 26–52.

Mühlberger, C., Jonas, E., Reiß, S., Jutzi, C., Kronbichler, M., & Klackl, J. (2024). Mentalizing in reactance: A functional magnetic resonance imaging study of freedom threats. *Motivation Science.*

Mühlberger, C., Klackl, J., Sittenthaler, S., & Jonas, E. (2020). The approach-motivational nature of reactance—Evidence from asymmetrical frontal cortical activation. *Motivation Science, 6(3),* 203–220.

Nezlek, J., & Brehm, J. W. (1975). Hostility as a function of the opportunity to counteraggress. *Journal of Personality, 43,* 421–433.

Palmgreen, P., Donohew, L., Lorch, E. P., Rogus, M., Helm, D., & Grant, N. (1991). Sensation seeking, message sensation value, and drug use as mediators of PSA effectiveness. *Health Communication, 3,* 217–227.

Proulx, T. (2012). Threat-compensation in social psychology: Is there a core motivation? *Social Cognition, 30,* 643–651.

Proulx, T., Inzlicht, M., & Harmon-Jones, E. (2012). Understanding all inconsistency compensation as a palliative response to violated expectations. *Trends in Cognitive Sciences, 16,* 285–291.

Quick, B. L. (2012). What is the best measure of psychological reactance?: An empirical test of two measures. *Health Communication, 27,* 1–9.

Quick, B. L. (2013). Perceived message sensation value and psychological reactance: A test of the dominant thought disruption hypothesis. *Journal of Health Communication, 18,* 1024–1038.

Quick, B. L., Bates, B. R., & Quinlan, M. M. (2009). The utility of anger in promoting clean indoor air policies. *Health Communication, 24,* 548–561.

Quick, B. L., Kam, J. A., Morgan, S. E., Montero Liberona, C. A., & Smith, R. A. (2015).

Prospect theory, discrete emotions, and freedom threats: An extension of psychological reactance theory. *Journal of Communication, 65*(1), 40–61.

Quick, B. L., & Kim, D. K. (2009). Examining reactance and reactance restoration with

South Korean adolescents: A test of psychological reactance within a collectivist culture. *Communication Research, 36,* 765–782.

Quick, B. L., Shen, L., & Dillard, J. P. (2013). Reactance theory and persuasion. In J. P. Dillard & L. Shen (Eds.), *The Sage handbook of persuasion: Developments in theory and practice* (2nd ed., pp. 167–183). Sage.

Rains, S. A. (2013). The nature of psychological reactance revisited: A meta-analytic review. *Human Communication Research, 39,* 47–73.

Rains, S. A., & Turner, M. M. (2007). Psychological reactance and persuasive health communication: A test and extension of the intertwined model. *Human Communication Research, 33,* 241–269.

Reynolds-Tylus, T. (2019). Psychological reactance and persuasive health communication: A review of the literature. *Frontiers in Communication, 4,* 56.

Reynolds-Tylus, T., Bigsby, E., & Quick, B. L. (2021). A comparison of three approaches for measuring negative cognitions for psychological reactance. *Communication Methods and Measures, 15*(1), 43–59.

Reynolds-Tylus, T., Smith, K. E., & Moore, M. E. (2022). Reducing psychological reactance to bystander intervention messages: Comparing preemptive and postscript mitigation strategies. *Communication Research Reports, 39*(5), 259–265.

Rhodewalt, F., & Marcroft, M. (1988). Type A behavior and diabetic control: Implications of psychological reactance for health outcomes. *Journal of Applied Social Psychology, 18,* 139–159.

Richards, A. S., & Banas, J. A. (2015). Inoculating against reactance to persuasive health messages. *Health Communication, 30,* 451–460.

Richards, A. S., Banas, J. A., & Magid, Y. (2017). More on inoculating against reactance to persuasive health messages: The paradox of threat. *Health Communication, 32,* 890–902.

Richards, A. S., Bessarabova, E., Banas, J. A., & Bernard, D. R. (2022). Reducing psychological reactance to health promotion messages: Comparing preemptive and postscript mitigation strategies. *Health Communication, 37*(3), 366–374.

Rosenberg, B. D., & Siegel, J. T. (2016). The effect of inconsistency appeals on the influence of direct-to-consumer prescription drug advertisements: An application of goal disruption theory. *Journal of Health Communication, 21,* 217–227.

Rosenberg, B. D., & Siegel, J. T. (2018). A 50-year review of psychological reactance theory: Do not read this article. *Motivation Science, 4*(4), 281–300.

Rosenberg, B. D., & Siegel, J. T. (2021). Threatening uncertainty and psychological reactance: are freedom threats always noxious? *Current Psychology: A Journal for Diverse Perspectives on Diverse Psychological Issues, 42*(5), 3968–3977.

Rotter, J. B. (1966). Generalized expectancies for internal versus external control of reinforcement. *Psychological Monographs: General and Applied, 80,* 1–28.

Sartre, J. P. (1956). *Being and nothingness.* Citadel Press. (Original work published 1943)

Schumpe, B. M., Bélanger, J. J., & Nisa, C. F. (2020). The reactance decoy effect: How including an appeal before a target message increases persuasion. *Journal of Personality and Social Psychology, 119*(2), 272–292.

Schumpe, B. M., & Leander, N. P. (2025). Rebels for a reason: How psychological reactance is goal-directed. *Motivation Science, 11*(2), 213–221.

Schüz, N., Schüz, B., & Eid, M. (2013). When risk communication backfires: Randomized controlled trial on self-affirmation and reactance to personalized risk feedback in high-risk individuals. *Health Psychology, 32,* 561–570.

Seligman, M. E. P. (1975). *Helplessness: On depression, development, and death.* W. H. Freeman/Times Books/Henry Holt.

Shen, L. (2010). Mitigating psychological reactance: The role of message-induced empathy in persuasion. *Human Communication Research, 36,* 397–422.

Shen, L. (2011). The effectiveness of empathy- versus fear-arousing antismoking PSAs. *Health Communication, 26,* 404–415.

Shen, L. (2015). Antecedents to psychological reactance: The impact of threat, message frame, and choice. *Health Communication, 30*(10), 975–985.

Shen, L., & Dillard, J. P. (2007). Reactance proneness assessment. Reactance proneness assessment. In R. A. Reynolds, R. Woods, J. D. Baker, R. A. Reynolds, R. Woods, & J. D. Baker (Eds.), *Handbook of research on electronic surveys and measurements* (pp. 323–329). Idea Group Reference/IGI Global.

Shoham, V., Bootzin, R. R., Rohrbaugh, M. J., & Urry, H. (1996). Paradoxical versus relaxation treatment for insomnia: The moderating role of reactance. *Sleep Research, 24,* 365.

Shoham, V., Trost, S. E., & Rohrbaugh, M. J. (2004). From state to trait and back again: Reactance theory goes clinical. In R. A. Wright, J. Greenberg, & S. S. Brehm (Eds.), *Motivational analyses of social behavior: Building on Jack Brehm's contributions to psychology* (pp. 167 185). Erlbaum.

Shoham-Salomon, V., Avner, R., & Neeman, R. (1989). You're changed if you do and changed if you don't: Mechanisms underlying paradoxical interventions. *Journal of Consulting and Clinical Psychology, 57,* 590–598.

Shoham-Salomon, V., & Rosenthal, R. (1987). Paradoxical interventions: A meta-analysis. *Journal of Consulting and Clinical Psychology, 55,* 22–28.

Siegel, J. T., & Rosenberg, B. D. (2025). When reactance begets more reactance: The reactive spiral. *Motivation Science, 11,* 222–233.

Silvia, P. J. (2006). A skeptical look at dispositional reactance. *Personality and Individual Differences, 40,* 1291–1297.

Sittenthaler, S., Jonas, E., & Traut-Mattausch, E. (2016). Explaining self and vicarious reactance: A process model approach. *Personality and Social Psychology Bulletin, 42,* 458–470.

Sittenthaler, S., Steindl, C., & Jonas, E. (2015a). Legitimate vs. illegitimate restrictions—A motivational and physiological approach investigating reactance processes. *Frontiers in Psychology, 6,* 632.

Sittenthaler, S., Traut-Mattausch, E., & Jonas, E. (2015b). Observing the restriction of another person: Vicarious reactance and the role of selfconstrual and culture. *Frontiers in Psychology, 6,* 1052.

Sittenthaler, S., Traut-Mattausch, E., Steindl, C., & Jonas, E. (2015c). Salzburger State Reactance Scale (SSR Scale): Validation of a scale measuring state reactance. *Zeitschrift fur Psychologie mit Zeitschrift fur Angewandte Psychologie, 223,* 257–266.

Sly, D. F., Hopkins, R. S., Trapido, E., & Ray, S. (2001). Influence of a counteradvertising media campaign on initiation of smoking: The Florida "truth" campaign. *American Journal of Public Health, 91,* 233–238.

Song, H., McComas, K. A., & Schuler, K. L. (2018). Source effects on psychological reactance to regulatory policies: The role of trust and similarity. *Science Communication, 40*(5), 591–620.

Soveri, A., Karlsson, L. C., Mäki, K. O., Holford, D., Fasce, A., Schmid, P., . . . Lewandowsky, S. (2024). Trait reactance as psychological motivation to reject vaccination: Two longitudinal studies and one experimental study. *Applied Psychology: Health and Well-Being, 16*(2), 597–614.

Sprengholz, P., Tannert, S., & Betsch, C. (2023). Explaining boomerang effects in persuasive health communication: How psychological reactance to healthy eating messages elevates attention to unhealthy food. *Journal of Health Communication, 28(6),* 384–390.

Staunton, T. V., Alvaro, E. M., & Rosenberg, B. D. (2022). A case for directives: Strategies for enhancing clarity while mitigating reactance. *Current Psychology, 41,* 611–621.

Steindl, C., & Jonas, E. (2015). The dynamic reactance interaction—How vested interests affect people's experience, behavior, and cognition in social interactions. *Frontiers in Psychology, 6,* 1752.

Steindl, C., Jonas, E., Sittenthaler, S., Traut-Mattausch, E., & Greenberg, J. (2015). Understanding psychological reactance: New developments and findings. *Zeitschrift fur Psychologie mit Zeitschrift fur Angewandte Psychologie, 223,* 205–214.

Sullivan, J. J., & Pallak, M. S. (1976). Effect of commitment and reactance on action-taking. *Personality and Social Psychology Bulletin, 2,* 179–182.

Swoboda, J. S., Dowd, E. T., & Wise, S. L. (1990). Reframing and restraining directives in the treatment of clinical depression. *Journal of Counseling Psychology, 37,* 254–260.

Tennen, H., Press, S., Rohrbaugh, M., & White, L. (1981). Reactance theory and therapeutic paradox: A compliance–defiance model. *Psychotherapy: Theory, Research, and Practice, 18,* 14–22.

Thomas, A., Donnell, A. J., & Buboltz, W. J. (2001). The Hong Psychological Reactance Scale: A confirmatory factor analysis. *Measurement & Evaluation in Counseling and Development, 34,* 2–13.

Tolman, E. (1932). *Purposive behavior in animals and men.* Appleton-Century.

Tormala, Z. L., & Clarkson, J. J. (2007). Assimilation and contrast in persuasion: The effects of source credibility in multiple message situations. *Personality and Social Psychology Bulletin, 33,* 559–571.

Tracey, T. J., Ellickson, J. L., & Sherry, P. (1989). Reactance in relation to different supervisory environments and counselor development. *Journal of Counseling Psychology, 36,* 336–344.

Tucker, R. K., & Byers, P. Y. (1987). Factorial validity of Merz's Psychological Reactance Scale. *Psychological Reports, 61,* 811–815.

Turner, M. M. (2007). Using emotion in risk communication: The anger activism model. *Public Relations Review, 33,* 114–119.

Vohs, K. D., & Baumeister, R. F. (Eds.). (2004). *Handbook of self-regulation: Research, theory, and applications.* Guilford Press.

Walster, E., & Festinger, L. (1962). The effectiveness of "overheard" persuasive communications. *Journal of Abnormal and Social Psychology, 65*(6), 395–402.

Waris, O., Karlsson, L., Antfolk, J., Karlsson, L., Karlsson, H., & Soveri, A. (2020). The factorial structure of the Hong Psychological Reactance Scale in two Finnish samples. *Nordic Psychology, 73(1)*, 68–90.

Wicklund, R. A. (1974). *Freedom and reactance.* Erlbaum.

Wicklund, R. A., & Brehm, J. W. (1968). Attitude change as a function of felt competence and threat to attitudinal freedom. *Journal of Experimental Social Psychology, 4,* 64–75.

Wicklund, R. A., Slattum, V., & Solomon, E. (1970). Effects of implied pressure toward commitment on ratings of choice alternatives. *Journal of Experimental Social Psychology, 6,* 449–457.

Worchel, S., & Brehm, J. W. (1970). Effect of threats to attitudinal freedom as a function of agreement with the communicator. *Journal of Personality and Social Psychology, 14,* 18–22.

Wortman, C. B., & Brehm, J. W. (1975). Response to uncontrollable outcomes: An integration of reactance theory and the learned helplessness model. In L. Berkowitz (Ed.), *Advances in experimental social psychology* (Vol. 8). Academic Press.

Wright, R. A. (2008). Refining the prediction of effort: Brehm's distinction between potential motivation and motivation intensity. *Social and Personality Psychology Compass, 2,* 682–701.

Wright, R. A., Agtarap, S. D., & Mlynski, C. (2015). Conversion of reactance motives into effortful goal pursuit: Implications of Brehm's theory of motivation intensity. *Zeitschrift fur Psychologie mit Zeitschrift fur Angewandte Psychologie, 223,* 267–276.

Zemack-Rugar, Y., Moore, S. G., & Fitzsimons, G. J. (2017). Just do it! Why committed consumers react negatively to assertive ads. *Journal of Consumer Psychology, 27,* 287–301.

Zucker, D., Hopkins, R. S., Sly, D. F., Urich, J., Kershaw, J. M., & Solari, S. (2000). Florida's "truth" campaign: A counter-marketing, antitobacco media campaign. *Journal of Public Health Management and Practice, 6,* 1–6.

CHAPTER 22

The Tyranny of Freedom

Choice Overload, Decision Fatigue, and the Meaning of Choice

Nathan N. Cheek

More than 50 years ago, futurist Alvin Toffler (1970/1990) published his now-classic volume *Future Shock*, detailing the overwhelming and chaotic society he saw emerging in the modern world. Toffler argued at the time that there was so much choice and such fragmentation of social life that people were becoming, ironically, *less* free than before:

> For there comes a time when choice, rather than freeing the individual, becomes so complex, difficult and costly, that it turns into its opposite. There comes a time, in short, when choice turns into overchoice and freedom into un-freedom. (p. 283)

Ballooning consumer wealth and economic growth were creating a larger and more diverse class of consumers at the same time that advancing technology enabled faster and more varied manufacturing across seemingly every domain of life. Car dealerships, bookstores, grocery stores—any number of everyday businesses were rapidly expanding their offerings, changing the landscape of Western consumption through the proliferation of choice. The days of constraint, much less scarcity, would soon be gone, replaced with the new problem of abundance: "the people of the future may suffer not from an absence of choice, but from a paralyzing surfeit of it" (Toffler, 1970/1990, p. 264).

We—at least those of us living in wealthy Western democracies—are living in Toffler's future. Some of Toffler's descriptions seem almost quaint by today's standards—how much more distressed would the "suburban matron" who lamented the difficulty of finding a book for her book club from the 30,000 books published per year in the United States (1970/1990, p. 279) be to learn that more than 100 times as many books are now published yearly across traditional and self-publishing formats (Kolmar, 2023)? In-person shopping can be overwhelming enough—even the grocery store in the small Midwestern college town of West Lafayette, Indiana, offers more than two dozen kinds of Triscuit crackers alone—but online shopping now provides basically anything a shopper could think of. A search for "shoes" on Amazon.com in August 2024 returned over 60,000 options; a search for "pants" returned over 100,000.

Moreover, people don't just have more options: They have more *choices*. In the course of human history, it is only relatively recently that a large number of people have acquired (or, in some cases, been legally granted) the choice of what to do for work, of where to live, of whom to marry, of how to raise a family, of how to navigate life, and even, with the growing availability of physician-assisted suicide, of how to navigate death. Social roles are becoming more flexible, and many societies' norms are loosening (albeit nonlinearly and not without resistance; e.g., Jackson et al., 2019; Richeson, 2020; Seamster & Ray, 2018), opening up still further new choices for people to make. Choices have also expanded because new reasons for making them have emerged—for example, marriages, once made for largely financial or practical arrangements, can now be made for love, and are, increasingly, made for self-actualization (Finkel, 2017). Maybe most importantly, people are freer than ever before to choose *who to be*.[1]

There is much to celebrate about this expansive freedom. In a narrow sense, abundant choice should let people better satisfy their preferences. With more shoes, or cars, or Triscuits to choose from, each person should be more likely to find the one that is just right for them. In a broader sense, freedom is often viewed as a moral imperative (Schwartz, 2000). People *should* be able to choose their jobs, their homes, their social networks, and their partners (if any)—they should, in short, have control over their own lives. In fact, people may *have to* have freedom to be healthy and happy: The vast self-determination literature has shown time and again that a feeling of autonomy is a fundamental human need (e.g., Deci & Ryan, 2000, 2002; Fischer & Boer, 2011; Ryan & Deci, 2000; Ryan et al., 2022; Vansteenkiste et al., 2020). This is true even in cultural contexts with conceptions of autonomy that are more interdependent than the personal freedoms prioritized by Western, independent cultural contexts (see, e.g., research in South Korea, Russia, Turkey, China, and Peru; Chen et al., 2015; Chirkov et al., 2003; Yu et al., 2018), though autonomy, choice, and freedom may look different in different cultural contexts (e.g., being free to make one's own choices versus being free to act in line with the choices of close others; Iyengar & DeVoe, 2003). Denying people choice and freedom can have profound negative consequences (Araki, 2024; Bone et al., 2014; Cheek et al., 2022; Hill et al., 2016), both for physical and mental well-being (e.g., Britton et al., 2014; Campbell et al., 2017; Cordeiro et al., 2016; Ng et al., 2012) and for behavior (e.g., lack of motivation, harmful behavioral reactance; Brehm, 1966; Deci & Ryan, 2000; Dillard & Shen, 2005).

So, freedom is a good thing. But, crucially, it is not only or always a good thing—it is not an unmitigated good (Cheek & Schwartz, 2025; Grant & Schwartz, 2011; Reutskaja & Hogarth, 2009; Schwartz, 2000, 2016). Increased freedom comes with costs, and those costs are the focus of this chapter. In what follows, I review some of the downsides of abundant choice and freedom, with a focus on three ways of conceptualizing freedom: freedom as the *number of options* people have, freedom as the *number of choices* people have, and freedom as the *type of choices* people have. In each of these cases, people can sometimes feel like they have *too much* freedom, at which point they may start to feel worse than they would with somewhat less freedom. I then explore some of the ways people attempt to manage or "escape from" (Fromm, 1941) excessive freedom, after which I conclude by highlighting the potential importance of achieving a balance between freedom and security for healthier and happier individuals and societies.

FREEDOM AS NUMBER OF OPTIONS: CHOICE OVERLOAD

One way that freedom and choice have been studied in the literature is in terms of how many options people have from which to choose, with the intuition that the more options people have, the more freedom they have (Cheek & Schwartz, 2025; Schwartz, 2000, 2016). Compared to having very limited options, having a moderate number of options can make people feel more decision freedom (Reibstein et al., 1975), can increase the perceived value of choice (Reutskaja et al., 2018), can increase satisfaction (Cheek et al., 2023), and can increase the likelihood that people will actually make a choice (Shah & Wolford, 2007). But three decades of consumer research has shown that these benefits diminish, and indeed reverse, when the number of options continues to grow, ultimately resulting in "choice overload"—the experience of having too much choice.

In a classic early study, Iyengar and Lepper (2000) documented *choice paralysis*—the failure to make any choice in the face of an overwhelming number of options. Even when people overcome paralysis to make a choice, having too many options may lead to worse outcomes (Schwartz, 2016). Large assortments make it harder to find the objectively best option, causing people to fail to identify even dominant alternatives (Bhargava et al., 2017)—sometimes with costly consequences, as when older adults face an overwhelming number of Medicare prescription drug plans and end up choosing more expensive or less comprehensive plans (Tanius et al., 2009). Abundant choice can also undermine subjective experiences—when people choose from larger choice sets, they feel more regret, greater uncertainty, greater disappointment, and less satisfaction, all while ruminating about the larger number of forgone alternatives they could have chosen (e.g., Botti & Iyengar, 2004; Hafner et al., 2012; Iyengar & Lepper, 2000; Schwartz, 2016).

There are some important moderators of choice overload (for reviews, see Chernev et al., 2015; Misuraca et al., 2020; see also Scheibehenne et al., 2010) and, in Chapter 23 of this volume, Reutskaja and Misuraca provide a much more extensive review of the choice overload literature. For the present purposes, the key insight is that, perhaps counterintuitively, there comes a point when having more options from which to choose becomes overwhelming to choosers, often harming rather than helping them. This is one sense in which freedom becomes costly—abundant options cause overload—but the effects of having too many options are compounded by the sheer number of choices people must make as they navigate daily life. One choice with a lot of options can already feel like too much freedom, but then people must continue making such demanding choices over and over again.

FREEDOM AS NUMBER OF CHOICES: DECISION FATIGUE

A second way to think about freedom and choice is in terms of how many choices people are afforded in daily life. There is a widespread claim in popular science writing that people make upward of 35,000 decisions every day (e.g., Graff, 2021; Hoomans, 2015; Marples, 2022). This statistic may well be apocryphal—it would mean, for instance, that people make about one decision every 2 seconds during waking hours (Krockow, 2018)—and none of these articles cites a source for this claim, but one reason why it persists may be that it resonates. People *feel* like they are making 35,000 daily decisions. And they certainly are making a lot of them, and more than ever before (Schwartz, 2016).

Each decision people make has a cost; even straightforward choices take some amount of cognitive effort. The costs of decision making can accumulate as people navigate the many choices that come with extensive freedom, ultimately resulting in "decision fatigue"—feelings of exhaustion and an impaired ability to make decisions as a result of repeated decision making (Levav et al., 2010; Pignatiello et al., 2020; Vohs et al., 2008). In addition to feeling burned out by having to make so many choices, people experiencing decision fatigue find decision making more unpleasant (Polman & Vohs, 2016); feel more uncertainty and less self-efficacy (Pignatiello et al., 2020); and are more likely to delay making additional decisions and to wish others would make decisions for them (Augenblick & Nicholson, 2016; Hickman et al., 2018). Fatigued decision makers are also more likely to rely on lower-effort heuristic strategies during decision making (e.g., sticking with the status quo or going with the easiest or least risky option; Allan et al., 2019; Augenblick & Nicholson, 2016; Baer & Schnall, 2021) and are more likely to make errors in decision making (Baer & Schnall, 2021; Busey et al., 2015; Hirshleifer et al., 2019; Hsiang et al., 2019).

Decision fatigue affects consumer decision making in everyday life, but perhaps even more concerning are instances of decision fatigue in high-stakes decision making. From forensic fingerprint analysts (Busey et al., 2015) and doctors (Linder et al., 2014) to air traffic control employees (Orasanu et al., 2012) and academic journal editors (Stewart et al., 2012), the exhausting number of choices people must make has been found to undermine decision making among professionals making potentially life-altering decisions. Putting a price tag on decision fatigue, one study found that a bank lost out on approximately half a million dollars in one month alone because of loan approval decisions made by employees who were decision fatigued (Baer & Schnall, 2021).

Decision fatigue is more likely when decisions are more difficult and more effortful (Oto, 2012), and thus choice overload exacerbates the already exhausting experience of having to make repeated decisions. Taken together, choice overload and decision fatigue mean that choice can be experienced as burdensome rather than freeing. In fact, people may often not want so much choice, and in particular may want less choice than often assumed by marketers and policymakers (Schwartz & Cheek, 2017; Sunstein, 2015). Research suggests, for instance, that people are less likely to want abundant options for high-stakes or complex choices (Reed et al., 2008), and may also prefer limited variety for functional, utilitarian, unexpressive choices (e.g., mops, vacuums; Cadario & Morewedge, 2022; Ratner & Kahn, 2002). Choice overload is felt especially when people are uncertain, such as when choices are difficult or when people have little familiarity with or knowledge about a choice domain (Chernev et al., 2015)—in such situations, people are often happy to forgo choice freedom and defer to others instead (Botti & McGill, 2011). And when people are forced to make tragic choices, such as life-or-death decisions for loved ones, choice feels particularly painful and fatiguing (Botti et al., 2009; Pignatiello & Hickman, 2019). This array of negative experiences with undesired choices has led some to argue that mandating choice can be understood, at least in some contexts, as a freedom-reducing form of paternalism: People may actually feel—and be—*less* free when they are overwhelmed by the choices they are forced to make (Schwartz & Cheek, 2017; Sunstein, 2015).

In sum, the large number of options people encounter and the large number of choices people make are two important dimensions of the modern environment of abundant freedom that can prove overwhelming and exhausting. The costs of freedom, however, emerge not only because people are making more choices with more options, but because they are making new *types* of choices. People are not just deciding what to eat for dinner or what to wear to work (though the preceding discussion suggests those could be difficult enough). They are also deciding who to be.

FREEDOM AS TYPES OF CHOICES: SELF-UNCERTAINTY AND THE BURDEN OF SELF-EXPRESSION

For the past several hundred years, the ongoing trend in Western cultural contexts has been a shift in sources of self-definition from *outside-in* to *inside-out* (Baumeister, 1986; Fromm, 1941; Taylor, 1989, 1992; Turner, 1976). Whereas institutions, authorities, castes, social roles, group identities, religious rules, family expectations, work obligations, and other external structures and constraints once formed the foundation of people's selves, unprecedented freedom now allows, and also requires, self-definition from within. People increasingly have the freedom to chart their own paths in life, choosing the careers, lifestyles, relationships, and passions they want (Jackson et al., 2019; Schwartz, 2000, 2016). But the cost of this freedom is the loss of the certainty and security that external constraints on selves used to provide, even as those constraints may also have had negative consequences (e.g., by forcing people into social roles and identities they did not want to inhabit). Individuation, Fromm (1941) argued, "creates a feeling of powerlessness and anxiety. . . . When one has become an individual, one stands alone and faces the world in all its perilous and overpowering aspects" (p. 29).

Having to navigate freedom and define oneself can thus spur stress and self-uncertainty (Cheek & Schwartz, 2025)—the self is not given but must be discovered and created. Such self-uncertainty is exacerbated by the potentially increased instability of selves when people are free to define and redefine themselves, and especially so when people find themselves with more choices and options than ever before. Choices are acts of meaning (Bruner, 1990) linked to the self: They can both express people's identities and change them (e.g., Bem, 1972; Goffman, 1959; Levy, 1959; Sirgy, 1982). And given the proliferation of choices inherent to modern freedom, there are a seemingly unlimited number of possible selves (Markus & Nurius, 1986) people could pursue through choice.

In fact, the proliferation of options may be turning even seemingly trivial choices into questions of identity. In a series of experiments manipulating choice set size, Cheek and colleagues (2023) randomly assigned participants to choose from either a smaller number of options or a larger number of options. They found that participants thought their choices were more self-expressive when they had more options, suggesting that having more options changes the meaning of choice by increasing its expressive value. Increases in perceived self-expression from larger choice sets were mediated by perceived preference matching—participants thought that having more options afforded a better opportunity to find the option that fit what they were looking for, and this predicted their perception that choices from larger sets took on more expressive value.

In some of Cheek and colleagues' (2023) studies, participants thought their choices were more self-expressive after choosing from larger assortments even when the additional options in the larger assortments did not objectively offer any better chance to match their preferences (i.e., when the additional options were all objectively lower quality than those in the smaller assortment). Just having additional unappealing options seems to create the *illusion* of better preference matching. It is worth noting that the choices in this research were mundane—for example, participants chose a drink they would want to consume or a short YouTube video to watch. Nonetheless, greater freedom through a larger number of options caused greater freedom through self-expression—even trivial choices started to be relevant to choosers' identities. YouTube videos were no longer *just* YouTube videos.

The increasing identity relevance of everyday choices connects back to Toffler's (1970/1990) argument that technological innovations and decreasing costs of production drive some of the overwhelming effects of freedom (see also Schwartz, 2000, 2016). Because many companies can more cheaply produce and market a varied line of products, they can more easily cause and then take advantage of the new self-defining choices people are increasingly forced to make. Reuseable water bottles, for instance, used to be more or less utilitarian tools—they helped people stay hydrated and that was about it. But in the last several years, water bottles have become identity accessories, so much so that people now buy many versions of the same bottle in different colors or styles, even though each one holds water as well as the next (Mull, 2019, 2024). This change in self-relevance is possible at least in part because of how many different kinds of water bottles there are; if there were only two kinds, they likely couldn't hold the same self-expressive meaning. But now that they do, it is difficult to opt out of a self-expressive choice—people will have a harder time just picking any water bottle, because even if they do not care what it looks like, those around them will. Freedom gives choices social meaning that shapes and expresses the self, adding another challenge for people to navigate alongside choice overload and decision fatigue.

To be clear, *some* self-expression is not bad—in fact, people often like to share information about themselves (Tamir & Mitchell, 2012) and self-expression can increase choice satisfaction when there are only a moderate number of options (Cheek et al., 2023). But when freedom overwhelms people by making so many choices self-relevant and by mandating self-expression, it becomes a burden. For instance, when choices are self-expressive, people may feel like they cannot make decisions they otherwise would because of concerns about how it would reflect on them (e.g., not canceling a rarely used gym membership to maintain a "health-conscious" self-concept or not using coupons to avoid appearing "cheap"; Ashworth et al., 2005; Savary & Dhar, 2020). Recent evidence even suggests that people have become less interested in or willing to express themselves over time (Chopik et al., 2024), perhaps as a response to the burden of frequently making identity-relevant choices.

Increased self-relevance also causes people to change their goals during choice. When choices become statements about the self, people are no longer happy to make a "good enough" choice—they need the best. Accordingly, increases in the self-expressiveness of choices increases *maximizing*—attempting to make the best possible choice by extensively searching for and comparing alternatives (Cheek et al., 2025; Cheek & Schwartz, 2016, 2025). Maximizing is a much more effortful and intensive approach to decision making, and also, ironically, often leads people to feel worse about their choice than if they had taken the easier path by aiming for a "good enough" option (Iyengar et al., 2006; Moyano-Díaz et al., 2014; Schwartz et al., 2002). The relation between self-relevance and maximizing illustrates how the different consequences of freedom—choice overload, decision fatigue, self-expressive burden—mutually reinforce one other. Larger choice sets increase the self-expressiveness of choices, which causes maximizing, and maximizing increases decision fatigue and heightens the negative effects of large choice sets (Dar-Nimrod et al., 2009). All three processes ultimately combine to turn excessive freedom into something that may hurt more than it helps.

FREEDOM HURTS

Fromm (1941) and other existentialists (e.g., Kierkegaard, 1844/1980) argued that extensive freedom would cause anxiety and loneliness, along with other harms to well-being. In line with this diagnosis, there is growing evidence that people in societies that emphasize extreme freedom are hurting, especially young people, who may feel freedom's burden most acutely as they try to figure out how to navigate life. Youth in the United States and many other countries are experiencing record rates of anxiety and other mental health concerns, such as depression and suicide (Goodwin et al., 2020; Jeffries & Unger, 2020; Keyes et al., 2019, 2024; Mojtabai et al., 2016; Thapar et al., 2022; Weinberger et al., 2018), and college campuses in the United States are encountering unprecedented levels of demand for counseling services amid this mental health crisis period (e.g., Center for Collegiate Mental Health, 2015; Lipson et al., 2019; Oswalt et al., 2020). There is also a "loneliness epidemic" (Office of the Surgeon General, 2023) as people suffer from what Fromm called the *aloneness* of individuation as a result of freedom.

Beyond these general trends, more specific evidence also links extreme freedom and lower well-being. Looking cross-culturally, research on the level of freedom in different societies (i.e., the tightness or looseness of cultural norms; Gelfand, 2018) has found that it is not just societies with very little freedom that are unhealthy—the citizens of societies with extremely high levels of freedom are also lower in well-being. Compared with nations with more moderate levels of freedom, nations with the highest levels of freedom have lower physical health, including higher rates of mortality from stress-related diseases such as cardiovascular disease and lower life expectancy, as well as lower mental health, including lower happiness and higher suicide rates (Harrington et al., 2015). At the extreme, these data suggest that freedom may literally be making people ill.

An alternative way to measure the amount of freedom people have beyond cultural tightness is in terms of individual wealth—generally speaking, the more money people have, the more freedom they have (indeed, Fromm [1941] explicitly argued freedom was most problematic for those with more money). Although people with more money tend to be healthier than those with less money, some research suggests that both people with very low incomes *and* people with very high incomes (i.e., those likely to feel the most freedom) are less healthy and less happy than those with sufficient but not extreme wealth (Korous et al., 2023; Luthar et al., 2013, 2020). If more money means more freedom, there may come a point at which the freedom money buys starts to hurt.

Finally, researchers have measured how much freedom people have by asking them directly. In one study, Reutskaja and colleagues (2022b) asked people to report how many options they had available to them both in mundane choice domains (e.g., soft drink options) and in higher-stakes domains (e.g., health care and housing). Participants who reported experiencing extreme freedom of choice in the sense of having many more options available to them than they wanted reported lower life satisfaction, especially in the United States, where there is particular cultural emphasis on choice and individual self-expression (e.g., Markus & Schwartz, 2010). In sum, various lines of research converge to validate the concerns of existentialists that too much freedom could be costly for well-being. Given this cost, the next section explores some of the ways people attempt to deal with the burden of freedom—or, as Fromm (1941) put it, how they attempt to "escape from" freedom.

ESCAPING FROM FREEDOM

Understanding how reckoning with freedom and its components like autonomy, choice, and free will beliefs drives people's behavior has been a major pursuit in existential psychology research (Koole et al., 2006). Fromm (1941), for example, viewed a conscious understanding of freedom and of its outcome (individuation of a self that must navigate an uncertain world) as a uniquely human experience—perhaps the defining one. A core tenet of his theorizing was that many maladaptive or harmful patterns of behavior (or "neuroses") could be traced back to people's attempts to escape from the anxieties and uncertainties of freedom. And because the primary path through which freedom inflicts suffering is, in his view, by atomizing society into isolated, anxious individuals who were stressed by their awareness of their aloneness, many attempts to escape freedom are attempts to escape the sense of the self as a separate entity adrift in an uncertain world: "*to get rid of the individual self, to lose oneself*; in other words, *to get rid of the burden of freedom*" (Fromm, 1941, p. 152, original emphasis).

Since the analyses of Fromm and other existential and psychodynamic theorists such as Kierkegaard (1844/1980) and Horney (1950/1991), a substantial amount of empirical psychological research has tackled the question of how people manage uncertainty and anxiety in the face of overwhelming freedom. This section briefly explores some of the paths people take, many of which are united by people's attempts to diminish the prominence of the individual self, such as by connecting to something else, be it other people, possessions, or ideas. Not all attempts to escape freedom are harmful, but, following Fromm's particular emphasis on acts of escape that are a problem for society, I begin with what is perhaps his most famous theorizing—support of authoritarianism as an escape.

Authoritarianism and Extremism

Fromm (1941) argued that authoritarianism offered an appealing escape from freedom by allowing people to submit the individual self to a powerful authority, thereby reducing uncertainty and anxiety, while also allowing people to enjoy the status of the powerful leader or group:

> By becoming part of a power which is felt as unshakably strong, eternal, and glamorous, one participates in its strength and glory. One surrenders one's own self and renounces all strength and pride connected with it, one loses one's integrity as an individual and surrenders freedom; but one gains a new security and a new pride in the participation in the power in which one submerges. One gains also security against the torture of doubt. (pp. 155–156)

Subsequent research supports the potential appeal of authoritarianism for those struggling with freedom; indeed, those who believe in free will are more likely to endorse right-wing authoritarian views (Costello et al., 2020). Authoritarianism, however, might be understood as one instance, and perhaps a particularly effective uncertainty-reducing instance, of the larger appeal of *extremism.* That is, people can reduce uncertainty in the face of freedom by finding something very certain, clear, and defined to cling to, and a potentially wide variety of extremist views and groups may be able to meet these criteria (Hogg, 2014). Conspiracy theories, populism, and terrorism can all attract people experiencing high levels of uncertainty and anxiety because of their clear descriptions and prescriptions of how the world works and how one should behave (e.g., Doosje et al., 2016; Douglas et al., 2017; Staub, 1989; van Prooijen, 2016).

Group Membership and Interpersonal Relationships

It is not only extremist leaders and groups that can offer relief from uncertainty and anxiety. Social identity theory (Tajfel, 1978; Tajfel & Turner, 1979; Turner et al., 1987) describes how groups can serve important identity functions for individuals, offering them a collective identity to incorporate into their self-definition, as well as norms and scripts to guide their behavior. Building on these insights, uncertainty–identity theory (Hogg, 2012) argues that uncertainty motivates people to find certainty, and given groups' ability to do so, people often join groups in an attempt to find a sense of certainty and meaning amid the anxieties of extensive freedom. While uncertainty–identity theory offers a formal explanation for the appeal of extremism described above (e.g., Hogg, 2014), groups do not need to be harmful or extreme to serve an uncertainty-reducing function. Teams, neighborhoods, families, classrooms, workplaces, and clubs can all serve to reduce individuals' uncertainty without necessarily leading to the harm of authoritarian or extremist groups.

In addition to providing certainty as groups, other people can also provide certainty in interpersonal relationships, including close friendships, family ties, and romantic relationships. Interpersonal relationships and group membership both involve expanding the self to incorporate others (Aron et al., 1991, Tropp & Wright, 2001), allowing people to construe the self more interdependently. Unlike overidentification and self-escape with authoritarianism or extremism, the potential adaptiveness of group memberships and interpersonal relationships, when they are balanced and healthy, may lie, as Fromm believed, in people's continued understanding of the self as an individual with a personal self as well as an individual *connected to others* with relational and collective selves. (There is also important cross-cultural variation in models of healthy and mature selves that goes beyond the scope of this chapter; e.g., Markus & Kitayama, 1991; Triandis, 1989). Group memberships and interpersonal relationships provide sources for self-definition and reduce uncertainty by allowing people to expand their identities beyond their individual selves to connect with other people.

Possessions

People are not the only entities external to the self that can provide relief from uncertainty—sometimes, people find certainty in material possessions. Consumer research shows that people may incorporate their possessions into their self-concept (e.g., Belk, 1988; Csikszentmihalyi & Rochberg-Halton, 1981) and that materialism—placing value on and potentially defining the self through material possessions—may arise from and function in part to reduce uncertainty (Richins, 2017). One's possessions, prized or even mundane, may be concrete representations of identity that can restore a sense of self-stability as people navigate an uncertain world defined by too much freedom (e.g., Rios Morrison & Johnson, 2011). Attempting to escape from freedom through materialism and inclusion of possessions in the self can sometimes lead to less adaptive responses, such as hoarding (e.g., Castriotta et al., 2019; Claes et al., 2016), and materialism may not offer the same solace that close relationships do, but it is also a less socially harmful path than authoritarianism or other forms of extremism.

The potential value of possessions in an uncertain world may also shed light on the appeal of beliefs and ideologies, whether extreme or moderate, in providing certainty to individuals confronted with the burden of freedom. Research suggests that people often think about their beliefs as possessions (Abelson, 1986; Abelson & Prentice, 1989) and thus holding onto and identifying with an attitude or worldview (e.g., a commitment to fairness or fighting for social justice) may be able to provide certainty and meaning through a cognitively similar path to the certainty and meaning provided by physical possessions (van den Bos & Miedema, 2000).

Self-Inflation

Sometimes people try to find a path to escaping freedom not in others or in their possessions, but in themselves. People may attempt to find certainty and relief from freedom through inflating their view of who they are (Bosson et al., 2008) or through striving for a level of perfection that wards off the anxieties of an unpredictable world of abundant choice (Graham et al., 2010). From a psychodynamic perspective, the former of these strategies can be conceptualized as narcissism, the latter as perfectionism. Fromm (1941) suggested that the feelings of "terror or aloneness and insignificance" can be "covered by compensatory feelings of eminence and perfection" (p. 151), and Horney (1950/1991) referred to narcissism and perfectionism as *expansive solutions,* where "the individual prevailingly identifies himself with his glorified self" (p. 191). Unfortunately, attempting to escape freedom through these forms of self-inflation often carries social and personal costs given the precarity of social status, the social stigma of self-entitlement, and the stress and impossibility of sustaining perfection (e.g., Callaghan et al., 2024; Carlson & DesJardins, 2015; Limburg et al., 2017).

Escaping the Self

Rather than inflating the self, people may use a variety of other absorbing behaviors to try to escape awareness of the self—or maybe even to destroy the self. Fromm (1941) described attempts such as seeking out pain or drinking alcohol as means of escaping the anxiety and uncertainty caused by self-awareness:

> If I can succeed in reducing my individual self to nothing, if I can overcome the awareness of my separateness as an individual, I may save myself . . . to be overwhelmed by pain and agony [is one way]; to be overcome by the effects of intoxication is another. The phantasy of suicide is the last hope if all other means have not succeeded in bringing relief from the burden of aloneness. (pp. 152–153)

Through this lens, a wide range of potentially self-destructive behaviors have been conceptualized as potential means of escaping the self, including alcohol and drug use, sex, extreme activities (e.g., potentially terrifying experiences like skydiving), violence, overconsumption (e.g., binge eating, spree shopping), nonsuicidal self-injury, and suicide (e.g., Baumeister, 1990, 1991; Donnelly et al., 2016; Jouhki & Oksanen, 2022). From an existential perspective, escaping the self through these kinds of behaviors may be a more common strategy of navigating the uncertainty of freedom for people who cannot find protection or defense in the self—that is, people with low self-esteem. Fitting with this theorizing, people with lower self-esteem are more likely to engage in many of these forms of self-escape (e.g., Dunkley & Grilo, 2007; Hull et al., 1983; Wisman et al., 2015).

Of course, not all attempts to escape the self are necessarily harmful. Leisure activities, for example, can be means of temporarily reducing self-awareness (Stenseng et al., 2012), as can volunteering in service to others (Meneghini, 2016). And, in moderation, drinking, say, or extreme recreational activities may offer temporary distraction without any long-term consequences. Most people want to escape the self at some point, but excessive freedom, and the uncertainty and anxiety it causes, may drive people to seek more frequent, more dangerous, and more maladaptive escapes.

Delegation to Surrogates

People do not always have to escape from or even change their sense of self in order to escape from the burden of freedom—not if they can instead escape from the *responsibility* of freedom. To do so, they can delegate decision making to a surrogate, such that another person or system (e.g., flipping a coin or using an algorithm) makes the decision for them. Delegation removes the cognitive costs of choice, such as information processing and determining reasons for or against different alternatives (Douneva et al., 2019; Jaffé et al., 2023), and people value delegation more when they are confused or undecided (Dwenger et al., 2018; Dykstra et al., 2022). Thus, delegation reduces the burden of choice in part by removing the effort required during choice, directly protecting people from choice overload and decision fatigue.

Beyond the immediate cognitive burden of choice, delegation also addresses the more existential burden of freedom. When another person takes over decision making, they also take on the responsibility for the choice and its consequences—responsibility has shifted and so too has the burden of uncertainty. Because in contexts of extensive freedom choices often have self-expressive meaning (Cheek & Schwartz, 2025), people feel stress when making decisions they could end up regretting or that could end up reflecting badly on them. Delegation avoids these concerns by passing the buck: People are especially willing to delegate decisions when they are concerned about how choices might reflect on them or when they are worried about making the wrong choice or about making a choice in a biased or unfair manner (Keren & Teigen, 2010; Lin & Reich, 2018). In this way, delegation shares some similarities with submission to authorities, in that people do not have to figure out their own path forward as individuals anymore, though delegation in everyday life need not come from the goal of fully escaping the self or be accompanied by a subsequent loss of self-awareness, unlike submitting to authoritarian rule. In interdependent cultural contexts, moreover, delegating to close others may especially align with people's sense of conjoint agency, increasing intrinsic motivation (Iyengar & DeVoe, 2003).

CONCLUSION: FINDING A BALANCE

Modern Western democracies often prize unlimited freedom as an unmitigated pragmatic good and moral right (Schwartz, 2000). To quote Toffler (1970/1990): "Maximum individual choice is regarded as the democratic ideal" (p. 263). Yet, freedom is a difficult thing. Existential psychology has long explored the uncertainty and anxiety of navigating extensive freedom, and the present chapter has highlighted how too much freedom can cause choice overload, decision fatigue, and the pressure of self-expression, leaving people exhausted, uncertain, anxious, and lonely. At the same time, freedom is important for well-being—people need some freedom to experience the autonomy and choice that are essential ingredients for happiness and health (e.g., Araki, 2024; Deci & Ryan, 2000, 2002; Ryan et al., 2022). People need enough freedom to flourish, but also enough security not to feel overwhelmed and alone. The existential challenge for individuals and for societies is finding the right balance between the two.

For individuals, one of the greatest sources of this balance may be connections to others. A large and robust literature in psychology has found that social relationships are one of the largest positive factors in well-being (e.g., Araki, 2024; Diener et al., 1999; Diener & Suh, 2001; Myers, 2000). Even relatively weak connections with others can make people happier (Sandstrom & Dunn, 2014). A core feature of relationships, however, is that they almost always reduce people's freedom. Individuals have to balance their wants and needs with others', and thus relationships constrain people's choices. Of course, in exchange for the loss of some freedom, people get love, joy, and security—not a bad trade. Healthy relationships that offer support without being overly controlling may be paradigmatic adaptive escapes from too much freedom (Fromm, 1941).

Cross-cultural research shows that the happiest and healthiest societies tend to be those that find a good balance between freedom and security, falling somewhere in the middle between extreme tightness (e.g., societies with strict norms that are harshly enforced) and extreme looseness (e.g., societies with lenient norms and little constraint; Harrington et al., 2015). Sometimes this balance may need to shift in one direction or the other—during crises and disasters, societies may need to increase security at the cost of freedom (Cheek et al., 2022), whereas during times of growth and innovation, shifting toward freedom at the cost of security may be more fruitful (Jackson et al., 2019). But the general principle holds—the relationship between choice, autonomy, and freedom on the one hand and well-being on the other takes the form of an inverted U, where moderate freedom leaves people better off than too little or too much (Gelfand, 2018; Grant & Schwartz, 2011; Harrington et al., 2015; Reutskaja & Hogarth, 2009; Reutskaja et al., 2022a; Schwartz, 2016; see also Reutskaja & Misuraca, Chapter 23, this volume).

The irony of freedom is that individuals are not always free to choose how much freedom they have. For people living in a society at one of the extremes on the tightness–looseness continuum, finding the balance between security and freedom will almost certainly be harder than for individuals living in one of the more moderate societies. Indeed, one of Fromm's (1941) main insights was to shift the focus from the individual to the individual-in-society, highlighting the burden of excessive externally imposed freedom. Since Fromm, a large body of psychology research, much of it reviewed in this chapter, has broadened and deepened Fromm's analysis, adding substantial empirical data to his theoretical claims. Having done so, the most pressing questions about freedom for the future of existential psychology may now be less about the effects of freedom and more about how to help individuals and societies achieve a better balance. How can individuals adaptively find security and constraints in their chaotic high-freedom environments? How can societies adjust to give their citizens the security of safety nets and infrastructure while preserving autonomy and choice? And how can behaviorally informed public policy help individuals and societies achieve these goals?

The science of existential psychology is well-poised to seek the answers to such questions.

NOTE

1. As I write this in 2024, it is salient to me that increased freedom is not universally or equally distributed, an injustice underlined by, among other ongoing disparities and crises, the overturning of *Roe v. Wade* in the United States; persistent racism and discrimination in education, housing, and health care; and new and old restrictions on voting rights. The focus of this chapter is on freedom, and in particular the increased freedom many have relative to the past, but it should be acknowledged that the experience of extensive freedom and its consequences (e.g., choice overload; Reutskaja et al., 2022a) are still often restricted to the most powerful and privileged people, and this chapter does not speak to the experience of having too little choice and too little freedom.

REFERENCES

Abelson, R. P. (1986). Beliefs are like possessions. *Journal for the Theory of Social Behaviour, 16,* 223–250.

Abelson, R. P., & Prentice, D. A. (1989). Beliefs as possessions: A functional perspective. In A. R. Pratkanis, S. J. Breckler, & A. G. Greenwald (Eds.), *Attitude structure and function* (pp. 361–381). Erlbaum.

Allan, J. L., Johnston, D. W., Powell, D. J. H., Farquharson, B., Jones, M. C., Leckie, G., & Johnston, M. (2019). Clinical decisions and time since rest break: An analysis of decision fatigue in nurses. *Health Psychology, 38,* 318–324.

Araki, S. (2024). The societal determinants of happiness and unhappiness: Evidence from 152 countries over 15 years. *Social Psychological and Personality Science, 15,* 603–615.

Aron, A., Aron, E. N., Tudor, M., & Nelson, G. (1991). Close relationships as including other in the self. *Journal of Personality and Social Psychology, 60,* 241–253.

Ashworth, L., Darke, P. R., & Shaller, M. (2005). No one wants to look cheap: Tradeoffs between social disincentives and the economic and psychological incentives to redeem coupons. *Journal of Consumer Psychology, 15,* 295–306.

Augenblick, N., & Nicholson, S. (2016). Ballot position, choice fatigue, and voter behaviour. *Review of Economic Studies, 83,* 460–480.

Baer, T., & Schnall, S. (2021). Quantifying the cost of decision fatigue: Suboptimal risk decisions in finance. *Royal Society Open Science, 8,* Article 201059.

Baumeister, R. F. (1986). *Identity: Cultural change and the struggle for self.* Oxford University Press.

Baumeister, R. F. (1990). Suicide as escape from self. *Psychological Review, 97,* 90–113.

Baumeister, R. F. (1991). *Escaping the self: Alcoholism, spirituality, masochism, and other flights from the burden of selfhood.* Basic Books.

Belk, R. W. (1988). Possessions and the extended self. *Journal of Consumer Research, 15,* 139–168.

Bem, D. J. (1972). Self-perception theory. In L. Berkowitz (Ed.), *Advances in experimental* social psychology (Vol. 6, pp. 1–62). Academic Press.

Bhargava, S., Loewenstein, G., & Sydnor, J. (2017). Choose to lose: Health plan choices from a menu with dominated option. *Quarterly Journal of Economics, 132,* 1319–1372.

Bone, S. A., Christensen, G. L., & Williams, J. D. (2014). Rejected, shackled, and alone: The impact of systemic restricted choice on minority consumers' construction of self. *Journal of Consumer Research, 41,* 451–474.

Bosson, J. K., Lakey, C. E., Campbell, W. K., Zeigler-Hill, V., Jordan, C. H., & Kernis, M. H. (2008). Untangling the links between narcissism and self-esteem: A theoretical and empirical review. *Social and Personality Psychology Compass, 2,* 1415–1439.

Botti, S., & Iyengar, S. S. (2004). The psychological pleasure and pain of choosing: When people prefer choosing at the cost of subsequent outcome satisfaction. *Journal of Personality and Social Psychology, 87,* 312–326.

Botti, S., & McGill, A. L. (2011). The locus of choice: Personal causality and satisfaction with hedonic and utilitarian choices. *Journal of Consumer Research, 37,* 1065–1078.

Botti, S., Orfali, K., & Iyengar, S. S. (2009). Tragic choices: Autonomy and emotional response to medical decisions. *Journal of Consumer Research, 36,* 337–352.

Brehm, J. W. (1966). *A theory of psychological reactance.* Academic Press.

Britton, P. C., Van Orden, K. A., Hirsch, J. K., & Williams, G. C. (2014). Basic psychological needs, suicidal ideation, and risk for suicidal behavior in young adults. *Suicide and Life-Threatening Behavior, 44,* 362–371.

Bruner, J. (1990). *Acts of meaning.* Harvard University Press.

Busey, T., Swofford, H. J., Vanderkolk, J., & Emerick, B. (2015). The impact of fatigue on latent print examinations as revealed by behavioral and eye gaze testing. *Forensic Science International, 251,* 202–208.

Cadario, R., & Morewedge, C. K. (2022). Why do people eat the same breakfast every day? Goals and circadian rhythms of variety seeking in meals. *Appetite, 168,* Article 105716.

Callaghan, T., Greene, D., Shafran, R., Lunn, J., & Egan, S. J. (2024). The relationship between perfectionism and symptoms of depression, anxiety and obsessive-compulsive disorder in adults: A systematic review and meta-analysis. *Cognitive Behaviour Therapy, 53,* 121–132.

Campbell, R., Tobback, E., Delesie, L., Vogelaers, D., Mariman, A., & Vansteenkiste, M. (2017). Basic psychological need experiences, fatigue, and sleep in individuals with unexplained chronic fatigue. *Stress and Health, 33,* 645–655.

Carlson, E. N., & DesJardins, N. M. L. (2015). Do mean guys always finish first or just say that they do? Narcissists' awareness of their social status and popularity over time. *Personality and Social Psychology Bulletin, 41,* 901–917.

Castriotta, N., Dozier, M. E., Taylor, C. T., & Mayes, T. (2019). Intolerance of uncertainty in hoarding disorder. *Journal of Obsessive-Compulsive and Related Disorders, 21,* 97–101.

Center for Collegiate Mental Health (CCMH). (2015). *Annual report.* https://ccmh.psu.edu/assets/docs/2015_CCMH_Report_1-18-2015-yq3vik.pdf.

Cheek, N. N., Reutskaja, E., & Schwartz, B. (2022). Balancing the freedom-security tradeoff during crises and disasters. *Perspectives on Psychological Science, 17,* 1024–1049.

Cheek, N. N., & Schwartz, B. (2016). On the meaning and measurement of maximization. *Judgment and Decision Making, 11,* 126–146.

Cheek, N. N., & Schwartz, B. (2025). Be careful what you wish for: The dark side of freedom. In P. J. Carroll, K. Rios, & K. C. Oleson (Eds.), *Handbook of the uncertain self* (2nd ed., pp 45–58). Routledge.

Cheek, N. N., & Schwartz, B., & Shafir, E. (2023). Choice set size shapes self-expression. *Personality and Social Psychology Bulletin, 49,* 267–281.

Cheek, N. N., Schwartz, B., & Shafir, E. (2025). *A self-expression-based account of choice overload.* Unpublished manuscript.

Chen, B., Vansteenkiste, M., Beyers, W., Boone, L., Deci, E. L., Van der Kaap-Deeder, . . . Verstuyf, J. (2015). Basic psychological need satisfaction, need frustration, and need strength across four cultures. *Motivation and Emotion, 39,* 216–236.

Chernev, A., Böckenholt, U., & Goodman, J. (2015). Choice overload: A conceptual review and meta-analysis. *Journal of Consumer Psychology, 25,* 333–358.

Chirkov, V., Ryan, R. M., Kim, Y., & Kaplan, U. (2003). Differentiating autonomy from individualism and independence: A self-determination theory perspective on internalization of cultural orientations and well-being. *Journal of Personality and Social Psychology, 84,* 97–110.

Chopik, W., Götschi, K., Carrillo, A., Weidmann, R., & Potter, J. (2024). Changes in need for uniqueness from 2000 until 2020. *Collabra: Psychology, 10,* Article 121937.

Claes, L., Müller, A., & Luyckx, K. (2016). Compulsive buying and hoarding as identity substitutes: The role of materialistic value endorsement and depression. *Comprehensive Psychiatry, 68,* 65–71.

Cordeiro, P., Paixão, P., Lens, W., Lacante, M., & Luyckx, K. (2016). The Portuguese validation of the basic psychological need satisfaction and frustration scale: Concurrent and longitudinal relations to well-being and ill-being. *Psychologica Bellica, 56,* 193–209.

Costello, T. H., Bowes, S. M., & Lilienfeld, S. O. (2020). "Escape from freedom": Authoritarianism-related traits, political ideology, personality, and belief in free will/determinism. *Journal of Research in Personality, 86,* Article 103957.

Csikszentmihalyi, M., & Rochberg-Halton, E. (1981). *The meaning of things: Domestic symbols and the self.* Cambridge University Press.

Dar-Nimrod, I., Rawn, C. D., Lehman, D. R., & Schwartz, B. (2009). The maximization paradox: The costs of seeking alternatives. *Personality and Individual Differences, 46,* 631–635.

Deci, E. L., & Ryan, R. M. (2000). The "what" and "why" of goal pursuits: Human needs and the self-determination of behavior. *Psychological Inquiry, 11,* 227–268.

Deci, E. L., & Ryan, R. M. (Eds.). (2002). *Handbook of self-determination research.* University of Rochester Press.

Diener, E. & Suh, E. M. (Eds.). (2001). *Subjective well-being across cultures.* MIT Press.

Diener, E., Suh, E. M., Lucas, R. E., & Smith, H. L. (1999). Subjective well-being: Three decades of progress. *Psychological Bulletin, 125,* 276–302.

Dillard, J. P., & Shen, L. (2005). On the nature of reactance and its role in persuasive health communication. *Communication Monographs, 72,* 144–168.

Donnelly, G. E., Ksendzova, M., Howell, R. T., Vohs, K. D., & Baumeister, R. F. (2016). Buying to blunt negative feelings: Materialistic escape from the self. *Review of General Psychology, 20,* 272–316.

Doosje, B., Moghaddam, F. M., Kruglanski, A. W., de Wolf, A., Mann, L., & Feddes, A. R. (2016). Terrorism, radicalization and de-radicalization. *Current Opinion in Psychology, 11,* 79–84.

Douglas, K. M., Sutton, R. M., & Cichocka, A. (2017). The psychology of conspiracy theories. *Current Directions in Psychological Science, 26,* 538–542.

Douneva, M., Jaffé, M. E., & Greifeneder, R. (2019). Toss and turn or toss and stop? A coin flip reduces the need for information in decision-making. *Journal of Experimental Social Psychology, 83,* 132–141.

Dunkley, D. M., & Grilo, C. M. (2007). Self-criticism, low self-esteem, depressive symptoms, and over-evaluation of shape and weight in binge eating disorder patients. *Behaviour Research and Therapy, 45,* 139–149.

Dwenger, N., Kübler, D., & Weizsäcker, G. (2018). Flipping a coin: Evidence from university applications. *Journal of Public Economics, 167,* 240–250.

Dykstra, H., Exley, C. L., & Niederle, M. (2022). *When do individuals give up agency?: The role of decision avoidance.* Working paper. www.hbs.edu/ris/Publication%20Files/DykstraExleyNIederle_Oct2022_58a4444b-d720-484d-b97f-37f13b21866a.pdf.

Finkel, E. J. (2017). *The all-or-nothing marriage: How the best marriages work.* Dutton.

Fischer, R., & Boer, D. (2011). What is more important for national well-being: Money or autonomy? A meta-analysis of well-being, burnout, and anxiety across 63 societies. *Journal of Personality and Social Psychology, 101,* 164–184.

Fromm, E. (1941). *Escape from freedom.* Rinehart & Co.

Gelfand, M. (2018). *Rule makers, rule breakers: How tight and loose cultures wire our world.* Scribner.

Goffman, E. (1959). *The presentation of self in everyday life.* Doubleday.

Goodwin, R. D., Weinberger, A. H., Kim, J. H., Wu, M., & Galea, S. (2020). Trends in anxiety among adults in the United States, 2008–2018: Rapid increases among young adults. *Journal of Psychiatric Research, 130,* 441–446.

Graff, F. (2021, August 13). *How many decisions do we make in one day?* PBS. www.pbsnc.org/blogs/science/how-many-decisions-do-we-make-in-one-day/.

Graham, A. R., Sherry, S. B., Stewart, S. H., Sherry, D. L., McGrath, D. S., Fossum, K. M., & Allen, S. L. (2010). The existential model of perfectionism and depressive symptoms: A short-term, four-wave longitudinal study. *Journal of Counseling Psychology, 57,* 423–438.

Grant, A. M., & Schwartz, B. (2011). Too much of a good thing: The challenge and opportunity of the inverted U. *Perspectives on Psychological Science, 6,* 61–76.

Hafner, R. J., White, M. P., & Handley, S. J. (2012). Spoilt for choice: The role of counterfactual thinking in the excess choice and reversibility paradoxes. *Journal of Experimental Social Psychology, 48,* 28–36.

Harrington, J. R., Boski, P., & Gelfand, M. J. (2015). Culture and national well-being: Should societies emphasize freedom or constraint? *PLOS One, 10,* e0127173.

Hickman, Jr., R. L., Pignatiello, G. A., & Tahir, S. (2018). Evaluation of the decision fatigue scale among surrogate decision makers of the critically ill. *Western Journal of Nursing Research, 40,* 191–208.

Hill, R. P., & Cunningham, D., & The Gramercy Gentlemen. (2016). Dehumanization and restriction inside a maximum security prison: Novel insights about consumer acquisition and ownership. *Journal of the Association for Consumer Research, 1,* 295–313.

Hirshleifer, D., Levi, Y., Lourie, B., & Teoh, S. H. (2019). Decision fatigue and heuristic analyst forecasts. *Journal of Financial Economics, 133,* 83–98.

Hogg, M. A. (2012). Uncertainty-identity theory. In P. A. M. Van Lange, A. W. Kruglanski, & E. T. Higgins (Eds.), *Handbook of theories of social psychology* (Vol. 2, pp. 62–80). Sage.

Hogg, M. A. (2014). From uncertainty to extremism: Social categorization and identity processes. *Current Directions in Psychological Science, 23,* 338–342.

Hoomans, J. (2015, March 20). 35,000 decisions: The great choices of strategic leaders.

The Leading Edge. https://go.roberts.edu/leadingedge/the-great-choices-of-strategic-leaders.

Horney, K. (1991). *Neurosis and human growth: The struggle toward self-realization*. Norton. (Original work published 1950)

Hsiang, E. Y., Mehta, S. J., Small, D. S., Rareshide, C. A. L., Snider, C. K., Day, S. C., & Patel, M. S. (2019). Association of primary care clinic appointment time with clinician ordering and patient completion of breast and colorectal cancer screening. *JAMA Network Open, 2*, Article e193403.

Hull, J. G., Levenson, R. W., Young, R. D., & Sher, K. J. (1983). Self-awareness-reducing effects of alcohol consumption. *Journal of Personality and Social Psychology, 44*, 461–473.

Iyengar, S. S., & DeVoe, S. E. (2003). Rethinking the value of choice: Considering cultural mediators of intrinsic motivation. In V. Murphy-Berman & J. Berman (Eds.), *Cross-cultural differences in perspectives on the self: Nebraska symposium on motivation* (Vol 49, pp. 146–191). University of Nebraska Press.

Iyengar, S. S., & Lepper, M. (2000). When choice is demotivating: Can one desire too much of a good thing? *Journal of Personality and Social Psychology, 79*, 995–1006.

Iyengar, S. S., Wells, R. E., & Schwartz, B. (2006). Doing better but feeling worse: Looking for the "best" job undermines satisfaction. *Psychological Science, 17*, 143–150.

Jackson, J. C., Gelfand, M., De, S., & Fox, A. (2019). The loosening of American culture over 200 years is associated with a creativity-order trade-off. *Nature Human Behaviour, 3*, 244–250.

Jaffé, M. E., Douneva, M., Bartlome, R., & Greifeneder, R. (2023). A million reasons or just one? How coin flips impact the number of relevant reasons for decisions. *European Journal of Social Psychology, 53*, 872–889.

Jeffries, P., & Ungar, M. (2020). Social anxiety in young people: A prevalence study in seven countries. *PLOS One, 15*, e0239133.

Jouhki, H., & Oksanen, A. (2022). To get high or to get out?: Examining the link between addictive behaviors and escapism. *Substance Use and Misuse, 57*, 202–211.

Keren, G., & Teigen, K. H. (2010). Decision by coin toss: Inappropriate but fair. *Judgment and Decision Making, 5*, 83–101.

Keyes, K. M., Gary, D., O'Malley, P. M., Hamilton, A., & Schulenberg, J. (2019). Recent increases in depressive symptoms among US adolescents: Trends from 1991 to 2018. *Social Psychiatry and Psychiatric Epidemiology, 54*, 987–996.

Keyes, K. M., Kreski, N. T., & Patrick, M. E. (2024). Depressive symptoms in adolescence and young adulthood. *JAMA Network Open, 7*, Article e2427748.

Kierkegaard, S. (1980). *The concept of anxiety: A simple psychologically orienting deliberation on the dogmatic issue of hereditary sin*. Princeton University Press. (Original work published 1844)

Kolmar, C. (2023, June 27). *23 gripping book industry statistics [2023]: How many books were published in 2022*. Zippia. www.zippia.com/advice/us-book-industry-statistics/.

Koole, S. L., Greenberg, J., & Pyszczynski, T. (2006). Introducing science to the psychology of the soul: Experimental existential psychology. *Current Directions in Psychological Science, 15*, 212–216.

Korous, K. M., Causadias, J. M., Bradley, R H., Levy, R., Cahill, K. M., Li, L., & Luthar, S. S. (2023). "More is better" or "better near the middle"? A U.S.-based individual participant data meta-analysis of socioeconomic status and depressive symptoms. *American Psychologist, 78*, 305–320.

Krockow, E. M. (2018, September 27). How many decisions do we make each day? *Psychology Today*. www.psychologytoday.com/us/blog/stretching-theory/201809/how-many-decisions-do-we-make-each-day.

Levav, J., Heitmann, M., Herrmann, A., & Iyengar, S. S. (2010). Order in product customization decisions: Evidence from field experiments. *Journal of Political Economy, 118*, 274–299.

Levy, S. J. (1959). Symbols for sale. *Harvard Business Review, July-August*, 117–124.

Limburg, K., Watson, H. J., Hagger, M. S., & Egan, S. J. (2017). The relationship between perfectionism and psychopathology: A meta-analysis. *Journal of Clinical Psychology, 73*, 1301–1326.

Lin, S. C., & Reich, T. (2018). To give or not to give? Choosing chance under moral conflict. *Journal of Consumer Psychology, 28*, 211–233.

Linder, J. A., Doctor, J. N., Friedberg, M. W., Reyes Nieva, H., Birks, C., Meeker, D., & Fox, C. R. (2014). Time of day and the decision to prescribe antibiotics. *JAMA Internal Medicine, 174*, 2029–2031.

Lipson, S. K., Lattie, E. G., & Eisenberg, D. (2019). Increased rates of mental health service utilization by U.S. college students: 10-year population-level trends (2007–2017). *Psychiatric Services, 70*, 60–63.

Luthar, S. S., Barkin, S. H., & Crossman, E. J. (2013). "I can, therefore I must": Fragility in the upper-middle classes. *Development and Psychopathology, 25*, 1529–1549.

Luthar, S. S., Kumar, N. L., & Zillmer, N. (2020). High-achieving schools connote risks for adolescents: Problems documented, processes implicated, and directions for interventions. *American Psychologist, 75,* 983–995.

Markus, H. R., & Kitayama, S. (1991). Culture and the self: Implications for cognition, emotion, and motivation. *Psychological Review, 98,* 224–253.

Markus, H., & Nurius, P. (1986). Possible selves. *American Psychologist, 41,* 954–969.

Markus, H. R., & Schwartz, B. (2010). Does choice mean freedom and well-being? *Journal of Consumer Psychology, 37,* 344–355.

Marples, M. (2022, April 22). *Decision fatigue drains you of your energy to make thoughtful choices. Here's how to get it back.* CNN. www.cnn.com/2022/04/21/health/decision-fatigue-solutions-wellness/index.html.

Meneghini, A. M. (2016). A meaningful break in a flat life: The motivations behind overseas volunteering. *Nonprofit and Voluntary Sector Quarterly, 45,* 1214–1233.

Misuraca, R., Reutskaja, E., Fasolo, B., & Iyengar, S. (2020). How much choice is "good enough"? Moderators of information and choice overload. In R. Viale (Ed.), *Routledge handbook of bounded rationality* (pp. 637–649). Routledge.

Mojtabai, R., Olfson, M., & Han, B. (2016). National trends in the prevalence and treatment of depression in adolescents and young adults. *Pediatrics, 138,* e20161878.

Moyano-Díaz, E., Martínez-Molina, A., & Ponce, F. P. (2014). The price of gaining: Maximization in decision-making, regret, and life satisfaction. *Judgment and Decision Making, 9,* 500–509.

Mull, A. (2019, February 12). How fancy water bottles became a 21st-century status symbol. *The Atlantic.* www.theatlantic.com/health/archive/2019/02/luxury-water-bottles/582595/.

Mull, A. (2024, January 19). It's just a water bottle. *The Atlantic.* www.theatlantic.com/technology/archive/2024/01/stanley-cups-valentines-day-target-starbucks/677190/.

Myers, D. (2000). *The American paradox.* Yale University Press.

Ng, J. Y. Y., Ntoumanis, N., Thøgersen-Ntoumani, C., Deci, E. L., Ryan, R. M., Duda, J. L., & Williams, G. C. (2012). Self-determination theory applied to health contexts: A meta-analysis. *Perspectives on Psychological Science, 7,* 325–340.

Office of the Surgeon General. (2023). *Our epidemic of loneliness and isolation.* www.hhs.gov/sites/default/files/surgeon-general-social-connection-advisory.pdf.

Orasanu, J., Parke, B., Kraft, N., Tada, Y., Hobbs, A., Anderson, B., . . . Dulchinos, V. (2012). *Evaluating the effectiveness of schedule changes for air traffic service (ATS) providers: Controller alertness and fatigue monitoring study.* Federal Aviation Administration Technical Report. https://humanfactors.arc.nasa.gov/publications/Orasanu_et_al_Controller_Alertness_Fatigue_Monitoring.pdf.

Oswalt, S. B., Lederer, A. M., Chestnut-Steich, K., Day, C., Halbritter, A., & Ortiz, D. (2020). Trends in college students' mental health diagnoses and utilization of services, 2009–2015. *Journal of American College Health, 68,* 41–51.

Oto, B. (2012). When thinking is hard: Managing decision fatigue. *EMS World, 41*(5), 46–50.

Pignatiello, G. A., & Hickman, R. L., Jr. (2019). Correlates of cognitive load in surrogate decision makers of the critically ill. *Western Journal of Nursing Research, 41,* 650–666.

Pignatiello, G. A., Martin, R. J., & Hickman, R. L., Jr. (2020). Decision fatigue: A conceptual analysis. *Journal of Health Psychology, 25,* 123–135.

Polman, E., & Vohs, K. D. (2016). Decision fatigue, choosing for others, and self-construal. *Social Psychological and Personality Science, 7,* 471–478.

Ratner, R. K., & Kahn, B. E. (2002). The impact of private versus public consumption on variety-seeking behavior. *Journal of Consumer Research, 29,* 246–257.

Reed, A. E., Mikels, J. A., & Simon, K. I. (2008). Older adults prefer less choice than younger adults. *Psychology and Aging, 23,* 671–675.

Reibstein, D., Youngblood, S., & Fromkin, H. (1975). Number of choices as a factor in consumer satisfaction: An empirical study. *Journal of Applied Psychology, 60,* 434–437.

Reutskaja, E., Cheek, N. N., Iyengar, S., & Schwartz, B. (2022a). Choice deprivation, choice overload, and satisfaction with choices across six nations. *Journal of International Marketing, 30,* 18–34.

Reutskaja, E., Cheek, N. N., Iyengar, S., & Schwartz, B. (2022b). *Choice deprivation, choice overload, and satisfaction with life across six nations.* [Unpublished raw data].

Reutskaja, E., & Hogarth, R. M. (2009). Satisfaction in choice as a function of the number of alternatives: When "goods satiate." *Psychology and Marketing, 26,* 197–203.

Reutskaja, E., Linder, A., Nagel, R., Andersen, R. A., & Camerer, C. F. (2018). Choice overload reduces neural signatures of choice set value in dorsal striatum and anterior cingulate cortex. *Nature Human Behaviour, 2,* 925–935.

Richeson, J. A. (2020). Americans are determined to believe in Black progress. *The*

Atlantic. www.theatlantic.com/magazine/archive/2020/09/the-mythology-of-racial-progress/614173/.

Richins, M. L. (2017). Materialism pathways: The processes that create and perpetuate materialism. *Journal of Consumer Psychology, 27,* 480–499.

Rios Morrison, K., & Johnson, C. S. (2011). When what you have is who you are: Self-uncertainty leads individualists to see themselves in their possessions. *Personality and Social Psychology Bulletin, 37,* 639–651.

Ryan, R. M., & Deci, E. L. (2000). Self-determination theory and the facilitation of intrinsic motivation, social development, and well-being. *American Psychologist, 55,* 68–78.

Ryan, R. M., Duineveld, J. J., Di Domenico, S. I., Ryan, W. S., Steward, B. A., & Bradshaw, E. L. (2022). We know this much is (meta-analytically) true: A meta-review of meta-analytic findings evaluating self-determination theory. *Psychological Bulletin, 148,* 813–842.

Sandstrom, G. M., & Dunn, E. W. (2014). Social interactions and well-being: The surprising power of weak ties. *Personality and Social Psychology Bulletin, 40,* 910–922.

Savary, J., & Dhar, R. (2020). The uncertain self: How self-concept structure affects subscription choice. *Journal of Consumer Research, 46,* 887–903.

Scheibehenne, B., Greifeneder, R., & Todd, P. M. (2010). Can there ever be too many options? A meta-analytic review of choice overload. *Journal of Consumer Research, 37,* 409–425.

Schwartz, B. (2000). Self-determination: The tyranny of freedom. *American Psychologist, 55,* 79–88.

Schwartz, B. (2016). *The paradox of choice: Why more is less* (2nd ed.). Ecco Press.

Schwartz, B., & Cheek, N. N. (2017). Choice, freedom, and well-being: Considerations for public policy. *Behavioural Public Policy, 1,* 106–121.

Schwartz, B., Ward, A., Monterosso, J., Lyubomirsky, S., White, K., & Lehman, D. R. (2002). Maximizing versus satisficing: Happiness is a matter of choice. *Journal of Personality and Social Psychology, 83,* 1178–1197.

Seamster, L., & Ray, V. (2018). Against teleology in the study of race: Toward the abolition of the progress paradigm. *Sociological Theory, 36,* 315–342.

Shah, A. M., & Wolford, G. (2007). Buying behavior as a function of parametric variation of number of choices. *Psychological Science, 18,* 369–370.

Sirgy, M. J. (1982). Self-concept in consumer behavior: A critical review. *Journal of Consumer Research, 9,* 287–300.

Staub, E. (1989). *The roots of evil: The psychological and cultural origins of genocide and other forms of group violence.* Cambridge University Press.

Stenseng, F., Rise, J., & Kraft, P. (2012). Activity engagement as escape from self: The role of self-suppression and self-expansion. *Leisure Sciences, 34,* 19–38.

Stewart, A. F., Ferriero, D. M., Josephson, S. A., Lowenstein, D. H., Messing, R. O., Oksenberg, J. R., . . . Hauser, S. L. (2012). Fighting decision fatigue. *Annals of Neurology, 71,* A5–A15.

Sunstein, C. R. (2015). *Choosing not to choose: Understanding the value of choice.* Oxford University Press.

Tajfel, H. (1978). The achievement of inter-group differentiation. In H. Tajfel (Ed.), *Differentiation between social groups* (pp. 77–100). Academic Press.

Tajfel, H., & Turner, J. C. (1979). An integrative theory of inter-group conflict. In W. G. Austin & S. Worchel (Eds.), *The social psychology of inter-group relations* (pp. 33–47). Brooks/Cole.

Tamir, D. I., & Mitchell, J. P. (2012). Disclosing information about the self is intrinsically rewarding. *Proceedings of the National Academy of Sciences, 109,* 8038–8043.

Tanius, B. E., Wood, S., Hanoch, Y., & Rice, T. (2009). Aging and choice: Applications to Medicare Part D. *Judgment and Decision Making, 4,* 92–101.

Taylor, C. (1989). *Sources of the self.* Harvard University Press.

Taylor, C. (1992). *The ethics of authenticity.* Harvard University Press.

Thapar, A., Eyre, O., Patel, V., & Brent, D. (2022). Depression in young people. *Lancet, 400,* 617–631.

Toffler, A. (1990). *Future shock.* Bantam Books. (Original work published 1970)

Triandis, H. C. (1989). The self and social behavior in differing cultural contexts. *Psychological Review, 96,* 506–520.

Tropp, L. R., & Wright, S. C. (2001). Ingroup identification as the inclusion of ingroup in the self. *Personality and Social Psychology Bulletin, 27,* 585–600.

Turner, J. C., Hogg, M. A., Oakes, P. J., Reicher, S. D., & Wetherell, M. S. (1987). *Rediscovering the social group: A self-categorization theory.* Blackwell.

Turner, R. H. (1976). The real self: From institution to impulse. *American Journal of Sociology, 81,* 989–1016.

van den Bos, K., & Miedema, J. (2000). Toward understanding why fairness matters: The influence of mortality salience on reactions to procedural fairness. *Journal of Personality and Social Psychology, 79,* 355–366.

van Prooijen, J.-W. (2016). Sometimes inclusion breeds suspicion: Self-uncertainty and belongingness predict belief in conspiracy theories. *European Journal of Social Psychology, 46,* 267–279.

Vansteenkiste, M., Ryan, R. M., & Soenens, B. (2020). Basic psychological need theory: Advancements, critical themes, and future directions. *Motivation and Emotion, 44,* 1–31.

Vohs, K. D., Baumeister, R. F., Schmeichel, B. J., Twenge, J. M., Nelson, N. M., & Tice, D. M. (2008). Making choices impairs subsequent self-control: A limited-resource account of decision making, self-regulation, and active initiative. *Journal of Personality and Social Psychology, 94,* 883–898.

Weinberger, A. H., Gbedemah, M., Martinez, A. M., Nash, D., Galea, S., & Goodwin, R. D. (2018). Trends in depression prevalence in the USA from 2005 to 2015: Widening disparities in vulnerable groups. *Psychological Medicine, 48,* 1308–1315.

Wisman, A., & Heflick, N., & Goldenberg, J. L. (2015). The great escape: The role of self-esteem and self-related cognition in terror management. *Journal of Experimental Social Psychology, 60,* 121–132.

Yu, S., Levesque-Bristol, C., & Maeda, Y. (2018). General need for autonomy and subjective well-being: A meta-analysis of studies in the US and East Asia. *Journal of Happiness Studies, 19,* 1863–1882.

CHAPTER 23

The Art of Choosing

Navigating the Benefits and Costs of Choice

Elena Reutskaja *and* Raffaella Misuraca

The concept of choice is fundamental to human decision making and is deeply ingrained in the fabric of modern society. It is often celebrated as a cornerstone of freedom and autonomy, allowing individuals to tailor their decisions to their preferences and needs. This perspective, embraced by existential psychologists such as Rollo May, Viktor Frankl, and Søren Kierkegaard, is particularly prominent in Western cultures, where an abundance of choice is equated with greater personal freedom and well-being (Schwartz, 2004). However, as existential psychology suggests, choice is a double-edged sword. On the one hand, it represents the freedom and the autonomy of an individual, but on the other, it brings with it the weight of responsibility and the potential for anxiety (May, 1950). In line with this existential view, a large body of modern research across various disciplines reveals that while choice can offer substantial benefits, it also comes with significant costs that can overwhelm and demotivate decision makers (Chernev et al., 2015; Iyengar & Lepper, 2000; Reutskaja et al., 2020). Moderate assortments of alternatives have been shown to be more motivating and satisfying for decision makers, and result in greater choice accuracy (Iyengar & Lepper, 2000; Jacoby, Speller, & Berning, 1974; Jacoby, Speller, & Kohn, 1974; Malhotra, 1982; Reutskaja & Hogarth, 2009; Reutskaja et al., 2018; Shah & Wolford, 2007). Research indicates that the relationship between the number of options and the net benefit to decision makers follows an inverted-U function: Too few choices can be as detrimental as too many, with the greatest net benefit occurring at a moderate number of options (Grant & Schwartz, 2011; Reutskaja & Hogarth, 2009).

This chapter explores the benefits and costs of choice, building on empirical evidence from psychology, economics, neuroscience, and marketing. We begin by discussing the numerous benefits of choice, including increased utility, competitive advantages, freedom, autonomy, personal control, authenticity, self-actualization, and psychological well-being. Next, we explore the costs associated with extensive choice, such as time, cognitive, and psychic burdens. We then present the conceptual model of the inverted-U function, supported by empirical evidence demonstrating that many choice outcomes follow this pattern. Finally, we discuss factors that influence the optimal assortment size and provide insights for choice architects on how to create environments that maximize satisfaction, motivation, and decision quality. Through this comprehensive examination, we aim to offer a balanced perspective on the complexity of choice, highlighting that while choice is essential for autonomy and well-being, it must be managed carefully to avoid the pitfalls of both deprivation and overload.

THE BENEFITS AND COSTS OF CHOICE

The Benefits of Choice

The provision of choice offers numerous benefits. As a thought experiment, imagine you have just traveled with your friends to a new country. You need to go grocery shopping. Besides purchasing items for the upcoming dinner and breakfast, you need to stock the apartment with necessities like soap, shampoo, and napkins for your stay over the few weeks. You discover that there are two grocery stores equally distant from your apartment. One store is small. It is neatly organized and clean but has a limited variety of products. There are only a few options in each product category: two or three types of soaps, three or four types of yogurt, two or three types of noodles and tomato sauces, three or four types of bakery products, three or four types of wines, and so on. The other store is large. It is also well-organized and clean but stocked with many different products and offers a vast variety of options within each category. The number of options per category is more than 15 and, depending on the category, it can range from 20–30 (for yogurt or soft drinks) to even hundreds (e.g., for wines). Which store would you choose?

Increased Likelihood of Matching Preferences

If you are like most people in the Western world, you would prefer the second store. There may be several reasons for this preference. First, there is a purely rational reason: Shoppers maximize their chances of finding a product that closely matches their preferences in a larger store. The probability of having exactly what you want and need available is simply higher in a larger store compared to a smaller one. In economic terms, people can maximize their utility and obtain the best option when the set of choices is large (Von Neumann & Morgenstern, 1944). If you are a white wine enthusiast, the chances that not only white wine but your favorite bottle is available are higher in the larger store. The likelihood that a shampoo with the right pH level, preferred smell, desired function (e.g., lightening, for flaky scalp or for curly hair), and from the preferred brand is available in the store is also higher in the larger store compared to the smaller one. The same logic would apply to almost any product category. Although the small store might carry a soap that is fully functional and "good enough," that soap might lack the perfect smell and moisturizing features that would make it an "ideal" soap you would love to have. In sum, one might prefer the larger store over the smaller one since the probability that the "ideal" soap, shampoo, or wine that perfectly matches your preferences is available is higher in the larger store.

Economic Benefits

Second, there is another compelling reason why larger stores are often preferred, rooted in economic principles. A higher number of choices promotes competition and benefits from economies of scale. When companies compete more intensively, they aim to attract customers by offering higher-quality products and services, and lower prices. These benefits of competition are fundamental to Western economies, where providing a variety of choices fosters a competitive market environment.

In larger stores, numerous competitive products within the same category are displayed side by side, enabling consumers to compare them simultaneously. Access to relevant information is highly valued by consumers (Jacoby, Speller, & Berning, 1974; Jacoby, Speller, & Kohn, 1974). Comparing products side by side enhances information transparency and, thus, the feeling of being informed.

As companies recognize that consumers can compare multiple products in large stores, they are incentivized to produce superior products, design attractive packaging, and offer competitive prices and promotions. These competitive advantages are more pronounced in larger stores compared to smaller ones. Smaller stores often carry a limited selection of products (e.g., budget options, well-known national brands, and intermediate products), reducing the incentive for producers to offer substantial promotions. Moreover, larger stores benefit from economies of scale, reducing costs associated with sales staff and space, and possessing greater negotiation power with producers. As a result, they are often better positioned to offer lower prices to their customers overall. Thus, customers frequently benefit from more competitive prices and promotions by shopping at larger stores, which offer greater choice, better prices, and higher-quality products compared to stores with limited alternatives.

However, on a broader scale, the economic benefits of increased product variety may extend far beyond the gains from competition and lower prices. Research has demonstrated that the benefits from increased product variety can generate higher consumer surplus than the efficiency gains derived from increased competition (Brynjolfsson et al., 2003). The authors estimated consumer welfare gains from increased product variety in online bookstores versus brick-and-mortar stores, finding that benefits from wider selection were 7–10 times larger than those from increased competition and lower prices.

Psychological Benefits

Third, there are numerous psychological benefits associated with large stores for consumers. Greater choice is simply psychologically more attractive than a limited selection. This attractiveness of larger assortments was demonstrated in a seminal experiment conducted in a grocery store in California (Iyengar & Lepper, 2000). In this study, researchers set up a tasting booth with two types of display of jams: In one setting, the tasting booth presented six different jams, while in the other setting, it displayed 24 different jams. The shoppers were free to stop by and taste any of the jams. They also received a $1 discount coupon for potential jam purchases.

The researchers found that when the booth displayed a larger array of options (24 jams), more shoppers (60%) stopped at the booth compared to when it offered only six jams (40%). This experiment offers evidence of an initial attractiveness to large assortments. In Western societies, people generally prefer having choice and find greater choice more attractive than limited options. Thus, when asked to choose between two different stores—a large one or a small one—individuals are likely to initially prefer the large store.

Research in psychology has also demonstrated that choice channels the positive feelings of freedom, autonomy, and control (Botti et al., 2023)—key existential concepts highly valued in Western societies. Choice itself, even a not very consequential choice such as selecting soap or detergent, can enhance positive feelings and happiness compared with situations where no choice is available. For example, a study by Langer and Rodin (1976) explored the impact of decision-making opportunities in nursing homes. Their research revealed that residents experienced enhanced happiness and satisfaction when they were allowed to make choices, even when those decisions were trivial or minor.

Research has also indicated that an increased number of options correlates with a heightened sense of decision freedom (Reibstein et al., 1975; Steiner, 1970; Walton & Berkowitz, 1979). In fact, in Western societies, choice has become almost synonymous with freedom (Markus & Schwartz, 2010). The ability to make decisions fosters a sense of autonomy and control over one's life, fulfilling a core existential need for personal agency and the creation of meaning. This relationship between choice and autonomy was well illustrated by existential psychologists such as Viktor Frankl (1946/2006), who argued that autonomy promotes intrinsic motivation, allowing individuals to engage more meaningfully with their lives (see also Deci & Ryan, 1985; Ryan & Deci, 2000; Zuckerman et al., 1978). In line with existential psychology, having a range of options also empowers individuals to make choices that align with their authentic values and beliefs, rather than merely conforming to societal pressures or external expectations. Heidegger (1927/1962), in his exploration of authenticity, emphasized that genuine decision making involves the freedom to choose in accordance with one's true self. Thus, the provision of choice extends beyond the specific act of choosing—it reinforces a sense of self-determination, authenticity, and personal growth, fostering an overall improvement in life satisfaction and well-being.

To summarize, expanded choice offers numerous benefits: It increases the likelihood that an option in the set will match individual preferences; it enhances information transparency and increases customer surplus through the benefits of competition and variety; and it also promotes autonomy, control, and freedom, which can lead to greater life satisfaction, personal growth, authenticity, and well-being, aligning with existential psychology's emphasis on the importance of freedom in shaping human experience.

The Costs of Choice

Despite the many benefits of choice, anyone who has visited a large department store to choose an item from a new product category (e.g., wall paint or curtains) can recognize that choosing among a large number of items is far from straightforward. Existential psychologists like Rollo May have long claimed that while choice provides freedom, it also comes with responsibility and anxiety over making the "right" decision (May, 1950). Recent research confirms that choice not only brings benefits but also incurs costs (Grant & Schwartz, 2011; Loewenstein, 1999; Reutskaja & Hogarth, 2009; Schwartz, 2000, 2004). We now examine these costs in more detail.

Time Costs

Greater choice usually implies increased time costs. Considering our previous example of choosing between a larger or smaller store for purchasing basic items for a vacation apartment, an individual will likely spend considerably more time choosing in the larger store compared to the smaller one, resulting in higher time costs when choosing from large assortments compared to smaller ones.

In many situations, people do not have well-established preferences beforehand and develop their preferences on the spot (Slovic, 1995). Without well-established preferences, uncertainty about which soap, shampoo, or wine to buy, coupled with decision making in a new store, can make choosing challenging. Aiming to choose "the best" item that potentially aligns with personal preferences requires the decision maker to do a lot of work: processing and examining all available options, evaluating the information on the alternatives' distinguishing attributes, making tradeoffs between the available alternatives, and finally deciding which item to purchase. As the number of options in the choice set increases, the time necessary to attend to and process the alternatives also increases, as does the time required to compare them and make a selection from them.

The temporal cost associated with excessive information and choice has been extensively researched. To consciously identify a visual object and consolidate it in short-term working memory before being able to start processing a second stimulus, an individual may require more than half a second (Marois & Ivanoff, 2005). When the quantity of options in the choice set is large, the time cost of just processing these options may be considerable. Indeed, a positive linear relationship has been observed between the total quantity of accessible information and the duration spent on its processing and evaluation (Jacoby, Speller, & Berning, 1974; Jacoby, Speller, & Kohn, 1974). However, some physiological evidence, specifically eye movement patterns, suggests that people can marginally reduce processing time per item as the choice set expands when pressed for time during decision making (Reutskaja et al., 2011). Nevertheless, overall time spent on selection increases significantly with choice set size. Thus, the total choice time typically grows with choice set size.

In addition to processing and evaluating alternatives, decision makers need to compare alternatives and make often challenging tradeoffs. The number of tradeoffs and comparisons an individual needs to make increases with available alternatives. Consider, for example, the number of comparisons necessary for four soaps in a smaller store versus 20 soaps in a larger store. Assuming the soaps differ on a single attribute, such as smell (i.e., the alternatives are "unidimensional"), and all other attributes like brand, price, or soap weight remain constant, a consumer needs to make six pairwise comparisons when comparing four soaps versus 190 comparisons when comparing 20 soaps. A customer confronted with 150 different choice items would need to make 11,175 pairwise comparisons. And this number of comparisons is only true if one assumes items differ on one dimension only. Thus, time costs associated with comparisons and tradeoffs may grow at an increasing rate if an individual examines and compares all alternatives. Previous research has consistently demonstrated that individuals require more time to reach a decision when presented with larger choice sets compared to smaller ones (Iyengar & Lepper, 2000). Furthermore, research has suggested that as the number of alternatives within a choice set grows, decision-making time escalates across the entire spectrum of task complexity (Hogarth, 1975; Loewenstein, 2000).

Time costs are likely to be higher for larger sets compared to smaller ones, even when people have strong and well-established preferences. Although in many situations people lack well-established preferences, in some cases individuals may have a clear idea of what to choose, which should facilitate decision making. For example, a shopper could enter a store with a specific shopping list on which all items to be purchased are clearly listed. However, one may argue that even in this situation, when individuals know which items from the shopping list they need to buy (assuming these items are available in both large and small stores), the shopping time would still likely be higher in the larger store compared to the smaller one.

This is likely due to higher search costs associated with larger versus smaller sets, meaning an individual still needs to locate that exact bottle of wine or specific shampoo appearing on their shopping list. As a thought experiment, imagine standing in front of wine shelves with only 15 different wines in a small store compared to 300 different wines in a large store. The mere exercise of finding your preferred bottle of wine among 300 different options would be significantly more time-consuming than finding this wine among 15 alternatives.

In the digital world, search time can decrease compared to brick-and-mortar stores. Nevertheless, it is still reasonable to assume that unless search algorithms are optimally built and decision makers are highly capable of creating precise prompts, search costs would be higher in larger online stores like Amazon, which carry millions of items, compared to a small digital store offering only hundreds.

To summarize, regardless of whether an individual has well-established preferences or not when choosing, time costs are likely to be higher for larger assortments compared to smaller ones.

Cognitive Costs

Another downside of excessive information and too much choice is that it imposes high cognitive costs on decision makers. These costs are closely connected to time costs, but they are cognitive in nature. Cognitive costs refer to mental resources necessary for attending to alternatives, processing information about choice options and their attributes, evaluating and comparing alternatives, and making a selection. While time costs are measured by the amount of time spent on decision making, cognitive costs are measured by the mental resources expended during choice and the number of errors decision makers commit.

In his classic paper "The Magic Number Seven, Plus or Minus Two," George Miller (1956) proposed that human abilities to receive, process, and remember information accurately are limited. Therefore, the amount of information provided to a decision maker as input may not equal the amount of information that is actually transmitted and processed. When the amount of information is low, it can be transmitted without errors, making the input and transmitted information equivalent. However, as the amount of input information increases, the number of errors humans make also rises. Consequently, the amount of transmitted information will plateau at some point and will not increase as the amount of input information continues to grow. That is, the amount of transmitted information is limited by the human capacity to process different types of information without errors. Miller referred to this capacity as "channel capacity." Channel capacity differs for different types of unidimensional stimuli;

nevertheless, it is surprisingly low. Miller argued that channel capacity is highest for visual stimuli, enabling decision makers to process 10–15 visual positions accurately. Beyond these numbers, individuals will start making errors. Channel capacity is lower for other types of stimuli: approximately four for tastes or six for tones and sounds. An individual can increase channel capacity by processing various dimensions of an item; however, the precision and accuracy for each dimension will decline.

This foundational research suggests that people would face fewer cognitive constraints when attending to, processing, and evaluating items in small sets. Large choice sets can impose high cognitive costs on decision makers. How large a choice set can be depends on the type of items an individual chooses from: It is presumably less cognitively costly to process larger choice sets with visual stimuli (e.g., fashion accessories) than with audio items (e.g., selections of songs).

Further research has expanded upon Miller's (1956) work, suggesting that larger amounts of information and choice impose cognitive costs on decision makers. Nobel laureate Herbert Simon elaborated on this idea, positing that people rarely make decisions considering all possible information (Simon, 1976). He suggested that people are "bounded" in their decision making by various constraints, including cognitive capacity and human processing abilities. Simon (1974) proposed that the brain possesses a "chunk" capacity, advising that short-term memory can retain approximately five to seven pieces of information. Thus, it is cognitively demanding for individuals to process excessively large choice assortments.

Measuring many covert processes and costs underlying decisions, such as attention, can be challenging. Recent studies have employed modern techniques such as eye tracking and brain imaging to investigate the choice overload phenomenon. Some research suggests that the brain's short-term memory capacity for simultaneously maintaining or monitoring information is relatively limited, with individuals typically able to process only about four objects simultaneously, regardless of the number of objects presented (Marois & Ivanoff, 2005). This supports previous research findings.

Eye-tracking research has also revealed that attention costs increase when individuals make choices from larger sets of alternatives under time constraints compared to smaller sets (Reutskaja et al., 2011). In an eye-tracking experiment, subjects chose snacks from different-sized choice sets. As the number of available snack options increased, the number of eye fixations—continuous looks at an object for 200–400 milliseconds—also increased. Eye fixations usually reflect the processing of and attention to different stimuli; consequently, a greater number of fixations for larger sets could indicate higher attention and processing costs compared to smaller choice sets. Furthermore, the number of options that participants looked at was higher when choosing from larger sets compared to smaller ones (though the percentage of items seen decreased with choice set size), indicating higher costs associated with larger versus smaller sets.

Another study investigating the mechanisms underlying the choice overload phenomenon used both eye-tracking and functional magnetic resonance imaging (fMRI) to monitor the eye-movements and brain activity of participants choosing landscape images from sets of different sizes (Reutskaja et al., 2018). Participants making selections from large choice sets of landscape images showed an increased number of eye movements and stronger activity in visual and sensorimotor brain areas compared with those choosing from smaller sets, which have previously been linked to movement planning and control, as well as visual scene processing. The greater number of eye movements and increased brain activity indicated that cognitive load—and thus cognitive costs—were greater for choice from large sets of alternatives compared to smaller sets.

To summarize, empirical evidence suggests that larger choice sets impose higher cognitive costs on decision makers compared to smaller choice sets. Additionally, choosing from extensive assortments is associated with greater perceived (self-reported) decision difficulty (Iyengar & Lepper, 2000; Reutskaja & Hogarth, 2009; Reutskaja et al., 2018). Thus, when an individual decides to go to a larger store rather than a small one, they should bear in mind that choosing from large assortments may be cognitively taxing.

Psychological (Psychic) Costs

Finally, making choices in a large store can be psychologically challenging. Reutskaja and Hogarth (2009) suggested that larger choice assortments impose higher psychic costs on decision makers (see also Loewenstein, 1999). Unlike cognitive costs, psychic costs are associated with affective states of decision makers either during the choice process or after the choice has been made. These psychic costs are emotional ("hot") rather than cognitive ("cold") in nature. These costs can manifest in several ways.

First, as many people lack stable preferences (Slovic, 1995), uncertainty about what to choose and lack of expertise can cause discomfort and emotional strain during choice, especially when faced with options that offer difficult tradeoffs (Loewenstein, 1999). The psychological costs associated with extensive choice can transform what should be a positive experience into a stressful one, converting the "freedom" of choice into a form of "tyranny" (Schwartz, 2000). Existential psychology echoes this perspective, as thinkers like Rollo May have argued that the freedom to choose inherently carries with it the burden of responsibility, which can lead to indecision and anxiety (May, 1950). As Sartre (1943/1956) argued, human beings are "condemned to be free," meaning that we are always faced with choices and the responsibility that comes with them.

Second, the decision-making process itself can create challenges. The act of decision making inherently encompasses an emotional tension that arises from the fundamental nature of choice, where selecting one option inevitably means forgoing others. Existentialists argue that this emotional burden reflects the human struggle with the weight of autonomy and the responsibility that accompanies freedom, as individuals must live with the consequences of their decisions. As Botti and Iyengar (2006) noted, this intrinsic tradeoff in the decision process can evoke conflicting emotions, as individuals must reconcile the positive aspects of their chosen option with the potential benefits they are forgoing from alternatives not selected. Moreover, as people closely examine available alternatives, they may develop an "attachment" to the options in the choice set, creating a feeling of ownership even when these items are not actually owned by the decision maker (Carmon et al., 2003). Consequently, decision makers might experience a sense of "loss" for the items they ultimately fail to select, which in turn creates negative emotional responses. This effect is amplified as the number of unselected options increases, leading to greater postchoice discomfort for decision makers when they choose from larger rather than smaller assortments.

Third, individuals may experience anxiety or regret about potentially making an incorrect decision (Loewenstein, 1999). The probability of "missing" the best option due to high search and cognitive costs increases with large assortments. People do not have unlimited time and lack cognitive resources to examine all alternatives and find their perfect option, and thus they might select a suboptimal option even when the perfect alternative is available in the choice set, a concern emphasized in existential psychology, where the responsibility of choice is often linked to anxiety and potential regret (May, 1950). In an eye-tracking study Reutskaja and colleagues (2011) demonstrated that the probability of picking the best item from the set of seen alternatives decreased as the choice set increased. While having expectations of finding a perfect shampoo in a large store, the failure to do so might lead to disappointment and negative feelings associated with the choice. Not being able to choose the perfect alternative can make people regret their choice afterward. Indeed, choice from large assortments is usually associated with lower confidence in one's decision (Lee & Lee, 2004; Malhotra, 1982).

Another psychic cost associated with choosing from large assortments is that the abundance of choice tends to elevate individuals' expectations regarding their decision outcomes (Schwartz, 2000). For example, in a notable study (Lenton et al., 2008), participants were presented with either a larger pool of 20–50 potential dating partners or a smaller set of four. Participants anticipated higher satisfaction with both their choice and selection process when choosing from larger sets versus limited choice. They also expected to feel less regret regarding their decision when choosing from the larger group of potential dating partners. However, when participants engaged in a simulated dating website scenario, they exhibited greater memory confusion and showed no significant improvement in their emotional states when selecting from 20 profiles compared to four. These results highlight the potential disconnect between predictions about the benefits of extensive choice and actual experiences when faced with such choices.

In sum, when an individual chooses whether to go to a larger or a smaller store to stock their apartment, they might initially feel strong inclinations to visit the larger store as the provision of choice offers positive feelings and benefits. People, especially in the Western world, like to have choice and even equate it with freedom. However, once in the store, they must face the detrimental consequences of choosing from larger assortments: Extensive choice can be cognitively and emotionally taxing, and choosing from large choice sets may be time-consuming and demotivating. To understand whether choice provision is beneficial overall, it is necessary to examine how the costs and benefits of choice are integrated. This is the focus on the next section of this chapter.

NET BENEFITS OF CHOICE FOLLOW AN INVERTED-U-SHAPED FUNCTION OF THE NUMBER OF ALTERNATIVES

As discussed previously, choice entails both benefits and costs. Previous research has suggested that both costs and benefits increase with the number of options available, but they do so at different rates. The benefits of choice are assumed to increase at a decreasing rate, consistent with the notion of diminishing marginal utility (Horowitz et al., 2007). This implies that adding one extra choice option generates a smaller increase in benefits than adding a previous choice item. However, the costs of choice are assumed to increase either linearly or at an increasing rate. Recall how the number of pairwise comparisons multiplies with the addition of one alternative to the set. Most importantly, as choice options increase, costs rise faster than benefits (Grant & Schwartz, 2011; Reutskaja & Hogarth, 2009).

One can derive a "net benefit" of choice by subtracting the costs from the benefits of choice. If the benefits of expanded choice grow at a diminishing rate, while the associated costs escalate more rapidly, the "net benefits" of choice would follow an inverted-U-shaped function relative to the number of alternatives, as illustrated in Figure 23.1.

This conceptual model yields two key insights. First, it suggests that individuals are likely to experience the highest net benefits from choice when selecting from assortments with a moderate number of options. Both larger and smaller sets are expected to provide fewer net benefits to decision makers than assortments with a moderate number of options.

The conceptual inverted-U model implies that when choice sets are relatively small, adding an extra alternative to the choice set would be beneficial, as the benefits of an additional choice alternative would exceed the costs of adding this item. Thus, initially, the net benefit curve is upward-sloping, and people are better off with more rather than less choice. The upward sloping part of the curve reflects "choice deprivation," or a feeling of having less choice than one would prefer to have "ideally."

However, at some point the net benefit curve reaches its peak and begins to level off. After this inflection point, adding extra alternatives to the choice set becomes counterproductive, as these new alternatives generate more costs for the decision maker than benefits, and the total net benefit decreases. When choosing from a large number of alternatives has detrimental consequences for decision makers, *choice overload* occurs. People stop appreciating the positive aspects of choice and become overwhelmed by the abundance of options.

The second implication of the inverted-U conceptual model is that shifts in perceived costs and benefits can alter the resulting "net benefit" curve and its peak. For example, when costs of choice increase (e.g., options become more complex) while the benefits remain constant, the peak of the resulting function is expected to shift leftward, and the optimal assortment size for the decision maker would become smaller than the original.

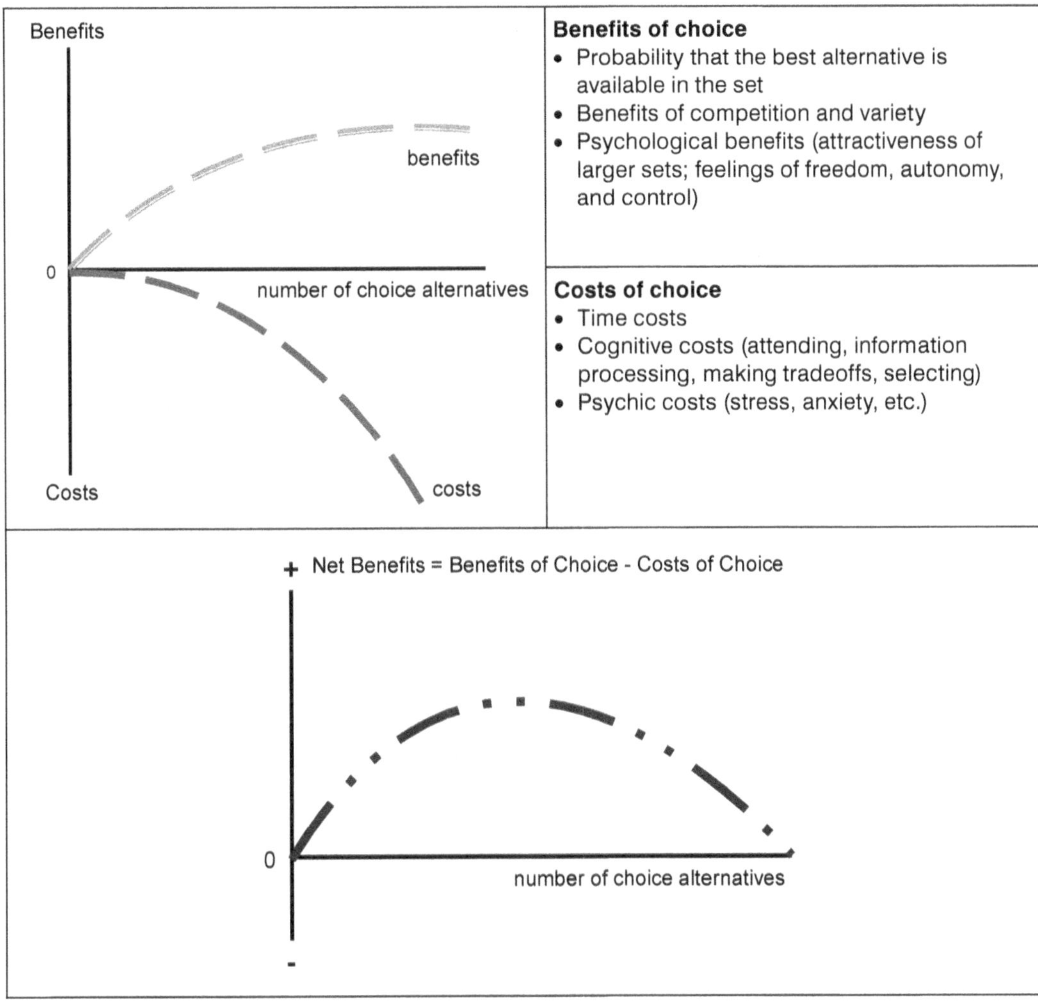

FIGURE 23.1. Net benefits of choice as a function of the number of alternatives in the choice set. Adapted from similar figures originally published in Reutskaja and Hogarth (2009).

There is no universally ideal choice set size. The optimal size of an assortment depends on various factors and, thus, should be assessed in each particular situation. Costs and benefits are influenced by the features of the decision environment and the individual characteristics of decision makers. Choice architects should carefully examine these factors to create optimal choice set sizes for specific situations.

We discuss both implications—the inverted-U curve and factors influencing costs and benefits—in more detail below.

EMPIRICAL EVIDENCE OF INVERTED-U-SHAPED FUNCTIONS OF NUMBER OF ALTERNATIVES

Numerous findings from previous research have consistently shown that several key variables—including decision motivation, choice quality, and satisfaction with both the choice process and the choice outcome—follow the pattern predicted by the conceptual model: Initially, the net benefit increases with the provision of choice, then it levels off. This empirical evidence reveals an inverted-U-shaped relationship between these key variables and the number of choice alternatives.

Motivation

First, the net benefit of choice can be measured as "motivation" for action, which includes motivation to choose, consume, buy, or engage in similar activities. Earlier empirical studies on choice have demonstrated that motivation increases with some choice and variety, as predicted by the conceptual model. For example, Rolls and colleagues (1981) demonstrated increased yogurt consumption when participants were presented with three visually distinct options compared to a single flavor. Kahn and Wansink (2004) further noted that both perceived and actual variety can boost consumption. This illustrates the upward-sloping part of the inverted-U-shaped function discussed earlier.

Conversely, excessive choice can be "demotivating." That is, motivation can decrease with more alternatives compared to fewer, consistent with the downward-sloping part of the inverted-U curve. The seminal "jam study" by Iyengar and Lepper (2000), which we discussed earlier, illustrated this paradox of choice: While more customers were attracted to a larger display of 24 jam flavors, fewer customers actually purchased jams when faced with the large assortment compared to a smaller display of six flavors.

The impact of excessive choice on crucial life decisions was further examined by Iyengar and colleagues (2004) in their study of U.S. 401(k) retirement plan participation. Analyzing plans offering between two and 59 investment choices, the researchers observed a consistent decline in participation as options increased. When only two fund options were available, plan enrollment reached its peak at 75%. However, this figure fell to 61% when participants faced an extensive array of 59 plan options. For each additional 10 options presented, the likelihood of individual participation in the 401(k) retirement plans decreased by approximately 1.5–2%. More choice demotivated employees from making a crucial decision that could positively affect their future well-being. These findings are consistent with the downward-sloping part of the curve representing the net benefits of choice.

Shah and Wolford (2007) examined buying behavior across a wide range of assortment sizes and empirically demonstrated that buying behavior follows an inverted-U function relative to the number of alternatives in the choice set. In their field experiment, participants could purchase pens from sets of varying sizes. The researchers found that participants bought more pens when presented with a set of 10 alternatives (intermediate sets), compared to sets containing two options (small sets) or 20 alternatives (larger sets). This finding suggests that, consistent with the inverted-U model, intermediate-sized choice sets are more effective at motivating purchases than either very limited or overly extensive arrays of options.

Interestingly, the inverted-U-shape phenomenon extends beyond observable behavior. Neuroimaging research has offered insights into the brain's response to choosing from different-sized assortments. A study employing fMRI revealed that brain activity in several decision-making regions—the striatum, associated with reward processing, and the anterior cingulate cortex (ACC), which balances costs and benefits—also exhibited an inverted-U function (Reutskaja et al., 2018). Consistent with behavioral studies, these regions showed peak activation when participants selected from choice sets of intermediate size (rather than small and large), which they also rated as having an optimal number of options, highlighting higher motivation and engagement in decision making when choosing from intermediate sets.

Choice Quality and Accuracy

Second, in addition to motivation, choice quality/accuracy—the ability to select the best option from the set—also exhibits an inverted-U pattern (Jacoby, Speller, & Berning, 1974; Jacoby, Speller, & Kohn, 1974). Several classic studies demonstrated that when participants chose a product (e.g., detergent) from sets of different sizes, each with varying amounts of information about each brand, decision quality initially increased but then decreased with the amount of information load (which was operationalized as a combination of the number of alternatives and attributes they differed on) resembling an inverted-U pattern.

Satisfaction

Additionally, satisfaction with both the decision-making process and the chosen option is affected by the assortment size. Malhotra (1982) and Iyengar and Lepper (2000) found that participants were less satisfied when they chose from larger rather than smaller arrays of options. Iyengar and colleagues (2006) observed that an abundance of choice could lead to reduced satisfaction, even when the outcomes were objectively superior. This evidence aligns again with the downward-sloping part of the net benefit function, suggesting that people are better off with fewer rather than more choice alternatives. Moreover, previous research has both theoretically proposed and empirically demonstrated that satisfaction with both the selection process and the final choice follows an inverted-U function relative to the number of alternatives in the assortment (Grant & Schwartz, 2011; Reutskaja, 2008; Reutskaja & Hogarth, 2009).

Finally, a recent large-scale cross-country study (Reutskaja et al., 2022) conducted in six different countries, representing almost half of the world's population, showed that satisfaction with choice follows a pattern consistent with the inverted-U model. The study demonstrated that when choice set sizes in natural settings matched participants' "ideal" set sizes, decision makers experienced the highest satisfaction. Both too little and too much choice negatively impacted satisfaction in noncontrolled, natural settings. However, the effect of too much and too little choice on satisfaction was not equivalent. In most countries a lack of choice had a much stronger negative impact on satisfaction than choice overload had. These findings suggest that the inverted-U function may be much steeper initially (left upward-sloping part of the curve in Figure 23.1) than on the choice overload side of the curve (right side of the curve in Figure 23.1).

To summarize, despite the main tenet of classical psychology and economic theory that more choice is always beneficial, research across different disciplines, including psychology, economics, neuroscience, management, and marketing, has documented that excessive choice may lead to detrimental consequences. Researchers have proposed and demonstrated that many choice outcomes—both objective and subjective—follow an inverted-U trend as the choice set size increases. Findings suggest that people are more motivated, make better quality choices, and experience higher satisfaction with both the decision-making process and choice outcome when choosing from intermediate rather than limited or extensive assortments. Both too few and too many choices negatively affect motivation, decision accuracy, and satisfaction. Moreover, the inverted-U curve may not be symmetrical. Preliminary empirical evidence suggests that the curve is steeper for too little choice than for too much choice, indicating that a lack of choice has a more harmful effect on satisfaction than excessive choice.

Overall, choice architects should aim to find the "peak" of the net benefit function to offer assortments with an "optimal" choice set to the public. However, the "optimal" assortment size depends on various factors, which we discuss in detail below.

FACTORS AFFECTING THE OPTIMAL ASSORTMENT SIZE

The second implication of the inverted-U conceptual model in Figure 23.1 is that the peak of the function is not static. It depends on the underlying costs and benefits of choice in each situation. Changes in perceived costs and benefits can shift the resulting "net benefit" curve and its peak. For instance, if the benefits of choice increase while costs remain constant, the net benefit curve may shift upward and/or the peak of the function may shift rightward. This means that when the benefits of choice increase and costs remain unchanged, individuals can handle larger assortments without feeling overloaded, thereby experiencing greater net benefits from choice overall. Conversely, if the benefits remain constant and the costs of choice rise, the opposite may occur: The peak of the function would shift downward and leftward, causing decision makers to feel overloaded with fewer alternatives than they originally were.

One of the main questions that has concerned both academics and practitioners is whether there is a universal "optimal" number of choices that would render people most satisfied and motivated. Empirical evidence so far indicates that the optimal number of choices is not universal. It depends on the environment in which decisions are made and individual characteristics of decision makers (for a more detailed review of different factors, see Chernev et al., 2015; Misuraca et al., 2020, 2021). These factors can affect the perceived benefits and costs of choice and, thus, determine the position of the peak of the resulting net benefit function. Below, we discuss empirical evidence regarding how different factors affect choice perceptions.

Choice Environment

Culture

It is important to note that most choice overload research discussed previously (with only few exceptions: e.g., Iyengar & Lepper, 1999; Reutskaja, 2008; Reutskaja et al., 2022; Savani et al., 2008) has been conducted in Western contexts and with WEIRD (Western, educated, industrialized, rich, and democratic) samples of participants. However, because choice has many meanings, and these meanings and their importance may vary across cultures (Markus & Schwartz, 2010), many researchers have emphasized the importance of considering cultural diversity when studying choice behavior and offered initial insights into how culture might affect perceptions of choice overload (Iyengar, 2010; Iyengar & Lepper, 1999; Savani et al., 2008).

So, how do people in different countries experience their everyday choices, and do they experience choice overload? A recent large study with more than 7,400 participants from six countries (Brazil, China, India, Japan, Russia, and the United States) where almost half of the world's population resides, assessed choice experiences across different domains (Reutskaja et al., 2022). It revealed an unexpected finding: Across the globe, participants reported experiencing choice deprivation—a sense of having fewer than the ideal number of options—more frequently (in 51% of the cases examined) than choice overload—a sense of having more options than ideally desired (14% of cases studied, see Figure 23.2). This was true for both unimportant and consequential domains. Thus, on average, people experience lack of choice rather than suffer from choice abundance.

Interestingly, there were significant country differences: Choice overload was more pronounced in the United States, where more than 60% of participants reported having too many choices of homes, for example, while in countries like China or Russia choice overload was experienced by less than 11% of participants across all domains. Similarly, in Brazil, choice deprivation was the most common experience in most of the domains studied. More intriguingly, this study further showed that, on average, people were most satisfied with choice sets that matched their ideal imaginary assortment size, and too little or too much choice negatively impacted satisfaction. However, even here, there were country differences that show that context matters: While in some countries, like the United States, too many choices was detrimental to satisfaction, in other countries, like Japan and China, an abundance of options beyond the desired amount did not necessarily correlate with decreased satisfaction. This suggests that what might be considered "overload" in some countries may not apply universally. In contrast to the impact of too much choice, choice deprivation consistently predicted dissatisfaction across all six countries studied, suggesting the negative impact of insufficient choice might be more universal.

Thus, it is important to recognize that choice overload is not a universal phenomenon, and whether it is experienced or how strongly it is experienced may depend significantly upon the specific context.

Choice Domain

The observation that choice overload perception is context-specific is further supported

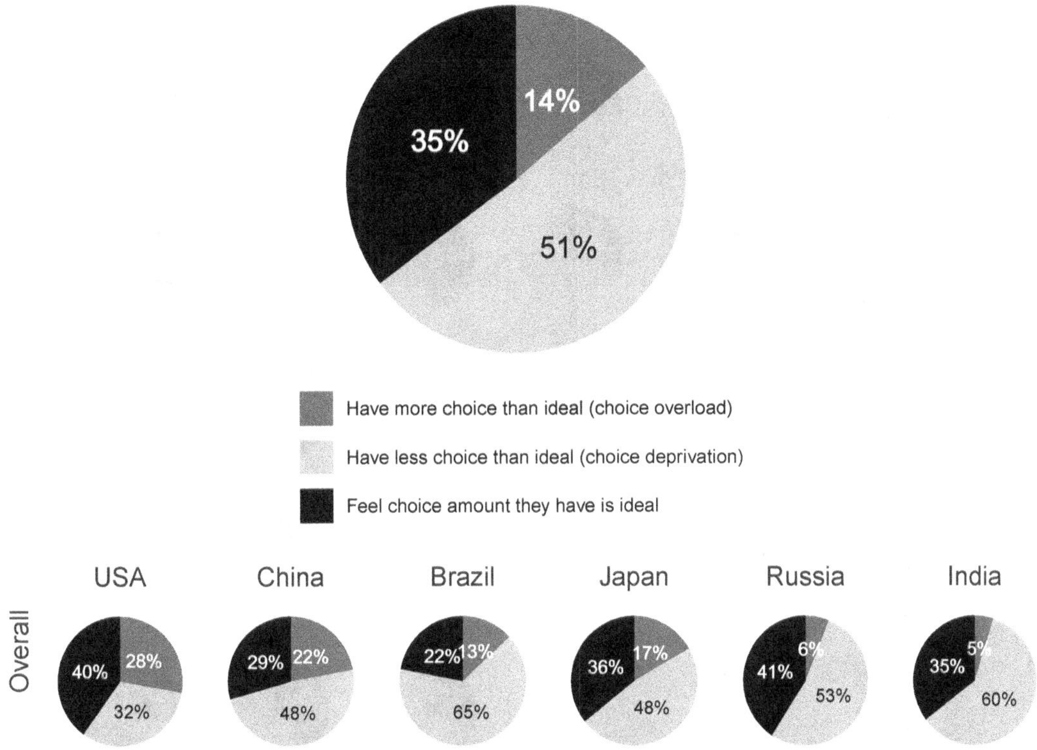

FIGURE 23.2. Percentage of people experiencing choice overload, choice deprivation, or believing they have "ideal" number of choice in their natural environment, overall and by country. Adapted from similar figures originally published in Reutskaja et al. (2022).

by additional findings in the Reutskaja and colleagues' (2022) study, where participants within the same country experienced choice differently across various choice domains (see Figure 23.3). For example, while most American participants reported being overloaded with choice of homes or soft drinks, they indicated too few job alternatives to choose from.

Similarly, previous research has found that in some domains, especially those that cause negative affect, people may find choice rather burdensome and stressful (Botti & Iyengar, 2006; Botti et al., 2009). Because negative psychic costs are high for unpleasant choices (e.g., increased stress and pressure of responsibility), it is possible that in such contexts the optimal number of choices would be smaller than in consumer domains where choice items evoke positive feelings and psychic costs are lower. Therefore, the amount of choice that is "enough" will depend on the domain in which the decision is made.

Choice Items

Related to choice domain, but slightly different in nature, are the characteristics of the choice items, which should also affect the costs and benefits choice. As discussed earlier, people's processing channel capacity differs for different types of stimuli (Miller, 1956) and is higher for visual compared to taste, odor, or sound stimuli. If the costs are lower for visual stimuli, it is likely that the optimal choice set size that decision makers can process without feeling overwhelmed would be larger for sets containing visual items (e.g., gift boxes) than for choices involving sounds (e.g., music tracks). Costs can be even more nuanced: Within the vi-

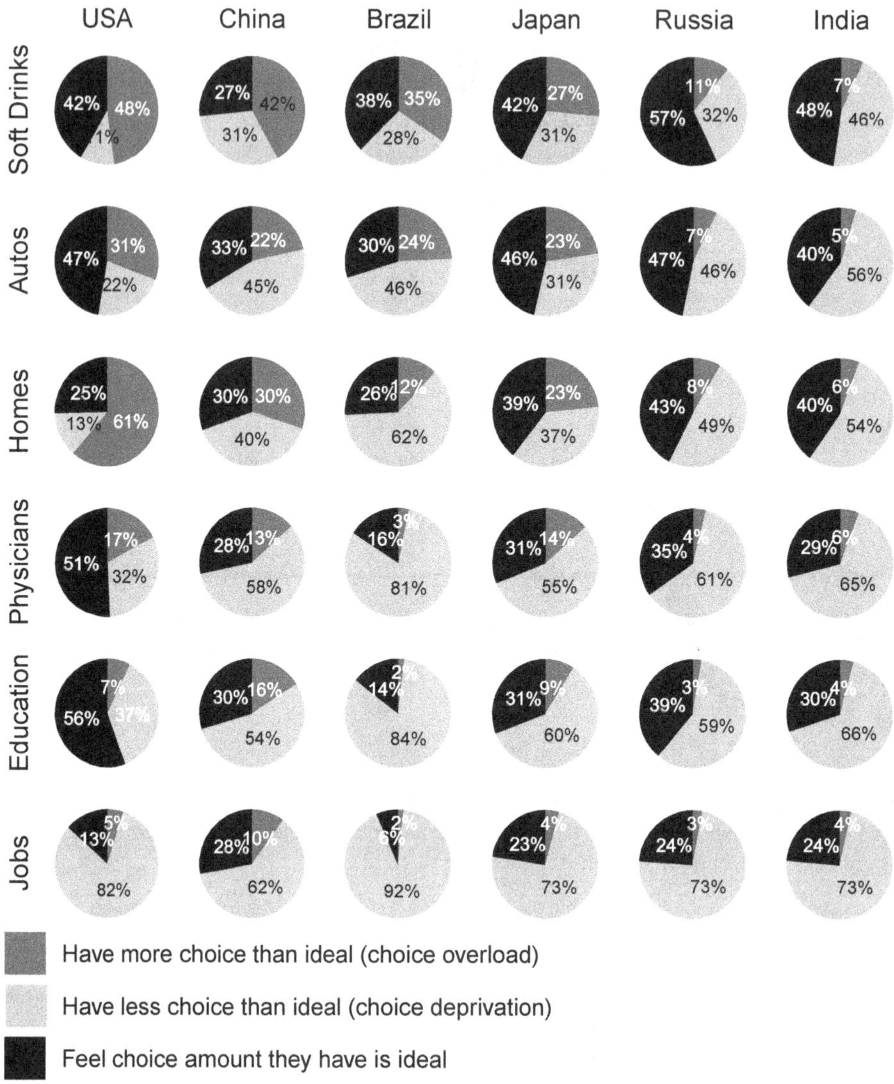

FIGURE 23.3. Percentage of people experiencing choice overload, choice deprivation, or believing they have "ideal" number of choice in their natural environment, by country and by choice domain. Adapted from similar figures originally published in Reutskaja et al. (2022).

sual stimuli category, some stimuli are more costly to process and evaluate than others. Therefore, the optimal set size for more-costly-to-process stimuli should be smaller than for less costly ones. For example, Reutskaja and Hogarth (2009) found that when consumers chose from different-sized sets of gift boxes that varied on one visual dimension only—color or shape—the "optimal" set size that was most satisfying for consumers was larger when they chose from sets of boxes that differed in color. This occurred because processing and evaluating different colors imposed lower costs on decision makers than processing shapes.

Chernev and colleagues (2015) also noted that choice complexity that encompassed four key factors—option attractiveness, presence of a dominant option, attribute alignability, and option complementarity—had a significant effect on people's experiences with number of choices, and thus should be considered when designing "optimal" assortments.

Presentation of Alternatives

Furthermore, extensive research has suggested that how alternatives are presented within a choice set can also affect perceptions of choice overload. Presentation of alternatives can affect both costs and benefits of choice, thereby influencing the position of the resulting net benefit function and its peak. For example, ordering alternatives (e.g., organizing clothes by colors) or presenting alternatives in certain chunks or categories (e.g., menu sections: meat, fish, desserts) should significantly decrease processing cost and, thus, may allow people to evaluate much larger assortments, shifting the peak of the net benefit function rightward. Previous research has provided empirical evidence that organization of information, including attribute order and chunking, can simplify processing and affect perceived variety especially for large sets (Kahn & Wansink, 2004; Levav et al., 2010; Miller, 1956). Moreover, aligning external product displays with consumers' internal schemas enhances perceived variety and satisfaction, particularly for familiar product categories (Morales et al., 2005). One could argue that congruency between internal consumer schemas and external choice alignment should decrease costs associated with choice and thus allow people to be satisfied with larger sets. Lastly, simultaneous presentation of options tends to yield higher satisfaction compared to sequential presentation, as it keeps decision makers focused on available choices rather than imagining potentially better alternatives (Mogilner et al., 2012).

Other contextual factors could affect people's experiences when choosing from large assortments, including time pressure (Dhar & Nowlis, 1999; Reutskaja et al., 2011), the medium where choice is offered (e.g., offline vs. online, Moser et al., 2017; also see Brynjolfsson et al., 2003), and the presence or absence of branding. Regarding the latter, Misuraca and colleagues (2019) demonstrated that choice overload is more likely to occur when a large number of options are presented without brand names. However, when brand names are included, even if unfamiliar, the negative effects of choice overload tend to disappear. This finding was originally observed in adults and later replicated with adolescents (Misuraca et al., 2021), suggesting that branding plays a similar role in mitigating choice overload across different age groups.

To summarize, the experience of choice overload varies significantly depending on the characteristics of the choice environment.

Individual Characteristics of Decision Makers

Previous research has shown that individual characteristics of decision makers, such as their demographic characteristics like gender and age, as well as their "maximizing" tendencies, also affect how choice is perceived. For example, costs and benefits of choice are perceived differently by different genders in various contexts. In a heterosexual dating context, men have a greater preference for variety, which could reflect higher benefits of choice for men than for women given the same cost of choosing. Thus, the optimal choice set size of potential dating mates for men is larger than that for women (Lenton et al., 2008). Conversely, in another decision context (choice of gift boxes), women appeared more satisfied than men when choosing over the entire range of choice sets (Reutskaja, 2008). This may result from lower costs of processing details for women compared to men. Gender differences in response to choice overload may stem from different information-processing strategies used by each gender. Meyers-Levy and Maheswaran (1991) found that women tend to focus more on details, while men prefer simpler information for quicker decisions and may not use all available information.

Individual tendencies, like being a "maximizer" (seeking the best outcome) or a "satisficer" (accepting "good enough") affect perceived choice costs and benefits. Maximizers face higher costs, especially with large assortments, as they must evaluate all options and make difficult tradeoffs. Satisficers stop searching once they find a satisfactory option, avoiding these extensive costs. Though maximizers typically find better alternatives, research shows they feel worse and are less satisfied with their outcomes than satisficers (Iyengar et al., 2006; Misuraca & Fasolo, 2018). Maximizing and satisficing tendencies are closely linked with age. Consequently, age has also been shown to influence perceptions of choice overload. For example, Misuraca and colleagues (2016) found that adolescents and adults suffer more from choice overload than do children and seniors, who experience less difficulty and maintain higher satisfaction levels when navigating large choices. This may be due to adults and adolescents employing similar maximizing strategies when choosing, while seniors are more likely to satisfice. Moreover, children likely experience lower costs of choosing because they use intuitive choice strategies and form strong preferences faster (Schlottmann & Wilkening, 2011).

Individual cognitive traits also play a crucial role in navigating choice abundance. Pilli and Mazzon (2016) observed that individuals with a higher need for cognition are less prone to choice overload and decision deferral. Other factors, including whether the goal was to browse rather than choose (Chernev & Hamilton, 2009; Reutskaja et al., 2018), choosing for others rather than oneself (Polman, 2012), choosing under positive affect (Spassova & Isen, 2013), or having articulated preferences before choice (Chernev et al., 2015), were shown to diminish the negative effects of large choice assortments.

To summarize, previous research has provided rich empirical evidence on how various factors influence individuals' choice experiences. While it is possible to intuitively predict how each individual factor would affect the costs and benefits of choice, and thus the net benefit function, we emphasize that determining the optimal choice set size in each situation requires empirical testing. While laboratory settings allow for the isolation of one factor and control for the influence of other variables, real-world conditions rarely permit such isolation. In real-world conditions, multiple factors interact and influence perceptions of choice simultaneously. Thus, based on the relative influence of each factor and the joint effect of all factors at play, choice architects must determine the optimal choice set size on a situation-specific basis. Choice architects also need to determine which sets would be considered choice depriving and which would be considered overwhelming in each particular situation. If they must err, previous research suggests it is better to offer an overwhelming rather than a depriving assortment (Reutskaja et al., 2022), as too little choice has more harmful consequences than too much choice.

CONCLUSION

In this chapter, we explored the benefits and costs of choice, revealing that while expanded choice offers several advantages, it also imposes significant costs on decision makers. The main advantages of a larger set of choices include:

- Increased likelihood of matching preferences: A larger set of choices enhances the probability that a product closely matching individual preferences is available.
- Economic benefits: More choices lead to higher-quality products and lower prices due to increased competition and economies of scale. Enhanced variety also increases consumer surplus.
- Psychological benefits: Larger assortments provide significant psychological benefits, as people find greater choice more attractive. Additionally, they foster feelings of freedom, autonomy, authenticity, and control—key concepts in existential psychology—which can enhance overall life satisfaction and well-being.

The main costs of expanded choice include:

- Time costs: Increased time spent processing, evaluating, and comparing numerous alternatives.
- Cognitive costs: Higher mental resources required to process large sets of information, leading to errors and cognitive strain.
- Psychic costs: Emotional strain and stress associated with making difficult tradeoffs, along with potential regret and anxiety over possibly making the wrong choice. As existential psychologists have claimed, freedom of choice brings with it feelings of anxiety and responsibility as individuals navigate the consequences of their decisions (May, 1950).

The conceptual model of an inverted-U-shaped function illustrates that the net benefits of choice initially increase with the number of alternatives but then level off and eventually decline as choice sets become excessively large. This model suggests that intermediate-sized choice sets yield the highest motivation, choice quality, and satisfaction with both the decision-making process and the chosen option, whereas both limited and extensive assortments negatively impact these key variables. This is in line with existential psychologists' idea that, while freedom and autonomy are essential for personal growth and psychological well-being, they also come with the weight of responsibility and the potential for existential anxiety. This perspective underscores the importance of balancing freedom with constraint, suggesting that optimal decision making occurs when individuals have enough choices to feel autonomous but not so many that they become overwhelmed by the possibilities.

Researchers have endeavored to determine the "ideal" number of alternatives to present to decision makers. As this chapter has demonstrated, there is no universal optimal number of choices, as the optimal choice set size depends on various factors, such as the environment in which decisions are made and the individual characteristics of decision makers.

Consequently, situation-specific assessment is crucial for determining the ideal assortment size. To identify the optimal point of the inverted-U curve and design choice environments that balance the benefits and costs of choice, choice architects should carefully consider the factors affecting choice perceptions in each particular situation. If errors are unavoidable, it is preferable to provide an overwhelming rather than a depriving assortment, as too little choice has more detrimental consequences than too much choice.

REFERENCES

Botti, S., & Iyengar, S. S. (2006). The dark side of choice: When choice impairs social welfare. *Journal of Public Policy and Marketing, 25*(1), 24–38.

Botti, S., Iyengar, S. S., & McGill, A. L. (2023). Choice freedom. *Journal of Consumer Psychology, 33*(1), 143–166.

Botti, S., Orfali, K., & Iyengar, S. S. (2009). Tragic choices: Autonomy and emotional responses to medical decisions. *Journal of Consumer Research, 36*(3), 337–352.

Brynjolfsson, E., Hu, Y., & Smith, M. D. (2003). Consumer surplus in the digital economy: Estimating the value of increased product variety at online booksellers. *Management Science, 49*(11), 1580–1596.

Carmon, Z., Wertenbroch, K., & Zeelenberg, M. (2003). Option attachment: When deliberating makes choosing feel like losing. *Journal of Consumer Research, 30*(1), 15–29.

Chernev, A., Böckenholt, U., & Goodman, J. (2015). Choice overload: A conceptual review and meta-analysis. *Journal of Consumer Psychology, 25*(2), 333–358.

Chernev, A., & Hamilton, R. (2009). Assortment size and option attractiveness in consumer choice among retailers. *Journal of Marketing Research, 46*(3), 410–420.

Deci, E. L., & Ryan, R. M. (1985). Cognitive evaluation theory. In E. L. Deci & R. M. Ryan (Eds.), *Intrinsic motivation and self-determination in human behavior* (pp. 43–85). Springer.

Dhar, R., & Nowlis, S. M. (1999). The effect of time pressure on consumer choice deferral. *Journal of Consumer Research, 25*(4), 369–384.

Frankl, V. E. (2006). *Man's search for meaning* (I. Lasch, Trans.). Beacon Press. (Original work published 1946)

Grant, A. M., & Schwartz, B. (2011). Too much of a good thing: The challenge and opportunity of the inverted U. *Perspectives on Psychological Science, 6*(1), 61–76.

Heidegger, M. (1962). *Being and time* (J. Macquarrie & E. Robinson, Trans.). Harper & Row. (Original work published 1927)

Hogarth, R. M. (1975). Decision time as a function of task complexity. In D. Wendt & C. A. Vliet (Eds.), *Utility, probability, and human decision making* (pp. 321–338). Springer.

Horowitz, J., List, J., & McConnell, K. (2007). A test of diminishing marginal value. *Economica, 74*(296), 650–663.

Iyengar, S. S. (2010). *The art of choosing.* Twelve Books.

Iyengar, S. S., Huberman, G., & Jiang, W. (2004). How much choice is too much?: Contributions to 401(k) retirement plans. In O. S. Mitchell & S. P. Utkus (Eds.), *Pension design and structure: New lessons from behavioral finance* (pp. 83–87). Oxford University Press.

Iyengar, S. S., & Lepper, M. R. (1999). Rethinking the value of choice: A cultural perspective on intrinsic motivation. *Journal of Personality and Social Psychology, 76*(3), 349–366.

Iyengar, S. S., & Lepper, M. R. (2000). When choice is demotivating: Can one desire too much of a good thing? *Journal of Personality and Social Psychology, 79*(6), 995–1006.

Iyengar, S. S., Wells, R. E., & Schwartz, B. (2006). Doing better but feeling worse: Looking for the "best" job undermines satisfaction. *Psychological Science, 17*(2), 143–150.

Jacoby, J., Speller, D. E., & Berning, C. K. (1974). Brand choice behavior as a function of information load: Replication and extension. *Journal of Consumer Research, 1*(1), 33–42.

Jacoby, J., Speller, D. E., & Kohn, C. A. (1974). Brand choice behavior as a function of information load. *Journal of Marketing Research, 11*(1), 63–69.

Kahn, B. E., & Wansink, B. (2004). The influence of assortment structure on perceived variety and consumption quantities. *Journal of Consumer Research, 30*(4), 519–533.

Langer, E. J., & Rodin, J. (1976). The effects of choice and enhanced personal responsibility for the aged: A field experiment in an institutional setting. *Journal of Personality and Social Psychology, 34*(2), 191–198.

Lee, B. K., & Lee, W. N. (2004). The effect of information overload on consumer choice quality in an on-line environment. *Psychology and Marketing, 21*(3), 159–183.

Lenton, A. P., Fasolo, B., & Todd, P. M. (2008). "Shopping" for a mate: Expected versus experienced preferences in online mate choice. *IEEE Transactions on Professional Communication, 51*(2), 169–182.

Levav, J., Heitmann, M., Herrmann, A., & Iyengar, S. S. (2010). Order in product customization decisions: Evidence from field experiments. *Journal of Political Economy, 118*(2), 274–299.

Loewenstein, G. (1999). Is more choice always better? *Social Security Brief,* 7.

Loewenstein, G. (2000). Emotions in economic theory and economic behavior. *American Economic Review, 90*(2), 426–432.

Malhotra, N. K. (1982). Information load and consumer decision making. *Journal of Consumer Research, 8*(4), 419–430.

Markus, H. R., & Schwartz, B. (2010). Does choice mean freedom and well-being? *Journal of Consumer Research, 37*(2), 344–355.

Marois, R., & Ivanoff, J. (2005). Capacity limits of information processing in the brain. *Trends in Cognitive Sciences, 9*(6), 296–305.

May, R. (1950). *The meaning of anxiety.* Ronald Press.

Meyers-Levy, J., & Maheswaran, D. (1991). Exploring differences in males' and females' processing strategies. *Journal of Consumer Research, 18*(1), 63–70.

Miller, G. A. (1956). The magical number seven, plus or minus two: Some limits on our capacity for processing information. *Psychological Review, 63*(2), 81–97.

Misuraca, R., Ceresia, F., Nixon, A. E., & Scaffidi-Abbate, C. (2021). When is more really more?: The effect of brands on choice overload in adolescents. *Journal of Consumer Marketing, 38*(2), 168–177.

Misuraca, R., Ceresia, F., Teuscher, U., & Faraci, P. (2019), The role of the brand on choice overload. *Mind and Society: Cognitive Studies in Economics and Social Sciences, 18,* 57–76.

Misuraca, R., & Fasolo, B. (2018). Maximizing versus satisficing in the digital age: Disjoint scales and the case for "construct consensus." *Personality and Individual Differences, 121,* 152–160.

Misuraca, R., Reutskaja, E., Fasolo, B., & Iyengar, S. S. (2020). How much choice is "good enough"? Moderators of information and choice overload. In R. Viale (Ed.), *Routledge handbook of bounded rationality* (pp. 637–649). Routledge.

Misuraca, R., Teuscher, U., & Faraci, P. (2016). Is more choice always worse?: Age differences in the overchoice effect. *Journal of Cognitive Psychology, 28*(2), 242–255.

Mogilner, C., Shiv, B., & Iyengar, S. S. (2012). Eternal quest for the best: Sequential (vs. simultaneous) option presentation undermines choice commitment. *Journal of Consumer Research, 39*(6), 1300–1312.

Morales, A., Kahn, B. E., McAlister, L., & Broniarczyk, S. M. (2005). Perceptions of assortment variety: The effects of congruency between consumers' internal and retailers' external organization. *Journal of Retailing, 81*(2), 159–169.

Moser, C., Phelan, C., Resnick, P., Schoenebeck, S. Y., & Reinecke, K. (2017). No such thing as too much chocolate: Evidence against choice overload in e-commerce. *Proceedings of the 2017 CHI Conference on Human Factors in Computing Systems,* pp. 4358–4369.

Pilli, L. E., & Mazzon, J. A. (2016). Information overload, choice deferral, and moderating role of need for cognition: Empirical evidence. *Revista de Administração, 51*(1), 36–55.

Polman, E. (2012). Effects of self–other decision making on regulatory focus and choice overload. *Journal of Personality and Social Psychology, 102*(5), 980–993.

Reibstein, D. J., Youngblood, S. A., & Fromkin, H. L. (1975). Number of choices and perceived decision freedom as a determinant of satisfaction and consumer behavior. *Journal of Applied Psychology, 60*(4), 434–437.

Reutskaja, E. (2008). *Experiments on the role of the number of alternatives in choice*. Doctoral thesis, Pompeu Fabra University.

Reutskaja, E., Cheek, N. N., Iyengar, S., & Schwartz, B. (2022). Choice deprivation, choice overload, and satisfaction with choices across six nations. *Journal of International Marketing, 30*(3), 18–34.

Reutskaja, E., & Hogarth, R. M. (2009). Satisfaction in choice as a function of the number of alternatives: When "goods satiate." *Psychology and Marketing, 26*(3), 197–203.

Reutskaja, E., Iyengar, S., Fasolo, B., & Misuraca, R. (2020). Cognitive and affective consequences of information and choice overload. In R. Viale (Ed.), *Routledge handbook of bounded rationality* (pp. 625–636). Routledge.

Reutskaja, E., Lindner, A., Nagel, R., Andersen, R. A., & Camerer, C. F. (2018). Choice overload reduces neural signatures of choice set value in dorsal striatum and anterior cingulate cortex. *Nature Human Behaviour, 2*(12), 925–935.

Reutskaja, E., Nagel, R., Camerer, C. F., & Rangel, A. (2011). Search dynamics in consumer choice under time pressure: An eye-tracking study. *American Economic Review, 101*(2), 900–926.

Rolls, B. J., Rowe, E. A., Rolls, E. T., Kingston, B., Megson, A., & Gunary, R. (1981). Variety in a meal enhances food intake in man. *Physiology and Behavior, 26*(2), 215–221.

Ryan, R. M., & Deci, E. L. (2000). Self-determination theory and the facilitation of intrinsic motivation, social development, and well-being. *American Psychologist, 55(*1), 68–78.

Savani, K., Markus, H. R., & Conner, A. L. (2008). Let your preferences be your guide?: Preferences and choices are more tightly linked for North Americans than for Indians. *Journal of Personality and Social Psychology, 95*(4), 861–876.

Sartre, J.-P. (1956). *Being and nothingness* (H. E. Barnes, Trans.). Washington Square Press. (Original work published 1943)

Schlottmann, A., & Wilkening, F. (2011). Judgment and decision making in young children. In M. Dhami, A. Schlottmann, & M. Waldmann (Eds.), *Judgment and decision-making as a skill: Learning, development, evolution* (pp. 55–83). Cambridge University Press.

Schwartz, B. (2000). Self-determination: The tyranny of freedom. *American Psychologist, 55*(1), 79–88.

Schwartz, B. (2004). *The paradox of choice: Why more is less*. Ecco.

Shah, A. M., & Wolford, G. (2007). Buying behavior as a function of parametric variation of number of choices. *Psychological Science, 18*(5), 369–370.

Simon, H. A. (1974). How big is a chunk? *Science, 183*(4124), 482–488.

Simon, H. A. (1976). From substantive to procedural rationality. In T. J. Kastelein, S. K. Kulpers, W. A. Nijenhuis, & G. R. Wagenaar (Eds.), *25 years of economic theory* (pp. 65–86). Martinus Nijhoff.

Slovic, P. (1995). The construction of preference. *American Psychologist, 50*(5), 364–371.

Spassova, G., & Isen, A. M. (2013). Positive affect moderates the impact of assortment size on choice satisfaction. *Journal of Retailing, 89*(4), 397–408.

Steiner, I. D. (1970). Perceived freedom. *Advances in Experimental Social Psychology, 5*, 187–248.

Von Neumann, J., & Morgenstern, O. (1944). *Theory of games and economic behavior*. Princeton University Press.

Walton, J. R., & Berkowitz, E. N. (1979). The effects of choice complexity and decision freedom on consumer choice behavior. *Advances in Consumer Research, 6*(1), 206–208.

Zuckerman, M., Porac, J., Lathin, D., & Deci, E. L. (1978). On the importance of self-determination for intrinsically-motivated behavior. *Personality and Social Psychology Bulletin, 4*(3), 443–446.

CHAPTER 24

Belief in Free Will, Moral Responsibility, and Personal Agency

Elizabeth Seto

Free will has been an alluring topic for scholars and laypersons for centuries. This is unsurprising given that concern for freedom, responsibility, and the will affect almost all facets of life. Existential philosophers were among the first theorists to offer their discerning perspectives on free will. For instance, Kierkegaard (1844/1981) believed that humans have freedom of choice and are thus entirely responsible for their own actions. Similarly, Sartre (1943/1974) argued that people have an active role in shaping their lives because they are afforded human freedom. Nietzsche (1886/2003), on the other hand, proposed that people do not possess free will; instead, free will is a concept used to falsely assign blame and responsibility for actions that may not be entirely within a person's control. While they may all have differed in the extent to which they believed people have free will, they all embraced the notion that free will serves an important function for the self and the social environment. These thought-provoking discussions have profoundly influenced how psychologists address the complexities of free will.

In the beginning, psychologists found themselves at the center of the free will debate. That is, they questioned whether free will was a possibility or impossibility. Seminal research in neuroscience found that brain activity seemed to precede voluntary actions, thus free will was ruled scientifically implausible given its incompatibility with brain processes (Libet et al., 1983). Research on mental causation suggested that free will is simply an illusion created by the brain and the mind (Wegner, 2004). Free will has also been called "mistaken causation" based on existing knowledge regarding conscious and unconscious processing (Bargh, 2008). While the question of whether free will exists remains dominant in scholarly conversations, a new and more fruitful approach to understanding free will has emerged over the past few decades. Specifically, psychologists have become less concerned about the reality of free will. Instead, their focus has turned to whether varying *belief* in free will has meaningful consequences (Baumeister & Brewer, 2012). This shift in scientific study has shown that free will beliefs influence much more than we realize and has inspired a plethora of research in existential psychology. This change also marks an essential return to original existential inquiries about the significance of belief in free will in everyday life.

In this chapter, I begin by defining belief in free will. Next, I examine a prominent view that free will beliefs exist to hold people morally responsible for their actions. Then, I propose that the importance of believing in free will extends beyond concerns about moral responsibility. Specifically, I argue that feelings of personal agency inherent in free will beliefs can immensely impact other social thoughts, feelings, and behaviors. Finally, I discuss major caveats in the belief in free will literature and considerations for future research.

WHAT IS BELIEF IN FREE WILL?

Scholars across disciplines tend to have different definitions of free will. To investigate belief in free will as a psychological concept, researchers have focused on how ordinary people understand free will. When asked directly what it means to have free will, people define it as a choice and as the ability to go against external pressures (Monroe & Malle, 2010). Content analyses of autobiographical narratives have also shown that people perceive free will as behaviors involving action control such as making progress toward achieving goals, engaging in conscientious decision making, and upholding moral values (Stillman et al., 2011). Free will has also been traditionally defined as a juxtaposition to determinism, which posits that every event is casually inevitable, and only one action and one outcome is possible; in contrast, free will means pursuing different actions that could result in different outcomes (Bergner & Ramon, 2013; MacKenzie et al., 2014). In the simplest conceptualization, the definition of belief in free will converges on the ability to make one's own choices and determine one's own outcomes free from constraints (Baumeister & Brewer, 2012).

The emergence of belief in free will as a construct of interest has prompted scholars to examine how it is distinct from other existing constructs in the psychological literature. Of particular relevance are locus of control and self-control. Locus of control describes how people attribute outcomes to internal or external causes (Rotter, 1966). Whereas locus of control is concerned with the perceived connection between actions and outcomes, belief in free will is focused on the perceived freedom of choice in one's actions (Feldman, 2017). Research has shown that belief in free will has a moderate, positive correlation with internal locus of control (Paulhus & Carey, 2011; Stillman et al., 2011), providing empirical support that they are relatively independent constructs. Self-control refers to the ability to overcome automatic impulses and desires (Vohs & Baumeister, 2004). Whereas self-control describes exerting effort to override constraints, belief in free will refers to the ability to override constraints (Feldman, 2017). Free will beliefs have been linked to the monitoring subprocess of self-control (Goto et al., 2018) and weakening free will beliefs have been shown to reduce self-control (Rigoni et al., 2012). This suggests that belief in free will may enable self-control. Although there are conceptual similarities between these constructs, free will beliefs are separate and unique. In fact, the experience of choice embedded in belief in free will influences a different set of important outcomes even when controlling for these related constructs (e.g., Crescioni et al., 2016, Feldman et al., 2016, Stillman et al., 2010).

Belief in free will is astonishingly widespread. The basic notion of free will develops between ages 4 and 6 (Kushnir et al., 2015; Nichols, 2004). Research has found that American and Chinese children believe that people can freely act against their desires, and the concept of choice tends to increase with age in early childhood (Wente et al., 2016). Belief in free will has also been demonstrated cross-culturally. People in the United States, Hong Kong, India, and Colombia generally believe that the world is indeterministic (Sarkissian et al., 2010). Furthermore, research has shown that most people believe in free will (Nahmias et al., 2005), and people believe they have more free will than others (Pronin & Kugler, 2011). In early research involving experimental manipulations of belief in free will, scholars investigated differences in psychological outcomes under pro-free will, anti-free will, and control conditions. Research has found that the condition designed to bolster free will beliefs has the same influence on psychological outcomes as the control condition (e.g., Alquist et al., 2013; Baumeister et al., 2009), implying that most people already espouse free will beliefs. These findings suggest that the vast majority of people believe in free will, but they do not directly address *why* this belief system is so prominent. While there are differing perspectives, the most common viewpoints are that free will beliefs invoke feelings of moral responsibility and promote personal agency.

Belief in Free Will and Moral Responsibility

Many theorists have proposed that free will is a prevailing belief system because people are motivated to hold others morally responsible for their actions and seek justification of punishment for wrongdoing (Clark et al., 2014, 2021; Nichols & Knobe, 2007; Pereboom, 2006). Belief in free will undoubtedly exists in the social and cultural framework of most societies. It is possible that societies recognize that people have freedom of choice, and belief in free will helps encourage people to exercise this freedom of choice in socially productive ways. Indeed, a common perspective is that the ability to inhibit automatic impulses and personal desires is the key to a harmonious society (Baumeister, 2008; Kane, 1996). Belief in free will seems to remind people that their freely chosen behaviors can have detrimental consequences for the self and their social environment if they violate the social contract of fostering cooperation and upholding the common good.

Moral responsibility is deeply embedded in people's lay understanding of free will. The very definition of free will implies that people have the opportunity to act in numerous ways in the same situation, and while there are presumably good or moral actions that one could make, there are also bad or immoral actions one could make. Nahmias and colleagues (2005) found that when judging the moral actions of a person in a hypothetically deterministic universe, people still ascribe moral responsibility for wrongdoing. This suggests that people have strong intuitions about free will and believe that people have the ability to choose socially desired behaviors even if explicitly told that the universe is deterministic. Additionally, research has found that greater free will beliefs are associated with having higher moral standards (Bergner & Ramon, 2013). This means that the more people espouse a capacity for choice, the stronger their moral convictions. Belief in free will is also related to belief in a just world (Carey & Paulhus, 2013), suggesting that people get what they deserve as a result of the good or poor choices they make. Similarly, belief in free will is linked to victim blaming (Genschow & Vehlow, 2021). Apparently, people attribute moral responsibility to victims even if circumstances are based on uncontrollable factors such as bad luck. Moreover, people who believe in free will tend to extract more meaningful lessons after reflecting on past misdeeds (Stillman & Baumeister, 2010), demonstrating that people do think about how they could have acted differently in morally complicated situations and consider how they can be more virtuous in the future. In sum, believing in free will also means believing in moral responsibility.

If belief in free will is a prerequisite for moral responsibility, then moral responsibility is a prerequisite for punishment. Free will beliefs describe unconstrained choices (Monroe & Malle, 2010), and moral responsibility describes accountability for choices (Malle et al., 2014). It follows that the repercussion for failing to exert moral responsibility is rightful punishment. The proposition that free will beliefs help justify punishment for wrongful actions is clearly reflected in moral and legal judgments. For example, contextual factors such as whether a person had the capacity to do otherwise in a given situation influences assignments of criminal punishment (Greene & Cohen, 2004). Many legal procedures also require proof that no formidable external pressures or neurological abnormalities impede on a person's free will to act otherwise (Burns & Bechara, 2007). Furthermore, research based on real crime rates has demonstrated a strong link between belief in free will and perceptions of punishment. In data garnered from 46 different countries, Martin and colleagues (2017) found that free will beliefs predicted greater intolerance of unethical behaviors. This was more pronounced for residents of countries with high and moderate institutional integrity where there were lower levels of corruption and more transparent governance. They also found that free will beliefs predicted greater support for criminal punishment regardless of institutional integrity. In a sample of 74 different countries, Clark and colleagues (2014) found that countries with higher homicide rates had higher free will beliefs compared to countries with lower homicide rates. Both findings suggest that belief in free will is strongly associated with the desire to punish criminal transgressions in the real world.

The robust influence of free will beliefs on punitive behavior has also been demonstrated in scientific investigations of moral judgments. Research has found that higher belief in free will is associated with greater punitiveness in hypothetical criminal scenarios (Carey & Paulhus, 2013) and greater endorsement of punishment including rehabilitation, retribution, and deterrence (Rakos et al., 2008). This shows that believing that people have control over their actions is related to assigning proportionate punishment for criminal behavior. Research has also found that the correspondence bias (or fundamental attribution error) mediates the relationship between belief in free will and prescribed punishment for negative behavior and prescribed reward for positive behavior (Genschow et al., 2017). As the correspondence bias reflects our tendency to make internal attributions as opposed to external attributions about a person's behavior, it follows that belief in free will strengthens one's personal responsibility for their actions. Furthermore, weakening belief in free will by inducing a mechanistic view of human nature has been shown to reduce retributive punishment (Shariff et al., 2014). Specifically, reading about the neural basis of behavior decreases the blameworthiness of an offender and reduces prison sentencing. Similarly, the presence of neurological abnormalities in an offender, such as a brain tumor (Stinnett & Alquist, 2022) or brain damage (Gil & Cerce, 2017), reduces the severity of punishment by lowering perceptions of free will. Perceiving transgressors' actions as freely chosen or not seems to shift culpability of behavior. Research has also found that boosting belief in free will alleviates punitive distress (Clark et al., 2017). While inflicting punishment can be psychologically distressing, believing that someone could have behaved differently helps justify this punishment. Finally, there is strong evidence of motivated free will attributions. Specifically, people consistently report greater belief in free will after reading about immoral actions than they do after reading about morally neutral actions (Clark et al., 2014, 2021). This suggests that when there is a desire to punish transgressors, people are motivated to believe in free will.

The extensive perception that belief in free will holds people morally responsible for their actions and justifies punishment for transgressions has instigated a growing niche of research focused on the influence of free will beliefs on moral behaviors. In explicating the importance of believing in free will, Vohs and Schooler (2008) proposed that undermining free will beliefs can have potentially devastating moral and societal consequences. Whereas belief in free will motivates people to behave according to high moral standards, disbelief in free will may encourage people to behave in more unconstrained, impulsive ways. Shariff and colleagues (2008) also contended that scientific acknowledgement of the illusion of free will may encourage the lay public to engage in moral leniency, and Smithdeal (2016) argued that we are better off believing in free will even if it is illusory. As social creatures, we live in a complex world where we need to temper our impulses and desires with others around us. Indeed, belief in free will has been characterized as procultural, helping to uphold societal rules and norms (Baumeister & Brewer, 2012). If free will does not exist, then people cannot be held responsible for their actions. Thus, believing in free will may serve society more than disbelieving in free will does.

The importance of belief in free will for moral behavior has been demonstrated across numerous lines of research. In early work examining the behavioral effects of free will beliefs, research found that inducing disbelief in free will reduces prosocial intentions, lowers helping behavior, and increases aggression toward others (Baumeister et al., 2009). Similarly, disbelief in free will decreases volunteerism; this effect was especially pronounced for individuals high in psychopathy, who lack empathy and inhibition (Stillman & Baumeister, 2010). These findings suggest that threatening free will beliefs diminishes the experience of choice, producing antisocial behaviors that would have been curtailed otherwise. Of course, there are boundary conditions to this complex relationship between belief in free will and moral behaviors.

For instance, research has found that disbelief in free will led people to donate less money to a group pot in an economic contribution game under time constraints; however, if people were given time to think about how much they wanted to contribute, they donated as much money as people who weren't exposed to anti-free will messaging (Protzko et al., 2016). Undermining free will beliefs also reduces charitable giving, but only among nonreligious people (Harms et al., 2017). Furthermore, in research examining whether people would choose to inflict an electric shock to another person in exchange for a small financial gain, inducing disbelief in free will actually led people to administer fewer shocks; this effect was notably only present for females (Caspar et al., 2017). While challenging belief in free will can elicit antisocial behavior, this relationship is more nuanced than expected. In some cases, disbelief in free will gives people the license to behave immorally. In other cases, it reduces punitiveness or may have little influence at all. Finally, while not a direct assessment of moral behavior, research has found that altering belief in free will changes perceptions of motivational sincerity (MacKenzie et al., 2014). Specifically, when people experience a reduction in free will beliefs, they also perceive benefactors as having less free will and do not feel as much gratitude for their prosocial behavior. This demonstrates that belief in free will influences moral actions as well as moral character.

Belief in free will is pervasive and meaningful because it fosters moral responsibility. It is widely assumed that people can freely choose prosocial or antisocial behaviors, and there are important consequences for the self and social environment when the exercise of free will is not constructive. Regardless of whether free will actually exists, scholars have found that belief in free will is essential to maintaining a moral and harmonious society.

Belief in Free Will and Personal Agency

While there is a predominant notion that belief in free will is important for cultivating moral responsibility, it also serves a broader purpose of invoking personal agency. Some scholars have proposed that believing in free will enables people to pursue their goals and desires (Dennett, 2003). In fact, the freedom to enact goals helps fuel goal achievement and foster personal growth (Sheldon & Goffredi, 2021). Belief in free will reminds people that they are active agents in the social world, capable of choosing their own actions and exercising control over the outcomes of a situation. As social creatures gifted with the freedom of choice, people can shape their lives to whatever they envision. While there are social and cultural norms (Baumeister & Brewer, 2012) or internal and external pressures (Feldman, 2017) that may limit the extent of our free will, believing that we have choices and recognizing that there is sense of authorship behind our actions helps us navigate our complex social environment.

Personal agency is acutely intertwined with free will beliefs. Believing that we have freedom of choice and can shape our own outcomes strengthens the perception that our actions emanate from us. Empirical research supports this proposition. In examining the foundations of belief in free will, Aarts and van den Bos (2011) found that free will beliefs increase when people engage in goal-directed behaviors. Specifically, when people perceive they are willfully producing chosen outcomes, they experience a form of "intentional binding." This intentional binding produces feelings of self-agency underlying free will beliefs. Research has also found that disbelief in free will reduces implicit components of self-agency (Lynn et al., 2014). Implicit self-agency refers to the prereflective stage of agency (Synofzik et al., 2008), thus suggesting that belief in free will can influence even the most basic processes of action control. Moreover, free will beliefs are positively associated with agentic traits such as self-efficacy (Crescioni et al., 2016) and internal locus of control (Paulhus & Carey, 2011). This means that the more people believe they have freedom of choice, the more they believe they can successfully execute goals and the more they perceive themselves as the cause of a particular outcome. Overall, believing in free will seems to remind us that we have ownership over our outcomes in life.

The impact of belief in free will extends beyond the moral domain, spilling over into other important facets of life where agency is pivotal. For instance, extensive research has investigated how free will beliefs influence different forms of social behavior. Alquist and colleagues (2013) found that inducing disbelief in free will increases conformity, reasoning that cues of determinism make people less motivated to think for themselves. In other words, the loss of agency from reduced belief in free will makes people more susceptible to social influence. Additionally, Kokkoris and colleagues (2019) found that belief in free will was related to lower indecisiveness, particularly for individuals who report high self-concept clarity. Free will beliefs seem to instill confidence in decision making because people perceive outcomes within their control. St Quinton and colleagues (2022) also found that people with greater belief in free will had lower intentions to gamble. This suggests that believing that one has choice and agency may insulate people from engaging in risky behaviors. Moreover, people who believe in free will tend to have better workplace evaluations (Stillman et al., 2010), achieve higher academic performance (Feldman et al., 2016), and have more perseverance for long-terms goals (Li et al., 2018). Because people see themselves as agents driven by freedom of choice, they are more likely to engage in positive, goal-directed behaviors.

Belief in free will has been widely examined in the social cognition literature. As free will beliefs emphasize agentic choice, it has the ability to influence judgments about ourselves and others. Research has found that bolstering belief in free will leads to more counterfactual thinking, especially upward counterfactuals and counterfactuals about the self (Alquist et al., 2015). Freedom of choice highlights the possibility of an alternate reality had another decision been made, signaling that people believe their actions can directly lead to different outcomes. Manipulating belief in free will also seems to change perceptions of our social positions in life. Research has shown that challenging belief in free will reduces subjective perceptions of social mobility such that climbing the socioeconomic ladder feels less feasible (Seto, 2024). When the experience of agency is diminished, people feel less confident about their ability to determine their own outcomes. Furthermore, belief in free will is linked to health stigmas such as obesity (Chandrashekar, 2020) and substance use (Ozkok et al., 2022). The perception that people have agency in their choices makes them more prone to stigmatize people who they believe lack willpower or control. Similarly, different physical states of health are associated with free will beliefs. For instance, greater feelings of tiredness and intense hunger are related to lower belief in free will (Ent & Baumeister, 2014), implying that our physical states can also reflect our immediate experience of agency. There is also research demonstrating how belief in free will can be altered by abating agency. Baldissarri and colleagues (2019) found that sexual objectification led to self-objectification and lower personal belief in free will. Specifically, women who experienced objectifying commentary came to see themselves more as instruments and less human, which in turn reduced their perceptions of freedom and choice in the world. This suggests that self and social judgments can impede on our experience of conscious choice and agency.

As belief in free will reflects our capacity for choice and exercise of personal agency, it is thought to promote psychological well-being. For example, the relationship between belief in free will and meaning has been examined across multiple lines of work. Research has found that inducing disbelief in free will led to lower meaning in life, and bolstering belief in free will led people to set more meaningful goals (Crescioni et al., 2016). Free will beliefs have also been shown to promote meaning in life through feelings of belongingness (Moynihan et al., 2017) and enhance psychological recovery after traumatic events through meaning-focused coping (Maffly-Kipp et al., 2022). Furthermore, counterfactual reflection has enhanced the meaningfulness of life events, particularly for people who espouse high free will beliefs, but not low free will beliefs (Seto et al., 2015). People have a fundamental need to experience meaning in their lives. The sense of agency underlying belief in free will helps highlight the significance of our freedom of choice. Research has also found that attenuating belief in free will led to greater feelings of self-alienation and lower perceptions of authenticity (Seto & Hicks, 2016), suggesting that our sense of agency is what gives rise to our sense of self. Additionally, belief in free will has a profound effect on our perception of time. Specifically, undermining free will beliefs led people to perceive that there is limited time to accomplish their goals (Seto et al., 2021). This suggests that belief in free will is used as an agentic tool, motivating one to pursue meaningful outcomes. Belief in free will is also a strong predictor of life satisfaction, self-efficacy, and job satisfaction (Crescioni et al., 2016; Feldman et al., 2018) and is associated with lower perceived life stress and greater positive affect (Crescioni et al., 2016; Li et al., 2017), implying that people believe they have a role in their own psychological health. The feeling of agency tied to belief in free will clearly contributes to our psychological well-being and quality of life.

The significance of belief in free will is not only due to its ties to moral responsibility. Free will beliefs are also prominent because they promote feelings of personal agency. The freedom to pursue our goals and desires is what helps us create a life worth living. Belief in free will reminds us that there is some degree of choice in our lives, and we should exercise our agency to create a meaningful existence.

Caveats and the Future of Belief in Free Will Research

Research on belief in free will ignited when Vohs and Schooler (2008) first found that threatening belief in free will, by exposing people to deterministic worldviews, led to greater dishonesty and cheating behavior. The implication that the absence of free will can potentially create a " 'why bother?' mentality" has incited almost two decades of investigation of this complex construct across the psychological sciences and other related fields (Vohs & Schooler, 2008, p. 54). These provocative findings, however, have undergone recent scrutiny. Some researchers have been unable to replicate these original findings (e.g., Buttrick et al., 2020; Nadelhoffer et al., 2020), and others have failed to find a general relationship between belief in free will and moral behavior (e.g., Crone & Levy, 2019). This has led to questions about whether the effects of threatening belief in free will have been inflated. Research has also found that perceptions about agent-specific choices, not general free will beliefs, influence moral judgments (Monroe et al., 2017), and one of the most widely used self-report measures of belief in free will may be confounding free will beliefs and moral responsibility beliefs (Stinnett et al., 2022), suggesting that the conceptualization of belief in free will may need to be examined more. Furthermore, a meta-analysis found that the psychological and behavioral consequences of altering belief in free will are relatively small at best (Genschow et al., 2023). As such, the urgency to examine the impact of free will beliefs becomes less clear.

While these findings may cast doubt about whether free will beliefs actually have important downstream consequences, to propose that belief in free will has no influence on our thoughts, feelings, and behaviors at all would be precarious. Inconsistent findings in the belief in free will literature can stem from limitations such as demographic characteristics of the sample, small sample sizes of early research, differences between laboratory and online data collection, variations in belief in free will scales, and the diversity of free will belief manipulations used in published research (Ewusi-Boisvert & Racine, 2018; Genschow et al., 2023). These limitations are not too different than critiques of other research in psychology and related fields. Additionally, inconsistent findings should not necessarily negate almost two decades of research on belief in free will. Instead, it should fuel scholars to engage in more thoughtful reflection of their research agenda, encourage them to be more meticulous when describing the implications of their findings, and inspire them to further explore circumstances under which belief in free will is particularly meaningful.

To obtain a better picture about the psychological consequences of belief in free will, it may be fruitful to engage in conceptual and direct replications of research. Scholars can conduct replications of their own research on free will beliefs to instill confidence in their findings. This would enhance the validity of the findings before research is disseminated across academic circles and the general public. Replications of particularly influential research in the belief in free will literature may also be worth pursuing. It may be the case that certain findings are the product of a specific time period. Successfully replicating research after a duration of time has passed since its initial publication will provide more insight into the resilience of the finding. It is also important to examine boundary conditions in replication research. In investigating a construct as complex as belief in free will, it is possible that the originally established causal relationships may be mediated or moderated by other variables. This is reflected in the niche of research examining the dynamic relationship between belief in free will and moral behaviors (e.g., Caspar et al., 2017; Harms et al., 2017; Protzko et al., 2016). Recent research has also found that political differences in belief in free will are associated with differences in moral judgment (Everett et al., 2021). It is clear that there is need for continued research in this important area of existential psychology to fully understand how belief in free will impacts our everyday lives.

SUMMARY AND CONCLUSION

In a diary entry on April 30, 1870, William James, a prominent philosopher and psychologist, wrote, "My first act of free will shall be to believe in free will" (Perry, 1935). Almost two decades of research in existential psychology attest to the importance of believing in free will. The perception that we do or do not have the freedom of choice profoundly influences how we make sense of the world and respond to the social environment. When the scientific investigation of belief in free will began, most scholars focused on the influence of free will beliefs on moral judgments and behavior. Beginning with the premise that free will exists to foster moral responsibility and justify punishment for wrongful actions, a wealth of research has generally found that altering free will beliefs influences how people assign punishment for transgressions. Perhaps more startling, people are less apt to behave in morally upstanding ways when belief in free will is threatened. To have free will implies that we have an obligation to create and maintain a harmonious society. Most people share the perspective that we must choose to engage in moral and virtuous behavior, as it provides order and stability to the world and has direct ramifications for our social and legal structures. Continuing to examine the moral consequences of the absence or diminished sense of free will is a worthwhile pursuit.

Research has now expanded to understanding how belief in free will influences outcomes beyond the moral domain. In some ways, this scholarly path may be the future of belief in free will research. Because belief in free will invokes personal agency, and agency impacts almost all facets of life, there is an abundance of questions ripe for scientific inquiry. Thus far, scholars have made strides in understanding how belief in free will affects various social behaviors, judgments about the self and others, and psychological well-being. Drawing from the perspective that free will exists to enable people to pursue their goals and desires, research has demonstrated the importance of exploring how perceptions of agency help us navigate a complex world and create a more meaningful life. Investigating belief in free will as an agentic tool to shape other psychological outcomes is a vital endeavor and should make its way to the greater landscape of the belief in free will literature.

REFERENCES

Aarts, H., & van den Bos, K. (2011). On the foundations of beliefs in free will: Intentional binding and unconscious priming in self-agency. *Psychological Science, 22*(4), 532–537.

Alquist, J. L., Ainsworth, S. E., & Baumeister, R. F. (2013). Determined to conform: Disbelief in free will increases conformity. *Journal of Experimental Social Psychology, 49*(1), 80–86.

Alquist, J. L., Ainsworth, S. E., Baumeister, R. F., Daly, M., & Stillman, T. F. (2015). The making of might-have-beens: Effects of free will belief on counterfactual thinking. *Personality and Social Psychology Bulletin, 41*(2), 268–283.

Baldissarri, C., Andrighetto, L., Gabbiadini, A., Valtorta, R. R., Sacino, A., & Volpato, C. (2019). Do self-objectified women believe themselves to be free?: Sexual objectification and belief in personal free will. *Frontiers in Psychology, 10.*

Bargh, J. A. (2008). Free will is un-natural. In J. Baer, J. C. Kaufman, & R. F. Baumeister (Eds.), *Are we free? Psychology and free will* (pp. 128–154). Oxford University Press.

Baumeister, R. F. (2008). Free will in scientific

psychology. *Perspectives on Psychological Science, 3*(1), 14–19.

Baumeister, R. F., & Brewer, L. E. (2012). Believing versus disbelieving in free will: Correlates and consequences. *Social and Personality Psychology Compass, 6*(10), 736–745.

Baumeister, R. F., Masicampo, E. J., & DeWall, C. N. (2009). Prosocial benefits of feeling free: Disbelief in free will increases aggression and reduces helpfulness. *Personality and Social Psychology Bulletin, 35*(2), 260–268.

Bergner, R. M., & Ramon, A. (2013). Some implications of beliefs in altruism, free will, and nonreductionism. *Journal of Social Psychology, 153*(5), 598–618.

Burns, K., & Bechara, A. (2007). Decision making and free will: A neuroscience perspective. *Behavioral Sciences and the Law, 25*(2), 263–280.

Buttrick, N. R., Aczel, B., Aeschbach, L. F., Bakos, B. E., Brühlmann, F., Claypool, H. M., . . . Wood, M. J. (2020). Many Labs 5: Registered replication of Vohs and Schooler (2008), Experiment 1. *Advances in Methods and Practices in Psychological Science, 3*(3), 429–438.

Carey, J. M., & Paulhus, D. L. (2013). Worldview implications of believing in free will and/or determinism: Politics, morality, and punitiveness. *Journal of Personality, 81*(2), 130–141.

Caspar, E. A., Vuillaume, L., Magalhães De Saldanha da Gama, P. A., & Cleeremans, A. (2017). The influence of (dis)belief in free will on immoral behavior. *Frontiers in Psychology, 8*. 1–9.

Chandrashekar, S. P. (2020). It's in your control: Free will beliefs and attribution of blame to obese people and people with mental illness. *Collabra: Psychology, 6*(1), 1–6.

Clark, C. J., Baumeister, R. F., & Ditto, P. H. (2017). Making punishment palatable: Belief in free will alleviates punitive distress. *Consciousness and Cognition: An International Journal, 51*, 193–211.

Clark, C. J., Luguri, J. B., Ditto, P. H., Knobe, J., Shariff, A. F., & Baumeister, R. F. (2014). Free to punish: A motivated account of free will belief. *Journal of Personality and Social Psychology, 106*(4), 501–513.

Clark, C. J., Winegard, B. M., & Shariff, A. F. (2021). Motivated free will belief: The theory, new (preregistered) studies, and three meta-analyses. *Journal of Experimental Psychology: General, 150*(7), e22–e47.

Crescioni, A. W., Baumeister, R. F., Ainsworth, S. E., Ent, M., & Lambert, N. M. (2016). Subjective correlates and consequences of belief in free will. *Philosophical Psychology, 29*(1), 41–63.

Crone, D. L., & Levy, N. L. (2019). Are free will believers nicer people? (Four studies suggest not). *Social Psychological and Personality Science, 10*(5), 612–619.

Dennett, D. C. (2003). The self as a responding—and responsible—artifact. *Annals of the New York Academy of Sciences, 1001*(1), 39–50.

Ent, M. R., & Baumeister, R. F. (2014). Embodied free will beliefs: Some effects of physical states on metaphysical opinions. *Consciousness and Cognition: An International Journal, 27*, 147–154.

Everett, J. A. C., Clark, C. J., Meindl, P., Luguri, J. B., Earp, B. D., Graham, J., . . . Shariff, A. F. (2021). Political differences in free will belief are associated with differences in moralization. *Journal of Personality and Social Psychology, 120*(2), 461–483.

Ewusi-Boisvert, E., & Racine, E. (2018). A critical review of methodologies and results in recent research on belief in free will. *Neuroethics, 11*(1), 97–110.

Feldman, G. (2017). Making sense of agency: Belief in free will as a unique and important construct. *Social and Personality Psychology Compass, 11*(1).

Feldman, G., Chandrashekar, S. P., & Wong, K. F. E. (2016). The freedom to excel: Belief in free will predicts better academic performance. *Personality and Individual Differences, 90*, 377–383.

Feldman, G., Farh, J.-L., & Wong, K. F. E. (2018). Agency beliefs over time and across cultures: Free will beliefs predict higher job satisfaction. *Personality and Social Psychology Bulletin, 44*(3), 304–317.

Genschow, O., Cracco, E., Schneider, J., Protzko, J., Wisniewski, D., Brass, M., & Schooler, J. W. (2023). Manipulating belief in free will and its downstream consequences: A meta-analysis. *Personality and Social Psychology Review, 27*(1), 52–82.

Genschow, O., Rigoni, D., & Brass, M. (2017). Belief in free will affects causal attributions when judging others' behavior. *Proceedings of the National Academy of Sciences, 114*(38), 10071–10076.

Genschow, O., & Vehlow, B. (2021). Free to blame?: Belief in free will is related to victim blaming. *Consciousness and Cognition: An International Journal, 88*.

Gill, M. J., & Cerce, S. C. (2017). He never willed to have the will he has: Historicist narratives, "civilized" blame, and the need to distinguish two notions of free will. *Journal of Personality and Social Psychology, 112*(3), 361–382.

Goto, T., Ishibashi, Y., Kajimura, S., Oka, R., & Kusumi, T. (2018). Belief in free will indirectly contributes to the strategic transition through

sympathetic arousal. *Personality and Individual Differences, 128,* 157–161.
Greene, J., & Cohen, J. (2004). For the law, neuroscience changes nothing and everything. *Philosophical Transactions of the Royal Society B: Biological Sciences, 359*(1451), 1775–1778.
Harms, J., Liket, K., Protzko, J., & Schölmerich, V. (2017). Free to help?: An experiment on free will belief and altruism. *PLOS One, 12*(3), 1–15.
Kane, R. (1996). *The significance of free will.* Oxford University Press.
Kierkegaard, S. (1981). *The concept of anxiety: A simple psychologically orienting deliberation on the dogmatic issue of hereditary sin.* Princeton University Press. (Original work published 1844)
Kokkoris, M. D., Baumeister, R. F., & Kühnen, U. (2019). Freeing or freezing decisions?: Belief in free will and indecisiveness. *Organizational Behavior and Human Decision Processes, 154,* 49–61.
Kushnir, T., Gopnik, A., Chernyak, N., Seiver, E., & Wellman, H. M. (2015). Developing intuitions about free will between ages four and six. *Cognition, 138,* 79–101.
Li, C., Wang, S., Zhao, Y., Kong, F., & Li, J. (2017). The freedom to pursue happiness: Belief in free will predicts life satisfaction and positive affect among Chinese adolescents. *Frontiers in Psychology, 7.*
Li, J., Zhao, Y., Lin, L., Chen, J., & Wang, S. (2018). The freedom to persist: Belief in free will predicts perseverance for long-term goals among Chinese adolescents. *Personality and Individual Differences, 121,* 7–10.
Libet, B., Gleason, C. A., Wright, E. W., & Pearl, D. K. (1983). Time of conscious intention to act in relation to onset of cerebral activity (readiness-potential) the unconscious initiation of a freely voluntary act. *Brain, 106,* 623–642.
Lynn, M. T., Muhle-Karbe, P. S., Aarts, H., & Brass, M. (2014). Priming determinist beliefs diminishes implicit (but not explicit) components of self-agency. *Frontiers in Psychology, 5.*
MacKenzie, M. J., Vohs, K. D., & Baumeister, R. F. (2014). You didn't have to do that: Belief in free will promotes gratitude. *Personality and Social Psychology Bulletin, 40*(11), 1423–1434.
Maffly-Kipp, J., Gause, C., Kim, J., Vess, M., & Hicks, J. A. (2022). Agentic meaning-making: Free will beliefs, sense-making, and psychological distress following collective traumas. *Current Research in Ecological and Social Psychology, 3.*
Malle, B. F., Guglielmo, S., & Monroe, A. E. (2014). A theory of blame. *Psychological Inquiry, 25*(2), 147–186.
Martin, N. D., Rigoni, D., & Vohs, K. D. (2017). Free will beliefs predict attitudes toward unethical behavior and criminal punishment. *Proceedings of the National Academy of Sciences, 114*(28), 7325–7330.
Monroe, A. E., Brady, G. L., & Malle, B. F. (2017). This isn't the free will worth looking for: General free will beliefs do not influence moral judgments, agent-specific choice ascriptions do. *Social Psychological and Personality Science, 8*(2), 191–199.
Monroe, A. E., & Malle, B. F. (2010). From uncaused will to conscious choice: The need to study, not speculate about people's folk concept of free will. *European Review of Philosophy, 1*(2), 211–224.
Moynihan, A. B., Igou, E. R., & van Tilburg, W. A. P. (2017). Free, connected, and meaningful: Free will beliefs promote meaningfulness through belongingness. *Personality and Individual Differences, 107,* 54–65.
Nadelhoffer, T., Shepard, J., Crone, D. L., Everett, J. A. C., Earp, B. D., & Levy, N. (2020). Does encouraging a belief in determinism increase cheating?: Reconsidering the value of believing in free will. *Cognition, 203,* 1–13.
Nahmias, E., Morris, S., Nadelhoffer, T., & Turner 1, J. (2005). Surveying freedom: Folk intuitions about free will and moral responsibility. *Philosophical Psychology, 18*(5), 561–584.
Nietzsche, F. (2003). *Beyond good and evil: Prelude to a philosophy of the future.* Penguin Books. (Original work published 1886)
Nichols, S. (2004). The folk psychology of free will: Fits and starts. *Mind and Language, 19*(5), 473–502.
Nichols, S., & Knobe, J. (2007). Moral responsibility and determinism: The cognitive science of folk intuitions. *Nous, 41*(4), 663–685.
Ozkok, H., Tatar, B. H., Ayyıldız, T. N., Eskin, M., Erdem, G., & Turan, B. (2022). To blame or not to blame: The role of belief in free will in substance use and suicide stigma. *International Journal of Mental Health and Addiction, 20*(6), 3301–3314.
Paulhus, D. L., & Carey, J. M. (2011). The FAD-Plus: Measuring lay beliefs regarding free will and related constructs. *Journal of Personality Assessment, 93*(1), 96–104.
Pereboom, D. (2006). *Living without free will.* Cambridge University Press.
Perry, R. B. (1935). *The thought and character of William James: Briefer version.* Harvard University Press.
Pronin, E., & Kugler, M. B. (2011). People be-

lieve they have more free will than others. *Proceedings of the National Academy of Sciences, 107*(52), 22469–22474.

Protzko, J., Ouimette, B., & Schooler, J. (2016). Believing there is no free will corrupts intuitive cooperation. *Cognition, 151*, 6–9.

Rakos, R. F., Laurene, K. R., Skala, S., & Slane, S. (2008). Belief in free will: Measurement and conceptualization innovations. *Behavior and Social Issues, 17*(1), 20–39.

Rigoni, D., Kühn, S., Gaudino, G., Sartori, G., & Brass, M. (2012). Reducing self-control by weakening belief in free will. *Consciousness and Cognition: An International Journal, 21*(3), 1482–1490.

Rotter, J. B. (1966). Generalized expectancies for internal versus external control of reinforcement. *Psychological Monographs: General and Applied, 80*(1), 1.

Sarkissian, H., Chatterjee, A., De Brigard, F., Knobe, J., Nichols, S., & Sirker, S. (2010). Is belief in free will a cultural universal? *Mind and Language, 25*(3), 346–358.

Sartre, J.-P. (1974). *Being and nothingness*. Citadel. (Original work published 1943)

Seto, E. (2024). Climbing the invisible ladder: Attenuating belief in free will reduces subjective perceptions of social mobility. *Social Psychological and Personality Science, 15*(1), 3–11.

Seto, E., & Hicks, J. A. (2016). Disassociating the agent from the self: Undermining belief in free will diminishes true self-knowledge. *Social Psychological and Personality Science, 7*(7), 726–734.

Seto, E., Hicks, J. A., Davis, W. E., & Smallman, R. (2015). Free will, counterfactual reflection, and the meaningfulness of life events. *Social Psychological and Personality Science, 6*(3), 243–250.

Seto, E., Kim, J., & Hicks, J. A. (2021). The illusion of time: Testing the bidirectional relationship between belief in free will and temporal horizons. *Social Psychological and Personality Science, 12*(2), 176–185.

Shariff, A. F., Greene, J. D., Karremans, J. C., Luguri, J. B., Clark, C. J., Schooler, J. W., . . . Vohs, K. D. (2014). Free will and punishment: A mechanistic view of human nature reduces retribution. *Psychological Science, 25*(8), 1563–1570.

Shariff, A. F., Schooler, J., & Vohs, K. D. (2008). The hazards of claiming to have solved the hard problem of free will. In J. Baer, J. C. Kaufman, & R. F. Baumeister (Eds.), *Are we free?: Psychology and free will* (pp. 181–204). Oxford University Press.

Sheldon, K. M., & Goffredi, R. (2021). Self-determination theory shows that free will matters. *Motivation Science, 7*(2), 119.

Smithdeal, M. (2016). Belief in free will as an adaptive, ungrounded belief. *Philosophical Psychology, 29*(8), 1241–1252.

St Quinton, T., Morris, B., & Crescioni, A. W. (2022). Beliefs in free will and determinism: Associations with social cognition and gambling behavior. *Addiction Research and Theory*.

Stillman, T. F., & Baumeister, R. F. (2010). Guilty, free, and wise: Determinism and psychopathy diminish learning from negative emotions. *Journal of Experimental Social Psychology, 46*(6), 951–960.

Stillman, T. F., Baumeister, R. F., & Mele, A. R. (2011). Free will in everyday life: Autobiographical accounts of free and unfree actions. *Philosophical Psychology, 24*(3), 381–394.

Stillman, T. F., Baumeister, R. F., Vohs, K. D., Lambert, N. M., Fincham, F. D., & Brewer, L. E. (2010). Personal philosophy and personnel achievement: Belief in free will predicts better job performance. *Social Psychological and Personality Science, 1*(1), 43–50.

Stinnett, A. J., & Alquist, J. L. (2022). Consider the tumor: Brain tumors decrease punishment via perceptions of free will. *Philosophical Psychology, 36*(1), 162–185.

Stinnett, A. J., Rodriguez, J. E., Littlefield, A. K., & Alquist, J. L. (2022). Distinguishing free will from moral responsibility when measuring free will beliefs: The FWS-II. *Philosophical Psychology, 37*(8), 2285–2311.

Synofzik, M., Vosgerau, G., & Newen, A. (2008). Beyond the comparator model: A multifactorial two-step account of agency. *Consciousness and Cognition: An International Journal, 17*(1), 219–239.

Vohs, K. D., & Baumeister, R. F. (2004). Understanding self-regulation: An introduction. In K. D. Vohs & R. F. Baumeister (Eds.), *Handbook of self-regulation: Research, theory, and applications* (pp. 1–9). Guilford Press.

Vohs, K. D., & Schooler, J. W. (2008). The value of believing in free will: Encouraging a belief in determinism increases cheating. *Psychological Science, 19*(1), 49–54.

Wegner, D. M. (2004). Précis of the illusion of conscious will. *Behavioral and Brain Sciences, 27*(5), 649–659.

Wente, A. O., Bridgers, S., Zhao, X., Seiver, E., Zhu, L., & Gopnik, A. (2016). How universal are free will beliefs?: Cultural differences in Chinese and US 4- and 6-year-olds. *Child Development, 87*(3), 666–676.

CHAPTER 25

Morality, the Self, and Self-Conscious Emotions

Jessica L. Tracy, Gabrielle C. Ibasco, *and* Ian Hohm

In one of the most famous scenes in Western literature, Lady Macbeth furiously scrubs her hands, desperately trying wash off the invisible blood she hallucinates covering them. Shakespeare uses this image, along with Lady Macbeth's immortal words ("out, out, damned spot!"), to convey the guilt she feels over her role in her husband's murderous behavior. In another well-known Shakespearean play, Hamlet struts and frets throughout his time upon the stage, over the shame he feels about his inability to avenge his father's death. Meanwhile, the moral crux of *Othello* is shaped by the titular king's hubristic pride, which allows him to believe that his wife was unfaithful. In all three tragedies, the story's narrative thrust thus relies on a tight connection between immoral behavior, moral decision making, and self-conscious emotions. These emotions, like guilt, shame, and pride, are regularly experienced in response to the self-reflection and self-evaluation that moral quandaries can cause, and they influence the moral and immoral behaviors that humans enact. As Shakespeare knew, a full understanding of human morality requires an understanding of self-conscious emotions and how they shape people's sense of self, and, as a consequence, the moral decisions they make.

The impact that these emotions have on people's identity, and the kind of person they see themselves becoming as they engage in moral or immoral behaviors, makes self-conscious emotions a critical part of existential psychology. Furthermore, being or becoming moral is one of the major ways in which people strive to make their lives meaningful, to belong, and to justify their existence. The intersection of self, emotions, and morality is thus a critical area of research in existential psychology.

Here, we review the extant literature on self-conscious emotions and morality, as well as broader links with moral identity. Although guilt and shame have been labeled *moral emotions* (Tangney & Fischer, 1995), few studies have directly examined the ways in which these emotions are integral to moral thinking or behavior. For the most part, research in moral psychology has proceeded separately from research on self-conscious emotions, and moral psychologists most often study emotions that shape judgments about others rather than self (e.g., Horberg et al., 2009). Although other-oriented emotions like disgust, anger, and contempt influence moral decision making and may underlie people's sense of what is and is not immoral (Schnall et al., 2008; Tracy et al.,

2019), these emotions do not typically influence the way that people view themselves.

In contrast, guilt, shame, and pride are elicited by our own morally relevant behavior, and motivate us to change our behavior to align with moral standards (e.g., Keltner & Buswell, 1997; Tangney & Tracy, 2012). People feel guilt or shame when they engage in immoral acts like lying, stealing, or cheating, and when they fail to engage in morally upstanding behaviors like helping or showing compassion for others (e.g., Leith & Baumeister, 1998; Tangney & Dearing, 2003). Conversely, behaving in a prosocial way, by avoiding temptation, donating to charity, or contributing to a shared pool of resources, can lead to feelings of pride (Dorfman et al., 2014; Hofmann & Fisher, 2012; Tracy & Ibasco, 2025). As a result, self-conscious emotions are intricately interconnected with morality, but only with those moral behaviors that elicit positive or negative evaluations of the self. Given that most moral or immoral acts cause individuals to self-reflect and self-evaluate, self-conscious emotions play a crucial role in human morality.

MORALITY AND THE SELF

Morality is central to the self-concept (e.g., Strohminger & Nichols, 2014), yet early research in moral psychology did not include the self in theories of moral judgments and decision making. Instead, initial work followed Kohlberg (1969), who emphasized the role of cognitive reasoning in shaping moral judgments. Most of this research focused on the moral judgments people make about others in hypothetical dilemmas (e.g., whether a husband should steal a drug to save his terminally ill wife; Rest et al., 1969), leaving open questions of how moral judgments influence people's own behavior. Although some studies found effects of moral judgments on behaviors (e.g., Bernardi et al., 2004), these associations tended to be weak or inconsistent (Blasi, 1980). This makes sense; even when people appraise a situation as morally wrong, there are many factors that might prevent them from acting to resolve it. However, theories emphasizing cognitive moral development have historically not accounted for the wide variation observed in enacted moral behaviors and reported moral intentions.

More recently, moral psychologists sought to address this gap between individuals' moral judgments and their behaviors by accounting for the role of the moral self-concept, defined as "a complex system of self-defining moral attributes involving moral beliefs, orientations, dispositions, and cognitive and affective capacities that engage regulatory focus toward moral behavior" (Jennings et al., 2015, p. 106). Researchers who incorporate the moral self still tend to include a role for cognitive reasoning but view the self as the primary anchor of moral processes, because it determines the criteria that shape whether an individual bears moral responsibility in a given situation (e.g., Aquino & Reed, 2002; Blasi, 1980). For example, a person whose moral identity is strongly tied to values of fairness might be particularly likely to intervene after witnessing a colleague being treated unfairly. As a result, individual differences in the moral self might explain the gap, or the association, between moral judgments and behavior (e.g., Patrick et al., 2018).

The Importance of the Moral Self

Studies have found that morality plays a central role in self-perceptions and occupies principal importance relative to other components of the self-concept like competence (e.g., Everett et al., 2020). Perceptions of oneself as a moral being start early in life; by age 8, children view moral beliefs as central to their self-understanding (Heiphetz et al., 2018). Among adults, moral identity is perhaps the most self-defining component of selfhood; one set of studies found that participants asked to imagine experiencing a permanent change to some aspect of their identity due to a traumatic event report the greatest identity change when moral traits are affected (Strohminger & Nichols, 2014).

From an evolutionary perspective, moral beliefs and the enforcement of moral norms emerged in human societies to promote harmonious group functioning, motivate cooperation, and minimize societal harm. A shared sense of morality allows people to live and work together in large groups (e.g., Curry et al., 2019; Gray & Kubin, 2024).

In this view, the moral self is adaptive because it is an internal representation of the extent to which a person is behaving in accordance with their society's moral norms. Holding a moral self, and desiring to maintain or increase the extent to which that self meets its moral values, facilitates each group member's ability to encode group norms and follow them (Aquino & Reed, 2002). Indeed, studies have found that people who view their ideal self as moral report a greater sense of purpose, social responsibility, and altruistic behavior, as well as lower levels of aggression (Hardy et al., 2014).

Moral Identity and Moral Behavior

Most extant empirical research on the moral self focuses on Aquino and Reed's (2002) concept of *moral identity*, defined as a self-concept organized around a collection of ideal moral traits. In the same way that social identities are formed based on traits, habits, or cultural beliefs people share with others in their society (Tajfel & Turner, 2004), moral identities form around a constellation of socially normative moral traits that others view as useful or aspire to possess. These identities, in turn, provide a framework that guides behavior, as people strive to behave consistently with their identity. Supporting this account, priming people to view themselves as morally good motivates them to engage in prosocial actions (Young et al., 2012).

Although moral identity is a central part of most people's self-concept, there are individual differences in the ways people think about these identities; these differences have been operationalized in terms of *internalization* and *symbolization*. Internalization captures the intrinsic importance of morality to the self, whereas symbolization captures the extrinsic, reputational aspect of identity (Aquino & Reed, 2002). Studies controlling for shared variance between internalization and symbolization have found that each dimension independently predicts moral outcomes (Jennings et al., 2015). Internalization tends to be the stronger and more positive predictor of prosocial moral behavior and attitudes, such as charitable donations (e.g., Aquino & Reed, 2002; see Hertz & Krettenauer, 2016, for a meta-analysis). Symbolization, in contrast, tends to predict moral behavior only in situations where individuals can gain public recognition for their actions (Winterich et al., 2013).

Nonetheless, moral decision making is regularly influenced by others, even for people low in symbolization. Indeed, when individuals are reminded that their moral judgments might influence how others perceive them, they are more likely to alter those judgments to align with social norms (Rom & Conway, 2018). Reputational concerns also contribute to engaging in moralistic third-party punishment against perceived offenders (e.g., Jordan & Kteily, 2023). However, for people who have a strongly internalized moral identity, moral behaviors tend to be less influenced by social or situational factors (Skarlicki & Rupp, 2010). For example, one study found that participants manipulated to feel powerful subsequently made more selfish decisions in a resource allocation task, but only if they were low in moral identity internalization. Overall, social cues and situations seem to be less reliable elicitors of moral behavior compared to holding a strong, core internalized moral identity (Krettenauer, 2022).

THE MORAL EMOTIONS

A growing number of studies have linked moral identity with behavior, but fewer have examined the specific self-relevant emotions likely to underlie these associations. Nonetheless, scholars have long suggested that self-conscious emotions like shame, guilt, and pride motivate moral behaviors, as these emotions are often elicited by situations appraised as congruent or incongruent with one's moral identity (Lewis, 1995; Tangney & Dearing, 2003; Tracy & Robins, 2004). For example, committing a social transgression (e.g., forgetting to call a friend on their birthday) that is incongruent with one's moral identity (e.g., being a good friend) is likely to promote feelings of guilt or shame (Tracy & Ibasco, 2025). These feelings, in turn, might motivate a compensatory response to address the incongruence (Tangney & Dearing, 2003). As a result, self-conscious emotions can be understood as serving a crucial moral-signaling function, informing individuals that the standards of their moral identity have been met or surpassed (eliciting moral pride) or violated (eliciting guilt or shame), and also a motivational function, prompting behavior to rectify the situation.

This account is consistent with the suggestion that moral identity influences behavior because people are intrinsically motivated to behave consistently with their identity (Aquino & Reed, 2002; Damon & Hart, 1992). Self-conscious emotions may provide an essential missing piece to this model, as they both inform individuals whether their behavior is consistent with their moral identity and motivate them to address any inconsistencies. A meta-analysis found that the self-rated importance of one's moral identity was positively correlated with experiencing self-conscious emotions (rs = 0.32–0.33; Lefebvre & Krettenauer, 2019).

Guilt, Shame, and Morality

According to a large body of research, individuals experience guilt when they focus on negative aspects of their behavior—"the thing done or undone"—and shame when they focus on negative aspects of themselves—the self who did or did not do it (Lewis, 1971, p. 30; Lewis, 2008; Tangney & Dearing, 2003; Tracy & Robins, 2006). In other words, both emotions are elicited by internal attributions, or blame to the self, but different kinds of internal attributions. The same negative self-relevant event, such as failure on an exam, tends to elicit greater guilt if attributed to unstable, controllable, and specific causes like the amount of effort a person put into studying, but greater shame if attributed to stable, uncontrollable, and global causes like general intelligence or ability (e.g., Brown & Weiner, 1984; Tracy & Robins, 2006).

Given this distinction, whether a person feels guilt or shame in response to a moral infraction depends at least in part on how the infraction is appraised. Both emotions follow appraisals of the self or the self's behavior as incongruent with moral identity standards (Tangney & Dearing, 2003). However, guilt is typically associated with self-blame for a specific moral transgression enacted, whereas shame entails appraisals of a flawed moral identity. Given this distinction, it is not surprising that shame is the far more painful emotion (Tangney & Dearing, 2003) and more difficult to address. Whereas feelings of guilt involve a sense of control over one's behavior and can motivate people to repair or compensate for their transgression (Graton & Ric, 2017), those who feel shame have no clear recourse, as there is no obvious way to fix a flawed moral identity.

Guilt thus tends to be the more morally adaptive and prosocial emotion, associated with reparations, concern for others, and cooperative behavior (e.g., de Hooge et al., 2007; Tangney & Dearing, 2003). Shame, in contrast, is associated with avoidance, externalizing blame, minimizing the negativity or impact of one's immoral actions, and attempts to deny or escape shame-inducing situations (de Hooge et al., 2007; Stuewig et al., 2010; Tangney & Dearing, 2003). Similarly, a tendency to experience guilt is associated with dispositional empathy and perspective taking, whereas trait shame-proneness is associated with a more egocentric focus on one's own negative feelings, along with reduced empathy and perspective taking (Joireman, 2004; Leith & Baumeister, 1998). Shame-proneness has also been found to motivate hostile, antisocial behaviors toward others, including verbal and physical aggression (e.g., Stuewig et al., 2010). Indeed, shame is strongly related to anger and aggression, at both the trait and state level (Heaven et al., 2009; Tangney et al., 2007). These externalizing responses are generally assumed to be attempts to counteract, suppress, and avoid painful feelings of shame (Tangney & Tracy, 2012; Tracy & Robins, 2006).

Although shame is clearly problematic for day-to-day moral functioning, it might nonetheless serve important moral functions at a more distal or ultimate evolutionary level. Although at a proximal level shame seems to promote morally problematic behaviors (e.g., avoidance, aggression), viewing shame from a distal perspective allows us to see how the emotion likely evolved to serve the crucial moral function of informing individuals that they have violated their group's moral norms, and motivating them to change course to avoid rejection (Beall & Tracy, 2020; Gilbert, 1998). Ancestral humans relied heavily on social groups for protection from external threats, and those without strong interpersonal connections would have failed to secure the benefits of shared cultural knowledge and resources. As a result, group membership and belongingness were crucial to survival (e.g., Henrich & Boyd, 1998). Functionalist accounts therefore suggest that shame is adaptive by virtue of helping individuals maintain their current social status and acceptance in the eyes of their group (Tracy & Robins, 2004).

Indeed, studies show that shame informs individuals of a discrepancy between their current and desired selves (Leary et al., 1995), and the resulting aversive emotional state pushes them to halt their unsuccessful status-seeking efforts and minimize further negative consequences of lowered status. A desire to avoid shame's unpleasant feelings may also provide an anticipatory incentive to avoid future status-lowering actions (Fessler, 2007). Like physical pain, which is aversive to experience but adaptive by virtue of promoting injury avoidance, shame feelings may have evolved as a kind of alarm system, warning individuals that a drop in social rank is imminent (or has already occurred; Fessler, 2007). Consistent with this account, Westerners asked to recount shame-eliciting events tend to list situations involving punishable moral transgressions; similar findings have emerged among members of a small-scale traditional village, suggesting that the propensity to feel shame in response to a moral deviation may be a human universal (Fessler, 2004).

Shame may be a particularly useful response to such transgressions; violating moral rules risks potentially dangerous reactions from others, such as anger or retaliation (Gilbert, 2007), and shame may help individuals avoid these penalties by motivating appeasement behaviors. Appeasing higher-status others is a cost-efficient way of dealing with conflict; though it may come at the cost of status, as it typically entails acknowledging one's transgression, appeasing a more formidable opponent saves valuable resources that might be lost from fighting (Keltner et al., 1997). In addition, the time and energy saved by submitting and appeasing rather than fighting can be used for other pursuits that enhance fitness, such as resource and mate acquisition and retention (Gangestad & Simpson, 2000).

Supporting this account, one study asked participants to read hypothetical scenarios about a fictitious CEO who apologized for an ecological incident caused by his company. Participants who learned that the CEO expressed feelings of shame while apologizing were more satisfied with the apology than were those who learned that he communicated guilt or no emotion (Giner-Sorolla et al., 2008). In another study, participants applied weaker penalties to fictitious offenders who were described as feeling ashamed compared to offenders who felt sad and remorseful, or no emotion (Proeve & Howells, 2006). According to Fessler (2007), expressions of shame reassure onlookers that, despite their misstep, the shamed individual is a morally upstanding, trustworthy group member who believes in and can behave in accordance with social norms.

Other research consistent with this account suggests that shame feelings directly correspond to—and therefore may inform individuals of—their social group's disapproval (Sznycer & Lukaszewski, 2019). Across several multinational studies, participants read scenarios about people engaging in socially undesirable behaviors (e.g., "He does a bad job taking care of children"), then rated either the extent to which they would devalue the behavior or feel shame if they were that person. Across countries, feelings of anticipatory shame were strongly correlated with others' likely devaluation (Sznycer et al., 2016). Extending these correlational findings, experiments have found that social exclusion causally increases shame due to increased feelings of devaluation (Robertson et al., 2018).

According to this interpersonal adaptiveness account, the proximal behaviors motivated by each self-conscious emotion are consistent with their distinctive distal-level evolved elicitors. Guilt motivates promotion-oriented behaviors, which ultimately increases a person's social value, and shame motivates escape or withdrawal from the triggering situation, which ultimately minimizes further social devaluation (Sznycer, 2019). Notably, although this perspective has been contrasted with the attributional perspective (see Landers et al., 2024), the two in fact complement one another. The suggestion that guilt leads people to focus on others whereas shame leads people to focus on themselves is consistent with H. B. Lewis's (1971) and Tangney and Dearing's (2003) original attributional distinction, given that attributions to specific wrongdoings promote greater attentiveness to the consequences suffered by others (guilt), whereas attributions to one's tarnished identity emerge with an egocentric concern for the self (shame). The two accounts may therefore be understood as two levels of explanation—distal and proximal—for the same set of effects and mental processes.

Interestingly, under the assumption that shame is a causal factor underlying one's awareness of their wrongdoing and corresponding desire to change, governments have historically used public shaming as a punitive means of curbing problematic behaviors that tend to violate moral rules (Jacquet, 2011). Such institutionally sanctioned shaming practices remain common; examples include the statewide issuance of marked license plates for individuals convicted of DUIs (Nussbaum, 2006) and online lists of noncompliant taxpayers (Jacquet, 2011). Supporting the use of these practices, researchers have found that the experience of shame motivates individuals to seek to improve their self-image (de Hooge et al., 2011) and that the threat of public shaming promotes greater contributions to a common good (Jacquet et al., 2011).

However, it is not clear that shame experienced about a particular wrongdoing promotes positive behavioral change relevant to *that* domain; in other words, whether the shame an individual feels from being forced to drive with a marked DUI license plate reduces that individual's future likelihood of drinking and driving, as opposed to deterring others from doing the same. In fact, feelings of shame for immoral or unhealthy behaviors are more often associated with continued problematic behaviors. One study found that the degree to which newly sober recovering alcoholics demonstrated behavioral displays of shame while discussing their past drinking significantly predicted subsequent declines in their physical and mental health, and, most importantly, positively predicted their likelihood of drinking again (Randles & Tracy, 2013). In sum, although shame may have evolved to serve adaptive moral functions, more research is needed to demonstrate its most adaptive consequences because, of all the emotions thought to be endemic to our species, shame seems to come with the most negative social and psychological outcomes (see Randles & Tracy, 2015).

Group-Based Guilt, Shame, and Morality

Interestingly, shame and guilt appear to be less clearly distinct when considered as group-based self-conscious emotions, or self-conscious emotions felt on behalf of one's social or group identities (e.g., nationality, race). People hold a sense of self at multiple levels of identity (Robins et al., 2008), such that they can feel shame, guilt, and pride in response to events enacted by others who share a self-relevant group identity (Lickel et al., 2007; Mackie et al., 2008). Correspondingly, studies have found that group-based guilt emerges in response to specific, controllable actions enacted by ingroup members, whereas group-based shame emerges in response to the perception that the group's moral identity is flawed (Branscombe et al., 2004; Lickel et al., 2004). In line with this attributional distinction, feelings of guilt for an ingroup's transgression motivate greater support for reparations, whereas group-based shame motivates avoidance of the issue, downplaying it, and even denying that a transgression occurred (e.g., Schmader & Lickel, 2006). However, other studies have found that group-based shame can be more predictive of support for reparations than group-based guilt (e.g., Allpress et al., 2014; Shepherd et al., 2013). A meta-analysis found that, overall, both group-based guilt and group-based shame are positive predictors of intergroup reparations (Hakim et al., 2021).

To address these mixed findings, and the apparent distinction between the outcomes of shame at the group versus individual level, scholars have made a distinction between two forms of group-based shame (Allpress et al., 2014). The first, labeled group-based *image shame,* is focused on how others perceive the ingroup's harmed reputation, and tends to preclude genuine moral culpability.

In contrast, group-based *moral shame* entails a focus on the group's tarnished moral identity, which has been internalized by the individual experiencing the emotion. After partialling out shared variance between group-based guilt, moral shame, and image shame, group-based moral shame tends to strongly predict a willingness to make institutional reparations for an ingroup's misdeeds, whereas group-based image shame predicts avoidance tactics (Allpress et al., 2014; Ibasco & Tracy, 2025) and has little-to-no effect on reparation intentions (Grigoryan et al., 2024). Furthermore, group-based guilt seems to only weakly predict support for reparations after controlling for group-based moral shame (e.g., Allpress et al., 2014; Ibasco & Tracy, 2025).

There are several possible explanations for the finding that group-based moral shame, compared to group-based guilt, seems more useful for promoting intergroup harmony even though, at intrapsychic and interpersonal levels, guilt tends to promote greater prosociality. First, individuals may be less desperate to protect themselves from group-based shame than personal shame, because ingroup identities tend to be several layers removed from the personal self, and efforts to repair the group identity do not rest on a single individual alone. As a result, individuals may be less defensive against, and thus more willing to experience, this form of shame. Second, shame may be the more relevant emotion to experience in response to group-level moral transgressions. Given that guilt is elicited by specific immoral actions, it is less likely to occur in response to group-based immorality, where experiencers are usually not directly involved in the problematic group actions (e.g., in the case of North Americans' feelings about their society's history of racism toward Indigenous populations). As a result, the more global and symbolic group identity that is the focus of group-based moral shame may be more relevant to culture- or country-level transgressions (e.g., Gausel et al., 2012).

Pride and Morality

Like shame and guilt, pride is elicited by internal attributions for a self-relevant event. However, in the case of pride, the event must be appraised as *congruent* with one's identity, rather than incongruent (Tracy & Robins, 2004). Moral pride therefore is elicited by events appraised as congruent with one's moral identity—behaving in ways that meet or exceed one's moral standards. Pride rewards morally upstanding behaviors, and a desire for pride motivates people to engage in such behaviors (Tracy & Robins, 2004). Indeed, although research on pride often emphasizes achievement-oriented activities, which tend to be amoral (e.g., academic or occupational achievements), pride is also an important component of moral judgments and decisions (Tangney et al., 2007).

The behaviors that give rise to pride are those that are socially valued (Sznycer et al., 2017), and individuals tend to be valued for acts that convey moral character, as they suggest that the individual is likely to be a cooperative social partner (Curry et al., 2019). As a result, pride plays an important role in the development of moral identity and in motivating moral behavior. Experience-sampling studies have found that pride felt in response to successful instances of self-control led to an increased ability to resist similar temptations in the future (Hofmann & Fisher, 2012). Similarly, considering future experiences of pride led to increased cooperation in economic games (Dorfman et al., 2014; van der Schalk et al., 2012). More specifically, anticipated pride increased fair decisions in bargaining, donations to public goods, and the perceived importance of cooperation.

However, in the same way that there are two distinct self-conscious emotions that occur in response to perceived incongruencies with one's identity (guilt and shame), a large body of research suggests that pride is not, in fact, a single unitary emotion. Instead, pride has two distinct components (Lewis, 2008; Tangney et al., 1989; Tracy & Robins, 2004; see Tracy et al., 2023, for a review). The first component, labeled "authentic pride," involves feelings such as "accomplished" and "confident," and fits with a prosocial, achievement-oriented, earned pride conceptualization. The second component, labeled "hubristic pride," involves feelings such as "arrogant" and "conceited," and fits with a more self-aggrandizing, egotistical, and undeserved pride conceptualization (Tracy & Robins, 2007).

Like shame and guilt, the two pride facets are different not only in their content but also in their implications for moral behavior. Authentic pride is positively related to prosocial traits like agreeableness, conscientiousness, and emotional stability, as well as humility (Tracy & Robins, 2007; Weidman et al., 2018). Furthermore, individuals high in dispositional authentic pride tend to be low in antisocial traits like hostility and aggression, and high in the tendency to support (and be supported by) others. In contrast, individuals high in hubristic pride tend to be disagreeable and unconscientious, regularly experience hostility, and engage in a range of antisocial misbehaviors (Tracy et al., 2009). Furthermore, although individuals high in agency are prone to experiencing both facets of pride, individuals high in communion—meaning those who tend to care for and be oriented toward others—are prone only to authentic pride; hubristic pride shows a negative relationship with communal traits (Cheng et al., 2010). Hubristic pride is also positively associated with psychopathy and Machiavellianism (Tracy et al., 2009), two traits that predict a range of immoral behaviors.

Both forms of pride have been found to promote social status or high rank (Tracy et al., 2023) but they seem to do so in different ways, with hubristic pride motivating people to engage in behaviors that are less moral or ethical in their status pursuits. For example, one set of studies found that people high in dispositional hubristic pride were more likely than those low in this emotional tendency to exaggerate their performance to a partner whom they knew had outperformed them (Mercadante & Tracy, 2022). These individuals were not more likely to lie in this manner if their partner had not outperformed them, suggesting that hubristic pride may facilitate immoral behavior specifically in the context of rank attainment. However, it is not associated with immoral activity or even false bragging more indiscriminately, in the way that psychopathy and narcissism might be. Pride therefore seems not to motivate general-purpose immoral behaviors but, rather, may be the affective mechanism that nudges people to take advantage of others when doing so is necessary to protect their own status.

Other research suggests that authentic pride may play an important role in another morally questionable trait: greed. Dispositional greed is defined as the desire to acquire more combined with the dissatisfaction of never having enough (Seuntjens et al., 2015). Although this personality trait has been associated with certain positive characteristics, it has more often been linked to unethical behaviors (e.g., Seuntjens et al., 2019). Until recently, however, it remained unclear why these individuals demonstrate the critical behavior that defines them as greedy: chronic acquisition. In other words, why are greedy people never satisfied with what they have, and always desiring more?

Across several longitudinal and cross-sectional studies, Mercadante and Tracy (2024) found that individuals high in dispositional greed experienced a sharp boost in authentic pride after a new acquisition. However, these feelings were short-lived, dissipating within a week, and thus required repeated boosting from more new acquisitions. The desire to increase feelings of authentic pride therefore may be a cause of greedy people's constant acquisitiveness. The additional finding that this pattern was particularly pronounced among those high in greed and low in self-esteem supports this account; greedy people with low self-esteem may be most in need of frequent upticks of authentic pride (the form of pride most closely related to self-esteem).

Several authors have argued that the pride felt in response to moral actions, or behaviors that directly benefit others, must be distinguished from a more generalized pride that can occur in response to morality or achievement (e.g., Etxebarria et al., 2015). These scholars argue that the standard authentic and hubristic pride scales (Tracy & Robins, 2007) are not ideal for capturing moral pride, given, for example, that participants are unlikely to report feeling "egotistical" or "snobbish" (two items on the hubristic pride scale) for prosocial behaviors. Instead, researchers have validated scenario-based measures that more directly target trait levels of authentic and hubristic moral pride (e.g., Ibasco & Tracy, 2025; Krettenauer & Casey, 2015). Similar to their broader counterparts, authentic moral pride occurs in response to appraisals of specific moral behaviors, whereas hubristic moral pride occurs in response to appraisals of an inflated moral character. In a study demonstrating the validity of these measures, authentic moral pride was associated with greater self-reported engagement in prosocial activity, whereas hubristic moral pride predicted fewer prosocial actions (Krettenauer & Casey, 2015).

In addition to motivating behaviors that fall within the moral domain of harm or care, pride also may influence attitudes relevant to the moral domain of fairness. Recent studies have identified two distinct moral values related to fairness: equality, or support for the equal distribution of resources, and proportionality, or support for resource distribution based on deservedness (Atari et al., 2023). In hierarchical social groups, a greater share of resources is typically allocated to those at the top (e.g., leaders) compared to those at the bottom (Brown & Maurer, 1986). Given that the unequal distribution of resources benefits those with high status, it is advantageous for high-status individuals to promote proportionality, rather than equality. A large body of evidence suggests that pride is elicited by achievements or other events that lead to status gains (see Tracy et al., 2023), so we might expect pride experiences to increase the value that individuals place on proportionality compared to equality.

There is evidence to support this prediction. First, nonverbal displays of pride communicate an individual's support for meritocracy, a form of proportionality in which resources are distributed based on merit (e.g., Horberg et al., 2013). When a target individual expresses pride, observers infer that the target endorses merit-based resource distributions over equality-based ones. This effect was mediated by observers' beliefs that proud targets were more self-interested and therefore likely to endorse ideologies that would benefit them. Other studies have shown that adherence to norms of equality is shaped by one's assigned role in a group. De Cremer and van Dijk (2005) found that leaders adhere less to equality values than followers do, and this effect is explained by leaders' feelings of entitlement and deservingness. Given that hubristic pride is associated with an increased sense of entitlement and dispositional traits that promote selfish behavior (e.g., Machiavellianism, narcissism), leaders high in hubristic pride may be particularly likely to shape their fairness values around proportionality rather than equality.

Given these findings, observers may attribute selfishness to those displaying pride. This expectation is consistent with research examining how needy targets' pride expressions influence observers' decisions about whether to help them. Tracy and colleagues (2018) coded the nonverbal displays shown by individuals in developing nations who used the website Kiva.org to request financial aid from donors in more economically developed countries. Requesters posted photos of themselves along with a short description of how they planned to use the funds. Across two preregistered studies, requesters who displayed pride in their photos received less aid, by 33–77%.

Group-Based Moral Pride

Few studies have examined group-based pride, let alone its moral relevance. However, new research has begun to explore the ways in which group-based pride might regulate group-based shame and guilt to promote moral outcomes. As noted above, studies have found that group-based guilt and moral shame have positive implications for intergroup reparations (Hakim et al., 2021). However, these emotions are aversive to experience, as they violate people's basic motivation to view their groups as morally good. As a result, individuals are often reluctant to feel group-based guilt and shame and tend to respond defensively when reminded of their group's current or past moral transgressions, denying or downplaying the immoral acts (Ferguson & Branscombe, 2014; Wohl et al., 2006).

New data, however, suggest that group-based moral pride might counteract this effect, increasing people's willingness to experience guilt and moral shame for their groups' moral transgressions (Ibasco & Tracy, 2025). Drawing on distinctions previously made between authentic and hubristic moral pride at the individual level, Ibasco and Tracy (2025) defined authentic group-based moral pride (AGMP) as involving a focus on specific, moral actions taken by ingroup members, and likely associated with low defensiveness. In contrast, hubristic group-based moral pride (HGMP) was expected to entail an aggrandized, inflated sense of the ingroup's moral character, and to motivate defensiveness against perceived threats to group character. Given this distinction, people experiencing or disposed to HGMP, compared to AGMP, should be less receptive to feeling or acknowledging group-based guilt or moral shame, and more likely to experience group-based image shame, in response to threats to the ingroup's morality.

A series of studies provided support for these hypotheses. Among non-Indigenous Canadian citizens, dispositional AGMP in Canada's moral prosocial history was associated with greater guilt and moral shame for Canada's historical genocide of Indigenous people. In contrast, dispositional HGMP in Canada's moral reputation was associated with greater image shame, but not group-based guilt or moral shame, for these historical atrocities. In subsequent experimental studies, non-Indigenous Canadians and White Americans were induced to feel AGMP in their respective countries, and this emotion manipulation led them to feel greater group-based guilt and moral shame for their countries' histories of racism. Moreover, elevated levels of group-based moral shame, caused by the AGMP induction, led to greater support for intergroup reparations, whereas elevated levels of group-based image shame mediated a relation between HGMP and a desire to avoid conversations about reparation (Ibasco & Tracy, 2025).

Other Self-Relevant Emotions and Morality

A number of emotions beyond pride, shame, and guilt contribute to individuals' self-perceptions. Although these emotions do not require self-evaluations and may not always influence the ways in which individuals see themselves, they often affect the self-concept and consequently influence moral behavior.

Awe

Awe is typically defined as the experience of vastness and accommodation (Keltner & Haidt, 2003), where vastness refers to an awareness of something much larger than oneself, either in physical or social size (e.g., fame); and accommodation refers to the adjustment of mental structures (e.g., knowledge, beliefs) that cannot make sense of (i.e., assimilate) the awe-inducing experience. Accommodation captures the confusion, disorientation, and, at times, fear that accompany experiences of awe. Studies show that the sense of vastness induced by awe leads to a sense of a smaller self (Campos et al., 2013; Piff et al., 2015). This changed self-perception can, in turn, influence moral behavior. As a result of their diminished self-focus, individuals experiencing awe become more inclined to define themselves in terms of larger social categories, rather than in purely individualistic terms (van Cappellen & Saroglou, 2012), which in turn allows for a greater focus on others and a motivation to engage with the collective group, promoting ethical decision making, generosity, and prosocial values more broadly (Piff et al., 2015).

Gratitude

Gratitude is defined as the positive emotional state that arises from a desired outcome that was partially or completely caused by another person (Emmons & McCullough, 2003). In other words, people feel grateful when someone else helps them achieve their goals. Grateful individuals, in turn, experience an enhanced sense of connectedness with others, humility, and indebtedness (Armenta et al., 2017). They may also feel heightened "elevation," a positive moral emotion elicited by perceptions of virtuosity and characterized by a warm feeling in the chest that motivates individuals to emulate others' virtuous behaviors (Haidt, 2003).

Gratitude seems to play an important role in facilitating moral behavior; it can promote self-improvement (Emmons & Mishra, 2011) and a broad range of prosocial behaviors (Ma et al., 2017). More specifically, people feeling gratitude show an increased desire to strengthen social bonds (Algoe, 2012); they tend to manage conflicts constructively and seek to spend more time with close others (e.g., Lambert & Fincham, 2011). Moreover, gratitude has been found to promote a "pay it forward" attitude, motivating increased kindness and upstream reciprocity that extends beyond one's benefactor toward improving society at large (e.g., Nowak & Roch, 2007).

Anger

According to evolutionary accounts, anger is experienced when an individual believes that their welfare is not sufficiently valued by others (Sznycer et al., 2022). Supporting this account, studies show that individuals' perceptions of their social value shape the extent to which they experience anger in response to transgressions (Sell et al., 2009). According to the recalibrational theory of anger (Sell et al., 2009), the emotion motivates behaviors like intimidation, threatening to impose costs (e.g., physical harm), and withholding benefits (e.g., not cooperating in the future), which function to incentivize the anger-eliciting target to recalibrate the angry individual's welfare (i.e., they come to see the angry person as more valuable). This recalibration, in turn, causes them to reconsider their anger-inducing behaviors.

One implication of this model is that a person's self-concept shapes their tendency to experience anger. Supporting this account, individuals who are more physically formidable, and thus able to inflict greater costs on others, are more prone to anger and more likely to use anger to effectively resolve conflicts (e.g., Wyckoff & Kirkpatrick, 2016). Similarly, individuals who are more physically attractive tend to be perceived as more valuable social partners (Langlois et al., 2000), allowing these individuals to withhold benefits from others (e.g., association with an attractive social partner). Purportedly as a result of this greater bargaining power, physically attractive people have also been found to be more prone to anger and more capable of using it to resolve conflicts (Sell et al., 2009). Individual differences in the propensity to experience anger, in turn, have important consequences for moral decision making. The most obvious moral consequence is a tendency to treat others with hostility and a willingness to engage in violence (Sell et al., 2009). However, anger also plays a role in generating the courage and moral outrage required to intervene when witnessing a moral violation (Salerno & Peter-Hagene, 2013).

Envy

An additional moral emotion that involves comparisons between the self and others is envy. In contrast to pride, which is experienced in response to one's own (potentially moral) accomplishment, envy is experienced in response to accomplishments of a competitor. It is defined as the negative emotional response to lacking a valuable possession, accomplishment, or quality that someone else has (Parrott & Smith, 1993). Like pride, envy has two distinct forms—benign and malicious—which promote distinct behaviors. In both cases, envy motivates people to bring an envied other closer to themselves in status or competence, but those who feel benign envy seek to raise their own status, to become as successful as the envied person; whereas those who feel malicious envy seek to lower the status of the envied person, to eliminate their advantage (Lange & Crusius, 2015). In either case, envy tends to occur only when individuals view themselves as similar to the envied person; a high-school basketball player is more likely to feel envious of a stronger player on their team than of Michael Jordan (Schaubroeck & Lam, 2004). As a result, a person's self-concept and self-evaluations influence which others become targets of envy.

Given its impact on interpersonal relationships, envy has substantial effects on moral behavior. It has been linked to the use of deception in ultimatum games, where an assigned proposer decides how to split a sum of money with a partner and the responder decides whether to accept the decision. If the responder declines, neither player receives any money, incentivizing proposers to make offers that will seem fair (Moran & Schweitzer, 2008). One study found that proposers who were made to feel envious of their responder partner were more likely to lie to them about the total sum available, increasing the likelihood that the responder would accept an unfair proposal. Envy also has been found to increase free riding in classic public goods dilemmas (Parks et al., 2002) and increase feelings of schadenfreude among male students who watched an academically superior male student experiencing a setback (Smith et al., 1996).

CONCLUSIONS AND FUTURE DIRECTIONS

The extant literature on moral identity and moral emotions suggests that certain emotions—especially those that are most intricately interconnected with people's sense of self—are important elicitors of moral and immoral behavior and even shape the extent to which individuals come to see their own behavior as moral or immoral. Nonetheless, the research literature integrating distinct emotions with moral behavior is in its infancy. Here, we mention several promising research directions.

First, in integrating the literature on moral identity and moral self-conscious emotions, a trend can be seen in the contrast between possessing an internal versus external motivation to behave morally and experiencing self-conscious emotions about one's immoral behavior or character versus one's moral reputation. Those who hold an internalized moral identity may be particularly likely to also show a nondefensive emotional profile, comprising emotions like guilt, moral shame, and authentic pride, which entail a genuine focus on moral accountability. In contrast, those who have a more external, symbolic moral identity tend to care most about appearing moral to others and therefore are likely to experience emotions reflecting defensiveness and an egocentric focus, such as image shame and hubristic moral pride. Studies are needed to test these emotion-specific hypotheses.

Future studies are also needed to parse the different functions of self-conscious emotions at different levels of the self. For example, although studies have produced mixed findings for the adaptive benefits of guilt and shame, results seem equivocal at the group level of identity, where both emotions tend to promote similar prosocial tendencies (see Hakim et al., 2021, for a meta-analysis). A growing body of work also suggests that group-based moral shame more strongly predicts prosocial intentions than group-based guilt does (e.g., Allpress et al., 2014; Grigoryan et al., 2024). Although theories offer possible explanations for these findings (e.g., Gausel et al., 2012), studies have yet to conclusively test either these accounts or the boundary conditions and mechanisms through which shame promotes more adaptive moral outcomes than guilt. Future work is therefore needed to examine whether interpersonal versus intergroup transgressions differently elicit feelings of guilt and shame or moderate the associations between each emotion and reparation intentions. It remains possible (and seems likely) that guilt, and not shame, is the emotion most predictive of reparations in response to interpersonal, but not intergroup transgressions.

Future research might also investigate how pride influences fairness judgments surrounding equality and proportionality. Previous research has shown that anticipated pride increases a motivation to abide by principles of equality (van der Schalk et al., 2012). However, other studies show that individuals displaying pride are assumed to value proportionality (Horberg et al., 2013). More research is needed to investigate these interrelations. These findings also raise questions for when pride displays are likely to be more or less functional. The extent to which equality (compared to proportionality) is valued varies between individuals and cultures (Atari et al., 2023). Given that pride displays communicate that the displayer values proportionality, these displays may be less adaptive in cultures that value equality. Supporting this expectation, villagers in a small-scale traditional society in Fiji were found to judge pride displays as less deserving of high status than happiness displays were, in contrast to the reverse pattern seen among North Americans (Tracy et al., 2014). Future research might investigate whether cross-cultural differences in equality (vs. proportionality) values contribute to this cultural distinction.

In summary, a substantial body of evidence supports the importance of self-conscious and self-relevant emotions to moral psychology. These emotions inform individuals of moral congruencies and incongruencies in their own behavior and motivate behavioral change (or consistency) to address these observations. We hope that this review serves as a useful starting point for scholars who wish to continue exploring the relevance of these emotions to the moral domain, perhaps eventually returning guilt, shame, and pride to their early status as "moral emotions."

REFERENCES

Algoe, S. B. (2012). Find, remind, and bind: The functions of gratitude in everyday relationships. *Social and Personality Psychology Compass, 6*(6), 455–469.

Allpress, J. A., Brown, R., Giner-Sorolla, R., Deonna, J. A., & Teroni, F. (2014). Two faces of group-based shame: Moral shame and image shame differentially predict positive and negative orientations to ingroup wrongdoing. *Personality and Social Psychology Bulletin, 40*(10), 1270–1284.

Aquino, K., & Reed, A., II. (2002). The self-importance of moral identity. *Journal of Personality and Social Psychology, 83,* 1423–1440.

Armenta, C. N., Fritz, M. M., & Lyubomirsky, S. (2017). Functions of positive emotions: Gratitude as a motivator of self-improvement and positive change. *Emotion Review, 9*(3), 183–190.

Atari, M., Haidt, J., Graham, J., Koleva, S., Stevens, S. T., & Dehghani, M. (2023). Morality beyond the WEIRD: How the nomological network of morality varies across cultures. *Journal of Personality and Social Psychology, 125*(5), 1157–1188.

Beall, A. T., & Tracy, J. L. (2020). Evolution of pride and shame. In L. Workman, W. Reader, & J. H. Barkow (Eds.), *The Cambridge handbook of evolutionary perspectives on human behaviour* (pp. 179–193). Cambridge University Press.

Bernardi, R. A., Metzger, R. L., Scofield Bruno, R. G., Wade Hoogkamp, M. A., Reyes, L. E., & Barnaby, G. H. (2004). Examining the decision process of students' cheating behavior: An empirical study. *Journal of Business Ethics, 50*(4), 397–414.

Blasi, A. (1980). Bridging moral cognition and moral action: A critical review of the literature. *Psychological Bulletin, 88*(1), 1–45.

Branscombe, N. B., Slugosky, B., & Kappen, D. M. (2004). The measurement of collective guilt: What it is and what it is not. In N. R. Branscombe & B. Doosje (Eds.), *Collective guilt: International perspectives* (pp. 16–34). Cambridge University Press.

Brown, J., & Weiner, B. (1984). Affective consequences of ability versus effort ascriptions: Controversies, resolutions, and quandaries. *Journal of Educational Psychology, 76*(1), 146–158.

Brown, J. H., & Maurer, B. A. (1986). Body size, ecological dominance and Cope's rule. *Nature, 324*(6094), 248–250.

Campos, B., Shiota, M. N., Keltner, D., Gonzaga, G. C., & Goetz, J. L. (2013). What is shared, what is different? Core relational themes and expressive displays of eight positive emotions. *Cognition and Emotion, 27*(1), 37–52.

Cheng, J. T., Tracy, J. L., & Henrich, J. (2010). Pride, personality, and the evolutionary foundations of human social status. *Evolution and Human Behavior, 31*(5), 334–347.

Curry, O. S., Jones Chesters, M., & Van Lissa, C. J. (2019). Mapping morality with a compass: Testing the theory of "morality-as-cooperation" with a new questionnaire. *Journal of Research in Personality, 78,* 106–124.

Damon, W., & Hart, D. (1992). Self-understanding and its role in social and moral development. In M. H. Bornstein & M. E. Lamb (Eds.), *Developmental psychology: An advanced textbook* (3rd ed., pp. 421–464). Erlbaum.

de Cremer, D., & van Dijk, E. (2005). When and why leaders put themselves first: Leader behaviour in resource allocations as a function of feeling entitled. *European Journal of Social Psychology, 35*(4), 553–563.

de Hooge, I. E., Nelissen, R., Breugelmans, S. M., & Zeelenberg, M. (2011). What is moral about guilt?: Acting "prosocially" at the disadvantage of others. *Journal of Personality and Social Psychology, 100*(3), 462–473.

de Hooge, I. E., Zeelenberg, M., & Breugelmans, S. M. (2007). Moral sentiments and cooperation: Differential influences of shame and guilt. *Cognition and Emotion, 21*(5), 1025–1042.

Dorfman, A., Eyal, T., & Bereby-Meyer, Y. (2014). Proud to cooperate: The consideration of pride promotes cooperation in a social dilemma. *Journal of Experimental Social Psychology, 55,* 105–109.

Emmons, R. A., & McCullough, M. E. (2003). Counting blessings versus burdens: An experimental investigation of gratitude and subjective well-being in daily life. *Journal of Personality and Social Psychology, 84*(2), 377–389.

Emmons, R. A., & Mishra, A. (2011). Why gratitude enhances well-being: What we know, what we need to know. In K. M. Sheldon, T. B. Kashdan, & M. F. Steger (Eds.), *Designing positive psychology: Taking stock and moving forward* (pp. 248–262). Oxford University Press.

Etxebarria, I., Ortiz, M.-J., Apodaca, P., Pascual, A., & Conejero, S. (2015). Pride as moral motive: Moral pride and prosocial behaviour. *Journal for the Study of Education and Development, 38*(4), 746–774.

Everett, J. A. C., Skorburg, J. A., & Savulescu, J. (2020). The moral self and moral duties. *Philosophical Psychology, 33*(7), 924–945.

Ferguson, M. A., & Branscombe, N. R. (2014). The social psychology of collective guilt. In C. Von Scheve & M. Salmela (Eds.), *Collective emotions: Perspectives from psychology, philosophy, and sociology* (pp. 251–262). Oxford University Press.

Fessler, D. (2004). Shame in two cultures: Implications for evolutionary approaches. *Journal of Cognition and Culture, 4*(2), 207–262.

Fessler, D. (2007). From appeasement to conformity. In J. L. Tracy, R. W. Robins, & J. P. Tangney (Eds.), *The self-conscious emotions: Theory and research* (pp. 174–193). Guilford Press.

Gangestad, S. W., & Simpson, J. A. (2000). The evolution of human mating: Trade-offs and strategic pluralism. *Behavioral and Brain Sciences, 23*(4), 573–587.

Gausel, N., Leach, C. W., Vignoles, V. L., & Brown, R. (2012). Defend or repair? Explaining responses to in-group moral failure by disentangling feelings of shame, rejection, and inferiority. *Journal of Personality and Social Psychology, 102*(5), 941–960.

Gilbert, P. (1998). What is shame? Some core issues and controversies. In P. Gilbert & B. Andrews (Eds.), *Shame: Interpersonal behavior, psychopathology, and culture* (pp. 3–38). Oxford University Press.

Gilbert, P. (2007). The evolution of shame as a marker for relationship security: A biopsychosocial approach. In J. L. Tracy, R. W. Robins, & J. P. Tangney (Eds.), *The self-conscious emotions: Theory and research* (pp. 283–309). Guilford Press.

Giner-Sorolla, R., Castano, E., Espinosa, P., & Brown, R. (2008). Shame expressions reduce the recipient's insult from outgroup reparations. *Journal of Experimental Social Psychology, 44*(3), 519–526.

Gratohn, A., & Ric, F. (2017). How guilt leads to reparation? Exploring the processes underlying the effects of guilt. *Motivation and Emotion, 41*(3), 343–352.

Gray, K., & Kubin, E. (2024). Victimhood: The most powerful force in morality and politics. *Advances in Experimental Social Psychology, 70*, 137–220.

Grigoryan, L., Ponizovskiy, V., Weißflog, M. I., Osin, E., & Lickel, B. (2024). Guilt, shame, and anti-war action in an authoritarian country at war. *Political Psychology.*

Haidt, J. (2003). Elevation and the positive psychology of morality. In C. L. M. Keyes & J. Haidt (Eds.), *Flourishing: Positive psychology and the life well-lived* (pp. 275–289). American Psychological Association.

Hakim, N., Branscombe, N., & Schoemann, A. (2021). Group-based emotions and support for reparations: A meta-analysis. *Affective Science, 2*(4), 363–378.

Hardy, S. A., Walker, L. J., Olsen, J. A., Woodbury, R. D., & Hickman, J. R. (2014). Moral identity as moral ideal self: Links to adolescent outcomes. *Developmental Psychology, 50*(1), 45–57.

Heaven, P. C. L., Ciarrochi, J., & Leeson, P. (2009). The longitudinal links between shame and increasing hostility during adolescence. *Personality and Individual Differences, 47*(8), 841–844.

Heiphetz, L., Strohminger, N., Gelman, S. A., & Young, L. L. (2018). Who am I? The role of moral beliefs in children's and adults' understanding of identity. *Journal of Experimental Social Psychology, 78*, 210–219.

Henrich, J., & Boyd, R. (1998). The evolution of conformist transmission and the emergence of between-group differences. *Evolution and Human Behavior, 19*(4), 215–241.

Hertz, S. G., & Krettenauer, T. (2016). Does moral identity effectively predict moral behavior? A meta-analysis. *Review of General Psychology, 20*(2), 129–140.

Hofmann, W., & Fisher, R. R. (2012). How guilt and pride shape subsequent self-control. *Social Psychological and Personality Science, 3*(6), 682–690.

Horberg, E. J., Kraus, M. W., & Keltner, D. (2013). Pride displays communicate self-interest and support for meritocracy. *Journal of Personality and Social Psychology, 105*(1), 24–37.

Horberg, E. J., Oveis, C., Keltner, D., & Cohen, A. B. (2009). Disgust and the moralization of purity. *Journal of Personality and Social Psychology, 97*(6), 963–976.

Ibasco, G. C., & Tracy, J. L. (2025). *The role of group-based moral pride in regulating guilt and shame for intergroup transgressions.* University of British Columbia.

Jacquet, J. (2011). *Is shame necessary?* Edge. www.edge.org/conversation/jennifer_jacquet-is-shame-necessary.

Jacquet, J., Hauert, C., Traulsen, A., & Milinski, M. (2011). Shame and honour drive cooperation. *Biology Letters, 7*(6), 899–901.

Jennings, P. L., Mitchell, M. S., & Hannah, S. T. (2015). The moral self: A review and integration of the literature. *Journal of Organizational Behavior, 36*(S1), S104–S168.

Joireman, J. (2004). Empathy and the self-absorption paradox II: Self-rumination and self-reflection as mediators between shame, guilt, and empathy. *Self and Identity, 3*(3), 225–238.

Jordan, J. J., & Kteily, N. S. (2023). How reputation does (and does not) drive people to punish without looking. *Proceedings of the National Academy of Sciences, 120*(28), 1–11.

Keltner, D., & Buswell, B. N. (1997). Embarrassment: Its distinct form and appeasement functions. *Psychological Bulletin, 122*(3), 250–270.

Keltner, D., & Haidt, J. (2003). Approaching awe, a moral, spiritual, and aesthetic emotion. *Cognition and Emotion, 17*(2), 297–314.

Keltner, D., Young, R. C., & Buswell, B. N. (1997). Appeasement in human emotion, social practice, and personality. *Aggressive Behavior, 23*(5), 359–374.

Kohlberg, L. (1969). Stage and sequence. The cognitive developmental approach to socialization. In D. Goslin (Ed.), *Handbook of socialization theory* (pp. 347–480). Rand McNally.

Krettenauer, T. (2022). When moral identity undermines moral behavior: An integrative framework. *Social and Personality Psychology Compass, 16*(3), e12655.

Krettenauer, T., & Casey, V. (2015). Moral identity development and positive moral emotions: Differences involving authentic and hubristic pride. *Identity: An International Journal of Theory and Research, 15*(3), 173–187.

Lambert, N. M., & Fincham, F. D. (2011). Expressing gratitude to a partner leads to more relationship maintenance behavior. *Emotion, 11*(1), 52–60.

Landers, M., Sznycer, D., & Durkee, P. (2024). Are self-conscious emotions about the self? Testing competing theories of shame and guilt across two disparate cultures. *Emotion.*

Lange, J., & Crusius, J. (2015). Dispositional envy revisited: Unraveling the motivational dynamics of benign and malicious envy. *Personality and Social Psychology Bulletin, 41*(2), 284–294.

Langlois, J. H., Kalakanis, L., Rubenstein, A. J., Larson, A., Hallam, M., & Smoot, M. (2000). Maxims or myths of beauty?: A meta-analytic and theoretical review. *Psychological Bulletin, 126*(3), 390–423.

Leary, M. R., Tambor, E. S., Terdal, S. K., & Downs, D. L. (1995). Self-esteem as an interpersonal monitor: The sociometer hypothesis. *Journal of Personality and Social Psychology, 68*(3), 518–530.

Lefebvre, J. P., & Krettenauer, T. (2019). Linking moral identity with moral emotions: A meta-analysis. *Review of General Psychology, 23*(4), 444–457.

Leith, K. P., & Baumeister, R. F. (1998). Empathy, shame, guilt, and narratives of interpersonal conflicts: Guilt-prone people are better at perspective taking. *Journal of Personality, 66*(1), 1–37.

Lewis, H. B. (1971). Shame and guilt in neurosis. *Psychoanalytic Review, 58*(3), 419.

Lewis, M. (1995). Self-conscious emotions. *American Scientist, 83*(1), 68–78.

Lewis, M. (2008). Self-conscious emotions: Embarrassment, pride, shame, and guilt. In M. Lewis, J. M. Haviland-Jones, & L. F. Barrett (Eds.), *Handbook of emotions* (3rd ed., pp. 742–756). Guilford Press.

Lickel, B., Schmader, T., & Barquissau, M. (2004). The evocation of moral emotions in intergroup contexts: The distinction between collective guilt and collective shame. In N. R. Branscombe & B. Doosje (Eds.), *Collective guilt: International perspectives* (pp. 35–55). Cambridge University Press.

Lickel, B., Schmader, T., & Spanovic, M. (2007). Group-conscious emotions: The implications of others' wrongdoings for identity and relationships. In J. L. Tracy, R. W. Robins, & J. P. Tangney (Eds.), *The Self-conscious emotions: Theory and research* (pp. 351–370). Guilford Press.

Ma, L. K., Tunney, R. J., & Ferguson, E. (2017). Does gratitude enhance prosociality?: A meta-analytic review. *Psychological Bulletin, 143*(6), 601–635.

Mackie, D. M., Smith, E. R., & Ray, D. G. (2008). Intergroup emotions and intergroup relations. *Social and Personality Psychology Compass, 2*(5), 1866–1880.

Mercadante, E. J., & Tracy, J. L. (2022). A paradox of pride: Hubristic pride predicts strategic dishonesty in response to status threats. *Journal of Experimental Psychology: General, 151*(7), 1681–1706.

Mercadante, E. J., & Tracy, J. L. (2024). How does it feel to be greedy?: The role of pride in avaricious acquisition. *Journal of Personality, 92*(2), 565–583.

Moran, S., & Schweitzer, M. E. (2008). When better is worse: Envy and the use of deception. *Negotiation and Conflict Management Research, 1*(1), 3–29.

Nowak, M. A., & Roch, S. (2007). Upstream reciprocity and the evolution of gratitude. *Proceedings. Biological Sciences, 274*(1610), 605–609.

Nussbaum, M. C. (2006). *Hiding from humanity: Disgust, shame, and the law.* Princeton University Press.

Parks, C. D., Rumble, A. C., & Posey, D. C. (2002). The effects of envy on reciprocation in a social dilemma. *Personality and Social Psychology Bulletin, 28*(4), 509–520.

Parrott, W. G., & Smith, R. H. (1993). Distinguishing the experiences of envy and jealousy. *Journal of Personality and Social Psychology, 64*(6), 906–920.

Patrick, R. B., Bodine, A. J., Gibbs, J. C., & Basinger, K. S. (2018). What accounts for prosocial behavior? Roles of moral identity, moral judgment, and self-efficacy beliefs. *Journal of Genetic Psychology, 179*(5), 231–245.

Piff, P. K., Dietze, P., Feinberg, M., Stancato, D. M., & Keltner, D. (2015). Awe, the small self, and prosocial behavior. *Journal of Personality and Social Psychology, 108*(6), 883–899.

Proeve, M. J., & Howells, K. (2006). Effects of remorse and shame and criminal justice experience on judgements about a sex offender. *Psychology, Crime and Law, 12*(2), 145–161.

Randles, D., & Tracy, J. L. (2013). Nonverbal displays of shame predict relapse and declining health in recovering alcoholics. *Clinical Psychological Science, 1*(2), 149–155.

Randles, D., & Tracy, J. L. (2015). Shame. In R. Segal K. & Stuckrad (Eds.), *Vocabulary for the study of religion* (pp. 339–343). Brill.

Rest, J., Turiel, E., & Kohlberg, L. (1969). Level of moral development as a determinant of preference and comprehension of moral judgments made by others. *Journal of Personality, 37*(2), 225–252.

Robertson, T. E., Sznycer, D., Delton, A. W., Tooby, J., & Cosmides, L. (2018). The true trigger of shame: Social devaluation is sufficient, wrongdoing is unnecessary. *Evolution and Human Behavior, 39*(5), 566–573.

Robins, R. W., Tracy, J. L., & Trzesniewski, K. H. (2008). Naturalizing the self. In O. P. John, R. W. Robins, & L. A. Pervin (Eds.), *Handbook of personality: Theory and research* (3rd ed., pp. 421–447). Guilford Press.

Rom, S. C., & Conway, P. (2018). The strategic moral self: Self-presentation shapes moral dilemma judgments. *Journal of Experimental Social Psychology, 74,* 24–37.

Salerno, J. M., & Peter-Hagene, L. C. (2013). The interactive effect of anger and disgust on moral outrage and judgments. *Psychological Science, 24*(10), 2069–2078.

Schaubroeck, J., & Lam, S. S. K. (2004). Comparing lots before and after: Promotion rejectees' invidious reactions to promotees. *Organizational Behavior and Human Decision Processes, 94*(1), 33–47.

Schmader, T., & Lickel, B. (2006). The approach and avoidance function of guilt and shame emotions: Comparing reactions to self-caused and other-caused wrongdoing. *Motivation and Emotion, 30*(1), 42–55.

Schnall, S., Haidt, J., Clore, G. L., & Jordan, A. H. (2008). Disgust as embodied moral judgment. *Personality and Social Psychology Bulletin, 34*(8), 1096–1109.

Sell, A., Tooby, J., & Cosmides, L. (2009). Formidability and the logic of human anger. *Proceedings of the National Academy of Sciences, 106*(35), 15073–15078.

Seuntjens, T. G., Zeelenberg, M., Breugelmans, S. M., & van de Ven, N. (2015). Defining greed. *British Journal of Psychology, 106*(3), 505–525.

Seuntjens, T. G., Zeelenberg, M., van de Ven, N., & Breugelmans, S. M. (2019). Greedy bastards: Testing the relationship between wanting more and unethical behavior. *Personality and Individual Differences, 138,* 147–156.

Shepherd, L., Spears, R., & Manstead, A. S. (2013). The self-regulatory role of anticipated group-based shame and guilt in inhibiting in-group favoritism. *European Journal of Social Psychology, 43*(6), 493–504.

Skarlicki, D. P., & Rupp, D. E. (2010). Dual processing and organizational justice: The role of rational versus experiential processing in third-party reactions to workplace mistreatment. *Journal of Applied Psychology, 95*(5), 944–952.

Smith, R. H., Turner, T. J., Garonzik, R., Leach, C. W., Urch-Druskat, V., & Weston, C. M. (1996). Envy and schadenfreude. *Personality and Social Psychology Bulletin, 22*(2), 158–168.

Strohminger, N., & Nichols, S. (2014). The essential moral self. *Cognition, 131*(1), 159–171.

Stuewig, J., Tangney, J. P., Heigel, C., Harty, L., & McCloskey, L. (2010). Shaming, blaming, and maiming: Functional links among the moral emotions, externalization of blame, and aggression. *Journal of Research in Personality, 44*(1), 91–102.

Sznycer, D. (2019). Forms and functions of the self-conscious emotions. *Trends in Cognitive Sciences, 23*(2), 143–157.

Sznycer, D., Al-Shawaf, L., Bereby-Meyer, Y., Curry, O. S., De Smet, D., Ermer, E., . . . Tooby, J. (2017). Cross-cultural regularities in the cognitive architecture of pride. *Proceedings of the National Academy of Sciences, 114*(8), 1874–1879.

Sznycer, D., & Lukaszewski, A. W. (2019). The emotion–valuation constellation: Multiple emotions are governed by a common grammar of social valuation. *Evolution and Human Behavior, 40*(4), 395–404.

Sznycer, D., Sell, A., & Dumont, A. (2022). How anger works. *Evolution and Human Behavior, 43*(2), 122–132.

Sznycer, D., Tooby, J., Cosmides, L., Porat, R.,

Shalvi, S., & Halperin, E. (2016). Shame closely tracks the threat of devaluation by others, even across cultures. *Proceedings of the National Academy of Sciences, 113*(10), 2625–2630.

Tajfel, H., & Turner, J. C. (2004). The social identity theory of intergroup behavior. In *Political psychology* (pp. 276–293). Psychology Press.

Tangney, J. P., & Dearing, R. L. (2003). *Shame and guilt.* Guilford Press.

Tangney, J. P., Dearing, R. L., Wagner, P. E., & Gramzow, R. (1989). *Test of Self-Conscious Affect–3.* George Mason University.

Tangney, J. P., & Fischer, K. W. (Eds.). (1995). *Self-conscious emotions: The psychology of shame, guilt, embarrassment, and pride.* Guilford Press.

Tangney, J. P., Stuewig, J., & Mashek, D. J. (2007). Moral emotions and moral behavior. *Annual Review of Psychology, 58,* 345–372.

Tangney, J. P., & Tracy, J. L. (2012). Self-conscious emotions. In M. R. Leary & J. P. Tangney (Eds.), *Handbook of self and identity* (pp. 446–480). Guilford Press.

Tracy, J. L., Steckler, C., Randles, D., & Mercadante, E. (2018). The financial cost of status signaling: Expansive postural displays are associated with a reduction in the receipt of altruistic donations. *Evolution and Human Behavior, 39,* 520–528.

Tracy, J. L., Cheng, J. T., Robins, R. W., & Trzesniewski, K. H. (2009). Authentic and hubristic pride: The affective core of self-esteem and narcissism. *Self and Identity, 8*(2–3), 196–213.

Tracy, J. L., & Ibasco, G. C. (2025). *The unexpected importance of expectations for self-conscious emotions.* University of British Columbia.

Tracy, J. L., Mercadante, E., & Hohm, I. (2023). Pride: The emotional foundation of social rank attainment. *Annual Review of Psychology, 74*(2023), 519–545.

Tracy, J. L., & Robins, R. W. (2004). Putting the self into self-conscious emotions: A theoretical model. *Psychological Inquiry, 15*(2), 103–125.

Tracy, J. L., & Robins, R. W. (2006). Appraisal antecedents of shame and guilt: Support for a theoretical model. *Personality and Social Psychology Bulletin, 32*(10), 1339–1351.

Tracy, J. L., & Robins, R. W. (2007). The psychological structure of pride: A tale of two facets. *Journal of Personality and Social Psychology, 92*(3), 506–525.

Tracy, J. L., Steckler, C. M., & Heltzel, G. (2019). The physiological basis of psychological disgust and moral judgments. *Journal of Personality and Social Psychology, 116*(1), 15–32.

Tracy, J. L., Weidman, A. C., Cheng, J. T., & Martens, J. P. (2014). Pride: The fundamental emotion of success, power, and status. In M. M. Tugade, M. N. Shiota, & L. D. Kirby (Eds.), *Handbook of positive emotions* (pp. 294–310). Guilford Press.

van Cappellen, P., & Saroglou, V. (2012). Awe activates religious and spiritual feelings and behavioral intentions. *Psychology of Religion and Spirituality, 4*(3), 223–236.

van der Schalk, J., Bruder, M., & Manstead, A. (2012). Regulating emotion in the context of interpersonal decisions: The role of anticipated pride and regret. *Frontiers in Psychology, 3.*

Weidman, A. C., Cheng, J. T., & Tracy, J. L. (2018). The psychological structure of humility. *Journal of Personality and Social Psychology, 114*(1), 153–178.

Winterich, K. P., Mittal, V., & Aquino, K. (2013). When does recognition increase charitable behavior?: Toward a moral identity-based model. *Journal of Marketing, 77*(3), 121–134.

Wohl, M. J. A., Branscombe, N. R., & Klar, Y. (2006). Collective guilt: Emotional reactions when one's group has done wrong or been wronged. *European Review of Social Psychology, 17*(1), 1–37.

Wyckoff, J. P., & Kirkpatrick, L. A. (2016). Direct and indirect aggression tactics as a function of domain-specific self-esteem. *Personality and Individual Differences, 92,* 135–142.

Young, L., Chakroff, A., & Tom, J. (2012). Doing good leads to more good: The reinforcing power of a moral self-concept. *Review of Philosophy and Psychology, 3*(3), 325–334.

SECTION IV

ISOLATION, UNCERTAINTY, AND SHARED REALITY

CHAPTER 26

Existential Isolation and I-Sharing

Theoretical and Empirical Contributions

Elif Bilal *and* Peter J. Helm

There are many ways people can be alone. Commonly studied forms include social isolation—an objective state in which a person lacks regular contact with others, such as when a person is physically alone (Child & Lawton, 2020)—and loneliness—a subjective and distressing feeling associated with dissatisfaction with one's social relationships (Mansfield et al., 2021; Peplau & Perlman, 1982). An existential perspective suggests an even more fundamental form of separation: existential isolation (Helm et al., 2019a; Pinel et al., 2017a). Yalom (1980) wrote that existential isolation "refers to an unbridgeable gulf between oneself and any other being. It refers, too, to an isolation even more fundamental—a separation between the individual and the world" (p. 355). Yalom was pointing out that because we cannot experience reality from another person's perspective, cannot read another person's inner thoughts, or be certain about another's inner feelings, we are inherently alone in our experiences of the world.

Yalom's (1980) definition describes what could be considered an existential reality of the human condition: a fundamental separation between the self and others (Moustakas, 1961; Mueller, 1834/1912). Yet people vary in the degree to which they notice and feel existentially isolated from others (Helm et al., 2019a; Pinel et al., 2017a), though qualitative studies suggest it is a common experience (McKenna-Plumley et al., 2023). Experiences of existential isolation commonly studied by psychologists and discussed in clinical settings refer to instances where an individual feels alone in their experience, as though no one else shares or understands their perspective (Helm et al., 2019a; Pinel et al., 2017a).

Conceptually, early theories about the nature of the self provide a framework for understanding the experience of existential isolation. William James (1890/1918) proposed that the self consists of two distinct aspects: the "Me" and the "I." The "Me" represents what contemporary psychologists refer to as our self-concept or self-as-object and includes all descriptive characteristics of a person including emotional evaluations, attitudes, memories, behaviors, and so forth. In contrast, the "I" represents our self-as-subject, or experiential self that "leaves a stream of consciousness" in its wake and is the aspect of the self that experiences reality in each given moment (James, 1890/1918).

The nature of our self-as-subject combined with natural perceptual limitations means that people are inherently separated from others, which renders us vulnerable to doubts about what is real and what is merely a product of our imaginations (Pinel et al., 2004). We can try to rely on others to verify and validate our perceptions, intuitions, and values (Swann et al., 1992) by attempting to infer the inner states of others from behavior (Wu et al., 2019), but these inferences are often inaccurate and misaligned with reality (e.g., Ross & Nisbett, 2011), making true validation and connection difficult.

KEY CONCERNS ASSOCIATED WITH FUNDAMENTAL ISOLATION

Awareness of our existentially isolated situation may be particularly problematic for a species that relies upon abstract symbolic representations of the world to sustain beliefs, meaning, and systems of value (Becker, 1973; Fonagy & Target, 2002), leading to both epistemic and affiliative uncertainty (Pinel et al., 2004).

Epistemic Uncertainty

Epistemic uncertainty refers to questions about whether we perceive reality as it really is, which subsequently affects the confidence in our beliefs (Higgins et al., 2021; Long et al., 2021; Swann & Bosson, 2010). Many theories highlight the importance of socially shared perspectives for making sense of and understanding the world around us (e.g., Asch, 1952; Becker, 1973; Festinger et al., 1954; Higgins et al., 2021). The motivation to share feelings, beliefs, and concerns about the world—the motivation to create a sense of shared reality—represents a fundamental motivation (Higgins et al., 2021) because shared understanding underlies self-knowledge and successful cooperation and is prevalent in developmental processes. For example, research suggests people use others to understand and define themselves (Vazire, 2010), rather than using introspection. People feel more confident in their beliefs when they are shared by others (Festinger et al., 1954) and will seek out others who will verify and confirm the ways in which they already feel (Swann, 1996). Those who feel their beliefs are validated more consistently tend to have better mental health and life satisfaction than those who do not feel validated (Çıkrıkçı & Gençdoğan, 2017).

Even in terms of our cultural beliefs, people rely on others to validate the ways in which they see and think about the world. For example, terror management theory (Arndt et al., 2013) argues that shared belief systems (i.e., cultural beliefs) function as an epistemological scaffold that structures meaning and ultimately buffers against awareness of mortality. In support of this proposition, after reminders of death, people tend to prefer others who confirm their preexisting cultural beliefs and values, and dislike those who challenge them (e.g., Greenberg et al., 1986), suggesting that social validation of beliefs underlies their protective function.

Affiliative Uncertainty

Affiliative uncertainty refers to questions about whether one belongs with a group (e.g., Baumeister & Leary, 1995; Ryan & Deci, 2000; Walton & Cohen, 2007). Motivation to satisfy this concern represents a fundamental human motivation (Allen et al., 2021; Baumeister & Leary, 1995). Low felt belonging is associated with poorer cognitive functioning (Baumeister et al., 2005) and worse physical and mental health (Ryff & Singer, 2000). When belonging and affiliative needs are met, people report higher self-esteem (Leary & Baumeister, 2000), higher life satisfaction (Diener et al., 1999), and better mental health (Kim & McKenry, 2002). Yet satisfaction of the belonging motive requires more than being physically present with others; it requires some degree of validation of one's sense of self or existential connection (Crocker & Canevello, 2008).

Taken together, a plethora of work underscores how social validation of experiences functions to satisfy fundamental epistemic and relational motives. Yet, feeling existentially isolated has the potential to thwart this process. If shared perspectives underly a sense of belonging, self-knowledge, cooperation, cultural beliefs, and defensive reactions after threat, then feeling alone in one's experience (i.e., existentially isolated) should undermine the connections one is able to make with others. Yalom (1980) wrote, "existential isolation impregnates the 'paste of things'" (p. 358) and because true validation of one's perspective is impossible, we are left vulnerable to doubts about whether we are correctly understanding others or whether we truly fit in with a group.

EMPIRICAL RESEARCH ON EXISTENTIAL ISOLATION

Research examining the experience of existential isolation has roots in early theories of loneliness (e.g., Moustakas, 1961), which posited loneliness to be "a fundamental truth of life" (Moustakas, 1961, p. ix). Yet only recently has empirical research begun to seriously examine the nature of this experience. These efforts have largely fallen into two camps: quantitative social psychological research (e.g., Helm et al., 2019a; Pinel et al., 2017a) and qualitative research (e.g., Bolmsjö et al., 2019; Ettema et al., 2010). Nevertheless, interest in the existential aspects of subjective disconnection has been receiving increased attention, as evidenced by recent efforts to review, describe, and differentiate the construct from other types of disconnection (e.g., Álvarez et al., 2023; Hadeei, 2023; van Tilburg, 2021).

The review below will primarily focus on quantitative inquiries into existential disconnection (see McAdams & Ture, Chapter 40, this volume, for a review of qualitative studies), though camps largely converge on the same core set of definitive features of the feelings of existential isolation. These features include (1) perceiving oneself as inherently separated from others and the world; (2) associations with negative reactions, attributions, and perceptions; and (3) that these feelings are distinct from other forms of subjective disconnection (e.g., loneliness, needs for belonging).

Pinel and colleagues (2017b) validated a six-item Existential Isolation Scale (EIS) assessing a generalized subjective sense of feeling alone in one's experiences. The EIS has been found to have small to moderate correlations with loneliness (Helm et al., 2020a, 2020b; Pinel et al., et al., 2017a), demonstrate relative stability over time (Pinel et al., 2017a), and show conceptually relevant concurrent and discriminant validity with related constructs (Helm et al., 2022a; Pinel et al., 2017a). Subsequently, a variety of empirical research has begun examining various ways an existential disconnection from others can stem from and affect a variety of psychological phenomena.

Helm and colleagues (2019a) published a theoretical model of existential isolation: the state–trait existential isolation model (STEIM). The STEIM posits that the experience of existential isolation can be conceptualized as stemming from in-the-moment and situational cues leading to short-term (or state) experiences, or stemming from sources that lead to a more chronically accessible (or trait) experience. A variety of studies lend support for these pathways.

Helm and colleagues (2019b) and Pinel and colleagues (2017a) have found that open-ended writing primes asking participants to recall instances of feeling alone in one's experiences (i.e., of existential isolation) have successfully increased in-the-moment feelings of existential isolation, suggesting that the construct is accessible in memory and can be elicited. Edwards and colleagues (2023) found that awe experiences via virtual reality or via a recall task indirectly led people to report higher existential isolation via feeling small and a lower sense of connectedness from others. Interestingly, awe experiences also led to feelings of vastness and greater connectedness, which predicted lower feelings of existential isolation, highlighting that in-the-moment experiences may in part be a consequence of general feelings of connectedness with others and with the attributions one makes about one's experiences.

Contextual references also appear to impact felt existential isolation. Helm and colleagues (2022b) asked Black and White participants to consider other White or other Black people when responding to the EIS. Black participants reported significantly higher existential isolation when considering White people than when considering other Black people. Conversely, White participants reported no difference in their self-reported existential isolation regardless of reference group. In a study assessing faith crises among current and former members of the Church of Jesus Christ of Latter-Day Saints (i.e., LDS or Mormon), Leavitt and Helm (2024) found that those who were actively doubting their faith tended to report relatively high levels of existential isolation compared to those who actively believed or who reported no longer believing in LDS teachings. Moreover, having many close friends who were active members of the LDS Church was associated with higher existential isolation among those who had left the LDS Church, but lower existential isolation among those who were still active. These findings converge on the idea that feelings of existential isolation can be influenced by context and upon salient groups with whom one compares their experiences.

Yalom (1980) wrote that feelings of "existential isolation produce a highly uncomfortable subjective state and . . . [this state] is not tolerated by the individual for long" (p. 362). Helm and colleagues (2019a) proposed these in-the-moment experiences should motivate an individual to seek ways to lessen their experience of existential isolation while leading to a variety of short-term consequences. While not directly testing a motivation to reduce the experience of existential isolation, Helm and colleagues (2022a) employed a correlational study during the early months of the COVID-19 pandemic lockdown in the United States and found that active social media use (i.e., actively posting, commenting, and participating on social media) was associated with lower in-the-moment existential isolation and subsequently higher meaning in life. If actively using social media offers opportunities to connect and share with like-minded others (Lee et al., 2018), and provides opportunities for confirmation bias (Ling, 2020), then perhaps actively engaging with others is a means to reduce existentially isolating feelings.

Relatedly, Oleskowicz and colleagues (2023) found frequency of alcohol consumption to be negatively correlated with existential isolation. This relationship was mediated by the desire to drink as a means to form existential connections. In a follow-up longitudinal study, increased alcohol consumption over time predicted decrease in existential isolation. These findings highlight that the experience of existential isolation may lead people to seek connection through confirmation biases, affiliating with likeminded individuals, and even through substance use.

While specific experiences and contexts may contribute to state feelings of existential isolation, regularly occurring and socialization experiences may contribute to chronically active, or trait, existential isolation. For example, Helm and colleagues (2020a) found insecure attachment, particularly avoidant attachment, to be associated with existential isolation. Attachment figures, in part, function to orient and validate people's subjective interpretations of reality (Fonagy & Target, 2002). Avoidant attachment, resulting from consistently unavailable caregivers, describes a distrustful orientation toward others and a discomfort with intimacy (Shaver & Mikulincer, 2007), mirroring theory proposing trait existential isolation to predict withdrawal from social activities. Thus, when a person's attachment needs are unmet, existential isolation may be a secondary consequence to developing insecure attachment.

Other socialization processes may also contribute to heightened trait existential isolation. For example, multiple studies have found men to report higher existential isolation than women (e.g., Park & Pinel, 2020; Pinel et al., 2017a), presumably because male gender norms do not emphasize expressing and sharing one's inner experiences. In support of this position, studies have found that controlling for other-focused orientations mediated sex differences in existential isolation (Helm et al., 2018; Park & Pinel, 2020). In a similar vein, multiple studies have found evidence that those from collectivistic cultural contexts (i.e., contexts that emphasize groups over individuals) tend to report less existential isolation than do those from individualistic contexts. For example, Park and Pinel (2020) found that South Korean participants reported less existential isolation than did American participants. Interestingly, no differences in existential isolation were found in a sample comparing bereaved German-speaking Swiss and Chinese participants (Zhou et al., 2023), perhaps suggesting that clinical samples may experience existential isolation more acutely regardless of their cultural orientation.

Other work has identified other sociocultural factors to be associated with existential isolation. For example, Pinel and colleagues (2021) found evidence that those with minoritized identities (e.g., participants of color, queer sexual identity, non-native English-speaking Americans) tend to report higher existential isolation than their majority-group counterparts (e.g., White participants, those with heterosexual identities, native English-speaking Americans). Similarly, those with multiracial identity (Carter et al., 2024) and transgender identity (Horner et al., 2023) reported higher existential isolation than their monoracial and cisgender counterparts, respectively.

Major life events may contribute to chronically accessible existential isolation. Events such as immigrating to another country (Olofsson et al., 2021), getting a cancer diagnosis (Sekse et al., 2010), leaving one's faith (Leavitt & Helm, 2024), and losing a loved one (Zhou et al., 2023) appear to be associated with higher feelings of existential isolation. Perhaps unsurprisingly, when life changes highlight how people's experiences differ from others, people tend to report elevated existential isolation.

Chronically elevated existential isolation has been found to be associated with a variety of negative outcomes. As described above, the experience of existential isolation threatens epistemic certainty. In support of this theoretical link, Pinel and colleagues (2021) asked Black participants to evaluate ambiguous but potentially racist situations and determine whether the situation reflected racism and to indicate their confidence of their determination. Existential isolation did not significantly predict determination of racism but did predict less confidence in one's attribution. Long and colleagues (2021) replicated and extended these findings and found that higher trait existential isolation predicted lower expectation that others would agree with one's views and less confidence in one's judgments. Importantly, this relationship was mediated by the expectation that others would not agree. Similarly, the expectation of being misunderstood and miscategorized by others explained the difference between multiracial and monoracial participant's existential isolation (Carter et al., 2024). These findings underscore that those who internalize being existentially isolated appear to expect others to perceive and react differently than them, and that this undermines their epistemic certainty.

One consequence of lacking self-confidence and not expecting others to understand is generalized distrust. In a study assessing clinical distress and experiences in mental health settings, higher existential isolation was associated with perceiving mental health professionals to be less competent, less satisfaction with current mental health providers, and lower intention of seeking future services (Constantino et al., 2019, 2023). Similarly, in a study assessing attitudes toward future but not yet available COVID-19 vaccines, higher existential isolation was associated with less trust in potential vaccines, even after controlling for a host of other predictors of vaccine hesitancy and mistrust (Galgali et al., 2023). Importantly, in a follow-up study a year after COVID-19 vaccines became available, higher existential isolation predicted a lower likelihood of having received a vaccine (Galgali et al., 2023), suggesting that existential isolation can influence important public health perceptions and behaviors. Perhaps unsurprisingly, these broader distrustful attitudes toward public health officials and mental health providers associated with higher existential isolation do not transfer to the distrust of all sources. Indeed, elevated existential isolation has been found to robustly correlate with holding conspiracy beliefs and a general orientation toward and trust in conspiratorial thinking (Galgali et al., 2023).

Beyond epistemic threats, elevated existential isolation has been associated with a host of psychosocial and mental health problems. For example, existential isolation has been found to be associated with lower self-esteem (Helm et al., 2018, 2020a), lower self-competence (Pinel et al., 2017a), higher death-thought accessibility (Helm et al., 2019b), and higher stress, anxiety, depression, and suicide ideation (Constantino et al., 2019; Helm et al., 2020b). Interestingly, existential isolation has been found to be negatively correlated with meaning in life, but only for those who have not had mystical-type experiences (Sielaff et al., 2022). Similarly, those endorsing quest religiosity reported lower existential isolation and subsequently greater well-being (Arrowood et al., 2021). These nuanced findings suggest existential disconnection's impact on negative outcomes may depend on past experiences and context.

Importantly, while there exists a broader existential reality of isolation (i.e., all humans are inherently alone in their subjective experiences), the reviewed findings above reflect subjective experiences of existential disconnection. Not all people feel this disconnect, situationally nor chronically. This highlights that it is possible to alleviate and quell threats engendered by existential isolation. The primary focus of research in this area has been on the construct of I-sharing.

I-SHARING

Given that existential isolation refers to the "unbridgeable gap" between the self and others (or the world), it inherently involves the sense that one's phenomenological experiences (e.g., thoughts, perceptions, reactions) are distinct from and unshared by others. As noted previously, in order to satisfy epistemic and affiliative needs, people rely upon inferences to validate their perspectives and experiences. I-sharing, as a unique form of connection, offers a potentially powerful solution by meeting both affiliative and epistemic needs (Pinel et al., 2006).

I-sharing refers to the belief that one has had "an identical, phenomenological, in-the-moment experience with at least one other person" (Pinel et al., 2020). The term draws from James's (1890) portrayal of the "I" as the self-as-subject, or aspect of self that experiences. Most interpersonal connection occurs via the "Me" or self-as-object. Numerous psychological theories draw upon liking via the self-as-object. For example, the similarity-attraction hypothesis (Byrne, 1971), the mere exposure effect (Bornstein & D'Agostino, 1992; Newell & Shanks, 2007; Zajonc, 1968), and the reward model of liking (Byrne & Clore, 1970) all suggest that people are generally attracted to those who share similarities regarding their values, beliefs, attitudes, and physical proximity.

In contrast, I-sharing represents a unique form of connection because it stems from the inference that one's experience of the world coincides with that of another. Importantly, I-sharing is an *inference* because, as noted above, given our existentially isolated situation, it is impossible to know whether an identical experience has actually occurred. This inference represents a form of existential connection, satisfying both epistemic needs (i.e., because one's sense of reality is validated by another) and affiliative needs (i.e., because one connects and shares in an experience). For example, if two people overhear a corny joke and both respond with "Ba Dum Tss" (imitating a snare drum and cymbal), they may experience an I-sharing moment. This occurs because they had a simultaneous and identical reaction (a specific imitation of an instrument) to the same stimulus (a corny joke). This experience may satisfy epistemic needs because both people interpreted the situation as an opportunity to give a specific response (and both people acted upon the opportunity), providing validation for their interpretation and reaction to the situation. Affiliation needs are met because their identical reaction implies they both belong to a group that responds to corny jokes with drum sounds.

This inference of identical experiences can occur with momentous events (e.g., crying at a wedding) or seemingly trivial day-to-day moments (e.g., two strangers smiling at a child's giggle in a grocery store).

Of course, sharing objective qualities with another may make a person more likely to assume I-sharing in ambiguous situations. For example, two people from the same country meet by chance in a foreign country and have the same reaction to a nearby sign promoting guided tours of their home country. They may assume they share subjective experience based on shared objective aspects of self (e.g., speaking the same language, shared ethnic identity) rather than the reaction itself. Moreover, it is plausible that they may infer that their objective similarities reflect a shared underlying existential connection (Pinel et al., 2020).

Manipulating I-Sharing

To manipulate I-sharing experiences in a laboratory setting, researchers typically utilize a computerized version of the board game Imaginiff (Pinel & Long, 2012). Participants are told that they will be paired with an ostensible online partner to complete an online task. This task asks the participant to imagine if a specific individual (e.g., Michael Jordan) were something else (e.g., a sea creature) and prompts them to respond with their gut reaction to a list of four possibilities of the provided category (e.g., octopus, dolphin, hammerhead shark, crab; Pinel et al., 2010). Immediately after submitting their answer, participants learn how their partners responded to the same question. In the I-sharing condition, they learn that one partner responded to these questions identically across most conditions (e.g., 8 out of 12 trials). In the no I-sharing condition, partners never respond identically as the participants. This task is sometimes administered using inkblots as the stimuli or includes multiple interaction partners, but largely follows the same procedures (e.g., Pinel et al., 2017b).

Importantly, this paradigm differentiates the experience of Me-sharing from I-sharing by making participants consider novel situations: it is unlikely many participants have imagined which sea creatures best represent various celebrities. Thus, this task is not likely to be activating cognitive mechanisms involving memory but instead activates a unique response for each participant. Combined with immediate feedback on partner responses, the task fosters an I-sharing experience when the ostensible interaction partner responds identically to the participant (Pinel et al., 2010).

I-sharing manipulations further distinguish I-sharing from Me-sharing by controlling for these experiences. Me-sharing typically includes the perception of sharing objective aspects of one's identity (e.g., race, country of origin, religion). In the experimental paradigm, Me-sharing is manipulated by making these aspects salient (e.g., when learning about the interaction partner, various demographic information is also shared). The task is set up such that in the I-sharing condition, demographic information about a participant's interaction partner suggests they are objectively dissimilar to the participant. In paradigms with multiple interaction partners, the ostensible partner who does not I-share with the participant is often objectively similar, thus allowing a direct comparison of liking between a Me-sharer and an I-sharer (Pinel et al., 2010, 2018).

Benefits of I-Sharing

Perhaps most strikingly, I-sharing consistently has positive intergroup ramifications. Participants appear to prefer those with whom they I-share over those with whom they have objective similarities (Pinel & Long, 2012; Pinel et al., 2022). This effect occurs even when the I-sharing partner is objectively dissimilar and conforms to outgroup stereotypes (Pinel et al., 2018). Pinel and colleagues (2017b) found that I-sharing mitigates outgroup dehumanization in the context of race. White participants interacted face-to-face with a Black or White confederate with whom they shared an I-sharing experience, or not. They then completed measures of humanization/dehumanization and of liking. Participants in general liked an I-sharing partner more than other conditions, but when White participants I-shared with a Black confederate, they also rated the confederate to be more human than when they did not I-share with them (Pinel et al., 2017b). In a follow-up study, mechanistic dehumanization (the tendency to attribute more machine-like qualities to another person), but not animalistic dehumanization (attributing less cultural sophistication to another), was particularly sensitive to I-sharing (Bastian & Haslam, 2010).

In similar work, heterosexual men tended to respond defensively (e.g., by derogating gay men) following a threat to gender status. However, following an I-sharing experience with a gay partner, gender threats no longer elicited defensive reactions from heterosexual men (Pinel et al., 2019). I-sharing has also been found to increase preference for outgroup members with different body mass indexes and socioeconomic statuses (Pinel et al., 2017b) and even appeared to foster openness toward those with opposing political beliefs (Pinel et al., 2022).

I-sharing has also been found to foster prosociality. In a resource-allocation task, participants tended to share more resources with an I-sharing partner than with a Me-sharing partner or a dissimilar other (Huneke & Pinel, 2016). In a second series of studies, participants were more likely to express desire to help their I-sharing partner relative to other conditions and reported that they believed their I-sharing partner would be similarly likely to help them (Pinel et al., 2018). I-sharing also appears to foster empathy and connection to others beyond the I-sharer. Cohabitating couples who I-shared with a stranger were subsequently more likely to reach consensus and express willingness to compromise with each other than were couples who did not I-share with a stranger (Gehman et al., 2022). Yet in another study, I-sharing promoted liking of a racial outgroup member, but did not reduce anxious behavior in a later interaction with a novel outgroup member (Gaither et al., 2016). Thus, the extent to which the palliative effects of I-sharing generalize beyond the context in which it occurs remains an open question.

I-Sharing as an Antidote to Existential Isolation

Our existentially isolated situation leaves us feeling vulnerable to questioning whether our experiences are real (epistemic uncertainty) and whether we belong with others (affiliative uncertainty). I-sharing, the inference of having a simultaneous and identical reaction to the same stimulus as another person, provides a sense of certainty that one *does* experience the world like others and that this other person is existentially connected with us. I-sharing soothes the existentially isolated by eliminating the feeling of being alone in one's own experience (Pinel, 2018; Pinel et al., 2004, 2006).

While people tend to prefer I-sharers in general, this preference becomes stronger when existential isolation is experimentally elevated (Pinel et al., 2006). In other work, those with chronically high existential isolation were found to report particularly high preferences for I-sharers (Pinel & Long, 2012; Pinel et al., 2018). Mediation analyses suggested that feeling existentially connected to the I-sharer partially explained the relationship between high trait existential isolation and preference for I-sharing (Pinel et al., 2018). In other words, one reason I-sharers are so appealing to the existentially isolated is because I-sharing fosters a sense of existential connection.

AREAS FOR FUTURE RESEARCH

While progress in the study of existential isolation is accelerating and garnering widespread interest (e.g., Álvarez et al., 2023; van Tilburg, 2021), there are numerous areas for future research.

The majority of research dedicated to existential isolation is correlational cross-sectional and qualitative. While both methodologies offer important insights and help establish the phenomenon, more experimental and longitudinal research is a necessary next step in understanding the nature of this experience. Specifically, more precise studies assessing the causal factors contributing to this experience (e.g., interpersonal conflict, major life events, unresolved loneliness, situational influences), and the mechanisms by which existential isolation undermines epistemic certainty (e.g., less confidence in public health officials) and contributes to mental health problems (e.g., depression and suicide ideation) are needed to pave the way for broader intervention and preventive efforts.

Most empirical studies assessing existential disconnection have also focused on chronic or trait versions of this experience. Future research would benefit from continuing to explore and assess differences between in-the-moment, contextual, and more chronic versions of this experience. For example, it is possible that state experiences of existential isolation are better captured by a sense of low shared reality (e.g., Higgins et al., 2021) or as a form of loneliness (e.g., van Tilburg, 2021) because the experience may be more fleeting, able to be suppressed or ignored, and not capture the deeper existential nature of isolation (e.g., Ettema et al., 2010). Conversely, trait experiences of existential isolation may be qualitatively different and more pervasive than situational experiences, leading to undermined affiliative and epistemic certainty. Additionally, almost all research in this area has studied this experience in the context of interpersonal relationships. Yet Yalom (1980) wrote that existential isolation also represents a disconnection "from the world." While this sentiment has been echoed by other researchers (e.g., Bolmsjö et al., 2019), little research has assessed this possibility (cf. Young & Bosson, 2023).

In the same vein of a deeper understanding of the construct, future research should seek to understand the degree to which this experience represents a condition, an experience, or a process (e.g., Ettema et al., 2010). As described, while existential isolation may represent an existential reality, it is studied as a subjective experience. Moreover, theoretical and empirical work highlights the potential for existentially isolating experiences to lead to positive growth and transformation (e.g., Mayers et al., 2005; Moustakas, 1961). Additionally, more clarity is needed to understand the extent to which the perception of being existentially isolated represents a cognitive appraisal or an emotional experience. The EIS (Pinel et al., 2017a) contains items using affective-free language, yet other work integrating existential concerns draws heavily upon emotional language (e.g., van Bruggen et al., 2017), as do scales assessing loneliness (e.g., van Tilburg, 2021). Thus, across current theoretical and empirical studies, existential isolation has been characterized and measured by numerous potentially nonoverlapping ways, which has important implications for interpreting results and developing interventions.

Another important area for future work is to expand research into less commonly studied populations. Most quantitative studies have utilized convenient samples of university students and crowdsourcing participants. Yet within these studies, findings suggest that those with less normative identities (e.g., Carter et al., 2024; Pinel et al., 2021) tend to be more vulnerable to existentially isolating feelings. Additional research is needed to understand if and how existentially isolating feelings are associated with psychosocial and health outcomes in these populations. For example, research highlights a robust relationship between loneliness and sleep problems (Hom et al., 2020). Yet in a recent study assessing social connectedness and sleep quality in an American Indian tribe, after controlling for anxiety and depression, existential isolation (but not loneliness or social isolation) was associated with poorer sleep health (John-Henderson et al., 2024), suggesting that existential disconnection may operate differently, or be particularly important, across different populations.

Addressing existential isolation across the lifespan would also be beneficial area for future research. One qualitative study found older adults felt their existential disconnection had gradually increased throughout their later life (Carr & Fang, 2023). Yet it is also a common experience among adolescents (McKenna-Plumley et al., 2023), and adolescents tend to report relatively high levels of disconnection in general (Franssen et al., 2020); thus, questions about when this experience is most likely to be prevalent remain open.

Future research on existential isolation would benefit from cross-disciplinary perspectives. As highlighted in this chapter and elsewhere (Álvarez et al., 2023), the quantitative and qualitative research groups have largely operated independently. While it is encouraging that findings are largely converging on the nature and consequences of this experience, integrative work would help progress understanding and facilitate future intervention work.

There are plenty of open areas of research for I-sharing and other potential ways to alleviate existential isolation. For example, I-sharing is conceptualized as an inferred shared experience between two people. Yet there may be other more collective experiences that facilitate a shared I. For example, religious and spiritual events have the potential to connect a person with larger groups (Pinel et al., 2020). Similarly, ideas of identity fusion (the sense of oneness with a group; Swann & Buhrmester, 2015) and "we-ness" (collective identification within a couple; Fergus & Reid, 2001) connote a dissolution of the self–other boundary, and thus they have the potential to satisfy existentially isolating concerns.

One potent study in this vein compared changes in existential isolation and other-focused compassion between people who completed a weeklong intensive silent Zen meditation and people who were on vacation for a week (Park & Pinel, 2023). Compared to vacationers, those who completed the retreat reported lower existential isolation and increased other-focused compassion. These findings mirror the effects of awe experiences (Edwards et al., 2023), and taken together, highlight the potential for collective experiences to quell existential disconnection.

These potential pathways for alleviating existential concerns mirror suggestions found in qualitative studies of existential disconnection. For example, older adults report coping with existential disconnection by reframing their situation and identifying new meaning in life (Chung et al., 2020), and adolescents report focusing on the positive relationships in their lives (Garnow et al., 2022). Other work highlights being acknowledged by others and being the focus of other's concerns (Sjöberg et al., 2019) may directly address feelings of existential disconnection.

Future research should also assess possibilities for connecting with collective entities, such as cultural identity (e.g., Americans connecting following the September 11, 2001, terrorist attacks; Pyszczynski et al., 2003) or in a collective experience (e.g., singing together; Zaroulia, 2013). Given I-sharing's positive impact on intergroup relations (Pinel et al., 2018, 2022), additional research into how collective experiences may foster I-sharing opens the potential for large-scale prosocial intergroup interventions.

CONCLUSION

Existential isolation reflects an existential reality for humans: the inherent disconnection between the self, others, and the world. Awareness of this experience undermines our epistemic and affiliative needs. Yet people vary in the degree to which they are aware of this reality, with some who have internalized a sense of separateness and others who only experience it during particular moments. Research utilizing a self-report measure finds the experience can be manipulated; those with minoritized or unique identities tend to report higher-than-average existential isolation, and higher existential isolation tends to be associated with worse well-being and mental health. I-sharing, a unique form of connection characterized by inferring the same inner state as another, appears to be especially palliating for the existentially isolated, and fosters prosocial orientations more generally. Future research in these areas would benefit from continuing to define the constructs, utilize multimethod approaches, and study a wider array of populations.

REFERENCES

Allen, K., Kern, M. L., Rozek, C. S., McInerney, D. M., & Slavich, G. M. (2021). Belonging: A review of conceptual issues, an integrative framework, and directions for future research. *Australian Journal of Psychology, 73*(1), 87–102.

Álvarez, M. G., Haugan, G., Larsson, H., Saarelainen, S., Duppen, D., & Dezutter, J. (2023). Mapping existential loneliness: A scoping review on existential loneliness/isolation conceptualizations and operationalizations. *Journal of Humanistic Psychology.*

Arndt, J., Landau, M. J., Vail, K. E., III, & Vess, M. (2013). An edifice for enduring personal value: A terror management perspective on the human quest for multilevel meaning. In K. D. Markman, T. Proulx, & M. J. Lindberg (Eds.), *The psychology of meaning* (pp. 49–69). American Psychological Association.

Arrowood, R. B., Cox, C. R., & Swets, J. A. (2021). Exploring associations between existential isolation, quest religiosity, and well-being. *Mental Health, Religion and Culture, 24*(10), 1101–1116.

Asch, S. E. (1952). Group forces in the modification and distortion of judgments. In S. E. Asch (Ed.), *Social psychology* (pp. 450–501). Prentice-Hall.

Bastian, B., & Haslam, N. (2010). Excluded from humanity: The dehumanizing effects of social ostracism. *Journal of Experimental Social Psychology, 46,* 107–113.

Baumeister, R. F., DeWall, C. N., Ciarocco, N. J., & Twenge, J. M. (2005). Social exclusion impairs self-regulation. *Journal of Personality and Social Psychology, 88,* 589–604.

Baumeister, R. F., & Leary, M. R. (1995). The need to belong. *Psychological Bulletin, 117,* 497–529.

Becker, E. (1973). *The denial of death.* Free Press.

Bolmsjö, I., Tengland, P. A., & Rämgård, M. (2019). Existential loneliness: An attempt at an analysis of the concept and the phenomenon. *Nursing Ethics, 26,* 1310–1325.

Bornstein, R. F., & D'Agostino, P. R. (1992). Stimulus recognition and the mere exposure effect. *Journal of Personality and Social Psychology, 63,* 545–552.

Byrne, D. (1971). *The attraction paradigm.* Academic Press.

Byrne, D., & Clore, G. L. (1970). A reinforcement model of evaluative responses. *Personality: An International Journal, 1,* 103–128.

Carr, S., & Fang, C. (2023). A gradual separation from the world: A qualitative exploration of existential loneliness in old age. *Ageing and Society, 43,* 1436–1456.
Carter, S., Helm, P. J., Jimenez, T., & Arndt, J. (2024). *All mixed up: Multiracial identity and existential isolation.* Manuscript under review.
Child, S., & Lawton, L. (2020). Personal networks and associations with psychological distress among young and older adults. *Social Science and Medicine, 246,* 112714.
Chung, B. P. M., Olofsson, J., Wong, F. K. Y., & Rämgård, M. (2020). Overcoming existential loneliness: A cross-cultural study. *BMC Geriatrics, 20,* 347–359.
Çıkrıkçı, Ö., & Gençdoğan, B. (2017). The effects of attachment styles and belongingness on life satisfaction among adolescents. *International Journal of Happiness and Development, 3,* 241.
Constantino, M. J., Gaines, A. N., Coyne, A. E., Boswell, J. F., & Kraus, D. R. (2023). Existential isolation as a correlate of mental health problems, predictor of treatment outcome, and moderator of a patient–therapist match effect. *Journal of Social and Clinical Psychology, 42,* 1–28.
Constantino, M. J., Sommer, R., Goodwin, B. J., Coyne, A. E., & Pinel, E. C. (2019). Existential isolation as a correlate of clinical distress, beliefs about psychotherapy, and experiences with mental health treatment. *Journal of Psychotherapy Integration, 29,* 389–399.
Crocker, J., & Canevello, A. (2008). Creating and undermining social support in communal relationships: The role of compassionate and self-image goals. *Journal of Personality and Social Psychology, 95,* 555–575.
Diener, E., Suh, E. M., Lucas, R. E., & Smith, H. L. (1999). Subjective well-being: Three decades of progress. *Psychological Bulletin, 125,* 276–302.
Edwards, M. E., Helm, P. J., Pratscher, S. D., Bettencourt, B. A., & Arndt, J. (2023). The impact of awe on existential isolation: Evidence for contrasting pathways. *Personality and Social Psychology Bulletin, 50*(5), 715–732.
Ettema, E., Derksen, L., & Van Leeuwen, E. (2010). Existential loneliness and end-of-life care: A systematic review. *Theoretical Medicine and Bioethics, 31,* 141–169.
Fergus, K. D., & Reid, D. W. (2001). The couple's mutual identity and reflexivity: A systemic-constructivist approach to the integration of persons and systems. *Journal of Psychotherapy Integration, 11,* 385–410.
Festinger, L., Torrey, J. W., & Willerman, B. (1954). Self-Evaluation as a function of attraction to the group. *Human Relations, 7,* 161–174.
Fonagy, P., & Target, M. (2002). Early intervention and the development of self-regulation. *Psychoanalytic Inquiry, 22,* 307–335.
Franssen, T., Stijnen, M., Hamers, F., & Schneider, F. (2020). Age differences in demographic, social, and health-related factors associated with loneliness across the adult life span (19–65 years): A cross-sectional study in the Netherlands. *BMC Public Health, 20,* 1118.
Gaither, S. E., Remedios, J. D., Schultz, J. R., Maddox, K. B., & Sommers, S. R. (2016). Examining the effects of I-sharing for future White–Black interactions. *Social Psychology, 47,* 125–135.
Galgali, M. S., Helm, P. J., & Arndt, J. (2023). Feeling too isolated to be vaccinated?: The contributing role of subjective interpersonal isolation factors towards COVID-19 vaccine hesitancy and resistance. *Social Science and Medicine, 323,* 115865.
Galgali, M. S., Helm, P. J., & Arndt, J. (2024). Isolated but not necessarily lonely: An exploratory analysis of subjective isolation and conspiracist ideation. *Journal of Individual Differences.*
Garnow, T., Garmy, P., Edberg, A., & Einberg, E. (2022). Deeply lonely in the borderland between childhood and adulthood: Experiences of existential loneliness as narrated by adolescents. *International Journal of Qualitative Studies on Health and Well-being, 17,* 2132653.
Gehman, R. M., Pinel, E. C., Johnson, L. C., & Grover, K. W. (2022). Emerging ideas. A ripple effect: Does I-sharing with a stranger promote compromise in cohabiting couples? *Family Relations: An Interdisciplinary Journal of Applied Family Studies, 72,* 794–801.
Greenberg, J., Pyszczynski, T., & Solomon, S. (1986). The causes and consequences of a need for self-esteem: A terror management theory. In R. F. Baumeister (Ed.), *Public self and private self* (pp. 189–212). Springer.
Hadeei, S. (2023). Development and validation of a new measurement scale for existential loneliness. *Assessment, 31*(5), 1100–1113.
Helm, P. J., Greenberg, J., Park, Y. C., & Pinel, E. C. (2019). Feeling alone in your subjectivity: Introducing the state trait existential isolation model (STEIM). *Journal of Theoretical Social Psychology, 3,* 146–157.
Helm, P. J., Jimenez, T., Bultmann, M. N., Lifshin, U., Greenberg, J., & Arndt, J. (2020a). Existential isolation, loneliness, and attachment in young adults. *Personality and Individual Differences, 159,* 109890.
Helm, P. J., Chau, R. F., & Greenberg, J. (2022a).

Existential isolation: Theory, empirical findings, and clinical considerations. In *Springer eBooks* (pp. 95–113). Springer.

Helm, P. J., Jimenez, T., Carter, S., & Arndt, J. (2022b). A phenomenological divide: Reference group consequences for existential isolation. *Personality and Social Psychology Bulletin, 00,* 1–15.

Helm, P. J., Jimenez, T., Galgali, M. S., Edwards, M. E., Vail, K. E., III, & Arndt, J. (2022c). Divergent effects of social media use on meaning in life during the coronavirus pandemic via loneliness and existential isolation. *Journal of Social and Personal Relationships, 39,* 1768–1793.

Helm, P. J., Lifshin, U., Chau, R. F., & Greenberg, J. (2019). Existential isolation and death thought accessibility. *Journal of Research in Personality, 82,* 103845.

Helm, P. J., Medrano, M. R., Allen, J. J. B., & Greenberg, J. (2020b). Existential isolation, loneliness, depression, and suicide ideation in young adults. *Journal of Social and Clinical Psychology, 39,* 641–674.

Helm, P. J., Rothschild, L., Greenberg, J., & Croft, A. (2018). Explaining sex differences in existential isolation research. *Personality and Individual Differences, 134,* 283–288.

Higgins, E. T., Rossignac-Milon, M., & Echterhoff, G. (2021). Shared reality: From sharing-is-believing to merging minds. *Current Directions in Psychological Science, 30,* 103–110.

Hom, M. A., Chu, C., Rogers, M. L., & Joiner, T. E. (2020). A meta-analysis of the relationship between sleep problems and loneliness. *Clinical Psychological Science, 8,* 799–824.

Horner, D. E., Sielaff, A., & Greenberg, J. (2023). Autonomy support for gender expression and managing existential concerns: An initial study among transgender individuals. *Journal of Humanistic Psychology,* 002216782211447.

Huneke, M., & Pinel, E. C. (2016). Fostering selflessness through I-sharing. *Journal of Experimental Social Psychology, 63,* 10–18.

James, W. (1918). *Principles of psychology.* General Publishing. (Original work published 1890)

John-Henderson, N., Henderson-Matthews, B., Helm, P. J., Gilham, S., Wood, Z., Heavy Runner, G., . . . Salois, E. (2024). Social connectedness and sleep in Blackfeet American Indian adults. *Sleep Health.*

Kim, H., & McKenry, P. C. (2002). The relationship between marriage and psychological well-being. *Journal of Family Issues, 23,* 885–911.

Leary, M. R., & Baumeister, R. F. (2000). The nature and function of self-esteem: Sociometer theory. *Advances in Experimental Social Psychology, 32,* 1–62.

Leavitt, P., & Helm, P. J. (2024). *Belief stage and social network composition predict existential isolation and loneliness among doubting and no-longer-believing LDS.* Manuscript under review.

Lee, C., Shin, J., & Hong, A. (2018). Does social media use really make people politically polarized?: Direct and indirect effects of social media use on political polarization in South Korea. *Telematics and Informatics, 35,* 245–254.

Ling, R. (2020) Confirmation bias in the era of mobile news consumption: The social and psychological dimensions. *Digital Journalism, 8,* 596–604.

Long, A. E., Pinel, E. C., Daily, J. R., & Costello, A. E. (2021). Existential isolation and the struggle for belief validation. *British Journal of Social Psychology, 61,* 491–509.

Mansfield, L., Chapot, V., Meads, C., Daykin, N., Tomlinson, A., Lane, J., . . . Golding, A. C. (2021). A conceptual review of loneliness in adults: Qualitative evidence synthesis. *International Journal of Environmental Research and Public Health, 18,* 11522.

Mayers, A. M., Naples, N. A., & Nilsen, R. D. (2005). Existential issues and coping: A qualitative study of low-income women with HIV. *Psychology and Health, 20,* 93–113.

McKenna-Plumley, P. E., Turner, R. N., Yang, K., & Groarke, J. M. (2023). "It's a feeling of complete disconnection": Experiences of existential loneliness from youth to older adulthood. *BMC Psychology, 11,* 1–14.

Moustakas, C. E. (1961). *Loneliness.* Prentice-Hall.

Mueller, J. (1912). Elements of physiology. In B. Rand (Ed.), *The classical psychologists: Selections illustrating psychology from Anaxagoras to Wundt* (pp. 530–544). Constable & Co. (Original work published 1834)

Newell, B. R., & Shanks, D. R. (2007). Recognising what you like: Examining the relation between the mere-exposure effect and recognition. *European Journal of Cognitive Psychology, 19,* 103–118.

Oleskowicz, T., Yawger, G. C., & Pinel, E. C. (2023). Not drinking and alone: Alcohol use and its implications for existential isolation. *Journal of Social and Clinical Psychology, 42,* 267–291.

Olofsson, J., Rämgård, M., Forss, K. S., & Bramhagen, A. (2021). Older migrants' experience of existential loneliness. *Nursing Ethics, 28,* 1183–1193.

Park, Y. C., & Pinel, E. C. (2020). Existential isolation and cultural orientation. *Personality and Individual Differences, 159,* 109891.

Park, Y. C., & Pinel, E. C. (2023). The effect of

a 7-day intensive Buddhist meditation on existential isolation, interpersonal isolation, and compassion among South Koreans. *Journal of Applied Social Psychology, 53,* 877–891.

Peplau, L. A., Perlman, D. (1982). Perspectives on loneliness. In L. A. Peplau & D. Perlman (Eds.), *Loneliness: A sourcebook of current theory, research and therapy* (pp. 1–18). Wiley.

Pinel, E. C. (2018). Existential isolation and I-sharing: Interpersonal and intergroup implications. *Current Opinion in Psychology, 23,* 84–87.

Pinel, E. C., Bronson, C. A., Zapata, J. P., & Bosson, J. K. (2019). I-sharing after a gender status threat and its implications for attitudes toward gay men. *Psychology of Men and Masculinity, 20,* 299–309.

Pinel, E. C., Fuchs, N. A., & Benjamin, S. (2022). I-sharing across the aisle: Can shared subjective experience bridge the political divide? *Journal of Applied Social Psychology, 52,* 407–413.

Pinel, E. C., Helm, P. J., Yawger, G. C., Long, A. E., & Scharnetzki, L. (2021). Feeling out of (existential) place: Existential isolation and nonnormative group membership. *Group Processes and Intergroup Relations, 25*(4), 990–1010.

Pinel, E. C., & Long, A. E. (2012). When I's meet: Sharing subjective experience with someone from the outgroup. *Personality and Social Psychology Bulletin, 38,* 296–307.

Pinel, E. C., Long, A. E., & Crimin, L. A. (2010). I-sharing and a classic conformity paradigm. *Social Cognition, 28,* 277–289.

Pinel, E. C., Long, A. E., Johnson, L., & Yawger, G. C. (2018). More about when I's meet: The intergroup ramifications of I-sharing, part II. *Personality and Social Psychology Bulletin, 44,* 1601–1614.

Pinel, E. C., Long, A. E., Landau, M. J., Alexander, K., & Pyszczynski, T. (2006). Seeing I to I: A pathway to interpersonal connectedness. *Journal of Personality and Social Psychology, 90,* 243–257.

Pinel, E. C., Long, A. E., Landau, M., & Pyszczynski, T. (2004). I-sharing, the problem of existential isolation, and their implications for interpersonal and intergroup phenomena. In Greenberg, J., S. Koole, & T. Pyszczynski (Eds.), *Handbook of experimental existential psychology* (pp. 352–368). Guilford Press.

Pinel, E. C., Long, A. E., Murdoch, E. Q., & Helm, P. J. (2017a). A prisoner of one's own mind: Identifying and understanding existential isolation. *Personality and Individual Differences, 105,* 54–63.

Pinel, E. C., Yawger, G. C., Long, A. E., Rampy, N., Brenna, R., & Finnell, S. K. (2017b). Human like me: Evidence that I-sharing humanizes the otherwise dehumanized. *British Journal of Social Psychology, 56,* 689–704.

Pinel, E. C., Yawger, G. C., & Park, Y. C. (2020). The holy grail of connection: I-sharing, existential isolation, and religion. In K. E. Vail III & C. Routledge (Eds.), *The science of religion, spirituality, and existentialism* (pp. 167–174). Elsevier Academic Press.

Pyszczynski, T., Solomon, S., & Greenberg, J. (2003). *In the wake of 9/11: The psychology of terror.* American Psychological Association.

Ross, L., & Nisbett, R. E. (2011). *The person and the situation: Perspectives of social psychology.* Pinter & Martin Publishers.

Ryan, R. M., & Deci, E. L. (2000). Intrinsic and extrinsic motivations: Classic definitions and new directions. *Contemporary Educational Psychology, 25,* 54–67.

Ryff, C. D., & Singer, B. (2000). Interpersonal flourishing: A positive health agenda for the new millennium. *Personality and Social Psychology Review, 4,* 30–44.

Sekse, R. J. T., Raaheim, M., Blaaka, G., & Gjengedal, E. (2010). Life beyond cancer: Women's experiences 5 years after treatment for gynaecological cancer. *Scandinavian Journal of Caring Sciences, 24,* 799–807.

Shaver, P. R., & Mikulincer, M. (2007). Adult attachment strategies and the regulation of emotion. In J. J. Gross (Ed.), *Handbook of emotion regulation* (pp. 446–465). Guilford Press.

Sielaff, A., Horner, D. E., & Greenberg, J. (2022). The moderating role of mystical-type experiences on the relationship between existential isolation and meaning in life. *Personality and Individual Differences, 186,* 111347.

Sjöberg, M., Edberg, A., Rasmussen, B. H., & Beck, I. (2019). Being acknowledged by others and bracketing negative thoughts and feelings: Frail older people's narrations of how existential loneliness is eased. *International Journal of Older People Nursing, 14,* e12213.

Swann, W. B. (1996). *Self-traps: The elusive quest for higher self-esteem.* Freeman/Times Books/Henry Holt.

Swann, W. B., & Bosson, J. K. (2010). Self and identity. In S. T. Fiske, D. T. Gilbert, & G. Lindzey (Eds.), *Handbook of social psychology* (5th ed., pp. 589–628). Wiley.

Swann, W. B., Jr., & Buhrmester, M. D. (2015). Identity fusion. *Current Directions in Psychological Science, 24*(1), 52–57.

Swann, W. B., Stein-Seroussi, A., & Giesler, R. B. (1992). Why people self-verify. *Journal of Personality and Social Psychology, 62*(3), 392.

van Bruggen, V., ten Klooster, P., Westerhof, G.,

Vos, J., de Kleine, E., Bohlmeijer, E., & Glas, G. (2017). The existential concerns questionnaire (ECQ): Development and initial validation of a new existential anxiety scale in a nonclinical and clinical sample. *Journal of Clinical Psychology, 0,* 1–12.

van Tilburg, T. G. (2021). Social, emotional, and existential loneliness: A test of the multidimensional concept. *The Gerontologist, 61,* e335–e344.

Vazire, S. (2010). Who knows what about a person?: The self–other knowledge asymmetry (SOKA) model. *Journal of Personality and Social Psychology, 98,* 281–300.

Walton, G. M., & Cohen, G. L. (2007). A question of belonging: Race, social fit, and achievement. *Journal of Personality and Social Psychology, 92,* 82–96.

Wu, W., Sheppard, E., & Mitchell, P. (2019). Interpreting signals in other people's behavior to sense things about them and to infer things about their world. *Social and Personality Compass, 13,* e12513.

Yalom, I. D. (1980). *Existential psychotherapy.* Basic Books.

Young, R. T., & Bosson, J. K. (2023). *From other and from world: Expanding the current model of existential isolation.* Paper presented at the International Society for the Science of Existential Psychology Preconference, Atlanta, GA.

Zajonc, R. B. (1968). Attitudinal effects of mere exposure. *Journal of Personality and Social Psychology, 9,* 1–27.

Zaroulia, M. (2013). "Sharing the moment": Europe, affect, and utopian performatives in the Eurovision Song Contest. In K. Fricker & M. Gluhovic (Eds.), *Performing the "new" Europe: Studies in international performance* (pp. 31–52). Palgrave Macmillan.

Zhou, N., Zhao, Y., Smith, K. V., Killikelly, C., Stelzer, E., Maercker, A., . . . Helm, P. J. (2023). Existential isolation and prolonged grief in bereaved people: The moderating role of culture. *Clinical Psychology and Psychotherapy, 30,* 862–872.

CHAPTER 27

Shared Reality

Matteo Masi *and* Gerald Echterhoff

Shared reality, defined as the subjective experience of common inner states (i.e., feelings, beliefs, or attitudes) about something with others, is an exquisitely human and ubiquitous experience (Echterhoff & Higgins, 2021; Echterhoff, Higgins, & Levine, 2009). Shared reality is exemplified by the experience of the feeling of being "on the same page" or "thinking the same thing" as someone else. For example, when people meet a new person in a social setting (e.g., at work), they tend to share their impressions with other people they trust around them (e.g., coworkers), and they feel more confident in their impressions if others agree. In other words, people tend to co-construct reality and validate each other's opinions. As argued elsewhere (Higgins, 2019), the research on the roots of human nature has mostly focused on the superior intelligence of humans compared to other animals rather than on social motivation, even though the development of human cognition is tightly intertwined with the motivation to communicate with others (Higgins, 2016; Wolf & Tomasello, 2023). As we elaborate here, people can fulfill basic existential needs, especially needs for meaning and social connection, in the process of creating and maintaining shared realities with others.

The concept of shared reality has been used and extended to touch on very different but interrelated fields, such as political, developmental, organizational, or comparative psychology, as exemplified by a special issue of *Current Opinion in Psychology* edited by Echterhoff and Higgins (2018). What these approaches have in common is the adoption of shared experiences to explain human cognition and behavior. Here, we focus on shared reality in interpersonal and intergroup relations and relevant recent studies rather than providing a comprehensive review of shared reality research (for which we refer to Echterhoff & Higgins, 2017, 2018, 2021; Higgins et al., 2021).

The key motivational principle of shared reality theory resonates well with basic tenets of existential psychology. For example, two of the most discussed needs in existential research are (1) the fear of isolation, which arises from the conflict between people's need to feel connected to others and the recognition of our own subjectivity, and (2) the need for meaning and understanding of issues and events in our world, especially those that challenge our existing concepts, wishes, and aspirations (Koole et al., 2006; see also Bilal & Helm, Chapter 26, this volume, and Bonarska et al., Chapter 28, this volume). By and large, these two concerns map onto relational and epistemic needs that have figured prominently in shared reality theory. Indeed, shared reality has been proposed to be a key avenue toward connecting with others, obtaining confident inner states about the world, and experiencing one's life as meaningful (Cornwell et al., 2017; Hardin & Conley, 2001).

In this chapter, we illustrate how creating a shared reality with others on a given topic satisfies basic human epistemic and relational needs. We then review experimental research on the behavioral markers of a generalized sense of shared reality in dyadic conversation. Additionally, we summarize recent findings linking the experience of shared reality in dyads to quality of life. Finally, we highlight potential avenues for future research.

CREATING SHARED REALITY: ACHIEVEMENT OF FUNDAMENTAL HUMAN NEEDS

One of the most satisfying human experiences in the social world is sharing inner states with someone else, whether beliefs about a movie, attitudes on pressing issues, or simple emotional and perceptual experiences. People value this experience highly, often feeling connected enough to form new groups based on minimal commonalities, such as a preference for one artist over another (Tajfel et al., 1971). Discovering commonalities with strangers helps dismantle social barriers, fulfilling the need for connection (Allen et al., 2021; Baumeister & Leary, 1995) and increasing social identification, which also boosts self-esteem (Abrams & Hogg, 1988).

However, the benefits of sharing extend beyond connection. Sharing our inner states with others aims to resolve uncertainties about various topics and issues, including existential ones, and elevate confidence in one's feelings or beliefs. This dual function—building connections and enhancing certainty—makes the act of sharing inner states profoundly meaningful and impactful in social interactions. Festinger (1957) argued that validation makes internal states objective rather than subjective. When validation is absent, as demonstrated in Asch's (1951) conformity studies, people feel uncertain and uncomfortable. Thus, others serve as sources of validation, especially in uncertain situations (Hillman et al., 2023; Kruglanski et al., 2010). By sharing our internal states with others, we seek meaningful connections (relational motives) and certainty about events (epistemic motives; Echterhoff & Higgins, 2021).

These motives work synergistically. Sharing states and beliefs with others validates subjective experiences, making them seem like truths about the world (Hardin & Higgins, 1996; Rossignac-Milon & Higgins, 2018a). Feeling connected to someone is also enhanced when inner states are shared (Echterhoff & Higgins, 2021; Shrauger & Jones, 1968). For instance, when an employee and a colleague share a confident impression of a newcomer at work, the employee feels more connected to the colleague. Conversely, when an employee aims to connect with a colleague by creating a shared impression of a newcomer and succeeds, the employee ends up with a more confident impression of the newcomer.

Thus, shared reality involves motivated connection (the *shared* in shared reality) and motivated cognition (the *reality* in shared reality; Echterhoff & Higgins, 2021; Higgins et al., 2021).

Shared Reality: Conceptualization

Communication enables us to share personal and other experiences (e.g., gossiping), connect with each other (Higgins, 1992, 2016), coordinate social and cultural activities, and establish common ground (Kashima et al., 2019; Lau et al., 2001). In addition, communication allows us to externalize our internal states and let others understand or "catch" them. Consider children pointing at an object, sharing their amusement or fear with their caregiver, expecting the caregiver to share their attention, and observing the caregiver's response (Liszkowski, 2018; Wolf & Tomasello, 2023; see Higgins, 2016, for shared reality development). This simple act of communication establishes the building blocks of shared reality (Higgins, 2019; Shteynberg et al., 2023). Without communication, one person might always assume that another person feels the same way about someone or something, but it is the very act of self-disclosure (not necessarily with spoken language) that creates the foundation for the experience of sharing (Echterhoff, Higgins, & Levine, 2009; Higgins, 2016).

Before proceeding, it is crucial to define *sharing*, which can have various meanings that may not directly relate to shared reality (Echterhoff & Higgins, 2021; Thompson & Fine, 1999). One interpretation of sharing involves simply conveying information to someone, such as through conversation. However, for shared reality to manifest, it is imperative that both individuals subjectively experience a commonality of opinions.[1] A second meaning refers to collaboration toward a shared goal, with tasks divided between individuals. Yet this form of sharing pertains to a common goal rather than shared opinions and thus is inadequate. A third interpretation arises when two individuals share an opinion without explicitly communicating it to each other. However, the objective evidence of their shared opinion still falls short of the achievement of shared reality. To meet our definition, individuals must not only hold objectively similar opinions but also subjectively experience this commonality. For instance, when Person A expresses their love for action movies and Person B reciprocates, a shared reality regarding action movies is established. Thus, shared reality transcends mere co-experiencing of events, requiring subjective acknowledgment (for further insights into shared knowledge, refer to Shteynberg et al., 2023).

Sharing-Is-Believing: Empirical Evidence of a Shared Reality Creation

Since its inception, the concept of shared reality has been studied using the saying-is-believing paradigm, which was developed by Higgins and Rholes (1978; see Echterhoff & Higgins, 2017, for a review). In this paradigm, a triadic relationship is established between participants (i.e., communicators) who are asked to communicate with a stranger (i.e., audience) about someone else (i.e., target person or object). Participants are first provided with evaluatively ambiguous descriptions of the target (a person who behaves in ways that can be interpreted either positively or negatively, for instance as stubborn or persistent). This ambiguity creates subjective uncertainty that motivates the creation of shared reality with the audience (Kopietz et al., 2010). Participants are then asked to describe the target to the audience, who has to recognize the target among other people based only on the participant's description.

Importantly, before describing the target to the audience, participants are told that the audience is positively or negatively biased toward the target person. This minimal information robustly triggers evaluative *audience tuning*: Participants "tune" or adapt their descriptions to their audience's attitude about a target person. For example, people describe a coworker more positively if they know that the audience's attitude toward that person was positive, thus emphasizing positive traits more than negative ones (Higgins & McCann, 1984; Higgins et al., 1982). A subsequent free-recall task for the target person's original behaviors typically reveals that the communicators' memory is also biased in the direction of the audience-tuned message and the audience's attitude (Echterhoff et al., 2005, 2009, 2013, 2017; Pinelli et al., 2022). Memory is the basis for many other cognitive processes, such as the formation of judgments, beliefs, and attitudes. Hence, the audience-tuning memory bias reflects a profound influence on how communicators construct their social reality (see Echterhoff & Higgins, 2017; Wyer & Srull, 1989).

The audience-congruent memory bias has been explained as a result of shared reality creation (for a review, see Echterhoff & Higgins, 2017): Indeed, a bulk of studies suggests that the memory bias emerges to the extent that communicators successfully create a reality about the target with the audience, a reality in which the target is believed to be a more positive than negative person (or vice versa). For instance, studies found that the memory bias is observed only when communicators have sufficient epistemic trust in their audience (Echterhoff et al., 2005, 2008, 2017) and when audience tuning is not motivated by alternative, non-shared reality goals such as politeness or obtaining incentives (Echterhoff et al., 2008). Hence, the paradigm has also been dubbed *sharing-is-believing* (Higgins et al., 2021).

In recent studies, validated scales were used to assess the subjective experience of the communicator's shared reality with the audience. Specifically, a measure of shared reality about a target (SR-T) was created for this purpose (Schmalbach et al., 2019). The scale allows a simple but effective assessment of perceived commonality about something between a person and a partner and includes five items—for example: "I think that partner X and I are on the same wavelength regarding target Y." In two studies, scale scores were strongly related to saying-is-believing memory tuning, supporting the idea that it is the subjective experience of commonality that explains such effects.

Several studies have found that audience tuning can influence social impressions using either written or visual information about a target (Hellman et al., 2011; Pierucci et al., 2014), attitudes toward controversial issues (Knausenberger et al., 2019), and acceptance of group stereotypes (Echterhoff & Higgins, 2021; Ye et al., 2021). In a recent experiment, Boytos and Costabile (2022) showed that audience-tuning effects extend to autobiographical recollections. Participants first wrote about valence-neutral topics (e.g., multitasking at work) and were then assigned to an audience condition with either a positive or negative attitude toward the topic. Participants' recollections aligned with the audience's attitude; a pattern strengthened when participants reported high shared reality. This evidence suggests that shared reality can shape not only immediate cognition but also self-related memories, demonstrating the broad scope of the phenomenon.

Motivated Connection: How Shared Reality Brings Us Closer

Audience tuning in the saying-is-believing paradigm is interpreted as evidence that a shared reality has been spontaneously created with a stranger. However, as argued above, shared reality is created for one reason: to satisfy basic human needs. Achieving a shared reality requires being motivated to connect with another person (Hardin & Conley, 2001). Schmalbach and colleagues (2019) found evidence that the SR-T, which measures the experience of commonality with another person, correlates positively with a measure of relational motivation (e.g., "I want to get along with person X") as well as with other measures related to relational needs (e.g., inclusion of the other in the self, shared identity), and its predictive power is higher than all of these constructs in explaining memory-tuning results.

Empirical studies have manipulated relational motives and measured whether audience tuning is affected. For example, the appearance of an audience can be systematically manipulated to modulate communication intentions with such an audience. If participants perceived an audience as less likeable, it would be difficult for a communicator to establish a connection, and thus shared reality-based outcomes should be disrupted. Pierucci and colleagues (2013) manipulated the facial appearance of the audience in a saying-is-believing experiment to increase or decrease motivation to relate to them. They found that the tuning effect was indeed significantly reduced when the presented faces were less (vs. more) pleasant, and the effect was associated with a measure of relational motivation, and not epistemic trust.

In addition, several experiments have varied the social identity of the audience as a way to manipulate affiliative motives. Social-identity similarity is relevant to shared reality because it may help communicators assume commonalities in their way of thinking or interpreting events. For example, when communicating with an outgroup audience (e.g., German students communicating with Turkish students at a German institution), participants showed evaluative audience tuning but not recall bias (e.g., Echterhoff et al., 2005, 2008, 2017; Kopietz et al., 2010; see also Skorinko & Sinclair, 2018). With an outgroup audience, evaluative tuning of one's message may be more strongly motivated by adherence to politeness or egalitarian norms than by shared reality creation. At the level of overt communication, participants apparently honored the outgroup audience's attitude; however, they did not internalize the audience-tuned message, as indicated by the lack of the audience-congruent memory bias.

Motivated Cognition: How Shared Reality Helps Us Understand Events

In synergy with relational motives, creating shared reality helps validate one's vision of the world and increase trust and confidence in one's inner states, in other words, fulfill epistemic motives. Echterhoff and Higgins (2017) proposed an epistemic process model to explain how a shared reality is created through communication. They considered three types of input that determine whether shared reality is created through communication in the saying-is-believing paradigm: judgment of the communicator (JC), judgment of the audience (JA), and message of the communicator (MC).

When JC is characterized by high self-confidence or self-reliance, there is less need to create a shared reality. Therefore, the need to seek the audience's opinion should be minimal. The result would be that communicators would not care about JA or MC if they believe they are their own epistemic authority (Kruglanski et al., 2010). This phenomenon is exemplified by a saying-is-believing study by Kopietz and colleagues (2010), in which participants were given false feedback about their ability to accurately form social impressions about others. When participants believed they had sufficient ability to judge others, their confidence increased and their tendency to create a shared reality decreased. As a result, they showed less memory bias toward the opinions of their audience. The opposite was found when participants were made to believe that their social-judgment abilities were below average, increasing their epistemic motivation to listen to and conform to the audience (see also Pierucci et al., 2014).

If, however, JC is more (vs. less) ambiguous, communicators are more likely to consider and follow JA for information that could guide their judgment. Thus, to increase reliance on JA and enable audience tuning, the audience must be perceived as a source of epistemic trust (Kruglanski et al., 2010). For example, one piece of information that people might use to assume that an audience is a trustworthy source is group identity, as people have higher epistemic trust in ingroup members than in outgroup members (Dovidio & Gaertner, 2010). By manipulating the group identity of the audience (ingroup vs. outgroup), studies have found that memory tuning is more likely to occur when there is an ingroup audience than when there is an outgroup audience (Echterhoff, Higgins, & Levine, 2009; Echterhoff et al., 2017). But is there a way to overcome this intergroup bias? Apparently, one way is to make the outgroup audience an expert on the target person. For example, when the target person was a member of the *audience's* ingroup rather than the communicator's group, the communicator's epistemic trust in the audience increased, and thus the recall bias occurred as expected (Echterhoff et al., 2017). Importantly, however, the audience must be perceived as an expert on the specific topic, not an expert on another topic (Knausenberger et al., 2019).

In most cases, message production (input MC) is a fundamental feature for establishing a shared reality, as suggested already by the first empirical demonstration of audience tuning (Higgins & Rholes, 1978). As argued above, message production can increase the sense that a newly formed opinion is true and valid (Echterhoff et al., 2008, 2013, 2017). What makes MC even more valid is receiving feedback from the audience. By default, communicators interpret silence in response to MC as a sign of message understanding and acceptance. However, when the audience gives feedback but then fails to identify the target, the creation of shared reality is interrupted. This has been demonstrated by Pinelli and colleagues (2022), who studied shared reality creation with multiple one-person audiences. Communicators can flexibly tune to the different opinions of the audience (Mata & Semin, 2020). However, there was no audience-congruent memory bias when the audience failed to identify the target.

Further evidence for the importance of shared reality regarding the achievement of epistemic and affiliative needs comes from lines of research on related concepts (e.g., Echterhoff & Higgins, 2018, 2021; Pinel et al., 2006), some of which are also reviewed in this volume (see Bilal & Helm, Chapter 26, this volume).

Shared Reality Generalizes Beyond the First Interaction

Most studies on shared reality focus on single interactions, but there is evidence that an established shared reality can extend to similar targets (Bebermeier et al., 2015). In Experiment 1, social verification of judgments about ambiguous social interactions was manipulated using pictures from the Multi-Motive Grid (Sokolowski et al., 2000). Participants received summaries of their own and their audience's judgments, which were either highly similar (high social verification) or dissimilar (low social verification). High social verification influenced opinions about a new, similarly ambivalent sexist target, even without audience feedback on the new target and without communication with the initial shared reality partner. Thus, a shared reality generalized more when participants received social verification. Experiment 2 found that an established shared reality continued to influence evaluations of a new target even after a 1-week delay. This effect occurred only when participants were prompted with several cues to recall the previously experienced shared reality, enhancing its cognitive accessibility (Eitam & Higgins, 2010).

Shared reality can also transfer to later interactions with the same partner (Schmalbach, 2019). In a series of experiments, participants received social verification (vs. no verification) of their decisions in a job-hiring task from a simulated partner. Participants chose between candidates with ambiguous profiles and then received feedback indicating high (identical choices) or low (different choices) social verification from their partner. High social verification led to increased epistemic trust, relational motivation, and an experience of shared reality as measured by SR-T. In a subsequent hiring task, participants decided whether to align with the partner's opinions, which they had previewed. Those who received high verification in the first task were more likely to align with the partner's decisions in the second task, while those who received low verification did not. This alignment was driven by increased epistemic trust and shared reality.

Thus, shared reality extends beyond single interactions, fostering trust and preparing individuals for future interactions with similar goals, regardless of the same target or partner's presence (Cosmides & Tooby, 2013; Fiske, 1992).

Generalized Shared Reality

The shared reality we have discussed thus far has been confined to one-shot interactions with one or more partners. However, people also share a general way of looking at the world with some people. Rossignac-Milon and colleagues (2021; Rossignac-Milon & Higgins, 2018b) proposed that for certain dyads, especially for romantic couples, this experience is an essential part of their daily life. Indeed, among adult relationships, romantic couples should be characterized by high levels of interdependence, trust, validation, and daily care for each other, epitomizing the phenomenon of "merged minds." To measure this new conceptualization, Rossignac-Milon and colleagues (2021) employed a novel tool assessing a generalized sense of shared reality (SR-G), which taps a dyad's shared perception of the world outside the relationship (i.e., shared reality across multiple topics and domains). The SR-G self-report questionnaire concerns, for example, the experience of regularly thinking about things at the same time.

In one study, the SR-G was tested on dyads of new acquaintances. They were asked to discuss their interpretation of ambiguous images about social situations. After the discussion, the SR-G questionnaire was administered, along with a variety of other constructs to establish validity (for details, see Rossignac-Milon et al., 2021). Participants with high SR-G scores reported feeling a deeper emotional closeness and a stronger rapport with their partner. They also described experiencing a genuine connection or sense of clicking with their partner and expressed a desire to continue the conversation. In addition, these participants believed they gained a clearer understanding of the images when discussing them with their partner and placed greater trust in their partner's insights regarding the content of the images. Thus, strangers experiencing high SR-G tend to increase their epistemic trust in their partner, who is likely to validate their worldview and increase their sense of certainty and connection. This is especially true when people perceive interaction and agreement as authentic and honest (Rossignac-Milon et al., 2024). Importantly, SR-G predicts these outcomes independently of SR-T, qualifying the two as distinct and complementary constructs that build shared reality in dyads (Rossignac-Milon et al., 2021).

Behavioral Signatures of Shared Reality in Dyadic Conversation

The initial wave of shared reality studies did not examine real-time communication and interaction behaviors (Echterhoff & Higgins, 2021). Recent studies have expanded the investigation scope by examining behavioral markers of shared reality in dyadic conversations.

Nonverbal behaviors constitute a significant part of our daily communication, occurring spontaneously with or without accompanying verbal communication (Burgoon et al., 1995; Hall et al., 2019). Observing and responding to the microdynamics of a conversation, such as turn-taking, nonverbal cues (e.g., nodding), and behavioral mimicry, can lead individuals to assume they are on the same wavelength (Koudenburg, 2018). Smooth turn-taking, close proximity, frequent eye contact, and smiling are interpreted as indicators of rapport (Burgoon et al., 1984, 1995). Similarly, behavioral mimicry increases when affiliative motives are enhanced (Lakin & Chartrand, 2003). For example, Templeton and colleagues (2022) asked dyads of friends or strangers to engage in a free conversation for 10 minutes and found that faster responses correlated with higher ratings of interpersonal connectedness. However, in conversations between friends, longer gaps in turn-taking also signaled enjoyment and connection (Templeton et al., 2023).

Expanding on the concept that behavioral cues can be indicative of shared reality, Rossignac-Milon and colleagues (2021) investigated pairs of strangers who met online discussing ambiguous social scenes from the Multi-Motive Grid. Using an instant messenger platform, participants' online behavior was coded based on behavioral signatures: vocalizing similar thoughts, expressing agreement on shared feelings, simultaneous or near-synchronous exclamations, and completing each other's sentences. Results showed that strangers engaging in such behaviors reported an increased sense of shared reality. Importantly, these behaviors predicted both relational and epistemic outcomes, such as feelings of closeness and certainty, especially when participants perceived them as indicative of shared reality. This suggests that although shared reality is subjectively experienced, it can be observed through interactional behaviors, offering a tangible basis for understanding this phenomenon.

Smooth interaction is often seen as an indication of mutual understanding (Burgoon et al., 1995). When conversations flow as expected, people feel socially validated and in agreement with their partner. However, disruptions in conversation, such as forced silence introduced by delays in computer-mediated communication, can lead to distress and negative affect (Koudenburg et al., 2011, 2013). Interestingly, studies on romantic couples, known for their strong connections, reveal a paradox: When conversation flow is disrupted, highly connected couples feel closer, not further apart (Koudenburg et al., 2014; Przybylinski & Andersen, 2015). This suggests that individuals in close relationships may be confident in their ability to quickly reestablish a threatened shared reality.

This assumption was tested by Rossignac-Milon and colleagues (2021) who observed 101 romantic couples in a laboratory experiment. Dyads received manipulated negative or positive reports on their similarities in interpreting sensory stimuli, potentially threatening their perceived sense of shared reality. Subsequently, when asked to discuss ambiguous images together, they exhibited more behavioral signatures of shared reality generation (SR-G), which were coded from the couple's recorded conversation. This behavior was interpreted as a mutual intention to reaffirm their closeness and reinforce their own reality when threatened by external influences, such as the experimenter. When external events challenge shared beliefs about how the world works, a couple can adapt by reaffirming the coherence and meaning they expect to find in their close relationship (Murray et al., 2018).

Consequences of Shared Reality in Dyadic Relationships

The previous discussion implies that creating and maintaining a shared reality with others can positively impact relationship satisfaction. When people around you provide validation and trust, feelings of being on the right track and pursuing the right goals are enhanced (Cornwell et al., 2017; Rossignac-Milon & Higgins, 2018b). Consequently, the motivation to create and maintain a shared reality can significantly influence life, especially when important issues and events are shared with significant others.

Although the theory has broad implications, shared reality has mostly been empirically investigated in laboratory studies focusing on cognitive, motivational, and interpersonal consequences (Echterhoff & Higgins, 2021). This focus may have created a disconnect between laboratory findings and real-world applications (Osborne-Crowley, 2020). Experimental lab approaches are fruitful for uncovering antecedents, underlying processes, and consequences of shared reality. However, research explicitly considering the consequences of shared reality in the external world represents an important extension. Recent studies address this gap by analyzing the resonance of shared reality experiences in real life, thereby enhancing ecological validity.

As we have argued, the perception of an established shared reality with close others acts as a protective factor against external threatening situations (Murray et al., 2018). The global spread of the SARS-CoV 2 virus, an unobservable and surreptitious threat, and increasing number of deaths from COVID-19 as well as vaccination debates created a great sense of uncertainty regarding maintenance of physical integrity and even the future of humanity (e.g., Baerg & Bruchmann, 2022). As noted, epistemic uncertainty is a chief condition that motivates the creation of a shared reality (Kopietz et al., 2010). Undoubtedly, one of the most affected social categories was that of frontline health care workers and, indirectly, their significant others. In times of distress, social support is much needed, especially with close partners and significant others (Bolger & Amarel, 2007; Girme et al., 2013).

Building on these considerations, Enestrom and Lydon (2021) investigated whether romantic partners' sense of shared reality could predict relationship satisfaction during uncertain and threatening times. The authors posited that shared reality should increase actual and perceived support from partners, thereby promoting greater relationship satisfaction. They recruited 155 couples, with one partner being a health care worker in contact with COVID-19 patients. They assessed shared reality with the SR-G, social support over the past 2 weeks (e.g., "My partner was helpful"), and relationship satisfaction. The results confirmed their expectations: Shared reality was associated with greater relationship satisfaction, mediated by the health care workers perceiving greater support from their partners.

These findings support the notion that the experience of stressful situations is influenced by whether two people have established a shared reality. In this study, the health care worker experienced the most stress, with their partner providing support. However, people sometimes face stressful situations together and respond jointly in real time. While it is well established that experiencing positive emotions together benefits couples' relationships and health (Brown & Fredrickson, 2021; Wells et al., 2022), the effect of jointly experiencing stressors is less clear. Shared reality might reduce the perceived negativity of a co-experienced stressor by creating shared feelings, validating perceptions, and providing bonding opportunities (e.g., Wagner et al., 2015). However, an alternative hypothesis suggests that the negative valence of co-experienced events could be reinforced, as emotional responses may become polarized through joint experiences (Boothby et al., 2014; Brown et al., 2022).

Goldring and colleagues (2022) conducted studies providing relevant data on these competing predictions. They demonstrated that experiencing a stressful event with a partner reduces anxiety due to achieved shared reality. In a laboratory experiment, 111 female undergraduates underwent the Trier Social Stress Task, inducing stress by impromptu speeches rated by trained raters. Before the speech, students rated its demandingness and were assigned one of three conditions: receiving feedback by the partner that was consistent with their perceptions, was inconsistent, or was ambiguous. As expected, consistent feedback increased perceived commonalities, epistemic trust, and relational motivation, while inconsistent or ambiguous feedback decreased them.

Participants' and confederates' physiological responses were monitored via electrocardiography during speeches and measured self-reported psychological distress. Results showed reduced distress when confederates perceived the task as equally demanding, with those participants exhibiting better stress control than those without validation. This provides remarkable evidence that shared reality induces positive physiological responses to stressful events.

In a follow-up study, Goldring and colleagues (2022) examined the generalizability of their prior findings with 102 heteronormative couples in a 14-day diary study. Participants rated common daily stressors identified the evening before completing the diary, their shared reality experience regarding the stressor using a subset of items from SR-T, and their psychological distress. The authors hypothesized that women, due to gender-related evolutionary, biological, and socialization differences, would be more sensitive to shared reality effects resulting from shared experiences. Specifically, women's tendencies toward befriending for survival, higher oxytocin levels during stress, and greater emotional expression were expected to influence their responses (Goldring et al., 2022). Results supported this hypothesis, with nearly all female participants (99%) experiencing reduced anxiety from daily shared reality. In contrast, less than half of male participants (42%) reported partial anxiety reduction.

Furthermore, longitudinal studies examining relational factors like responsiveness and physical presence shed light on their interplay with shared reality and satisfaction. Bar-Shachar and Bar-Kalifa (2021) conducted a 4-week longitudinal study where participants reported their partner's perceived responsiveness to social events. In relationships, partners anticipate responses to disclosures about social events (Reis & Gable, 2015). Responsive reactions, whether positive or negative, signal care and validation, bolstering shared reality and meaning (Rossignac-Milon & Higgins, 2018b). The researchers found that sharing a personal event and responding to a partner's disclosure was related to daily shared reality (SR-G), particularly when partners shared negative and uncertain events. This highlights the importance of receiving validation during uncertain times, which is consistent with the idea that uncertainty drives seeking of validation through shared reality (Echterhoff & Higgins, 2021; Murray et al., 2018).

Enestrom and colleagues (2023) conducted a study examining the long-term effects of shared reality in romantic couples. Over a 4-week period, participants completed online diary assessments, reporting their shared reality experience with their partner and relationship satisfaction. They also noted their partner's presence during survey completion, reflecting spatial proximity. Psychological closeness with loved ones is promoted by spatial proximity, and partner presence may be important also for shared reality (Niedenthal et al., 2005; Przybylinski & Andersen, 2015). Results indicated that partner physical presence was associated with same-day shared reality and predicted an increase in shared reality compared to the previous day. These findings remained consistent after controlling for reported conflict, shared daily activities, and concurrent survey completion. Interestingly, increases in relationship satisfaction over time were more related to shared reality than to physical presence.

Taken together, these results show that shared reality represents a remarkable source of achieving existential human needs in our daily lives. This is particularly true when reality is shared with a close other, helping increase life satisfaction when the world threatens mental and physical health.

TRENDS IN SHARED REALITY RESEARCH: WHAT NOW?

In this outlook, we summarize recent trends in shared reality research and discuss implications from neighboring theories regarding existential needs. A chronological analysis of the theory's development reveals a shift from early work, which focused on uncovering the mechanism of shared reality and its relation to epistemic and relational needs (Echterhoff & Higgins, 2017; Echterhoff, Higgins, & Levine, 2009), to more recent observational and dyadic perspectives that study the evolution of shared reality over time (e.g., Bar-Shachar & Bar-Kalifa, 2021; Enestrom & Lydon, 2021; Goldring et al., 2022; Rossignac-Milon et al., 2021). Utilizing advanced techniques like ecological momentary assessment via smartphone notifications appears promising for testing the predictive power of the theory.

Complementary considerations have been given to the behavioral features of conversation that might signal commonality of states. Although we have presented some of this work, much remains to be discovered. Key questions include how the behavioral signatures of shared reality evolve over time, what early signs predict a stronger future shared reality, and how these behaviors might differ by topic. For instance, do people signal shared reality differently when discussing political issues compared to everyday experiences like a café visit? Verbal and nonverbal communication is influenced by numerous overlapping factors (Burgoon et al., 1995; Hall et al., 2019), and research on behavioral signatures of shared reality is still in its infancy. Exploring these dimensions could provide deeper insights into the mechanisms and manifestations of shared reality in various contexts.

A second direction that has not yet been explored is observing shared reality in action within digital and online social environments. People spend increasing amounts of time on social media, with over 90% of internet users having a social media identity and spending an average of 2.5 hours daily on these platforms (Kemp, 2024). Social media use affects life satisfaction, loneliness, and depression (Verduyn et al., 2022), though the impact may not be as significant as assumed (Appel et al., 2020).

Social media offers unique opportunities for field studies that can reach vast numbers of people (Mosleh et al., 2021, 2022). Unlike correlational studies, these field studies randomly assign conditions and observe responses. For instance, experimenters could create profiles that express specific views on political or social events and measure interaction rates, such as follow-backs or message responses. Analyzing these behaviors can reveal the willingness to create a shared reality with these profiles.

People are aware of the impact online interactions can have on their perception of reality (Bowe & Wohn, 2015), suggesting they might achieve a shared reality on these platforms. Private messages can be used to measure the sense of shared reality through validated scales or by examining behavioral signatures during interactions. This methodology can investigate the interplay between shared reality theory and phenomena typical of social media, such as the creation of echo chambers and polarization of beliefs, characterized by significant information selection bias (Cinelli et al., 2021; Jost et al., 2018; Sharot & Sunstein, 2020; Stern & Ondish, 2018). The motivation to create a shared reality can bring people closer but also exacerbate existing differences, especially in unrestricted online environments (Higgins, 2019).

A further step for shared reality theory involves testing it across various cultural settings. Experimental studies conducted in Eastern countries have addressed relevant issues and replicated or extended previous findings (e.g., Ye et al., 2021), suggesting the theory's potential beyond WEIRD (Western, educated, industrialized, rich, democratic) populations. Understanding whether the motivation to share with others is culturally influenced is essential for a comprehensive theory.

We know that collectivistic versus individualistic cultural backgrounds can moderate social attunement effects (Skorinko & Sinclair, 2018). However, cultural differences extend beyond this dimension. For instance, tight and loose cultures, as described by Gelfand and colleagues (2011) and Uz (2015), may vary in their motivation to create a shared reality with strangers. Tight cultures, which arise from threatening environmental conditions and repressive societies, are characterized by low tolerance for deviations from norms and high uncertainty avoidance compared to loose cultures (i.e., although this is not necessarily always the case; Uz, 2015). In high uncertainty-avoidance societies, individuals believe strict rules make life more predictable and less stressful (Minkov & Hofstede, 2014), which may translate into high epistemic needs for control or understanding, especially under high perceived social threat (Kashima et al., 2022).

In tight cultures, motivation to create a shared reality might increase but primarily toward nondeviant ingroup members, seen as epistemically reliable, rather than outgroup members. This inclination reflects a need to reinforce social norms and reduce uncertainty. Conversely, loose cultures, with their higher tolerance for deviations and lower uncertainty avoidance, might display a more inclusive motivation for shared reality, extending beyond close ingroup members to include a broader range of social interactions. Exploring these cultural differences in shared reality is crucial. It involves examining how cultural norms, environmental threats, and social structures influence the creation and maintenance of shared realities, providing deeper insights into the universality and variability of this psychological phenomenon.

CONCLUSION

In this chapter, we have provided a comprehensive overview of both classic and recent findings within the shared reality literature. Emphasizing the dual and synergistic nature of shared reality motivation, we have underscored its significance in both understanding events and fostering connections with others. Our overview revealed consistent findings on shared reality stemming from controlled laboratory experiments, as well as emerging evidence from longitudinal and observational studies related to relationship quality.

Furthermore, we outlined several potential avenues for future research, spanning various psychology subfields. Overall, our examination suggests that shared reality theory remains vibrant and dynamic. There is still much to uncover about the intricacies of shared reality and its far-reaching implications, making it an exciting and fertile area for ongoing investigation.

NOTE

1. Tacit agreement from Person B could indeed create an initial sense of shared reality by implying that Person B shares the same opinion. Studies support that explicit feedback is not always required to establish shared reality with someone's opinion (Echterhoff et al., 2017). However, conceptually, the unilateral act of Person A communicating with Person B does not guarantee that Person A will perceive a commonality with Person B, hence the importance of making this distinction clear.

REFERENCES

Abrams, D., & Hogg, M. A. (1988). Comments on the motivational status of self-esteem in social identity and intergroup discrimination. *European Journal of Social Psychology, 18*(4), 317–334.

Allen, K. A., Kern, M. L., Rozek, C. S., McInerney, D. M., & Slavich, G. M. (2021). Belonging: A review of conceptual issues, an integrative framework, and directions for future research. *Australian Journal of Psychology, 73*(1), 87–102.

Appel, M., Marker, C., & Gnambs, T. (2020). Are social media ruining our lives?: A review of meta-analytic evidence. *Review of General Psychology, 24*(1), 60–74.

Asch, S. E. (1951). Effects of group pressure upon the modification and distortion of judgments. In H. S. Guetzkow (Ed.), *Groups, leadership and men* (pp. 177–190). Carnegie Press.

Baerg, L., & Bruchmann, K. (2022). COVID-19 information overload: Intolerance of uncertainty moderates the relationship between frequency of internet searching and fear of COVID-19. *Acta Psychologica, 224,* 103534.

Bar-Shachar, Y., & Bar-Kalifa, E. (2021). Responsiveness processes and daily experiences of shared reality among romantic couples. *Journal of Social and Personal Relationships, 38*(11), 3156–3176.

Baumeister, R. F., & Leary, M. R. (1995). The need to belong: Desire for interpersonal attachments as a fundamental human motivation. *Psychological Bulletin, 117,* 497–529.

Bebermeier, S., Echterhoff, G., Bohner, G., & Hellmann, J. H. (2015). The generalization of shared reality: When communication about one target shapes evaluations of other targets. *European Journal of Social Psychology, 45*(5), 623–640.

Bolger, N., & Amarel, D. (2007). Effects of social support visibility on adjustment to stress: Experimental evidence. *Journal of Personality and Social Psychology, 92*(3), 458–475.

Boothby, E. J., Clark, M. S., & Bargh, J. A. (2014). Shared experiences are amplified. *Psychological Science, 25*(12), 2209–2216.

Bowe, B. J., & Wohn, D. Y. (2015). Are there generational differences?: Social media use and perceived shared reality. *Proceedings of the 2015 International Conference on Social Media and Society, 17,* 1–5.

Boytos, A. S., & Costabile, K. A. (2022). Social influence and autobiographical recall: Shared reality and epistemic trust shape perceptions of autobiographical events. *Social Cognition, 40*(5), 411–437.

Brown, C. L., Chen, K.-H., Wells, J. L., Otero, M. C., Connelly, D. E., Levenson, R. W., & Fredrickson, B. L. (2022). Shared emotions in shared lives: Moments of co-experienced affect, more than individually experienced affect, linked to relationship quality. *Emotion, 22*(6), 1387–1393.

Brown, C. L., & Fredrickson, B. L. (2021). Characteristics and consequences of co-experienced positive affect: Understanding the origins of social skills, social bonds, and caring, healthy communities. *Current Opinion in Behavioral Sciences, 39*, 58–63.

Burgoon, J. K., Buller, D. B., Hale, J. L., & de Turck, M. A. (1984). Relational messages associated with nonverbal behaviors. *Human Communication Research, 10*(3), 351–378.

Burgoon, J. K., Stern, L. A., & Dillman, L. (1995). *Interpersonal adaptation: Dyadic interaction patterns*. Cambridge University Press.

Cinelli, M., De Francisci Morales, G., Galeazzi, A., Quattrociocchi, W., & Starnini, M. (2021). The echo chamber effect on social media. *Proceedings of the National Academy of Sciences, 118*(9), e2023301118.

Cornwell, J. F. M., Franks, B., & Higgins, E. T. (2017). Shared reality makes life meaningful: Are we *really* going in the right direction? *Motivation Science, 3*(3), 260–274.

Cosmides, L., & Tooby, J. (2013). Evolutionary psychology: New perspectives on cognition and motivation. *Annual Review of Psychology, 64*, 201–229.

Dovidio, J. F., & Gaertner, S. L. (2010). Intergroup bias. In S. T. Fiske, D. T. Gilbert, & G. Lindzey (Eds.), *Handbook of social psychology* (5th ed., pp. 1084–1121). Wiley.

Echterhoff, G., & Higgins, E. T. (2017). Creating shared reality in interpersonal and intergroup communication: The role of epistemic processes and their interplay. *European Review of Social Psychology, 28*, 175–226.

Echterhoff, G., & Higgins, E. T. (2018). Editorial: Shared reality. *Current Opinion in Psychology, 23*, vii–xi.

Echterhoff, G., & Higgins, E. T. (2021). Shared reality: Motivated connection and motivated cognition. In P. A. M. van Lange, E. T. Higgins, & A. W. Kruglanski, *Social psychology: Handbook of basic principles* (3rd ed., pp. 181–201). Guilford Press.

Echterhoff, G., Higgins, E. T., & Groll, S. (2005). Audience-tuning effects on memory: The role of shared reality. *Journal of Personality and Social Psychology, 89*, 257–276.

Echterhoff, G., Higgins, E. T., Kopietz, R., & Groll, S. (2008). How communication goals determine when audience tuning biases memory. *Journal of Experimental Psychology: General, 137*, 3–21.

Echterhoff, G., Higgins, E. T., & Levine, J. M. (2009). Shared reality: Experiencing commonality with others' inner states about the world. *Perspectives on Psychological Science, 4*, 496–521.

Echterhoff, G., Kopietz, R., & Higgins, E. T. (2013). Adjusting shared reality: Communicators' memory changes as their connection with their audience changes. *Social Cognition, 31*(2), 162–186.

Echterhoff, G., Kopietz, R., & Higgins, E. T. (2017). Shared reality in intergroup communication: Increasing the epistemic authority of an out-group audience. *Journal of Experimental Psychology: General, 146*(6), 806–825.

Echterhoff, G., Lang, S., Krämer, N., & Higgins, E. T. (2009). Audience-tuning effects on communicators' memory: The role of audience status in sharing reality. *Social Psychology, 40*, 150–163.

Eitam, B., & Higgins, E. T. (2010). Motivation in mental accessibility: Relevance of a representation (ROAR) as a new framework. *Social and Personality Psychology Compass, 4*(10), 951–967.

Enestrom, M. C., Bar-Kalifa, E., Bar-Shachar, Y., & Lydon, J. E. (2023). Spatial proximity in relationships research methods: The effect of partner's presence during survey completion on shared reality in romantic couples' daily lives. *Journal of Social and Personal Relationships, 40*(6), 1943–1960.

Enestrom, M. C., & Lydon, J. E. (2021). Relationship satisfaction in the time of COVID-19: The role of shared reality in perceiving partner support for frontline health-care workers. *Journal of Social and Personal Relationships, 38*(8), 2330–2349.

Festinger, L. (1957). *A theory of cognitive dissonance*. Stanford University Press.

Fiske, S. T. (1992). Thinking is for doing: Portraits of social cognition from Daguerreotype to laserphoto. *Journal of Personality and Social Psychology, 63*(6), 877–889.

Gelfand, M. J., Raver, J. L., Nishii, L., Leslie, L. M., Lun, J., Lim, B. C., . . . Yamaguchi, S. (2011). Differences between tight and loose cultures: A 33-nation study. *Science, 332*(6033), 1100–1104.

Girme, Y. U., Overall, N. C., & Simpson, J. A. (2013). When visibility matters: Short-term versus long-term costs and benefits of visible and invisible support. *Personality and Social Psychology Bulletin, 39*(11), 1441–1454.

Goldring, M. R., Pinelli, F., & Bolger, N. (2022). Shared reality can reduce stressor reactivity. *Frontiers in Psychology, 13*, 853750.

Hall, J. A., Horgan, T. G., & Murphy, N. A. (2019). Nonverbal communication. *Annual Review of Psychology, 70*, 271–294.

Hardin, C. D., & Conley, T. D. (2001). A relational approach to cognition: Shared experience and relationship affirmation in social cognition. In G. B. Moskowitz (Ed.), *Cognitive social psychology: The Princeton Symposium on the legacy and future of social cognition* (pp. 3–17). Erlbaum.

Hardin, C. D., & Higgins, E. T. (1996). Shared reality: How social verification makes the subjective objective. In R. M. Sorrentino & E. T. Higgins (Eds.), *Handbook of motivation and cognition: The interpersonal context* (Vol. 3, pp. 28–84). Guilford Press.

Hellmann, J. H., Echterhoff, G., Kopietz, R., Niemeier, S., & Memon, A. (2011). Talking about visually perceived events: Communication effects on eyewitness memory. *European Journal of Social Psychology, 41*(5), 658–671.

Higgins, E. T. (1992). Achieving "shared reality" in the communication game: A social action that creates meaning. *Journal of Language and Social Psychology, 11,* 107–131.

Higgins, E. T. (2016). Shared-reality development in childhood. *Perspectives on Psychological Science, 11,* 466–495.

Higgins, E. T. (2019). *Shared reality: What makes us strong . . . and tears us apart.* Oxford University Press.

Higgins, E. T., & McCann, C. D. (1984). Social encoding and subsequent attitudes, impressions, and memory: "Context-driven" and motivational aspects of processing. *Journal of Personality and Social Psychology, 47*(1), 26–39.

Higgins, E. T., McCann, C. D., & Fondacaro, R. (1982). The "communication game": Goal-directed encoding and cognitive consequences. *Social Cognition, 1*(1), 21–37.

Higgins, E. T., & Rholes, W. S. (1978). "Saying is believing": Effects of message modification on memory and liking for the person described. *Journal of Experimental Social Psychology, 14,* 363–378.

Higgins, E. T., Rossignac-Milon, M., & Echterhoff, G. (2021). Shared reality: From sharing-is-believing to merging minds. *Current Directions in Psychological Science, 30*(2), 103–110.

Hillman, J. G., Fowlie, D. I., & MacDonald, T. K. (2023). Social verification theory: A new way to conceptualize validation, dissonance, and belonging. *Personality and Social Psychology Review, 27*(3), 309–331.

Jost, J. T., van der Linden, S., Panagopoulos, C., & Hardin, C. D. (2018). Ideological asymmetries in conformity, desire for shared reality, and the spread of misinformation. *Current Opinion in Psychology, 23,* 77–83.

Kashima, E. S., Ochoa, D. P., Nicolas, G., Ah Gang, G. C., Du, H., Klackl, J., . . . Fiske, S. T. (2022). Exploring the adaptive role of core social motives in perceived societal threats. *Asian Journal of Social Psychology, 25*(2), 249–266.

Kashima, Y., Bain, P. G., & Perfors, A. (2019). The psychology of cultural dynamics: What is it, what do we know, and what is yet to be known? *Annual Review of Psychology, 70,* 499–529.

Kemp, S. (2024, January 31). *The time we spend on social media.* https://datareportal.com/reports/digital-2024-deep-dive-the-time-we-spend-on-social-media.

Knausenberger, J., Wagner, U., Higgins, E. T., & Echterhoff, G. (2019). Epistemic authority in communication effects on memory: Creating shared reality with experts on the topic. *Journal of Applied Research in Memory and Cognition, 8*(4), 439–449.

Koole, S. L., Greenberg, J., & Pyszczynski, T. (2006). Introducing science to the psychology of the soul: Experimental existential psychology. *Current Directions in Psychological Science, 15*(5), 212–216.

Kopietz, R., Hellmann, J. H., Higgins, E. T., & Echterhoff, G. (2010). Shared-reality effects on memory: Communicating to fulfill epistemic needs. *Social Cognition, 28,* 353–378.

Koudenburg, N. (2018). Regulating shared reality with micro-dynamics in the form of conversation. *Current Opinion in Psychology, 23,* 47–51.

Koudenburg, N., Gordijn, E. H., & Postmes, T. (2014). "More than words": Social validation in close relationships. *Personality and Social Psychology Bulletin, 40*(11), 1517–1528.

Koudenburg, N., Postmes, T., & Gordijn, E. H. (2011). Disrupting the flow: How brief silences in group conversations affect social needs. *Journal of Experimental Social Psychology, 47*(2), 512–515.

Koudenburg, N., Postmes, T., & Gordijn, E. H. (2013). Resounding silences: Subtle norm regulation in everyday interactions. *Social Psychology Quarterly, 76*(3), 224–241.

Kruglanski, A. W., Orehek, E., Dechsne, M., & Pierro, A. (2010). Lay epistemic theory: The motivational, cognitive, and social aspects of knowledge formation. *Social and Personality Psychology Compass, 4,* 939–950.

Lakin, J. L., & Chartrand, T. L. (2003). Using nonconscious behavioral mimicry to create affiliation and rapport. *Psychological Science, 14*(4), 334–339.

Lau, I. Y., Chiu, C. Y., & Lee, S. L. (2001). Communication and shared reality: Implications for the psychological foundations of culture. *Social Cognition, 19*(3), 350–371.

Liszkowski, U. (2018). Emergence of shared reference and shared minds in infancy. *Current Opinion in Psychology, 23,* 26–29.

Mata, A., & Semin, G. R. (2020). Multiple shared realities: The context sensitivity of the saying-is-believing effect. *Social Cognition, 38*(4), 354–366.

Minkov, M., & Hofstede, G. (2014). A replication of Hofstede's uncertainty avoidance dimension across nationally representative samples from Europe. *International Journal of Cross Cultural Management, 14*(2), 161–171.

Mosleh, M., Martel, C., Eckles, D., & Rand, D. G. (2021). Shared partisanship dramatically increases social tie formation in a Twitter field experiment. *Proceedings of the National Academy of Sciences, 118*(7), e2022761118.

Mosleh, M., Pennycook, G., & Rand, D. G. (2022). Field experiments on social media. *Current Directions in Psychological Science, 31*(1), 69–75.

Murray, S. L., Lamarche, V., & Seery, M. D. (2018). Romantic relationships as shared reality defense. *Current Opinion in Psychology, 23,* 34–37.

Niedenthal P. M., Barsalou L. W., Winkielman P., Krauth-Gruber S., & Ric F. (2005). Embodiment in attitudes, social perception, and emotion. *Personality and Social Psychology Review, 9*(3), 184–211.

Osborne-Crowley, K. (2020). Social cognition in the real world: Reconnecting the study of social cognition with social reality. *Review of General Psychology, 24*(2), 144–158.

Pierucci, S., Echterhoff, G., Marchal, C., & Klein, O. (2014). Creating shared reality about ambiguous sexual harassment: The role of stimulus ambiguity in audience-tuning effects on memory. *Journal of Applied Research in Memory and Cognition,* 3, 300–306.

Pierucci, S., Klein, O., & Carnaghi, A. (2013). You are the one I want to communicate with! Relational motives driving audience-tuning effects on memory. *Social Psychology, 44,* 16–25.

Pinel, E. C., Long, A. E., Landau, M. J., Alexander, K., & Pyszczynski, T. (2006). Seeing I to I: A pathway to interpersonal connectedness. *Journal of Personality and Social Psychology, 90,* 243–257.

Pinelli, F., Davachi, L., & Higgins, E. T. (2022). Shared reality effects of tuning messages to multiple audiences. *Social Cognition, 40*(2), 172–183.

Przybylinski, E., & Andersen, S. M. (2015). Systems of meaning and transference: Implicit significant-other activation evokes shared reality. *Journal of Personality and Social Psychology, 109*(4), 636.

Reis, H. T., & Gable, S. L. (2015). Responsiveness. *Current Opinion in Psychology, 1,* 67–71.

Rossignac-Milon, M., Bolger, N., Zee, K. S., Boothby, E. J., & Higgins, E. T. (2021). Merged minds: Generalized shared reality in dyadic relationships. *Journal of Personality and Social Psychology, 120*(4), 882–911.

Rossignac-Milon, M., & Higgins, E. T. (2018a). Beyond intrapersonal cognitive consistency: Shared reality and the interpersonal motivation for truth. *Psychological Inquiry, 29,* 86–93.

Rossignac-Milon, M., & Higgins, E. T. (2018b). Epistemic companions: Shared reality development in close relationships. *Current Opinion in Psychology, 23,* 66–71.

Rossignac-Milon, M., Pillemer, J., Bailey, E. R., Horton, C. B., Jr., & Iyengar, S. S. (2024). Just be real with me: Perceived partner authenticity promotes relationship initiation via shared reality. *Organizational Behavior and Human Decision Processes, 180,* 104306.

Schmalbach, B. (2019). *The experience of shared reality.* Unpublished doctoral thesis.

Schmalbach, B., Hennemuth, L., & Echterhoff, G. (2019). A tool for assessing the experience of shared reality: Validation of the German SR-T. *Frontiers in Psychology, 10,* 438954.

Sharot, T., & Sunstein, C. R. (2020). How people decide what they want to know. *Nature Human Behaviour, 4*(1), 14–19.

Shrauger, J. S., & Jones, S. C. (1968). Social validation and interpersonal evaluations. *Journal of Experimental Social Psychology, 4*(3), 315–323.

Shteynberg, G., Hirsh, J. B., Wolf, W., Bargh, J. A., Boothby, E. B., Colman, A. M., . . . Rossignac-Milon, M. (2023). Theory of collective mind. *Trends in Cognitive Sciences, 27*(11), 1019–1031.

Skorinko, J. L., & Sinclair, S. (2018). Shared reality through social tuning of implicit prejudice. *Current Opinion in Psychology, 23,* 109–112.

Sokolowski, K., Schmalt, H. D., Langens, T. A., & Puca, R. M. (2000). Assessing achievement, affiliation, and power motives all at once: The Multi-Motive Grid (MMG). *Journal of Personality Assessment, 74*(1), 126–145.

Stern, C., & Ondish, P. (2018). Political aspects of shared reality. *Current Opinion in Psychology, 23,* 11–14.

Tajfel, H., Billig, M. G., Bundy, R. P., & Flament, C. (1971). Social categorization and intergroup behaviour. *European Journal of Social Psychology, 1*(2), 149–178.

Templeton, E. M., Chang, L. J., Reynolds, E. A., Cone LeBeaumont, M. D., & Wheatley, T. (2022). Fast response times signal social connection in conversation. *Proceedings of the National Academy of Sciences, 119*(4), e2116915119.

Templeton, E. M., Chang, L. J., Reynolds, E. A., Cone LeBeaumont, M. D., & Wheatley, T. (2023). Long gaps between turns are awkward for strangers but not for friends. *Philosophical Transactions of the Royal Society B, 378*(1875), 20210471.

Thompson, L., & Fine, G. A. (1999). Socially shared cognition, affect, and behavior: A review and integration. *Personality and Social Psychology Review, 3,* 278–302.

Uz, I. (2015). The index of cultural tightness and looseness among 68 countries. *Journal of Cross-Cultural Psychology, 46*(3), 319–335.

Verduyn, P., Gugushvili, N., & Kross, E. (2022). Do social networking sites influence well-being?: The extended active-passive model. *Current Directions in Psychological Science, 31*(1), 62–68.

Wagner, U., Galli, L., Schott, B. H., Wold, A., van der Schalk, J., Manstead, A. S., . . . Walter, H. (2015). Beautiful friendship: Social sharing of emotions improves subjective feelings and activates the neural reward circuitry. *Social Cognitive and Affective Neuroscience, 10*(6), 801–808.

Wells, J. L., Haase, C. M., Rothwell, E. S., Naugle, K. G., Otero, M. C., Brown, C. L., . . . Fredrickson, B. L. (2022). Positivity resonance in long-term married couples: Multimodal characteristics and consequences for health and longevity. *Journal of Personality and Social Psychology, 123*(5), 983–1003.

Wolf, W., & Tomasello, M. (2023). A shared intentionality account of uniquely human social bonding. *Perspectives on Psychological Science, 20*(2), 264–275.

Wyer, R. S., & Srull, T. K. (1989). *Memory and cognition in its social context.* Erlbaum.

Ye, J., Zhao, L., Huang, Z., & Meng, F. (2021). The audience-tuning effect of negative stereotypes in communication. *Frontiers in Psychology, 12,* 663814.

CHAPTER 28

Navigating Uncertainty

Cognitive Closure, Information Processing, Epistemic Authority in the Pursuit of Knowledge

Karolina Bonarska, Jakub Cacek, Małgorzata Kossowska, *and* Ewa Szumowska

The quest for understanding oneself and the world emerges as an existential pursuit that has piqued human curiosity throughout history. Knowledge forms the foundation for individuals and societies to understand and navigate existence. The formation and transmission of knowledge both shape how individuals perceive the world and interact with others. Knowledge is essential for personal and societal development, progress, and well-being.

The quest for knowledge involves complexity and ambiguity, especially when addressing philosophical and metaphysical dilemmas. This pursuit often engenders a deeper sense of wonder and humility in the face of the complexity of existence. Beyond being solely an individual endeavor, the pursuit of truth is also a collective venture characterized by dialogue, discourse, and shared exploration. Through ongoing engagement in this collective quest, individuals strive to enhance their understanding of both themselves and the world around them (Higgins et al., 2021).

Kruglanski (1989) conceptualized knowledge as belief rather than absolute truth, with its formation being thought of as subjective and naive. People often rely on their own subjective understanding of how they can best go about gathering and interpreting information. These subjective understandings, often termed *naive theories,* serve as the basis for formulating and testing hypotheses about observed phenomena. Contrary to popular belief, individuals tend to adhere to structured patterns influenced by their prior knowledge and subjective interpretations.

Knowledge acquisition is motivated (Kruglanski, 1989). Naturally, curiosity drives individuals to explore, inquire, and learn about their surroundings (Lauriola et al., 2015; Szumowska & Kruglanski, 2020). Indeed, nurturing curiosity and offering discovery opportunities can unlock human potential and drive progress. However, the pursuit of knowledge may also be a response to the challenges posed by the complexity of the world and its inherent uncertainty (Kruglanski, 2004, 2023), further intensified by

---

Karolina Bonarska and Jakub Cacek played a lead role in conceptualization, write-up of the first draft, and discussions on the original draft of this chapter. Małgorzata Kossowska and Ewa Szumowska played a supporting role in conceptualization and in write-up reviews and edit of the manuscript.

the daily deluge of incoming information (Chowdhury et al., 2011). Moreover, the proliferation of misinformation compounds this challenge, spanning from mundane decision making to profound existential uncertainties (Vaccari & Chadwick, 2020). Navigating this overabundance of information poses a daunting task, requiring individuals to discern the reliability of sources and sift through reams of complex data in order to obtain firm and valid knowledge (Roets et al., 2015).

This chapter delves into the quest for knowledge about oneself and the world. It examines the motivations driving knowledge acquisition, focusing on the need for cognitive closure and its impact on knowledge formation, attitudes, social judgments, interpersonal communication, and group relations and dynamics. It also explores how knowledge is processed, considering factors such as the subjective relevance of information, cognitive demands, and psychological resources. In addition, it investigates the role of epistemic authority and trusted sources in shaping and transmitting knowledge. Lastly, this chapter discusses the implications of these processes on the intergenerational transmission of traditions, systems of meaning, and attitudes toward those with differing beliefs.

THE "WHY" OF KNOWLEDGE ACQUISITION AND TRANSMISSION

People seek knowledge, understanding, and certainty with regard to the world around them (e.g., Fiske, 2003; Kruglanski, 2004) and what motivates them to gather this information and resolve uncertainties is the wish to gain a sense of comprehension (e.g., Chaiken & Trope, 1999; Kruglanski, 1989; Petty et al., 1981). Their motivations typically stem from specific epistemic needs—these include the "thirst" for knowledge and cognitive coherence (see Festinger, 1957; Kruglanski et al., 2010; Neuberg & Newsom, 1993). While these motives are discussed across research traditions, they can be categorized into two main classes: the *need for specific closure* (i.e., to confirm specific knowledge) and the *need for nonspecific closure* (i.e., to form any sort of certain knowledge whatsoever) (Kruglanski & Thompson, 1999). Although it is generally true to say that people are motivated by specific or nonspecific closure, in certain instances, they may instead seek to actively avoid any closure, particularly specific closure, due to a perception that the process of attaining closure will turn out to be a stressor (Otto et al., 2016). This avoidance behavior can also manifest in situations where the absence of closure is perceived as advantageous, such as fostering independence, preserving a sense of mystery, or anticipating surprises (Snyder & Wicklund, 1981; Todor, 2014).

The Motivation to Defend Prior Knowledge

The need for specific closure is the desire for concrete knowledge on a subject, leading to definitive judgments or opinions (Dunning, 1999; Kunda, 1990). This phenomenon is not simply about forming beliefs but is also about defending them. Prior beliefs shape how people interpret new information, leading them to seek out and process information that conforms to their beliefs, with more of a focus on content that reinforces their previously held viewpoints (Kappes et al., 2020; Ling, 2020). This biased processing can lead to overconfidence in their beliefs and resistance to alternative perspectives (e.g., Ottati et al., 2015).

Conversely, people with a need for specific closure often avoid information that might challenge their beliefs, especially on highly significant issues such as abortion rights or gun control (e.g., Kunda, 1990; Lodge & Taber, 2013; Nickerson, 1998). This bias intensifies as ideological differences widen, making people reluctant to consider alternative stances (Wason, 1960). Once their opinions have hardened, individuals defend them and hunt down evidence supporting their beliefs (Lilienfeld et al., 2009; Nickerson, 1998), selectively exposing themselves to aligned media and steering clear of countervailing information (Hart et al., 2009; Knobloch-Westerwick, 2014; Smith et al., 2008). This bias also includes processing information in favorable ways, such as emphasizing supportive evidence or disregarding contradictory facts (Hart et al., 2009; Lilienfeld et al., 2009; Lodge & Taber, 2013).

The Motivation to Form Certain Knowledge

Let us now turn our attention to the need for nonspecific closure, which is the drive to acquire *any* valid knowledge whatsoever that provides some measure of certainty and sufficiency to enable one to describe a given phenomenon (Kruglanski, 1989). It involves the urge to grasp any opinion or belief that furnishes a sense of security, even if it is not necessarily accurate. This type of motivation leads people to streamline their information processing, focusing on familiar stereotypes and general knowledge (Webster & Kruglanski, 1994). It can also lead to a state of heightened alertness so as to identify threats, react impulsively, and make rapid decisions (Kossowska & Bar-Tal, 2013). People motivated by this need for nonspecific closure tend to latch on to the first morsels of information they encounter (the primacy effect) and then use these as anchors to influence their understanding of subsequent information (Kruglanski, 2004; Kruglanski & Webster, 1996). What is more, they often exhibit risk aversion, selective attention toward threatening stimuli, and impaired performance on tasks requiring working memory and decision-making skills (Kruglanski et al., 1993; Kruglanski & Webster, 1991, 1996; Otto et al., 2016). In completing tasks or making decisions, they may rely on stereotypes and heuristics, opting for a simplistic type of cognition that prioritizes speed over accuracy (Chirumbolo et al., 2014; Dijksterhuis et al., 1998; Kruglanski & Webster, 1991; Pierro et al., 2003; Shah et al., 1998; Wiersema et al., 2012). This preference for simplicity and familiarity can influence how people seek, interpret, and even shun new information, as they strive to maintain a sense of certainty in an uncertain world (see Kossowska et al., 2020; Kruglanski & Webster, 1991; Webster & Kruglanski, 1997).

Although the pursuit of certainty can give rise to biased, narrow, and closed-minded thinking, some studies have put forward a more nuanced picture (Kossowska et al., 2018; Roets et al., 2015). In particular situations, people seeking knowledge may actively seek and incorporate new information to improve their understanding and predictive abilities, fostering a more open-minded approach. This occurs, for instance, when the act of challenging preexisting beliefs actually serves their goals; in these cases, individuals motivated by the need for closure were shown to be more attuned to the instrumental aspect of cognitive strategies and the information received (Kossowska et al., 2018).

Another factor influencing a willingness to embrace more intricate cognitive strategies is people's perception of their own existing knowledge and prior experience. Individuals motivated by the need for closure tend to use simpler strategies when they perceive their knowledge to be fixed, unchangeable, and difficult to undermine (Kossowska, et al., 2018), leading to more stereotypical information processing. However, when their knowledge is somewhat in doubt, they are more likely to resort to complex and open-minded decision-making strategies (Jaśko et al., 2015; Kossowska & Bar-Tal, 2013; Kossowska et al., 2018), indicating that an encounter with uncertainty has the power to prompt deeper cognitive processing.

Individuals motivated by the need for closure tend to opt for elaborate cognitive strategies and a "more is better" heuristic, leading them to seek out more information and explore multiple options. Uncertainty can be triggered by conflicting information, challenging problem-solving tasks (Kossowska et al., 2015; Szumowska et al., 2017), or discrepancies in expertise between oneself and others (Jensen & Hurley, 2012). Hence, it is clear that when the usual mental framework of people motivated by the need for closure fails to provide direction on how to proceed, this predicament prompts individuals to explore more precise and complex cognitive strategies.

Interpersonal Phenomena

In the interpersonal realm, those with a high need for closure are more eager to encounter people more similar to themselves (Growiec & Szumowska, 2024). They are also more sensitive to normative cues and more compliant with social and cultural norms, rules, and expectations in contrast to those with a low need for closure (e.g., Jia et al., 2014).

More broadly, people greatly motivated to attain a sense of closure were also found to exhibit attribution biases characteristic of the culture (Chiu et al., 2000) and conform to cultural norms in respect to conflict judgements (Fu et al., 2007). What these intriguing findings highlight is that the need for closure affects crucial aspects of how people form ties and interact with others and with their culture, as well as influencing their relations within and between groups.

Groups as Certainty Providers

In the context of groups, it has been shown that the motivation to reduce uncertainty via the formulation of certain knowledge predisposes individuals to identify with a particular group and maintain a shared social reality within these groupings. Such a motivation also fosters a preference for decisions that reinforce the ingroup's identity over other groups (Kruglanski, Pierro, et al., 2006). These effects have been demonstrated in both minimal group settings, where individuals exhibited a bias toward their ingroup when faced with subjective uncertainty (Hogg & Grieve, 1999), and in real contexts, in which individuals grappling with uncertainty about themselves were more prone to affiliate with extremist groups (Hogg, 2021; Kruglanski et al., 2013).

When individuals seek shared understandings and a shared sense of reality to reduce uncertainty and foster cohesion, this is known as collective closure (Dugas & Kruglanski, 2018). The advantage of this shared reality is that it reassures individuals that their opinions are valid through the mechanism of social proof (Heiphetz, 2018; Higgins et al., 2021). Collective agreement on beliefs and norms also serves to help individuals navigate ambiguity and establish a sense of cast-iron certainty in a shape-shifting world. This shared consensus within the group then functions as a form of social validation, confirming each individual's beliefs, and offers a sense of predictability and stability, allowing individuals to bolster their confidence in their right understanding of the world (Hardin & Higgins, 1996; Higgins, 2019).

Notwithstanding these advantages, it transpires that not all groups provide certainty equally effectively. Individuals facing uncertainty gravitate toward groups they view as autonomous, united, and exceptionally competent (Brewer et al., 2004). Such groups offer the reassurance of decisive action, prompting individuals to find solace in collective thinking and comfort in collective endeavors. Indeed, studies have demonstrated that under conditions of uncertainty, some are inclined to join extremist groups (Hogg, 2021), since these groups offer a robust social identity and a solid sense of certainty, which in turn underpins individuals' sense of self-worth. While Hogg (2021) emphasized the cohesive nature of extremist groups, as well as their internal uniformity and common destiny, Kruglanski and colleagues (2022) put forward an additional reason for this tendency: Extremist groups typically exhibit unwavering dedication to their central goal. This intense focus provides individuals with an enhanced sense of personal value, which is a boon for those whose self-worth has previously been undermined by feelings of uncertainty.

Group identification can go further by mitigating the adverse effects of uncertainty on an individual's perceptions of others (Hogg & Mahajan, 2018). Moreover, by idealizing the group itself as a whole, individuals gain a sense of being shielded from uncertainty (Cichocka, 2016; Cichocka et al., 2016; Golec de Zavala et al., 2009). This phenomenon, termed *collective narcissism*, involves an inflated positive evaluation of one's group, and can lead to negative outcomes, including hostility, hypersensitivity to threats against the group's positive image, exaggerated reactions to criticism (Golec de Zavala et al., 2016), and selective historical memory (Kofta & Bilewicz, 2011). The latter magnifies the sense of how others wronged "our group" while downplaying the injustices perpetrated by their own group on others.

Research indicates that groups often organize themselves hierarchically across cultures and contexts (Berger et al., 1980; Chase et al., 2002; Gould, 2002; Magee & Galinsky, 2008; Sidanius & Pratto, 2003) and that this tendency strengthens during times of crisis and political instability (Doty et al., 1991; McCann, 1997, 1999; Peterson et al., 1993; Peterson & Gerstein, 2005;

Sales, 1972, 1973). In fact, people prefer not only hierarchical solutions but also strong leaders to restore order in times of chaos (Adorno, 1950; Feldman, 2003; Feldman & Stenner, 1997; McCann, 2008; Rickert, 1998; Stenner, 2005). Nevertheless, support for authoritarian systems and governance is contingent upon multiple conditions, namely, their perceived effectiveness, alignment with individual interests, and freedom from corruption (Kay et al., 2008).

To compound matters further, when groups are composed of people with a high need for closure, these individuals lean toward autocratic decision making and reject divergent opinions. Due to their preference toward ingroup consensus, pressure for uniformity, and reliance on commonly available information (Kruglanski et al., 2006b; Shah et al., 1998), this can lead to the stability of norms, despite changes in membership (Livi et al., 2015; Manchi Chao et al., 2010).

Shared perspectives foster a sense of belonging and facilitate communication between people, serving as a bonding mechanism (Greenaway et al., 2015). Moreover, it has been found that when people tailor their descriptions to align with their communication partner's attitudes, this also helps people share a sense of reality and underscore the delineation of ingroup and outgroup distinctions (Higgins et al., 2021). This predisposition toward ingroup solidarity is accentuated by the phenomenon of group centrism, wherein individuals rely on their group's norms and values to navigate social interactions and establish their own identity (Kruglanski et al., 2006b; Shah et al., 1998). Group centrism is usually characterized by a uniformity of opinions, autocratic leadership, ingroup partiality, and resistance to change (Kruglanski et al., 2006b). It may result in the glorification of the ingroup, support for extreme measures against perceived enemies (Dugas & Kruglanski, 2018), and more stereotypical perceptions of social groups, along with increased ingroup favoritism and outgroup derogation (Shah et al., 1998).

In summary, group membership contributes in manifold ways to individuals' feelings of certainty and security within a group context by providing shared beliefs, social validation, consensus building, group identity, authority figures, and social support networks.

The Quest for Certainty in Collective Narratives

People manage uncertainty through narrative creation and storytelling (Szumowska et al., 2020) and although collective narratives may not align with consensual reality, they fulfil a yearning for security, meaning, and significance. Still, it turns out some narratives assuage uncertainty better than others (Hogg & Adelman, 2013; Hogg et al., 2013; Proulx & Inzlicht, 2012; Saroglou, 2002; Szumowska et al., 2020); for example, conservative and religious ideologies often provide more comfort than liberal or atheist perspectives provide (Szumowska et al., 2020). Religious narratives also serve existential, epistemic, and identity-related functions (Szumowska et al., 2020) by providing an untestable system of knowledge. What is more, they offer moral guidance, helping individuals understand life's purpose and navigate its challenges (Barnes, 1978). Conservative values promote social identity and a sense of a shared reality (Jost et al., 2007, 2018), while right-wing ideologies, with their resistance to change and acceptance of hierarchy, offer simple solutions as a bulwark against uncertainty (Jost et al., 2018).

When levels of uncertainty become even more greatly heightened, individuals are often galvanized to seek out "the truth" by whatever means necessary. This impetus might go some way toward explaining the growing prevalence of conspiracy theories and conspiratorial thinking (Douglas et al., 2015; van Prooijen, 2016, 2019). Subscribing to conspiracy-driven "explanations" delivers more straightforward, seemingly quite reasonable, interpretations of complex topics (Douglas et al., 2015; Marchlewska et al., 2018), bringing order, predictability, and meaning to life's vagaries, while providing a sense of certainty, control, and connection with others. Indeed, research suggests a correlation between a need for closure and a tendency to embrace conspiracy-led explanations (Marchlewska et al., 2018; Staszak et al., 2022), findings that may account for the escalating popularity of conspiratorial theorizing around the COVID-19 pandemic and changes in global climate, to take two recent examples.

THE "HOW" OF KNOWLEDGE FORMATION

The quest for certainty drives people's search for knowledge, but how is this knowledge formed? To answer this question, lay epistemics theory (Kruglanski, 1989; Kruglanski et al., 2009) and the unimodel of social judgment (Kruglanski et al., 2006a, 2007) have drawn parallels between knowledge acquisition and the systematic approach implemented on the path to scientific discovery (see also Popper, 1959). Unlike qualified scientists, who possess specialized knowledge in gathering objective data, individuals often rely on their subjective and occasionally naive understanding of how to optimally gather and interpret information. Nonetheless, research indicates that this process is not entirely haphazard; it follows logical rules akin to "if–then" reasoning, leading from premises to conclusions (Erb et al., 2003; Kruglanski, 1989; Kruglanski & Thompson, 1999). The outcome of this sort of reasoning process is some kind of knowledge—an opinion, conviction, or judgment—regardless of the quality of the information acquired. More specifically, knowledge formation can be understood as a syllogism comprising a major and minor premise: The major premise connects evidence to a conclusion ("If *E*, then *C*"); the minor premise relates to this conclusion via people's observations or salient information. For instance, if someone believes people holding doctoral degrees are intelligent (major premise) and then learns that person X has a doctorate (minor premise), they may conclude that person X is smart. However, a single piece of information may not suffice by itself to change a belief: If someone does not subscribe to the notion that individuals with doctoral degrees are intelligent, information about an academic title may not affect their judgment.

It is clear that when forming knowledge, individuals learn the relationship between evidence and conclusions through experience in various contexts (Kruglanski & Gigerenzer, 2011), influenced by the frequency with which they encounter the association. Within a given context, rule acquisition also depends on sources of epistemic authority (see the later section in this chapter on the "who" of knowledge formation), stemming from figures such as parents or teachers in childhood. Hence, we know that infants may learn to avoid touching a hot pan without having to experience the associated pain firsthand, and this mode of learning extends into adulthood as individuals continue to acquire beliefs. For example, during the acculturation process, individuals assimilate stereotypes about different social groups, which may vary across cultures. According to lay epistemics theory, using evidence to infer rules is a method of knowledge acquisition that frequently occurs unconsciously (Kruglanski et al., 2009). Thereafter, well-established rules are applied automatically, without the requirement for conscious cognitive control (Logan, 1992).

When Evidence Leads to Judgment

Judgment formation depends on parameters such as (1) subjective relevance, (2) the difficulty of the judgment task itself, and (3) the availability of cognitive resources (Kruglanski et al., 2009). The first parameter, subjective relevance, is the strength of an individual's belief in the association between the evidence and a given rule (Kruglanski et al., 2009) and is more on a continuum than strictly dichotomous. For instance, when forming an opinion on global climate change, an individual may receive reports from different sources. On hearing climate researchers asserting its reality, their clear expertise grants their perspective a degree of relevance. Later, this same person may come across a video of a personal trainer disputing global warming, citing recent snowfall as evidence. The individual's perception of each source's relevance is influenced by personal beliefs: Those who trust scientists may value their expert viewpoint more, while those skeptical of global warming might prefer the personal trainer's perspective.

The second parameter affecting judgment formation is the difficulty of the judgment task, which itself is shaped by three factors (Kruglanski et al., 2009). First, connecting evidence with rules is feasible when a rule is accessible in memory, which depends on the history of its use (Higgins, 1996). Second, individuals must recognize a matchup between the evidence and the rule (Kruglanski et al., 2009), making the saliency of information crucial to overcome any background noise. Third, the manner in which the information is presented affects the difficulty of judgment. For example, the amount of information can vary in length and complexity, and this can have an impact. Pierro and colleagues (2012) showed that lengthy information only influenced highly motivated participants when the source was presented as an expert. In contrast, succinct information was persuasive for participants with low involvement, but again, only when the source was presented as an expert. In addition, the sequencing of the information influences the difficulty of judgment. Presenting relevant information earlier made it more persuasive for all participants. When the order was reversed, only highly motivated participants utilized the later, relevant information (Pierro et al., 2004). Lastly, difficulty of judgment also depends on processing ease, which hinges on how consistent the newly presented information is with a person's beliefs. Aligned information is easier to process than incongruent information, as demonstrated in a study by Plaks and colleagues (2001) where participants paid more attention to information that matched their mindsets than to information that opposed their beliefs.

The third parameter for judgment formation is cognitive resource availability. Information processing depends on the amount of cognitive resources available (Kruglanski et al., 2009). Limited resources make people rely on easier-to-process information or peripheral cues, such as relying on information about the source of the message rather than the message content itself. This might be mainly attributable to the information concerning the source being briefer and easier to handle than the message itself. However, processing lengthy information demands more resources, so only motivated individuals make use of it in forming their judgments (Kruglanski & Thompson, 1999). Even if processing lengthy information requires cognitive resources, it does not imply that being in possession of these resources leads to better judgments. Both easy rules and complex rules can be equally accurate, depending on the situation (Kruglanski & Gigerenzer, 2011). What is critical when making judgments is selecting a rule that is fit for the purpose vis-à-vis a given context.

In summary, knowledge is constructed from evidence and is represented in the syllogistic form of "if 'evidence,' then 'conclusion'." People acquire judgmental rules from their experience, those around them, and their cultural milieu. As for knowledge formation, three parameters must be taken into account: subjective relevance, the difficulty of the task, and the cognitive resources available.

THE "WHO" OF KNOWLEDGE TRANSMISSION

Knowledge acquisition is influenced by the opinions of people one respects, known as epistemic authority, referring to a trusted source from whom individuals seek knowledge across various topics (Kruglanski, 1989). Researchers have striven to define the criteria that make a source of information reliable, only to discover that objective characteristics matter less than the attribution of substantive reliability (Kruglanski et al., 2005). Epistemic authority can be ascribed to individuals, groups, or even entities like TV shows or online discussion forums that line up with one's own perspectives (Echterhoff et al., 2017; Kruglanski et al., 2005). Individuals can also bestow epistemic authority upon themselves by trusting in their own knowledge and capabilities (Ellis & Kruglanski, 1992). However, there are several downsides to this level of self-belief: It can limit a person's willingness to test hypotheses, hindering the acquisition of new knowledge, and it may also lead them to reject information that is not in accordance with what they know, especially when the information pertains to the self (Szumowska et al., 2022).

Perceiving epistemic authority is a social process partially influenced by the perceived gap between one's own and other people's epistemic authority. Raviv and colleagues (1993) discovered that people may adjust their self-ascribed epistemic authority when comparing themselves to various groups. When they perceive their reference group as more competent, they may underestimate their own epistemic authority, and vice versa. The larger the perceived authority gap, the more important the source is perceived to be (Kruglanski et al., 2009).

Self-ascribed epistemic authority also involves the use of prior knowledge to evaluate a source's reliability (Hämäläinen et al., 2021). Nonetheless, it is insufficient for an individual to merely recognize their lack of knowledge; it is also essential for them to be adequately informed and sufficiently experienced to be able to ascertain which epistemic authority to best refer to. This evaluative task is becoming increasingly challenging in light of the overabundance of online sources of knowledge, disinformation, and fake news.

Research indicates that individuals who perceive themselves as an epistemic authority tend to lean heavily on their own expertise (Kruglanski et al., 2010), avoiding external knowledge sources (Kruglanski et al., 2005). Furthermore, when assessing the need for closure, it has been shown that, when coupled with high self-ascribed epistemic authority, the higher the need for closure, the lower the tendency there was to engage in any external seeking of information. Instead, individuals exhibited a greater reliance on themselves as the primary sources of epistemic authority.

Epistemic authority has risen to prominence as skepticism toward traditional sources of information escalates (Pittinsky, 2015). Despite the ongoing trust in scientists by most people (see Cologna et al., 2025), there is a growing distrust in science as a reliable source of knowledge (Rutjens et al., 2018). This skepticism persists even in the face of extensive scientific consensus on issues like global climate change and vaccination efficacy, which many people remain unconvinced about, revealing a notable disparity between scientific evidence and public opinion (Antonio & Brulle, 2011; Scruggs & Benegal, 2012). Access to the web has engendered a democratization of knowledge acquisition, granting virtually anyone the ability to acquire specialized knowledge across various fields. By enabling individuals to acquire new competencies, individuals thereby assume the role of strategic arbiters of expertise and knowledge. As a result, their own self-ascribed epistemic authority may be considerably enhanced.

However, the reliability of information sources varies significantly, presenting a formidable challenge in discerning credible sources from unreliable ones. The complexity of specialist knowledge further complicates the comprehension of scientific explanations, posing a serious barrier to clear understanding. This difficulty in grasping scientific concepts to their full extent may fuel, in part, the upswelling in popularity of conspiracy theories. For instance, conspiracy theories have exerted tangible repercussions on our reality, especially evident in contexts such as the COVID-19 pandemic and global climate change (Staszak et al., 2022; Ylä-Anttila, 2018). The prevalence of conspiracy theories is often linked to "populist knowledge," which surfaces in anti-elitist discourses, and rejects established epistemic authorities, including scientific expertise and the mainstream media. Instead, it is more likely to rely on emotions and sentiments (Ylä-Anttila, 2018).

Paradoxically, the internet's ubiquity entails heightened uncertainty by exposing individuals to vast unknowns on the one hand, while offering a trove of knowledge on the other. Individuals enjoy unprecedented access to highly specialized and detailed information sources across all domains currently known to humankind. Navigating this minefield of information requires preexisting knowledge on how to verify information, interpret it, and identify trustworthy sources. The accessibility of online knowledge amplifies the perception of information overload, compelling individuals to actively verify what they encounter. This awareness of one's knowledge gaps represents a contemporary phenomenon that is quite distinct from the preceding decades. In earlier times, the pressure of not knowing was far less pronounced, and individuals did not experience such a pervasive sense of urgency across diverse spheres of life. Thus, the paradox is that the internet plays a dual role as both a source of uncertainty and a means to alleviate it, impacting how individuals interact with and seek knowledge in today's information-rich environments. Moreover, these vast databases of information draw individuals into dedicating hours researching specific topics independently, accelerated and warped by social media algorithms that recommend content based on past interactions, and connected with previously seen materials, thereby creating informational bubbles (Vancompernolle Vromman & Fouss, 2021) and potentially amplifying conspiracy thinking even further (Douglas & Sutton, 2018). Conspiracy theories, populist knowledge, and distorted perspectives from self-ascribed epistemic authorities contribute to a further erosion of trust in the media and specialists. Socially and politically, there exists an unprecedented challenge to established epistemic authorities, accompanied by a surge in distrust in experts. This trend is exacerbated by the adulteration caused by fake news, propaganda, and disinformation, creating an informational environment where distinguishing between genuine facts and falsehoods becomes increasingly arduous.

INTERGENERATIONAL KNOWLEDGE TRANSMISSION

Knowledge formation serves as a cornerstone in both the preservation and the transmission of cultural traditions across successive generations. As individuals learn about their cultural heritage, including customs, rituals, and values, they maintain these traditions within their familial and communal contexts. Through socialization processes like storytelling, education, and cultural practices, younger generations internalize and uphold the beliefs and practices of their elders. Consequently, knowledge formation emerges as a vital conduit for ensuring the intergenerational continuity of cultural identity and heritage.

Beyond its role in cultural transmission, knowledge formation profoundly shapes individuals' understanding of the world and their interpretation of events. As people acquaint themselves with societal norms, cultural values, and historical narratives, they construct systems of meaning that furnish frameworks for comprehending their surroundings and guiding their conduct. The transmission of these systems of meaning occurs across generations through familial bonds, educational institutions, media outlets, and religious establishments. The formation of shared meanings fosters social cohesion and collective identity within communities, thereby influencing individuals' perceptions, attitudes, and behaviors.

Regrettably, such knowledge formation processes can also give rise to challenges such as ethnocentrism, prejudice, and discriminatory attitudes toward those with differing beliefs or cultural backgrounds. When knowledge acquisition concerning one's cultural identity lacks nuance, it may foster a sense of cultural superiority and jaundiced beliefs, perpetuating negative stereotypes and discriminatory behaviors. The intergenerational transmission of biased beliefs can deepen and exacerbate social divisions and marginalize minority groups within society. Recognizing the impact of knowledge formation on these phenomena is critical for promoting cultural diversity, nurturing intercultural understanding, and combating prejudice and discrimination.

CONCLUSIONS

In this chapter, we have delved into lay epistemic cognition and its intersection with the existential, generational, and informational dimensions of modern life. We encountered the imperative for cognitive closure, underscoring the drive to mitigate uncertainty, and the pursuit of knowledge. Exploring invaluable frameworks (such as Kruglanski's unimodel of social judgment), we shed light on how knowledge is formed and synthesized from evidence. Additionally, we directed our attention toward epistemic authority, accentuating the meta-cognitive aspects of knowledge acquisition and the strategies employed for identifying trustworthy sources.

By presenting a comprehensive, coherent, and interlocking array of findings, explanations, and theories, we hope to enrich the comprehension of knowledge acquisition at an individual and a collective level. These insights enable us to grasp the epistemic behaviors exhibited by both laypeople and specialists on a broad scale. Leveraging theories such as Kruglanski's (1989; Kruglanski et al., 2007, 2009) lay epistemics theory and the unimodel of social judgment (Kruglanski et al., 2006a), both of which are particularly well suited to the contemporary context, we can make strides in outlining the process of knowledge acquisition. This progression begins with its motivational foundations, proceeds to strategies for acquiring knowledge, and culminates in examining the roles of various sources of knowledge and experience, including our own cognitive functioning as epistemic tools in recognizing reliable sources.

In our current epistemic environment, where individuals are confronted by a cornucopia of sources and myriad domains of expertise, amid an informational landscape bustling with AI chatbots and self-proclaimed epistemic authorities, theoretical frameworks such as these stand out as invaluable paradigms, supporting individuals and societies in more adeptly navigating the tumult, complexities, and uncertainties inherent in our present existence.

ACKNOWLEDGMENT

Preparation of this chapter has been supported by a grant from the Priority Research Area (Future Society: Behavior in Crisis Lab—Flagship Project) under the Strategic Programme Excellence Initiative at Jagiellonian University.

REFERENCES

Adorno, T. W. (1950). *The authoritarian personality.* Harper & Brothers.

Antonio, R. J., & Brulle, R. J. (2011). The unbearable lightness of politics: Climate change denial and political polarization. *Sociological Quarterly, 52*(2), 195–202.

Barnes, D. (1978). Charisma and religious leadership: An historical analysis. *Journal for the Scientific Study of Religion, 17*(1), 118.

Berger, J., Rosenholtz, S. J., & Zelditch, M., Jr. (1980). Status organizing processes. *Annual Review of Sociology, 6*(1), 479–508.

Brewer, M. B., Hong, Y. Y., & Li, Q. (2004). Dynamic entitavity. In V. Yzerbyt, C. M. Judd, & O. Corneille (Eds.), *The psychology of group perception: Perceived variability, entitativity, and essentialism* (pp. 19–29). Psychology Press.

Chaiken, S., & Trope, Y. (Eds.). (1999). *Dual-process theories in social psychology.* Guilford Press.

Chase, I. D., Tovey, C., Spangler-Martin, D., & Manfredonia, M. (2002). Individual differences versus social dynamics in the formation of animal dominance hierarchies. *Proceedings of the National Academy of Sciences, 99*(8), 5744–5749.

Chirumbolo, A., Brizi, A., Mastandrea, S., & Mannetti, L. (2014). "Beauty is no quality in things themselves": Epistemic motivation affects implicit preferences for art. *PLOS ONE, 9*(10), e110323.

Chiu, C., Morris, M. W., Hong, Y., & Menon, T. (2000). Motivated cultural cognition: The impact of implicit cultural theories on dispositional attribution varies as a function of need for closure. *Journal of Personality and Social Psychology, 78,* 247–259.

Chowdhury, S., Gibb, F., & Landoni, M. (2011). Uncertainty in information seeking and retrieval: A study in an academic environment. *Information Processing and Management, 47*(2), 157–175.

Cichocka, A. (2016). Understanding defensive and secure in-group positivity: The role of collective narcissism. *European Review of Social Psychology, 27*(1), 283–317.

Cichocka, A., Marchlewska, M., & De Zavala, A. G. (2016). Does self-love or self-hate predict conspiracy beliefs? Narcissism, self-esteem, and the endorsement of conspiracy theories. *Social Psychological and Personality Science, 7*(2), 157–166.

Cologna, V., Mede, N. G., Berge, S., Besley, J., Brick, C., Joubert, M., . . . Miller, J. (2025). Trust in scientists and their role in society across 67 countries. *Nature Human Behavior, 9,* 713–730.

Dijksterhuis, A., Spears, R., Postmes, T., Stapel, D., Koomen, W., Knippenberg, A. V., & Scheepers, D. (1998). Seeing one thing and doing another: Contrast effects in automatic behavior. *Journal of Personality and Social Psychology, 75*(4), 862–871.

Doty, R. M., Peterson, B. E., & Winter, D. G. (1991). Threat and authoritarianism in the United States, 1978–1987. *Journal of Personality and Social Psychology, 61*(4), 629.

Douglas, K. M., & Sutton, R. M. (2018). Why conspiracy theories matter: A social psychological analysis. *European Review of Social Psychology, 29*(1), 256–298.

Douglas, K. M., Sutton, R. M., Jolley, D., & Wood, M. J. (2015). The social, political, environmental, and health-related consequences of conspiracy theories: Problems and potential solutions. In M. Bilewicz, A. Cichocka, & W. Soral (Eds.), *The psychology of conspiracy* (pp. 183–200). Routledge/Taylor & Francis Group.

Dugas, M., & Kruglanski, A. W. (2018). Shared reality as collective closure. *Current Opinion in Psychology, 23,* 72–76.

Dunning, D. (1999). A newer look: Motivated social cognition and the schematic representation of social concepts. *Psychological Inquiry, 10*(1), 1–11.

Echterhoff, G., Kopietz, R., & Higgins, E. T. (2017). Shared reality in intergroup communication: Increasing the epistemic authority of an out-group audience. *Journal of Experimental Psychology: General, 146*(6), 806–825.

Ellis, S., & Kruglanski, A. W. (1992). Self as an epistemic authority: Effects on experiential and instructional learning. *Social Cognition, 10*(4), 357–375.

Erb, H. P., Kruglanski, A., Chun, W. Y., Pierro, A., Mannetti, L., & Spiegel, S. (2003). Searching for commonalities in human judgement: The parametric unimodel and its dual mode alternatives. In W. Stroebe & M. Hewstone (Eds.), *European review of social psychology* (Vol. 14, pp. 1–47). Psychology Press/Taylor & Francis.

Feldman, S. (2003). Enforcing social conformity: A theory of authoritarianism. *Political Psychology, 24*(1), 41–74.

Feldman, S., & Stenner, K. (1997). Perceived threat and authoritarianism. *Political Psychology, 18*(4), 741–770.

Festinger, L. (1957). *A theory of cognitive dissonance.* Stanford University Press.

Fiske, S. T. (2003, January). Five core social motives, plus or minus five. In M. P. Zanna & J. M. Olson (Eds.), *Motivated social perception: The Ontario Symposium* (Vol. 9, p. 233–246). Psychology Press.

Fu, J. H., Morris, M. W., Lee, S., Chao, M., Chiu, C., & Hong, Y. (2007). Epistemic motives and cultural conformity: Need for closure, culture, and context as determinants of conflict judgments. *Journal of Personality and Social Psychology, 92,* 191–207.

Golec de Zavala, A., Peker, M., Guerra, R., & Baran, T. (2016). Collective narcissism predicts hypersensitivity to in-group insult and direct and indirect retaliatory intergroup hostility. *European Journal of Personality, 30*(6), 532–551.

Golec de Zavala, A. G., Cichocka, A., Eidelson, R., & Jayawickreme, N. (2009). Collective narcissism and its social consequences. *Journal of Personality and Social Psychology, 97*(6), 1074–1096.

Gould, R. V. (2002). The origins of status hierarchies: A formal theory and empirical test. *American Journal of Sociology, 107*(5), 1143–1178.

Greenaway, K. H., Wright, R. G., Willingham, J., Reynolds, K. J., & Haslam, S. A. (2015). Shared identity is key to effective communication. *Personality and Social Psychology Bulletin, 41*(2), 171–182.

Growiec, K., & Szumowska, E. (2024). *Building bridges and bonds in the context of cognitive motivation: The relation between Heterophilous and Homophilous interactions and need for cognitive closure.* Manuscript submitted for publication.

Hämäläinen, E. K., Kiili, C., Räikkönen, E., & Marttunen, M. (2021). Students' abilities to evaluate the credibility of online texts: The role of internet-specific epistemic justifications. *Journal of Computer Assisted Learning, 37*(5), 1409–1422.

Hardin, C. D., & Higgins, E. T. (1996). Shared reality: How social verification makes the subjective objective. In R. M. Sorrentino & E. T. Higgins (Eds.), *Handbook of motivation and cognition: Vol. 3. The interpersonal context* (pp. 28–84). Guilford Press.

Hart, W., Albarracín, D., Eagly, A. H., Brechan, I., Lindberg, M. J., & Merrill, L. (2009). Feeling validated versus being correct: A meta-analysis of selective exposure to information. *Psychological Bulletin, 135*(4), 555–588.

Heiphetz, L. (2018). The development and importance of shared reality in the domains of opinion, morality, and religion. *Current Opinion in Psychology, 23,* 1–5.

Higgins, E. T. (1996). Knowledge activation: Accessibility, applicability and salience. In E. T. Higgins & A. W. Kruglanski (Eds.), *Social psychology: Handbook of basic principles* (pp. 133–168). Guilford Press.

Higgins, E. T. (2019). *Shared reality: What makes us strong and tears us apart.* Oxford University Press.

Higgins, E. T., Rossignac-Milon, M., & Echterhoff, G. (2021). Shared reality: From sharing-is-believing to merging minds. *Current Directions in Psychological Science, 30*(2), 103–110.

Hogg, M. A. (2021). Self-uncertainty and group identification: Consequences for social identity, group behavior, intergroup relations, and society. In B. Gawronski (Ed.), *Advances in experimental social psychology* (Vol. 64, pp. 263–316). Elsevier Academic Press.

Hogg, M. A., & Adelman, J. (2013). Uncertainty-identity theory: Extreme groups, radical behavior, and authoritarian leadership. *Journal of Social Issues, 69,* 436–454.

Hogg, M. A., & Grieve, P. (1999). Social identity theory and the crisis of confidence in social psychology: A commentary, and some research on uncertainty reduction. *Asian Journal of Social Psychology, 2*(1), 79–93.

Hogg, M. A., Kruglanski, A. W., & Van den Bos, K. (2013). Uncertainty and the roots of extremism. *Journal of Social Issues, 69*, 407–418.

Hogg, M. A., & Mahajan, N. (2018). Domains of self-uncertainty and their relationship to group identification. *Journal of Theoretical Social Psychology, 2*(3), 67–75.

Jaśko, K., Czernatowicz-Kukuczka, A., Kossowska, M., & Czarna, A. Z. (2015). Individual differences in response to uncertainty and decision making: The role of behavioral inhibition system and need for closure. *Motivation and Emotion, 39*(4), 541–552.

Jensen, J. D., & Hurley, R. J. (2012). Conflicting stories about public scientific controversies: Effects of news convergence and divergence on scientists' credibility. *Public Understanding of Science, 21*(6), 689–704.

Jia, L., Hirt, E. R., & Evans, D. N. (2014). Putting the freeze on priming: The role of need for cognitive closure on the prime-norm dynamic. *Personality and Social Psychology Bulletin, 40*(7), 931–942.

Jost, J. T., Napier, J. L., Thorisdottir, H., Gosling, S. D., Palfai, T. P., & Ostafin, B. (2007). Are needs to manage uncertainty and threat associated with political conservatism or ideological extremity? *Personality and Social Psychology Bulletin, 33*(7), 989–1007.

Jost, J. T., van der Linden, S., Panagopoulos, C., & Hardin, C. D. (2018). Ideological asymmetries in conformity, desire for shared reality, and the spread of misinformation. *Current Opinion in Psychology, 23*, 77–83.

Kappes, A., Harvey, A. H., Lohrenz, T., Montague, P. R., & Sharot, T. (2020). Confirmation bias in the utilization of others' opinion strength. *Nature Neuroscience, 23*(1), 130–137.

Kay, A. C., Gaucher, D., Napier, J. L., Callan, M. J., & Laurin, K. (2008). God and the government: Testing a compensatory control mechanism for the support of external systems. *Journal of Personality and Social Psychology, 95*(1), 18–35.

Knobloch-Westerwick, S. (2014). *Choice and preference in media use: Advances in selective exposure theory and research*. Routledge.

Kofta, M., & Bilewicz, M. (2011). The demons of anti-Semitism. *ACADEMIA: The Magazine of the Polish Academy of Sciences*, pp. 28–31.

Kossowska, M., & Bar-Tal, Y. (2013). Need for closure and heuristic information processing: The moderating role of the ability to achieve the need for closure. *British Journal of Psychology, 104*(4), 457–480.

Kossowska, M., Dragon, P., & Bukowski, M. (2015). When need for closure leads to positive attitudes towards a negatively stereotyped outgroup. *Motivation and Emotion, 1*, 88–98.

Kossowska, M., Szumowska, E., Dragon, P., Jaśko, K., & Kruglanski, A. W. (2018). Disparate roads to certainty processing strategy choices under need for closure. *European Review of Social Psychology, 29*(1), 161–211.

Kossowska, M., Szumowska, E., & Szwed, P. (2020). *Tolerance in uncertain times*. Routledge.

Kruglanski, A. (2023). *Uncertain: How to turn your biggest fear into your greatest power*. Michael Joseph.

Kruglanski, A. W. (1989). The psychology of being "right": The problem of accuracy in social perception and cognition. *Psychological Bulletin, 106*(3), 395–409.

Kruglanski, A. W. (2004). *The psychology of closed mindedness*. Psychology Press.

Kruglanski, A. W., Atash, M. N., De Grada, E., Mannetti, L., & Pierro, A. (2013). Need for Closure Scale (NFC). Measurement instrument database for the social science. *Journal of Personality and Social Psychology, 73*, 1005–1016.

Kruglanski, A. W., Chen, X., Pierro, A., Mannetti, L., Erb, H. P., & Spiegel, S. (2006a). Persuasion according to the unimodel: Implications for cancer communication. *Journal of Communication, 56*, 105–122.

Kruglanski, A. W., Dechesne, M., Orehek, E., & Pierro, A. (2009). Three decades of lay epistemics: The why, how, and who of knowledge formation. *European Review of Social Psychology, 20*(1), 146–191.

Kruglanski, A. W., & Gigerenzer, G. (2011). Intuitive and deliberative judgements are based on common principles. *Psychological Review, 118*, 97–109.

Kruglanski, A. W., Kopetz, C., & Szumowska, E. (Eds.). (2022). *The psychology of extremism: A motivational perspective*. Routledge/Taylor & Francis Group.

Kruglanski, A. W., Orehek, E., Dechesne, M., & Pierro, A. (2010). Lay epistemic theory: The motivational, cognitive, and social aspects of knowledge formation. *Social and Personality Psychology Compass, 4*(10), 939–950.

Kruglanski, A. W., Pierro, A., Mannetti, L., & De Grada, E. (2006b). Groups as epistemic providers: need for closure and the unfolding of group-centrism. *Psychological Review, 113*(1), 84–100.

Kruglanski, A. W., Pierro, A., Mannetti, L., Erb, H. P., & Chun, W. Y. (2007). On the parameters of human judgment. *Advances in Experimental Social Psychology, 39*, 255–303.

Kruglanski, A. W., Raviv, A., Bar-Tal, D., Raviv, A., Sharvit, K., Ellis, S., & Mannetti, L.

(2005). Says who?: Epistemic authority effects in social judgment. *Advances in Experimental Social Psychology, 37*(37), 345–392.

Kruglanski, A. W., & Thompson, E. P. (1999). Persuasion by a single route: A view from the unimodel. *Psychological Inquiry, 10*(2), 83–109.

Kruglanski, A. W., & Webster, D. M. (1991). Group members' reactions to opinion deviates and conformists at varying degrees of proximity to decision deadline and of environmental noise. *Journal of Personality and Social Psychology, 61*(2), 212–225.

Kruglanski, A. W., & Webster, D. M. (1996). Motivated closing of the mind: "Seizing" and "freezing." *Psychological Review, 103,* 263–283.

Kruglanski, A. W., Webster, D. M., & Klem, A. (1993). Motivated resistance and openness to persuasion in the presence or absence of prior information. *Journal of Personality and Social Psychology, 65*(5), 861–876.

Kunda, Z. (1990). The case for motivated reasoning. *Psychological Bulletin, 108*(3), 480–498.

Lauriola, M., Litman, J. A., Mussel, P., De Santis, R., Crowson, H. M., & Hoffman, R. R. (2015). Epistemic curiosity and self-regulation. *Personality and Individual Differences, 83,* 202–207.

Lilienfeld, S. O., Ammirati, R., & Landfield, K. (2009). Giving debiasing away: Can psychological research on correcting cognitive errors promote human welfare? *Perspectives on Psychological Science, 4*(4), 390–398.

Ling, R. (2020). Confirmation bias in the era of mobile news consumption: the social and psychological dimensions. *Digital Journalism, 8*(5), 596–604.

Livi, S., Kruglanski, A. W., Pierro, A., Mannetti, L., & Kenny, D. A. (2015). Epistemic motivation and perpetuation of group culture: Effects of need for cognitive closure on trans-generational norm transmission. *Organizational Behavior and Human Decision Processes, 129,* 105–112.

Lodge, M., & Taber, C. S. (2013). *The rationalizing voter.* Cambridge University Press.

Logan, G. D. (1992). Attention and preattention in theories of automaticity. *American Journal of Psychology, 105,* 317–339.

Magee, J. C., & Galinsky, A. D. (2008, November). *The self-reinforcing nature of social hierarchy: Origins and consequences of power and status.* Paper presented at the 21st annual conference of the IACM.

Manchi Chao, M., Zhang, Z. X., & Chiu, C. Y. (2010). Adherence to perceived norms across cultural boundaries: The role of need for cognitive closure and ingroup identification. *Group Processes and Intergroup Relations, 13*(1), 69–89.

Marchlewska, M., Cichocka, A., & Kossowska, M. (2018). Addicted to answers: Need for cognitive closure and the endorsement of conspiracy beliefs. *European Journal of Social Psychology, 48*(2), 109–117.

McCann, E. J. (1999). Race, protest, and public space: Contextualizing Lefebvre in the US city. *Antipode, 31*(2), 163–184.

McCann, S. J. (1997). Threatening times, "strong" presidential popular vote winners, and the victory margin, 1824–1964. *Journal of Personality and Social Psychology, 73*(1), 160–170.

McCann, S. J. H. (2008). Societal threat, authoritarianism, conservatism, and U.S. state death penalty sentencing (1977–2004). *Journal of Personality and Social Psychology, 94*(5), 913–923.

Neuberg, S. L., & Newsom, J. T. (1993). Personal need for structure: Individual differences in the desire for simpler structure. *Journal of Personality and Social Psychology, 65*(1), 113–131.

Nickerson, R. S. (1998). Confirmation bias: A ubiquitous phenomenon in many guises. *Review of General Psychology, 2*(2), 175–220.

Ottati, V., Price, E. D., Wilson, C., & Sumaktoyo, N. (2015). When self-perceptions of expertise increase closed-minded cognition: The earned dogmatism effect. *Journal of Experimental Social Psychology, 61,* 131–138.

Otto, A. S., Clarkson, J. J., & Kardes, F. R. (2016). Decision sidestepping: How the motivation for closure prompts individuals to bypass decision making. *Journal of Personality and Social Psychology, 111*(1), 1–16.

Peterson, B. E., Doty, R. M., & Winter, D. G. (1993). Authoritarianism and attitudes toward contemporary social issues. *Personality and Social Psychology Bulletin, 19*(2), 174–184.

Peterson, B. E., & Gerstein, E. D. (2005). Fighting and flying: Archival analysis of threat, authoritarianism, and the North American comic book. *Political Psychology, 26*(6), 887–904.

Petty, R. E., Cacioppo, J. T., & Goldman, R. (1981). Personal involvement as a determinant of argument-based persuasion. *Journal of Personality and Social Psychology, 41*(5), 847–855.

Pierro, A., Mannetti, L., De Grada, E., Livi, S., & Kruglanski, A. W. (2003). Autocracy bias in informal groups under need for closure. *Personality and Social Psychology Bulletin, 29*(3), 405–417.

Pierro, A., Mannetti, L., Erb, H. P., Spiegel, S., & Kruglanski, A. W. (2004). Informational length and order of presentation as determinants of persuasion. *Journal of Experimental Social Psychology, 41*(5), 458–469.

Pierro, A., Mannetti, L., Kruglanski, A. W., Klein, K., & Orehek, E. (2012). Persistence of attitude change and attitude–behavior correspondence based on extensive processing of source information. *European Journal of Social Psychology, 42*(1), 103–111.

Pittinsky, T. L. (2015). America's crisis of faith in science. *Science, 348*, 511–512.

Plaks, J. E., Stroessner, S. J., Dweck, C. S., & Sherman, J. W. (2001). Person theories and attention allocation: preferences for stereotypic versus counterstereotypic information. *Journal of Personality and Social Psychology, 80*(6), 876–893.

Popper, K. R. (1959). *The logic of scientific discovery*. Basic Books.

Proulx, T., & Inzlicht, M. (2012). The five "A"s of meaning maintenance: Finding meaning in the theories of sense-making. *Psychological Inquiry, 23*, 317–335.

Raviv, A., Bar-Tal, D., Raviv, A., & Abin, R. (1993). Measuring epistemic authority: Studies of politicians and professors. *European Journal of Personality, 7*(2), 119–138.

Rickert, E. J. (1998). Authoritarianism and economic threat: Implications for political behavior. *Political Psychology, 19*(4), 707–720.

Roets, A., Kruglanski, A. W., Kossowska, M., Pierro, A., & Hong, Y. Y. (2015). The motivated gatekeeper of our minds: New directions in need for closure theory and research. *Advances in Experimental Social Psychology, 52*, 221–283.

Rutjens, B. T., Sutton, R. M., & van der Lee, R. (2018). Not all skepticism is equal: Exploring the ideological antecedents of science acceptance and rejection. *Personality and Social Psychology Bulletin, 44*(3), 384–405.

Sales, S. M. (1972). Economic threat as a factor in authoritarianism: The case of the Great Depression. *Proceedings of the Annual Convention of the American Psychological Association, 7*(Pt. 1), 249–250.

Sales, S. M. (1973). Threat as a factor in authoritarianism: An analysis of archival data. *Journal of Personality and Social Psychology, 28*(1), 44–57.

Saroglou, V. (2002). Religion and the five factors of personality: A meta-analytic review. *Personality and Individual Differences, 32*(1), 15–25.

Scruggs, L., & Benegal, S. (2012). Declining public concern about climate change: Can we blame the great recession? *Global Environmental Change, 22*(2), 505–515.

Shah, J. Y., Kruglanski, A. W., & Thompson, E. P. (1998). Membership has its (epistemic) rewards: Need for closure effects on in-group bias. *Journal of Personality and Social Psychology, 75*(2), 383–393.

Sidanius, J., & Pratto, F. (2003). Social dominance theory and the dynamics of inequality: A reply to Schmitt, Branscombe, & Kappen and Wilson & Liu. *British Journal of Social Psychology, 42*(2), 207–213.

Smith, S. M., Fabrigar, L. R., & Norris, M. E. (2008). Reflecting on six decades of selective exposure research: Progress, challenges, and opportunities. *Social and Personality Psychology Compass, 2*(1), 464–493.

Snyder, M. L., & Wicklund, R. A. (1981). Attribute ambiguity. *New Directions in Attribution Research, 3*, 197–221.

Staszak, S., Maciejowska, J., Urjasz, W., Misiuro, T., & Cudo, A. (2022). The relationship between the need for closure and coronavirus fear: The mediating effect of beliefs in conspiracy theories about COVID-19. *International Journal of Environmental Research and Public Health, 19*(22), 14789.

Stenner, K. (2005). *The authoritarian dynamic*. Cambridge University Press.

Szumowska, E., Czernatowicz-Kukuczka, A., Kossowska, M., Król, S., & Kruglanski, A. W. (2020). Truth and significance: A 3N Model (needs, narratives, networks) perspective on religion. In K. E. Vail III & C. Routledge (Eds.), *The science of religion, spirituality, and existentialism* (pp. 225–242). Academic Press.

Szumowska, E., & Kruglanski, A. W. (2020). Curiosity as end and means. *Current Opinion in Behavioral Sciences, 35*, 35–39.

Szumowska, E., Szwed, P., Kossowska, M., & Wright, R. (2017). Multifaceted effects of need for cognitive closure on effort: A cardiovascular response study. *Motivation Science, 3*, 369–382.

Szumowska, E., Wójcik, N., Szwed, P., & Kruglanski, A. W. (2022). Says who?: Credibility effects in self-verification strivings. *Psychological Science, 33*(5), 699–715.

Todor, I. (2014). Need for closure and cognitive inhibition of unwanted or irrelevant information. *Procedia-Social and Behavioral Sciences, 141*, 712–717.

Vaccari, C., & Chadwick, A. (2020). Deepfakes and disinformation: Exploring the impact of synthetic political video on deception, uncertainty, and trust in news. *Social Media+ Society, 6*(1).

van Prooijen, J. W. (2016). Sometimes inclusion breeds suspicion: Self-uncertainty and belongingness predict belief in conspiracy theories. *European Journal of Social Psychology, 46*(3), 267–279.

Van Prooijen, J. W. (2019). An existential threat model of conspiracy theories. *European Psychologist, 25*(1), 16–25.

Vancompernolle Vromman, F., & Fouss, F. (2021, December). Filter bubbles created by collaborative filtering algorithms themselves, fact or fiction?: An experimental comparison. *Proceedings of the IEEE/WIC/ACM International Conference on Web Intelligence and Intelligent Agent Technology*, pp. 153–159.

Wason, P. C. (1960). On the failure to eliminate hypotheses in a conceptual task. *Quarterly Journal of Experimental Psychology, 12*(3), 129–140.

Webster, D. M., & Kruglanski, A. W. (1994). Individual differences in need for cognitive closure. *Journal of Personality and Social Psychology, 67*(6), 1049–1062.

Webster, D. M., & Kruglanski, A. W. (1997). Cognitive and social consequences of the need for cognitive closure. *European Review of Social Psychology, 8*(1), 133–173.

Wiersema, D. V., Van Der Schalk, J., & van Kleef, G. A. (2012). Who's afraid of red, yellow, and blue? Need for cognitive closure predicts aesthetic preferences. *Psychology of Aesthetics, Creativity, and the Arts, 6*(2), 168–174.

Ylä-Anttila, T. (2018). Populist knowledge: "Post-truth" repertoires of contesting epistemic authorities. *European Journal of Cultural and Political Sociology, 5*(4), 356–388.

CHAPTER 29

Uncertainty and Social Identity

Benjamin J. Anjewierden, Kathryn M. Kincaid, Amber M. Gaffney, *and* David E. Rast III

The desire to understand ourselves and the world around us defines the core of human existence. In a world filled with uncertainty, this is no easy task. René Descartes (1899) famously said, "And as I observed that this truth, I think, therefore I am, was so certain and of such evidence that no ground of doubt, however extravagant, could be alleged by the Sceptics capable of shaking it" (p. 35). Descartes desperately attempted to find anything he could truly be certain of. He reasoned that he could not be certain of his own senses, perceptions, or about anything or anyone around him. The only thing he could be truly certain of was that he existed because he doubted the certainty of anything in the first place: "I think, therefore I am" (p. 35).

We can take two important points from Descartes' struggle for certainty. First, virtually everything is uncertain. We can never truly be certain of anything about ourselves, others, or the world. *We can only be more or less uncertain.* We will never be able to answer such questions as "How smart am I?"; "Am I a good parent?"; "Where is our country headed?"; and "What will happen when I die?" with complete certainty. We can only strive to be less uncertain about these things. A second point from Descartes' meditations is that people are highly motivated to reduce uncertainty. When people question who they are, their existence, and their place in this world and the next, they are engaged in existential meaning-making. Whereas Descartes engaged in deep philosophical thinking over a long period, there are less laborious ways to reduce uncertainty. Here, we focus on uncertainty reduction through group identification (Hogg, 2007, 2012, 2014, 2021a).

UNCERTAINTY REDUCTION AND SOCIAL IDENTITY MOTIVES

General Motives of Social Identity

Uncertainty reduction is one of three motives of group identification established under the social identity framework (Hogg & Abrams, 1988; Tajfel & Turner, 1979; Turner et al., 1987). By some conceptualizations, processes related to uncertainty reduction temporally precede those related to other motives of group identification (Anjewierden et al., 2024). However, the other two of these motives: self-enhancement (Tajfel & Turner, 1979) and optimal distinctiveness (Brewer, 1991; Leonardelli et al., 2010), precede uncertainty reduction in their establishment in the social identity literature.

The enhancement motive has been present since the inception of the social identity theory of intergroup relations (Tajfel & Turner, 1979). People derive a portion of their self-concept (understanding of self) from their social groups. In other words, the groups with which we identify are extensions of the self and provide a sense of social or collective identity. Given that our social groups directly reflect who we are, we are motivated to enhance, protect, or maintain their statuses to achieve a positive social identity. Tajfel and Turner treated status as a subjective social construct, rather than some finite resource. "High status" is established through favorable comparisons with other relevant groups.

Concern with ingroup status underlies certain intergroup phenomena. Those who strongly identify with their ingroup engage in outgroup derogation and endorse social inequality toward outgroups who threaten ingroup status (Branscombe & Wann, 1994; Morrison et al., 2009). Threats to ingroup status can also come from within. Ingroup members who deviate from important group and societal standards threaten the ingroup's positive identity, which often results in social control mechanisms such as derogation of deviants (e.g. Marques et al., 1998; Pinto et al., 2010). In addition, members of low-status groups can engage in behaviors in the interest of obtaining a positive social identity, such as psychologically or actually exiting their groups in favor of entering a higher-status group (individual mobility), making creative comparisons with outgroups that shed a positive light on the ingroup (social creativity; van Bezouw et al., 2021), or collectively acting to raise the ingroup's social standing (social change).

Although enhancement was a focus of early social identity research, optimal distinctiveness emerged as a complementary motivation for group identification (Brewer, 1991; Leonardelli et al., 2010). Optimal distinctiveness theory posits that people prefer groups that optimally satisfy competing needs for assimilation (inclusion) and differentiation (uniqueness). People tend to favor groups that provide them with a level of inclusiveness that effectively balances feelings of belonging with feelings of uniqueness in a given social context.

Uncertainty Reduction as a Motive of Social Identity

The uncertainty-reduction motive of group identification emerged most recently in the social identity literature. Independent of self-enhancement and optimal distinctiveness, uncertainty–identity theory (UIT; Hogg, 2007, 2021a) posits that when people feel uncertain about their self-concepts, they are motivated to identify with groups that effectively reduce the uncertainty. Social psychologists have identified different types of uncertainty related to the self (e.g., Marigold et al., 2009; McGregor et al., 2001; van den Bos, 2009); however, UIT focuses specifically on how uncertainty motivates group identification. UIT defines uncertainty surrounding one's self-concept (self-conceptual uncertainty) as a feeling of a deficit of information, knowledge, or clarity about self. We can be uncertain about how we should act, think, and feel, but also about broader questions such as "Who am I?"; "What is my place in the world?"; and "What do I stand for?" Such uncertainty is generally aversive—it threatens existential meaning-making and reduces our ability to effectively plan our behavior or predict how others will treat us (van den Bos, 2009). An important point for this chapter: Uncertainty, as a cognition, is both conceptually and empirically different from a drive for self and collective enhancement, which means it should occupy a quantitatively and qualitatively different space in the existential literature than work on self-esteem, belonging, and enhancement. Participants experiencing low uncertainty identify more strongly with high-status rather than low-status groups; however, under high uncertainty, this preference disappears (Reid & Hogg, 2005). This suggests that when people question their self-concepts, uncertainty reduction takes precedence. Once this epistemic drive is fulfilled, people are free to satisfy enhancement needs by identifying with high-status groups (see Anjewierden et al., 2024).

"Self" is not static—it is dynamic and context-dependent. Brewer and Gardner (1996) defined the self at three levels: personal, relational, and collective. Sometimes, we view ourselves as individuals, defined by personal traits and idiosyncrasies (e.g., "I am nice"; "I like to play video games"). Other times we view ourselves in relation to specific others (e.g., "I am a son"; "I am a partner"). At other times still, we define ourselves according to social groups (e.g., "I am an academic"; "I am a YouTuber"). Although the level of self-definition is context-dependent, self-uncertainty may arise across all levels of self (e.g., Hogg & Mahajan, 2018).

Although one's sensitivity to uncertainty may be dispositional (Webster & Kruglanski, 1994) or culturally bound (Sorrentino et al., 2008), feelings of self-uncertainty are reactions to social context. Uncertainty may be prompted by events such as becoming an "empty nester," organizational mergers, feeling like an outsider in important ingroups (Hohman et al., 2017), personal experiences that cause self-reflection, or thoughts about death and uncertainty about the afterlife (Hohman & Hogg, 2011). Several factors produce uncertainty across multiple dimensions of self, thus UIT posits that identifying with a group provides an overarching means of self-conceptual uncertainty reduction (Choi & Hogg, 2020; Hogg, 2007; Hogg & Mahajan, 2018). Uncertainty felt on personal or relational levels of self can be addressed at the collective level. For instance, adolescents experiencing high levels of uncertainty about their changing relationships with parents and their sense of individuality may be inclined to reduce uncertainty by identifying strongly with their friend groups (Cruwys et al., 2017).

Wagoner and colleagues (e.g., 2017; Wagoner & Chur, 2024) identified social identity uncertainty (feeling uncertain about what one's group stands for or feeling uncertain about one's place in a social group) as separate from self-uncertainty. Indeed, different levels of self-uncertainty have unique ramifications for group identification (e.g., feeling uncertain about what it means to be a group member can motivate disidentification from that group). However, we take the position that because the *self*-concept is composed of idiosyncratic personal aspects along with the knowledge gleaned from interpersonal relationships and membership in social groups, self-uncertainty occurs at all levels of self. At the collective level, it produces disidentification, but at personal and interpersonal levels, it promotes group identification. Our focus, and the focus of UIT as detailing a motivational force for social identity, is *self*-uncertainty.

Uncertainty Reduction through Group Identification

The theoretical explanation for how group identification reduces uncertainty is firmly rooted in self-categorization theory (SCT; Turner, 1982, 1985; Turner et al., 1987). Whereas social identity theory emphasizes the consequences of social groups being an extension of self, SCT emphasizes the processes by which we see groups as an extension of self in the first place. These two theories examine the same underlying theme (the role of social groups in the self-concept) at different points of the internalization process, forming the social identity framework.

SCT posits that in a given social context, we cognitively recognize ourselves and others as members of groups. For example, a marine biology student may categorize the students living in their natural sciences dorm as marine biology, wildlife, or forestry majors. This is a socially adaptive process. Categorization allows people to make cognitive shortcuts as they navigate social environments (Hogg, 2006a). Knowing the major of fellow undergraduates may provide important insight into things such as what conversation topics they enjoy, whether they would prefer to go for a walk on the beach or in the forest, or if they could be helpful with marine biology homework. Without categorization, this student would need to ascertain the answers to situationally specific questions from each individual interaction, expending exhaustive amounts of cognitive effort.

Categorization requires some cognitive energy to determine the appropriate categories from which to draw the best information about the self and others. When an appropriate categorization becomes salient, people *depersonalize* such that they view the self and others as interchangeable representatives of their respective groups. (Turner et al., 1987). How we perceive a depersonalized other is guided by the knowledge that we hold of their group, rather than knowledge of the individual. The amalgamation of knowledge we hold of a given group is the group's prototype. Prototypes are cognitive schemata—collections of features that most effectively describe a group and differentiate its members from other groups (Hogg, 2006b). As an example, the prototypical features that separate weightlifters from nonweightlifters are attributes such as being physically muscular, having gym time, eating "clean," and tracking progress. When we categorize and depersonalize a weightlifter to their prototype, we automatically view them as embodying these characteristics and thus derive a degree of understanding about what we can expect from them.

Self and social categorization reduces self-uncertainty (Hogg, 2007). When depersonalizing *ourselves,* we draw from ingroup prototypes as a framework of knowledge from which to reduce uncertainty about our own actions, thoughts, and feelings. If we begin to spend extended amounts of time at the gym and become increasingly muscular, we may find it appropriate to categorize ourselves as a weightlifter, depersonalize ourselves to the weightlifter prototype, and deduce that we ought to "eat clean" and closely track our training progress. This deduction of what we *ought* to do by nature of being a weightlifter highlights the prescriptive nature of prototypes. They do not solely describe what group members do; they also prescribe what group members *ought* to do. This is the essence of how group identification reduces uncertainty. Ingroup prototypes dictate prescriptive standards for individual actions, thoughts, and behaviors (Abrams et al., 2001; Hogg & Turner, 1987; Turner, 1982).

Characteristics of Uncertainty-Reducing Groups

Not all groups are equally equipped to reduce uncertainty. Uncertainty reduction through depersonalization depends on the degree to which people can clearly and easily understand prototypical features. People prefer to identify with groups with structured, understandable prototypes when they experience uncertainty. Simply put, uncertainty creates a preference for *entitative* groups (Hogg et al., 2007).

Entitativity is the degree to which a group is viewed as a distinct, real entity (Campbell, 1958), rather than a collection of individuals. At the most basic level, individuals must first recognize the existence of a group before self or social categorization processes occur. Entitativity is characterized by shared goals, similarity, and interactivity among group members; clear-cut intergroup boundaries; and established group history (Blanchard et al., 2020). Groups vary in their entitativity (Lickel et al., 2000). A Special Weapons and Tactics (SWAT) team is a small unit of specially trained law enforcement officers who must work interdependently to address crises. SWAT teams are more likely to be perceived as entitative than are people who simply live on the same street. Groups high in entitativity clearly represent what comprises "us" as a group, and thus provide clear, uncertainty-reducing information about group membership. Threats to a group's entitativity can cause members to experience uncertainty about the group, which is related to disidentification (e.g., Jung et al., 2019).

Entitativity is related to the meta-contrast principle (Turner et al., 1987), which postulates that collections of individuals are perceived as distinct entities to the degree that they accentuate intergroup differences and minimize intragroup differences. Entitativity captures "minimizing intragroup differences" with ingroup member similarity and shared goals and captures "accentuating intergroup differences" with clear intergroup boundaries. The principle of meta-contrast defines prototypes, which are composed of shared group characteristics that differentiate the ingroup from a relevant outgroup. Entitativity is thus the degree to which a prototype effectively does what a prototype is "supposed to do."

The meta-contrast principle is represented mathematically with meta-contrast ratios (MCRs), which are numeric representations of how well a group or individual group members maximize intragroup similarity and create distance from an outgroup (Turner et al., 1987). MCRs are calculated for groups by taking the mean of the absolute distances of all individual outgroup members from the mean ingroup position and dividing this value by the mean of the absolute distances of all individual ingroup members from the mean ingroup position. More simply, this is dividing intergroup differences by intragroup differences. Larger MCRs represent greater adherence to the meta-contrast principle at the group level. Groups with high MCR values display a marked distance between the ingroup and the outgroup on one or more denotative domains (e.g., abortion policy in the United States clearly defines Republicans and Democrats) and display high levels of intragroup consensus—two features of highly entitative groups.

MCRs can also be calculated for individual group members. These represent how well *individual* positions within an ingroup effectively abide by the meta-contrast principle. In other words, the value of MCRs for individuals is a measure of their prototypicality (how well a group member is aligned with their group's prototype) in comparison to other group members.

MCRs calculated for groups and individuals are employed as predictor variables in social identity research. For example, Di Bernardo and colleagues (2021) calculated MCRs for each student in a high school class. Students who perceived the student with the highest MCR as engaging in collective action on behalf of a disadvantaged group reported high intentions to engage in collective action themselves (a clever demonstration that prototypical group members drive influence in groups). Hogg and colleagues (1990) computed MCRs to show group polarization, and Haslam and Turner (1995) calculated MCRs to serve as a tool for theoretically modeling extremism. Recently, Anjewierden and colleagues (2024) used MCRs as a proof of concept to demonstrate how the presence of normative deviance in a group can polarize, depolarize, and shape group composition. Their model details the importance of the epistemic motive for group identification, by illustrating social contexts in which the ingroup can provide epistemic fulfillment through uncertainty reduction (i.e., when there is high intragroup consensus and high intergroup distance) and when this is threatened. These calculations are important for understanding how uncertainty drives group identification and the groups people find informative of their self-concepts.

CONSEQUENCES OF UNCERTAINTY

Uncertainty, despite being cognitively negotiated at the individual level, is strongly tied to several broad phenomena, including social influence (e.g., Gaffney & Hogg, 2017), leadership (Guillén et al., 2023; Rast et al., 2012), extremism (Hogg & Adelman, 2013; McGregor, 2006; McGregor et al., 2001), and polarization (e.g., Gaffney et al., 2014).

Uncertainty, Leadership, and Social Influence

The social identity perspective on leadership treats leadership as a reciprocal process between leaders and followers that depends on group composition and social context (Haslam, Gaffney, et al., 2022; Haslam et al., 2011; Hogg, 2001; Hogg et al., 2012; Hogg & van Knippenberg, 2003). Leaders both shape their groups and are shaped by both their groups and the intergroup context. Almost 30 years of research conducted under the social identity framework (Haslam et al., 2022a) demonstrates that people desire leaders to represent the essence of their group to the world at large, to stand up for them, and to work toward the group's betterment (see Steffens et al., 2014). Experimental and correlational evidence establish a "prototypical leader advantage," such that people find prototypical leaders (those who best embody the core attributes of their group's prototype) more effective than nonprototypical leaders (Barreto & Hogg, 2017; Steffens et al., 2020). Group members look to prototypical others in their groups for important cues about their social identities. This makes leaders the source of group-based influence. Prototypical leaders capture group members' attention as members look to them for cues to prescribe group norms. This gives prototypical leaders the ability to mold and shape their groups' prototypes (see Reicher et al., 2005). This shaping of prototypes occurs even when leaders transgress societal norms (Abrams et al., 2018; Davies et al., 2024) or engage in deviant acts (Syfers et al., 2022). Simply put, when leaders are prototypical, their actions dictate what is group normative, and their deviance is often accepted as a legitimate feature of the group prototype.

Prototypical leaders can stand as figureheads and literal faces of their groups (see Crano & Gaffney, 2021), which acts to clarify the group's prototype. For example, Syfers and colleagues (2024) demonstrated that as people's perceptions of their leaders' prototypicality increased (Democrats' and Republicans' perceptions of Biden and Trump, respectively, and Bolsonaro and De Silva supporters' perceptions of Bolsanaro's and De Silva's prototypicality, respectively), so did their beliefs that their Party or voting group was highly entitative. The presence of a prototypical leader galvanizes a group's entitativity.

When people experience self-uncertainty, the prototypical leader advantage can weaken or disappear. In both within- and between-subjects designs, Rast and colleagues (2012) demonstrated that university students low in uncertainty preferred a prototypical to a nonprototypical leader. However, among those high in uncertainty, the prototypical leadership advantage disappeared. Presumably, when people experience self-uncertainty, they desire leadership per se, rather than focusing on the leader's prototypicality. This relationship (in part) appears to be qualified by the need for cognition, such that among those low in need for cognition, uncertainty strengthens the prototypical leader advantage, with participants preferring a prototypical to a nonprototypical leader. However, among participants high in need for cognition, who presumably enjoy scrutinizing new information, uncertainty weakens the prototypical leader advantage. Rast and colleagues (2015) reasoned that prototypicality operates as a peripheral cue; thus, those low in need for cognition rely only on the cue to make decisions regarding leadership.

Incumbent leaders are known entities, but prospective leaders present a gambling-like situation (unknowns). In line with the findings of Rast and colleagues (2012), incumbent leaders appear to enjoy a prototypical leader advantage when their followers are low in uncertainty, which is weakened when followers experience uncertainty. However, prospective leaders experience the prototypical leader advantage under high but not low uncertainty (Ouyang et al., 2024).

Drastic changes to group identity can promote collective uncertainty and change resistance. However, Syfers and colleagues (2021, 2024) demonstrated in both student samples and samples of Canadian partisans that leaders can promote group-level changes, even among members who experience uncertainty, to the extent that leaders rhetorically describe the group identity as holding to core principles from the past, to the present, and into the future. Social identity continuity rhetoric mitigates the experience of uncertainty because it provides a coherent and temporally consistent source of social identity. Holding knowledge of the group's permanence and its ability to provide a continuous source of epistemic fulfillment, opens people to change. Thus, leaders can rhetorically define their groups in such a way that allows them to (1) keep and build membership and (2) wield influence.

Leaders play a critical role in social identity processes by providing a literal face for their movements and creating follower engagement (see Haslam et al., 2022b). The presence of leadership clarifies and molds the group prototype and shapes the way members view themselves as respective members of their groups. Two longitudinal studies showed that from a few weeks before to a few weeks after the 2020 election, Republicans' ratings of Trump's prototypicality in the Party decreased. As perceptions of Trump's prototypicality decreased, Republicans' self-prototypicality in the Party decreased, which predicted an increase in self-uncertainty (Kuljian et al., 2023). These studies operationalized Trump's prototypicality in terms of felt perceptions of his prototypicality (Study 1) and through modified MCRs (Study 2) and demonstrated consistent findings in two large samples. The findings strongly imply ramifications for followers' self-concepts when their leader no longer holds their post and thus does not wield prototypicality in their group. Specifically, if their once-prototypical leader is no longer at the helm, followers may question their own prototypicality and question who they are as group members and individuals. It is unlikely that this effect held long for Republicans, as there is evidence that Trump and his followers regained significant influence in the Republican Party (see Haslam et al., 2022b) and that Trump is currently the face of the Republican Party.

The desire for uncertainty reduction makes groups with tight systems, clear norms, and rigid structures desirable (Hogg, 2014). Such groups are often led by autocrats. For example, mortality salience and existential uncertainty help explain why some individuals gravitate toward autocratic leaders (e.g., Harms et al., 2018; Padilla et al., 2007; Schoel et al., 2011). One study found that mortality salience[1] and reminders of 9/11 terrorism increased support for U.S. President George Bush and his counterterrorism policies (Landau et al., 2004).

People residing in democracies typically desire shared governance and democratic leadership; however, as self-uncertainty increases, so does the desire for autocratic leadership (Hogg, 2021b; Rast et al., 2013). Reicher and Haslam (2006) reconceptualized the Stanford Prison Study (Haney et al., 1973; Zimbardo, 1989; Zimbardo et al., 1999) in their BBC Prison Study. Rather than conceptually replicating the Stanford Prison Study's findings, Reicher and Haslam found that support for tyranny and autocratic rule only arose when the social systems the "guards" and "prisoners" negotiated broke down and the "guard" identity was not a recognized or valuable source of information in the context of the "prison." These observations strongly implicate the role of social and societal confusion and destruction in the desire for autocratic leadership. Chaotic contexts give space for leadership that dictates the boundaries of group identity and tells people precisely how to "fix" their current predicaments. The aftermath of populism, in an overthrown system of governance, can give rise to authoritarian regimes led by strict autocrats (Crano & Gaffney, 2021; Hogg & Gøtzsche-Astrup, 2021). Indeed, in nations experiencing democratic backsliding (or full assaults on democracy) leaders who build a rigid structure and definition of national identity that excludes minority groups and who enact isolationist policies (e.g., Modi in India, Orban in Hungary, Netanyahu in Israel) show no sign of relinquishing their grips on their respective nations' reins.

Uncertainty, Polarization, and Extremism

Categorizing oneself as a member of a clearly defined group is epistemically fulfilling. Although not all entitative groups are radicalized extremist organizations, all radicalized groups are entitative. The very nature of being extremist makes them highly entitative. Gangs, terrorist organizations, cults, conspiratorial groups, and the like, are composed of members who share interdependent and common goals, have high member similarity, and operate as a unit. People on the extremes and members of radicalized groups hold deep convictions and do not waver in their worldviews (Zwicker et al., 2020). The lure of uncertainty reduction can be a powerful carrot to entice individuals to join extremist groups and radicalize them in the process.

Groups characterized by high intragroup consensus, in which members display similarity to one another and agree on relevant aspects of their group's prototype, and by high differentiation from a relevant outgroup are satisfying because they provide a significant amount of uncertainty-reducing information by telling members both who they are and who they are not (see Anjewierden et al., 2024). As a result, when people experience uncertainty in an intergroup context, the group members and/or factions with the highest MCRs should wield the most influence and drive the trajectory of intergroup polarization. Hogg and colleagues' (1990) work on polarization demonstrated that group prototypes (computed by MCRs) polarize away from a relevant outgroup in an intergroup context but remain moderate when an outgroup isn't implicated. Gaffney and colleagues (2014) showed this in a political context. They primed moderate conservatives with high or low uncertainty and then exposed them to an ingroup minority group (Tea Party) message. When the message was ostensibly presented to Republicans, participants were unmoved by the message. However, among participants experiencing high uncertainty, the Tea Party message was viewed as attractive when the message was presented to a *true* outgroup (Democrats), and participants' attitudes aligned with the Tea Party message, effectively polarizing away from Democrats. This work implies that when people experience uncertainty, they desire their groups to polarize away from relevant outgroups because the ingroup can then provide them with an unambiguous definition of self that exists in contradistinction to an outgroup.

Group polarization is a precursor to intergroup violence (Piazza, 2023). Group members who view the outgroup as irreconcilably different from their ingroup tend to dehumanize outgroup members and support threats of violence against them (Kleinfeld, 2023). Political and religious violence is on the rise (van den Bos, 2018), particularly in countries such as the United States (Kleinfeld, 2022). Whereas some acts of mass violence are committed by "lone wolves," the bulk of political and religious violence is committed on behalf of collectives (see Ellenberg & Kruglanski, 2024).

Experimentally and correlationally, Hogg and colleagues (2010b) showed that self-uncertainty encourages identification with radicalized groups that support violent campus protests. Similarly, self-uncertainty appears to weaken identification with moderate groups and strengthen it with radicalized groups (see Hogg et al., 2013). Moreover, because uncertainty creates a reliance on a salient social category if that social category promotes risky behaviors, people often adopt these behaviors. Across two studies, Syfers and colleagues (2023) showed that self-uncertain conservatives reported symbolic threats from the COVID-19 pandemic (e.g., threat to the values of U.S. citizens), which in turn predicted risky social behaviors amid a pandemic (e.g., unwillingness to social distance), in line with fellow conservatives.

The uncertainty–identity approach posits that religious groups are particularly well suited for uncertainty reduction, as they prescribe clear doctrines that manage adherents' thoughts, feelings, and behaviors (Hogg et al., 2010a). Religious groups confer meaning and purpose to existence, and they provide consensual validation of an ideological worldview that addresses questions about the nature of existence and the afterlife. Such qualities make religious groups particularly effective in reducing existential uncertainty (e.g., Hunsberger & Jackson, 2005; Inzlicht et al., 2009; Silberman, 2005).

Religion on its own does not have to precipitate violence; however, deeply held belief systems, embedded within entitative groups that fully encompass and prescribe adherers' behaviors, form a context ripe for extremism. Strongly religious people tend to react with anger toward antireligious statements that violate their religious belief system when they experience uncertainty (van den Bos et al., 2006). Similarly, non-Muslims who experience uncertainty derogate Islam, and uncertainty increases religious zeal and support for war to defend one's own religious beliefs (McGregor et al., 2008). Reacting to uncertainty with zeal or extremism (e.g., related to opinions, values, or group identifications) effectively reduces the subjective salience of unrelated personal uncertainty (McGregor, 2006; McGregor & Marigold, 2003).

The work on uncertainty and extremism is vast; however, most scholars agree that the experience of uncertainty can make extremist groups with rigid ideological structures attractive. Providing individuals who feel marginalized in society with a way to feel significant and getting them to view political and social systems as procedurally fair would go a long way toward reducing the attractiveness of groups that go against these systems or seek to destroy them (van den Bos, 2001). The problem then becomes twofold: creating structural change at a societal level while finding a way to counteract conspiratorial and untruthful narratives from leaders who wish to delegitimize democratic systems.

Uncertainty and Mortality Salience

Uncertainty appears to play a role in mortality salience alongside a significant body of research linking self-enhancement to existential anxiety (see Lifshin et al., 2021). Terror management theory researchers have reliably shown that when humans' mortality is salient, they seek to bolster both their collective worldviews and their self-esteem. Death anxiety results in a need to defend important groups, relationships, and worldviews that leave a real or symbolic legacy after death. Directly relevant to self-uncertainty, Hohman and Hogg (2011) showed that mortality salience *produces* self-uncertainty, presumably because not knowing how and when we die or what happens after death produces existential uncertainty. Van den Bos and colleagues (2005) provide empirical evidence that uncertainty is a stronger predictor of worldview defense than mortality salience.

We view the basic tenet of terror management theory (people use cultural worldviews to achieve symbolic mortality, make meaning out of their lives, and feel good about their lives) as compatible with our position that collective enhancement and uncertainty reduction are two primary and separate motives for social identity. When mortality salience produces existential uncertainty, people must make sense of the purpose of their lives by seeking information from important cultural and social institutions and groups that establish clearly defined worldviews. This suggests that uncertainty surrounding death causes people to identify with groups that have uncertainty-reducing features. Groups with clearly defined ideological structures and worldviews provide epistemic fulfillment for existential uncertainty. In turn, people then seek ways to feel good about themselves via those groups and defend those groups from outside threats.

NEXT STEPS IN STUDYING UNCERTAINTY AND GROUPS

Conspiracy Groups

Conspiracy theory research has ventured into the realm of group-based motivations for endorsing conspiracies but has focused on how conspiracy theories create, maintain, and protect a positive identity (see van Prooijen, 2024) rather than an informative, uncertainty-reducing identity. Although researchers have made clear connections between self-uncertainty and conspiracy beliefs (e.g. van Prooijen, 2015; van Prooijen & Jostmann, 2012), identification with conspiracy groups motivated by uncertainty reduction using a UIT framework has not yet been explored.

Conspiracy groups by nature are extreme and thus embody the same attractive, uncertainty-reducing characteristics as any extreme group. However, conspiracy groups may have advantages over other extremist groups in how attractive they are for uncertainty reduction. Belief in a particular conspiracy theory can form the basis of a social identity (van Prooijen, 2024), giving socially validated structure and meaning to a circumstance that otherwise lacks it (Douglas et al., 2017). Given that people draw from their groups to inform their thoughts, feelings, and behaviors, groups formed based on sense-making (as opposed to common interests or shared social categories) may be especially inviting. Conspiracy groups may also be better equipped than other groups to reduce uncertainty about how to act, think, and feel in emergent contexts. For example, "anti-vaxx" groups who either dismissed COVID-19 vaccines or espoused their dangers, may have attracted interest and attention in early 2020 due to the pandemic creating a unique circumstance rife with uncertainty. In most contexts, anti-vaxx conspiracy groups do not provide relevant information to reduce uncertainty but they did so in the context of COVID-19. Because conspiracy groups possess features relevant to uncertainty reduction beyond even those of other extreme groups, these particular dimensions of conspiracy groups warrant empirical investigation.

Modeling Using MCRs

Recent theoretical and methodological ideas open the door to novel investigation of numerous group phenomena through the lens of uncertainty reduction. Anjewierden and colleagues (2024) outlined a method of observing features indicative of the epistemic value of a group by plotting group member MCRs on a given normative dimension (e.g., an attitude score) in a given intergroup context while accounting for the composition of each group and the difference between the groups. This method of plotting MCRs for ingroup positions and creating an "MCR distribution" allows for simple observation and comparison of how well groups provide a clear prototypical ingroup position that group members can easily understand and emulate. These distributions can also show which group members are leaders in occupying the most prototypical positions, how much deviant group members undermine the structure of their group, and even how changes to the group composition may provide attractive or aversive alternative group positions. This method helps us understand and make predictions about the properties of the group and the members who best satisfy or threaten epistemic and existential needs. Currently, these ideas are extensions of the theory, but with the potential to shed light on a variety of social identity processes in a novel fashion, they warrant empirical testing. of how and why groups provide individuals information that allows for daily functioning.

Uncertainty surrounding one's self-concept (individual, interpersonal, or collective) is aversive. We live in a world where we cannot exist without experiencing uncertainty, and much of it is existential. Wars, famines, divorces, career changes, and simply the reality of human disagreement all guarantee that uncertainty is a ubiquitous cognitive experience. No one is ever completely correct. We will always operate with some degree of uncertainty. As scientists, we can continue to uncover new methods for studying and measuring uncertainty's impact on groups and apply science to reducing its negative consequences.

NOTE

1. Note that it is impossible to discern mortality salience from intergroup threat in this design.

REFERENCES

Abrams, D., Travaglino, G. A., Marques, J. M., Pinto, I., & Levine, J. M. (2018). Deviance credit: Tolerance of deviant ingroup leaders is mediated by their accrual of prototypicality and conferral of their right to be supported. *Journal of Social Issues, 74*(1), 36–55.

Abrams, D., Wetherell, M., Cochrane, S., Hogg, M. A., & Turner, J. C. (2001). Knowing what to think by knowing who you are: Self-categorization and the nature of norm formation, conformity and group polarization. In M. A. Hogg & D. Abrams (Eds.), *Intergroup relations: Essential readings* (pp. 270–288). Psychology Press.

Anjewierden, B. J., Syfers, L., Pinto, I. R., Gaffney, A. M., & Hogg, M. A. (2024). Group responses to deviance: Disentangling the motivational roles of collective enhancement and self-uncertainty reduction. *Group Processes and Intergroup Relations, 27*(5), 1170–1187.

Barreto, N. B., & Hogg, M. A. (2017). Evaluation of and support for group prototypical leaders: A meta-analysis of twenty years of empirical research. *Social Influence, 12*(1), 41–55.

Blanchard, A. L., Caudill, L. E., & Walker, L. S. (2020). Developing an entitativity measure and distinguishing it from antecedents and outcomes within online and face-to-face groups. *Group Processes and Intergroup Relations, 23*(1), 91–108.

Branscombe, N. R., & Wann, D. L. (1994). Collective self-esteem consequences of outgroup derogation when a valued social identity is on trial. *European Journal of Social Psychology, 24*(6), 641–657.

Brewer, M. B. (1991). The social self: On being the same and different at the same time. *Personality and Social Psychology Bulletin, 17*(5), 475–482.

Brewer, M. B., & Gardner, W. (1996). Who is this "we"?: Levels of collective identity and self-representation. *Journal of Personality and Social Psychology, 71*(1), 83–93.

Campbell, D. T. (1958). Common fate, similarity, and other indices of the status of aggregates of persons as social entities. *Behavioral Science, 3*(1), 14–25.

Crano, W. D., & Gaffney, A. M. (2021). Populism in the west as a form of influence. In J. P. Forgas, K. Fiedler, & W. D. Crano (Eds.), *The psychology of populism: The tribal change to liberal democracy. Sydney Symposium of Social Psychology* (pp. 297–318). Psychology Press.

Cruwys, T., Gaffney, A. M., & Skipper, Y. (2017). Uncertainty in transition: The influence of group cohesion on learning. In K. I. Mavor, M. J. Platow, & B. Bizumic (Eds.), *Self and social identity in educational contexts* (pp. 193–208). Routledge/Taylor & Francis Group.

Choi, E. U., & Hogg, M. A. (2020). Self-uncertainty and group identification: A meta-analysis. *Group Processes and Intergroup Relations, 23*(4), 483–501.

Davies, B., Abrams, D., & Leicht, C. (2024). Why leaders can be bad: Linking rigor with relevance using machine learning analysis to test the transgression credit theory of leadership. *Group Processes and Intergroup Relations, 27*(5), 1068–1087.

Descartes, R. (1899). *Discourse on the method of rightly conducting the reason, and seeking*

truth in the sciences (J. Veitch, Trans.). Open Court Publishing.
Di Bernardo, G. A., Cocco, V. M., Paolini, S., Vezzali, L., Stathi, S., Rubin, M., & Subašić, E. (2021). Following the best of us to help them: Group member prototypicality and collective action. *Group Processes and Intergroup Relations, 26*(1), 243–260.
Douglas, K. M., Sutton, R. M., & Cichoka, A. (2017). The psychology of conspiracy theories. *Current Directions in Psychological Science, 26*(6), 538–542.
Ellenberg, M., & Kruglanski, A. W. (2024). Power of the network and power from the network: Group processes and radicalization. *Group Processes and Intergroup Relations, 27*(5), 990–1001.
Festinger, L. (1954a). Motivation leading to social behavior. In M. R. Jones (Ed.), *Nebraska symposium on motivation* (Vol. 2, pp. 121–218). University of Nebraska Press.
Festinger, L. (1954b). A theory of social comparison processes. *Human Relations, 7,* 117–140.
Gaffney, A. M., & Hogg, M. A. (2017). Social identity and social influence. In S. Harkins, K. D. Williams, & J. Burger (Eds.), *The Oxford handbook of social influence* (pp. 259–273). Oxford University Press.
Gaffney, A. M., Rast, D. E., Hackett, J. D., & Hogg, M. A. (2014). Further to the right: Uncertainty, political polarization and the American "Tea Party" movement. *Social Influence, 9*(4), 272–288.
Guillén, L., Jacquart, P., & Hogg, M. A. (2023). To lead, or to follow?: How self-uncertainty and the dark triad of personality influence leadership motivation. *Personality and Social Psychology Bulletin, 49*(7), 1043–1057.
Haney, C., Banks, C., & Zimbardo, P. (1973). A study of prisoners and guards in a simulated prison. *Naval Research Review, 9,* 1–17 [Reprinted in E. Aronson (Ed.), *Readings about the social animal* (3rd ed., pp. 52–67). Freeman].
Harms, P. D., Wood, D., Landay, K., Lester, P. B., & Lester, G. V. (2018). Autocratic leaders and authoritarian followers revisited: A review and agenda for the future. *Leadership Quarterly, 29*(1), 105–122.
Haslam, S. A., Gaffney, A. M., Hogg, M. A., Rast, D. E., III, & Steffens, N. K. (2022a) Reconciling identity leadership and leader identity: A dual-identity framework. *Leadership Quarterly, 33*(4), 101620.
Haslam, S. A., Reicher, S. D., & Platow, M. J. (2011). *The new psychology of leadership: Identity, influence and power.* Psychology Press.
Haslam, S. A., Reicher, S. D., Selvanathan, H. P., Gaffney, A. M., Steffens, N. K., Packer, D., . . . Platow, M. J. (2022b). Examining the role of Donald Trump and his supporters in the 2021 assault on the U.S. Capitol: A dual-agency model of identity leadership and engaged followership. *Leadership Quarterly, 34*(2), 101622.
Haslam, S. A., & Turner, J. C. (1995). Context-dependent variation in social stereotyping: III. Extremism as a self-categorical basis for polarized judgment. *European Journal of Social Psychology, 25*(3), 341–371.
Hogg, M. A. (2001). A social identity theory of leadership. *Personality and Social Psychology Review, 5*(3), 184–200.
Hogg, M. A. (2006a). Social categorization, depersonalization, and group behavior. In M. A. Hogg & R. S. Tindale (Eds.), *Blackwell handbook of social psychology: Group processes* (pp. 56–85). Blackwell.
Hogg, M. A. (2006b). Social identity theory. In P. J. Burke (Ed.), *Contemporary social psychological theories* (pp. 287–314). Stanford University Press.
Hogg, M. A. (2007). Uncertainty–identity theory. In M. P. Zanna (Ed.), *Advances in experimental social psychology* (Vol. 39, pp. 69–126). Elsevier Academic Press.
Hogg, M. A. (2012). Uncertainty–identity theory. In P. A. M. Van Lange, A. W. Kruglanski, & E. T. Higgins (Eds.), *Handbook of theories of social psychology* (pp. 62–80). Sage.
Hogg, M. A. (2014). From uncertainty to extremism: Social categorization and identity processes. *Current Directions in Psychological Science, 23*(5), 338–342.
Hogg, M. A. (2021a). Self-uncertainty and group identification: Consequences for social identity, group behavior, intergroup relations, and Society. *Advances in Experimental Social Psychology, 65,* 263–316.
Hogg, M. A. (2021b). Uncertain self in a changing world: A foundation for radicalization, populism and autocratic leadership. *European Review of Social Psychology, 32*(2), 235–268.
Hogg, M. A., Abrams, D. (1988). *Social identifications: A social psychology of intergroup relations and group processes.* Taylor & Francis/Routledge.
Hogg, M. A., & Adelman, J. (2013). Uncertainty–identity theory: Extreme groups, radical behavior, and authoritarian leadership. *Journal of Social Issues, 69*(3), 436–454.
Hogg, M. A., Adelman, J. R., & Blagg, R. D. (2010). Religion in the face of uncertainty: An uncertainty-identity theory account of religiousness. *Personality and Social Psychology Review, 14*(1), 72–83. Hogg, M. A., & Gøtzsche-Astrup, O. (2021). Self-uncertainty

and populism: Why we endorse populist ideologies, identify with populist groups, and support populist leaders. In J. P. Forgas, W. D. Crano, & K. Fiedler (Eds.), *The psychology of populism: The tribal challenge to liberal democracy* (pp. 197–218). Routledge/Taylor & Francis Group.

Hogg, M. A., Kruglanski, A., & van den Bos, K. (2013). Uncertainty and the roots of extremism. *Journal of Social Issues, 69*(3), 407–418.

Hogg, M. A., & Mahajan, N. (2018). Domains of self-uncertainty and their relationship to group identification. *Journal of Theoretical Social Psychology, 2*(3), 67–75.

Hogg, M. A., Meehan, C., & Farquharson, J. (2010). The solace of radicalism: Self-uncertainty and group identification in the face of threat. *Journal of Experimental Social Psychology, 46*(6), 1061–1066.

Hogg, M. A., Sherman, D. K., Dierselhuis, J., Maitner, A. T., & Moffitt, G. (2007). Uncertainty, entitativity, and group identification. *Journal of Experimental Social Psychology, 43*(1), 135–142.

Hogg, M. A., & Turner, J. C. (1987). Social identity and conformity: A theory of referent informational influence. In W. Doise & S. Moscovici (Eds.), *Current issues in European social psychology* (Vol. 2, pp. 139–182). Cambridge University Press.

Hogg, M. A., Turner, J. C., & Davidson, B. (1990). Polarized norms and social frames of reference: A test of the self-categorization theory of group polarization. *Basic and Applied Social Psychology, 11*(1), 77–100.

Hogg, M. A., & van Knippenberg, D. (2003). Social identity and leadership processes in groups. *Advances in Experimental Social Psychology, 35,* 1–52.

Hogg, M. A., van Knippenberg, D., & Rast, D. E., III. (2012). The social identity theory of leadership: Theoretical origins, research findings, and conceptual developments. *European Review of Social Psychology, 23*(1), 258–304.

Hohman, Z. P., Gaffney, A. M., & Hogg, M. A. (2017). Who am I if I am not like my group?: Self-uncertainty and feeling peripheral in a group. *Journal of Experimental Social Psychology, 72,* 125–132.

Hohman, Z. P., & Hogg, M. A. (2011). Fear and uncertainty in the face of death: The role of life after death in group identification. *European Journal of Social Psychology, 41*(6), 751–760.

Hunsberger, B., & Jackson, L. M. (2005). Religion, meaning, and prejudice. *Journal of Social Issues, 61*(4), 807–826.

Inzlicht, M., McGregor, I., Hirsh, J. B., & Nash, K. (2009). Neural markers of religious conviction. *Psychological Science, 20*(3), 385–392.

Jung, J., Hogg, M. A., Livingstone, A. G., & Choi, H. (2019). From uncertain boundaries to uncertain identity: Effects of entitativity threat on identity-uncertainty and emigration. *Journal of Applied Social Psychology, 49*(10), 623–633.

Kleinfeld, R. (2022). *The rise in political violence in the United States and damage to our democracy.* Carnegie Endowment for International Peace. https://carnegieendowment.org/2022/03/31/rise-in-political-violence-in-united-states-and-damage-to-our-democracy-pub-87584.

Kleinfeld, R. (2023). *Polarization, democracy, and political violence in the United States: What the research says.* Carnegie Endowment for International Peace. https://carnegieendowment.org/2023/09/05/polarization-democracy-and-political-violence-in-united-states-what-research-says-pub-90457.

Kuljian, O. R., Hohman, Z. P., & Gaffney, A. M. (2023). Who are we if we do not know who our leader is? Perceptions of leaders' prototypicality affects followers' self-prototypicality and uncertainty. *Social Psychological and Personality Science, 14*(5), 599–609.

Landau, M. J., Solomon, S., Greenberg, J., Cohen, F., Pyszczynski, T., Arndt, J., . . . Cook, A. (2004). Deliver us from evil: The effects of mortality salience and reminders of 9/11 on support for President George W. Bush. *Personality and Social Psychology Bulletin, 30*(9), 1136–1150.

Leonardelli, G. J., Pickett, C. L., & Brewer, M. B. (2010). Optimal distinctiveness theory: A framework for social identity, social cognition, and intergroup relations. In M. P. Zanna & J. M. Olson (Eds.), *Advances in Experimental Social Psychology* (Vol. 43, pp. 63–113). Academic Press.

Lickel, B., Hamilton, D. L., Wieczorkowska, G., Lewis, A., Sherman, S. J., & Uhles, A. N. (2000). Varieties of groups and the perception of group entitativity. *Journal of Personality and Social Psychology, 78*(2), 223–246.

Lifshin, U., Horner, D. E., Helm, P. J., Solomon, S., & Greenberg, J. (2021). Self-esteem and immortality: Evidence regarding the terror management hypothesis that high self-esteem is associated with a stronger sense of symbolic immortality. *Personality and Individual Differences, 175,* 110712.

Marigold, D. C., McGregor, I., & Zanna, M. P. (2009). Defensive conviction as emotion regulation: Goal mechanisms and interpersonal implications. In R. M. Arkin, K. C. Oleson, & P. J. Carroll (Eds.), *Handbook of the uncertain self* (pp. 232–248). Psychology Press.

Marques, J., Abrams, D., Paez, D., & Martinez-Taboada, C. (1998). The role of categorization and in-group norms in judgments of groups and their members. *Journal of Personality and Social Psychology, 75*(4), 976–988.

McGregor, I. (2006). Offensive defensiveness: Toward an integrative neuroscience of compensatory zeal after mortality salience, personal uncertainty, and other poignant self-threats. *Psychological Inquiry, 17*(4), 299–308.

McGregor, I., Haji, R., Nash, K. A., & Teper, R. (2008). Religious zeal and the uncertain self. *Basic and Applied Social Psychology, 30*(2), 183–188.

McGregor, I., & Marigold, D. C. (2003). Defensive zeal and the uncertain self: What makes you so sure? *Journal of Personality and Social Psychology, 85*(5), 838.

McGregor, I., Zanna, M. P., Holmes, J. G., & Spencer, S. J. (2001). Compensatory conviction in the face of personal uncertainty: Going to extremes and being oneself. *Journal of Personality and Social Psychology, 80*(3), 472–488.

Morrison, K. R., Fast, N. J., & Ybarra, O. (2009). Group status, perceptions of threat, and support for Social Inequality. *Journal of Experimental Social Psychology, 45*(1), 204–210.

Ouyang, Y., Kincaid, K. M., Rast, D. E., Gaffney, A. M., & Hogg, M. A. (2024). Incumbency and self-uncertainty: when prototypical leaders lose their advantage. *Journal of Social Psychology*, 1–18.

Padilla, A., Hogan, R., & Kaiser, R. B. (2007). The toxic triangle: Destructive leaders, susceptible followers, and conducive environments. *Leadership Quarterly, 18*(3), 176–194.

Piazza, J. A. (2023). Political polarization and political violence. *Security Studies, 32*(3), 476–504.

Pinto, I. R., Marques, J. M., Levine, J. M., & Abrams, D. (2010). Membership status and subjective group dynamics: Who triggers the black sheep effect? *Journal of Personality and Social Psychology, 99*, 107–119.

Rast, D. E., III, Gaffney, A. M., Hogg, M. A., & Crisp, R. J. (2012). Leadership under uncertainty: When leaders who are non-prototypical group members can gain support. *Journal of Experimental Social Psychology, 48*(3), 646–653.

Rast, D. E., III, Hogg, M. A., & Giessner, S. R. (2013). Self-uncertainty and support for autocratic leadership. *Self and Identity, 12*(6), 635–649.

Rast, D. E., III, Hogg, M. A., & Tomory, J. J. (2015). Prototypical leaders do not always get our support: Impact of self-uncertainty and need for cognition. *Self and Identity, 14*(2), 135–146.

Reicher, S., & Haslam, S. A. (2006). Rethinking the psychology of tyranny: The BBC prison study. *British Journal of Social Psychology, 45*(1), 1–40.

Reicher, S., Haslam, A. S., & Hopkins, N. (2005). Social identity and the dynamics of leadership: Leaders and followers as collaborative agents in the transformation of social reality. *Leadership Quarterly, 16*, 547–568.

Reid, S. A., & Hogg, M. A. (2005). Uncertainty reduction, self-enhancement, and ingroup identification. *Personality and Social Psychology Bulletin, 31*(6), 804–817.

Schoel, C., Bluemke, M., Mueller, P., & Stahlberg, D. (2011). When autocratic leaders become an option—Uncertainty and self-esteem predict implicit leadership preferences. *Journal of Personality and Social Psychology, 101*(3), 521.

Silberman, I. (2005). Religion as a meaning system: Implications for the new millennium. *Journal of Social Issues, 61*(4), 641–663.

Sorrentino, R. M., Nezlek, J. B., Yasunaga, S., Kouhara, S., Otsubo, Y., & Shuper, P. (2008). Uncertainty orientation and affective experiences: Individual differences within and across cultures. *Journal of Cross-Cultural Psychology, 39*(2), 129–146.

Steffens, N. K., Haslam, S. A., Reicher, S. D., Platow, M. J., Fransen, K., Yang, J., . . . Boen, F. (2014). Leadership as social identity management: Introducing the Identity Leadership Inventory (ILI) to assess and validate a four-dimensional model. *Leadership Quarterly, 25*(5), 1001–1024.

Steffens, N. K., Munt, K. A., van Knippenberg, D., Platow, M. J., & Haslam, S. A. (2020). Advancing the social identity theory of leadership: A meta-analytic review of leader group prototypicality. *Organizational Psychology Review, 11*(1), 35–72.

Syfers, L., Gaffney, A. M., Rast, D. E., III, & Estrada, D. A. (2022). Communicating group norms through election results. *British Journal of Social Psychology, 61*(1), 300–321.

Syfers, L., Jaurique, A., Anjewierden, B., Burke, S. E., Hackett, J. D., & Gaffney, A. M. (2023). Self-uncertainty and conservatism during the COVID-19 pandemic predict perceived threat and engagement in risky social behaviors. *Group Processes and Intergroup Relations, 27*(3), 619–638.

Syfers, L., Rast, D. E., & Gaffney, A. M. (2021). Leading change by protecting group identity in the 2019 Canadian general election. *Analyses of Social Issues and Public Policy, 21*(1), 415–438.

Syfers, L., Royer, Z., Anjewierden, B., Rast, D. E., III, & Gaffney, A. M. (2024). Our group is worth the fight: Group cohesion is embedded in willingness to fight or die for relatively deprived political groups during national elections. *Translational Issues in Psychological Science, 10*(1), 7–20.

Tajfel, H., & Turner, J. C. (1979). An integrative theory of intergroup conflict. In S. Worchel & W. G. Austin (Eds.), *The social psychology of intergroup relations* (pp. 33–47). Brooks/Cole.

Turner, J. C. (1982). Towards a cognitive redefinition of the social group. In H. Tajfel (Ed.), *Social identity and intergroup relations*. Cambridge University Press.

Turner, J. C. (1985). Social categorization and the self-concept: A social cognitive theory of group behaviour. In E. J. Lawler (Ed.), *Advances in group processes: Theory and Research* (Vol. 2, pp. 77–122). JAI Press.

Turner, J. C., Hogg, M. A., Oakes, P. J., Reicher, S. D., & Wetherell, M. S. (1987). *Rediscovering the social group: A self-categorization theory*. Basil Blackwell.

van Bezouw, M. J., van der Toorn, J., & Becker, J. C. (2021). Social creativity: Reviving a social identity approach to social stability. *European Journal of Social Psychology, 51*(2), 409–422.

van den Bos, K. (2001). Uncertainty management: The influence of uncertainty salience on reactions to perceived procedural fairness. *Journal of Personality and Social Psychology, 80*(6), 931–941.

van den Bos, K. (2009). Making sense of life: The existential self trying to deal with personal uncertainty. *Psychological Inquiry, 20*(4), 197–217.

van den Bos, K. (2018). *Why people radicalize: How unfairness judgments are used to fuel radical beliefs, extremist behaviors, and terrorism*. Oxford University Press.

van den Bos, K., Poortvliet, P. M., Maas, M., Miedema, J., & Van den Ham, E. J. (2005). An enquiry concerning the principles of cultural norms and values: The impact of uncertainty and mortality salience on reactions to violations and bolstering of cultural worldviews. *Journal of Experimental Social Psychology, 41*(2), 91–113.

van den Bos, K., Van Ameijde, J., & Van Gorp, H. (2006). On the psychology of religion: The role of personal uncertainty in religious worldview defense. *Basic and Applied Social Psychology, 28*(4), 333–341.

van Prooijen, J. (2015). Sometimes inclusion breeds suspicion: Self-uncertainty and belongingness predict belief in conspiracy theories. *European Journal of Social Psychology, 46*(3), 267–279.

van Prooijen, J.-W. (2024). Group-oriented motivations underlying conspiracy theories. *Group Processes and Intergroup Relations, 27*(5), 1050–1067. Wagoner, J. A., Belavadi, S., & Jung, J. (2017). Social identity uncertainty: Conceptualization, measurement, and construct validity. *Self and Identity, 16*(5), 505–530.

van Prooijen, J., & Jostmann, N. B. (2012). Belief in conspiracy theories: The influence of uncertainty and perceived morality. *European Journal of Social Psychology, 43*(1), 109–115.

Wagoner, J. A., Belavadi, S., & Jung, J. (2017). Social identity uncertainty: Conceptualization, measurement, and construct validity. *Self and Identity, 16*(5), 505–530.

Wagoner, J. A., & Chur, M. (2024). Domains of uncertainty, identification processes, and exit intentions. *Group Processes and Intergroup Relations, 27*(7), 1541–1568.

Webster, D. M., & Kruglanski, A. W. (1994). Individual differences in need for cognitive closure. *Journal of Personality and Social Psychology, 67*(6), 1049–1062.

Zimbardo, P. (1989). *Quiet rage: The Stanford Prison Study video*. Stanford University.

Zimbardo, P. G., Maslach, C., & Haney, C. (1999). Reflections on the Stanford prison experiment: Genesis, transformations, consequences. In T. Blass (Ed.), *Obedience to authority: Current perspectives on the Milgram paradigm* (pp. 193–237). Erlbaum.

Zwicker, M. V., van Prooijen, J.-W., & Krouwel, A. P. M. (2020). Persistent beliefs: Political extremism predicts ideological stability over time. *Group Processes and Intergroup Relations, 23*(8), 1137–1149.

CHAPTER 30

How Meaningful Values Supplant Reactive Approach Motivation for Hostile Worldview Extremes

Ian McGregor

Freud claimed people use "excessively intense" and "extreme" thoughts to keep unwanted worries and conflicts out of awareness—"the reactive thought keeps the objectionable one under repression by means of a certain surplus of intensity" (Gay, 1989, p. 200). He compared such extremes to bouncers who eject unruly guests from consciousness and then bar the door (Freud, 1910). Neoanalytic theorists like Fromm and Adorno adapted this idea to blame personal uncertainties and conflicts for the authoritarian hate and conformity that fueled World War II—extremes help people hide from their bewildered selves. Through Lewin and Festinger, this conflict-to-extremes hypothesis moved into the lab to help launch the field of experimental social psychology after the war (Patnoe, 1988). Over the next 80 years, versions of the conflict-to-extremes idea tumbled along, as premise or foil, in a proliferation of threat and defense theories in experimental social psychology (Jonas et al., 2014). This chapter traces how this seminal idea evolved into a theoretically resonant and empirically stable, reactive approach motivation (RAM) account of why hostile extremes are rewarding, and how personally meaningful values can supplant them. In doing so it lends integrative theoretical hope for a balanced way forward in areas of experimental social psychology that have been challenged by the methods revolution and replication concerns (e.g., Klein et al., 2022; Viadis et al., 2024; Vohs et al., 2021). It concludes with discussion of how RAM theory might inform interventions to quell the kinds of extremes that experimental social psychology arose to confront in the first place.

Psychodynamic ideas about unconscious conflicts causing defensive extremes were popular with scientists and intellectuals suffering under the fascist populism that fueled World War II. Nobel laureate Ivan Pavlov seems to have agreed that intrapsychic conflicts could cause hostile extremes, even in dogs. Around when he was publicly condemning Stalin's fascism, he reoriented his research program toward experiments showing how motivational conflicts and uncertainties about food or pain could make his laboratory dogs "hysterical," "neurotic," and inclined toward extremes—losing balance between excitatory enthusiasm and inhibition-linked worry (Pavlov, 1927). Referencing these demonstrations, he suggested Soviet extremes were driven by the same motivational mechanics: "inhibition is eliminated, there remains only excitation . . . [that] produces all sorts of excesses in the realms of desire, thought, and behavior" (Todes, 1995, pp. 385–395). The prevailing idea was that people, dogs, and countries were going to extremes as a way to repress the conflicts and uncertainties that swirled around and within them. Even Einstein seems to have seen some promise in such psychodynamic explanations. He sent an open letter to Freud with the title "why war?" (Einstein, 1932).

Meanwhile, Lewin's early experiments were showing how uncertainties and conflicts could cause restless tension and antisocial extremes in groups of children (e.g., Lewin, 1933, 1935; Lewin et al., 1939); and frustration–aggression theorists were forwarding the idea that people and animals use aggression as a way to diffuse discomfort arising from frustrating conflicts (Dollard et al., 1939). Around the same time, neoanalytic theorists, informed by existential philosophical ideas about how difficult it is for humans to manage uncertainty about life choices, converged on the premise that conflict or uncertainty was the "worst of all pains" that motivated "escape from freedom" extremes of conformity, authoritarianism, rigidity, and hate (Adorno et al., 1950; Fromm, 1941, p. 35). Importantly, they also endorsed the corollary idea that "fascist" tendencies could be supplanted by "an increase in people's capacity to see themselves and to be themselves" (e.g., Adorno et al., p. 975). This core neoanalytic idea was elaborated by the likes of Adler, Erikson, Allport, Maslow, and Frankl, who all promoted, in various ways, the importance of authentic commitment to prosocial values as the basis for magnanimous character.

The field of experimental social psychology grew from this zeitgeist, with an initial focus on psychological causes of the intergroup conflicts and fascist extremes that animated World War II (Patnoe, 1988). Lewin was exposed to Freud, Fromm, and Adorno in Berlin and at the Frankfurt School before he was forced to flee Nazi Germany, and his own ideas shared an emphasis on vicissitudes of goal conflict and uncertainty. Like Pavlov, Lewin tried to understand extremes from the perspective of normal goal regulation gone awry. He noticed that it was normal for focus on one "psychical system" to block out awareness of others: "This sometimes astoundingly complete segregation . . . extreme exclusion . . . exclusive connection . . . with one special region of inner tensions makes ordered action possible" (Lewin, 1935, p. 55). From there he claimed that to relieve the uncomfortable state of tension arising from motivational conflicts, people defensively mobilize this palliative capacity for single-mindedness by turning to delusional fantasy, compensatory substitution, deference to authority, obduracy, affective outbursts, and fits of rage (Lewin, 1933, pp. 609–610; Lewin, 1935, pp. 103, 145). In 1945 he founded his Research Center for Group Dynamics at MIT to illuminate causes of intergroup hostility. There, Festinger's theory about the irrational and worldview defensive consequences of cognitive conflict gathered momentum. Since those early days, thousands of studies have continued to investigate how cognitive dissonance and other varieties of conflict and uncertainty can cause extreme reactions that are self-serving, rigid, aggressive, and worldview defensive (reviewed in McGregor et al., 2019; Xu & McGregor, 2018).

From the early emphasis on conflicts and cognitive dissonance as noxious causes of reactive extremes, two branches of experimental social psychology led to the main ideas advanced in this chapter. One focused on how diverse threats can all cause the same family of defensive reactions. For example, hundreds of experiments demonstrate that confronting research participants with diverse threats, from dissonance and uncertainty to failure, rejection, or death reminders, can interchangeably cause various forms of hostility, self-enhancement, worldview defense, or compensatory conviction about personal opinions (reviewed in Jonas et al., 2014; McGregor, 2006; McGregor et al., 2019). The other branch focused on how proactive focus on personal values, or other kinds of self-affirmations that make people feel good about themselves, can make people immune to distress and free from defensive reactions after threats (e.g., Sherman, 2013). Together, these two branches roughly mirror the Adorno and colleagues (1950) claims that threats cause defensive extremes, and that capacity to see and be oneself can supplant the allure of such defensive extremes.

Why are such diverse threats capable of interchangeably causing an array of defensive reactions, far from the topic or domain of the eliciting threat? Forty years of theorizing in social psychology ran with Allport's (1943) "fluid compensation" idea that the various threats on the one hand and defenses/affirmations on the other must somehow respectively deplete or replenish a reservoir of some central need—for example, for cognitive consistency, esteem, control, integrity, immortality, relational security/belonging, or meaning maintenance (Hart et al., 2005; Heine et al., 2006; Kay et al., 2009; McGregor et al., 2001; Solomon et al., Chapter 6, this volume; Steele et al., 1988; Tesser, 2000; reviewed in Jonas et al., 2014). As these various need-reservoir accounts competed with each other in the literature, the broadest definitions of the central need had the explanatory advantage that diverse threats, defenses, and values could most easily fit under their canopies. For example, Steele (1988, p. 262) proposed that threats undermine, and defenses or affirmations restore "perceived adequacy or integrity of the self." Such broad reservoir metaphors have been generative, but the premise of this chapter is that they could be even more so with further understanding of how they map onto neuromotivational processes that underlie them.

Continuing where Pavlov left off, this chapter attributes threat, defense, and value-affirmation dynamics to output from primitive motivational systems that evolved to facilitate goal regulation. Normally, any kind of threat that renders goal progress uncertain activates the anxiety-linked goal/behavioral inhibition system (G/BIS) that evolved to help vertebrates "look out" and get ready to disengage and reorient toward more viable opportunities. When goals start going well again, the G/BIS subsides and the "lock-in" goal/behavioral approach system (G/BAS) rivets enthusiastic focus to engagement in the more viable goal. BIS and BAS (Gray & McNaughton, 1982/2000) were recently renamed as GIS and GAS (McNaughton & Gray, 2024) to account for their applicability to goal-related intentions and values as well as to behaviors. The main idea in this chapter is that joint dynamics of the G/BIS and G/BAS systems are what drive threat, defense, and value-affirmation processes (Jonas et al., 2014; McGregor, 2006).

WORLDVIEW DEFENSE AS DYSREGULATION OF G/BAS "LOCK-IN" AND G/BIS "LOOK-OUT" MODES

At least since Pavlov's ideas about his dogs' excitatory and inhibitory tendencies, motivational and personality theorists have proposed that goals are jointly regulated by modes that either lock organisms in when goals are going well or help them disengage and switch when goals get impeded by conflict, uncertainty, or worry about possible danger. Theory and research on G/BAS and G/BIS brain systems (McNaughton & Gray, 2024) evolved directly from Pavlov's/Eysenck's ideas about traits and states related to excitation/extraversion and inhibition/neuroticism (Corr & Perkins, 2006). G/BAS activation bolsters goal commitment and locked-in attentional engagement free from distractions and is rewarded by dopaminergically mediated feelings of vitality and strength (see also, Carver & White, 1994; Domachowska et al., 2016; Harmon-Jones et al., 2009). In contrast, G/BIS activation mediated by septo-hippocampal neural activity weakens tenacity and helps organisms look out with diffuse vigilance beyond the current goal (i.e., in the environment or self) in order to find a way to adjust course or disengage when they face impedance from possible threats, conflicts, or uncertainties. G/BIS-arousal undermines engagement by making people feel less confident and more anxious (and bored and tired; see Britton, 2023; Hockey, 2013; Inzlicht et al., 2015; Mercer-Lynn et al., 2014). It also mutes the incentive value of ongoing goals, directly inhibits G/BAS engagement, and at the same time heightens diffuse scanning for problems or alternative opportunities. Activation of either G/BIS or G/BAS mutes activation of the other system (evidence reviewed in Jonas et al., 2014), which is how G/BAS–G/BIS toggling in response to changing circumstances normally sustains engagement in viable goals.

Crucially, however, a feature of human cognition and motivation with profound implications for human coexistence is that idealistic extremes and anger are G/BAS activating (Carver & Harmon-Jones, 2009; Jonas et al., 2014) and so can be directly rewarding by way of the vitality they animate and indirectly rewarding by way of the BIS-related distress they mute. Seizing on hostile worldviews can accordingly be a potent way to activate G/BAS for palliative relief from G/BIS-mediated malaise. Doing so also narrows perspective around the focal view—the lock-in feature of G/BAS activation (Harmon-Jones & Gable, 2009). Such extreme and constricted perspectives can become overly confident and oblivious to others' perspectives and interpersonal cues (as in mania; Harmon-Jones et al., 2002). In such circumstances, imagined consensus inflates as it becomes increasingly difficult to imagine how anyone could disagree with one's own extreme perspective (McGregor et al., 2005; cf. Horney, 1950, p. 184). Such extreme and blinkered states are unwise and maladaptive insofar as they are out of touch with reality (Grossman et al., 2020), but they are palliative (G/BIS muting) and so are reinforced (McGregor et al., 2012).

Hijacking normal G/BIS–G/BAS dynamics to maintain the palliative benefits of G/BAS activation can be especially alluring for humans due to our evolved capacity for radical (G/BIS-activating) uncertainty, as highlighted in existential philosophy. For humans, any concrete goal can become mired in uncertainty by merely asking increasingly more abstract "why" questions. Multiple alternative selves can also be imagined at the abstract level of priorities and values, with potential for chronic uncertainty and BIS-linked distress about the interrelated questions of what to do and who to be. The main idea in this chapter is that either rigid defenses conducive to authoritarian worldviews or authentic values can help resolve such distress via the G/BAS-linked vigor they arouse and the BIS-linked distress that G/BAS activation can quell. Either way, the key to understanding the power and allure of ideological or idealistic values is to understand them as abstract goals (Sagiv & Schwartz, 2022) that are especially potent because they can be reliably engaged by mere contemplation (cf. Klinger, 1977). Enthusiastic commitment to them, or the worldviews that carry them, can activate G/BAS by reflection or devotion. From this perspective, authentic commitment to identity-consolidating values (a.k.a. seeing and being oneself; Adorno et al., 1950) can supplant hostile worldview extremes because authentic identities and worldview extremes are alternative ways to cope with the G/BIS activation endemic to the human condition (see Figure 30.1). They serve the same purpose. Either can reliably spur G/BAS-activated relief via approach of the values (abstract goals) they promote. Moreover, augmenting them with anger can further fan the G/BAS flames, because anger also promotes G/BAS activation (Carver & Harmon-Jones, 2009).

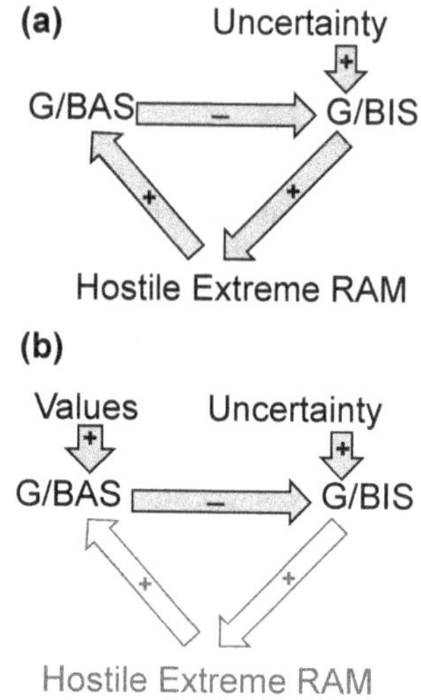

FIGURE 30.1. (a) Hostile extreme RAM or (b) preemptive values supplant RAM.

CONFIDENCE FROM CONSENSUS

Echoing classic sociological ideas about how social consensus helps bolster commitment to values, Festinger's first theory (before dissonance) emphasized that confidence in abstract ideas requires social consensus because abstractions lack objective criteria (Festinger, 1954; see also Hardin & Higgins, 1996). People reflexively turn to consensus as a way to bolster personal confidence in the priorities that abstract values represent. This kind of confidence about abstract values is crucial because goal regulation is guided by identity-related boundaries that constrain the potential for chronic G/BIS-linked anxiety from unlimited capacity to imagine conflicting possibilities for action (Hirsh et al., 2012). Beyond the bolstered *intra*personal confidence and freedom from uncertainty that consensus brings, other sociologically informed theories in social psychology emphasize how value-related consensus in shared reality also functions to bind groups together, conferring the adaptive capacity for enthusiastic collective and personal action (Elnakouri et al., 2023; Gómez et al., 2024; Graham & Haidt, 2010). Beyond these pragmatic personal-confidence-consolidating and social-cooperation-facilitating functions of values, this chapter emphasizes an immediate palliative reward that confident commitment to authoritarian or authentic values can confer—of vigor from G/BAS activation and distress-relief from downregulation of the BIS.

The neoanalytic theories of personal development that gained traction after World War II focused mostly on the palliative allure of consensus. They incorporated the existentialists' idea that fascist conformity, guarded by hate, is a kind of foreclosure that saves people from agonizing personal uncertainty about what they might authentically value. In power-vaunting and vulnerability-shaming environments, the prolonged uncertainty/vulnerability required to notice authentic preferences from the bottom up can feel too humiliating, especially when such attunement reveals vulnerable yearnings for acceptance and closeness with others. Foreclosing on coercive top-down norms of powerful groups provides immediate G/BAS relief from G/BIS-activating vulnerability. Authoritarian zeal operates as a kind of militant superego that represses vulnerability, leaving no room for uncertainty and no cracks of weakness. In G/BAS and G/BIS terms, the power, status, and certainty that can come from identification with powerful groups is alluring because it can activate G/BAS for immediate G/BIS relief (Jonas et al., 2014; cf. Fritsche, 2022; Hogg, 2021).

The clear distinction between bottom-up authenticity and top-down authoritarianism is not so clear-cut in reality, however. Shared worldviews are not always just gateways to authoritarian conformity. They can also scaffold authentic and prosocial identity by providing thematic support for the "stories we live by" (McAdams, 1993; Taylor, 1989). Even so, the challenge of integrating idiosyncratic preferences with consensual worldview templates still makes relatively authoritarian hostility alluring as a path toward immediately confident, G/BAS-activated relief for uncertainty-laced identities.

DEFENSIVE EXTREMES, AND HOW AUTHENTIC VALUES CAN SUPPLANT THEM

Over 80 years of experiments since Lewin show that diverse, vulnerability-inducing threats can cause various forms of hostile extremes and worldview defenses (reviewed in Jonas et al., 2014). Most of that evidence is from pre-2012 studies, however, and advances in statistical and methodological research practices have made it clear that conclusions from this foundational work should be reassessed with new evidence from preregistered studies with larger samples and fewer experimenter degrees of freedom. In what remains I emphasize newer research that supports the foundational claims that (1) people defend against the anxious uncertainty aroused by various threats by going to extremes; (2) salience of authentic personal values can supplant the reactive extremes; and (3) defensive extremes and effects of values are mediated by dynamics of G/BIS and G/BAS activation, as illustrated in Figure 30.1. Authentic values supplant reactive worldview extremes because they serve the same G/BAS-activating and G/BIS-muting function.

From Early Work to Preregistered, Large-N Evidence for a G/BIS–G/BAS View of Threat–Defense Dynamics

The ideas in Figure 30.1a help make sense of research on reactions to experimental manipulations of dissonance, ego depletion, and personal uncertainty, all of which confront participants with predicaments that hinge on conflict between or among actions, goals, and preferences. The first cognitive dissonance experiments manipulated this kind of conflict by subtly inducing participants to freely do things that conflicted with their opinions or preferences (e.g., to argue persuasively for points they disagreed with). To quell the discomfort arising from this hypocrisy-related conflict, the standard finding was that participants would claim to have had initial opinions or preferences that were in line with what they had done. This kind of motivated attitude change lowers feelings of being bothered, uneasy, and uncomfortable and appears to happen without awareness, as a kind of nonconscious rationalization. Evidence that such defenses are mediated by a shift from conflict-induced G/BIS to G/BAS activation comes from the action model of dissonance (Harmon-Jones et al., 2009) research with self-report and neural evidence for G/BIS activation being aroused after conflicts and G/BAS activation after reactive resolution.

The same motivational dynamics may also account for how another kind of action-based conflict disrupts motivation and judgment. Manipulations in "ego-depletion" research require participants to follow boring and/or tedious instructions that go against their predilections to do something else. Hundreds of experiments have found that such manipulations can cause subsequent malaise and various forms of dysregulation and hostility in unrelated domains (Baumeister & Vohs, 2016). From the basic motivational perspective of this chapter these demonstrations that action-based conflicts can cause dysregulation in unrelated domains extends the range of effects typically found in cognitive dissonance experiments. New cognitive dissonance research justifies the theoretical merger of dissonance and ego-depletion literatures into a single category of action-based conflicts by showing that in classic cognitive dissonance paradigms, simply following instructions to act against one's preferences (regardless of free choice) can be enough to cause subsequent discomfort and defensive rationalization (Viadis et al., 2024).

Ego-depletion manipulations, such as having to follow complicated instructions to do a tedious task (e.g., crossing out some of the letter-*e* instances in a boring article, or having to write stories without using letters *A* or *N*, or having to watch an evocative film without showing emotion) cause generalized malaise characterized by fatigue, behavioral passivity, inability to persevere on difficult tasks, and a seemingly lazy lack of initiative in problem solving or goal pursuit (Baumeister & Vohs, 2016). Such malaise is consistent with characteristics of G/BIS activation that include direct inhibition and muted incentive value of ongoing goals (Hockey, 2013; McNaughton & Gray, 2024). Beyond causing such seemingly G/BIS-related states, depletion manipulations also heighten behavioral volatility and reduce one's ability to control impulsive indulgences in G/BAS-activating experiences. For example, depletion manipulations have heightened subsequent prejudice, aggression, boasting, sexual license, ethical risk-taking, and indulgences with money, food, addictive substances, extremes, greed, selfish choices, and wishful thinking (Baumeister & Vohs, 2016).

Evidence that these categories of response may represent a G/BIS-motivated shift toward G/BAS activation comes from results indicating that in addition to the malaise they initially can cause, depletion manipulations orient people toward approach-motivation-related cues—for example, noticing money cues more quickly, making riskier monetary bets, or reporting more enthusiasm for incentives in general (Schmeichel et al., 2010). There is also neural evidence for reactive G/BAS activation after depletion manipulations (Schmeichel et al., 2016; relative left frontal cortical activation, the same neural shift as with dissonance reduction, Harmon-Jones et al., 2009). Loss of self-control after depletion manipulations could accordingly arise directly from residual G/BIS-induced inhibition and feelings of fatigue, or also indirectly from reactive BAS-induced impulsiveness. The role of G/BIS in either case is supported by evidence from a multilab project (N = 3,531) in which ego-depletion manipulations caused self-reported fatigue that moderated the tendency to give up on a subsequent task that required concentrated effort (Vohs et al., 2021). Like some other recent efforts to replicate ego-depletion findings, this multilab project by Vohs and colleagues (2021) failed to support its focal, main-effect hypothesis, that common depletion manipulations (e.g., letter-*e*-crossing) would cause common depletion outcomes (loss of persistence on an impossible line-tracing task). Intriguingly, however, the fatigue-moderation finding is theoretically consistent with the proposed role of BIS activation because a kind of fatigue (bored malaise and loss of enthusiasm for goals) is a cardinal feature of BIS activation (Britton, 2023; Hockey, 2013; McNaughton & Gray, 2024).

Dozens of experiments have found that direct personal uncertainty manipulations can have the same kinds of effects as dissonance and ego depletion on G/BIS and RAM for personal or group-based extremes (reviewed in Jonas et al., 2014; see also Hogg, 2021; Randles et al., 2015). Similarities between effects of personal uncertainty and depletion manipulations were highlighted in a preregistered study (N = 337; Alquist et al., 2018). Experimentally manipulated uncertainty, induced by having participants ruminate about a real-life dilemma versus writing about a clear, high-value one, increased self-reported affect related to dissonance and G/BIS activation (e.g., bothered, uneasy, uncertain, torn, confused, anxious; cf. Franchina et al., 2024; Harmon-Jones et al., 2009). Importantly, this specific affect then mediated the standard ego-depletion effect of taking longer to complete a word-puzzle task. Participants in the uncertainty condition were also over three times more likely than participants in the clear value condition to impulsively quit the study before completion.

Other kinds of threats that have caused extreme reactions in past research also caused evidence of BIS activation and depletion-like loss of self-control. For example, in a preregistered within-subjects experiment, writing about relationship problems (vs. desires or values) heightened BIS-related affect (torn, confused, indecisive, uncertain, chaotic, conflicted) that mediated feelings of boredom and decreased self-control (anticipated) at the thought of completing the rest of the study materials (Britton, 2023, Study 7). Similarly, in a preregistered, between-subjects experiment (Britton, 2023, Study 2 and preregistered replication Study 3, collapsed, total N = 819), writing about personal death for a few minutes (vs. dental pain) specifically heightened the same G/BIS-related affect (i.e., torn, confused, indecisive, uncertain, chaotic, conflicted; but not generalized negative affect). Moreover, the G/BIS affect that was aroused by what the participants had written about serially mediated feelings of boredom and loss of self-control for real-life personal projects (as preregistered). The G/BIS-related affect aroused by writing about personal death also serially mediated (as preregistered) boredom and lost self-control on a speeded data-entry task that participants had pledged to fully engage without checking their phones (they entered fewer characters and checked their phones more). These findings are consistent with other evidence that mortality salience is an initially G/BIS-activating threat that can make people apathetic and impulsive (reviewed in Jonas et al., 2014; see also Hayes et al., 2016). Given that mortality salience (and salience of relationship troubles) have also caused hostile worldview defense extremes and/or G/BAS-linked RAM in dozens of previous experiments (reviewed in Jonas et al., 2014), this new evidence connects G/BIS with G/BAS evidence to support the idea that threats cause extremes, for the reasons depicted in Figure 30.1a.

Other new experimental research on defensive extremes after diverse psychological threats is increasingly finding evidence for both G/BIS and G/BAS involvement. Two preregistered experiments (N = 1,252; Willardt & Schmid, 2024) found that powerlessness-related threats caused G/BIS-linked (anxious) affect, which mediated more extremely partisan allegiances to political and football-fan ingroups (i.e., elevated perceptions of ingroup entitativity, homogeneity, and consensus). Other preregistered experiments (N = 432; Leota et al., 2023) found that experimentally manipulated worries about academic competence caused money-losing recklessness in a task in which participants could earn money by fully pumping up but not popping balloons (students in the worries condition impulsively popped more). Importantly, G/BIS affect (anxious, confused, uncertain, frustrated, insecure) mediated the recklessness, and the recklessness effect was most pronounced among participants with high G/BAS-trait scores, presumably because they had readier access to use of G/BAS states to use for G/

BIS-muting purposes. Results from a second experiment reported in the same research conceptually replicated this result with the same balloon-popping measure of recklessness and the same G/BAS-trait measure, but with a different experimentally induced threat (economic uncertainty) and an electroencephalographic (EEG) measure (medial right frontal theta) instead of self-report measure of G/BIS activation. Together, these recent results from preregistered and large-*N* studies give some cause for continued confidence in conclusions from the first generation of research on RAM reactions to G/BIS-activating threats (reviewed in Jonas et al., 2014).

One limitation of RAM research is that the dependent variables have tended to focus on either demonstrating reactive G/BAS activation in personal goals and neural measures, or on demonstrating effects on specific kinds of extremes related to elements of hostile worldview defense (e.g., exaggerated certainty, conviction, or consensus about opinions). The logic has been that these various elements help push the lever people use to flip motivation from G/BIS to G/BAS. However, studies rarely assessed the motivational substrates together with composite-dependent measures related to hostile worldview defense (e.g., ethnocentrism). This limitation has been recently addressed by three experiments ($N = 1{,}078$; Klackl et al., 2024) in which false feedback about poor scores on an academic achievement test (in two of the studies) or mortality salience (in the third) caused especially extreme ethnocentrism and derogation of foreigners among participants with high G/BIS and high G/BAS scores. This new evidence for involvement of high G/BIS and high G/BAS replicates the few small studies that had previously suggested that effects of mortality salience on worldview defense were jointly modulated by G/BIS activation and G/BAS reactions (reviewed in Jonas et al., 2014).

This new work is important because mortality salience effects on worldview-related extremes were the most common demonstrations of defensive zeal in the experimental social psychological literature in the 1990s and 2000s. The terror management theory interpretation of such results is that worldview defenses after mortality salience that emphasize personal connection to cultural meanings help make people feel symbolically immortal and thereby buffered from anxiety (Solomon et al., Chapter 6, this volume). The Klackl and colleagues results (2024, Study 3, from reanalysis of data from a multilab attempt to replicate the effect of mortality salience on worldview defense) are consistent with the interpretation that the potential for anxiety aroused by mortality salience (Greenberg et al., 2003) is G/BIS-linked. They are also consistent with the interpretation that feelings of symbolic immortality and immunity from mortality-related anxiety may arise from the G/BAS that meaningful worldview defenses activate. People with high trait scores related to G/BAS are especially inclined to defensively mobilize both state-G/BAS activation, and worldview defenses after mortality salience (Jonas et al., 2014; McGregor, 2006). High trait and experimentally manipulated state G/BAS also predict perceptions of meaning in life (Elnakouri, 2018; Elnakouri et al., 2022) that robustly predict self-control, hope, self-esteem, self-compassion, and freedom from boredom, stress, and depression (correlations between $r = .4$ and $r = .6$, McGregor, unpublished data, 2024, $N > 700$).

Additional new evidence linking mortality salience effects on worldview defense to the more general RAM interpretation illustrated in Figure 30.1a comes from three new experimental results ($N = 683$; Stollberg et al., 2024) showing that mortality salience, relationship uncertainties, and loss of control (vs. more neutral topics) can cause discrepancies that elevate G/BIS affect (e.g., worried, nervous, afraid, inhibited, scared, jittery) and also cause reactive value extremes that elevate G/BAS affect (e.g., determined, strong, active, alert). In these studies, the value extremes were not necessarily antisocial, and the study design did not allow for assessment of whether or not the reactive G/BAS muted the G/BIS that catalyzed the reaction in the first place. Evidence for specifically antisocial extremes activating G/BAS and muting G/BIS can be found in two other recent experiments (Elnakouri et al., 2022; $N = 762$; Study 2 preregistered) in which experimentally manipulated collective hate caused more G/BAS affect (determined, enthusiastic, eager) and less G/BIS affect (confused, conflicted, uncertain). This finding extends past work on anger as a G/BAS-activating state (Carver & Harmon-Jones, 2009) and helps make sense of why worldview extremes can so easily become hateful—extremes and hate can both converge on similarly confident (G/BAS) states that are rewarded by (G/BIS) relief.

Meaningful Values, G/BIS–G/BAS Dynamics, and Freedom from Defensive Extremes (Figure 30.1b)

A hopeful note arising from the previously described Stollberg and colleagues (2024) studies is that RAM reactions to various threats are not necessarily hostile. When faced with anxious predicaments, people need potent and reliable cues to lean into, as a lever for G/BAS-activating relief. As reviewed in Jonas and colleagues (2014), after various threats people will become either more hostile or magnanimous, depending on which kind of social cues are most salient. If personal ideals and values are highly salient, threatened people will tend to lean more strongly into them. These kinds of findings (e.g., Jonas et al., 2008; Schumann et al., 2014; but see the Schindler et al., 2023, call for preregistered replications) are compatible with the early neoanalytic speculation that authentic identity commitments revolving around prosocial and generative values can shield people from fascist reactions to conflict and uncertainty, either by providing an alternative (and less antisocial) lever for RAM, or by supplanting the need for RAM in the first place, with proactive value focus.

If prosocial values are central to core identity commitments, then they will be chronically accessible for use to fortify G/BAS and shield against G/BIS in anxious circumstances. Developmentally, frustration–aggression-like reactions to anxious uncertainty may be normative before prosocial identities are consolidated. Anger, resentment, and aggression are always readily available to reliably activate G/BAS for short-term G/BIS relief in stressful circumstances and such indulgences require no vulnerability, soul-searching, or moral commitment. They are immediately rewarding insofar as they provide G/BAS-activated G/BIS relief. Over time, hostile reactions and syndromes of cynicism and resentment are conducive to downward spirals of dysfunction and alienation, however (Allen et al., 2018; Stavrova, 2020). In contrast, habitually turning toward identity-congruent highest values may more likely get positively reinforced over time, not just by immediate G/BAS-activating and G/BIS-muting relief, but also by upward spirals of resilience, adaptive functioning, and social rewards (Crocker et al., 2008, 2017).

Prosocial values are not the only viable basis for a meaningful identity, however. In the preregistered Elnakouri and colleagues (2022) research in which collective hate caused higher G/BAS and lower G/BIS, those motivational shifts jointly mediated perceptions of more meaning in life. If meaningful identities and values usually revolved around hate, then that would negate Figure 30.1b effects. Importantly, however, when people are asked about their highest values in life, they usually nominate self-transcendent ones related to loving and helping (McGregor et al., 2022b; Sagiv & Schwartz, 2022, in 63 societies tested). Moreover, love-related (vs. self-enhancing) values are especially good at making people less defensive under threat (Burson et al., 2012; Crocker et al., 2008; Shnabel et al., 2013) and so are presumably most likely to be reinforced over time by the effectiveness they promote and the BIS activation they mute (cf. Creswell et al., 2005). Finally, prosocial values appear especially effective at sustaining meaning (Bojanowska & Piotrowski, 2021), perhaps because they are rated by observers as especially virtuous (King & Napa, 1998; Twenge & King, 2005), which may stabilize and bolster them with easy-to-garner validation and consensus.

Incorporating such prosocial values into the fabric of daily lives and personal projects has long been associated with meaning in life and higher BAS and lower BIS (McGregor & Little, 1998; McGregor et al., 2012). Moreover, a series of preregistered experiments (total N = 740) demonstrates that the causal effect of highest-value focus on meaning is jointly mediated by elevated BAS and muted BIS (McGregor, 2024, unpublished data). These results are consistent with the finding that, especially among meaning-oriented people, prosocial value focus increases G/BAS activation (see McGregor et al., 2022b, for converging self-report and EEG evidence; Kang et al., 2018, for functional magnetic resonance imaging [fMRI] evidence). Together, these results are consistent with Adorno and colleagues' (1950) and other neoanalytic theorists' seminal claim that rigid and hostile worldview defenses can be ameliorated by authentic identity commitments to prosocial values. Prosocial value salience supplants antisocial worldview defenses because they are alternative routes to the same motivational state (see Figure 30.1b).

Empirical support for this claim comes from two experiments ($N = 677$; McGregor et al., 2022b) in which all participants were confronted by BIS-arousing uncertainties and conflicts. Writing about highest values, compassionate actions, or spirituality (as compared to other values, power, or desire) supplanted participants' tendency to react with hostile and ideological extremes, that is, with severe punishments for moral transgressors or with partisan hostility about religious allegiances. Importantly, the extremism-reducing effects of the values and related phenomena were mediated by the higher G/BAS activation aroused while writing about them. Results were consistent across the two experiments, regardless of whether the G/BAS activation was assessed with a self-report or a neural (EEG) measure of G/BAS-linked relative left prefrontal activation.

These findings complement past evidence from hundreds of experiments showing that proactive focus on highest personal values can quell distress and defensiveness after threats by "untethering" people from preoccupation with "a state of vigilance in which the threat commands their attention" (Sherman et al., 2021, p. 71). They support a clear G/BIS–G/BAS account for *how* the untethering occurs, and advance understanding of for whom value affirmations should be most effective. In both studies, effects occurred only among participants with relatively high trait meaning-search scores that reflect an orientation toward finding meaning in life. This moderation replicates the past finding that value affirmations caused fMRI evidence of BAS activation that mediated freedom from defensiveness about lifestyle choices, but only among participants oriented toward self-transcendent meaning (Kang et al., 2018).

Converging evidence for the defensiveness-relieving power of prosocial value commitments comes from three studies on how anxious distress interacts with personality traits related to prosocial value commitments to predict RAM-related extremism (McGregor et al., 2022a; $N = 1{,}163$). In the first, experimentally manipulated focus on real-life anxious uncertainties about relationships or economic viability (vs. benign topics) caused more extreme endorsement of religious zeal scale items such as "if I was convinced God wanted me to do something extreme, I would do it," and "God makes me powerful." A RAM interpretation of the results is bolstered by the findings that the effects occurred only among participants with high scores on a BAS-related trait (as in the Klackl et al. [2024] and the Leota et al. [2023] studies; see discussion of similar BAS-trait moderation in research reviewed in Jonas et al., 2014). Crucially, there was also a three-way interaction such that the reactive religious extremes were only present among participants with relatively low scores on a trait that reflects identity commitment to personally meaningful values, that is, referring to focus on hopes, aspirations, ideals, ambitions, and identity integrity (Lockwood et al., 2002). This three-way interaction indicates that, as in studies showing a reduction in defensive extremism after experimentally manipulated value affirmation, there is also an apparent reduction in reactive extremism when values are chronically salient among people with strong identity commitments to them (see McGregor et al., 2015, for further discussion of how weak identity moderates religious radicalization). The second experiment in this series conceptually replicated the finding with the same moderator variables but a different threat (mortality salience) and a different measure of reactive extremism (punitive reactions to moral deviants). The third did the same with measured stress instead of manipulated threat, and with authoritarianism and social dominance orientation as the dependent variables. These authentic-identity/value findings are consistent with evidence from hundreds of experiments with smaller sample sizes and weaker methods, from the 1970s to the 2010s, showing proactive focus on highest personal values can make people less stressed and less defensive after various threats (reviewed in Cohen & Sherman, 2014).

DISCUSSION

The RAM perspective on threat, defense, and affirmation provides an integrative theoretical account for the many guises of threat and defense dynamics in the experimental social psychology literature. The underlying motivational account described here does not "explain away" the more metaphorical accounts. Rather, it helps ground them in neuromotivational processes that have been on psychological scientists' radar since Pavlov tried to test the Freudian premise that conflicts cause reactive extremes. For example, according to the RAM account, proactive and prosocial focus on highest personal values arouses G/BAS activation. It mutes G/BIS activation in stressful circumstances, thereby making it unnecessary to use hostile extremes for the same purpose. A cardinal output of G/BIS activation is that it increases vigilant attention to the domain of the threat (McNaughton & Gray, 2024). Dissolving G/BIS activation via G/BAS activation accordingly provides a simple explanation for *how* highest-value focus can "untether" the self-concept from stressful experiences (cf. Crichter & Dunning, 2015). As another example of how a basic process model might help clarify more metaphorical theorizing, terror management theory contends that worldview defenses like derogating cultural outgroup members provide an anxiety buffer via the symbolic immortality conferred by defending and identifying with cultural standards of value (Solomon et al., Chapter 6, this volume). Understanding worldview defenses as convictions people seize on for G/BIS-muting G/BAS activation provides a simple way to understand *how* they buffer mortality-related anxiety.

The field of experimental social psychology began as an effort to understand motivation for the fascist and hostile extremes that propelled the intergroup conflicts around World War II. Inspired by psychodynamic theory, Pavlov (1927) and Lewin (e.g., 1933) proposed that motivational and cognitive conflicts were to blame. Dogs, toddlers, and people react to such conflicts by having tantrums and going to extremes to relieve the distress arising from the conflicts. Since those early days and in the 80 years since the dawn of experimental social psychology with Lewin's research group at MIT, thousands of experiments have found that conflicts and various other kinds of uncertainty-related psychological threats and frustrations do indeed cause people to go to extremes that often seem far removed from the topics of the threats. The RAM understanding forwarded in this chapter brings the general explanation for this tendency back full circle to Pavlov's speculation about his dogs reacting to uncertainties (G/BIS) by becoming extremely excitatory (G/BAS), and Lewin's ideas about fantasy and rage serving to exclude motivational tensions from awareness. The G/BIS evolved specifically to respond to motivational conflicts and uncertainties with anxious distress and vigilance (McNaughton & Gray, 2024). Anything that downregulates the G/BIS in such circumstances should accordingly be reinforced. G/BAS can do so (reviewed in Jonas et al., 2014), which is why hostile defenses that activate it (anger, hate, extremes, worldview convictions) can become habitual in threatening circumstances.

The key to understanding how values or worldviews that carry them can activate G/BAS is that values are abstract goals that can spur enthusiastic approach motivation (self-report, EEG, and fMRI evidence reviewed in McGregor et al., 2022b). People who are oriented toward finding meaning in life can readily activate G/BAS states by merely thinking about their high values, that is, even more readily than from thinking about concrete goals related to power or desire (McGregor et al., 2022b). Due to their abstract nature, however, they can require some consensual social or cultural support for confidence, because these high values are difficult to justify objectively. Consensual worldviews are accordingly useful vehicles for reliable mobilization of confident values to palliate

G/BIS-linked distress. Given the G/BAS-activating power of anger and hate, however, it is also easy for hostility to taint worldviews for an especially potent anxiety-buffer.

The present chapter illuminates why worldviews laced with anger, hate, and extremes can be so alluring in frustrating and uncertain circumstances. The reemergence of far-right politics in countries across the globe highlights this potent cocktail of rewarding ingredients—jingoism, cynical resentment, punitive blame, and fascist ideology—that can activate the G/BAS and mute the G/BIS by mere identification. While some people might be talked down from addiction to this cocktail by appeals to reasonable and practical alternatives, it is not always effective to treat addictions with appeals to rationality. Addictions can be irrationally mediated by G/BAS-linked, dopaminergic "wanting," even when the addict is well aware that they no longer really even like what they want (Berridge & Robinson, 2016; cf. Dixon et al., 2018, on "dark flow"). From this perspective, a more effective strategy could be to find something else to powerfully and reliably activate the wanting system, to supplant interest in the angry addiction. It is now clear that focusing on highest personal values can do that. Like hateful worldview extremes, values can activate the G/BAS, thereby supplanting the allure of angry extremes by way of a kind of "higher power" (McGregor et al., 2022b). As illustrated in Figure 30.1b, the self-transcendent, prosocial values that most people spontaneously identify with when focusing on their highest values can be an effective antidote to defensive extremes. This capacity of value focus to relieve G/BIS-linked anxious distress and defensive extremes in domains far removed from the value focus is not mediated by pragmatic consideration or reasonableness. Rather, it is a nonconsciously mediated switcheroo. The values make the extremes motivationally redundant.

Analogous approaches are increasingly guiding deradicalization programs. A conventional approach to deradicalization policy emphasizes reeducation with a focus on pragmatic and economic benefits of deradicalizing (e.g., Public Safety Canada, 2024). Sociologists who have infiltrated terror groups, however, see avenues for prosocial self-transcendence as vital for successful deradicalization. Radicalization often arises from profound uncertainties that make the vigorous moral engagement of self-righteous anger and religious extremism appealing (Atran, 2015; Dawson & Amarasingam, 2017; McGregor et al., 2015; cf. Hogg, 2021; Kruglanski et al., 2014). The findings in this chapter are compatible with Atran's (2015) conclusion that for successful deradicalization, "sacred value must be fought with other sacred values. . . . violent extremism represents not the resurgence of traditional cultures, but their collapse, as young people unmoored from millennial traditions flail about in search of a social identity that gives personal significance and glory."

All religions, at their best, promote the idea that humans have a vulnerability toward selfish and hostile habits, and that salvation can come from orienting toward tenets of the faith that include commitment to prosocial values. This theme was present in the first known human story, of King Gilgamesh (Mitchell, 2004), whose "restless heart" drove him to hostile and self-serving extremes until an experience of graceful hospitality, compassionately purveyed by the immortal Utnapishtim, oriented him toward generativity, at which point the anxiety and extremes receded. The Buddhist eightfold path similarly emphasizes disciplined orientation toward prosocial virtue as the way to liberate oneself from the anxious dukkha of ignorant craving, clinging, and hostility (Bodhi, 2010). Greek moral philosophy presents a variation on this theme most evident with Plato, but also detectable with Pythagoras, Aristotle, and the Stoics (Tarnas, 1991). Turning toward the light of ideals or attempting to actualize one's essence through virtue can support true well-being (eudaimonia) and liberation from the shadowy chains of ignorance and despair (e.g., as illustrated in Plato's allegory of the cave). Liberal/metaphorical interpretations of Christianity similarly interpret redemption as a psychological shift from anxiety-provoking preoccupation with getting and winning to a new identity focused on self-transcendent values focused on compassion and service (e.g., Borg, 2009).

This chapter suggests at least part of the way "religious rapture" and "moral enthusiasm" unify the "discordant self" and make the "sand and grit of self-hood incline to disappear" (James, 1902/1958 pp. 58, 240, 399) is through the G/BAS-activating power of the self-transcendent value commitments that religious and moral enthusiasms promote. In the same way RAM theory can help specify mechanisms beneath metaphorical theories in psychology, it could do the same for religions (McGregor et al., 2022b; Schumann et al., 2014). Such an approach could inform ecumenical and religious reeducation efforts by furnishing an alternative and more tolerant way to understand how the power of religious faith can be something that "redeems and vivifies the interior world which otherwise would be an empty waste" (James, 1902/1958, p. 58). Such an understanding could help distinguish and disentangle the prosocial parts from the rigid extremes and hostilities that can so easily colonize religions, because prosocial values, extremes, anger, and hate run on the same G/BAS-activating and G/BIS-muting motivational platform. It could also help explain why it can be so intuitive to attribute the power of religion to some external agency from another realm. The G/BAS boost of vitality that can come from mere consideration of elevating abstract values (McGregor et al., 2012; cf. Van de Vyver & Abrams, 2017; amplified by the "collective effervescence" of consensus, Rimé & Páez, 2023) is so paradoxical and surprising it can feel like an infusion of grace and inspiration from beyond the usual realm of cause and effect (see Thrash & Elliot, 2004, for the approach motivational substrate of inspiration).

This chapter proposes that the often mysterious and closely connected powers of good and evil do indeed arise from a different realm—a neurobiological one we share with other vertebrates, of basic motivational processes that evolved before capacities for conscious awareness. Ideas and metaphors in myth, religion, philosophy, psychodynamic theory, and experimental social psychology have been revolving around dynamics of these processes for millennia. We may now be able to understand them in a more biologically based and connected way.

REFERENCES

Adorno, T. W., Frenkel-Brunswik, E., Levinson, D. J., & Sanford, R. N. (1950). *The authoritarian personality.* Harpers.

Allen, J. J., Anderson, C. A., & Bushman, B. J. (2018). The general aggression model. *Current Opinion in Psychology, 19,* 75–80.

Allport, G. W. (1943). The ego in contemporary psychology. *Psychological Review, 50,* 451–478.

Alquist, J. L., Baumeister, R. F., McGregor, I., Core, T. J., Benjamin, I., & Tice, D. M. (2018). Personal conflict impairs performance on an unrelated self-control task: Lingering costs of uncertainty and conflict. *Journal of Experimental Social Psychology, 74,* 157–160.

Atran, S. (2015). *The role of youth in countering violent extremism and promoting peace.* Address to the United Nations Security Council. International Centre for Muslim and Non-Muslim Understanding.

Baumeister, R. F., & Vohs, K. D. (2016). Strength model of self-regulation as limited resource: Assessment, controversies, update. In J. M. Olson & M. P. Zanna (Eds.), *Advances in experimental social psychology* (pp. 67–127). Elsevier/Academic Press.

Berridge, K. C., & Robinson, T. E. (2016). Liking, wanting, and the incentive-sensitization theory of addiction. *American Psychologist, 71,* 670.

Bodhi, B. (2010). *The noble eightfold path: The way to the end of suffering.* Buddhist Publication Society.

Bojanowska, A., & Piotrowski, K. (2021). Two levels of personality: Temperament and values and their effects on hedonic and eudaimonic well-being. *Current Psychology, 40,* 1185–1194.

Borg, M. J. (2009). *The heart of Christianity: Rediscovering a life of faith.* HarperCollins.

Britton, E. M. (2023). *The uncertainty model of boredom and self-control failure: How ambient uncertainty influences affect and behaviour during unrelated goal pursuit.* Doctoral dissertation, University of Waterloo.

Burson, A., Crocker, J., & Mischkowski, D. (2012). Two types of value-affirmation: Implications for self-control following social exclusion. *Social Psychological and Personality Science, 3,* 510–516.

Carver, C. S., & Harmon-Jones, E. (2009). Anger is an approach-related affect: Evidence and implications. *Psychological Bulletin, 135*(2), 183–204.

Carver, C. S., & White, T. L. (1994). Behavioral inhibition, behavioral activation, and affective responses to impending reward and punishment: The BIS/BAS Scales. *Journal of Personality and Social Psychology, 67,* 319–333.

Cohen, G. L., & Sherman, D. K. (2014). The psychology of change: Self-affirmation and social psychological intervention. *Annual Review of Psychology, 65,* 333–371.

Corr, P. J., & Perkins, A. M. (2006). The role of theory in the psychophysiology of personality: From Ivan Pavlov to Jeffrey Gray. *International Journal of Psychophysiology, 62,* 367–376.

Creswell, J. D., Welch, W. T., Taylor, S. E., Sherman, D. K., Gruenewald, T. L., & Mann, T. (2005). Affirmation of personal values buffers neuroendocrine and psychological stress responses. *Psychological Science, 16,* 846–851.

Critcher, C. R., & Dunning, D. (2015). Self-affirmations provide a broader perspective on self-threat. *Personality and Social Psychology Bulletin, 41*(1), 3–18.

Crocker, J., Canevello, A., & Brown, A. A. (2017). Social motivation: Costs and benefits of selfishness and otherishness. *Annual Review of Psychology, 68,* 299–325.

Crocker, J., Niiya, Y, & Mischkowski, D. (2008). Why does writing about important values reduce defensiveness?: Self-affirmation and the role of positive other-directed feelings. *Psychological Science, 19,* 740–747.

Dawson, L. L., & Amarasingam, A. (2017). Talking to foreign fighters: Insights into the motivations for Hijrah to Syria and Iraq. *Studies in Conflict & Terrorism, 40*(3), 191–210.

Dixon, M. J., Stange, M., Larche, C. J., Graydon, C., Fugelsang, J. A., & Harrigan, K. A. (2018). Dark flow, depression and multiline slot machine play. *Journal of Gambling Studies, 34,* 73–84.

Dollard, J., Doob, L. W., Miller, N. E., Mowrer, O. H., & Sears, R. R. (1939). *Frustration and aggression.* Yale University Press.

Domachowska, I., Heitmann, C., Deutsch, R., Goschke, T., Scherbaum, S., & Bolte, A. (2016). Approach-motivated positive affect reduces breadth of attention: Registered replication report of Gable and Harmon-Jones (2008). *Journal of Experimental Social Psychology, 67,* 50–56.

Einstein, A. (1932, July 30). [Letter from Albert Einstein to Sigmund Freud.] UNESCO. https://en.unesco.org/courier/may-1985/why-war-letter-albert-einstein-sigmund-freud.

Elnakouri, A. (2018). *Approach motivation gives rise to meaning in life.* Master's thesis, University of Waterloo.

Elnakouri, A., Hubley, C., & McGregor, I. (2022). Hate and meaning in life: How collective, but not personal, hate quells threat and spurs meaning in life. *Journal of Experimental Social Psychology, 98,* Article 104227.

Elnakouri, A., Rossignac-Milon, M., Krueger, K. L., Forest, A. L., Higgins, E. T., & Scholer, A. A. (2023). In it together: Shared reality with instrumental others is linked to goal success. *Journal of Personality and Social Psychology, 125*(5), 1072–1095.

Festinger, L. (1954). A theory of social comparison processes. *Human Relations, 7,* 117–140.

Franchina, V., Klackl, J., & Jonas, E. (2024). The reinforcement sensitivity theory affects questionnaire (RST-AQ). A validation study of a new scale targeting affects related to anxiety, approach motivation and fear. *Current Psychology, 43,* 5193–5205.

Freud, S. (1910). The origin and development of psychoanalysis. *American Journal of Psychology, 21,* 181–218.

Fromm, E. (1941). *Escape from freedom.* Farrar & Rinehart.

Fritsche, I. (2022). Agency through the we: Group-based control theory. *Current Directions in Psychological Science, 31,* 194–201.

Gay, P. (1989). *The Freud reader.* Norton.

Gómez, A., Vázquez, A., Alba, B., Blanco, L., Chinchilla, J., Chiclana, S., & Swann, W. B., Jr. (2024). Feeling understood fosters identity fusion. *Journal of Personality and Social Psychology.*

Graham, J., & Haidt, J. (2010). Beyond beliefs: Religions bind individuals into moral communities. *Personality and Social Psychology Review, 14,* 140–150.

Gray, J. A., & McNaughton, N. (2000) *The neuropsychology of anxiety: An inquiry into the functions of the septo-hippocampal system* (2nd ed.). Oxford University Press. (Original work published 1982)

Greenberg, J., Martens, A., Jonas, E., Eisenstadt, D., Pyszczynski, T., & Solomon, S. (2003). Psychological defense in anticipation of anxiety: Eliminating the potential for anxiety eliminates the effect of mortality salience on worldview defense. *Psychological Science, 14,* 516–519.

Grossmann, I., Weststrate, N. M., Ardelt, M., Brienza, J. P., Dong, M., Ferrari, M., . . . Vervaeke, J. (2020). The science of wisdom in a polarized world: Knowns and unknowns. *Psychological Inquiry, 31*(2), 103–133.

Hardin, C. D., & Higgins, E. T. (1996). Shared reality: How social verification makes the subjective objective. In R. M. Sorrentino & E. T. Higgins (Eds.), *Handbook of motivation and cognition: Vol. 3. The interpersonal context* (pp. 28–84). Guilford Press.

Harmon-Jones, E., Abramson, L. Y., Sigelman, J., Bohlig, A., Hogan, M. E., & Harmon-Jones, C. (2002). Proneness to hypomania/mania symptoms or depression symptoms and asymmetrical frontal cortical responses to an anger-evoking event. *Journal of personality and Social Psychology, 82,* 610.

Harmon-Jones, E., Amodio, D. M., & Harmon-Jones, C. (2009). Action-based model of dissonance: A review, integration, and expansion of conceptions of cognitive conflict. In M. P. Zanna (Ed.), *Advances in experimental social psychology* (Vol. 41, pp. 119–166). Elsevier/Academic Press.

Harmon-Jones, E., & Gable, P. A. (2009). Neural activity underlying the effect of approach-motivated positive affect on narrowed attention. *Psychological Science, 20,* 406–409.

Hart, J., Shaver, P. R., & Goldenberg, J. L. (2005). Attachment, self-esteem, worldviews, and terror management: evidence for a tripartite security system. *Journal of Personality and Social Psychology, 88*(6), 999.

Hayes, J., Ward, C. L., & McGregor, I. (2016). Why bother?: Death, failure, and fatalistic withdrawal from life. *Journal of Personality and Social Psychology, 110*(1), 96.

Heine, S. J., Proulx, T., & Vohs, K. D. (2006). The meaning maintenance model: On the coherence of social motivations. *Personality and Social Psychology Review, 10*(2), 88–110.

Hirsh, J. B., Mar, R. A., & Peterson, J. B. (2012). Psychological entropy: A framework for understanding uncertainty-related anxiety. *Psychological Review, 119,* 304.

Hockey, R. (2013). *The psychology of fatigue: Work, effort and control.* Cambridge University Press.

Hogg, M. A. (2021). Self-uncertainty and group identification: Consequences for social identity, group behavior, intergroup relations, and society. In B. Gawronski (Ed.), *Advances in experimental social psychology* (Vol. 64, pp. 263–316). Academic Press.

Horney, K. (1950). *Neurosis and human growth: The struggle toward self-realization.* Norton.

Inzlicht, M., Bartholow, B. D., & Hirsh, J. B. (2015). Emotional foundations of cognitive control. *Trends in Cognitive Sciences, 19,* 126–132.

James, W. (1958). *The varieties of religious experience.* Mentor. (Original work published 1902)

Jonas, E., Martens, A., Kayser, D. N., Fritsche, I., Sullivan, D., & Greenberg, J. (2008). Focus theory of normative conduct and terror-management theory: The interactive impact of mortality salience and norm salience on social judgment. *Journal of Personality and Social Psychology, 95,* 1239–1251.

Jonas, E., McGregor, I., Klackl, J., Agroskin, D., Fritsche, I., Holbrook, C., . . . Quirin, M. (2014). Threat and defense: From anxiety to approach. In J. M. Olson & M. P. Zanna (Eds.), *Advances in experimental social psychology* (Vol. 49, pp. 219–286). Academic Press.

Kang, Y., Cooper, N., Pandey, P., Scholz, C., O'Donnell, M. B., Lieberman, M. D., . . . Falk, E. B. (2018). Effects of self-transcendence on neural responses to persuasive messages and health behavior change. *Proceedings of the National Academy of Sciences, 115*(40), 9974–9979.

Kay, A. C., Whitson, J. A., Gaucher, D., & Galinsky, A. D. (2009). Compensatory control: Achieving order through the mind, our institutions, and the heavens. *Current Directions in Psychological Science, 18*(5), 264–268.

King, L. A., & Napa, C. K. (1998). What makes a life good? *Journal of Personality and Social Psychology, 75,* 156–165.

Klackl, J., Lüders, A., & Jonas, E. (2024). Q: What is the recipe for defense? A: Threat, anxiety, and approach motivation. *Motivation Science, 10,* 63–77.

Klein, R. A., Cook, C. L., Ebersole, C. R., Vitiello, C., Nosek, B. A., Hilgard, J., . . . Ratliff, K. A. (2022). Many Labs 4: Failure to replicate mortality salience effect with and without original author involvement. *Collabra: Psychology, 8*(1), 35271.

Klinger, E. (1977). *Meaning and void: Inner experience and the incentives in people's lives.* University of Minnesota.

Kruglanski, A. W., Gelfand, M. J., Bélanger, J. J., Sheveland, A., Hetiarachchi, M., & Gunaratna, R. (2014). The psychology of radicalization and deradicalization: How significance quest impacts violent extremism. *Political Psychology, 35,* 69–93.

Leota, J., Nash, K., & McGregor, I. (2023). Reactive risk-taking: Anxiety regulation via approach motivation increases risk-taking behavior. *Personality and Social Psychology Bulletin, 49*(1), 81–96.

Lewin, K. (1933). Environmental forces. In C. Murchison (Ed.), *A handbook of child psychology* (2nd ed., pp. 590–625). Clark University Press.

Lewin, K. (1935). *A dynamic theory of personality.* McGraw-Hill.

Lewin, K., Lippitt, R., & White, R. K. (1939). Patterns of aggressive behavior in experimentally created "social climates." *Journal of Social Psychology, 10,* 271–299.

Lockwood, P., Jordan, C. H., & Kunda, Z.

(2002). Motivation by positive or negative role models: regulatory focus determines who will best inspire us. *Journal of Personality and Social Psychology, 83,* 854–864.

McAdams, D. P. (1993). *The stories we live by: Personal myths and the making of the self.* William Morrow.

McGregor, I. (2006). Offensive defensiveness: Toward an integrative neuroscience of compensatory zeal after mortality salience, personal uncertainty, and other poignant self-threats. *Psychological Inquiry, 17,* 299–308.

McGregor, I., Britton, E., Elnakouri, A., & Sharpinskyi, K. (2022). *Weak personal ideals incline proud people towards religious radicalization in anxious circumstances.* Canadian Network for Research on Terrorism, Security, and Society.

McGregor, I., Hayes, J., & Prentice, M. (2015). Motivation for aggressive religious radicalization: Goal regulation theory and a personality × threat × affordance hypothesis. *Frontiers in Psychology, 6,* 1325.

McGregor, I., & Little, B. R. (1998). Personal projects, happiness, and meaning. On doing well and being yourself. *Journal of Personality and Social Psychology, 74,* 494–512.

McGregor, I., Nail, P. R., Marigold, D. C., & Kang, S.-J. (2005). Defensive pride and consensus: Strength in imaginary numbers. *Journal of Personality and Social Psychology, 89,* 978–996.

McGregor, I., Newby-Clark, I. R., & Zanna, M. P. (2019). Dissonance now: How accessible discrepancies moderate distress and diverse defensive reactions. In E. Harmon-Jones & J. Mills (Eds.), *Cognitive dissonance: Perspectives on a pivotal theory in social psychology* (2nd ed., pp. 117–138). American Psychological Association.

McGregor, I., Prentice, M., & Nash, K. (2012). Approaching relief: Compensatory ideals relieve threat-induced anxiety by promoting approach-motivated states. *Social Cognition, 30*(6), 689–714.

McGregor, I., Tran, A., Auger, E., Britton, E., Hayes, J., Elnakouri, A., . . . Nash, K. (2022b). Higher power dynamics: How meaning search and self-transcendence inspire approach motivation and magnanimity. *Journal of Experimental Social Psychology, 102,* 104350.

McGregor, I., Zanna, M. P., Holmes, J. G., & Spencer, S. J. (2001). Compensatory conviction in the face of personal uncertainty: Going to extremes and being oneself. *Journal of Personality and Social Psychology, 80*(3), 472–488.

McNaughton, N., & Gray, J. A. (2024). *The neuropsychology of anxiety: An inquiry into the functions of the septo-hippocampal system* (3rd ed.). Oxford University Press. (Original work published 1982)

Mercer-Lynn, K. B., Bar, R. J., & Eastwood, J. D. (2014). Causes of boredom: The person, the situation, or both? *Personality and Individual Differences, 56,* 122–126.

Mitchell, S. (2004). *Gilgamesh: A new English version.* Simon & Schuster.

Patnoe, S. (1988). *A narrative history of experimental social psychology: The Lewin tradition.* Springer-Verlag.

Pavlov, I. (1927). Lecture 17: *The different types of nervous system. Pathological disturbances of the cortex, result of functional interferences.* York University. https://psychclassics.yorku.ca/Pavlov/lecture17.htm.

Public Safety Canada. (2024). *National strategy on countering radicalization to violence.* www.publicsafety.gc.ca/cnt/rsrcs/pblctns/ntnl-strtg-cntrng-rdclztn-vlnc/index-en.aspx#s1.

Randles, D., Inzlicht, M., Proulx, T., Tullett, A. M., & Heine, S. J. (2015). Is dissonance reduction a special case of fluid compensation?: Evidence that dissonant cognitions cause compensatory affirmation and abstraction. *Journal of Personality and Social Psychology, 108,* 697.

Rimé, B., & Páez, D. (2023). Why we gather: A new look, empirically documented, at Émile Durkheim's theory of collective assemblies and collective effervescence. *Perspectives on Psychological Science, 18*(6), 1306–1330.

Sagiv, L., & Schwartz, S. H. (2022). Personal values across cultures. *Annual Review of Psychology, 73,* 517–546.

Schindler, S., Hilgard, J., Fritsche, I., Burke, B., & Pfattheicher, S. (2023). Do salient social norms moderate mortality salience effects?: A (challenging) meta-analysis of terror management studies. *Personality and Social Psychology Review, 27,* 195–225.

Schmeichel, B. J., Crowell, A., & Harmon-Jones, E. (2016). Exercising self-control increases relative left frontal cortical activation. *Social Cognitive and Affective Neuroscience, 11,* 282–288.

Schmeichel, B. J., Harmon-Jones, C., & Harmon-Jones, E. (2010). Exercising self-control increases approach motivation. *Journal of Personality and Social Psychology, 99*(1), 162–173.

Schumann, K., McGregor, I., Nash, K. A., & Ross, M. (2014). Religious magnanimity: reminding people of their religious belief system reduces hostility after threat. *Journal of Personality and Social Psychology, 107,* 432–453.

Sherman, D. K. (2013). Self-affirmation: Understanding the effects. *Social and Personality Psychology Compass, 7*(11), 834–845.

Sherman D. K., Lokhande, M., Muller, T., & Cohen, G. L. (2021). Self-affirmation interventions. In G. M. Walton & A. J. Crum (Eds.), *Handbook of wise interventions* (pp. 63–99). Guilford Press.

Shnabel, N., Purdie-Vaughns, V., Cook, J. E., Garcia, J., & Cohen, G. L. (2013). Demystifying values-affirmation interventions: Writing about social belonging is a key to buffering against identity threat. *Personality and Social Psychology Bulletin, 39*(5), 663–676.

Stavrova, O., Ehlebracht, D., & Vohs, K. D. (2020). Victims, perpetrators, or both?: The vicious cycle of disrespect and cynical beliefs about human nature. *Journal of Experimental Psychology: General, 149,* 1736–1754.

Steele, C. M. (1988). The psychology of self-affirmation: Sustaining the integrity of the self. In L. Berkowitz (Ed.), *Advances in experimental social psychology* (pp. 261–302). Academic Press.

Stollberg, J., Klackl, J., & Jonas, E. (2024). Empirical test of a general process model of threat and defense: A systematic examination of the affective-motivational processes underlying proximal and distal reactions to threat. *Journal of Experimental Social Psychology, 110,* 1–14.

Tarnas, R. (1991). *The passion of the Western mind: Understanding the ideas that have shaped our world view.* Ballantine.

Taylor, C. (1989). *Sources of the self: The making of the modern identity.* Harvard University Press.

Tesser, A. (2000). On the confluence of self-esteem maintenance mechanisms. *Personality and Social Psychology Review, 4,* 290–299.

Thrash, T. M., & Elliot, A. J. (2004). Inspiration: Core characteristics, component processes, antecedents, and function. *Journal of Personality and Social Psychology, 87*(6), 957–973.

Todes, D. P. (1995). Pavlov and the Bolsheviks. *History and Philosophy of the Life Sciences,* 379–418.

Twenge, J. M., & King, L. A. (2005). A good life is a personal life: Relationship fulfillment and work fulfillment in judgments of life quality. *Journal of Research in Personality, 39,* 336–353.

Van de Vyver, J., & Abrams, D. (2017). Is moral elevation an approach-oriented emotion? *Journal of Positive Psychology, 12*(2), 178–185.

Viadis, D., Sleegers, W., van Leeuwen, F., Demarree, K., Sætrevik, B., Ross, R., . . . Priolo, D. (2024). A multilab replication of the induced-compliance paradigm of cognitive dissonance. *Advances in Methods and Practices in Psychological Science, 7*(1), 1–26.

Vohs, K. D., Schmeichel, B. J., Lohmann, S., Gronau, Q. F., Finley, A. J., Ainsworth, S. E., . . . Albarracín, D. (2021). A multisite preregistered paradigmatic test of the ego-depletion effect. *Psychological Science, 32*(10), 1566–1581.

Willardt, R., & Schmid, P. C. (2024). The threat of powerlessness: Consequences for affect and (social) cognition. *Journal of Experimental Social Psychology, 111,* 104576.

Xu, X., & McGregor, I. (2018). Motivation, threat, and defense: Perspective from social psychology. *Psychological Inquiry, 29,* 32–37.

CHAPTER 31

An Attachment Perspective on the Management of Existential Concerns and Cultivation of Personal Growth

Mario Mikulincer *and* Phillip R. Shaver

In this chapter, we focus on the role that security dynamics play in shaping the ways we think, experience, and cope with such existential concerns as mortality, lack of freedom, and meaninglessness. Specifically, we deal with and review evidence concerning three core aspects of security dynamics associated with existential concerns. First, people tend to react to existential threats and worries by seeking the proximity and support of competent and benevolent others (e.g., parents, lovers, therapists, social groups or organizations, religious/spiritual figures). Second, the availability of loving and responsive others and the resulting felt security help a person effectively navigate existential concerns. Third, beyond mitigating these concerns, cultivating a sense of attachment security allows a person to experience authentic senses of autonomy, self-continuity, and meaning.

OVERVIEW OF SECURITY DYNAMICS

The Search for Social Sources of Protection and Support

According to attachment theory (Bowlby, 1982), human beings are born with an evolved psychobiological system (*attachment behavioral system*) that motivates them to seek proximity to supportive others (*attachment figures*) in times of need for the sake of protection, distress management, and personal growth. Attachment figures are special individuals or social entities (e.g., groups) that are perceived to be benevolent and competent and therefore to be potential providers of a *safe haven* (i.e., which alleviates fears and distress) and a *secure base* from which to explore, learn, and thrive in a confident manner (Ainsworth, 1991). Bowlby (1988) believed that the search for a safe haven and secure base, which is critical for survival during infancy, continues to operate throughout life, as indicated by adults' needs for affection, support, and encouragement, especially when facing threats or challenges (Zeifman & Hazan, 2016).

Although the need for a safe haven and a secure base is important across the lifespan (Bowlby, 1988), the identity of targeted attachment figures tends to change with development. During infancy, primary caregivers (usually parents or parent substitutes) typically occupy the role of attachment figures (Ainsworth, 1991). However, during adolescence and adulthood, research indicates that close friends and romantic partners also become potential attachment figures (Zeifman & Hazan, 2016). In addition, a wide variety of people can be targeted as potential sources of support and encouragement in particular contexts, such as teachers, coaches, and mentors in educational and recreational settings, managers in work settings, officers in the military, therapists in clinical settings, health care workers in medical settings, clergy in religion-related settings, and leaders in social and political organizations. Research indicates that children, adolescents, and adults tend to rely on one or more of these people, depending on circumstances, for obtaining a safe haven and secure base (e.g., Mallinckrodt et al., 2009; Mayseless & Popper, 2019; Sabol & Pianta, 2012). There is also evidence that other individuals and social entities can be recruited as potential attachment figures, including groups, social organizations, and God (e.g., Granqvist, 2020; Mayseless & Popper, 2007; Smith et al., 1999).

Attachment-Figure Responsiveness, Felt Security, and Insecure Forms of Attachment

According to Bowlby (1973), interactions with attachment figures who are sensitive and responsive to one's bids for proximity and support and who effectively provide the needed safe haven and secure base promote a sense of attachment security and contribute to positive mental representations (*working models*) of self as worthy and competent and of others as kind, caring, and trustworthy. In contrast, interactions with attachment figures who behave in a rejecting or neglectful manner disrupt one's sense of safety and security, foster more negative working models of self and others, and promote insecure attachment styles or orientations (i.e., relatively stable patterns of relational expectations, emotions, and behaviors). These orientations are conceptualized and measured along two continuous and roughly orthogonal dimensions (Brennan et al., 1998). *Attachment anxiety* is organized around worries about one's lovability and reliance on overly demanding, intrusive, and even coercive attempts to attain others' care. *Attachment-related avoidance* is defined by distrust of others' goodwill, resistance to relational closeness, and effortful attempts to maintain independence and self-reliance within personal and social relationships.

A person's general attachment orientation (i.e., general location in the two-dimensional anxiety-by-avoidance space) can be viewed as the top node in a complex network of attachment representations, some of which apply only to specific people and relationships and others of which apply only in certain relational contexts (Mikulincer & Shaver, 2016). These more specific mental representations can be activated by actual or imagined encounters with supportive or unsupportive others, even if these representations are incongruent with the dominant attachment orientation, and can then temporarily shift a person's cognitions, emotions, and behaviors (Mikulincer & Shaver, 2016). For example, the presence of a supportive figure can create a momentary sense of security (which we have called *security priming*; Mikulincer & Shaver, 2016) even on the part of chronically insecure people and lead them to think and behave more like a secure person (see Gillath et al., 2022, for a systematic review and meta-analyses).

Bowlby (1988) summarized the adaptive benefits of a well-functioning, effective attachment system. First, interactions with a security-enhancing attachment figure help a person downregulate negative emotions and maintain stability in times of need or stress (Bowlby, 1973). Second, such interactions facilitate the cultivation of personal skills and talents, because a child or adult who feels adequately protected and supported has greater courage and more conflict-free attentional resources to engage in free play, curiously investigate objects and environments, and develop affiliative relationships with peers (Bowlby, 1988). Following this reasoning, it is easy to understand why the search for social sources of protection and support and the attainment of felt attachment security are crucial for the effective management of existential concerns and the maintenance of emotional equanimity despite constant reminders of our biological fragility and life's uncertainty and potential absurdity.

According to several social psychological theories, life events or circumstances that remind us of the fragility of our existence, our biological finitude, or our inability to predict and control life's course are major sources of existential anxiety (concerning death, uncertainty, or lack of control) and a powerful trigger of psychological defenses (e.g., Fritsche et al., 2013; Pyszczynski et al., 2019). From an attachment perspective, these existential concerns are likely to automatically activate the attachment system and energize a person's attempts to seek and rely upon social sources of care, protection, and safety (Hart et al., 2005). If these proximity- and support-seeking bids regularly elicit accepting and caring responses from responsive attachment figures, a person learns that support will be available when needed (felt security) and that they are not alone and vulnerable in dealing with existential threats. In this way, this emerging sense of attachment security may provide an effective psychological shield against existential concerns and assist people in restoring feelings of safety, continuity, meaning, relatedness, and autonomy, thereby rendering other symbolic defenses less necessary. In contrast, lack of available, responsive, and supportive attachment figures may cause people to rely on other forms of defense against existential concerns (Hart et al., 2005).

EXISTENTIAL CONCERNS AND THE SEARCH FOR SOCIAL SOURCES OF PROTECTION AND SUPPORT

In our model of attachment system functioning in adulthood (Mikulincer & Shaver, 2003), the search for social sources of protection and support in times of need involves two stages. In the first stage, threats and challenges automatically trigger preconscious attachment-related mental representations. This process involves heightened access to representations (not necessarily conscious) of supportive relationship partners, groups, or organizations; episodic memories of comforting interactions with these figures; and thoughts and images related to closeness, warmth, and love. In the second stage, if the eliciting conditions are sufficiently robust, this preconscious activation can alter a person's motivational strivings and subjective feelings and elicit cognitive and behavioral tactics aimed at increasing proximity to, and gaining support from, an attachment figure. In young children, preconscious activation typically gives way quickly to behavioral enactment, because preconscious thought of an action tends to trigger the action unless there is restraint or inhibition. In adults, there may be many steps between thoughts and actions, and proximity seeking may take place only intrapsychically, with or without awareness.

Following this reasoning, existential concerns may not only activate actual behavioral attempts to seek or maintain proximity to supportive relationship partners, groups, or organizations; they may also automatically increase mental access to comforting attachment-related cognitions and feelings and can cause people to selectively retrieve memories of positive attachment experiences. From an attachment perspective, these positive preconscious and conscious images, memories, and thoughts are intrapsychic means of sustaining emotional equanimity while coping with existential concerns. They allow people to deal with existential threats in a more relaxed and mindful manner and take more effective steps to mitigate the resulting distress and learn new things about themselves and others in the context of challenging, life-altering experiences.

This kind of mental activation has been observed, for example, in Mikulincer and colleagues' (2000) study of contextual triggers of attachment-related representations. In this study, participants were subliminally exposed to the word *death* or a neutral word (for 22 milliseconds) in each of several trials of a lexical decision task in which they were asked to identify whether a string of letters was a word or a non-word. The target words included ones related to attachment security (e.g., *love*, *hug*, *closeness*), attachment-unrelated positive words, and neutral words. Findings indicated that words related to attachment security became more available for processing (as indicated by faster reaction times in the lexical decision task) following the death prime (compared with the neutral prime). The word *death* had no effect on the mental accessibility of attachment-unrelated positive or neutral words. Similar effects have been reported in a study of symbolic proximity seeking to God, an omnipotent source of protection (Granqvist et al., 2012). Specifically, as compared to implicit exposure to a neutral word, Israeli Jewish believers reacted to the word *death* with faster recognition of words expressing a close relationship with God (e.g., *prayer, devotion*). However, Gruneau Brulin and colleagues (2018) failed to replicate this effect among Swedish and American Christians, perhaps indicating some cultural or religious differences in believers' symbolic proximity-seeking to God when faced with the threat of biological finitude.

Preconscious activation of attachment-related cognitions can sometimes be followed by intentional memory retrieval of past comforting interactions with a current caring relationship partner (or other loving figures), which can revive feelings of safety, protection, and comfort originally experienced in the recalled circumstances. In other words, people facing existential threats may engage in nostalgic reveries, which, according to Wildschut and colleagues (2006), involve mental reactivation of past positive and comforting social experiences and relationships. Indeed, there is experimental evidence that, as compared to neutral conditions, reminding participants of their biological finitude (mortality) or inducing threats to their sense of identity and meaning in the laboratory heighten engagement in nostalgic reveries (e.g., Juhl et al., 2010; Sedikides et al., 2015; van Tilburg et al., 2013).

Beyond mental activation of attachment-related cognitions, existential concerns often lead to effortful actions aimed at gaining actual proximity to, and support from, currently available relationship partners, groups, organizations, or spiritual/religious figures. In the context of romantic relationships, terror management studies have revealed that laboratory reminders of one's death heighten proximity seeking to a romantic partner (for reviews, see Mikulincer et al., 2003; Plusnin et al., 2018). In a pioneering study, Florian and colleagues (2002) randomly assigned participants to write about either their own death (the mortality salience condition) or a neutral topic and then assessed participants' personal commitment to their romantic partner (e.g., "I am completely devoted to my partner") and their moral commitment to the institution of marriage (e.g., "Marriages are supposed to last forever"). Compared to the neutral condition, mortality salience increased personal commitment to a romantic partner but had no effect on moral commitment to the institution of marriage. It seems that existential concerns increase the desire to stay close to a romantic partner but not the adherence to cultural norms concerning marriage.

Subsequent studies have extended Florian and colleagues' (2002) findings to other motivational, cognitive, and behavioral manifestations of proximity seeking within romantic relationships. For example, exposure to a death reminder (vs. a neutral condition) heightens both interest in forming a new romantic relationship and desire for intimacy within such a relationship (e.g., Hoppe et al., 2018; Silveira et al., 2014). Moreover, as compared to a control condition, mortality salience increases the tendency to make compromises in study participants' mate selection criteria to secure a long-term mate (e.g., Hirschberger et al., 2002). Death reminders have also been found to increase study participants' desire for emotional intimacy with a romantic partner even after this partner has disapproved of or criticized them. It seems that death awareness makes people willing to pay the price of diminished self-esteem to maintain proximity to a romantic partner (Hirschberger et al., 2003).

In the context of group relationships, existential concerns might be expected to lead people to turn for protection and support from the social group to which they belong (ingroup). This group-level proximity seeking can be manifested in heightened emotional connection to, and identification with, the group, and the resulting tendencies of accepting, valuing, and endorsing the goals, beliefs, values, and prototypical traits and behaviors of the group. These kinds of proximity-seeking bids might also result in positive attitudes toward other group members and preference for ingroup over outgroup members, group loyalty, and wearing or using objects (e.g., clothes, flags) that are visible reminders of group membership.

In a series of surveys, a dramatic increase in patriotism (love of country, ingroup solidarity) and identification with national symbols (e.g., flag, anthem) were found among American adults immediately after the 9/11 terrorist attacks (e.g., Li & Brewer, 2004). For example, more Americans were flying

U.S. flags shortly after 9/11 than prior to the terrorist attack. A similar increase in patriotism was reported recently by Sibley and colleagues (2020) among New Zealanders immediately following the COVID-19 outbreak (compared to a matched prepandemic group).

People also tend to strengthen their psychological connection to an ingroup when facing threats to their sense of control and agency (Fritsche et al., 2013). Experimental reminders of lack of personal control over life events have been found to increase ingroup identification, mainly when groups are framed as strong and competent (Stollberg et al., 2015). These reminders have also been found to increase positive appraisals of ingroups (Fritsche et al., 2013) and conformity with salient ingroup (but not outgroup) norms (Stollberg et al., 2017).

Terror management studies provide some of the best evidence that existential concerns (i.e., death reminders) activate proximity-seeking inclinations in relation to a group. For example, Castano and colleagues (2002) found that, as compared to Italian participants in a control condition, Italians exposed to death reminders displayed stronger identification with Italians, perceived themselves to share more common characteristics with Italians, and held more positive attitudes toward Italians (vs. Germans). Moreover, mortality salience has been found to increase self-group overlap, causing people to conform to an ingroup's beliefs and overestimate their similarity to ingroup members in both psychological traits and opinions (Pyszczynski et al., 1996; Watanabe & Karasawa, 2012).

Mortality salience also increases positive attitudes toward ingroup members. In one of the early terror management studies, Greenberg and colleagues (1990) found that Christians who were reminded of their mortality gave more positive evaluations of Christians but more negative evaluations of Jews. This finding was conceptually replicated when ingroups and outgroups were arbitrarily formed in the context of a lab experiment (using the minimal group paradigm; Harmon-Jones et al., 1996). Moreover, as compared to a control condition, participants exposed to death reminders tend to report more interest in interacting with an ingroup rather than an outgroup member (e.g., Frischlich et al., 2015).

There is also some evidence supporting the idea that existential concerns increase citizens' tendency to rely on social institutions (e.g., government, army) for protection and support. Longitudinal surveys conducted in the United States and Switzerland indicate that people expressed greater trust in government and public health agencies during the H1N1 pandemic than in a prepandemic assessment (Bangerter et al., 2012; Quinn et al., 2013). Similar findings were reported by Sibley and colleagues (2020), who examined the effects of a nationwide lockdown in response to the COVID-19 outbreak by comparing matched samples of New Zealanders assessed before and during the first 18 days of lockdown. People in the pandemic/lockdown group reported more trust in the government and in the police, and they expressed more positive attitudes toward them than was the case before the pandemic.

Experimentally induced reminders of one's biological finitude and lack of personal control also seem to heighten reliance on governmental services and foster more positive attitudes toward social organizations. For example, Kay and colleagues (2008) found that, relative to a control condition, a threat to personal control (created by a memory task that required participants to recall uncontrollable events) increased explicit requests for help from the government. Prusova and Gulevich (2019) found that a mortality salience manipulation caused Russian students to give government more responsibility and control over their lives, and Jonas and colleagues (2011) reported that participants exposed to death reminders were more likely to endorse aspects of their workplace culture (i.e., heightened positive evaluations of symbols, mottos, or products representing their organization) than participants in a control condition were. Beyond these experimental findings, a cross-national survey conducted in 67 countries found that people who felt less control over their lives were more likely than those who felt more control to turn to their government in times of need (Kay et al., 2008).

The search for protection and support in times of need may also be directed at social or political leaders. Popper and Mayseless

(2003) proposed that desire for a strong leader tends to arise in times of personal or collective crisis, trauma, or uncertainty. During demanding and challenging periods, people wish to feel close to, and rely upon, a leader who can protect them. This tendency was first documented in 1970 by John Mueller, a political scientist who found that sudden international crises during the Cold War led Americans to rally behind their leaders and increase their trust in American presidents. In a subsequent review, Baker and Oneal (2001) suggested that military crises, mainly if they are sudden, dramatic, and international in scope, can in and of themselves trigger heightened support for a president. Indeed, dramatic increases in support for American presidents were found following the attack on Pearl Harbor in 1941, the Bay of Pigs crisis in 1962, the entry of the United States into the Gulf War in 1991, the 9/11 terrorist attacks in 2001, and the invasion of Iraq in 2003 (Lambert et al., 2011). This "rally behind the leader" tendency was also found in laboratory studies: As compared to a control condition, American participants who were reminded of the 9/11 attacks (by watching a short video clip) expressed more favorable attitudes toward then-President George W. Bush (Lambert et al., 2011).

Within the context of religious/spiritual relationships, there is extensive evidence that existential threats lead believers to turn to God and to strengthen their emotional connection to this protective figure by praying, the most prototypical proximity-seeking behavior in relation to God (Granqvist, 2020). In early studies of prayer, Stouffer (1949) observed that combat soldiers pray frequently before, during, and after battle. And subsequent studies have shown, as we know from personal observations and experience, that prayer is a common practice used by believers to cope with physical illnesses and injuries (see Koenig et al., 2012, for a review).

Believers might also be expected to react to existential threats by heightening their endorsement of religious beliefs and engagement in religious practices, thereby strengthening their emotional connection to God. Indeed, studies conducted with patients diagnosed with a serious physical illness have reported these people's more frequent attendance at religious services, increased desire for closeness to God, and greater tendency to ask for God's protection and support during the illness (e.g., Keefe et al., 2001). Similar increases in religious faith have been found among people who were directly affected by the 2011 Christchurch earthquake in New Zealand (Sibley & Bulbulia, 2012) and among Louisiana flood survivors (Davis et al., 2019).

Heightened emotional connection with God can also be observed following experimental inductions of existential threats in the laboratory. Kay and colleagues (2008) found, for example, that, as compared to a control condition, participants who were asked to recall an uncontrollable personal event were more likely to say they believed in God's existence and power. In addition, terror management studies have found stronger endorsement of religious beliefs following a mortality salience manipulation than following neutral inductions among Christians, Muslims, and Agnostics (e.g., Vail et al., 2012).

Although the search for protection and support from one's social or religious group, institutions, or leaders might, under ideal conditions, result in the provision of a safe haven and secure base and a renewal of the sense of attachment security, it can create two important societal problems under less optimal conditions. First, this search can contribute to the rise of autocratic leaders or dictators who promise to restore order and security at the price of eroding personal freedom and trampling on democratic values and practices. Indeed, Gelfand (2018) found that people in United States and France who were more fearful about social threats (e.g., illegal immigration, unemployment, crime, terrorism) were more supportive of autocratic candidates (e.g., Donald Trump, Marine Le Pen) who offered simple solutions to these complex problems. Second, manipulative leaders can take advantage of people's need for security and deliberately emphasize the imminence and severity of external threats as a way to increase people's reliance on their leadership. In a 2020 article, Bar-Tal provided examples of authoritarian leaders intentionally attempting to evoke fear and insecurity among their followers as a method of increasing dependence, conformity, and obedience. From our attachment-theory perspective, autocratic leadership involves a cynical manipulation of security dynamics in order to amplify followers' search for protection from, and dependence on, a leader,

Similarly dangerous dynamics can be observed in religious/spiritual relationships. Placing one's problems in God's hands can put emotionally troubled people at risk of being exploited by manipulative and deceptive religious leaders, who promise redemption and inner peace at the price of giving up individuality and autonomy. As a result, believers can be entrapped in a self-exacerbating cycle of dependence, self-dissolution, fanatic adherence to a faith, and blind merger with the religious group, leader, and cause. This process might be particularly characteristic of attachment-anxious believers, who may be overly dependent on their religious faith and leaders (Granqvist, 2020). However, this dark side of attachment to God might be avoided by a solid sense of attachment security, which sustains and promotes more mature forms of spirituality, curious exploration of others' religious beliefs, and the ability to disengage from religious/spiritual groups, leaders, and institutions that threaten one's individuality and autonomy (Mikulincer & Shaver, 2016).

FELT SECURITY, ATTACHMENT INSECURITIES, AND COPING WITH EXISTENTIAL CONCERNS

According to attachment theory, interactions with attachment figures who are sensitive and responsive to one's proximity- and support-seeking bids in times of need can move a person toward greater felt security, with positive repercussions for emotion regulation and mental health (Bowlby, 1973, 1988). This sense of security is associated with positive working models of self (as worthy and competent) and others (as trustworthy and benevolent) and with constructive, flexible, and reality-attuned emotion-regulation strategies (e.g., positive reappraisals, support seeking), which promote distress alleviation and bolster personal adjustment (Mikulincer & Shaver, 2023). In this way, felt security may allow people to remain relatively unperturbed and well-regulated in the face of existential threats. In contrast, nonresponsive attachment figures as well as the attachment insecurities (anxiety, avoidance) they arouse can leave a person vulnerable to anxieties about mortality, meaninglessness, isolation, and lack of freedom, causing the person to adopt less constructive ways of coping with these existential concerns.

In support of this theoretical view, several studies have found that individual differences in the sense of attachment security are highly relevant for explaining the ways people experience and manage death-related concerns. For example, Mikulincer and Florian (2000) and Mikulincer and colleagues (1990) found that attachment security is associated with lower levels of death-related thoughts and fear of death measured by self-report scales, projective tests (narrative responses to Thematic Apperception Test [TAT] cards), and cognitive tasks (completion of death-related word fragments). In contrast, attachment anxiety is associated with heightened fear of death as measured by both self-reports and TAT responses, and with greater accessibility of death-related thoughts even when no death reminder is present. Attachment-related avoidance is related to lower self-reported fear of death, but with a higher level of death-related thoughts and anxiety in TAT responses. That is, avoidant individuals tend to suppress death concerns and exhibit dissociation between their conscious and unconscious thoughts about death.

Attachment insecurities are also involved in the ways people subjectively construe their fear of personal death (Florian & Mikulincer, 1998; Mikulincer et al., 1990). Whereas attachment-anxious people tend to attribute this fear to the loss of social identity after death (e.g., "People will forget me"), attachment-avoidant people tend to attribute it to the unknown nature of the hereafter (e.g., "uncertainty about what to expect"). These findings are compatible with the emotion regulation strategies associated with attachment anxiety and avoidance. Attachment-anxious people tend to regulate their insecurities and distress by inflating and overemphasizing worries about rejection and abandonment and tend to view death as yet another relational setting in which they can be abandoned or forgotten.

Attachment-avoidant people tend to regulate their insecurities and distress by sustaining self-reliance and strong personal control, which might lead them to be afraid of the uncertain and unknown aspects of death that compromise their sense of mastery.

Individual differences in felt security and attachment insecurities are also relevant in explaining the ways people manage death-related concerns. Although validation of dominant cultural worldviews has been considered the normative defense against existential threats (Pyszczynski et al., 2019), there is evidence that this response is more characteristic of insecure than of secure individuals. For example, experimentally induced death reminders produced more severe judgments and punishments of moral transgressors, greater willingness to die for a political cause, and more support for a conservative presidential candidate only among attachment-insecure people (Caspi-Berkowitz et al., 2019; Mikulincer & Florian, 2000; Weise et al., 2008). More secure individuals were less affected by death reminders. Moreover, the experimental priming of attachment security buffered the effects of mortality salience on increased support for violent measures against terrorists (Weise et al., 2008) and increased support for the war in Iraq and harsh foreign policy toward North Korea (Gillath & Hart, 2010).

Some studies have revealed ways in which secure people react to death reminders. Mikulincer and Florian (2000) found that secure people reacted to mortality salience with an increased sense of symbolic immortality—a constructive, transformational strategy that, while not solving the unsolvable problem of death, leads people to invest in their children's care and to engage in creative, growth-oriented activities whose products live on after death. Secure people also reacted to mortality salience with a heightened seeking of relational closeness—a more intense desire for intimacy in close relationships (Mikulincer & Florian, 2000), heightened reliance on others in times of need (Cox et al., 2008), and greater willingness to engage in social interactions (Taubman Ben-Ari et al., 2002). In addition, Yaakobi and colleagues (2014) found that childless young adults who scored lower on attachment avoidance (i.e., were more secure) reported a greater desire to become a parent following death reminders, perhaps relying on biological continuity as a buffer against death anxiety.

Secure individuals also tend to react to death reminders by strengthening their desire to care for others. In Caspi-Berkowitz and colleagues' (2019) study, people read hypothetical scenarios in which a relationship partner was in danger of death; the participants were then asked about their willingness to endanger their own life to save their partner's life. Secure individuals reacted to death reminders with heightened willingness to sacrifice themselves. Insecure people were generally averse to self-sacrifice and reacted to death reminders with less willingness to save others' lives. It's notable that insecure individuals, who seem more ready than secure ones to die for their self-enhancing cultural worldviews, are more reluctant to sacrifice themselves for a particular other person.

THE EXISTENTIAL BENEFITS OF FELT SECURITY

Beyond mitigating existential concerns, felt security can assist people in attaining authentic senses of autonomy, self-continuity, and meaning. These positive outcomes seem to be mediated by the formation of a positive and cohesive self-structure, which allows secure individuals to confidently pursue their own interests and realize their ideals, aspirations, and talents, which is crucial for autonomous growth and self-actualization (Mikulincer & Shaver, 2023). This is the way in which attachment theory integrates well with positive and humanistic approaches to psychology (e.g., Maslow, 1971; Ryan & Deci, 2017; Seligman, 2002).

Beginning in infancy, soothing and empowering interactions with responsive caregivers and the resulting felt security allow children to develop a positive and cohesive self-structure, which in turn allows them to confidently venture out from their safe haven and explore the world on their own (reinforced by confidence that they can return to the safe haven and secure base when needed). These exploratory and learning activities allow secure children to practice and improve their evolving executive functions (working memory, response inhibition, cognitive flexibility) and organizational skills (e.g., setting goals and priorities, means–end planning), which then enable them to accomplish adaptive tasks throughout life (e.g., constructing and sustaining a personal identity, choosing and managing a career, establishing rewarding social relationships). In this way, secure children, adolescents, and adults are more likely than their insecure counterparts to satisfy the three basic psychological needs postulated by self-determination theory (Ryan & Deci, 2017)—relatedness, competence, and autonomy—and therefore experience higher levels of life satisfaction, purpose, and meaning.

One important aspect of the self that develops from interactions with a responsive attachment figure is a set of positive beliefs about personal value and strength. These beliefs are derived from the way secure people see and evaluate themselves during supportive interactions. Secure people can view themselves as valuable and special thanks to actually being valued, loved, and accepted by a caring attachment figure. Moreover, they can feel strong, competent, and successful, because the responsive attachment figure expresses confidence in their abilities while providing a secure base for exploration, validates their aspirations, and celebrates their achievements. During interactions with a responsive attachment figure, secure individuals also realize that they can mobilize this figure's support when needed as well as venture away from them while exploring, learning, or working or playing alone. In support of this view, hundreds of cross-sectional and longitudinal studies conducted with children, adolescents, and adults have found strong associations between measures of attachment security and higher scores on scales measuring self-esteem and self-efficacy (see Mikulincer & Shaver, 2016, for a review).

The experimental priming of mental representations of secure attachment (security priming) has also been found to heighten positive self-views. For example, Dandeneau and colleagues (2007) primed felt security for 5 consecutive days. Each day, a sample of telemarketers performed an attention-training task and were asked to detect an accepting/smiling target face in a 4 × 4 matrix of otherwise negative faces, thereby increasing attention to signs of others' responsiveness. In the control condition, participants had to find a five-petaled flower in a 4 × 4 array of seven-petaled flowers. Before the study and at the end of each day, participants completed a measure of state self-esteem. By the end of the study, the self-esteem of the participants in the security-priming group had increased significantly. No such change occurred among participants in the control condition. These findings support the notion that priming security-related mental representations can increase state self-esteem.

Another set of self-beliefs that derives from security-enhancing interactions and resulting felt security concerns a person's sense of autonomy and self-direction. Responsive attachment figures who provide a reliable secure base for exploration and learning encourage, support, celebrate, and empower a person's strivings for exploration, competence, and self-expansion without conditioning their support on the person's acceptance of their demands and self-interest. In this way, a person becomes confident that support and encouragement will be available when needed no matter what they decide to do, what honest mistakes they may make, and what failures and setbacks they experience in pursuing personal goals. In this kind of accepting and supportive social context, people feel autonomous in pursuing what they want and feel that their actions are determined through an *inner compass*—the self-routine or self-component that explicitly conveys what is truly important and desirable to a person (Assor, 2012).

In support of this view, self-reports of attachment security in close relationships have been found associated with a stronger sense of self-direction (as opposed to feelings of pressure and coercion; e.g., van Petegem et al., 2013). Research also suggests that felt security contributes to a more reality-attuned system of ideals and values, and that secure individuals seem to feel comfortable with this system. In studies of perfectionism, adolescents and adults who hold a stronger sense of attachment security tend to score higher on measures of adaptive forms of goal setting (maintaining demanding but achievable personal standards). In contrast, attachment-insecure individuals are more likely to endorse maladaptive forms of perfectionism, including the setting of unrealistically high standards, ruminating about mistakes, and feeling pressured by others to be perfect (see Hewitt et al., 2017, for a review). Chen and colleagues (2012) also found that adolescents who felt more secure in close relationships were less likely to be focused on actively defending a supposed "perfection" and did not have problems in revealing their perceived imperfections.

Research also indicates that felt security is associated with higher scores on measures of self-authenticity (e.g., "I am true to myself in most situations"; Lopez et al., 2015). In addition, security-priming interventions have been found to increase state authenticity and to reduce dishonesty (lying to and cheating on a romantic partner; Gillath et al., 2010). In contrast, attachment insecurities are associated with a tendency to modify one's behavior to meet others' expectations (Fuglestad et al., 2020) and with feelings of *impostorism*—feeling that one's achievements are "fake" and undeserved or illusory (Bachem et al., 2020). It seems that attachment-insecure people find it difficult to live up to their unrealistic self-standards (perhaps rooted in early experiences with critical, disapproving, ambivalent, or unsupportive parents). This unfortunate situation can, understandably, lead to psychological problems ranging from defensive narcissism to depression (Hewitt et al., 2017).

Beyond holding positive self-views, secure individuals are expected theoretically to hold a strong sense of self-continuity—"a sense of persistent cross-temporal identity wherein the present self is seen as overlapping with past and future selves" (Sokol & Serper, 2019, p. 157). Theoretically, positive interactions with a responsive attachment figure are foundational for creating a sense of self-continuity. The ability of this figure to help one understand important experiences, whether positive or negative, and weave them into a coherent and positive life narrative, is helpful in building a strong, coherent, and continuous sense of self. Moreover, learning that others' support will be available when needed implies that vulnerability and dependence are temporary states and that one can confidently expect to return to exploratory ventures that sometimes get interrupted by threats and failures. Who and what one was in the past is not lost because of these interruptions, and getting through a troubled period with the help of an attachment figure allows one to link positive coping experiences with confidence in one's ability to move confidently into the future.

Unfortunately, to date no research has been conducted to examine associations between measures of attachment security and measures of perceived self-continuity. However, there is some evidence that engagement in nostalgic reveries, which bring to mind comforting memories of loving and caring others, temporarily increases a person's sense of self-continuity (see Sedikides & Wildschut, 2019, for a review). For example, as compared with control conditions, asking participants to reflect on and write about past events or periods that they miss raises their scores on a self-continuity index (Sedikides et al., 2015). This effect seems to be mediated by momentarily enhanced feelings of belongingness and acceptance (Sedikides et al., 2016). That is, engagement in nostalgic reveries increases feelings of relational closeness and felt security, which in turn enhance the sense of self-continuity.

Felt security also has positive implications for perceptions of life's meaning. There is evidence that feelings of closeness and social support (which are aspects of felt security) are associated with a heightened sense of life's meaning (e.g., Hicks & King, 2009; Steger et al., 2008). Similarly, Lambert and colleagues (2010) reported that perceived closeness to family members and support from them was associated with greater meaning in life among young adults, even when self-esteem, feelings of autonomy and competence, and social desirability were statistically controlled. Moreover, implicit priming of relational closeness increased the perception of life's meaning when participants were in a bad mood (Hicks & King, 2009). In contrast, experimental manipulations of rejection, social exclusion, and loneliness (which are related to attachment insecurity) reduce people's sense that life is meaningful (e.g., Hicks et al., 2010; Stillman et al., 2009; Williams, 2007).

Mikulincer and Shaver (2005) reported a preliminary study examining the impact of security priming on perception of life's meaning. Participants who had previously completed a self-report attachment measure were primed with representations of either a security provider (thinking about a supportive other) or a person who did not serve attachment functions. They then completed a self-report measure of the extent to which they perceived the world as understandable and life as "making sense." Lower scores on attachment anxiety and avoidance scales (i.e., greater attachment security) were associated with higher levels of meaning and coherence in life. Moreover, compared to neutral priming, security priming increased the sense of meaning even among dispositionally insecure participants.

CONCLUDING REMARKS

Considering the research reviewed here, it's interesting to reflect on the fact that existential philosophy originally focused on the subjective thoughts and feelings of isolated adult individuals (Camus's stranger, Kierkegaard's fictional versions of himself, Sartre's view that "hell is other people"). In contrast, attachment theory is rooted in psychoanalytic, social, and developmental theories and research, and it emphasizes the gradual creation of a secure or insecure individual through social interactions and relationships with other people. Attachment theory views meaning and self-confidence as rooted in social relationships and the mental residues of such relationships, including projections of these residues onto leaders and religious figures such as God. The creation of meaning does not happen in a vacuum, and it does not arise mainly through introspection; it occurs in activities and projects undertaken with other people. When a project is undertaken with other people whose needs and goals are perceived as legitimate and valuable, the project has meaning. The meaning is not necessarily grand or all encompassing, but it is a focus of commitment and shared effort. When an individual feels disconnected from and unsupported by others (perhaps including societal leaders and God), it is much easier for them to perceive life as worthless and meaningless.

REFERENCES

Ainsworth, M. D. S. (1991). Attachment and other affectional bonds across the life cycle. In C. M. Parkes, J. Stevenson-Hinde, & P. Marris (Eds.), *Attachment across the life cycle* (pp. 33–51). Routledge.

Assor, A. (2012). Allowing choice and nurturing an inner compass: Educational practices supporting students' need for autonomy. In S. L. Christenson, A. L. Reschly, & C. Wylie (Eds.), *Handbook of research on student engagement* (pp. 421–439). Springer.

Bachem, R., Mikulincer, M., & Solomon, Z. (2020). Interpersonal manifestations of attachment avoidance: The moderating role of impostorism. *Personality and Individual Differences, 154,* Article 109669.

Baker, W. D., & Oneal, J. R. (2001). Patriotism or opinion leadership?: The nature and origins of the "rally 'round the flag" effect. *Journal of Conflict Resolution, 45,* 661–687.

Bangerter, A., Krings, F., Mouton, A., Gilles, I., Green, E. G. T., & Clémence, A. (2012). Longitudinal investigation of public trust in institutions relative to the 2009 H1N1 pandemic in Switzerland. *PLOS One, 7,* Article e49806.

Bar-Tal, D. (2020). Creating fear and insecurity for political goals. *International Perspectives in Psychology: Research, Practice, Consultation, 9,* 5–17.

Bowlby, J. (1973). *Attachment and loss: Vol. 2. Separation: Anxiety and anger.* Basic Books.

Bowlby, J. (1982). *Attachment and loss: Vol. 1. Attachment* (2nd ed.). Basic Books.

Bowlby, J. (1988). *A secure base: Clinical applications of attachment theory.* Routledge.

Brennan, K. A., Clark, C. L., & Shaver, P. R. (1998). Self-report measurement of adult attachment: An integrative overview. In J. A. Simpson & W. S. Rholes (Eds.), *Attachment theory and close relationships* (pp. 46–76). Guilford Press.

Caspi-Berkowitz, N., Mikulincer, M., Hirschberger, G., Ein-Dor, T., & Shaver, P. R. (2019). To die for a cause but not for a companion: Attachment-related variations in the terror management function of self-sacrifice. *Journal of Personality and Social Psychology, 117,* 1105–1126.

Castano, E., Yzerbyt, V., Paladino, M.-P., & Sacchi, S. (2002). I belong, therefore, I exist: Ingroup identification, ingroup entitativity, and ingroup bias. *Personality and Social Psychology Bulletin, 28,* 135–143.

Chen, C., Hewitt, P. L., Flett, G. L., Cassels, T. G., Birch, S., & Blasberg, J. S. (2012). Insecure attachment, perfectionistic self-presentation, and social disconnection. *Personality and Individual Differences, 52,* 936–941.

Cox, C. R., Arndt, J., Pyszczynski, T., Greenberg, J., Abdollahi, A, & Solomon, S. (2008). Terror management and adults' attachment to their parents: The safe haven remains. *Journal of Personality and Social Psychology, 94,* 696–717.

Dandeneau, S. D., Baldwin, M. W., Baccus, J. R., Sakellaropoulo, M., & Pruessner, J. C. (2007). Cutting stress off at the pass: Reducing vigilance and responsiveness to social threat by manipulating attention. *Journal of Personality and Social Psychology, 93,* 651–666.

Davis, E. B., Kimball, C. N., Aten, J. D., Hamilton, C., Andrews, B., Lemke, A., . . . Chung, J. (2019). Faith in the wake of disaster: A longitudinal qualitative study of religious attachment following a catastrophic flood. *Psychological Trauma: Theory, Research, Practice, and Policy, 11,* 578–587.

Florian, V., & Mikulincer, M. (1998). Symbolic immortality and the management of the terror of death: The moderating role of attachment style. *Journal of Personality and Social Psychology, 74,* 725–734.

Florian, V., Mikulincer, M., & Hirschberger, G. (2002). The anxiety buffering function of close relationships: Evidence that relationship commitment acts as a terror management mechanism. *Journal of Personality and Social Psychology, 82,* 527–542.

Frischlich, L., Rieger, D., Dratsch, T., & Bente, G. (2015). Meet Joe Black?: The effects of mortality salience and similarity on the desire to date in-group versus out-group members online. *Journal of Social and Personal Relationships, 32,* 509–528.

Fritsche, I., Jonas, E., Ablasser, C., Beyer, M., Kuban, J., Manger, A.-M., & Schultz, M. (2013). The power of we: Evidence for group-based control. *Journal of Experimental Social Psychology, 49,* 19–32.

Fuglestad, P. T., Leone, C., & Drury, T. (2020). Protective and acquisitive self-monitoring differences in attachment anxiety and avoidance. *Self and Identity, 19,* 219–234.

Gelfand, M. (2018). *Rule makers, rule breaker: How tight and loose cultures wire our world.* Scribner.

Gillath, O., & Hart, J. (2010). The effects of psychological security and insecurity on political attitudes and leadership preferences. *European Journal of Social Psychology, 40,* 122–134.

Gillath, O., Karantzas, G. C., Romano, D., & Karantzas, K. M. (2022). Attachment security priming: A meta-analysis. *Personality and Social Psychology Review, 26,* 183–241.

Gillath, O., Sesko, A. K., Shaver, P. R., & Chun, D. S. (2010). Attachment, authenticity, and honesty: Dispositional and experimentally induced security can reduce self- and other-deception. *Journal of Personality and Social Psychology, 98,* 841–855.

Granqvist, P. (2020). *Attachment in religion and spirituality.* Guilford Press.

Granqvist, P., Mikulincer, M., Gurwitz, V., & Shaver, P. R. (2012). Experimental findings on God as an attachment figure: Normative processes and moderating effects of internal working models. *Journal of Personality and Social Psychology, 103,* 804–818.

Greenberg, J., Pyszczynski, T., Solomon, S., Rosenblatt, A., Veeder, M., Kirkland, S., & Lyon, D. (1990). Evidence for terror management theory II: The effects of mortality salience on reactions to those who threaten or bolster the cultural worldview. *Journal of Personality and Social Psychology, 58,* 308–318.

Gruneau Brulin, J., Hill, P. C., Laurin, K., Mikulincer, M., & Granqvist, P. (2018). Religion vs. the welfare state: The importance of cultural context for religious schematicity and priming. *Psychology of Religion and Spirituality, 10,* 276–287.

Harmon-Jones, E., Greenberg, J., Solomon, S., & Simon, L. (1996). The effects of mortality salience on intergroup bias between minimal groups. *European Journal of Social Psychology, 26,* 677–681.

Hart, J., Shaver, P. R., & Goldenberg, J. L. (2005). Attachment, self-esteem, worldviews, and terror management: Evidence for a tripartite security system. *Journal of Personality and Social Psychology, 88,* 999–1013.

Hewitt, P. L., Flett, G. L., & Mikail, S. F. (2017). *Perfectionism: A relational approach to conceptualization, assessment, and treatment.* Guilford Press.

Hicks, J. A., & King, L. A. (2009). Positive mood and social relatedness as information about meaning in life. *Journal of Positive Psychology, 4,* 471–482.

Hicks, J. A., Schlegel, R. J., & King, L. A. (2010). Social threats, happiness, and the dynamics of meaning in life judgments. *Personality and Social Psychology Bulletin, 36,* 1305–1317.

Hirschberger, G., Florian, V., & Mikulincer, M. (2002). The anxiety buffering function of close relationships: Mortality salience effects on the readiness to compromise mate selection standards. *European Journal of Social Psychology, 32,* 609–625.

Hirschberger, G., Florian, V., & Mikulincer, M. (2003). Strivings for romantic intimacy following partner complaint or partner criticism:

A terror management perspective. *Journal of Social and Personal Relationships, 20,* 675–687.

Hoppe, A., Fritsche, I., & Koranyi, N. (2018). Romantic love versus reproduction opportunities: Disentangling the contributions of different anxiety buffers under conditions of existential threat. *European Journal of Social Psychology, 48,* 269–284.

Jonas, E., Kauffeld, S., Sullivan, D., & Fritsche, I. (2011). Dedicate your life to the company! A terror management perspective on organizations. *Journal of Applied Social Psychology, 41,* 2858–2882.

Juhl, J., Routledge, C., Arndt, J., Sedikides, C., & Wildschut, T. (2010). Fighting the future with the past: Nostalgia buffers existential threat. *Journal of Research in Personality, 44,* 309–314.

Kay, A. C., Gaucher, D., Napier, J. L., Callan, M. J., & Laurin, K. (2008). God and the government: Testing a compensatory control mechanism for the support of external systems. *Journal of Personality and Social Psychology, 95,* 18–35.

Keefe, F. J., Affleck, G., Lefebvre, J., Underwood, L., Caldwell, D. S., Drew, J., . . . Pargament, K. (2001). Living with rheumatoid arthritis: The role of daily spirituality and daily religious and spiritual coping. *Journal of Pain, 2,* 101–110.

Koenig, H. G., King, D. E., & Carson, V. B. (Eds.). (2012). *Handbook of religion and health* (2nd ed.). Oxford University Press.

Lambert, A. J., Schott, J. P., & Scherer, L. (2011). Threat, politics, and attitudes: Toward a greater understanding of rally-'round-the-flag effects. *Current Directions in Psychological Science, 20,* 343–348.

Lambert, N. M., Stillman, T. F., Baumeister, R. F., Fincham, F. D., Hicks, J. A., & Graham, S. M. (2010). Family as a salient source of meaning in young adulthood. *Journal of Positive Psychology, 5,* 367–375.

Li, Q., & Brewer, M. B. (2004). What does it mean to be an American?: Patriotism, nationalism, and American identity after 9/11. *Political Psychology, 25,* 727–739.

Lopez, F. G., Ramos, K., Nisenbaum, M., Thind, N., & Ortiz-Rodriguez, T. (2015). Predicting the presence and search for life meaning: Test of an attachment theory-driven model. *Journal of Happiness Studies, 16,* 103–116.

Mallinckrodt, B., Daly, K., & Wang, C.-C. D. C. (2009). An attachment approach to adult psychotherapy. In J. H. Obegi & E. Berant (Eds.), *Attachment theory and research in clinical work with adults* (pp. 234–268). Guilford Press.

Maslow, A. H. (1971). *The farther reaches of human nature.* Viking.

Mayseless, O., & Popper, M. (2007). Reliance on leaders and social institutions: An attachment perspective. *Attachment and Human Development, 9,* 73–93.

Mayseless, O., & Popper, M. (2019). Attachment and leadership: Review and new insights. *Current Opinion in Psychology, 25,* 157–161.

Mikulincer, M., Birnbaum, G., Woddis, D., & Nachmias, O. (2000). Stress and accessibility of proximity-related thoughts: Exploring the normative and intraindividual components of attachment theory. *Journal of Personality and Social Psychology, 78,* 509–523.

Mikulincer, M., & Florian, V. (2000). Exploring individual differences in reactions to mortality salience: Does attachment style regulate terror management mechanisms? *Journal of Personality and Social Psychology, 79,* 260–273.

Mikulincer, M., Florian, V., & Hirschberger, G. (2003). The existential function of close relationships: Introducing death into the science of love. *Personality and Social Psychology Review, 7,* 20–40.

Mikulincer, M., Florian, V., & Tolmacz, R. (1990). Attachment styles and fear of personal death: A case study of affect regulation. *Journal of Personality and Social Psychology, 58,* 273–280.

Mikulincer, M., & Shaver, P. R. (2003). The attachment behavioral system in adulthood: Activation, psychodynamics, and interpersonal processes. In M. P. Zanna (Ed.), *Advances in experimental social psychology* (Vol. 35, pp. 53–152). Academic Press.

Mikulincer, M., & Shaver, P. R. (2005). Mental representations of attachment security: Theoretical foundation for a positive social psychology. In M. W. Baldwin (Ed.), *Interpersonal cognition* (pp. 233–266). Guilford Press.

Mikulincer, M., & Shaver, P. R. (2016). *Attachment in adulthood: Structure, dynamics, and change* (2nd ed.). Guilford Press.

Mikulincer, M., & Shaver, P. R. (2023). *Attachment theory expanded: Security dynamics in individuals, dyads, groups, and societies.* Guilford Press.

Mueller, J. E. (1970). Presidential popularity from Truman to Johnson. *American Political Science Review, 64,* 18–34.

Plusnin, N., Pepping, C. A., & Kashima, E. S. (2018). The role of close relationships in terror management: A systematic review and research agenda. *Personality and Social Psychology Review, 22,* 307–346.

Popper, M., & Mayseless, O. (2003). Back to basics: Applying a parenting perspective to transformational leadership. *Leadership Quarterly, 14,* 41–65.

Prusova, I., & Gulevich, O. (2019). *The effect of mortality salience on attitudes toward national outgroups.* Higher School of Economics Research Paper No. WP BRP 105/PSY/2019.

Pyszczynski, T., Kesebir, P., & Lockett, M. (2019). A terror management theory perspective on human motivation. In R. M. Ryan (Ed.), *The Oxford handbook of human motivation* (2nd ed., pp. 67–88). Oxford University Press.

Pyszczynski, T., Wicklund, R. A., Floresku, S., Koch, H., Gauch, G., Solomon, S., & Greenberg, J. (1996). Whistling in the dark: Exaggerated consensus estimates in response to incidental reminders of mortality. *Psychological Science, 7,* 332–336.

Quinn, S. C., Parmer, J., Freimuth, V. S., Hilyard, K. M., Musa, D., & Kim, K. H. (2013). Exploring communication, trust in government, and vaccination intention later in the 2009 H1N1 pandemic: Results of a national survey. *Biosecurity and Bioterrorism, 11,* 96–106.

Ryan, R. M., & Deci, E. L. (2017). *Self-determination theory: Basic psychological needs in motivation, development, and wellness.* Guilford Press.

Sabol, T. J., & Pianta, R. C. (2012). Recent trends in research on teacher–child relationships. *Attachment and Human Development, 14,* 213–231.

Sedikides, C., & Wildschut, T. (2019). The sociality of personal and collective nostalgia. *European Review of Social Psychology, 30,* 123–173.

Sedikides, C., Wildschut, T., Cheung, W.-Y., Routledge, C., Hepper, E. G., Arndt, J., . . . Vingerhoets, A. J. J. M. (2016). Nostalgia fosters self-continuity: Uncovering the mechanism (social connectedness) and consequence (eudaimonic well-being). *Emotion, 16,* 524–539.

Sedikides, C., Wildschut, T., Routledge, C., & Arndt, J. (2015). Nostalgia counteracts self-discontinuity and restores self-continuity. *European Journal of Social Psychology, 45,* 52–61.

Seligman, M. E. P. (2002). *Authentic happiness: Using the new positive psychology to realize your potential for lasting fulfillment.* Free Press.

Sibley, C. G., & Bulbulia, J. (2012). Faith after an earthquake: A longitudinal study of religion and perceived health before and after the 2011 Christchurch New Zealand earthquake. *PLOS One, 7,* e49648.

Sibley, C. G., Greaves, L. M., Satherley, N., Wilson, M. S., Overall, N. C., Lee, C. H. J., . . . Barlow, F. K. (2020). Effects of the COVID-19 pandemic and nationwide lockdown on trust, attitudes toward government, and well-being. *American Psychologist, 75,* 618–630.

Silveira, S., Graupmann, V., Agthe, M., Gutyrchik, E., Blautzik, J., Demirçapa, I., . . . Hennig-Fast, K. (2014). Existential neuroscience: Effects of mortality salience on the neurocognitive processing of attractive opposite-sex faces. *Social Cognitive and Affective Neuroscience, 9,* 1601–1607.

Smith, E. R., Murphy, J., & Coats, S. (1999). Attachment to groups: Theory and management. *Journal of Personality and Social Psychology, 77,* 94–110.

Sokol, Y., & Serper, M. (2019). Experimentally increasing self-continuity improves subjective well-being and protects against self-esteem deterioration from an ego-deflating task. *Identity, 19,* 157–172.

Steger, M. F., Kashdan, T. B., Sullivan, B. A., & Lorentz, D. (2008). Understanding the search for meaning in life: Personality, cognitive style, and the dynamic between seeking and experiencing meaning. *Journal of Research in Personality, 42,* 660–678.

Stillman, T. S., Baumeister, R. F., Lambert, N. M., Crescioni, A. W., DeWall, C. N., & Fincham, F. D. (2009). Alone and without purpose: Life loses meaning following social exclusion. *Journal of Experimental Social Psychology, 45,* 686–694.

Stollberg, J., Fritsche, I., & Bäcker, A. (2015). Striving for group agency: Threat to personal control increases the attractiveness of agentic groups. *Frontiers in Psychology, 6,* Article 649.

Stollberg, J., Fritsche, I., & Jonas, E. (2017). The groupy shift: Conformity to liberal in-group norms as a group-based response to threatened personal control. *Social Cognition, 35,* 374–394.

Stouffer, S. A. (1949). *The American soldier: Vol. 2. Combat and its aftermath.* Princeton University Press.

Taubman Ben-Ari, O., Findler, L., & Mikulincer, M. (2002). The effects of mortality salience on relationship strivings and beliefs: The moderating role of attachment style. *British Journal of Social Psychology, 41,* 419–441.

Vail, K. E. III, Arndt, J., & Abdollahi, A. (2012). Exploring the existential function of religion and supernatural agent beliefs among Christians, Muslims, Atheists, and Agnostics. *Personality and Social Psychology Bulletin, 38,* 1288–1300.

van Petegem, S., Beyers, W., Brenning, K., & Vansteenkiste, M. (2013). Exploring the association between insecure attachment styles and adolescent autonomy in family decision making: A differentiated approach. *Journal of Youth and Adolescence, 42,* 1837–1846.

van Tilburg, W. A. P., Igou, E. R., & Sedikides, C. (2013). In search of meaningfulness: Nostalgia as an antidote to boredom. *Emotion, 13,* 450–461.

Watanabe, T., & Karasawa, K. (2012). Self-ingroup overlap in the face of mortality salience. *Japanese Journal of Experimental Social Psychology, 52,* 25–34.

Weise, D. R., Pyszczynski, T., Cox, C. R., Arndt, J., Greenberg, J., & Solomon, S. (2008). Interpersonal politics: The role of terror management and attachment processes in shaping political preferences. *Psychological Science, 19,* 148–155.

Wildschut, T., Sedikides, C., Arndt, J., & Routledge, C. (2006). Nostalgia: Content, triggers, functions. *Journal of Personality and Social Psychology, 91,* 975–993.

Williams, K. D. (2007). Ostracism. *Annual Review of Psychology, 58,* 425–452.

Yaakobi, E., Mikulincer, M., & Shaver, P. R. (2014). Parenthood as a terror management mechanism: The moderating role of attachment orientations. *Personality and Social Psychology Bulletin, 40,* 762–774.

Zeifman, D., & Hazan, C. (2016). Pair bonds as attachments: Mounting evidence in support of Bowlby's hypothesis. In J. Cassidy & P. R. Shaver (Eds.), *Handbook of attachment: Theory, research, and clinical applications* (3rd ed., pp. 416–434). Guilford Press.

CHAPTER 32

Ostracism as an Existential Threat

Sydney G. Wicks, Sarah Mohammadi, Natasha R. Wood, *and* Andrew H. Hales

Ostracism is defined as being excluded and ignored (Williams, 2009). This phenomenon, commonly encountered in various social contexts, has significant consequences for individuals' well-being. Human beings, as inherently social animals, possess a profound instinct to belong, a crucial element for survival and successful reproduction (Baumeister & Leary, 1995). Deeply rooted in our evolutionary history, those who were oblivious to cues of ostracism faced a distinct disadvantage in terms of survival (Wesselmann et al., 2012). This (hyper-)sensitivity to ostracism is not merely a by-product of evolution; it also reflects a fundamental aspect of our existence.

Ostracism is an experience that can be observed in different situations and relationships, and most individuals have experienced it at some point in their lives. Research suggests that this experience may occur at least once a week (Bernstein et al., 2021), but may even occur daily (Nezlek et al., 2012). While the effect of ostracism is most often examined from the perspective of the target (the person being ostracized), it is also shown to have some negative impact on the sources of ostracism. For instance, Legate and colleagues (2013) show that individuals experience negative affect and thwarted needs (e.g., self-esteem) both when they themselves are ostracized *and* when engaging in the act of ostracizing others. Further, the responsive theory of social exclusion supports this notion that both parties (the source and the target) are negatively impacted by social exclusion and fare better when explicit rejection is used (Freedman et al., 2016). Ostracism may also negatively impact third-party observers in which audience members experience vicarious ostracism (e.g., Paolini et al., 2017; Wesselmann et al., 2013b)

Although a negative experience, ostracism may serve as a way to protect individuals from threat, to signal that an individual's behavior needs to be adjusted, and to permanently remove deviant group members (Hales et al., 2017). Ultimately, this indicates both the costs and benefits associated with the act of ostracism, at least from the source's perspective. Though ostracizing others may initially provide a sense of control, the ostracizer (i.e., source of ostracism) may eventually find themselves just as helpless in the situation as the target (Zadro & Gonsalkorale, 2014).

The consequences of ostracism (and other social threats) extend beyond only the immediate social discomfort. Individuals subjected to ostracism may also experience a profound sense of insignificance, feeling that their existence lacks meaning to others (Williams, 2009; Williams & Zadro, 2001). Research by Hames and colleagues (2018) and Legate and colleagues (2013) further emphasizes the profound impact of ostracism, showing that both those who experienced and those who administered ostracism suffered negative psychological effects (e.g., threatened needs). Poulsen and Kashy (2012) also found that more severe forms of exclusion led to more significant negative outcomes.

In this chapter, we first provide a brief overview of ostracism, as well as how it poses an existential threat and how it is studied. Next, we discuss the leading theoretical model for understanding the consequences of ostracism: the temporal need–threat model. Finally, we discuss the use of ostracism as a conformity tool and how individuals may feel ostracized from a variety of sources.

OVERVIEW OF OSTRACISM

In its broadest definition, ostracism encompasses both severe and dramatic instances of being ignored and excluded (e.g., excommunication from the church; Hales et al., 2020) as well as even its subtlest forms (e.g., gender-exclusive language, like using a generic *he;* Stout & Dasgupta, 2011) and everyday behaviors like cell-phone use during a social interaction (phubbing; Hales et al., 2018). Similarly, ostracism may vary in intensity, from partial (e.g., lack of eye contact from a virtual confederate; Dvir et al., 2021; Wirth et al., 2010) to complete exclusion. This variability in ostracism is crucial to understanding its wide-ranging effects (Hales et al., 2017). Notably, it has been demonstrated that even brief encounters with ostracism, such as those involving strangers with no expectation of future interactions, may be capable of producing significant negative reactions (Goodwin et al., 2010). As such, this broad approach has been instrumental in examining ostracism in both controlled laboratory settings and naturalistic settings.

Ostracism as an Existential Psychological Threat

The consequences of social threats, such as ostracism, extend beyond immediate social discomfort. Ostracism (and other social threats) appears to lead people to confront major existential concerns of death, isolation, identity, freedom, and meaning (Koole et al., 2006; Yalom, 1980). For instance, ostracism has commonly been referred to as a social death (e.g., Bauman, 1992; Williams, 2007) and may also be equated with death itself (Case & Williams, 2004; Hales, 2018; but see Taggert et al., 2024, for limits on this connection). Further emphasizing the critical role of social connections in human survival, a social death evolutionarily equates to a physical (literal) death. From an evolutionary perspective, the human brain may have evolved to process social exclusion as a threat to survival, triggering responses similar to those evoked by the threat of physical harm or death (MacDonald & Leary, 2005; Spoor & Williams, 2007). As evidence of the connection between ostracism and death, an absence of positive relationships has been shown to be a risk factor in mortality, similar to that of other factors, such as cigarette smoking (Holt-Lunstad et al., 2010). Additionally, ostracism is one reason why people may experience *both* social (interpersonal) isolation (feeling isolated from others; Williams & Nida, 2022) and existential isolation (feeling isolated in one's experiences or from reality; Pinel et al., 2017). Identity may be threatened by ostracism through inducing feelings of self-uncertainty. Moments of uncertainty, such as concerns for what the future holds as well as ambiguity of one's exclusion, may also invoke a sense of (social) isolation (Hales et al., 2021). Ostracized individuals may also search for the reasons and rationale for *why* they were excluded, which may lead them to invoke negative internal attributions, lowering their self-esteem (e.g., Liu, 2019). The loss of control (autonomy) associated with ostracism may also represent a threat to concerns of free will and freedom. For instance, ostracized individuals (compared to included individuals) reported feeling less autonomous (e.g., feeling *less* like they were free to decided for themsevels how to act; Legate et al., 2013). Similarly, research suggests that individuals subjected to ostracism may be linked with a profound sense of insignificance (Park & Pinel, 2020), feeling that their existence lacks meaning to others (Williams, 2009; Williams & Zadro, 2001).

Beyond its analogy to death, ostracism is associated with existential anxiety (Zamperini et al., 2020). For instance, Steele and colleagues (2015) emphasized the role of social connections in keeping existential threats at bay. They found that ostracism induced a state of insignificance and increased mental accessibility to thoughts of death (although findings of the latter have been mixed (Taggart et al., 2024). In line with this thinking, ostracism can lead to deep reflections on one's meaning, importance, and even existence (e.g., Hales, 2018). In extreme forms of ostracism—such as receiving the silent treatment from loved ones or close others for long periods of time—one experiences a glimpse of what life would be like if one did not exist, watching others carry on as if one were not there (Williams et al., 2000a; Zadro et al., 2008).

Even seemingly minor instances of ostracism elicit transient feelings of invisibility and a painful sense of lacking worth, purpose, or meaning (Williams, 2012), during which ostracized people have pinched themselves in order to test their environment and mere existence. Indicating a decrease in one's relational value (Leary, 2005), this impact goes beyond conventional aversive behaviors, as ostracism uniquely threatens existential needs related to recognition and worthiness of attention. For instance, the consequences of social ostracism extend to questioning one's purpose, self-worth, value, and the ability to control goals and outcomes (Jiang & Chen, 2020a; Stillman et al., 2009; Zadro et al., 2006). By examining the language individuals use after being ostracized, research has shown that when compared to a control group, ostracized individuals used function words (e.g., pronouns and articles) that indicated greater self-focus and worsened mood (Klauke & Kauffeld, 2020). Additionally, studies have confirmed that ostracism typically leads to feelings of meaninglessness and reminders of mortality (Steele et al., 2015; Stillman et al., 2009).

How We Study Ostracism

The most commonly used experimental paradigm to study ostracism is Cyberball, in which participants play an online ball-tossing game with preprogrammed avatars who they are led to believe are other participants (Williams et al., 2000b; Williams & Jarvis, 2006). In a typical game, people in the inclusion (comparison) condition receive the ball about an equal number of times as the other players. Participants in the ostracism condition receive the ball twice at the beginning of the game but never again and, instead, have to watch the ball being passed between the other players. A meta-analysis of 120 Cyberball studies shows that—despite the deliberately minimal features of the game—ostracism has a large effect on basic psychological needs, and this effect decreases over time, supporting the notion that people begin to recover quickly (Hartgerink et al., 2015). A benefit of Cyberball is that aspects of the game can be altered, including the number of players, the names of the players and what they look like, and the presence of an audience. A newly developed Social Ball paradigm seems to be a promising avenue to vary yet more features of the game, and do so in a more immersive virtual setting (Meral et al., 2022).

There are many other ways to measure and manipulate ostracism: autobiographical reliving paradigm (e.g., Hales et al., 2018; Pickett et al., 2004), self-reported chronic ostracism with the Ostracism Experiences Scale (Carter-Sowell, 2010), or momentary assessments of real-world experiences of exclusion (e.g, Bernstein et al., 2021; Nezlek et al., 2012). But we expand upon two additional commonly used experimental paradigms: the Future Life paradigm and the Ostracism Online paradigm. In the Future Life paradigm (Twenge et al., 2001), participants first complete a personality assessment. They are then told false feedback about their future social network that is supposedly based on the results of the assessment: They will have rewarding relationships throughout life (included condition), they will end up alone later in life (excluded condition), or they will be accident-prone later in life (control condition). Interestingly, while Cyberball leads to *pain hypersensitivity*, the Future Life paradigm leads to a *numbing* effect, potentially because Cyberball is relatively less severe (Bernstein & Claypool, 2012).

In an increasingly digital age, online platforms offer an environment for individuals to also be ostracized. To investigate dynamics in this setting, researchers developed the Ostracism Online paradigm, whereby participants interact with other avatars (believed to be real people but actually preprogrammed) in a social media–like website (Wolf et al., 2015). After creating a "profile" with an avatar and personal bio introducing themselves to the rest of the group, participants can like/dislike other people's profiles and receive attention (in the form of likes or dislikes) from others. In the inclusion condition, participants typically receive six likes (and no dislikes). In the ostracism condition, participants receive one like and one dislike at the beginning of the task and then are ignored for the remainder of the time. This paradigm has also been further developed to include a dislike button and an explicit rejection condition whereby participants receive no likes and six dislikes (Lutz & Schneider, 2020). Ostracism Online similarly threatens basic psychological needs (ostracism vs. inclusion) compared to Cyberball (Wolf et al., 2015), and it may be particularly useful when studying online phenomenon, such as the spread of misinformation (e.g., Wicks et al., 2023) or certain extremist groups (e.g., incels).

The Hurt of Ostracism

In line with theories such as pain-overlap theory (Eisenberger, 2012), research has established that social exclusion not only emotionally hurts but also activates brain areas associated with physical pain (Eisenberger et al., 2003). This pain can be more serious and long-lasting than physical pain, potentially suggesting a deep-rooted evolutionary basis for this response (Chen et al., 2008). The severe impact of the social pain of ostracism is likely due to the ease of it being reexperienced compared to that of physical pain (Meyer et al., 2015). The human species, dependent on social relationships for survival, has likely evolved to be particularly sensitive to any cues of social exclusion, with some researchers referring to this as an ostracism detection system (Kerr & Levine, 2008; Spoor & Williams, 2007; Wesselmann et al., 2012).

Ostracism also has severe mental health consequences that are especially relevant to its role as a—sometimes literal—existential threat, including increasing suicidal thoughts (Chen et al., 2020). Similarly, belongingness theory suggests that social exclusion triggers anxiety due to the perceived loss of belonging (Baumeister & Leary, 1995). Notably, ostracism directly impacts self-worth and identity, posing a threat to one's sense of meaningful existence (Chen et al., 2020; Steele et al., 2015).

Finally, even minimal ostracism experiences, such as not receiving the ball in a brief Cyberball game, can cause significant emotional distress and perceived threats to fundamental needs like belonging and self-esteem (Wesselmann et al., 2012). In fact, even when the game is arranged so that being *included* increases one's chances of a sort of symbolic death—through a version called "Cyberbomb" in which the ball is replaced with a virtual bomb set to detonate—ostracism still hurts (van Beest et al., 2011). This underscores the potent psychological impact of ostracism, regardless of its form or duration.

The notion that ostracism is painful, regardless of its form, is supported by a range of research. Studies have shown that participants in Cyberball experiments feel ostracized and experience lower levels on psychological needs, even under conditions where they are told that the exclusion is not personal, such as being informed that their computer is not connected to others (Eisenberger et al., 2003; Jauch et al., 2022; Zadro et al., 2004). Additionally, research shows that even when inclusion is financially costly, being ostracized still hurts (van Beest & Williams, 2006). This suggests that the pain of ostracism is not mitigated by knowing the intentionality of the ostracism or knowing that it offers other benefits.

THE TEMPORAL NEED–THREAT MODEL OF OSTRACISM

The *temporal need–threat model* outlines how responses to ostracism unfold in three distinct stages upon detection: the reflexive, reflective, and resignation stages (Williams, 2009).

Stage 1: Reflexive Stage

First, individuals very quickly detect that they are being ostracized. Immediately upon detection, they enter the *reflexive* stage, in which they experience social pain, negative emotions, and harmful consequences of having their fundamental psychological needs threatened. These needs include belonging, self-esteem, control, and meaningful existence (e.g., Baumeister & Leary, 1995; Williams & Zadro, 2001). These psychological needs map onto the existential concerns previously mentioned, such as a loss (even if temporarily) of control in social interactions also threatening concerns of free will and freedom. In addition to threatening these four needs, research has shown the detrimental effect of ostracism on one's need for certainty (both for themselves and their surroundings; Hales & Williams, 2018), and the theory has been updated to include this need (Hales & Williams, 2021). Upon experiencing ostracism, individuals often report a range of negative outcomes that may also include physiological reactions typical of perceived threats, such as increased secretion of cortisol stress hormones (Bernstein, 2016; McDonald & Brent Donnellan, 2012; Williams, 2009). Additionally, individuals may also experience emotional responses, such as distress, anger, sadness, even in response to minimal ostracizing experiences (Carter-Sowell et al., 2008).

Because these immediate negative effects are theorized to be *reflexive* (i.e., automatic and nondeliberate), they should occur even in situations where one would expect ostracism to logically have no effect. This is the case in the original minimal Cyberball game where the players are strangers one will never meet, and yet needs are still thwarted (Williams et al., 2000b). Beyond this, efforts to identify situations where ostracism is not hurtful have been surprisingly difficult to identify. Ostracism still hurts even when one would logically expect it not to. For example, even when ostracism is known to be from a despised group (e.g., the Ku Klux Klan), the immediate reactions are still distressful (Fayant et al., 2014; Gonsalkorale & Williams, 2007). As mentioned earlier, financial incentives have been shown to be ineffective in alleviating ostracism-induced distress. For instance, participants who were charged money for each ball thrown to them in a variant of Cyberball, called €yberball, still felt as badly ostracized as in a nonmonetary version of the game (van Beest & Williams, 2006).

Stage 2: Reflective Stage

In the *reflective* stage, ostracized individuals focus their attention on improving these needs and regaining some sense of connection—be it from the sources of the ostracism or from entirely new individuals. Recovery is suggested to begin soon after the initial effects of ostracism (Goodwin et al., 2010). Within this reflective stage, there are numerous factors that may impact the extent in which individuals recover, such as attributions ostracized individuals make about their exclusion and the tools they have available to help cope with the experience. It is during the reflective stage when people attend to, appraise, and make attributions for their exclusion, as well as attempt to replenish their previously lost needs. Because needs can be replenished in a variety of ways (e.g., Paravati et al., 2021), reactions to ostracism generally begin to vary, particularly in terms of the rate in which they recover from the experience and behavioral responses (e.g., Zadro et al., 2006).

Recovery from Ostracism

According to the need–threat model, while ostracism may reflexively hurt most people the same, people vary in the rate at which they recover. It is during this stage where people try to make sense of their exclusion and aim to replenish their previously lost needs. Just as meaning-making may be helpful in response to disasters in life (e.g., Park, 2016), attributions made about reasons for one's exclusion can change the rate at which one recovers from the experience. For instance, Wirth and Williams (2009) showed that ostracized individuals who attributed their exclusion to permanent group identities (e.g., gender) recovered slower than those who attributed their exclusion to more temporary identities (e.g., random group assignment). Similarly, when individuals interpreted their exclusion to be racially motivated, ostracized individuals recovered at a slower rate (Goodwin et al., 2010). Along the same lines, the impact of ostracism on identity may be seen in the way experiences of ostracism distort perceptions of the self, such as interrupting self-continuity (Jiang et al., 2021) and increasing self-malleability

(Richman et al., 2015). Furthermore, feeling uncertain of one's identity has been shown to motivate people to increase ingroup behaviors (Hohman et al., 2017) and even be more open to groups they were not previously a part of, with a preference for highly entitative groups (e.g., extreme groups; Hales & Williams, 2018; Hogg & Adelman, 2013) as attempts to appease this existential threat.

To help recover from experiences of social exclusion, individuals may explore various types of strategies. For example, the social surrogacy hypothesis suggests that individuals can transform common technologies into temporary substitutes (referred to as surrogates) for social connection, thus providing an experience of belonging (Derrick et al., 2009; Gabriel & Valenti, 2017). Examples of social surrogates have ranged from one's pets (McConnell et al., 2011), to favorite fictional characters, (Gabriel & Young, 2011), and even comfort foods (Troisi & Gabriel, 2011). In addition to obtaining benefits from familiar surrogates (e.g., one's favorite TV character), there is growing evidence that even unfamiliar surrogates (such as being presented with preselected consumer products or music) may also be effective in helping people feel better after exclusion (Mourey et al., 2017; Wicks & Hales, 2023). According to a systematic review of 119 studies, using media tools to cope with social exclusion was found to be more effective than ineffective (Lutz et al., 2022). In addition to those previously mentioned, strategies such as prayer (Hales et al., 2016) and viewing pictures of nature (Poon et al., 2016) can also aid in exclusion recovery. Contrastingly, one strategy that has been shown to be counterproductive is ruminating about one's experience. As such, strategies that reduce rumination may, in turn, improve recovery (e.g., Hales et al., 2016; Wesselmann et al., 2013a).

Behavioral Responses

Exclusion may also lead people to be more sensitive to social cues and have a stronger craving for social interaction (Pickett et al., 2004). After being excluded, people may act prosocially as a means of being desirable to others and reincluded. This behavior may help them restore all threatened needs, but particularly belonging and self-esteem, referred to as the *inclusionary* need cluster (Williams, 2009). Excluded people contribute more to a group (Williams & Sommer, 1997), are more compliant to social influence (Carter-Sowell et al., 2008), and obey an authority figure even when the request is undesirable (Riva et al., 2014). More specifically, prosocial behavior is more likely if the potential target is innocent (i.e., not the exclusion source; Gerber & Wheeler, 2009).

Although it seems counterintuitive to the goal of reinclusion, people may also act antisocially after being excluded in order to help them restore their thwarted needs of control and meaningful existence, or the *power and provocation* need cluster (Williams, 2009). In other words, exclusion can lead to aggression (Leary et al., 2006; Ren et al., 2018), particularly when prioritizing restoring a need for control (Warburton et al., 2006). In the lab, aggressive behavioral responses to exclusion manifest as greater likelihood to administer a painful noise (e.g., Twenge et al., 2001) and give other people more hot sauce (e.g., Warburton et al., 2006). People may choose to act aggressively because they feel less constrained by social norms after being excluded (Poon & Teng, 2017; Twenge et al., 2001); have fewer perceived costs of aggression (Poon & Wong, 2019); or as a result of negative emotion, such as relative deprivation (Jiang & Chen, 2020b), malicious envy (Poon et al., 2023), or anger (Chow et al., 2008).

Finally, a third and more recently identified behavioral response to ostracism is *withdrawal*. Research suggests that people are more willing to seek solitude after being excluded (Ren, 2016). After the painful experience of being excluded, people may wish to avoid it happening again by withdrawing from social interactions during which others could have the opportunity to exclude them again (Sunami et al., 2019). Indeed, ostracism leads to greater desire for solitude (Ren et al., 2016, 2021). Interestingly, people are more willing to ostracize those with higher dispositional preference for solitude (Ren & Evans, 2021), suggesting that the relationship between exclusion and solitude may be cyclical. Thus, exclusion is capable of driving individuals toward and away from both human and nonhuman agents (e.g., Epley et al., 2008). Attributions as well as the perceived possibility of being (re-)included influence whether individuals will have more prevention-focused (e.g., solitude-seeking) or promotion-focused (e.g., reengagement) responses to exclusion (Maner et al., 2007; Molden et al., 2009).

Stage 3: Resignation Stage

If social connection cannot be (re-)established, ostracized individuals may give up and further alienate themselves (Williams, 2009). This may take the form of separating from others and deciding to no longer seek connection, serving as the final stage of the need–threat model: *resignation*. Continuous experiences of ostracism may accumulate and lead to a state of insecurity, whereby the prolonged loss of each type of need is suggested to result in a severe negative outcome specific to that need: alienation (belonging need), depression (self-esteem need), learned helplessness (control need), and unworthiness (meaningful existence need). These hypotheses cannot be tested experimentally for ethical and logistical reasons, but existing correlational and longitudinal research is consistent with these predictions (Riva et al., 2017; Rudert et al., 2021). Similarly, although research has shown that ostracism may also induce feelings of uncertainty, the equivalent outcome associated with prolonged, exclusion-induced uncertainty is currently unknown, thus offering an avenue for future research.

THE USE OF OSTRACISM AS A TOOL FOR SOCIAL INFLUENCE

Recognized as a universally applied tactic of social control, ostracism can play an important role in influencing individual behavior and fostering group conformity (e.g., Hales et al., 2017; Riva et al., 2014). Conforming to group norms and expectations can help people feel accepted and maintain a sense of belonging. This conformity can be seen as a defensive mechanism against the existential threat of ostracism—helping people feel connected and meaningful in their social groups. Extensive research spanning over two decades underscores the effectiveness of ostracism in exerting social influence (e.g, Hales et al., 2017). Individuals, upon perceiving ostracism, tend to adjust their behaviors to regain acceptance into the group, often becoming highly susceptible to social influence (Carter-Sowell et al., 2008).

Even the mere threat of ostracism can have a profound impact, suppressing deviant behaviors that pose a threat to group cohesion and survival (Ouwerkerk et al., 2005). The need to belong and maintain self-esteem compels ostracized individuals to conform to group norms (Williams et al., 2000b).

Ostracized individuals are also more likely to comply with requests, such as for financial donations, under different compliance tactics (Carter-Sowell et al., 2008). For instance, women who experienced ostracism during a ball-tossing game displayed heightened efforts in a subsequent collective task, showcasing a form of social compensation (Williams & Sommer, 1997). As a social (rather than physical) death, instances of ostracism can be reversed, thus allowing for a "social resurrection" as individuals are reintegrated into a group (Hales, 2018; Zamperini et al., 2020). After being ostracized, individuals often engage in more behaviors aimed at readmission to the group, demonstrating an increased susceptibility to social influence and a tendency to conform to group norms (DeWall, 2010; Nezlek et al., 2015; Williams et al., 2000b). For instance, ostracism has been shown to increase interest in extreme groups. Indeed, Hales and Williams (2018) found that ostracized (vs. included) individuals were more willing to attend a meeting of an activist campus organization and expressed greater openness toward gang membership, suggesting that social exclusion increases susceptibility to new—even deviant—groups.

Ostracism is not only a tool used against individuals deviating from group norms; it also serves as a means to prompt corrective behaviors and motivate prosocial actions for regaining standing within the group (Hales et al., 2017). As a corrective measure, ostracism signals that a member's behavior requires modification, leading to a heightened desire to belong among individuals who experience ostracism. This desire enhances these individuals' adaptability and openness to social influence, making them more susceptible to conformity, a key aspect of social influence.

SOURCES OF OSTRACISM

In addition to ostracism being a powerful tool for social influence, there are different ways in which one may feel ostracized by others. From being excommunicated from a church to receiving the silent treatment from a loved one, ostracism may be enacted by a variety of sources (Williams, 2001). Because people can feel ostracized from a variety of sources, these same sources also pose a threat to one's existence. Particularly, we focus on sources at the institution-level, those at the individual-level, and those that are nonhuman agents.

Feeling Ostracized from Groups, Institutions, and Systems

Institutional ostracism occurs when someone feels excluded through policies and structures (Sherman et al., 2022). For example, someone in the United States who does not have children might feel they are being excluded by their work or government through policies such as time off for maternity leave (there is not a child-free alternative) or the Child Tax Credit (receiving additional tax benefit if one has children age 17 or younger; there is not a child-free alternative). A public figure being "canceled" (i.e., losing fame, credibility, or power) due to unfavorable behavior is also an example of institutional ostracism. Empirical work has yet to directly investigate the effects of institutional ostracism, but it is theorized to be similar to institutional prejudice/discrimination (Murphy et al., 2018), though differs by not always being based on group membership. Systems are usually concrete and enduring, suggesting that it most closely resembles the resignation stage of interpersonal ostracism. Thus, it not only thwarts basic psychological needs, but also leads to hopelessness, depression, and overall lower well-being. Overall, this creates dysfunction and imbalance in one's life, further threatening existential well-being (Galanaki et al., 2023).

In addition to the behavioral responses to interpersonal exclusion, when being ostracized by an institution, people might try to leave the system. This is often possible on a small scale, such as someone quitting a job if they feel excluded by their employer. However, this response may be difficult on a large scale, such as feeling excluded by the legal system in one's country. While someone can attempt to disengage from the system, it may be difficult (e.g., financially) or undesirable (e.g., due to losing close others still in the system). Additionally, people might try to change the system from which they are being excluded, such as through protesting or organizing counter movements. In turn, thwarted psychological needs might be bolstered (e.g., finding a new group to belong with).

Feeling Ostracized from Individuals and Close Others

Severe forms of ostracism often originate from close relationships and endure for a significant period, making them particularly harmful (Hales et al., 2017). Studies indicate that participants feel worse and experience greater threats to their psychological needs when ostracized by closer others compared to strangers (Nezlek et al., 2012). One reason for this may be due to having higher expectations of the partner. Contrastingly, some research suggests that ostracism from strangers is more painful than when ostracized by close others, because the preexisting relationship may act as a buffer (Iannone et al., 2014). Although ostracism is more commonly reported in the context of acquaintances or strangers, ostracizers report feeling increased control in these situations, unlike when ostracizing close friends (Nezlek et al., 2015).

A prevalent form of ostracism in close relationships is the "silent treatment," which poses significant psychological consequences. Targets of this form of ostracism experience heightened threats to their sense of belonging and self-esteem, particularly when they cannot attribute the ostracism to a specific cause (Sommer et al., 2001). Qualitative interviews reveal that targets of ostracism in close relationships express feelings indicative of threatened primary needs, which become internalized due to prolonged or repeated experiences (Zadro et al., 2008). The involvement of a partner in the act of exclusion significantly affects need satisfaction and relationship evaluations, more so than when ostracism involves only strangers, due to people having greater relational expectations (Arriaga et al., 2014). Furthermore, a study investigating the impact of ostracism on children revealed that both complete and partial ostracism have strong negative effects, with the presence of a single ally reducing distress (Sandstrom et al., 2017). This underscores the importance of understanding ostracism in various contexts, including its impact on vulnerable populations such as children.

Feeling Ostracized from Nonhuman Agents

Just as nonhuman agents may be able to offer social connection, they may also be capable of inducing social exclusion. Individuals can feel excluded from agents without a physical shape (e.g., nonhuman or supernatural agents), particularly by those with whom they share a symbolic (i.e., parasocial) relationship. For instance, while prayer may be effective in helping people recover from social ostracism (e.g., Hales et al., 2016; Wesselmann & Williams, 2010), exposure to Bible passages of God's exclusion (e.g., that God would abandon them) may have negative impacts on one's well-being (George et al., 2021; van Beest & Williams, 2011). Likewise, research has shown that divine struggle—feeling anger toward or punished/abandoned by God (e.g., questioning God's love)—is linked with decreased life satisfaction, poor psychological functioning, and greater emotional distress (e.g., higher anxiety rating, greater depressive symptoms; Exline et al., 2014; Wilt et al., 2016). Additionally, one's perceptions of God influence the type of divine struggle one may experience: Viewing God as cruel has been associated with greater anger toward God while viewing God as distant has been related with greater feelings of abandonment and doubts of God's existence (Exline et al., 2015). Thus, similar to how individuals may feel hurt when excluded by human agents, exclusion from nonhuman, supernatural agents such as God may also yield detrimental consequences.

As evidence of technological advancement, human–robot interactions provide another opportunity for individuals to feel ostracized by nonhuman agents. Even when people know they are interacting with a computer programmed to exclude them, the experience of this exclusion still hurts (Zadro et al., 2004). One reason for this robust finding may lie in people's tendency to anthropomorphize nonhuman agents, imbuing these agents with human-like qualities (Jauch et al., 2022). These experiences are becoming more common and intense as technology continues to advance. For instance, in a physical adaptation of Cyberball where participants played a ball-tossing game with two nonhumanoid robots, people still felt excluded when they did not receive the ball even when knowing that the other players were robots (Erel et al., 2021). Similarly, this (over-)sensitivity to detect ostracism is also present when people observed two robots interact while believing the robots were communicating through robotic language (e.g., beeps and clicks) rather than natural language (i.e., that which can be understood by humans). Indeed, Rosenthal-von Der Pütten and Bock (2023) found that when hearing robots transmit information through robotic language, people felt ostracized by being out of the loop. Due to the associations between ostracism and mortality, even slight experiences of ostracism, regardless of source, may serve as an existential threat and a reminder of one's mortality.

SUMMARY

Ostracism is an event capable of causing pain, negative affect, and thwarted basic psychological needs. The experience of ostracism serves as an existential threat, exacerbating existential concerns of death, isolation, freedom, identity, and meaninglessness. There are three distinct stages that unfold in the need–threat model of ostracism. The reflexive stage consists of immediate reactions to ostracism. The reflective stage involves the attribution and appraisal of ostracism as well as the restoration of needs. Lastly, following chronic experiences of ostracism, people may enter the resignation stage. Although research has primarily focused on the reflexive and reflective stages of the model, research is continuing to grow surrounding the consequences of chronic ostracism. While being a negative experience, ostracism is an extremely powerful tool of conformity, capable of being enacted by various sources.

ACKNOWLEDGMENT

This work was supported in part by the National Science Foundation Graduate Research Fellowship Program under Grant No. 2235036 to Wicks. Any opinions, findings, and conclusions, or recommendations expressed do not necessarily reflect the views of the National Science Foundation.

REFERENCES

Arriaga, X. B., Capezza, N. M., Reed, J. T., Wesselmann, E. D., & Williams, K. D. (2014). With partners like you, who needs strangers?: Ostracism involving a romantic partner. *Personal Relationships, 21*(4), 557–569.

Bauman, Z. (1992). *Mortality, immortality, and other life strategies.* Stanford University Press.

Baumeister, R. F., & Leary, M. R. (1995). The need to belong: Desire for interpersonal attachments as a fundamental human motivation. *Psychological Bulletin, 117*(3), 497–529.

Bernstein, M. J. (2016). Research in social psychology: Consequences of short-and long-term social exclusion. In P. Riva & J. Eck (Eds.), *Social exclusion: Psychological approaches to understanding and reducing its impact* (pp. 51–72). Springer Nature.

Bernstein, M. J., & Claypool, H. M. (2012). Social exclusion and pain sensitivity: Why exclusion sometimes hurts and sometimes numbs. *Personality and Social Psychology Bulletin, 38*(2), 185–196.

Bernstein, M. J., Neubauer, A. B., Benfield, J. A., Potter, L., & Smyth, J. M. (2021). Within-person effects of inclusion and exclusion on well-being in daily life. *Personal Relationships*, pere.12399.

Carter-Sowell, A. R. (2010). *Salting a wound, building a callous, or throwing in the towel?: The measurement and effects of chronic ostracism experiences.* Doctoral dissertation, Purdue University. ProQuest Dissertations Publishing.

Carter-Sowell, A. R., Chen, Z., & Williams, K. D. (2008). Ostracism increases social susceptibility. *Social Influence, 3*(3), 143–153.

Case, T. I., & Williams, K. D. (2004). Ostracism: A metaphor for death. In J. Greenberg, S. L. Koole, & T. Pyszczynski (Eds.), *Handbook of experimental existential psychology* (pp. 336–351). Guilford Press.

Chen, Z., Poon, K. T., DeWall, C. N., & Jiang, T. (2020). Life lacks meaning without acceptance: Ostracism triggers suicidal thoughts. *Journal of Personality and Social Psychology, 119*(6).

Chen, Z., Williams, K. D., Fitness, J., & Newton, N. C. (2008). When hurt will not heal: Exploring the capacity to relive social and physical pain. *Psychological Science, 19*(8), 789–795.

Chow, R. M., Tiedens, L. Z., & Govan, C. L. (2008). Excluded emotions: The role of anger in antisocial responses to ostracism. *Journal of Experimental Social Psychology, 44*(3), 896–903.

Derrick, J. L., Gabriel, S., & Hugenberg, K. (2009). Social surrogacy: How favored television programs provide the experience of belonging. *Journal of Experimental Social Psychology, 45*(2), 352–362.

DeWall, C. N. (2010). Forming a basis for acceptance: Excluded people form attitudes to agree with potential affiliates. *Social Influence, 5*(4), 245–260.

Dvir, M., Kelly, J. R., Tyler, J. M., & Williams, K. D. (2021). I'm up here!: Sexual objectification leads to feeling ostracized. *Journal of Personality and Social Psychology, 121*(2), 332–353.

Eisenberger, N. I. (2012). Broken hearts and broken bones: A neural perspective on the similarities between social and physical pain. *Current Directions in Psychological Science, 21*(1), 42–47.

Eisenberger, N. I., Lieberman, M. D., & Williams, K. D. (2003). Does rejection hurt?: An fMRI study of social exclusion. *Science, 302*(5643), 290–292.

Epley, N., Waytz, A., Akalis, S., & Cacioppo, J. T. (2008). When we need a human: Motivational determinants of anthropomorphism. *Social Cognition, 26*(2), 143–155.

Erel, H., Cohen, Y., Shafrir, K., Levy, S. D., Vidra, I. D., Shem Tov, T., & Zuckerman, O. (2021). Excluded by robots: Can robot-robot-human interaction lead to ostracism? *Proceedings of the 2021 ACM/IEEE International Conference on Human-Robot Interaction*, pp. 312–321.

Exline, J. J., Grubbs, J. B., & Homolka, S. J. (2015). Seeing God as cruel or distant: Links with divine struggles involving anger, doubt, and fear of God's disapproval. *International Journal for the Psychology of Religion, 25*(1), 29–41.

Exline, J. J., Pargament, K. I., Grubbs, J. B., & Yali, A. M. (2014). The Religious and Spiritual Struggles Scale: Development and initial validation. *Psychology of Religion and Spirituality, 6*(3), 208–222.

Fayant, M. P., Muller, D., Hartgerink, C. H. J., & Lantian, A. (2014). Is ostracism by a despised outgroup really hurtful?: A replication and extension of Gonsalkorale and Williams (2007). *Social Psychology, 45*(6), 489–494.

Freedman, G., Williams, K. D., & Beer, J. S. (2016). Softening the blow of social exclusion: The responsive theory of social exclusion. *Frontiers in Psychology, 7.*

Gabriel, S., & Valenti, J. (2017). Social surrogates and rejection: How reading, watching TV, and eating comfort food can ease the pain of social isolation. In K. D. Williams & S. A. Nida (Eds.), *Ostracism, exclusion, and rejection* (pp. 156–171). Routledge.

Gabriel, S., & Young, A. F. (2011). Becoming a vampire without being bitten: The narrative collective-assimilation hypothesis. *Psychological Science, 22*(8), 990–994.

Galanaki, E. P., Nelson, L. J., & Antoniou, F. (2023). Social withdrawal, solitude, and existential concerns in emerging adulthood. *Emerging Adulthood, 11*(4), 1006–1021.

George, A. R., Wesselmann, E. D., Hilgard, J., Young, A. I., & van Beest, I. (2021). The effect of thinking about being excluded by God on well-being: A replication and extension. *International Journal for the Psychology of Religion, 31*(2), 138–148.

Gerber, J., & Wheeler, L. (2009). On being rejected: A meta-analysis of experimental research on rejection. *Perspectives on Psychological Science, 4*(5), 468–488.

Gonsalkorale, K., & Williams, K. D. (2007). The KKK won't let me play: Ostracism even by a despised outgroup hurts. *European Journal of Social Psychology, 37*(6), 1176–1186.

Goodwin, S. A., Williams, K. D., & Carter-Sowell, A. R. (2010). The psychological sting of stigma: The costs of attributing ostracism to racism. *Journal of Experimental Social Psychology, 46*(4), 612–618.

Hales, A. (2018). Death as a metaphor for ostracism: Social invincibility, autopsy, necromancy, and resurrection. *Mortality, 23*(4), 366–380.

Hales, A. H., Dvir, M., Wesselmann, E. D., Kruger, D. J., & Finkenauer, C. (2018). Cell phone-induced ostracism threatens fundamental needs. *Journal of Social Psychology, 158*(4), 460–473.

Hales, A. H., Ren, D., & Williams, K. D. (2017). Protect, correct, and eject: Ostracism as a social influence tool. In S. G. Harkins, K. D. Williams, & J. Burger (Eds.), *The Oxford handbook of social influence* (Vol. 1). Oxford University Press.

Hales, A. H., Wesselmann, E. D., & Williams, K. D. (2016). Prayer, self-affirmation, and distraction improve recovery from short-term ostracism. *Journal of Experimental Social Psychology, 64,* 8–20.

Hales, A. H., Wesselmann, E. D., & Williams, K. D. (2020). Social ostracism, religion, and existential concerns. In K. E. Vail III & C. Routledge (Eds.), *The science of religion, spirituality, and existentialism* (pp. 153–166). Elsevier.

Hales, A. H., & Williams, K. D. (2018). Marginalized individuals and extremism: The role of ostracism in openness to extreme groups. *Journal of Social Issues, 74*(1), 75–92.

Hales, A. H., & Williams, K. D. (2021). Social ostracism: Theoretical foundations and basic principles. In P. A. M. Van Lange, E. T. Higgins, & A. W. Kruglanski (Eds.), *Social psychology: Handbook of basic principles* (3rd ed., pp. 337–349). Guilford Press.

Hales, A. H., Wood, N. R., & Williams, K. D. (2021). Navigating COVID-19: Insights from research on social ostracism. *Group Processes and Intergroup Relations, 24*(2), 306–310.

Hames, J. L., Rogers, M. L., Silva, C., Ribeiro, J. D., Teale, N. E., & Joiner, T. E. (2018). A social exclusion manipulation interacts with acquired capability for suicide to predict self-aggressive behaviors. *Archives of Suicide Research, 22*(1), 32–45.

Hartgerink, C. H. J., Van Beest, I., Wicherts, J. M., & Williams, K. D. (2015). The ordinal effects of ostracism: A meta-analysis of 120 Cyberball studies. *PLOS One, 10*(5), e0127002.

Hogg, M. A., & Adelman, J. (2013). Uncertainty-identity theory: Extreme groups, radical behavior, and authoritarian leadership. *Journal of Social Issues, 69*(3), 436–454.

Hohman, Z. P., Gaffney, A. M., & Hogg, M. A. (2017). Who am I if I am not like my group?: Self-uncertainty and feeling peripheral in a group. *Journal of Experimental Social Psychology, 72,* 125–132.

Holt-Lunstad, J., Smith, T. B., & Layton, J. B. (2010). Social relationships and mortality risk: A meta-analytic review. *PLOS Medicine, 7*(7), e1000316.

Iannone, N. E., McCarty, M. K., Kelly, J. R., & Williams, K. D. (2014). Friends with each other but strangers to you: Source relationship softens ostracism's blow. *Group Dynamics: Theory, Research, and Practice, 18*(4), 349–356.

Jauch, M., Rudert, S. C., & Greifeneder, R. (2022). Social pain by non-social agents: Exclusion hurts and provokes punishment even if the excluding source is a computer. *Acta Psychologica, 230,* 103753.

Jiang, T., & Chen, Z. (2020a). Meaning in life accounts for the association between long-term ostracism and depressive symptoms: The moderating role of self-compassion. *Journal of Social Psychology, 160*(5), 535–547.

Jiang, T., & Chen, Z. (2020b). Relative deprivation: A mechanism for the ostracism–aggression link. *European Journal of Social Psychology, 50*(2), 347–359.

Jiang, T., Chen, Z., Wang, S., & Hou, Y. (2021). Ostracism disrupts self-continuity. *Personality and Social Psychology Bulletin, 47*(9), 1390–1400.

Kerr, N. L., & Levine, J. M. (2008). The detection of social exclusion: Evolution and beyond. *Group Dynamics: Theory, Research, and Practice, 12*(1), 39–52.

Klauke, F., & Kauffeld, S. (2020). Does it matter what I say?: Using language to examine reactions to ostracism as it occurs. *Frontiers in Psychology, 11*, 558069.

Koole, S. L., Greenberg, J., & Pyszczynski, T. (2006). Introducing science to the psychology of the soul: Experimental existential psychology. *Current Directions in Psychological Science, 15*(5), 212–216.

Leary, M. R. (2005). Sociometer theory and the pursuit of relational value: Getting to the root of self-esteem. *European Review of Social Psychology, 16*(1), 75–111.

Leary, M. R., Twenge, J. M., & Quinlivan, E. (2006). Interpersonal rejection as a determinant of anger and aggression. *Personality and Social Psychology Review, 10*(2), 111–132.

Legate, N., DeHaan, C. R., Weinstein, N., & Ryan, R. M. (2013). Hurting you hurts me too: The psychological costs of complying with ostracism. *Psychological Science, 24*(4), 583–588.

Liu, C. (2019). Ostracism, attributions, and their relationships with international students' and employees' outcomes: The moderating effect of perceived harming intent. *Journal of Occupational Health Psychology, 24*(5), 556–571.

Lutz, S., Schneider, F. M., & Reich, S. (2022). Media as powerful coping tools to recover from social exclusion experiences?: A systematic review on need restoration and emotion regulation through using media. *Media Psychology, 26*(4), 388–413.

Lutz, S., & Schneider, F. M. (2020). Is receiving dislikes in social media still better than being ignored?: The effects of ostracism and rejection on need threat and coping responses online. *Media Psychology, 24*(6), 741–765.

MacDonald, G., & Leary, M. R. (2005). Why does social exclusion hurt?: The relationship between social and physical pain. *Psychological Bulletin, 131*(2), 202–223.

Maner, J. K., DeWall, C. N., Baumeister, R. F., & Schaller, M. (2007). Does social exclusion motivate interpersonal reconnection?: Resolving the "porcupine problem." *Journal of Personality and Social Psychology, 92*(1), 42–55.

McConnell, A. R., Brown, C. M., Shoda, T. M., Stayton, L. E., & Martin, C. E. (2011). Friends with benefits: On the positive consequences of pet ownership. *Journal of Personality and Social Psychology, 101*(6), 1239–1252.

McDonald, M. M., & Brent Donnellan, M. (2012). Is ostracism a strong situation?: The influence of personality in reactions to rejection. *Journal of Research in Personality, 46*(5), 614–618. h

Meral, E. O., Rosenbusch, H., Kip, A., Ren, D., Dijk, E., & Beest, I. (2022). *Social Ball: An immersive research paradigm to study social ostracism.* PsyArXiv Preprints. https://osf.io/preprints/psyarxiv/v8kwx_v1.

Meyer, M. L., Williams, K. D., & Eisenberger, N. I. (2015). Why social pain can live on: Different neural mechanisms are associated with reliving social and physical pain. *PLOS One, 10*(6), e0128294.

Molden, D. C., Lucas, G. M., Gardner, W. L., Dean, K., & Knowles, M. L. (2009). Motivations for prevention or promotion following social exclusion: Being rejected versus being ignored. *Journal of Personality and Social Psychology, 96*(2), 415–431.

Mourey, J. A., Olson, J. G., & Yoon, C. (2017). Products as pals: Engaging with anthropomorphic products mitigates the effects of social exclusion. *Journal of Consumer Research, 44*(2), 414–431.

Murphy, M. C., Kroeper, K. M., & Ozier, E. M. (2018). Prejudiced places: How contexts shape inequality and how policy can change them. *Policy Insights from the Behavioral and Brain Sciences, 5*(1), 66–74.

Nezlek, J. B., Wesselmann, E. D., Wheeler, L., & Williams, K. D. (2012). Ostracism in everyday life. *Group Dynamics: Theory, Research, and Practice, 16*(2), 91–104.

Nezlek, J. B., Wesselmann, E. D., Wheeler, L., & Williams, K. D. (2015). Ostracism in everyday life: The effects of ostracism on those who ostracize. *Journal of Social Psychology, 155*(5), 432–451.

Ouwerkerk, J. W., Kerr, N. L., Gallucci, M., & Lange, P. A. (2005). Avoiding the social death penalty. In K. D. Williams, J. P. Forgas, & W. von Hippel (Eds.), *The social outcast: Ostracism, social exclusion, rejection, and bullying* (pp. 321–332). Psychology Press.

Paolini, D., Pagliaro, S., Alparone, F. R., Marotta, F., & Van Beest, I. (2017). On vicarious ostracism. Examining the mediators of observers' reactions towards the target and the sources of ostracism. *Social Influence, 12*(4), 117–127.

Paravati, E., Naidu, E., & Gabriel, S. (2021). From "love actually" to love, actually: The sociometer takes every kind of fuel. *Self and Identity, 20*(1), 6–24.

Park, C. L. (2016). Meaning making in the context of disasters. *Journal of Clinical Psychology, 72*(12), 1234–1246.

Park, Y. C., & Pinel, E. C. (2020). Existential isolation and cultural orientation. *Personality and Individual Differences, 159,* 109891.

Pickett, C. L., Gardner, W. L., & Knowles, M. (2004). Getting a cue: The need to belong and enhanced sensitivity to social cues. *Personality and Social Psychology Bulletin, 30*(9), 1095–1107.

Pinel, E. C., Long, A. E., Murdoch, E. Q., & Helm, P. (2017). A prisoner of one's own mind: Identifying and understanding existential isolation. *Personality and Individual Differences, 105,* 54–63.

Poon, K. T., & Teng, F. (2017). Feeling unrestricted by rules: Ostracism promotes aggressive responses. *Aggressive Behavior, 43*(6), 558–567.

Poon, K. T., To, N., Lo, W. Y., Wong, N. H. L., Jiang, Y., & Chan, R. S. (2023). Green with envy: Ostracism increases aggressive tendencies. *Current Psychology, 42,* 32314–32323.

Poon, K. T., & Wong, W.-Y. (2019). Turning a blind eye to potential costs: Ostracism increases aggressive tendency. *Psychology of Violence, 9*(6), 634–643.

Poon, K.-T., Teng, F., Wong, W.-Y., & Chen, Z. (2016). When nature heals: Nature exposure moderates the relationship between ostracism and aggression. *Journal of Environmental Psychology, 48,* 159–168.

Poulsen, J. R., & Kashy, D. A. (2012). Two sides of the ostracism coin: How sources and targets of social exclusion perceive themselves and one another. *Group Processes and Intergroup Relations, 15*(4), 457–470.

Ren, D. (2016). *Solitude seeking: The good, the bad, and the balance.* Doctoral dissertation, Purdue University. ProQuest Dissertations Publishing.

Ren, D., & Evans, A. M. (2021). Leaving the loners alone: Dispositional preference for solitude evokes ostracism. *Personality and Social Psychology Bulletin, 47*(8), 1294–1308.

Ren, D., Wesselmann, E. D., & Van Beest, I. (2021). Seeking solitude after being ostracized: A Replication and beyond. *Personality and Social Psychology Bulletin, 47*(3), 426–440.

Ren, D., Wesselmann, E., & Williams, K. D. (2016). Evidence for another response to ostracism: Solitude seeking. *Social Psychological and Personality Science, 7*(3), 204–212.

Ren, D., Wesselmann, E. D., & Williams, K. D. (2018). Hurt people hurt people: Ostracism and aggression. *Current Opinion in Psychology, 19,* 34–38.

Richman, S. B., Slotter, E. B., Gardner, W. L., & DeWall, C. N. (2015). Reaching out by changing what's within: Social exclusion increases self-concept malleability. *Journal of Experimental Social Psychology, 57,* 64–77.

Riva, P., Montali, L., Wirth, J. H., Curioni, S., & Williams, K. D. (2017). Chronic social exclusion and evidence for the resignation stage: An empirical investigation. *Journal of Social and Personal Relationships, 34*(4), 541–564.

Riva, P., Williams, K. D., Torstrick, A. M., & Montali, L. (2014). Orders to shoot (a camera): Effects of ostracism on obedience. *Journal of Social Psychology, 154*(3), 208–216.

Rosenthal-von Der Pütten, A., & Bock, N. (2023). Seriously, what did one robot say to the other?: Being left out from communication by robots causes feelings of social exclusion. *Human-Machine Communication, 6,* 117–134.

Rudert, S. C., Janke, S., & Greifeneder, R. (2021). Ostracism breeds depression: Longitudinal associations between ostracism and depression over a three-year-period. *Journal of Affective Disorders Reports, 4,* 100118.

Sandstrom, M. J., Deutz, M. H., Lansu, T. A., Noorden, T. H., Karremans, J. C., & Cillessen, A. H. (2017). Unanimous versus partial rejection: How the number of excluders influences the impact of ostracism in children. *Aggressive Behavior, 43*(2), 190–203.

Sherman, J., Benson-Greenwald, T., & Bernstein, M. J. (2022). *Scaling up ostracism: A theory of institutional ostracism.* PsyArXiv Preprints. https://osf.io/preprints/psyarxiv/jea9n_v1.

Sommer, K. L., Williams, K. D., Ciarocco, N. J., & Baumeister, R. F. (2001). When silence speaks louder than words: Explorations into the intrapsychic and interpersonal consequences of social ostracism. *Basic and Applied Social Psychology, 23*(4), 225–243.

Spoor, J. R., & Williams, K. D. (2007). The evolution of an ostracism detection system. In J. P. Forgas, M. Haselton, & W. von Hippel (Eds.), *Evolution and the social mind: Evolutionary psychology and social cognition* (pp. 279–292). Routledge/Taylor & Francis.

Steele, C., Kidd, D. C., & Castano, E. (2015). On social death: Ostracism and the accessibility of death thoughts. *Death Studies, 39*(1), 19–23.

Stillman, T. F., Baumeister, R. F., Lambert, N. M., Crescioni, A. W., DeWall, C. N., & Fincham, F. D. (2009). Alone and without purpose: Life loses meaning following social exclusion. *Journal of Experimental Social Psychology, 45*(4), 686–694.

Stout, J. G., & Dasgupta, N. (2011). When he doesn't mean you: Gender-exclusive language as ostracism. *Personality and Social Psychology Bulletin, 37*(6), 757–769.

Sunami, N., Nadzan, M. A., & Jaremka, L. M. (2019). The bi-dimensional rejection taxonomy: Organizing responses to interpersonal rejection along antisocial–prosocial and engaged–disengaged dimensions. *Social and Personality Psychology Compass, 13*(9), 12497.

Taggart, R. S., Dvir, M., Kelly, J. R., Bradley, E. S., & Williams, K. D. (2024). Death of the social self?: Comparing the effects of ostracism to mortality salience. *Social Influence, 19*(1), 2342308.

Troisi, J. D., & Gabriel, S. (2011). Chicken soup really is good for the soul: "Comfort food" fulfills the need to belong. *Psychological Science, 22*(6), 747–753.

Twenge, J. M., Baumeister, R. F., Tice, D. M., & Stucke, T. S. (2001). If you can't join them, beat them: Effects of social exclusion on aggressive behavior. *Journal of Personality and Social Psychology, 81*(6), 1058–1069.

van Beest, I., & Williams, K. D. (2006). When inclusion costs and ostracism pays, ostracism still hurts. *Journal of Personality and Social Psychology, 91*(5), 918–928.

van Beest, I., & Williams, K. D. (2011). "Why Hast thou forsaken me?": The effect of thinking about being ostracized by God on well-being and prosocial behavior. *Social Psychological and Personality Science, 2*(4), 379–386.

van Beest, I., Williams, K. D., & van Dijk, E. (2011). Cyberbomb: Effects of being ostracized from a death game. *Group Processes & Intergroup Relations, 14*(4), 581–596.

Warburton, W. A., Williams, K. D., & Cairns, D. R. (2006). When ostracism leads to aggression: The moderating effects of control deprivation. *Journal of Experimental Social Psychology, 42*(2), 213–220.

Wesselmann, E. D., Nairne, J. S., & Williams, K. D. (2012). An evolutionary social psychological approach to studying the effects of ostracism. *Journal of Social, Evolutionary, and Cultural Psychology, 6*(3), 309–328.

Wesselmann, E. D., Ren, D., Swim, E., & Williams, K. (2013a). Rumination hinders recovery from ostracism. *International Journal of Developmental Sciences, 7*, 33–39.

Wesselmann, E. D., & Williams, K. D. (2010). The potential balm of religion and spirituality for recovering from ostracism. *Journal of Management, Spirituality and Religion, 7*(1), 31–49.

Wesselmann, E. D., Williams, K. D., & Hales, A. H. (2013b). Vicarious ostracism. *Frontiers in Human Neuroscience, 7.*

Wicks, S. G., & Hales, A. H. (2023). *Examining the impact of music on ostracism recovery.* Poster presentation at the annual conference of the Society of Southeastern Social Psychologists, Charlotte, NC.

Wicks, S. G., Hales, A. H., & Hennes, E. P. (2023). Does disseminating (mis)information restore social connection during a global pandemic? *Social and Personality Psychology Compass*, e12825.

Williams, K. D. (2001). *Ostracism: The power of silence.* Guilford Press.

Williams, K. D. (2007). Ostracism: The kiss of social death. *Social and Personality Psychology Compass, 1*(1), 236–247.

Williams, K. D. (2009). Ostracism: A temporal need-threat model. In M. Zanna (Ed.), *Advances in experimental social psychology* (Vol. 41, pp. 275–314). Elsevier/Academic Press.

Williams, K. D. (2012). Ostracism: The impact of being rendered meaningless. In P. R. Shaver & M. Mikulincer (Eds.), *Meaning, mortality, and choice: The social psychology of existential concerns.* (pp. 309–323). American Psychological Association.

Williams, K. D., Bernieri, F. J., Faulkner, S. L., Gada-Jain, N., & Grahe, J. E. (2000a). The Scarlet Letter Study: Five days of social ostracism. *Journal of Personal and Interpersonal Loss, 5*(1), 19–63.

Williams, K. D., Cheung, C. K. T., & Choi, W. (2000b). Cyberostracism: Effects of being ignored over the Internet. *Journal of Personality and Social Psychology, 79*(5), 748–776.

Williams, K. D., & Jarvis, B. (2006). Cyberball: A program for use in research on interpersonal ostracism and acceptance. *Behavior Research Methods, 38*(1), 174–180.

Williams, K. D., & Nida, S. A. (2022). Ostracism and social exclusion: Implications for separation, social isolation, and loss. *Current Opinion in Psychology, 47,* 101353.

Williams, K. D., & Sommer, K. L. (1997). Social ostracism by coworkers: Does rejection lead to loafing or compensation? *Personality and Social Psychology Bulletin, 23*(7), 693–706.

Williams, K. D., & Zadro, L. (2001). Ostracism: On being ignored, excluded, and rejected. *Interpersonal Rejection,* 21–53.

Wilt, J. A., Exline, J. J., Grubbs, J. B., Park, C. L., & Pargament, K. I. (2016). God's role in suffering: Theodicies, divine struggle, and mental health. *Psychology of Religion and Spirituality, 8*(4), 352–362.

Wirth, J. H., Sacco, D. F., Hugenberg, K., & Williams, K. D. (2010). Eye gaze as relational evaluation: Averted eye gaze leads to feelings of ostracism and relational devaluation. *Personality and Social Psychology Bulletin, 36*(7), 869–882.

Wirth, J. H., & Williams, K. D. (2009). "They don't like our kind": Consequences of being ostracized while possessing a group membership. *Group Processes and Intergroup Relations, 12*(1), 111–127.

Wolf, W., Levordashka, A., Ruff, J. R., Kraaijeveld, S., Lueckmann, J. M., & Williams, K. D. (2015). Ostracism online: A social media ostracism paradigm. *Behavior Research Methods, 47*(2), 361–373.

Yalom, I. D. (1980). Existential psychotherapy. *Existential Psychotherapy, xii,* 524.

Zadro, L., Arriaga, X. B., & Williams, K. D. (2008). Relational ostracism. *Social Relationships: Cognitive, Affective, and Motivational Processes,* 305–320.

Zadro, L., Boland, C., & Richardson, R. (2006). How long does it last?: The persistence of the effects of ostracism in the socially anxious. *Journal of Experimental Social Psychology, 42*(5), 692–697.

Zadro, L., & Gonsalkorale, K. (2014). Sources of ostracism: The nature and consequences of excluding and ignoring others. *Current Directions in Psychological Science, 23*(2), 93–97.

Zadro, L., Williams, K. D., & Richardson, R. (2004). How low can you go?: Ostracism by a computer is sufficient to lower self-reported levels of belonging, control, self-esteem, and meaningful existence. *Journal of Experimental Social Psychology, 40*(4), 560–567.

Zamperini, A., Menegatto, M., Mostacchi, M., Barbagallo, S., & Testoni, I. (2020). Loss of close relationships and loss of religious belonging as cumulative ostracism: From social death to social resurrection. *Behavioral Sciences, 10*(6), 99.

CHAPTER 33

Existential Loneliness and Aging

Phoebe E. McKenna-Plumley *and* Jenny M. Groarke

LONELINESS: A PRIMER

Writing in 1961, Clark Moustakas suggested that loneliness is "as much organic to human existence as the blood is to the heart" and constitutes "a dimension of human life whether existential, sociological, or psychological" (Moustakas, 1961, p. 34). In recent years, loneliness has become a common topic of media thinkpieces (e.g., Michelle Cottle's 2023 opinion piece in the *New York Times* that suggested that the cure to male loneliness may lie "on the pickleball court," spawning a wealth of commentary and memes). These conversations became particularly prominent in light of the COVID-19 pandemic, which kept people physically isolated from one another. You might have found yourself in conversations about loneliness: Maybe you moved to college and felt left out in your classes, like you were the only person without a group of close friends, or worried about one of your family members feeling lonely after a loved one died. Perhaps you've found yourself on Reddit's r/Lonely forum, which describes itself as "A community for all the lonely people" and includes over 370,000 members, making it comparable in size to subreddits devoted to plants, working out, feminism, and many major cities.

This interest in loneliness has brought a swell of policy aiming to raise awareness, decrease stigma, and reduce loneliness. England devoted over £20 million to manage loneliness via charities and community groups in 2018, in a move that has been followed in countries such as Scotland, the Netherlands, and Australia. Similarly, U.S. Surgeon General Dr. Vivek Murthy described loneliness as an urgent public health problem (U.S. Department of Health and Human Services, 2023), putting forward a national strategy to promote social connection. This has led to the creation of the World Health Organization Commission on Social Connection to address loneliness and social isolation, which plans to advance solutions for loneliness and measure their effectiveness. But what, exactly, is loneliness?

The most common description stems from the cognitive discrepancy model, which characterizes loneliness as a distressing experience that occurs when there is a mismatch between the social relations a person has and the ones they desire (Perlman & Peplau, 1981). Breaking this down further, we might think of loneliness in terms of different types of lonely experiences: Sociologist Robert Weiss described loneliness as "a response to the absence of some particular relational provision" (1973, p. 17); loneliness comes about when we lack something that a relationship can provide, like attachment, social integration, reassurance of our worth, or the opportunity to nurture others. Weiss distinguished between social and emotional loneliness, where social loneliness derives from the perception that one's social network is lacking, whereas emotional loneliness comes about in light of inadequate intimate attachments. A developing body of research focuses on social and emotional loneliness, indicating distinct developmental pathways, correlates, and consequences (DiTommaso & Spinner, 1997; O'Súilleabháin et al., 2019; Salo et al., 2020). There is also an increasing body of empirical work on existential loneliness, which is the focus of this chapter.

Existential loneliness stems from one of what Yalom (1980, p. 8) referred to as the "givens of existence," or ultimate facts of human life: death, isolation, meaninglessness, and freedom. Isolation, in this sense, refers to the fact that we ultimately enter and leave life alone—we cannot fully close the gap between ourselves and other people despite our desire for connection and community. Each of us is having a unique experience: Our understandings of the world and our place within it depend on other people and are validated by them, but we can never fully see inside another person's mind or be fully known by them. These concerns are relevant from the cradle to the grave and, similarly, it seems that loneliness is common at various life stages. Children as young as 5 describe and report loneliness (Cassidy & Asher, 1992), while research indicates that most 7-year-olds can comprehend the difference between the objective experience of being alone and the subjective feeling of being lonely (Galanaki, 2004). Meanwhile, when people are asked how often during the past week they felt lonely, particularly high levels are observed in younger and older adulthood, with lower levels from around 30 to 60 years old (Victor & Yang, 2012; Yang & Victor, 2011). Other research shows the highest levels of loneliness as occurring in younger adulthood (Barreto et al., 2021; Office for National Statistics, 2023). Less research has focused specifically on the experience of existential loneliness in relation to the lifespan, even though existential concerns have enduring relevance to loneliness: We are born alone, die alone, and are often alone in important moments of life, such as when facing serious illness or loss.

Previous chapters and a growing body of empirical research have discussed existential isolation, which is often defined in existential psychological literature as "feeling as though one differs, either chronically or acutely, with respect to one's subjective experience" (Pinel et al., 2017, p. 56). In this chapter, we focus on the empirical literature on experiences of *existential loneliness*, described as a subjective feeling of distress that a person experiences when they feel profoundly or fundamentally separate from all other people. These experiences likely parallel one another and crossover; indeed, the conceptual overlap between existential isolation and existential loneliness operationalizations has been noted (Gil Álvarez et al., 2023; McKenna-Plumley et al., 2023b). While Yalom (1980) distinguished between interpersonal isolation (which he characterized as being generally experienced as loneliness) and existential isolation (the fundamental gap between a person and the wider world), he also suggested that the two experiences overlap and may essentially feel the same: The existential awareness of our fundamental isolation can be experienced as a form of subjective loneliness. It can be particularly valuable to attend to the experience of loneliness that stems from our fundamental separation, given that loneliness (above and beyond objective social isolation) is associated with a host of poor physical and mental health outcomes, particularly when it is enduring (Hawkley & Cacioppo, 2010; Lim et al., 2016; Shiovitz-Ezra & Ayalon, 2010). Indeed, Clark Moustakas suggested that there is an "emotional climate of existential loneliness" (1961, p. 33), which is brought about by the awareness of our ultimate isolation. This chapter therefore draws on quantitative literature from social, developmental, and existential psychology, as well as the body of qualitative evidence on existential loneliness stemming from nursing, gerontology, and health psychology traditions.

In particular, this chapter discusses our knowledge of existential loneliness across the lifespan: How, and to what degree, do people experience existential loneliness at different life stages? To do this, we look at research using a variety of methodologies, including quantitative, qualitative, and evidence synthesis methods.

LONELINESS: A SUBJECTIVE EXPERIENCE, AN EXISTENTIAL REALITY

As outlined in the previous section, *loneliness* is a subjective experience of distress that occurs when we feel that our social world is inadequate (for example, that we have too few connections or that they are lacking in some way). Fay Bound Alberti (2018) suggested that the use of the word *loneliness* in printed texts emerged in the 1800s, but there was a general dearth of academic exploration into loneliness until much more recently. Indeed, in 1959, Frieda Fromm-Reichmann suggested that loneliness was poorly conceptualized as a psychological experience partly because it is "such a painful, frightening experience that people will do practically everything to avoid it" (p. 305).

Through the 1970s and 1980s, loneliness became the focus of more empirical research following interest from researchers including Robert Weiss, Letitia Anne Peplau, Daniel Perlman, and Jenny de Jong Gierveld. This research has touched on the harmful impacts that loneliness can have on health (Hawkley & Cacioppo, 2010; Lim et al., 2016) and mortality (Holt-Lunstad et al., 2015), as well as potential mechanisms underlying these effects. It also shows that the feeling of loneliness is separable from the objective situation of social isolation, where a person has few or infrequent social contacts (de Jong Gierveld et al., 2016). While loneliness commonly occurs alongside social isolation, a person might feel disconnected despite having ample social connections. This might be because they miss a specific person—for example, college students in long-distance relationships have reported loneliness due to being separated from their boyfriends (Firmin et al., 2014). It might also be due to missing a certain type of relationship, like a romantic partner (Rönkä et al., 2018) or a friend from the same culture (Cela & Fokkema, 2017), despite having other satisfying relationships. In synthesizing the qualitative literature on experiences of loneliness (McKenna-Plumley et al., 2023a), it seems that this perceived lack of specific relationships or relationship types can bring about loneliness. However, for some people, loneliness appears to be more pervasive.

For some, this overarching feeling of loneliness could be existential. Our fundamental aloneness might be an existential reality: We can never completely share our thoughts and experiences with another person; we are limited to trying to convey them through language and other means. We might be more or less aware of this gap between ourselves and others. Indeed, research indicates that people differ in the degree to which they experience existential isolation: For example, it appears that men (Helm et al., 2018) and people with minoritized identities such as people who are not White, heterosexual, or native English speakers in the United States (Pinel et al., 2022) felt more strongly that others tend not to share their thoughts and subjective experiences. Similarly, people may vary in terms of how troubling or distressing they find this essential barrier between themselves and other people. Just like two socially isolated people may differ in the degree of social loneliness they experience, two people who are both fundamentally separate may differ in the degree of existential loneliness they feel. For some, this may be a neutral reality, or something they are relatively unaware of; for others, it may constitute a distressing source of loneliness.

In qualitative research including descriptions of existential loneliness from 175 adults from 16 to 72 years old, the findings appeared to support this idea (McKenna-Plumley et al., 2023b). When definitions of existential loneliness were provided, a proportion of respondents stated that they had never experienced it. However, other respondents gave rich descriptions of these experiences, indicating that existential loneliness is experienced as a deeper form of loneliness involving a feeling of profound disconnection that is longer lasting and harder to resolve than other forms of loneliness. For one participant, existential loneliness felt like being "alone in a void," while others described it as "debilitating" and "like a punch in the gut" (p. 415). Compared to other, more directly social forms of loneliness, existential loneliness appears to constitute an upsetting feeling of profound aloneness and separation from others that may be more challenging to resolve. These experiences involved negative emotions like fear and dread, as well as cognitive elements such as overthinking about life, death, and aloneness.

Less research has focused on this existential dimension of loneliness with respect to the lifespan, but there are important reasons to look at the experience of existential loneliness at different life stages. We know that people differ in the extent to which they feel existentially isolated (Pinel et al., 2022), and there appear to be certain life stages at which loneliness is generally more common: namely adolescence, early adulthood, and later life (Barreto et al., 2021; Victor & Yang, 2011). Existential loneliness is also suggested to be universal (McGraw, 1995) but may be prompted by life events that are linked to certain life stages. With this in mind, the next section focuses on older adulthood and ill health, which have driven much of the qualitative literature on existential loneliness.

EXISTENTIAL LONELINESS IN OLDER AGE AND ILL HEALTH

When discussing what we know about the experience of existential loneliness across the lifespan, it makes sense to begin toward the end, rather than the beginning. This is because much of what we know about existential loneliness comes from qualitative literature carried out with older adults, often specifically focusing on older people who are experiencing frailty, ill health, and/or living in residential care. This focus on older adults is echoed in much of the scientific literature on loneliness, which has often focused on later life. This may be due to the assumption that older adulthood often involves events that trigger loneliness, such as bereavement, a restricted social circle, and issues with health and functional ability that might limit the ability to socialize. People of all ages—including older adults—tend to overestimate the seriousness of loneliness in later life (Abramson & Silverstein, 2006), but there are common features of older adulthood that might bring about loneliness or its existential counterpart.

Particularly with respect to existential loneliness, the type of drastic experiences that are described as inciting it by Moustakas (1961) may be particularly likely to occur in later life. Experiencing the illness and death of loved ones and the "torturous pain or the isolation of disease" (p. 34) are more likely, as one's social networks are often aging and health may be jeopardized. These urgent experiences, often referred to as "boundary situations" (as formalized by Karl Jaspers in his 1919 *Psychologie der Weltanschauungen*), confront us with ultimate concerns about life, including the nature of our aloneness (Grieder, 2009; Yalom, 1980). Awareness of death may constitute the ultimate boundary situation (Yalom, 1980), and aging may bring increased awareness of the inevitability of death; research shows that viewing photos of older people can make thoughts about death more accessible (Martens et al., 2004). It has been suggested that this may be one mechanism by which ageism comes about (Greenberg et al., 2017). Indeed qualitative research suggests that older-old adults (ages 95 to 101 years old) described themselves as having a heightened awareness of death because many of their peers had died (Fleming et al., 2016). Moreover, the loss of loved ones such as spouses can contribute to feelings of existential loneliness in later life (Carr & Fang, 2021).

While many of these studies involved samples for whom older age is complicated by ill health or residential living (and we can't assume that they represent existential loneliness purely in relation to chronological age), we have gained important insights into existential loneliness from this qualitative research. It is clear that existential loneliness is perceived as relevant by people who are near the end of life. This makes sense given that mortality salience (our awareness that death is inevitable) may make concerns about fundamental separation more prominent. Indeed, older people suggest that existential loneliness comes alongside feelings of wanting to share their life stories and culture with others; for older migrants, these feelings could occur when this sort of sharing was not possible (Olofsson et al., 2021). While much of this qualitative research with older adults has been carried out in Scandinavian countries, it appears that existential loneliness may be experienced in similar ways across cultures: For example, Chung and colleagues (2020) found that Chinese and Swedish older people described existential loneliness in similar ways, although

Chinese participants tended to define themselves more through their place in the family and Swedish participants more through friendships and individual needs and accomplishments.

Moreover, this research tells us how people experience existential loneliness. What does it feel like? Research with older adults and people experiencing ill health suggests that existential loneliness is related to one's social world, as we might expect: It comes about when older people have lost close attachments (Carr & Fang, 2021), lack family or people with similar experiences to belong with (Olofsson et al., 2021), feel distant from others (Chung et al., 2020), and have no one with whom they can share their life, experience intimacy, and have meaningful exchanges of thoughts and feelings (Sjöberg et al., 2019). Eddie, a participant in Chung and colleagues (2020), stated, "Have you ever been in a situation when you felt like your words couldn't get through, not being understood even talking to your own children and to your close relatives? Like you were expressing yourself over and over again, yet you were being misunderstood by your loved ones? . . . I was miserable, upset, woke up at four in the morning and looking at the ceiling" (p. 352). It appears likely that these feelings often overlap with other forms of loneliness, which may make it challenging to disentangle these experiences. On the other hand, the qualitative literature allows us to view the richness of existential loneliness experiences, including the feelings with which they co-occur, without oversimplifying them. Although there is little quantitative research focusing on existential loneliness in later life, studies with Dutch older adults also indicate that social network characteristics are relevant. Not living with a partner and having a smaller social network were associated with existential loneliness for older adults (van Tilburg, 2021). It appears that older people feel existentially lonely when they feel like they don't belong, lack close attachments with similar others, and cannot meaningfully connect with other people. However, underlining that these experiences may not be specific to older age, Tarbi and Meghani (2019) noted similar feelings in people with advanced cancer diagnoses.

Existential loneliness experiences also involve meaninglessness, where older people describe feeling insignificant and struggling to identify a purpose in living (Chung et al., 2020; Olofsson et al., 2021; Sjöberg et al., 2018). The relevance of poor health, frailty, and oncoming death is clear in these samples as participants discussed how existential loneliness can arise in light of deteriorating cognitive and physical health that separates them from others and makes it challenging to manage daily activities, creating frustration, alienation, and a lack of autonomy (Carr & Fang, 2021; Sjöberg et al., 2018). These issues may also make mortality particularly salient and contribute to awareness of one's fundamental aloneness, bringing about these feelings of loneliness. This mechanism is perceived by some older people who described the loss of functional abilities as causing a realization that death is inevitable (Sjöberg et al., 2018). In systematically reviewing the literature on existential loneliness, Ettema and colleagues (2010) suggested that death is a key feature: Though existential loneliness is not specific to the end of life, they are intertwined.

While insights about remedies for existential loneliness are scarce, it is clear that older people aim to resolve these feelings (Carr & Fang, 2021). Some older people have suggested that sharing meaningful connections with other people, being treated kindly and with care, exchanging physical touch, and discussing meaningful topics can manage existential loneliness (Sjöberg et al., 2019). Others have indicated that it can help to think positively, try to accept their feelings, distract themselves, and draw strength from life experiences and memories (Sjöberg et al., 2019). Older adults may be more adept at engaging in these forms of loneliness management, as the ability to regulate emotions improves with age (Carstensen et al., 2003). However, research suggests that this type of emotion-focused coping, where people try to change the way they feel about a stressful situation, is less effective at managing loneliness than problem-focused coping, where people try to change their circumstances (Deckx et al., 2018). This emotion-oriented strategy may not actually be the best approach, but choosing it may be related to beliefs about what kind of options are available; Schoenmakers and colleagues (2012) found that older adults were more likely to suggest emotion-focused coping strategies (like lowering their expectations) and less likely to suggest problem-focused methods (like trying to improve their relationships) to older people.

It is important to bear in mind the limitations of what this qualitative literature on older adults can tell us. The studies reviewed above were conducted in relatively specific contexts, aside from age. There is little research on existential loneliness in older people living outside of care settings and experiencing generally good health. It appears that a lack of belonging and intimacy, declining health and functional ability, and their impact on meaning in life are involved in experiences of existential loneliness in this age group. However, it is possible that existential loneliness is felt differently by older people who are experiencing more functional independence and better health.

Moreover, while this qualitative literature is instrumental to learn how existential loneliness is experienced, there is little quantitative evidence focusing on older adults, making it challenging to compare levels, predictors, and consequences of existential loneliness at this life stage. Moreover, research using general measures of loneliness (not specific to the existential dimension) indicates that older adults can be remarkably resilient to loneliness. Much of the research suggests that younger adults experience loneliness more than older people (Barreto et al., 2021). With this in mind, the following section reviews findings from qualitative and quantitative literature on existential loneliness in earlier life.

EXISTENTIAL LONELINESS ACROSS THE LIFESPAN

While much of the qualitative research on existential loneliness focuses on older people, we also have insights into the experience of existential loneliness at other life stages from theory and research. The following sections focus on childhood, emerging adulthood, and middle age.

Existential Loneliness in Childhood

When we are born, we are entirely reliant on other people for care and safety. However, as we begin to develop psychologically, we generally become aware that we are separate from other people and have different knowledge, desires, and points of view from others. As shown in classic developmental psychology studies, very young children are generally unable to understand that another person will have different knowledge or points of view from them. For example, in the false-belief task, children are presented with a story where an object has been moved without a character in the story being aware of this movement. Children at 3 and 4 years old tend to claim that the character will think the object is in its new location (where the child knows it is); they are seemingly unable to differentiate their own point of view from other people's. Children over the age of 4 are typically able to complete this task, recognizing the different points of view (Wimmer & Perner, 1983).

The ability to manage physical separation from others and the realization of loneliness also develops through childhood. Jacobs (2006) suggested that the capacity to be alone is "a vital developmental achievement" (p. 217), as is the ability to separate from parental bonds to engage fully with other people. Similarly, psychoanalyst Donald Winnicott (1958) suggested that the ability to tolerate being alone is "one of the most important signs of maturity in emotional development" (p. 416). It is evident that children can understand and experience loneliness after they become aware that they are separate from others. Cassidy and Asher (1992) noted that children as young as 5 can accurately report and describe loneliness (e.g., "When you're alone, and you feel kinda sad"; p. 355). Moreover, being rejected and feeling lonely can be separate experiences in children under the age of 10; some children are rejected but not lonely and others feel lonely even though they are accepted by peers (Qualter & Munn, 2002). It appears that children begin to wonder about existential concerns; Pramling and Johansson (1995) found that children ask existential questions in early childhood, many of which focus on togetherness.

In exploring childhood loneliness, Kristensen (1995) identified existential isolation, where children experienced loneliness as "a radical separateness not related to a particular situation" including quotes from 8- to 10-year-olds, such as "You feel like you're the only person in the world" (p. 129). Although there is a lack of studies directly investigating existential loneliness in childhood, studies of adults indicate that its roots may sometimes extend back to the early years of life. Carr and Fang (2021) included older adults whose existential loneliness related to unresolved issues from childhood. For example, one 80-year-old participant described how "from an early childhood, I learned that I was a bad person," which made it hard to forgive those who had hurt them. These findings indicate that existential loneliness can be subjectively related to childhood experiences and may be felt during childhood by some people.

Additionally, boundary situations in childhood may also be pertinent to later existential loneliness. Boundary situations certainly occur in childhood, to the extent that children experience serious illness, loss, and trauma. Grieder (2009) suggested that these events may not be experienced as constituting boundary situations in early childhood, but it is clear that traumatic and life-altering experiences in childhood can provoke loneliness. Earlier exposures to trauma are more strongly associated with later-life loneliness than exposures at older ages, even though older-age traumatic events are more temporally proximate (Palgi et al., 2012). Indeed, experiences such as childhood neglect and maltreatment are implicated in existential loneliness by adults (McKenna-Plumley et al., 2023b).

Children can experience loneliness (Cassidy & Asher, 1992; Qualter & Munn, 2002), and Kristensen (1995) provided evidence that children as young as 8 to 10 years old may feel existentially lonely. It also appears that adverse childhood experiences may precipitate existential loneliness in adulthood. While direct explorations of existential loneliness in childhood are lacking, these findings indicate the relevance of childhood experiences to feelings of existential separation.

Existential Loneliness in Adolescence and Emerging Adulthood

In adolescence and early adulthood, loneliness appears to be particularly common. In the BBC Loneliness Experiment (2018), which included over 50,000 people around the world, 40% of 16- to 24-year-olds reported feeling lonely often or very often, relative to just 27% of people over 75. In adolescence, people gain more autonomy over social interactions and begin to create close relationships based on shared values rather than simply playing side by side (Heinrich & Gullone, 2006; Qualter et al., 2015). Additionally, this is a common life stage for the experience of transitions in education, leaving the family home, and potentially moving to another area or country. Young people describe loneliness as normative in this period, as they have to grow up, make new friends, and adjust to life transitions (Kirwan et al., 2023). Existential loneliness has been suggested to emerge in this phase of life as identity and meaning in life become more relevant (Brennan, 1982).

Adolescence and early adulthood may also be an important time for the development or experience of existential loneliness. Research identifies existential isolation among this age group, with higher levels in those who report avoidant or anxious attachment (Helm, Jimenez, et al., 2020). This is suggested to potentially constitute a causal path, where being avoidantly attached makes a person more likely to feel that their subjective experience is different and unknowable to other people. Alternatively, Helm and colleagues (2020) suggested that secure attachment may allow people to accept their fundamental separation from others and experience meaningful connection regardless, buffering them against existential loneliness. Indeed, research suggests that insecure attachment is associated with higher levels of other loneliness dimensions, such as loneliness in relation to romantic relationships, family, and wider social connections (DiTommaso et al., 2003).

Interviews with 21- to 27-year-old men indicated that they experienced existential concerns and felt like it was hard to talk to others about how they felt, making them feel distanced from others (Lundvall et al.,

2020). In interviews with 16- to 25-year-old women, these feelings were expressed in terms of struggling to create meaning in life while constrained by social norms around young womanhood, and wanting to be vulnerable with others without experiencing rejection (Lundvall et al., 2019). Research with adolescents and young adults suggests that existential loneliness involves a reluctance to share one's inner life in case that sharing leads to rejection, and that this loneliness is experienced when they feel like they do not fit in and cannot be understood (Garnow et al., 2022). Age appears relevant here, as young people suggested that existential loneliness came about in light of the in-betweenness of this life stage, where they felt both young and old in the face of approaching adulthood and responsibility. These feelings may have problematic outcomes in this age group; while existential isolation and general loneliness both predict depression and suicidal ideation among undergraduate students, it appears that those who are both lonely and existentially isolated experience higher levels of depression (Helm, Medrano, et al., 2020). Likewise, qualitative research with participants at a range of ages suggests that existential loneliness is felt in times of poor mental health (McKenna-Plumley et al., 2023b).

Quantitative work examining existential loneliness specifically in younger adults shows that existential loneliness is predicted by being left out, having an avoidant approach to social interaction, and experiencing less intimacy and closeness (Galanaki et al., 2023). These results are somewhat consistent with research showing relationships between avoidant attachment, existential isolation, and loneliness in younger adulthood (DiTommaso et al., 2003; Helm, Jimenez, et al., 2020). Moreover, younger and middle-aged adults have been found to experience higher levels of existential loneliness than older adults (McKenna-Plumley, 2024), which is supported by qualitative work in which some older people suggested that existential loneliness was primarily a feature of younger life (McKenna-Plumley et al., 2023b).

Existential loneliness appears to be a relevant aspect of younger adulthood, potentially in relation to social transitions, burgeoning autonomy and identity formation, insecure attachment, and feelings of not fitting in. This may be particularly concerning given that there are indications of problematic associations with mental health and related outcomes at this life stage.

Existential Loneliness in Midlife

There is a general lack of research examining loneliness in midlife, which extends into the existential loneliness and isolation literature. As mentioned previously, the majority of qualitative existential loneliness literature focuses on older and seriously ill adults, with some exceptions including young adults and wider age ranges, while most quantitative existential isolation research focuses on younger adults. However, midlife brings about a number of changes that may be pertinent to existential loneliness.

Many people in midlife face social transitions such as children leaving home or the decline or death of their own parents. These transitions might promote a focus on existential concerns. Becker (2006) described how the frailty and death of important social contacts such as parents and changes within the family home may make existential isolation more salient in midlife. He noted that developmental terms that describe midlife often touch on the inherent isolation of this life stage. While loneliness appears to be generally low in midlife relative to earlier and later ages, slight increases have been observed from age 40 to 60 (Luhmann & Hawkley, 2016), suggesting that this may be an important life stage for the development of loneliness.

Additionally, one's own aging process may make mortality more salient. Many people may enter a phase where they begin to notice signs of physical aging, and these physical reminders can increase their awareness of mortality (Martens et al., 2004). These sorts of changes, alongside declines in health and vitality, may bring existential concerns to the fore. Indeed, Jaques described the "compulsive attempts, in many men and women reaching middle age, to remain young, the hypochondriacal concern over health and appearance" as constituting "attempts at a race against time" (in Yalom, 1980) in light of a heightened awareness of their own death.

The often-described "midlife crisis" may also be relevant with respect to existential loneliness. In a so-called midlife crisis, people reassess their life choices, identity, and relationships to better understand their life's meaning. While research on the veracity of the midlife crisis is mixed, recent research suggests a midlife peak around age 50 in sleeping issues, suicide, depression, and other issues in rich nations (Giuntella et al., 2023). Additionally, around 26% of Americans described themselves as having experienced a midlife crisis in one study (Wethington, 2000), characterizing them as caused by an awareness that they were aging and time was passing. Concerns about mortality also decline after midlife (Fortner & Neimeyer, 1999), indicating that existential concerns and accompanying feelings may be particularly relevant during middle age. Relationships that may be pertinent to loneliness are also shifting at this time; in the United Kingdom, for example, divorce is most common in men and women at midlife ages. In 2013, over 42,000 men and women ages 40 to 44 years old got divorced (as did around 68,000 30- to 39-year-olds and 44,000 people in their 50s), compared to approximately 16,000 25- to 29-year-olds and 9,000 60- to 64-year-olds (Office for National Statistics, 2015).

McKenna-Plumley (2024) found significantly lower levels of existential loneliness in later life relative to earlier stages of adulthood. Existential loneliness was slightly lower in middle-aged adults than younger adults in this study, although the difference was marginal and not statistically significant. This finding suggests that despite the relative focus on older and younger adults in this literature, middle adulthood is a life stage at which existential loneliness is experienced. This may occur in light of social and personal changes that make existential concerns more relevant. Moreover, specific experiences like boundary situations may bring existential loneliness to the fore at this life stage: In one study, health care professionals observed that younger and middle-aged patients had a stronger need to discuss loneliness and existential concerns than older patients did and suggested that existential loneliness at the end of life was more common for middle-aged patients than for older people (Sundström et al., 2019).

Evidently, although much of the qualitative existential loneliness literature focuses on older adults and much of the quantitative research on existential isolation concerns younger adults, the experience of existential loneliness is relevant at various life stages. It may be the case that common features of different life stages predict loneliness, rather than chronological age itself (Luhmann & Hawkley, 2016). However, these findings provide insights into how existential loneliness might be relevant at stages across the lifespan.

A PERSONAL ISSUE, A PUBLIC PROBLEM

As suggested in the previous sections, existential loneliness is, in many respects, a highly personal experience that can be relevant at various life stages. People feel existentially lonely when they feel like there is a profound disconnection between themselves and everyone else. Indeed, existential loneliness can make a person feel like they are "completely alone in the world" (McKenna-Plumley et al., 2023b, p. 416). However, loneliness is increasingly positioned as a public health problem for which national and international solutions must be found (Cacioppo & Cacioppo, 2018). Indeed, in the United Kingdom and other locations, efforts like social prescribing have been put forward to manage loneliness, poor mental health, and long-term health conditions. These schemes pair lonely people with link workers, who work with them to address the social and emotional needs that impact their health and well-being by connecting them with activities, services, and resources in their communities. Social-prescribing schemes have received investment on the scale of millions of pounds in England (U.K. Department of Health and Social Care, 2018) and have been rolled out in other countries including Ireland, Australia, Denmark, and the United States (Morse et al., 2022). A consideration of existential loneliness within this work is needed, given the evidence reviewed above showing that it is a relevant aspect of loneliness experiences. With an increasing call to address loneliness within these public efforts, how might large-scale approaches "tackle" existential loneliness?

It is not encouraging that the literature reviewed here includes indications that existential loneliness is harder to resolve than other forms of loneliness (McKenna-Plumley et al., 2023b). However, these studies and others suggest that there are ways of managing and ameliorating these feelings. Although they may be less effective for loneliness, emotion-focused methods are often used. Younger adults described trying to avoid these thoughts and feelings, although they acknowledged that this may not be a helpful approach (Garnow et al., 2022). Older adults also attempted to distract themselves and accept their situation when faced with existential loneliness (Sjöberg et al., 2019). Finding effective ways to manage these feelings is important, particularly in light of evidence that young people may resort to deleterious behaviors such as self-medicating with alcohol (Garnow et al., 2022).

Within qualitative work, it has been suggested that positive thinking, gratitude, and shared experiences with others may help reduce feelings of existential loneliness (McKenna-Plumley et al., 2023b). Similarly, participants in Sjöberg and colleagues' (2019) study suggested that being meaningfully listened to could ease existential loneliness. While Yalom (1980) suggested that no relationship can fully manage our existential isolation, it seems that experiences of sincere connection may momentarily help. Moustakas (1961) and Yalom suggested that this can be best achieved when a person is at peace or has accepted their fundamental isolation; indeed, Moustakas suggested that this acceptance is the only real solution to loneliness. Many loneliness interventions focus on creating social connections, like befriending (Fakoya et al., 2020), or changing cognitions, for example by reducing perceptions of social threat (Riddleston et al., 2023), but approaches to existential loneliness might usefully consider ways to provide shared perspective and meaning at various life stages.

While interventions focusing on existential loneliness are rare, there are a number of studies suggesting potential strategies for managing it. Logotherapy, developed by Viktor Frankl, aims to foster meaning in life based on the understanding that humans long to experience meaning and that this is possible even under challenging circumstances (Schulenberg et al., 2008). A randomized controlled trial of patients with advanced cancer showed that those who took part in 10 weeks of group logotherapy experienced a significant reduction in existential loneliness, a reduction that was not observed in the control condition; this was also the case for anxiety about death (Heidary et al., 2023). There is also evidence that a 7-day course of Buddhist Zen meditation, which focuses on adopting a nonjudgmental awareness of the present moment, is effective at reducing existential isolation relative to a control condition (Park & Pinel, 2023). There are therefore indications for policymakers and clinicians of methods that may be effective at reducing existential loneliness, alongside common approaches to managing loneliness, such as addressing social cognitive biases, providing social connection, and engaging people in activities (Eccles & Qualter, 2021; Masi et al., 2011).

Yalom (1980) suggested the value of group therapy to allow people to learn and test new ways of connecting. Other routes of shared activity may also be beneficial. Pinel and colleagues (2017) suggested that cultivating shared subjective experiences, for example playing an engaging game together, may ease feelings of existential isolation. This sort of shared experience, where people feel that their subjective experiences of a situation are the same, is described as "I-sharing" and is suggested to promote existential connection by heightening people's sense that their perception of the world is accurate and that they belong (Pinel et al., 2006). Relationships that foster these feelings may be helpful (Helm et al., 2019). Yalom also suggested that an "invisible bond" (p. 398) exists between people participating in the same experience, like being part of a shared audience. "Arts on prescription," where people are referred to participation in creative and arts activities to improve health and well-being (Stickley & Eades, 2013), could serve as a route to providing existential connection and easing loneliness.

While loneliness is often catastrophized and communicated as an epidemic (Nicioli, 2023) and public health crisis (Holt-Lunstad, 2021), it is also worth noting that positive outcomes of existential loneliness have been suggested. For example, the negative experience of existential loneliness may be transformed into a positive one (Ettema et al., 2010), constituting the start of a journey toward more insight, growth, and meaning (Frankl, 1959; Moustakas, 1961). In this case, the picture might not be quite so bleak for people who are able to transition from existential loneliness toward a place of peace: Learning who manages to achieve this, and how, is an important target for the intersection of existential psychology and loneliness research and practice.

SUMMARY

Existential loneliness may be relevant at various stages across the lifespan, although the majority of qualitative evidence focuses on people who are older, frail, or experiencing serious illness. However, there is evidence that the distressing feeling of being profoundly separate and disconnected from other people is felt in midlife, younger adulthood, adolescence, and perhaps even childhood. Empirical research using quantitative and qualitative approaches sheds light on the subjective experience, correlates, and outcomes of these experiences, although more research is needed to establish how and under what circumstances existential loneliness can be ameliorated.

REFERENCES

Abramson, A., & Silverstein, M. (2006). *Images of aging in America 2004.* American Association of Retired Persons. https://assets.aarp.org/rgcenter/general/images_aging.pdf.

Barreto, M., Victor, C., Hammond, C., Eccles, A., Richins, M. T., & Qualter, P. (2021). Loneliness around the world: Age, gender, and cultural differences in loneliness. *Personality and Individual Differences, 169,* 110066.

BBC Loneliness Experiment. (2018). *Who feels lonely?: The results of the world's largest loneliness study.* BBC. www.bbc.co.uk/programmes/articles/2yzhfv4DvqVp5nZyxBD8G23/who-feels-lonely-the-results-of-the-world-s-largest-loneliness-study.

Becker, D. (2006). Therapy for the middle-aged: The relevance of existential issues. *American Journal of Psychotherapy, 60*(1), 87–99.

Bound Alberti, F. (2018). This "modern epidemic": Loneliness as an emotion cluster and a neglected subject in the history of emotions. *Emotion Review, 10*(3), 242–254.

Brennan, T. (1982). Loneliness at adolescence. In L. A. Peplau & D. Perlman (Eds.), *Loneliness: A sourcebook of current theory, research and therapy* (pp. 269–290). Wiley.

Cacioppo, J. T., & Cacioppo, S. (2018). The growing problem of loneliness. *Lancet, 391*(10119), 426.

Carr, S., & Fang, C. (2021). A gradual separation from the world: A qualitative exploration of existential loneliness in old age. *Ageing and Society,* 1–21.

Carstensen, L. L., Fung, H. H., & Charles, S. T. (2003). Socioemotional selectivity theory and the regulation of emotion in the second half of life. *Motivation and Emotion, 27*(2), 103–123.

Cassidy, J., & Asher, S. R. (1992). Loneliness and peer relations in young children. *Child Development, 63*(2), 350–365.

Cela, E., & Fokkema, T. (2017). Being lonely later in life: A qualitative study among Albanians and Moroccans in Italy. *Ageing and Society, 37*(6), 1197–1226.

Chung, B. P. M., Olofsson, J., Wong, F. K. Y., & Rämgård, M. (2020). Overcoming existential loneliness: A cross-cultural study. *BMC Geriatrics, 20*(1), 347.

Cottle, M. (2023, July 19). Is the cure to male loneliness out on the pickleball court? *New York Times.* https://www.nytimes.com/2023/07/19/opinion/male-loneliness.html.

de Jong Gierveld, J., van Tilburg, T. G., & Dykstra, P. A. (2016). New ways of theorizing and conducting research in the field of loneliness and social isolation. In A. Vangelisti & D. Perlman (Eds.), *The Cambridge handbook of personal relationships* (2nd ed., pp. 1–30). Cambridge University Press.

Deckx, L., van den Akker, M., Buntinx, F., & van Driel, M. (2018). A systematic literature review on the association between loneliness and coping strategies. *Psychology, Health and Medicine, 23*(8), 899–916.

DiTommaso, E., Brannen-McNulty, C., Ross, L., & Burgess, M. (2003). Attachment styles, social skills and loneliness in young adults. *Personality and Individual Differences, 35*(2), 303–312.

DiTommaso, E., & Spinner, B. (1997). Social and emotional loneliness: A re-examination of

Weiss' typology of loneliness. *Personality and Individual Differences, 22*(3), 417–427.

Eccles, A. M., & Qualter, P. (2021). Review: Alleviating loneliness in young people—A meta-analysis of interventions. *Child and Adolescent Mental Health, 26*(1), 17–33.

Ettema, E. J., Derksen, L. D., & van Leeuwen, E. (2010). Existential loneliness and end-of-life care: A systematic review. *Theoretical Medicine and Bioethics, 31*(2), 141–169.

Fakoya, O. A., McCorry, N. K., & Donnelly, M. (2020). Loneliness and social isolation interventions for older adults: A scoping review of reviews. *BMC Public Health, 20*(1), 129.

Firmin, M., Firmin, R., & Lorenzen, K. (2014). A qualitative analysis of loneliness dynamics involved with college long-distance relationships. *College Student Journal, 1,* 57–71.

Fleming, J., Farquhar, M., Cambridge City Over-75s Cohort (CC75C) Study Collaboration, Brayne, C., & Barclay, S. (2016). Death and the oldest old: Attitudes and preferences for end-of-life care—Qualitative research within a population-based cohort study. *PLOS One, 11*(4), e0150686.

Fortner, B. V., & Neimeyer, R. A. (1999). Death anxiety in older adults: A quantitative review. *Death Studies, 23*(5), 387–411.

Frankl, V. E. (1959). *Man's search for meaning: An introduction to logotherapy.* Washington Square Press.

Fromm-Reichmann, F. (1959). Loneliness. *Psychiatry, 22*(1), 1–15.

Galanaki, E. P. (2004). Are children able to distinguish among the concepts of aloneness, loneliness, and solitude? *International Journal of Behavioral Development, 28*(5), 435–443.

Galanaki, E. P., Nelson, L. J., & Antoniou, F. (2023). Social withdrawal, solitude, and existential concerns in emerging adulthood. *Emerging Adulthood, 11*(4), 1006–1021.

Garnow, T., Garmy, P., Edberg, A.-K., & Einberg, E.-L. (2022). Deeply lonely in the borderland between childhood and adulthood—Experiences of existential loneliness as narrated by adolescents. *International Journal of Qualitative Studies on Health and Well-Being, 17*(1), 2132653.

Gil Álvarez, M., Haugan, G., Larsson, H., Saarelainen, S.-M., Duppen, D., & Dezutter, J. (2023). Mapping existential loneliness: A scoping review on existential loneliness/isolation conceptualizations and operationalizations. *Journal of Humanistic Psychology.*

Giuntella, O., McManus, S., Mujcic, R., Oswald, A. J., Powdthavee, N., & Tohamy, A. (2023). The midlife crisis. *Economica, 90*(357), 65–110.

Greenberg, J., Helm, P., Maxfield, M., & Schimel, J. (2017). How our mortal fate contributes to ageism: A terror management perspective. In T. D. Nelson (Ed.), *Ageism: Stereotyping and prejudice against older persons* (pp. 105–132). MIT Press.

Grieder, A. (2009). What are boundary situations?: A Jaspersian notion reconsidered. *Journal of the British Society for Phenomenology, 40*(3), 330–336.

Hawkley, L. C., & Cacioppo, J. T. (2010). Loneliness matters: A theoretical and empirical review of consequences and mechanisms. *Annals of Behavioral Medicine, 40*(2), 218–227.

Heidary, M., Heshmati, R., & Hayes, J. (2023). Effect of group logotherapy on anxiety about death and existential loneliness in patients with advanced cancer: A randomized controlled trial. *Cancer Nursing, 46*(1). https://journals.lww.com/cancernursingonline/Fulltext/2023/01000/Effect_of_Group_Logotherapy_on_Anxiety_About_Death.13.aspx.

Heinrich, L. M., & Gullone, E. (2006). The clinical significance of loneliness: A literature review. *Clinical Psychology Review, 26*(6), 695–718.

Helm, P. J., Rothschild, L. G., Greenberg, J., & Croft, A. (2018). Explaining sex differences in existential isolation research. *Personality and Individual Differences, 134*, 283–288.

Helm, P. J., Greenberg, J., Park, Y. C., & Pinel, E. C. (2019). Feeling alone in your subjectivity: Introducing the State Trait Existential Isolation Model (STEIM). *Journal of Theoretical Social Psychology, 3*(3), 146–157.

Helm, P. J., Jimenez, T., Bultmann, M., Lifshin, U., Greenberg, J., & Arndt, J. (2020). Existential isolation, loneliness, and attachment in young adults. *Personality and Individual Differences, 159,* 109890.

Helm, P. J., Medrano, M. R., Allen, J. J. B., & Greenberg, J. (2020). Existential isolation, loneliness, depression, and suicide ideation in young adults. *Journal of Social and Clinical Psychology, 39*(8), 641–674.

Holt-Lunstad, J. (2021). Loneliness and social isolation as risk factors: The power of social connection in prevention. *American Journal of Lifestyle Medicine, 15*(5), 567–573.

Holt-Lunstad, J., Smith, T. B., Baker, M., Harris, T., & Stephenson, D. (2015). Loneliness and social isolation as risk factors for mortality: A meta-analytic review. *Perspectives on Psychological Science, 10*(2), 227–237.

Jacobs, M. (2006). *The presenting past: The core of psychodynamic counselling and therapy* (3rd ed.). Open University Press.

Jaspers, K. (1919). *Psychologie der weltanschauungen.* Springer.

Kirwan, E. M., O'Súilleabháin, P. S., Burns, A., Ogoro, M., Allen, E., & Creaven, A.-M. (2023). Exploring loneliness in emerging adulthood: A qualitative study. *Emerging Adulthood.*

Kristensen, K. L. (1995). The lived experience of childhood loneliness: A phenomenological study. *Issues in Comprehensive Pediatric Nursing, 18*(2), 125–137.

Lim, M., Rodebaugh, T. L., Zyphur, M. J., & Gleeson, J. F. M. (2016). Loneliness over time: The crucial role of social anxiety. *Journal of Abnormal Psychology, 125,* 620–630.

Luhmann, M., & Hawkley, L. C. (2016). Age differences in loneliness from late adolescence to oldest old age. *Developmental Psychology, 52*(6), 943–959.

Lundvall, M., Hörberg, U., Palmér, L., Carlsson, G., & Lindberg, E. (2020). Young men's experiences of living with existential concerns: "Living close to a bottomless darkness." *International Journal of Qualitative Studies on Health and Well-Being, 15*(1), 1810947.

Lundvall, M., Lindberg, E., Hörberg, U., Carlsson, G., & Palmér, L. (2019). Lost in an unknown terrain: A phenomenological contribution to the understanding of existential concerns as experienced by young women in Sweden. *International Journal of Qualitative Studies on Health and Well-Being, 14*(1), 1658843.

Martens, A., Greenberg, J., Schimel, J., & Landau, M. J. (2004). Ageism and death: Effects of mortality salience and perceived similarity to elders on reactions to elderly people. *Personality and Social Psychology Bulletin, 30*(12), 1524–1536.

Masi, C. M., Chen, H.-Y., Hawkley, L. C., & Cacioppo, J. T. (2011). A meta-analysis of interventions to reduce loneliness. *Personality and Social Psychology Review, 15*(3), 219–266.

McGraw, J. G. (1995). Loneliness, its nature and forms: An existential perspective. *Man and World, 28*(1), 43–64.

McKenna-Plumley, P. E. (2024). *Conceptualising and measuring loneliness across the lifespan: A multidimensional approach.* Unpublished doctoral thesis, Queen's University Belfast.

McKenna-Plumley, P. E., Turner, R. N., Yang, K., & Groarke, J. M. (2023a). Experiences of loneliness across the lifespan: A systematic review and thematic synthesis of qualitative studies. *International Journal of Qualitative Studies on Health and Well-Being, 18*(1), 2223868.

McKenna-Plumley, P. E., Turner, R. N., Yang, K., & Groarke, J. M. (2023b). "It's a feeling of complete disconnection": Experiences of existential loneliness from youth to older adulthood. *BMC Psychology, 11*(1), 408.

McKenna-Plumley. P. E., Turner, R. N., Yang, K., & Groarke, J. M. (2024). The Brief Scale of Existential Loneliness: Scale development and psychometric evaluation. *Current Psychology, 43,* 1–14.

Morse, D. F., Sandhu, S., Mulligan, K., Tierney, S., Polley, M., Chiva Giurca, B., . . . Husk, K. (2022). Global developments in social prescribing. *BMJ Global Health, 7*(5), e008524.

Moustakas, C. E. (1961). *Loneliness.* Prentice-Hall.

Nicioli, T. (2023). *The loneliness epidemic: Nearly 1 in 4 adults feel lonely, new survey finds.* CNN. https://edition.cnn.com/2023/10/24/health/lonely-adults-gallup-poll-wellness/index.html.

Office for National Statistics. (2015). *Divorces in England and Wales by age, marital status before marriage and reason: Historical data* [dataset]. www.ons.gov.uk/peoplepopulationandcommunity/birthsdeathsandmarriages/divorce/datasets/divorcesinenglandandwalesnumberofdivorcesageatdivorceandmaritalstatusbeforemarriage.

Office for National Statistics. (2023). *Public opinions and social trends, Great Britain: How often do you feel lonely? November 2022 to February 2023.* https://www.ons.gov.uk/peoplepopulationandcommunity/wellbeing/adhocs/15615publicopinionsandsocialtrendsgreatbritainhowoftendoyoufeellonelynovember2022tofebruary2023.

Olofsson, J., Rämgård, M., Sjögren-Forss, K., & Bramhagen, A.-C. (2021). Older migrants' experience of existential loneliness. *Nursing Ethics, 28*(7–8), 1183–1193.

O'Súilleabháin, P. S., Gallagher, S., & Steptoe, A. (2019). Loneliness, living alone, and all-cause mortality: The role of emotional and social loneliness in the elderly during 19 years of follow-up. *Psychosomatic Medicine, 81*(6).

Palgi, Y., Shrira, A., Ben-Ezra, M., Shiovitz-Ezra, S., & Ayalon, L. (2012). Self- and other-oriented potential lifetime traumatic events as predictors of loneliness in the second half of life. *Aging and Mental Health, 16*(4), 423–430.

Park, Y. C., & Pinel, E. C. (2023). The effect of a 7-day intensive Buddhist meditation on existential isolation, interpersonal isolation, and compassion among South Koreans. *Journal of Applied Social Psychology, 53*(9), 877–891.

Perlman, D., & Peplau, L. A. (1981) Toward a social psychology of loneliness. In R. Gilmour & S. Duck (Eds.), *Personal relationships: Relationships in disorder* (pp. 31–56). Academic Press.

Pinel, E. C., Long, A. E., Landau, M. J., Alexander, K., & Pyszczynski, T. (2006). Seeing I to I: A pathway to interpersonal connectedness.

Journal of Personality and Social Psychology, 90(2), 243–257.
Pinel, E. C., Long, A. E., Murdoch, E. Q., & Helm, P. (2017). A prisoner of one's own mind: Identifying and understanding existential isolation. *Personality and Individual Differences, 105,* 54–63.
Pinel, E. C., Helm, P. J., Yawger, G. C., Long, A. E., & Scharnetzki, L. (2022). Feeling out of (existential) place: Existential isolation and nonnormative group membership. *Group Processes & Intergroup Relations, 25*(4), 990–1010.
Pramling, I., & Johansson, E. (1995). Existential questions in early childhood programs in Sweden: Teachers' conceptions and children's experience. *Child and Youth Care Forum, 24*(2), 125–146.
Qualter, P., & Munn, P. (2002). The separateness of social and emotional loneliness in childhood. *Journal of Child Psychology and Psychiatry, 43*(2), 233–244.
Qualter, P., Vanhalst, J., Harris, R., Van Roekel, E., Lodder, G., Bangee, M., . . . Verhagen, M. (2015). Loneliness across the life span. *Perspectives on Psychological Science, 10*(2), 250–264.
Riddleston, L., Bangura, E., Gibson, O., Qualter, P., & Lau, J. Y. F. (2023). Developing an interpretation bias modification training task for alleviating loneliness in young people. *Behaviour Research and Therapy, 168,* 104380.
Rönkä, A. R., Taanila, A., Rautio, A., & Sunnari, V. (2018). Multidimensional and fluctuating experiences of loneliness from childhood to young adulthood in Northern Finland. *Advances in Life Course Research, 35,* 87–102.
Salo, A.-E., Junttila, N., & Vauras, M. (2020). Social and emotional loneliness: Longitudinal stability, interdependence, and intergenerational transmission among boys and girls. *Family Relations, 69*(1), 151–165.
Schoenmakers, E. C., van Tilburg, T. G., & Fokkema, T. (2012). Coping with loneliness: What do older adults suggest? *Aging and Mental Health, 16*(3), 353–360.
Schulenberg, S. E., Hutzell, R. R., Nassif, C., & Rogina, J. M. (2008). Logotherapy for clinical practice. *Psychotherapy: Theory, Research, Practice, Training, 45*(4), 447–463.
Shiovitz-Ezra, S., & Ayalon, L. (2010). Situational versus chronic loneliness as risk factors for all-cause mortality. *International Psychogeriatrics, 22*(3), 455–462.
Sjöberg, M., Beck, I., Rasmussen, B. H., & Edberg, A.-K. (2018). Being disconnected from life: Meanings of existential loneliness as narrated by frail older people. *Aging and Mental Health, 22*(10), 1357–1364.
Sjöberg, M., Edberg, A.-K., Rasmussen, B. H., & Beck, I. (2019). Being acknowledged by others and bracketing negative thoughts and feelings: Frail older people's narrations of how existential loneliness is eased. *International Journal of Older People Nursing, 14*(1), e12213.
Stickley, T., & Eades, M. (2013). Arts on prescription: A qualitative outcomes study. *Public Health, 127*(8), 727–734.
Sundström, M., Blomqvist, K., Edberg, A.-K., & Rämgård, M. (2019). The context of care matters: Older people's existential loneliness from the perspective of healthcare professionals—A multiple case study. *International Journal of Older People Nursing, 14*(3), e12234.
Tarbi, E. C., & Meghani, S. H. (2019). A concept analysis of the existential experience of adults with advanced cancer. *Nursing Outlook, 67*(5), 540–557.
U.K. Department of Health and Social Care. (2018). *Social prescribing schemes across England to receive £4.5 million.* www.gov.uk/government/news/social-prescribing-schemes-across-england-to-receive-45-million.
U.S. Department of Health and Human Services. (2023). *Our epidemic of loneliness and isolation: The U.S. Surgeon General's Advisory on the Healing Effects of Social Connection and Community.* Office of the U.S. Surgeon General. www.hhs.gov/sites/default/files/surgeon-general-social-connection-advisory.pdf.
van Tilburg, T. G. (2021). Social, emotional, and existential loneliness: A test of the multidimensional concept. *The Gerontologist, 61*(7), e335–e344.
Victor, C. R., & Yang, K. (2012). The prevalence of loneliness among adults: A case study of the United Kingdom. *Journal of Psychology, 146*(1–2), 85–104.
Weiss, R. S. (1973). *The experience of emotional and social isolation.* MIT Press.
Wethington, E. (2000). Expecting stress: Americans and the "midlife crisis." *Motivation and Emotion, 24*(2), 85–103.
Wimmer, H., & Perner, J. (1983). Beliefs about beliefs: Representation and constraining function of wrong beliefs in young children's understanding of deception. *Cognition, 13*(1), 103–128.
Winnicott, D. W. (1958). The capacity to be alone. *International Journal of Psycho-Analysis, 39,* 416.
Yalom, I. (1980). *Existential psychotherapy.* Basic Books.
Yang, K., & Victor, C. R. (2011). Age and loneliness in 25 European nations. *Ageing & Society, 31*(8), 1368–1388.

SECTION V

CULTURE, SELF, AND IDENTITY

CHAPTER 34

The Cultural Pursuit of Meaning

Steven J. Heine *and* Michael B. Mask

Jean-Paul Sartre (1947/2003) offered, "Life has no meaning a priori. . . . It is up to you to give it a meaning, and value is nothing but the meaning that you choose" (p. 8). Sartre recognized that so much of what makes life meaningful rests upon the individual's perspective and the choices that they make; the meanings in people's lives are up to them to find for themselves. However true this may be, it is important to emphasize that people are not alone in their quests to find meaning. We are not a collection of isolated individuals, disconnected from everything around us, but rather our lives are intertwined by the shared cultural meanings that we regularly exchange with each other. Humans are a cultural species (e.g., Boyd et al., 2011; Fox, 1970), and everything we do is shaped by the meanings we learn from our cultures. These meanings not only guide our quotidian concerns, such as what we should eat or what social scripts we should follow, but they also play a key role in shaping our own understanding of what is valued, what is significant, what is purposeful, and what kinds of lives we should lead. To be able to have a rich understanding of how we as individuals can find meaning in our lives, we need to consider the cultural fabric that our lives are made from.

One of the central topics pursued by existential psychologists is to understand what makes life meaningful (King & Hicks, 2021). A life that is bereft of meaning has little to offer, and people bear substantial costs to their well-being if they are unable to appreciate what is meaningful in their own lives (Kleiman & Beaver, 2013; Ostafin & Proulx, 2020; Steger et al., 2009). But it is not at all straightforward to identify what leads to a meaningful life, and many ancient wisdom traditions from around the world have grappled with this question over the centuries. While there is much that can be learned by turning to these philosophical and religious texts directly, the field of existential psychology has made efforts to provide a very different perspective on this question. Using the tools of science, existential psychology has sought to uncover an empirical foundation of a meaningful life. Over the past few decades, researchers have strived to identify what distinguishes meaningful lives from meaningless ones. In this chapter we consider the arguments and evidence that these efforts have produced, and how they speak to the role of culture in people's pursuits of a meaningful life.

MEANING IS CONNECTION

To understand how people go about pursuing meaningful lives we first need to consider what precisely is *meaning*. The study of meaning in psychology has generally been pursued in two related and overlapping literatures: *meaning* and *meaning in life*. In the first section of the chapter, we explore in detail the literature on meaning, before returning later in the chapter to the literature on meaning in life.

Since at least the time of Jerome Bruner, who, in the cognitive revolution of the 1950s, strove to establish "meaning as the central concept of psychology" (1990, p. 2), a large literature has focused on what Baumeister and Landau (2018) referred to as "denotative meaning." Denotative meaning (*meaning* hereafter) refers to how people understand any concept, event, or object in terms of what kinds of ideas people expect to connect to them (Heine et al., 2006; Park, 2010; Steger, 2012). For example, Baumeister (1991) defined *meaning* as a "mental representation of possible relationships among things, events, and relationships" (p. 15). Similarly, Heintzelman and King (2014a) referred to *meaning* as the detection of reliable associations in the environment, and Hicks and colleagues (2010) defined *meaning* as the perceived coherence among stimuli. These various definitions converge on identifying meaning as being ultimately about connections.

For example, consider what someone's job might mean to them. It means all of the ideas that people intuitively associate with their jobs. This includes their relations with their boss, the kinds of tasks they do on a regular basis, their commute to and from work, the struggles they experience there, the feelings they get when they do their job well, their regular lunches with their colleagues, the promotion they are working toward, and so on. If any of these expected relations change in a significant manner, then the meaning of their job would also change. Some of these expected connections would largely be perceived similarly by everyone, and these would reflect consensually agreed upon meanings. In contrast, other kinds of meanings could be uniquely perceived by an individual, reflecting personal aspects to meaning. But all of these instances of meaning share in common that they are based on the connections that people perceive.

The many connections people perceive around everything they encounter are organized into broad networks of associations. Various terminologies that have been adopted to refer to these networks of associations include schemas, scripts, paradigms, mental models, worldviews, meaning frameworks, and narratives. What they have in common is that they all refer to meaning as being made up of the many associations that surround any idea.

In many ways, people interact with events in the world in terms of what those events mean to them, and they are thus highly dependent upon perceiving their meaning frameworks as stable and coherent. Sometimes people encounter information that may stand at odds with their meaning frameworks, which can be disorienting. In response to such kinds of violations of their meaning frameworks, people turn to a number of different responses in order to feel they are able to continue to make sense of their worlds (Heine et al., 2006). One response is that an individual may be able to identify the anomaly and they then work toward modifying their meaning framework to account for the violation—Piaget (1953) described this process as accommodation. Accommodation involves the creation of new meaning as meaning frameworks are altered to accommodate the anomalous information. This is the ultimate goal people have when they encounter things that do not make sense, as it is surely more adaptive when people's simulations of the world align with reality—the more accurate their meaning frameworks, the more likely they should be to successfully navigate their worlds (although minor departures from reality may sometimes have some benefits for well-being; Taylor & Brown, 1988). As adaptive as it may be to accommodate violations to one's meaning frameworks, achieving such conscious reorganizing of one's meaning frameworks may involve a great deal of effort, cognitive resources, and time (Proulx & Heine, 2010). For example, Thomas Kuhn (1962/1996) noted that scientists are frequently unable to adjust their theories to accommodate anomalous observations and may remain steadfastly opposed to acknowledging these violations, often to the end of their careers.

Given the substantial cognitive resources that may be required to accommodate violations to one's meaning frameworks, people may often engage in another response to meaning threats: They may change how they view the problematic information such that it appears to fit with their meaning frameworks through the process of assimilation (Piaget, 1953). For example, when Bruner and Postman (1949) presented participants with doctored playing cards that had their colors reversed, thereby violating the expected associations that people had about the cards, participants typically reacted by "seeing" the cards as they originally imagined them to be, such as seeing a red 6 of spades as a 6 of hearts. However, these attempts at assimilation are rarely complete and people often continue to have the sense that something remains not quite right. For example, in Bruner and Postman's study, they noted that a majority of their participants experienced a "disruption" in response to seeing the doctored cards, where they would "lose confidence" and become "perceptually confused" (p. 218)—indeed, some of their participants became quite agitated. People's efforts to assimilate broken meaning frameworks thus appear to serve as temporary strategies to manage the meaning threat by failing to consciously recognize it.

Festinger's (1957) cognitive dissonance theory is perhaps the most influential account of how people respond to information that is at odds with their meaning frameworks. The theory has led to a large body of research showing numerous ways people can regain a sense of meaning when they encounter anomalous information that they are unable to make sense of (for a review, see McGrath, 2017). It posits that people respond to inconsistencies that threaten meaning with strategies to reduce the perceived dissonance. Some kinds of responses, such as trivializing an inconsistency (e.g., Simon et al., 1995), are consistent with assimilation, as the problematic anomaly is largely discounted. In contrast, other kinds of responses to dissonance, such as insufficient justification (e.g., Aronson & Mills, 1959), or post-choice dissonance reduction (e.g., Brehm, 1956; Heine & Lehman, 1997), require the addition of cognitions to create new meaning, which is consistent with accommodation.

Heine and colleagues (2006), however, proposed a third response, which occurs when people encounter information that conflicts with their meaning frameworks that was not anticipated by cognitive dissonance theory: They may instead try to distract themselves by committing themselves to alternative meaning frameworks that remain intact. In the face of a meaning violation that they are unable to make sense of, people may instead become more committed to their other beliefs. For example, religious people may become more religious (Randles et al., 2015), liberals and conservatives may become more polarized (Randles et al., 2017), and people become even more committed to defending the status quo (Proulx & Heine, 2008). These efforts to affirm alternative meaning frameworks do not solve the problem of the meaning threat that was encountered; however, they do seem to temporarily dispel the uncomfortable arousal that the anomaly elicited (Benjamin & Heine, 2023). These affirmations allow people to feel that the world makes sense again, and they enable them to return to reflect on their meaningless experiences from a more grounded and less anxious perspective. These diverse kinds of responses to occasions where people experience anomalies to their meaning frameworks highlight how important it is for people to feel that their meaning frameworks are accurate simulations of reality. People are dependent upon their meaning frameworks for making sense of, and functioning within, the worlds around them, and they engage in considerable cognitive efforts to preserve the sense that their perceptions of the world are accurate.

HUMANS LIVE IN ECOLOGIES OF MEANING

Meaning is central to people's psychological worlds, as humans have evolved to live in ecologies of meaning (e.g., Heine et al., 2024). That is, humans live in the contexts of cultures that are constituted of meanings that are shared among cultural members. These environments of shared meanings arise because people find it rewarding to share their inner experiences with others (Tamir & Mitchell, 2012), thereby providing people with some awareness of how others are perceiving their worlds. Some evidence for just how much people tend to share their experiences can be seen in analyses of conversations revealing that approximately one-third of everyday speech consists of people sharing their private experiences or personal relationships (Dunbar et al., 1997), and up to 80% of posts on X (Twitter) are announcements about one's personal experiences (Naaman et al., 2010). By regularly sharing what individuals think about what is happening around them, people can see how their own views align with those of others. Over time, these interactions, and the meanings that are communicated, accumulate into edifices of shared meanings (Tomasello et al., 1993), which result in the creation of norms and the perception of a shared reality (e.g., Baumeister, 2022; Berger & Luckmann, 1967; Sherif, 1937). These shared realities constitute the complex cultures that all humans live within (Heine, 2025).

Human cultures are vast meaning frameworks that include shared understandings about norms that dictate the kinds of behavior that are valued, shunned, tolerated, or encouraged (see e.g., Becker, 1962). For example, these norms guide the decisions people make regarding what foods they should eat, how they should dress, how they should interact with others, how they should strive to attract a mate, which gods they should worship, and the kinds of lifestyles they value. The shared meanings that we learn from others come to govern all of our behaviors—there really aren't domains of life that are not shaped by cultural learning (e.g., Heine, 2020). The cultures we exist in do not take long to form; for instance, field studies have revealed the creation of differentiated subcultures in as little as a few months (Cullum & Harton, 2007; Ricart-Huguet & Paluck, 2023), as people come to adapt to the norms they detect among those around them. Despite that new cultures can be created so quickly (also see Talhelm & Dong, 2024), once formed, cultural norms can be very resistant to change, and can continue to persist for many centuries, as new members of the culture are enculturated to the existing norms, thereby perpetuating them (e.g., Nunn & Wantchekon, 2011; Putnam et al., 1993). People thus do not experience reality just from their own perspective but also consider events in their world in terms of how others in their culture understand them. The meaning frameworks of their cultures influence how people interpret what is happening around them.

Cultures can be highly distinct from each other, yet at the same time, humans everywhere share a similar set of basic needs, such as needs for physiological resources, self-protection, belongingness, status, mate acquisition and retention, and parenting (e.g., Kenrick et al., 2010). While these basic needs may constitute human universals, people go about satisfying these needs in culturally determined ways—that is, the ways that people go about achieving status, making friends, finding a mate, raising their children, and so forth, can vary enormously across cultures (e.g., Heine, 2020). This means that people's abilities to satisfy their fundamental needs are contingent upon them acquiring and utilizing local cultural meanings. In this way, we can see how humans have long been dependent upon mastering cultural meanings in order to survive and to pursue fulfilling lives (Heine, 2025).

Living in an ecology of meanings requires humans to engage with cultural meanings in order to thrive. They could more effectively accomplish this to the extent that cultural meanings were easily accessible to them, such that their default reactions would largely be aligned with cultural meanings. Baumeister, Maranges, and Vohs (2018) have proposed that the human self evolved as a means to make these meanings more accessible. The self-concept internalizes, consolidates, and organizes the various meanings of an individual's culture to facilitate an individual's abilities to act in ways that are aligned with their culture's meanings. By internalizing the surrounding culture's meanings, an individual's default interpretations and reactions to events should be aligned with local cultural meanings, rather than in opposition to them. In this way, cultures and selves become mutually constituted (Markus & Kitayama, 2010; Shweder, 1990). Moreover, as individuals participate in multiple overlapping kinds of subcultures, such as the cultures of their country, local region, religion, ethnicity, sexual orientation, occupation, hobbies, and so forth, their self-concepts also have multiple overlapping identities that correspond to each of these subcultures (Hong et al., 2000). People's self-concepts are what connect them to each of these cultural meaning frameworks. Or, as Baumeister (2022, p. 4) put it, "The self exists at the interface between the human animal body and the complicated social structures that we call society and culture." This perspective suggests that to understand an individual's self, and how this informs their primary life concerns, one needs to consider the cultural contexts that it is connected with.

PEOPLE FARE BETTER WHEN MEANINGS IN THE SELF ARE ALIGNED WITH CULTURAL MEANINGS

Though the meanings of selves and cultures are connected and mutually constitute each other, this does not imply that people who share the same culture will largely share the same selves. Rather, cultures are made up of the interactions among their members who may differ from each other in myriad ways that influence how they will respond to the shared cultural meanings they encounter. For example, within any given culture, people differ from each other in that they each have a one-of-a-kind genome, they each have unique life histories that they narrate in individual ways, and they each belong to a particular collection of overlapping subcultures, which results in a great deal of diversity of the self-concepts among people living within any culture. The diversity of individual self-concepts within all cultures results in a situation where some people's selves are necessarily closer to the dominant culture's prototypical self-concept than are others. This tendency for people to vary in the degree to which they approximate the prototypes of their cultures is termed "cultural fit" (e.g., De Leersnyder et al., 2014; Götz et al., 2018). People with greater cultural fit are more closely connected with the meanings of their cultures, and this is of much consequence for how people come to lead their lives (Heine et al., 2024).

People whose selves fit more closely with the dominant culture should be able to act more efficaciously because they are more closely connected with cultural meanings. On average, their selves would largely be aligned with the ways that their culture encourages, in contrast to "cultural misfits" who may often feel that their preferred ways of acting are at odds with the dominant culture. The greater degree of connections between the self-concepts and the meanings of the dominant culture among people with greater cultural fit should enable them to act more effectively and thereby experience greater well-being. In recent years, much research has revealed the importance of having good cultural fit. For example, research has found that people whose emotional repertoire is more similar to those in the surrounding culture tend to have more satisfying relationships (De Leersnyder et al., 2014), personality fit predicts greater well-being (Götz et al., 2018), religious fit predicts longevity (Ebert et al., 2020), self-concept fit predicts healthier lifestyles (Levine et al., 2016), and people whose sleep durations more closely approximate cultural norms have better health (Ou et al., 2025). When people's self-concepts are aligned with dominant cultural meanings, they experience less friction in living their lives, and their actions are facilitated by the surrounding culture. Moreover, we have found that people who have better subjective cultural fit report leading more meaningful lives (Mask & Heine, 2025). That is, when people feel that their ways of living are more connected to the norms they perceive around them, their lives come to feel richer in meaning. Below we now consider the kinds of connections that provide the foundation of a meaningful life.

AS WITH MEANING, MEANING IN LIFE IS ALSO ABOUT CONNECTIONS

While the above review focused on the central role that *meaning* occupies in people's lives, we now turn to consider the related construct of *meaning in life*, or what Baumeister and Landau (2018) called "existential meaning." Typically, meaning in life has been understood as people's sense that their lives are sufficiently worthwhile or significant. Discussions of meaningful lives in Western culture date back at least to Aristotle's consideration of eudaimonia (Aristotle, fourth century B.C.E./1986), in which he viewed the good life to be lived in accordance with internal virtues, and this topic was a primary concern of the existential philosophers (e.g., Camus, 1955; Sartre, 1947/2003). However, considerations of meaningful lives have a more recent history in psychology. Earlier investigations of meaning in life by psychologists largely relied upon people's intuitions about what this was referring to, so there was little consensus across researchers with respect to what meaning in life consisted of (e.g., Antonovsky, 1993; Crumbaugh & Maholick, 1964; Ryff, 1989). The field gained traction when researchers started to operationalize meaning in life by using a questionnaire created by Steger and colleagues (2006), which has since become the most widely used measure to assess it (Schutte et al., 2023).

Similar to the concept of meaning discussed above, meaning in life can also be understood in terms of connections, specifically the kinds of connections that people have with respect to their thoughts of their own lives (Heine et al., 2024). In this respect meaning in life may be understood as a more specific category of meaning. There are a variety of different types of connections that are importantly linked to the feeling that one's life is meaningful.

First, people's connections with others are especially important for their sense that their life is meaningful (e.g., Hicks & King, 2009; Martela et al., 2018). Anthropologists describe humans as an ultrasocial species (e.g., Richerson & Boyd, 2005; Tomasello, 2014), where our degree of sociality transcends that of other species of primates, in terms of our dependence upon others and the size of the social networks that we maintain (Dunbar, 1992). Baumeister and Leary (1995) explored the many ways people demonstrate a homeostatic drive to maintain a sufficient degree of close relationships. They proposed that human's drive for belongingness represents a full-fledged need, and their survival is threatened when those needs are not met—a notion that has received much support in the health literature (Hakulinen et al., 2018; Holt-Lunstad et al., 2010). But more recent research has shown that people's interpersonal relationships constitute one of the stronger foundations of the sense that life is meaningful. When people are feeling lonely and out of touch with their relationships, they feel less meaning in life (Hicks et al., 2010; Mwilambwe-Tshilobo et al., 2019), and this relation emerges reliably across cultures (Mask & Heine, 2025). Arguably, family relationships are the category of relationships that are most connected with people's meaning in life (Lambert et al., 2010); indeed, people from 17 countries nominated "family and children" as the variable that provided their lives with the most meaning (Silver et al., 2021). Family relationships may be such potent sources of meaning as they are also linked with people's feelings of identity, they remain some of the most significant relationships across different life stages, and they are the basis of much social support. Relationships in which one takes on a caretaker role, especially having children, feel more purposeful, and they are also tightly linked with feelings of meaning in life (Baumeister et al., 2013; Shim et al., 2013). The relationships people have with their communities are also importantly associated with greater meaning in life (Lambert et al., 2013; Stavrova & Luhmann, 2016). The fact that people in many societies have been increasingly struggling with being able to maintain sufficient close relationships in their lives, as highlighted in a recent report from the U.S. Surgeon General (2023), does not bode well for people having their existential needs satisfied.

People's connections with their work also predict meaning in life (Duffy & Sedlacek, 2010). For example, after Studs Terkel (1997) had interviewed hundreds of Americans about their careers, he concluded that work is about a search "for daily meaning as well as daily bread." More than half of Americans report that their jobs provide them with a key source of identity (Gallup, 2014), and people's jobs also provide them with a sense of purpose, self-worth, and typically a social network (Baumeister, 1991). These connections between one's work and one's sense that life is meaningful have been observed across diverse cultures (Mask & Heine, 2025).

People's connections to a transcendent realm via their religious and spiritual beliefs are particularly strong predictors of meaning in life (e.g., Hood et al., 2018; Stroope et al., 2013). People's spiritual beliefs can connect them to teleological values that transcend their daily concerns. We can see evidence for the existential benefits of these connections in a variety of ways. For example, an investigation into the differences among American and British samples of religious believers, nonbelievers, and those who identified as "spiritual but not religious," found that meaning in life was distinctly lower among nonbelievers compared to the other groups, and these differences were mediated by a variety of different kinds of mystical beliefs (Jettinghoff et al., in press; also see Krok, 2015). Likewise, across four different cultures Mask and Heine (2025) found that people who reported a diverse set of transcendent connections, such as experiencing a greater spiritual relationship with nature (ecospirituality; Billet et al., 2023), having more transcendent ineffable mystical experiences (see Hanley et al., 2018), experiencing awe in their everyday lives (see Shiota et al., 2006), being more religious (see Hoge, 1972), and praying and meditating, all reported greater meaning in life.

There are a number of explanations for why these transcendent connections seem to be so closely linked with feelings of meaning in life. First, people's spiritual beliefs provide them with a worldview that aids them in making sense of the events around them. Whatever suffering a person may experience, they may derive some consolation from feeling that their difficulties may make sense in the grander scheme of things. However, it is not the case that just any kind of worldview makes one's life feel more meaningful. For example, while a scientifically materialistic worldview can offer an explanation for the events in the world, this worldview tends to be negatively associated with meaning in life, even among scientists (Folk et al., 2025). Furthermore, spiritual beliefs may allow individuals to see greater significance in their suffering (Frankl, 1959; Prinzing et al., 2021; Stephens et al., 2012). These beliefs may also enhance a sense of meaning by providing a sense of structure, thereby reducing the apparent randomness of the world (Hood et al., 2018; Laurin & Kay, 2017; Park & Edmonson, 2012). Moreover, transcendent connections may help combat people's existential anxieties by providing the sense that one's existence will continue even after one has died (Becker, 1973; Vail et al., 2012). In sum, people's transcendent connections are reliably linked with heightened feelings of meaning in life, and this may be what enables religions to help assuage people's anxieties (Inzlicht et al., 2009).

The role of connections is also evident when we consider how meaning in life is enhanced when people feel their current lives are integrated with their pasts and futures (George & Park, 2016; McAdams & Olson, 2010). Research on nostalgia finds that people's nostalgic memories from the past are existentially grounding and predict greater feelings of meaning in life (Routledge et al., 2011; Sedikides & Wildschut, 2018). When people are feeling that their lives are particularly low in meaning, such as when they are bored or feeling lonely (Sedikides et al., 2018; van Tilburg et al., 2013), they are especially likely to consider past episodes of their lives, reflecting on how these nostalgic connections serve to shore up a sense of meaning. People's sense of identity is bolstered when they are able to see how their present lives are connected to the many past episodes they have experienced.

The key role of connections in meaning in life can also be seen in the tripartite model of meaning in life (George & Park, 2016). Recently, the tripartite model of meaning in life has offered much insight into the predictors of a meaningful life. This model has identified three kinds of connections that are importantly related to feelings of meaning in life. First, meaning in life is strongly associated with feelings of *purpose*. Individuals' lives feel more meaningful when they feel that their actions are guided by a sense of purpose and they are able to understand why they are doing what they are doing. *Coherence* has been identified as another core facet of meaning in life, and this reflects how well organized the various connections across one's life are. One's life is more likely to feel meaningful if it feels that it makes sense. And, third, *mattering*, reflects that one's life has implications for others (Prinzing et al., 2023), and for the universe (e.g., George & Park, 2017; Krause & Hayward, 2014). In one study, mattering was identified as the strongest facet of meaning in life (Costin & Vignoles, 2020)—participants seemed to be most likely to feel that their lives were meaningful when they felt that their existence was of consequence to others.

The tripartite model of meaning in life holds up well across cultures, and research has found that people across 17 different countries around the world show a remarkably similar ratio of endorsing each of coherence, purpose, and mattering (Russo-Netzer et al., 2023). On average, across all countries, purpose was endorsed the most strongly, followed by coherence, with mattering endorsed the least. This pattern was largely consistent within each country.

PEOPLE'S PURSUIT OF A MEANINGFUL LIFE IS ALSO GROUNDED IN THEIR CULTURES

As a cultural species, virtually everything people do is grounded in shared meaning frameworks. Accordingly, people pursue meaningful lives in ways that are shaped by their cultures. People are regularly sizing themselves up alongside standards for what their cultures inform them regarding what is an appropriate, commendable, and meaningful life. While meaning in life is surely a concern for people in all cultures, there has been a broad consensus that the field had been relying too much on Western samples to explore such existential questions (Heintzelman & King, 2014b; Heintzelman et al., 2020; Schutte et al., 2023). However, more recently there has been a trend of growing research with samples from other parts of the world. This is facilitated by the finding by Schutte and colleagues (2023) that the most commonly used measure of meaning in life, the Meaning in Life Questionnaire (Steger et al., 2006), has largely robust psychometric properties across 17 different cultures. The authors concluded that the striking degree of measurement invariance of the presence of meaning in life across such a wide variety of cultures suggests that the experience of meaning in life may constitute a human universal.

In support of Schutte and colleagues' (2023) contention that experiencing meaningful lives may be a human universal, Heintzelman and King (2014b) pointed out that meaning in life is a common occurrence, with participants in diverse samples and countries often selecting above the scale midpoint for various meaning in life related scales. More strikingly, in a large cross-cultural Gallup World Poll, Oishi and Diener (2014) reported that 91% of all individuals surveyed in 132 countries responded "yes" to the question "Do you feel your life has an important purpose or meaning?" In this same dataset, no countries had fewer than 60% of participants reporting that life felt meaningful. The observation of how prevalent meaning in life appears to be prompted Heintzelman and King (2014b) to posit that meaning in life may even be evolutionarily adaptive. Indeed, much research has found that meaning in life is a predictor of mental well-being across diverse samples (for reviews, see King et al., 2016; Steger, 2012). In a large meta-analysis spanning 22 countries, He and colleagues (2023) found that meaning in life was negatively related to psychological distress (i.e., depression, suicidal ideation, anxiety, and negative affect) in every country included in the meta-analysis. Furthermore, the presence of meaning in life had an overall moderate negative correlation with psychological distress. Meaning in life thus seems to be universally protective against various kinds of psychological distress, lending support to the notion that it is adaptive.

CROSS-CULTURAL DIFFERENCES AND SIMILARITIES IN PREDICTORS OF MEANINGFUL LIVES

While the above research suggests that meaningful lives may well be universally associated with well-being, it is not clear whether the predictors of meaningful lives are similar across cultures. On the one hand, the fact that people's lives and various psychological processes are shaped so much by culture would lead one to expect much cultural variation in the bases of meaningful lives. On the other hand, the stark similarity in degrees of meaning in life across cultures, and their associations with psychological distress, would suggest that meaning in life might look very similar around the world. A number of recent investigations have explored what predicts meaning in life in a variety of different cultures.

One aspect of a culture that seems to predict greater meaning in life is, ironically, poverty. Oishi and Diener (2014) examined Gallup data from around the world that had included the question "Do you feel your life has an important purpose or meaning?" Strikingly, meaning in life was far lower in countries with higher per-capita GDP. This was the precise opposite relation that was found in the same dataset between per-capita GDP and life satisfaction. National wealth thus seems to be associated with more life satisfaction, but lower levels of meaning. This pattern aligns with Baumeister's (1991, p. 3) claim that "desperate people do not ponder the meaning of life. When survival is at stake . . . life's meaning is irrelevant. The meaning of life is a problem for people who are not desperate, people who can count on survival, comfort, security, and some measure of pleasure." Further evidence that links suffering with meaning in life can be seen in the findings from Baumeister and colleagues (2013), who found that the more negative events a person had experienced, as well as the degree of stress and worrying they felt about those events, positively predicted the residual of meaning in life after controlling for happiness. Moreover, there is extensive literature on posttraumatic growth that finds that people's sense of meaning in life often grows after experiences with tragedy as they become more dependent on their close relationships for support, and they may get more involved in charitable work (George & Park, 2022; Tedeschi & Calhoun, 2004). Likewise, victims of trauma often become more religious (Park, 2005; Tedeschi & Calhoun, 2004).

The link between suffering and religiosity may largely be responsible for the finding that meaning in life is higher in poorer countries. After controlling for religiosity, Oishi and Diener (2014) reported that the national-level association between per-capita GDP and meaning in life disappears. However, a multilevel analysis revealed that people in poorer countries remained higher in meaning in life after controlling for religiosity, suggesting that there remains something beyond religiosity that is responsible for the association between per-capita GDP and meaning in life.

Another cultural factor that seems plausibly linked to cultural differences in meaning in life is individualism, given the important role social connection plays in augmenting perceptions that life is meaningful (Heintzelman et al., 2020; Hofer et al., 2014; Oishi & Westgate, 2022). Since individualism is typically construed as entailing a greater focus on how the self is distinct from others, whereas collectivism emphasizes one's social interconnection with others (Oyserman et al., 2002), it might follow that meaning in life should be higher in collectivistic countries. A variety of investigations have provided support for this prediction.

For instance, Russo-Netzer and colleagues (2023) found that, with a few exceptions, people from more individualistic societies tended to report lower levels of the three facets of meaning in life from the tripartite model: coherence, purpose, and mattering. Likewise, an investigation across 17 countries found that, on average, participants from more individualistic societies tended to report lower levels of meaning in life (Schutte et al., 2023). In addition, in their examination of Gallup World Poll data, Oishi and Diener (2014) also found that individualism correlated moderately negatively with meaning in life, although this relation disappeared after controlling for religiosity and GDP per capita. To the extent that the relation between individualism and meaning in life is robust, the trend of increasing individualism that has been identified in many countries around the world (e.g., Santos et al., 2017) does not bode well for global levels of meaning in life.

Other cultural traits may also differentially relate to meaning in life. For example, the concept of face (面子) is a prominent value in East Asian societies, believed to have its roots in Confucianism (Heine, 2005; Monkhouse et al., 2013). *Face* refers to maintaining one's public image and living up to the expectations others have for one's social role (Ho, 1976). Likewise, an important cultural concept in Indian society, *izzat*, is similar to face (Baig et al., 2014). Mask and Heine (2025) found that face concerns positively predicted meaning in life in Japan and India, where these are especially valued. In contrast, in the United States and Poland, where cultural elaborations about face maintenance are less pronounced, face concerns were not related to meaning in life. This is some initial evidence to suggest that culturally valued traits may predict meaning in life differently across cultures.

While the above review points to some ways that cultures differ in what leads to a meaningful life, there is much evidence that meaning in life is based on similar sources across countries. For example, Heintzelman and colleagues (2020) found that participants from eight different countries provided quite similar responses regarding which of six different possible sources of meaning were important to them. They found that social relationships and happiness were endorsed as the two most important sources in almost all countries, and that religion was endorsed the least in seven out of eight countries (with Angola being the exception). However, although religion was rated as the least important source of meaning in most countries, it had the highest correlations with meaning in life in Germany, Norway, and the United States.

Similarly, the Pew Research Center asked participants from 17 countries with advanced economies what made their lives meaningful (Silver et al., 2021). Family was the source of meaning that was most often referenced (ranked #1 in 14 countries), while occupation was also a commonly referenced source of meaning, ranking in the top 5 in 15 of the countries. Friends, health, and material well-being were also among the top-ranked cross-cultural sources of meaning in life. Likewise, Oishi and Westgate (2022) asked participants in four nations (United States, Japan, India, and Angola) to provide descriptions of the ideal life in a free-response format. Family and occupation were listed in the top 5 most common descriptions of the ideal life in each country.

In addition, Mask, Folk, and Heine (in press) investigated the kinds of purposes people say are guiding their lives. Participants in four cultures (United States, Poland, India, and Japan) rated how important 16 different kinds of purpose were for them, and their rank-order of these purposes was highly similar across cultures. For instance, participants in all countries endorsed family, pursuing happiness, and becoming self-sufficient more strongly than they did other kinds of purpose, whereas religiosity and pursuing recognition were consistently ranked among the least-endorsed kinds of purpose for each country. Moreover, as with Heintzelman and colleagues (2020), despite that religiosity was less commonly endorsed as an important purpose in life, religiosity was among the most strongly correlated with participants' well-being.

A consideration of what predicts meaningful lives among older participants (age 60+) in Cameroon, the Czech Republic, Hong Kong, and Germany, revealed that concerns for generativity, and offering guidance and support to younger generations (Erickson, 1963) predicted meaning in life in all four countries (Hofer et al., 2014). Additionally, reminiscing on the past and teaching others were also predictive of a meaningful life across cultures.

Personality traits also tend to predict meaningful lives similarly across cultures. Oishi and Westgate (2022) correlated traits from the five-factor model of personality with meaning in life across the United States, India, and South Korea. In all three countries, openness to experience, conscientiousness, extraversion, and agreeableness (with the exception of South Korea) were positively related to meaning in life and neuroticism was negatively associated with meaning in life. A similar pattern of results was obtained in another investigation among American, Polish, Japanese, and Indian samples (Mask & Heine, 2025). Thus, it appears that across cultures, with a few exceptions, perceiving life to be meaningful tends to positively relate to openness, conscientiousness, extraversion, and agreeableness and negatively with neuroticism.

People's beliefs about meaning in life also share many similarities across cultures. Heintzelman and colleagues (2020) explored what ordinary people believe about meaning in life by asking people in eight different countries around the world whether they thought that meaning in life required hard work in order to achieve, and whether it was important, mysterious, rare, or common. With the curious exception of Singapore, participants in all countries reported that it required hard work to live a meaningful life, that it was important for people to live meaningful lives, that meaning in life was mysterious, and that meaningful lives were common. By contrast, participants in Singapore reported that experiencing meaning in life was neither important, mysterious, common, nor requiring hard work to attain. Across all eight countries, people rejected the idea that meaningful lives were rare. In sum, there is much agreement across countries (with the exception of Singapore) on people's ideas about some attributes of meaningful lives. In a number of respects, the predictors of meaningful lives are quite cross-culturally robust.

CONCLUSION

Our review of research on meaningful lives points to a number of conclusions. First, we submit that in order to have a rich understanding of what makes life meaningful, we first need to direct our attention to clarifying what *meaning* itself is. As several researchers have underscored, meaning is based on *connections;* that is, the ideas people connect to any object, event, or person ultimately determines what those mean to them. These various connections are combined and organized into meaning frameworks, and these frameworks determine how people make sense of what is happening around them. Because people are always interacting with the world through the interface of their meaning frameworks, they are highly dependent upon these meaning frameworks and they are motivated to defend them, using a number of different strategies that ensure people feel they can make sense of what is happening to them. And because humans are a cultural species, their meaning frameworks are importantly shaped by the meanings that are provided by their cultures, which can themselves be understood as vast networks of shared meanings. Everything people encounter in their lives is made meaningful in accordance with shared cultural meaning frameworks. Furthermore, the meanings in people's cultures come to shape the meanings that exist within people's selves, such that cultures and selves can be said to be mutually constituted. However, cultures are made up of distinct individuals with different self-concepts, and people will tend to experience less friction and difficulty in their lives when the meanings between an individual's self and the dominant culture are aligned, and the individual experiences good cultural fit.

This recognition that meaning is ultimately based on connections, including shared connections among people living in a culture, sheds some important light on the nature of meaningful lives. Just as with meaning more generally, lives are made meaningful by the connections they are based on. Research has identified a number of kinds of connections that are especially important for building meaningful lives. People's connections with their closest relationships, whether those are with friends, family members, or communities, are reliably associated with feelings that life is meaningful. In addition, people's connections with their work and with their transcendent beliefs and experiences are also associated with more meaningful lives. Moreover, research on the tripartite model of meaning underscores that meaningful lives tend to have more organized connections (coherence), they are connected to a sense of purpose that guides them, and they are connected to the world beyond themselves, such that people feel that their lives are impactful and matter in the grand scheme of things.

Recently, a growing body of research has explored the question of how meaningful lives compare across cultures. In general, this research has found that lives tend to be experienced as less meaningful, on average, in cultures that are more individualistic, and in wealthier cultures, where people don't have to struggle to meet their basic needs and may consequently be less religious (Norenzayan, 2013). On the other hand, much research has highlighted that despite cultures differing from each other in so many ways, there is a striking amount of agreement across cultures in terms of what predicts meaningful lives. People from diverse cultures largely agree on the sources that make their lives meaningful, they identify many of the same purposes as guiding their lives, and similar kinds of personality traits and beliefs about meaning are predictive of meaningful lives. While there may be many different ways people experience how life is made meaningful, the paths that lead to meaningful lives in different cultures cross much of the same kinds of terrain.

REFERENCES

Antonovsky, A. (1993). The structure and properties of the sense of coherence scale. *Social Sciences and Medicine, 36,* 725–733.

Aristotle. (1986). *Nicomachean ethics.* Macmillan. (Original work published fourth century B.C.E.)

Aronson, E., & Mills, J. (1959). The effect of severity of initiation on liking for a group. *Journal of Abnormal and Personality Psychology, 59,* 177–181.

Baig, N., Ting-Toomey, S., & Dorjee, T. (2014). Intergenerational narratives on face: A South Asian Indian American perspective. *Journal of International and Intercultural Communication, 7*(2), 127–147.

Baumeister, R. F. (1991). *Meanings of life.* Guilford Press.

Baumeister, R. F. (2022). *The self explained.* Guilford Press.

Baumeister, R. F., & Landau, M. J. (2018). Finding the meaning of meaning: Emerging insights on four grand questions. *Review of General Psychology, 22,* 1–10.

Baumeister, R. F., & Leary, M. R. (1995). The need to belong: Desire for interpersonal attachments as a fundamental human motivation. *Psychological Bulletin, 117,* 497–529.

Baumeister, R. F., Maranges, H. M., & Vohs, K. D. (2018). Human self as information agent: Functioning in a social environment based on shared meanings. *Review of General Psychology, 22,* 36–47.

Baumeister, R. F., Vohs, K. D., Aaker, J. L., & Garbinsky, E. N. (2013). Some key differences between a happy life and a meaningful life. *Journal of Positive Psychology, 8,* 505–516.

Becker, E. (1962). *The birth and death of meaning.* Free Press.

Becker, E. (1973). *The denial of death.* Free Press.

Benjamin, R. F., & Heine, S. J. (2023). From Freud to Androids: Constructing a scale of uncanny feelings. *Journal of Personality Assessment, 105,* 121–133.

Berger, P. L., & Luckmann, T. (1967). *The social construction of reality.* Anchor Books.

Billet, M. I., Baimel, A., Sahakari, S. S., Schaller, M., & Norenzayan, A. (2023). Ecospirituality: The psychology of moral concern for nature. *Journal of Environmental Psychology, 87,* 102001.

Boyd, R., Richerson, P. J., & Henrich, J. (2011). The cultural niche: Why social learning is essential for human adaptation. *Proceedings of the National Academy of Sciences, 108*(Suppl. 2), 10918–10925.

Brehm, J. (1956). Postdecision changes in the desirability of alternatives. *Journal of Abnormal and Social Psychology, 52,* 384–389.

Bruner, J. (1990). *Acts of meaning.* Harvard University Press.

Bruner, J., & Postman, L. (1949). On the perception of incongruity: A paradigm. *Journal of Personality,* 18, 206–223.

Camus, A. (1955). *An absurd reasoning: The myth of Sisyphus and other essays* (pp. 3–49). Vintage Books.

Costin, V., & Vignoles, V. L. (2020). Meaning is about mattering: Evaluating coherence, purpose, and existential mattering as precursors of meaning in life judgments. *Journal of Personality and Social Psychology, 118*(4), 864.

Crumbaugh, J. C., & Maholick, L. T. (1964). An experimental study in existentialism: The psychometric approach to Frankl's concept of noogenic neurosis. *Journal of Clinical Psychology, 20,* 200–207.

Cullum, J. G., & Harton, H. C. (2007). Cultural evolution: Importance and the development of shared attitudes in college residence halls. *Personality and Social Psychology Bulletin, 33,* 1327–1339.

De Leersnyder, J., Mesquita, B., Kim, H., Eom, K., & Choi, H. (2014). Emotional fit with culture: A predictor of individual differences in relational well-being. *Emotion, 14,* 241–245.

Duffy, R. D., & Sedlacek, W. E. (2010). The salience of a career calling among college students: Exploring group differences and links to religiousness, life meaning, and life satisfaction. *Career Development Quarterly, 59,* 27–41.

Dunbar, R. I. M. (1992). Neocortex size as a constraint on group size in primates. *Journal of Human Evolution, 20,* 469–493.

Dunbar, R. I. M., Duncan, N. D. C., & Marriott, A. M. (1997). Human conversational behavior. *Human Nature, 8*(3), 231–246.

Ebert, T., Gebauer, J. E., Talman, J. R., & Rentfrow, P. J. (2020). Religious people only live longer in religious cultural contexts: A gravestone analysis. *Journal of Personality and Social Psychology, 119,* 1–6.

Erickson, E. H. (1963). *Childhood and society.* Norton.

Festinger, L. (1957). *A theory of cognitive dissonance.* Stanford University Press.

Folk, D., Rutjens, B. T., Van Elk, M., & Heine, S. J. (2025). Dare to know!: The existential costs

of a faith in science. *Journal of Positive Psychology, 20,* 31–42.
Fox, R. (1970). The cultural animal. *Social Science Information, 9,* 7–25.
Frankl, V. E. (1959). *Man's search for meaning.* Washington Square Press.
Gallup. (2014). *In U.S., 55% of workers get sense of identity from their job.* https://news.gallup.com/poll/175400/workers-sense-identity-job.aspx.
George, L. S., & Park, C. L. (2016). Meaning in life as comprehension, purpose, and mattering: Toward integration and new research questions. *Review of General Psychology, 20*(3), 205–220.
George, L. S., & Park, C. L. (2017). The multidimensional existential meaning scale: A tripartite approach to measuring meaning in life. *Journal of Positive Psychology, 12*(6), 613–627.
George, L. S., & Park, C. L. (2022). Do violations of global beliefs and goals drive distress and meaning making following life stressors? *Illness, Crisis, and Loss, 30,* 378–395.
Götz, F. M., Ebert, T., & Rentfrow, P. J. (2018). Regional cultures and the psychological geography of Switzerland: Person-environment-fit in personality predicts subjective well-being. *Frontiers in Psychology, 9,* 517.
Hakulinen, C., Pulkki-Raback, L., Virtanen, M., Jokela, M., Kivimaki, M., & Elovainio, M. (2018). Social isolation and loneliness as risk factors for myocardial infarction, stroke and mortality: UK Biobank cohort study of 479,054 men and women. *Heart, 104,* 1536–1542.
Hanley, A. W., Nakamura, Y., & Garland, E. L. (2018). The Nondual Awareness Dimensional Assessment (NADA): New tools to assess nondual traits and states of consciousness occurring within and beyond the context of meditation. *Psychological Assessment, 30*(12), 1625–1639.
He, X.-X., Wang, X., Steger, M. F., Ji, L.-J., Jing, K., Liu, M., & Ye, B. (2023). Meaning in life and psychological distress: A meta-analysis. *Journal of Research in Personality, 104,* 104381.
Heine, S. J. (2005). Constructing good selves in Japan and North America. In R. M. Sorrentino, D. Cohen, J. M. Olson, & M. P. Zanna (Eds.), *Culture and social behavior: The Tenth Ontario symposium* (pp. 95–116). Erlbaum.
Heine, S. J. (2020). *Cultural psychology* (4th ed.) Norton.
Heine, S. J. (2025). *Start making sense.* Basic Books.
Heine, S. J., Folk, D. P., Guan, K. W., Benjamin, R., Bahng, J. M., & Proulx, T. (2024). An ecology of meaning: An integrative framework for understanding human motivations. *Advances in Motivation Science, 11,* 75–121.
Heine, S. J., & Lehman, D. R. (1997). Culture, dissonance, and self-affirmation. *Personality and Social Psychology Bulletin, 23,* 389–400.
Heine, S. J., Proulx, T., & Vohs, K. D. (2006). The meaning maintenance model: On the coherence of social motivations. *Personality and Social Psychology Review, 10*(2), 88–110.
Heintzelman, S. J., & King, L. A. (2014a). (The feeling of) meaning-as-information. *Personality and Social Psychology Review, 18*(2), 153–167.
Heintzelman, S. J., & King, L. A. (2014b). Life is pretty meaningful. *American Psychologist, 69*(6), 561–574.
Heintzelman, S. J., Mohideen, F., Oishi, S., & King, L. A. (2020). Lay beliefs about meaning in life: Examinations across targets, time, and countries. *Journal of Research in Personality, 88,* 104003.
Hicks, J. A., & King, L. A. (2009). Positive mood and social relatedness as information about meaning in life. *Journal of Positive Psychology, 4,* 471–482.
Hicks, J. A., Schlegel, R. J., & King, L. A. (2010). Social threats, happiness, and the dynamics of meaning in life judgments. *Personality and Social Psychological Bulletin, 36,* 1305–1317.
Ho, D. Y. F. (1976). On the concept of face. *American Journal of Sociology, 81,* 867–884.
Hofer, J., Busch, H., Au, A., Poláčková Šolcová, I., Tavel, P., & Wong, T. (2014). For the benefit of others: Generativity and meaning in life in the elderly in four cultures. *Psychology and Aging, 29*(4), 764–775.
Hoge, R. (1972). A validated intrinsic religious motivation scale. *Journal for the Scientific Study of Religion,* 369–376.
Holt-Lunstad, J., Smith, T. B., & Layton, J. B. (2010). Social relationships and mortality risk: A meta-analytic review. *PLOS Medicine, 7* (7), e1000316.
Hong, Y., Morris, M. W., Chiu, C., & Benet-Martinez, V. (2000). Multicultural minds: A dynamic constructivist approach to culture and cognition. *American Psychologist, 55,* 705–720.
Hood, R. W., Jr., Hill, P. C., & Spilka, B. (2018). *The psychology of religion: An empirical approach.* Guilford Press.
Inzlicht, M., McGregor, I., Hirsh, J. B., & Nash, K. (2009). Neural markers of religious conviction. *Psychological Science, 20,* 385–392.
Jettinghoff, W., Folk, D., Radjaee, P., Willard, A., Norenzayan, A., & Heine, S. J. (in press).

The varieties of nonreligious experience: Meaning in life among believers, nonbelievers, and the spiritual but not religious. *Religion, Brain, & Behavior.*
Kenrick, D. T., Griskevicius, V., Neuberg, S. L., & Schaller, M. (2010). Renovating the pyramid of needs: Contemporary extensions built upon ancient foundations. *Perspectives in Psychological Science, 5,* 292–314.
King, L. A., & Hicks, J. A. (2021). The science of meaning in life. *Annual Review of Psychology, 72,* 561–584.
King, L. A., Heintzelman, S. J., & Ward, S. J. (2016). Beyond the search for meaning: The contemporary science of meaning in life. *Current Directions in Psychological Science, 25,* 211–216.
Kleiman, E. M., & Beaver, J. K. (2013). A meaningful life is worth living: Meaning in life as a suicide resiliency factor. *Psychiatry Research, 210,* 934–939.
Krause, N., & Hayward, R. D. (2014). Assessing stability and change in a second-order confirmatory factor model of meaning in life. *Journal of Happiness Studies, 15,* 237–253.
Krok, D. (2015). Striving for significance: The relationships between religiousness, spirituality, and meaning in life. *Implicit Religion, 18*(2), 233–257.
Kuhn, T. (1996). *The structure of scientific revolutions.* University of Chicago Press. (Original work published 1962)
Lambert, N. M., Stillman, T. F., Baumeister, R. F., Fincham, F. D., Hicks, J. A., & Graham, S. (2010). Family as a salient source of meaning in young adulthood. *Journal of Positive Psychology, 5,* 367–376.
Lambert, N. M., Stillman, T. F., Hicks, J. A., Kamble, S., Baumeister, R. F., & Fincham, F. D. (2013). To belong is to matter: Sense of belonging enhances meaning in life. *Personality and Social Psychology Bulletin, 39,* 1418–1427.
Laurin, K., & Kay, A. C. (2017). The motivational underpinnings of belief in God. *Advances in Experimental Social Psychology, 56,* 201–257.
Levine, C. S., Miyamoto, Y., Markus, H. R., Rigotti, A., Boylan, J. M., Park, J., . . . Ryff, C. D. (2016). Culture and healthy eating: the role of independence and interdependence in the United States and Japan. *Personality and Social Psychology Bulletin, 42,* 1335–1348.
Markus, H. R., & Kitayama, S. (2010). Cultures and selves: A cycle of mutual constitution. *Perspectives on Psychological Science, 5,* 420–430.
Martela, F., Ryan, R. M., & Steger, M. F. (2018). Meaningfulness as satisfaction of autonomy, competence, relatedness, and beneficence: Comparing the four satisfactions and positive affect as predictors of meaning in life. *Journal of Happiness Studies, 19,* 1261–1282.
Mask, M. B., & Heine, S. J. (2025). *Cross-cultural predictors of meaning in life.* Manuscript in preparation.
Mask, M. B., Folk, D. P., & Heine, S. J. (in press). How sources of purpose predict meaning in life, happiness and psychological richness across cultures. *Journal of Positive Psychology.*
McAdams, D. P., & Olson, B. D. (2010). Personality development: Continuity and change over the life course. *Annual Review of Psychology, 61,* 517–542.
McGrath, A. (2017). Dealing with dissonance: A review of cognitive dissonance reduction. *Social and Personality Psychology Compass, 11*(12), e12362.
Monkhouse, L. L., Barnes, B. R., & Hanh Pham, T. S. (2013). Measuring Confucian values among East Asian consumers: A four country study. *Asia Pacific Business Review, 19*(3), 320–336.
Mwilambwe-Tshilobo, L., Ge, T., Chong, M., Ferguson, M. A., Misic, B., Burrow, A. L., . . . Spreng, R. N. (2019). Loneliness and meaning in life are reflected in the intrinsic network architecture of the brain. *Social Cognitive and Affective Neuroscience, 14,* 423–433.
Naaman, M., Boase, J., & Lai, C. H. (2010). Is it really about me?: Message content in social awareness streams. *Proceedings of the 2010 ACM Conference on Computer Supported Cooperative Work*, pp. 189–192.
Norenzayan, A. (2013). *Big gods: How religion transformed cooperation and conflict.* Princeton University Press.
Nunn, N., & Wantchekon, L. (2011). The slave trade and the origins of mistrust in Africa. *American Economic Review, 101,* 3221–3252.
Oishi, S., & Diener, E. (2014). Residents of poor nations have a greater sense of meaning in life than residents of wealthy nations. *Psychological Science, 25*(2), 422–430.
Oishi, S., & Westgate, E. C. (2022). A psychologically rich life: Beyond happiness and meaning. *Psychological Review, 129*(4), 790–811.
Ostafin, B. D., & Proulx, T. (2020). Meaning in life and resilience to stressors. *Anxiety, Stress and Coping, 33,* 603–622.
Ou, C., Lou, N. M., Maheshka, C., Shi, M., Takemura, K., Cheung, B. Y., . . . Heine, S. J. (2025). Healthy sleep durations appear to vary across cultures. *Proceedings of the National Academy of Sciences, 122*(19), e2419269122.
Oyserman, D., Coon, H. M., & Kemmelmeier, M. (2002). Rethinking individualism and col-

lectivism: Evaluation of theoretical assumptions and meta-analyses. *Psychological Bulletin, 128*(1), 3–72.

Park, C. L. (2005). Religion as a meaning-making framework in coping with life stress. *Journal of Social Issues, 61,* 707–729.

Park, C. L. (2010). Making sense of the meaning literature: An integrative review of meaning making and its effects on adjustment to stressful life events. *Psychological Bulletin, 136,* 257–301.

Park, C. L., & Edmondson, D. (2012). Religion as a source of meaning. In P. R. Shaver & M. Mikulincer (Eds.), *Meaning, mortality, and choice: The social psychology of existential concerns* (pp. 145–162). American Psychological Association.

Piaget, J. (1953). *The origin of intelligence in the child.* Routledge & Kegan Paul.

Prinzing, M. M., Sappenfield, C. A., & Fredrickson, B. L. (2023). What makes me matter?: Investigating how and why people feel significant. *Journal of Positive Psychology, 18,* 995–1011.

Prinzing, M., Van Cappellen, P., & Fredrickson, B. L. (2021). More than a momentary blip in the universe?: Investigating the link between religiousness and perceived meaning in life. *Personality and Social Psychology Bulletin.*

Proulx, T., & Heine, S. J. (2008). The case of the transmogrifying experimenter: Reaffirmation of moral schemas following implicit change detection. *Psychological Science, 19,* 1294–1300.

Proulx, T., & Heine, S. J. (2010). The frog in Kierkegaard's beer: Finding meaning in the threat-compensation literature. *Social and Personality Psychology Compass, 4,* 889–905.

Putnam, R. D., Leonardi, R., & Nanetti, R. Y. (1993). *Making democracy work.* Princeton University Press.

Randles, D., Heine, S. J., Poulin, M., & Cohen-Silver, R. (2017). Experienced adversity in life is associated with polarized and affirmed political attitudes. *Social Psychological and Personality Science, 8,* 652–659.

Randles, D., Inzlicht, M., Proulx, T., Tullett., A., & Heine, S. J. (2015). Is dissonance reduction a special case of fluid compensation?: Evidence that dissonant cognitions cause compensatory affirmation and abstraction. *Journal of Personality and Social Psychology, 108,* 697–710.

Ricart-Huguet, J., & Paluck, E. L. (2023). When the sorting hat sorts randomly: A natural experiment on culture. *Quarterly Journal of Political Science, 18,* 39–73.

Richerson, P. J., & Boyd, R. (2005). *Not by genes alone.* University of Chicago Press.

Routledge, C., Arndt, J., Wildschut, T., Sedikides, C., Hart, C. M., Juhl, J., . . . Schlotz, W. (2011). The past makes the present meaningful: Nostalgia as an existential resource. *Journal of Personality and Social Psychology, 101,* 638–652.

Russo-Netzer, P., Niemiec, R. M., & Tarrasch, R. (2023). Developmental, genderial and cross-cultural aspects of meaning. *Journal of Happiness Studies.*

Ryff, C. D. (1989). Happiness is everything, or is it?: Explorations on the meaning of psychological well-being. *Journal of Personality and Social Psychology, 57,* 1069–1081.

Santos, H. C., Varnum, M. E. W., & Grossmann, I. (2017). Global increases in individualism. *Psychological Science, 28,* 1228–1239.

Sartre, J.-P. (2003). *Existentialism is a humanism.* Yale University Press. (Original work published 1947)

Schutte, L., Brdar, I., Wissing, M. P., Tončić, M., Araujo, U., Carlquist, E., . . . Delle Fave, A. (2023). Measurement invariance of the meaning in life questionnaire across 17 countries. *Applied Research in Quality of Life, 18*(3), 1491–1519.

Sedikides, C., Cheung, W. Y., Wildschut, T., Hepper, E. G., Baldursson, E., & Pedersen, B. (2018). Nostalgia motivates pursuit of important goals by increasing meaning in life. *European Journal of Social Psychology, 48,* 209–216.

Sedikides, C., & Wildschut, T. (2018). Finding meaning in nostalgia. *Review of General Psychology, 22,* 48–61.

Sherif, M. (1937). An experimental approach to the study of attitudes. *Sociometry, 1,* 90–98.

Shim, B., Barroso, J., Gillis, C. L., & Davis, L. L. (2013). Finding meaning in caring for a spouse with dementia. *Applied Nursing Research, 26,* 121–126.

Shiota, M. N., Keltner, D., & John, O. P. (2006). Positive emotion dispositions differentially associated with Big Five personality and attachment style. *Journal of Positive Psychology, 1*(2), 61–71.

Shweder, R. A. (1990). Cultural psychology: What is it? In J. W. Stigler, R. A. Shweder, & G. Herdt (Eds.), *Cultural psychology: Essays on comparative human development* (pp. 1–43). Cambridge University Press.

Silver, L., Kessel, P. V., Huang, C., Clancy, L., & Gubbala, S. (2021, November 18). *What makes life meaningful?: Views from 17 advanced economies.* Pew Research Center. www.pewresearch.org/global/2021/11/18/what-makes-life-meaningful-views-from-17-advanced-economies/.

Simon, L., Greenberg, J., & Brehm, J. (1995).

Trivialization: The forgotten mode of dissonance reduction. *Journal of Personality and Social Psychology, 68,* 247–260.

Stavrova, O., & Luhmann, M. (2016). Social connectedness as a source and consequence of meaning in life. *Journal of Positive Psychology, 11,* 470–479.

Steger, M. F. (2012). Experiencing meaning in life: Optimal functioning at the nexus of spirituality, psychopathology, and well-being. In P. T. P. Wong (Ed.), *The human quest for meaning: Theories, research, and applications* (2nd ed., pp. 165–184). Routledge.

Steger, M. F., Frazier, P., Oishi, S., & Kaler, M. (2006). The meaning in life questionnaire: assessing the presence of and search for meaning in life. *Journal of Counseling Psychology, 53*(1), 80.

Steger, M. F., Oishi, S., & Kashdan, T. B. (2009). Meaning in life across the life span: Levels and correlates of meaning in life from emerging adulthood to older adulthood. *Journal of Positive Psychology, 4,* 43–52.

Stephens, N. M., Fryberg, S. A., Markus, H. R., & Hamedani, M. G. (2012). Who explains Hurricane Katrina and the Chilean earthquake as an act of God?: The experience of extreme hardship predicts religious meaning-making. *Journal of Cross-Cultural Psychology, 44*(4), 606–619.

Stroope, S., Draper, S., & Whitehead, A. L. (2013). Images of a loving God and sense of meaning in life. *Social Indicators Research, 111*(1), 25–44.

Talhelm, T., & Dong, X. (2024). People quasi-randomly assigned to farm rice are more collectivistic than people assigned to farm wheat. *Nature Communications, 15,* 1782.

Tamir, D. I., & Mitchell, J. P. (2012). Disclosing information about the self is intrinsically rewarding. *Proceedings of the National Academy of Sciences, 109,* 8038–8043.

Taylor, S. E., & Brown, J. D. (1988). Illusion and well-being: A social psychological perspective on mental health. *Psychological Bulletin, 103,* 193–210.

Tedeschi, R. G., & Calhoun, L. G. (2004) Posttraumatic growth: Conceptual foundations and empirical evidence. *Psychological Inquiry, 15,* 1–18.

Terkel, S. (1997). *Working.* New Press.

Tomasello, M. (2014). The ultra-social animal. *European Journal of Social Psychology, 44,* 187–194.

Tomasello, M., Kruger, A. C., & Ratner, H. H. (1993). Cultural learning. *Behavioral and Brain Sciences, 16,* 495–552.

U.S. Surgeon General. (2023). *Our epidemic of loneliness and isolation: The U.S. Surgeon General's advisory on the healing effects of social connection and community.* www.hhs.gov/sites/default/files/surgeon-general-social-connection-advisory.pdf.

Vail, K. E. III, Arndt, J., & Abdollahi, A. (2012). Exploring the existential function of religion and supernatural agent beliefs among Christians, Muslims, atheists, and agnostics. *Personality and Social Psychology Bulletin, 38,* 1288–1300.

van Tilburg, W. A. P., Igou, E. R., & Sedikides, C. (2013). In search of meaningfulness: Nostalgia as an antidote to boredom. *Emotion, 13,* 450–461.

CHAPTER 35

Metaphor Shapes Existential Cognition

Mark J. Landau, Amy P. Kenny, *and* Young-Ju Ryu

In an essay collection titled *Existential Psychology* (1968), theorist Rollo May shared his hope for a new approach to understanding human beings. At that time, mainstream psychology cast the individual in terms of universal drives and discrete mechanisms. May cautioned that this reductionist approach ignored essential aspects of individuals' experience, such as the insecurities, desires, and conflicts that shape how they make sense of their lives and relate to the world. He called for an existential psychology sensitized to these dynamics, though he worried that many psychologists would reject existential terms as vague and untestable. Were he alive today, he would be gratified to see that existential psychology has matured into a vibrant research area shared among researchers worldwide, many of whom are contributors to this handbook.

Heeding May's call, we start with one of existentialism's central tenets: Individuals are motivated to view themselves as significant members of a meaningful world. Some researchers focus on the "whys" of this motive, such as the distal goal served by meaning in life. We tackle some "how" questions: What makes it generally so difficult to form and maintain confident conceptions of life's meaning and significance? What cognitive processes do people use to overcome this epistemic hurdle and make sense of their lives and human life in general?

Our answer to the first question is that perceiving life as meaningful and significant requires getting a handle on existentially relevant concepts, such as *belonging*, *tragedy*, and *authenticity*, that are inherently abstract and thus difficult to grasp. Our answer to the second question builds on an observation gleaned from cross-disciplinary studies of communication: Across cultural and historical contexts, people communicate about existential concepts *metaphorically* in terms of superficially dissimilar ideas (Forceville & Urios-Aparisi, 2009; Gibbs, 2008; Kövecses, 2005). For example, when talking about the abstract idea of belonging to a larger social entity, such as a political movement or a romantic relationship, an English speaker might say, "I'm *moving toward* socialism these days," while a Korean speaker might say, "애써 그 사람을 그리워하는 마음을 밀어냈다" (translation: "With much effort I *pushed away* my longing for him"). As another example, people worldwide talk about abstract notions of personal agency and responsibility in terms of a tangible object's integrity/fragmentation: "I'm *all over the place*; *falling apart*; I need to *get it together*." However familiar, none of these expressions makes any sense when interpreted in a strict literal sense.

If we zoom out from language to consider other modes of communication, we see metaphors expressed in cultural practices, ceremonies, artwork, and artifacts. To mention just a few examples, across cultures we see people fabricate images and objects depicting *good/evil* as *light/dark* (Eliade, 1996); stage ritual performances that establish physical *boundaries* between the *sacred* (ordered, clean) and the *profane* (disordered, dirty; Douglas, 1966); produce images and pageantry depicting *death* as an anthropomorphized *person* (Guthke, 1999); and represent (e.g., in iconography) the fate of their groups (e.g., the outcome of military campaigns) in terms of *fertility* and regeneration (Stookey, 2004).

Seen through the lens of conceptual metaphor theory (CMT), such metaphoric communications are not merely colorful garnishes on the plate of human nature. Rather, they reflect people's use of metaphor at a cognitive level to think about (and not "just" talk about) an existential concept in terms of another concept—one that is superficially unrelated but relatively more concrete and easier to grasp. This perspective implies that metaphorical thinking is essential to how people understand existential concepts and, as a result, plays an integral role in the diverse existential psychological dynamics discussed in this handbook.

To explore this possibility, we first unpack our assumptions about what existential concepts are and why they are so hard to comprehend. We then summarize CMT and review three empirical strategies that researchers use to experimentally test whether and when people use metaphor to think. With that theoretical and empirical background in place, we circle back to review preliminary evidence that metaphors shape how people understand and relate to three existential concepts: *self-continuity*, *self-esteem*, and *authenticity*. We conclude by discussing avenues for researching metaphors' potential role in other existential concepts.

How does our perspective satisfy Rollo May's call for a mature existential psychology? One way is highlighted by Abraham Maslow, who, in response to May's essay, wrote that existentialism's primary contribution to psychology lies in illuminating "that human predicament presented by the gap between human aspirations and human limitations—between what the human being *is*, what he would *like* to be, and what he *could* be" (1968, p. 54). Toward that end, we aim to demonstrate that appreciating conceptual metaphor's role in existential cognition provides a fresh look at the collision between human aspirations and limitations: Humans are intent on viewing themselves as significant members of a meaningful world, but they are limited in their ability to comprehend abstract concepts related to existence. They overcome this limitation by using an imaginative, uniquely human ability to mentally scaffold existential concepts around superficially dissimilar ideas. As poet Wallace Stevens (1967, p. 179) put it, "Reality is a cliché from which we escape by metaphor."

EXISTENTIAL CONCEPTS AND THE CHALLENGE OF ABSTRACTNESS

As noted earlier, existential theorists generally agree that people are motivated to view themselves as significant members of a meaningful world. Unlike other creatures, humans have the special capacity to step back and survey themselves, and they are constantly reflecting on how they (and other people) are living their lives. Think of the enormous quantities of energy, risk, and intense concern an ordinary person devotes to their health, their public image, their success and failure, and the quality of their relationships. Supporting evidence shows that when people encounter circumstances or entertain thoughts that undermine their confidence in sources of meaning and significance, they feel distressed and take efforts to restore that confidence (Shaver & Mikulincer, 2012).

Some researchers approach this motive by characterizing life's perceived meaning and significance as a global subjective evaluation. From there, they operationalize it as a unidimensional self-report construct, assessing people's agreement with statements like, "I have a good sense of what makes my life meaningful" (Steger et al., 2006). We take a complementary approach, proposing that an individual's global picture of life's meaning and significance is based on several *existential concepts*, which we define as concepts related to the "big" questions about existence. In contrast to mundane concepts like *lawn care* and *student credit hours*, existential concepts are central to most people's efforts to define their personal and collective identity; explore and explain the nature of the physical environment, the mysteries of creation, death, and the afterlife; imbue their sense of reality with order and permanence; and reproduce shared conceptions of life's significance within history, society, and the cosmos. Here are some existential concepts highlighted in classic existential theorizing and throughout the current handbook:

- *Human specialness/creatureliness*: As a human, am I special in some way that sets me apart from the countless critters out there?
- *Self-continuity*: Do the separate parts of my life—my personal history, current actions, and envisioned future—fit into a coherent whole?
- *Connection/isolation*: Do I belong to something bigger than myself, or am I essentially on my own?
- *Self-esteem*: Am I a good person? Do I have esteemed qualities? Am I doing enough?
- *Purpose/pointlessness*: Are my day-to-day experiences oriented toward some worthwhile end that I'm making progress toward, or are they pointless?
- *Desire*: What do I want? Why am I never satisfied for long with what I have?
- *Truth/relativism*: Is there one correct way to view the world and lead one's life, or does truth depend on the person?
- *Fairness* and *tragedy*: Do I inhabit a world where good people get ahead while bad people are punished?
- *Authenticity*: Is there a "real" me that is different from the person that I present to others? Am I faking it?
- *Agency* and *responsibility*: Am I in control of my thoughts, emotions, and actions? Am I acting in accordance with my beliefs and values?
- *Time*: What is "my" time as opposed to time that's out of my control? How should I best use my time?
- *Divinity* and *spirituality*: Are there agents, forces, or dimensions that operate outside of my everyday awareness? Can I engage with them?

In their quest to view their lives as globally meaningful and significant, individuals need to form and maintain a subjectively confident understanding of these (and other) existential concepts. They need a clear mental image of what makes them special, what it means to belong, how to negotiate their public image, how to ensure a lasting personal legacy beyond death, and so on.

Our next theoretical assumption is so baked into existential scholarship that researchers rarely bother to spell it out: Understanding existential concepts is *hard*. For most people, these concepts do not present themselves in any direct, self-evident way. Instead, confident understanding is something that one must actively find or create and is under constant assault from intimations of life's meaningless (Flanagan, 2009; Shaver & Mikulincer, 2012). Even the intellectual elite struggle to comprehend these concepts. Pick any concept from the list above—or others like *happiness* and *anxiety*—and you'll find thousands of scholarly analyses wrestling with its exact meaning.

What makes existential concepts so difficult to get a handle on? Although many factors likely play a role, we propose that the challenge is largely due to these concepts' inherent abstractness. Such abstractness results when thinking about entities, forces, and relations that cannot be directly observed, and which seem removed from the practical realities of daily life (Trope & Liberman, 2010). To illustrate this abstractness, consider Riley's struggle with *self-continuity*. Riley stands to form a confident understanding of self-continuity by appreciating how events from her past summer (e.g., the lake trip that started out awesome but ended in a terminated friendship) reflect the person she used to be, and how they set the stage for the person she is becoming. But this requires that she create causal links between events and identities separated in time—links that are not clearly determined and may seem arbitrary. Riley could also view experiences separated in time as cohering around a self-defining trait or a recurring theme (e.g., loyalty), but because the mental images thus formed are not present to the senses, she may be unsure whether they are based in reality or her imagination.

There is plenty of evidence that abstractness interferes with confident understanding. People have lower confidence in abstract causal relations compared to relatively more concrete relations in which causes have directly observable and immediate consequences (Michotte, 1946/1963). They also struggle to understand and remember messages expressed in abstract language that prevents them from forming vivid mental images (Kosslyn et al., 2006).

The question then becomes: How do people manage this abstractness to get a firm(er) grasp on existential concepts? One answer is provided by CMT. The next section takes a detour from existential concepts to unpack this theory and the research it has inspired.

CMT AND RESEARCH

As far back as Aristotle, *metaphor* is traditionally defined as a figure of speech that uses a term for one thing to describe another. The thing is called the metaphor's *target* and the "something else" is the metaphor's *source*. For example, in the sentence "We need to scrub the internet clean of all this pornographic filth," we see two linked metaphors: one compares explicit content (target) to physical dirt (source); the other compares censorship (target) to cleansing (source).

Prominent philosophers like Hobbes and Locke backed this traditional definition and treated metaphor as a colorful but essentially useless (and even deceptive) embellishment to "normal" language. But even Aristotle suspected that metaphor is about more than words. He said, "it is from metaphor that we can best get hold of something fresh" (ca. 330 B.C.E.; trans. 1924; 1.1410). Going further, theorists outside philosophy's mainstream claimed that metaphor profoundly shapes how individuals and cultures experience reality, not just how they talk. Nietzsche, Julian Jaynes, Susanne Langer, and others claimed that people *think* they have a direct grasp of abstractions like *time*, *truth*, *causation*, *emotion*, and *divinity*, but they're actually grounding these concepts in sensorimotor experiences (e.g., putting objects in containers), stereotyped knowledge of the natural world (e.g., plant growth; meteorological events), or schemas for cultural products and activities (e.g., building construction; marketplace transactions).

Building on these early views, linguists Lakoff and Johnson (1980) explained how metaphorical thinking operates at a process level. In what has come to be known as CMT, they said that metaphor creates a *conceptual mapping*, defined as a set of systematic associations between bits of knowledge about a target (e.g., its salient features, causal relations) and analogous bits of knowledge about a source. By accessing this mapping, people can draw on their source knowledge as a template or framework to think about a target, even though the two concepts are unrelated on the surface (Kövecses, 2010, provides a more thorough introduction).

To illustrate, imagine your friend Claire says, "I've *come a long way* in my academic career. I'm *on the right path* now, and I'm *going places*. I appreciate you *moving me* in the right *direction*." Claire's career is not a trip or a journey in any literal sense, so why does she talk this way? Perhaps she's simply using clichéd expressions that reveal nothing interesting about her cognition. CMT offers a more provocative answer: Claire struggles to form a mental image that ties together career-defining events and identities from her past, present, and anticipated future. She compensates by using metaphor to mentally map those abstract ideas onto analogous bits of knowledge about goal-directed motion along a path—knowledge that she acquired over years of routine bodily activity. This mapping, depicted in Figure 35.1, enables Claire to represent herself as a *traveler* and her career goal as an intended *destination*. She can identify her career's *starting point* and evaluate events and people as creating *obstacles* or moving her *forward*. She can easily visualize *branching paths* and use that image to decide what the priorities among her various aims should be. Moreover, Claire can perform this mapping while plopped in her La-Z-Boy recliner—more precisely, without her concurrently experiencing a bodily state associated with traveling. That's because she's mentally borrowing a well-structured schema to scaffold her target understanding.

A few points about this mapping process: It is *partial*, meaning that not every bit of target and source knowledge participates. Claire knows many things about journeys (e.g., airport security line etiquette) that she's not using to visualize her career. Mapping is also *selective*, meaning that mapping a target onto different sources will highlight and downplay different sets of target knowl-

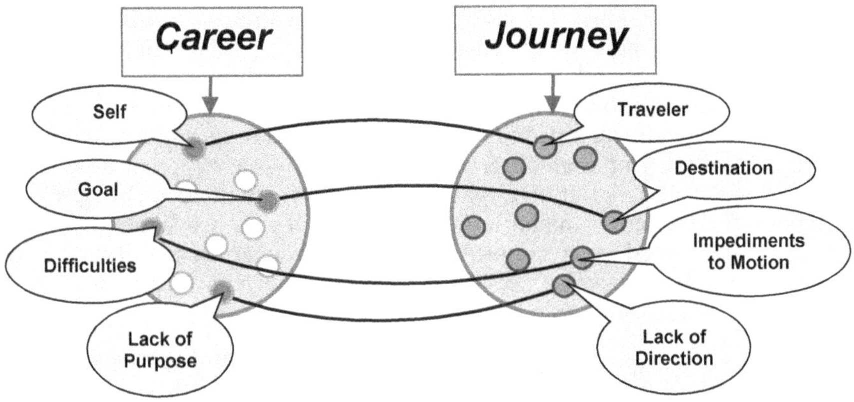

FIGURE 35.1. Thinking about a professional career metaphorically as a physical journey creates a mapping between analogous elements of the two concepts.

edge, which in turn changes how people interpret, evaluate, and act with relation to the target. To illustrate, if Claire believes that journeys are more pleasant with travel companions than alone, then mapping her career onto a journey will prompt her to infer that a satisfying career requires strong connections with co-workers. If, alternatively, she mapped her career onto her schema for *military combat*, she would be more likely to infer, for example, that reaching her career goals requires competition and endurance of suffering.

A third point is that metaphor use is an *intermediary step* to understanding abstract targets. People think using metaphor because they have difficulty comprehending a target as a whole or some significant aspects of it. And yet, for the target to participate in a metaphor's mapping, it needs some degree of structural delineation. For Claire to access a *career is a journey* mapping, she first needs to identify her career's salient parts (e.g., goals, decisions). Otherwise, there would be nothing to map onto analogous elements of a journey. Nevertheless, Claire still feels that something about her career is vague or elusive, and the metaphor offers a coherent mental image.

CMT presents a provocative view of how people understand abstractions, but is it true? Some evidence comes from linguistic analyses (Gibbs, 2008; Kövecses, 2010). The big finding is that conventional metaphoric linguistic expressions "cluster" in ways that would be expected if they reflected an underlying mapping, and that would be unlikely if each expression were an isolated cliché. For example, by positing that people map *ideas* onto *food*, linguists can explain why various expressions about ideas correspond to common knowledge about food: You *devour* a book, *chew on* its ideas, and *regurgitate* those ideas when asked; some ideas may be *half-baked* and hard to *digest* or *swallow*. Positing a mapping also explains why people effortlessly understand expressions they've never heard but that correspond analogously to their source knowledge (e.g., "For years I *shoved my face* with postmodernism").

Linguistic evidence also comes from cross-cultural analyses that reveal remarkable parallels across languages in the particular linguistic metaphors that people use to talk about the same target (Kövecses, 2005). Whether you're looking at English, Hungarian, Zulu, Wolof, Japanese, or Tunisian Arabic, you'll hear people talk about *happiness* as *up* ("*lift* my spirits"); *understanding* as *seeing* ("*shed some light* on this issue because I'm *in the dark*"); *importance* as *size* ("this album's way *bigger* than their last"); *intensity* as *heat* ("the competition is *heating up*"); *intimacy* as *closeness* ("why do I feel a *distance* between us?"), and *social systems* as *buildings* ("their marriage is *falling into ruins*"). If metaphoric linguistic expressions were merely isolated, arbitrary figures of speech, then we wouldn't expect these cross-cultural similarities.

Although intriguing, it must be recognized that these lines of linguistic evidence are indirect, impressionistic, and unconvincing to some researchers. No one denies that metaphoric expressions cluster into culturally widespread families, but that observation alone cannot dispel a deflationary alternative explanation: Even if metaphoric expressions were motivated by a cognitive mapping *at some point in time*, people today employ those expressions as a matter of convention without necessarily accessing some underlying cognitive mapping between target and source. To overcome this limitation, researchers in social psychology have in recent years developed empirical strategies that can be used to experimentally test metaphoric influences on social-cognitive processes (Landau, 2017).

Metaphoric Transfer Strategy

Researchers reasoned that if people understand a target by mapping it on a source, as CMT claims, then manipulating their experience of that source should transfer across that mapping and produce analogous changes in target processing. If, instead, there was no mapping shaping target understanding, then there would be no reason to expect such effects, because people's representations of the target would not be systematically structured around the source.

Many studies using this strategy show that manipulating source experiences (e.g., sensations, movements, proprioceptive states) changes how people process (e.g., reason about, evaluate, remember) a target in directions suggested by the linguistic metaphors linking those concepts, even in contexts where metaphoric language is not made salient. For example, consistent with linguistic metaphors linking importance to physical weight ("that's a *heavy* topic"; "*lighten* up"), studies show that holding a heavy versus light object (e.g., a 2.29-pound clipboard vs. a 1.45-pound clipboard) increases judgments of importance. This effect holds for judgments of community issues (Jostmann et al., 2009; Zestcott et al., 2017), a job applicant's seriousness (Ackerman et al., 2010), the severity of a disease (Kaspar, 2013), and a book's literary significance (Chandler et al., 2012).

The metaphoric transfer strategy presupposes that the mapping of interest is chronically accessible—always there, on the periphery of consciousness. That is why we expect that experimentally induced variations in source experience will transfer over to produce analogous changes in target processing. There are likely to be other cases, though, where the situation determines whether a given mapping is accessible.

Metaphoric Framing Strategy

In these cases, researchers can experimentally prime a mapping. The most common way this priming has been operationalized is exposing participants to a *metaphoric framing*—a message that uses language or imagery to compare a target and a source. Participants in comparison conditions receive an equivalent message framing the same target in literal terms or comparing it to an alternative source. Participants are then assessed on their attitudes toward aspects of the target that were not explicitly mentioned in the metaphoric framing but are theorized to participate in the mapping of interest. If exposure to a metaphoric framing primes a mapping, then it should prompt recipients to interpret those unmentioned aspects of the target in ways that correspond to their source knowledge, even if they are not consciously aware of thinking by analogy to the source.

In one illustrative study (Morris et al., 2007), participants read commentaries that compared trends in the stock market to either living agents (e.g., "This afternoon the Nasdaq starting *climbing* upward") or inanimate objects (e.g., "This afternoon the Nasdaq was *swept* upward"; emphasis added). Next, participants were asked to predict what would happen to those trends the following day. People generally know that living agents, unlike inanimate objects, move with the intention of reaching destinations. Thus, we can predict that people exposed to agent-metaphoric framing will transfer this knowledge and infer that the price trends will continue along their current trajectories. This is exactly what was found, suggesting that metaphoric framing exposure primed a mapping that led recipients to interpret its target in ways that correspond to its source. Other studies (reviewed in Landau, 2017) show that metaphoric framing exposure produces source-consistent effects on target problem solving, attribution, decision making, and memory, to name just a few processes studied.

Is incidental exposure to metaphoric framing always sufficient to prompt a mapping between disparate concepts? Probably not. Insight into moderating factors comes from CMT's functional analysis of metaphorical thinking.

Target Certainty Strategy

From a CMT perspective, metaphors do not just sit there; instead, they support a sense of confident target understanding. That analysis creates a direct line with social psychological perspectives on the motivation for certain knowledge. Among the most influential of these is Kruglanksi's (2004) lay epistemology theory, which posits a need for "nonspecific closure"—a motive to seize on the first available judgment or decision without extensive effort to minimize unpleasant feelings of uncertainty. When this motive is high (e.g., in response to salient uncertainty), people do not have a strong preference for one interpretation over another; instead, they desire a simple, concrete understanding regardless of the specific conclusions they reach.

Integrating these theoretical insights suggests another strategy for testing metaphoric influences: Researchers can cross metaphoric framing exposure (or any other operationalization of metaphor activation) with experimental manipulations of subjective target certainty. They can use situational inductions designed to get people to perceive a target to be unfamiliar, abstract, complex, unstable, or obscure. The resulting desire to restore a sense of understanding will increase the appeal of a provided metaphoric framing that compares that target to sources perceived as familiar, concrete, simple, consistent, or discernable. This should make them more reliant on source knowledge as a framework for interpreting the target. Those who are instead situationally induced to feel certain in their target understanding will be less likely to seize on a provided metaphor.

Jia and Smith (2013) tested this interaction hypothesis, building on evidence that people construe ideas in a more abstract manner when those ideas are psychologically distant—that is, removed from the immediate experience of the self in the here and now (Trope & Liberman, 2010). They reasoned that increasing a target's psychological distance, and hence perceived abstractness, would encourage greater reliance on a provided metaphoric framing to interpret that target. Replicating Morris and colleagues (2007), they showed that when participants read commentaries framing the stock market as an autonomous agent (vs. an alternate framing), their market forecasts were higher for days that showed an upward trend. Participants seem to have inferred that price trends would continue along their current trajectory in a manner that is analogous to the way that intentional agents move deliberately toward destinations. However, this effect held only for participants previously primed to construe the stock market as remote and hence abstract. The same agent-metaphoric framing was inert when the stock market was made to seem near and hence concrete.

Researchers are beginning to apply these empirical strategies to examine metaphor's potential role in existential concepts. Empirical attention has thus far focused on three basic aspects of the self: self-continuity, self-esteem, and authenticity. We review representative studies in the following sections and return in the Conclusion to the potential relevance of a metaphor-enriched perspective for studying how people make sense of other existential concepts.

SELF-CONTINUITY

"In the end, each life is no more than the sum of contingent facts, a chronicle of chance intersections, of flukes, of random events that divulge nothing but their own lack of purpose" (Auster, 1990, p. 256). Novelist Paul Auster contended that if a person were to scrutinize their experience and see the transient states of consciousness for what they are, they would not find anything that persists over time and defines their identity.

But that's not how most people want to view themselves or their lives. As adolescents they're preoccupied with envisioning future identities; in midlife they ponder alternative lifestyles; and in old age they review their personal history for patterns (Butler, 1963; Erikson, 1968). These strivings toward self-continuity, or a coherent sense of self-in-time, are not in vain: Dispositionally high and experimentally increased self-continuity predict stronger meaning in life (Sani, 2008).

When people think about self-continuity, what does it look like in their mind's eye? One clue comes from how they talk about it. They compare it to various things that it is not: a *story*, a *game*, a *fabric*, and so on. But by far the most common source is a *journey*. Lakoff and Johnson's (1980) influential analysis of journey-metaphoric expressions led many researchers to hypothesize that people (unconsciously) borrow knowledge about the physical act of traveling along bounded paths toward destinations to construe the otherwise abstract relations between activities, events, and identities separated in time.

Inspired by these linguistic analyses, Keefer and colleagues (2011) used the target certainty strategy to test whether people employ a provided journey metaphor to interpret their lives, and whether this effect holds particularly when they desire a confident understanding of themselves (i.e., when the need for nonspecific closure is high). They randomized participants to think about self-relevant uncertainty or pain experiences (an aversive topic for comparison with uncertainty). Half were then induced to visualize separate events from their past as locations along a physical path, while the other participants organized past events without a provided metaphor. All participants then evaluated how influential their past was in shaping the person they are today. Compared to participants in the other conditions, those made uncertain about themselves and exposed to a journey-metaphoric framing of past events viewed their past as especially formative of their current identity (Figure 35.2).

In addition to connecting past and present, a journey metaphor can reinforce continuity between one's current identity and a possible future identity. Landau and colleagues (2014) had college freshmen jot down a few words to imagine themselves in the future as an academically accomplished graduate.

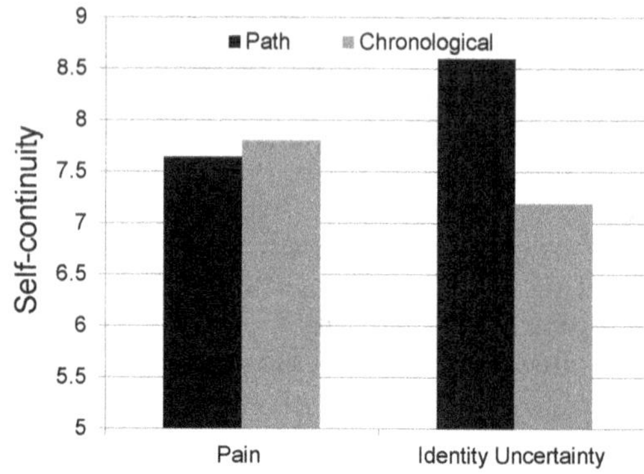

FIGURE 35.2. Framing past events as steps in a journey bolstered continuity between personal history and current identity, but only when participants felt uncertain about who they are (Keefer et al., 2011).

The rest of the page displayed an image of a path extending forward from their vantage and labeled progressively with the four undergrad years. In one comparison condition, freshmen likewise wrote about their future academic identity, but the rest of the page was blank. In a second comparison condition, they saw the same journey image but described themselves as achieving great social status in their graduating year. In this way, the researchers tested the unique effect of activating an academic future identity and a journey metaphor in conjunction. Participants primed with a journey-metaphoric framing of their academic future identity perceived a stronger connection between their current self and the academic superstar they imagined being in the future.

How exactly does a journey metaphor tie together the present and future? Theoretically, exposure to journey-metaphoric framing prompts people to draw on their knowledge of journeys, even if they are not consciously aware of doing so. And one thing people likely know from their bodily experience is that, when they move forward along a path toward a destination, the visible stretch of path in front of them affords a clear procedure, or sequence of steps, that they take to move from here (current location) to there (destination). Using that knowledge as a scaffold, people can visualize how their current goal-directed efforts (metaphorically, the steps taken now) fit into a sequence of actions necessary to attain a possible future identity—even though none of these ideas occupy physical space in any literal sense.

Based on this analysis, Landau and colleagues (2014) hypothesized that priming a journey metaphor would strengthen current–future identity connection by boosting confidence that one knows the procedure for realizing a future identity. They asked all of the college freshmen in their sample to imagine their academic possible identity as a destination ahead of them. Half were then guided through a visualization induction portraying them as an avatar walking forward over labeled stretches of college's road toward that destination (top image sequence [A], Figure 35.3). The others were induced to visualize themselves as passengers riding a vehicle moving along college's road toward that destination (lower image sequence [B], Figure 35.3). In this latter "vehicle" variant of the journey metaphor, the traveler is passively carried along following a predetermined route. This implies that the traveler reaches their destination without being aware of how current activities fit into a procedure for getting there. They simply arrive.

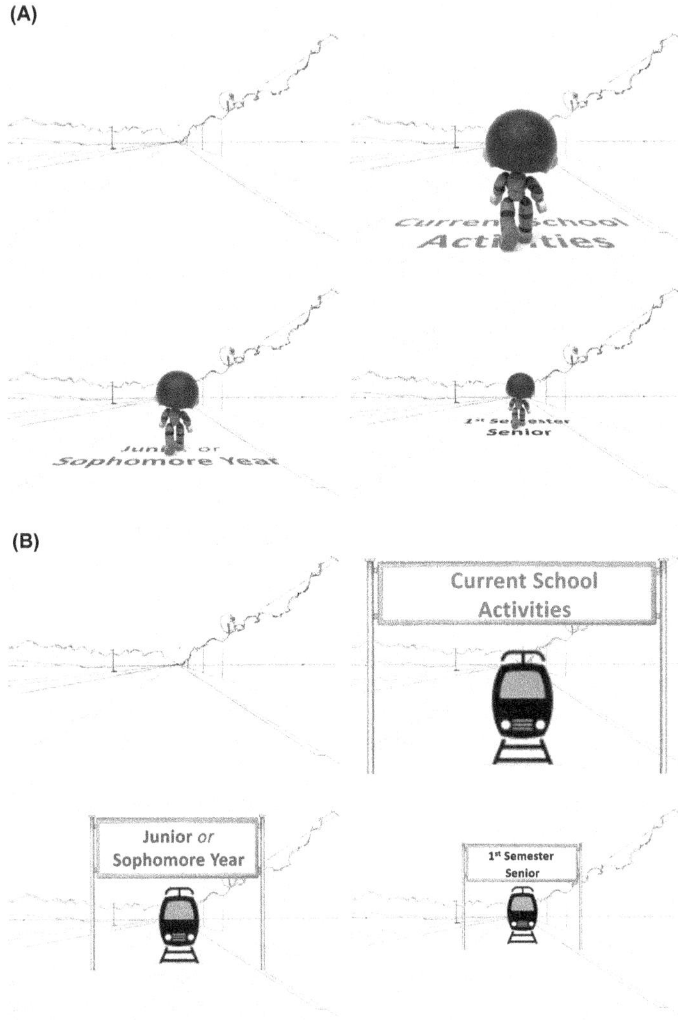

FIGURE 35.3. Visualization induction used to manipulate active versus passive journey metaphor salience (Landau et al., 2014).

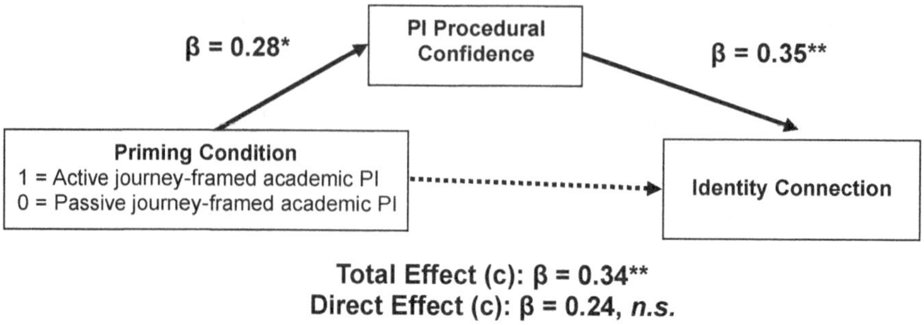

FIGURE 35.4. A possible identity (PI) framed metaphorically as an active (vs. passive) journey felt more connected to a current identity by means of bolstering confidence that current activities fit into a procedure for realizing that future goal (Landau et al., 2014).

As predicted, participants who visualized actively (vs. passively) moving along a path toward a possible identity reported feeling stronger procedural confidence—put simply, they appreciated that their academic activities in the present (e.g., an hour of flash cards this afternoon) determine whether or not they attain long-term academic goals. This procedural confidence in turn predicted a stronger perceived connection between their current identity and possible academic identity (Figure 35.4). These findings suggest that a salient journey metaphor bolsters self-continuity by calling up a concrete schema for goal-directed motion along a path, which helps one visualize how current actions fit into a procedure by which the self changes over time.

More work is clearly needed to test whether other metaphors help people create and maintain a continuous sense of identity over time. If we look at how people talk about life, an obvious candidate for future work is the metaphor of a self-narrative, or life story, which casts the self as the main character in a unique and interesting drama complete with chapters, plot twists, conflicts, and their resolutions (McAdams, 2001).

SELF-ESTEEM

Theorists working across existential and humanistic traditions, such as Ernest Becker, Rollo May, and Carl Rogers, emphasized that a confident sense of personal value, or self-esteem, is integral for viewing life as globally meaningful and significant. Accordingly, research described elsewhere in this handbook points to self-esteem's importance in various existential psychological phenomena. The question we pose is: How do people represent self-esteem at a basic cognitive level? Because *value* is an abstract concept, people may struggle to form a clear mental image of what self-esteem is, how to attain it, and whether they have "enough."

We propose that they compensate for this abstractness by conceptualizing self-esteem metaphorically in terms of concrete ideas. Observations of ordinary language strongly suggest this is the case, as people everywhere describe their own and other's value in terms like *hard/soft*, *firm/flakey*, *clean/dirty*, *solid/fragile*, *well balanced*, *warm/cool/cold*, and *big/small* (Kövecses, 2010). As we've discussed, however, analyses of language provide only indirect tests of metaphor's role in thought. Researchers are therefore examining self-esteem metaphors using the empirical strategies reviewed earlier.

Some research focuses on the metaphor *good is up/bad is down*. This metaphor is so common in language that it can appear literal. People talk of being in *high* spirits; at the *top* of their game; *climbing* the corporate *ladder* (before *hitting the glass ceiling*); *shooting up* in status like a *rising star*; feeling *down*; *falling* from grace; and *sinking into* a *depression*. Depending on a group's *upward* mobility, they're considered *high*, *middle*, or *low* class. Individuals diagnosed with major depressive disorder customarily describe their self-esteem issues in *up/down* terms (McMullen & Conway, 2002). Social psychologists similarly use terms like *upward/downward* social comparison.

The *up/down* metaphor also pervades cultural products and practices intended to communicate value-related ideas like power and morality. To mention just a few examples, the caste system in Nepal codifies an institutional arrangement of value along a vertical dimension, starting at the bottom with the nobodies and ascending up to social, political, or economic elite; *tree of life* models, which dominated biology in its early days and continue to guide thinking to this day (Gould, 1994), depict humankind as the supreme fruit of creation, not an evolutionary accident; and Olympic medal ceremonies use podiums of varying heights to express accomplishment.

Inspired by these patterns in communication, researchers have used the metaphoric transfer strategy to experimentally test the effects of perceptual and motoric verticality cues on value judgments (Landau, 2017). Studies show, for example, that increasing the vertical, but not the horizontal, distance between pictorial representations of a manager and subordinates led participants to view the manager as more powerful (Giessner & Schubert, 2007; Lakens et al., 2011). Examining potential effects on memory, Casasanto and Dijkstra (2010) presented participants with open-ended prompts like "recall something that happened yesterday." Meanwhile, in an ostensibly unrelated task, participants moved marbles upward or downward. Simply performing upward motions prompted them to bring to mind self-enhancing memories.

Related studies by Keefer and colleagues (2011) used the target certainty strategy to test the hypothesis that up/down cues affect self-relevant evaluations particularly when people feel uncertain about personal value. They asked college freshmen to write about one of three topics: uncertainties about the value of their college experience, physical pain, or mundane experiences shelving books. Participants were then asked to think back to their decision to attend their current university rather than another college or university. They were handed a worksheet with six vertically arranged lines and asked to list the factors behind that decision in an upward or downward orientation. Specifically, those in the "up" condition summarized the earliest factor on the bottom line, a subsequent factor on the next line up, and so forth, with the most recent factor at the top. Their "down" counterparts listed their decision factors downward from the earliest (top line) to the most recent (bottom line). Finally, participants were asked how satisfied they were with their decision. Arranging decision factors on a vertical axis influenced decision satisfaction in line with the linguistic metaphor *good is up/bad is down*, but only when target uncertainty was high (Figure 35.5). As important, participants not made uncertain about college's value did not rely on the up/down cues to inform their judgment. These findings suggest metaphor is not a built-in feature of our cognition, but rather a tool that comes in handy for giving structure to vague ideas.

Other lines of research focus on metaphoric construal of personal value as a number. People commonly describe abstractions metaphorically as though they were numbers. For example, government officials attempt to legitimize military aggression by comparing enemy casualties to points in a game (Lakoff, 1992). People similarly talk about ideas related to personal value in terms of scores along metrics: professional worth is salary; scientific impact is number of publications; sexual prowess is number of partners; physi-

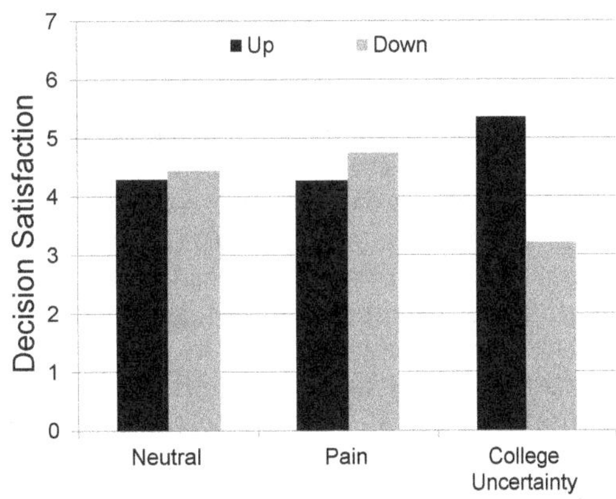

FIGURE 35.5. Priming *up/down* affected satisfaction with one's university choice only when uncertainties about college were salient (Keefer et al., 2011).

cal fitness is number of "steps"; and philanthropy is years spent volunteering or dollars donated.

Unlike such quantitative representations, qualitative representations are malleable, meaning that the person can shift their definitions and standards to view themselves in a positive light (e.g., a "good" friend always has your side *or* tells it like it is). So, why would people prefer to equate their value to a rigid number? One answer is that quantitative information is generally perceived to be certain and precise (von Winterfeldt & Edwards, 1986). This finding led Rothschild and colleagues (2011) to hypothesize that people would seize on quantitative (over qualitative) self-esteem representations when they are motivated to maintain *certain* knowledge of their value, independent of their motivation to increase their self-esteem *level.*

The researchers asked participants to complete a card-matching task purported to assess their visual intelligence. In one condition, the task had unclear performance contingencies. That means that, based on immediate performance feedback, participants couldn't tell how much success and failure outcomes reflected their ability or some external factor, such as luck. In an ostensibly unrelated part of the study, they were presented with two indices of their verbal intelligence. The indices were equally flattering, but one represented their intelligence as a number, the other in qualitative terms. How did participants feel about them?

Participants exposed to unclear (versus clear) performance contingencies experienced a drop in their global self-esteem certainty (but not level), and they compensated by identifying with the quantitative index of their value on the second task. Furthermore, this effect was specific to participants with a high dispositional desire for well-structured knowledge—those known to respond to uncertainty-arousing situations with compensatory efforts to restore certainty. Metaphor can help people get some purchase on the notion of personal value, independent of its utility for increasing one's level of self-esteem.

Related lines of research examine how sources of self-esteem are grounded in superficially dissimilar concepts. For example, self-esteem is for many people contingent on one's sense of social support, and research reveals a metaphoric connection between felt social support and the concepts *warm/cold* (IJzerman & Semin, 2009). Other studies examine the metaphoric link between value and physical cleanliness, showing, for example, that the act of cleaning allayed people's worries about the value of their major decisions (Lee et al., 2024).

In addition to studying the metaphors used to construe value itself, researchers have begun studying how metaphor use serves to compensate for threats to self-esteem. Sullivan and colleagues (2014) built on Erving Goffman's depiction of everyday social life as a stage play—what is often called the *dramaturgical perspective.* In this metaphor, people are *actors* who adopt shifting *roles* when sharing different *stages* with rotating sets of other *characters*, and they emerge from *backstage* in *costume* to enact their *performances* in the hope of gaining *applause.*

Sullivan and colleagues proposed that people would be motivated to embrace this metaphor when they feel they are somehow falling short of standards of value. Viewing life as an elaborate stage play may be desirable because it allows them to discount *all* social roles and activities as theatrical constructions. Put another way, people may experience feelings of inadequacy in a variety of different areas—in the workplace, in their knowledge of art and culture, in their physical appearance, and so on. To defend their sense of personal adequacy in *any* of these domains, they may adopt the *theater* metaphor, reassuring themselves that life is just one big theatrical production and one's performance in a given role does not indicate the self's ultimate value. One is simply crafting an identity by trying on roles and masks.

Supporting studies show that college students told they were performing poorly in school endorsed an essay expressing the *theater* metaphor, but not an essay trivializing the value of the student role, suggesting that understanding life as a play is distinct from trivializing a threatened role. Another study showed that exposure to this metaphor (vs. a nonmetaphoric description of life) buffered participants from a threat to their self-esteem. By interpreting life through a theatrical metaphor, viewing all social roles as essentially artificial dramatic performances, people can brush off threats to their performance in any given role or domain.

AUTHENTICITY

Our discussion of "masks" points to people's broader existential concern with when and how to express their "true" or authentic self. For instance, individuals might struggle to find a career path that balances their genuine interests and talents with other people's expectations and standards for success, or they might feel pressure to conceal their authentic attitudes when they suspect that others will judge them harshly. From these experiences, people form an *intrinsic self-concept*—an understanding of who they truly are that is not conditioned by or dependent upon social approval. The more people feel they are expressing their intrinsic self-concept, the more they feel that life is meaningful and satisfying (Schlegel et al., 2009; Sedikides et al., 2017).

Despite its implications for a sense of existential significance, the intrinsic self-concept is one of the less easily definable aspects of the self. How do people wrap their head around it? They conventionally *talk* about it metaphorically as a core-like physical entity lodged inside of an external casing or shell: "I *found* who I am *deep down*, beneath the *surface*." The inner core stands for their "essence," while the external layer corresponds to the extrinsic self that they assume in society, and which is not always consistent with the true self.

Speakers of diverse languages extend this *entity* metaphor to describe the enhanced expression of their intrinsic self in terms of their inner core expanding or emerging. Students in the United States and Switzerland describe self-development, but not other self-aspects, with expressions like "I am *growing* inside" and "My true self is really *coming out*" (Moser, 2007). In Japanese, intrinsic self-expression is likened to entity emergence, as in the expression "Kare-wa mettani hontōno jibun-o dasa-na-i," which translates as "He rarely *puts out* (his) real self" (Lakoff & Johnson, 1999, p. 286). These expressions reflect a picture in which a person's private, truthful self—called *hone*—is situated internally in the stomach area (*hara*), whereas *tatemae* is the external face one puts on when the situation demands that one "hide" the innermost self and conform to social standards of conduct. Existentially oriented theorists like Carl Rogers similarly characterized the intrinsic self metaphorically as an "inner core" that expands (under facilitating conditions) to express its true nature and responds to social threats by seeking shelter behind external "facades."

Of course, these expressions are senseless when interpreted literally. There is no core lodged in your body that bursts forth like the creature in the movie *Alien*. Are they simply figures of speech? Perhaps, but a more interesting possibility is that they offer a window into how people represent intrinsic self-expression. People know that many physical objects increase in strength and influence as they expand in size. By means of metaphor, they can apply that knowledge to conceptualize the enhanced influence of their intrinsic self in terms of entity expansion. This leads to a testable hypothesis: Priming individuals with the expansion of a physical entity will facilitate expression of the intrinsic self in self-perceptions and behavior.

Landau and colleagues (2011) tested this hypothesis using the metaphoric transfer strategy. Participants completed a neutral word task on the computer. In between trials, a sequence of different-sized squares flashed on the screen for about one second. In the *expansion* condition, the squares progressed from small to large; in the *stasis* condition, the large square reappeared; in the *fragmentation* condition the squares expanded but fragmented into an array of progressively smaller pieces (the *inner core* metaphor conventionally refers to an *integral* entity, not one that "falls apart"). Participants exposed to an expanding entity later reported feeling less concerned with others' approval.

In a follow-up study, participants were presented with an expanding entity, a static entity, or a contracting entity, and were next asked to evaluate abstract paintings. Using a subtle ruse, the researchers arranged it so that participants could see the evaluations ostensibly made by former participants. It was clear which paintings their peers liked and despised. Those flashed with images of entity expansion felt more comfortable expressing their genuine preferences rather than conforming to popular opinion.

CONCLUSION

Our goal in this chapter was to advance existential psychology by integrating CMT's perspective on the cognitive processes that people ordinarily use to understand and relate to abstract concepts. We reviewed CMT's explanation of how metaphor, traditionally dismissed as a figure of speech, operates at a cognitive level to structure abstractions around knowledge of superficially dissimilar concepts that are relatively more concrete and easier to grasp. We described empirical strategies that have proven useful for experimentally testing metaphor's influence on perception, attitudes, and behavior. We reviewed a small but growing body of research that applies these empirical strategies to test whether, when, and how metaphor shapes people's understanding of concepts that are central to their existential quest to feel like significant members of a meaningful world.

Although this work is in its infancy, it supports our "take-home" point: To develop a complete account of the meanings people give to existential concepts, research needs to model how people structure those concepts around ideas that, on the surface, are very different.

Although our literature review focused on just three self-aspects, we hope the reader appreciates the utility of a metaphor-enriched perspective for inspiring research into how people understand and relate to other existential concepts, such as those listed earlier in this chapter and featured in other chapters of this handbook. Finding, maintaining, and losing a sense of meaning and value in life depends on one's understanding of several existential concepts, and although the relevant experimental tests are lacking, analyses of communication suggest that many of them are construed metaphorically.

In addition to zooming in on other existential concepts, future research should consider why people gravitate toward one or another metaphor for the same existential concept. Consider, for example, that American and Swiss students spontaneously described themselves using metaphoric expressions that clustered around 20 sources as diverse as military combat, weight, economics, sports, law, technology, and art (Moser, 2007). What factors—both individual difference and situational—determine which sources people prefer to map a given target on?

To answer this question, researchers can draw on CMT's abovementioned claim that metaphorical thinking functions not only to support comprehension (satisfying nonspecific closure) but also to put a particular spin on a target—satisfying what lay epistemology theory calls the need for specific closure (Kruglanski, 2004). Mapping a target onto one source directs attention to certain bits of target knowledge while pushing others to the periphery of awareness. Hence, individuals motivated to maintain a particular interpretation of a target may strategically map it onto select sources.

We close with an example of an existential concept ripe for studying motivated metaphor preference: people's conception of death. Consider a podcast in which a 22-year-old man diagnosed with cystic fibrosis reflected on his mortality: "Death is a deadline: You have to finish everything you wanna do before then." This metaphor highlights the comforting idea that death, like a term paper deadline, is set to take place at a predictable time. By the same coin, it downplays the unsettling idea that one's death can occur at any moment from random sources of misfortunate that are impossible to fully anticipate or control.

In this vein, perhaps the most culturally widespread and comforting metaphor for death likens it to a person. Art forms such as image making and dance employ metaphor to transform the meaning of death from an abstract and unpredictable eventuality into an anthropomorphized agent—a witch, reaper, thief (Guthke, 1999). Putting a memorable face on death likely allays mortality-related anxiety. After all, if death were a person, it could be reasoned with, bargained with, tricked, or overwhelmed by one's own powers or those of a supernatural intercessor. Even such prosaic metaphors as those comparing death to sleep, or the afterlife to a "place" where people (or their souls) "go," reflect a profoundly motivated urge to not only give tangible form to death but also bolster faith in the validity of an anxiety-buffering conception of death and one's ultimate fate.

Future research could test motivated metaphorization of death by manipulating factors known to activate people's desire to affirm specific ideologies and self-views that are consistent with their death-denying worldview. For example, situationally salient reminders of personal mortality should make people more eager to embrace metaphors that downplay the possibility that death represents the self's total annihilation and highlight the possibility that death is merely a chapter in the epic story of *me*.

REFERENCES

Ackerman, J., Nocera, C., & Bargh, J. (2010). Incidental haptic sensations influence social judgments and decisions. *Science, 328,* 1712–1715.

Aristotle. (1924). Rhetorica (W. Roberts, Trans.). In W. Ross (Ed.), *The works of Aristotle* (Vol. 11). Clarendon Press. (Original work written ca. 330 B.C.E.)

Auster, P. (1990). *The New York trilogy.* Penguin.

Butler, R. (1963). The life review: An interpretation of reminiscence in the aged. *Psychiatry, 26,* 65–76.

Casasanto, D., & Dijkstra, K. (2010). Motor action and emotional memory. *Cognition, 115,* 179–185.

Chandler, J., Reinhard, D., & Schwarz, N. (2012). To judge a book by its weight you need to know its content: Knowledge moderates the use of embodied cues. *Journal of Experimental Social Psychology, 48,* 948–952.

Douglas, M. (1966). *Purity and danger: An analysis of concepts of pollution and taboo.* Penguin.

Eliade, M. (1996). *Patterns in comparative religion.* University of Nebraska Press.

Erikson, E. (1968). *Identity: Youth and crisis.* Norton.

Flanagan, O. (2009). *The really hard problem: Meaning in a material world.* MIT Press.

Forceville, C., & Urios-Aparisi, E. (Eds.). (2009). *Multimodal metaphor.* Mouton De Gruyter.

Gibbs, R. W. (Ed.). (2008). *The Cambridge handbook of metaphor and thought.* Cambridge University Press.

Giessner, S., & Schubert, T. (2007). High in the hierarchy: How vertical location and judgments of leaders' power are interrelated. *Organizational Behavior and Human Decision Processes, 104,* 30–44.

Gould, S. (1994, October). The evolution of life on earth. *Scientific American, 271,* 84.

Guthke, K. (1999). *The gender of death: A cultural history in art and literature.* Cambridge University Press.

IJzerman, H., & Semin, G. (2009). The thermometer of social relations: Mapping social proximity on temperature. *Psychological Science, 20,* 1214–1220.

Jia, L., & Smith, E. (2013). Distance makes the metaphor grow stronger: A psychological distance model of metaphor use. *Journal of Experimental Social Psychology, 49,* 492–497.

Jostmann, N., Lakens, D., & Schubert, T. (2009). Weight as an embodiment of importance. *Psychological Science, 20,* 1169–1174.

Kaspar, K. (2013). A weighty matter: Heaviness influences the evaluation of disease severity, drug effectiveness, and side effects. *PLOS One, 8,* e78307.

Keefer, L., Landau, M. J., Sullivan, D., & Rothschild, Z. (2011). Exploring metaphor's epistemic function: Uncertainty moderates metaphor-consistent priming effects on social perceptions. *Journal of Experimental Social Psychology, 47,* 657–660.

Kosslyn, S., Thompson, W., & Ganis, G. (2006). *The case for mental imagery.* Oxford University Press.

Kövecses, Z. (2005). *Metaphor in culture: Universality and variation.* Cambridge University Press.

Kövecses, Z. (2010). *Metaphor: A practical introduction.* Oxford University Press.

Kruglanski, A. (2004). *The psychology of closed mindedness.* Taylor & Francis.

Lakens, D., Semin, G., & Foroni, F. (2011). Why your highness needs the people: Comparing the absolute and relative representation of power in vertical space. *Social Psychology, 42,* 205–213.

Lakoff, G. (1992). Metaphors and war: The metaphor system used to justify war in the Gulf. In M. Putz (Ed.), *Thirty years of linguistic evolution* (pp. 463–481). John Benjamins.

Lakoff, G., & Johnson, M. (1980). *Metaphors we live by.* University of Chicago Press.

Lakoff, G., & Johnson, M. (1999). *Philosophy in the flesh.* Basic Books.

Landau, M. J. (2017). *Conceptual metaphor in social psychology: The poetics of everyday life.* Routledge.

Landau, M. J., Oyserman, D., Keefer, L., & Smith, G. (2014). The college journey and academic engagement: How metaphor use enhances identity-based motivation. *Journal of Personality and Social Psychology, 106,* 679–698.

Landau, M. J., Vess, M., Arndt, J., Rothschild, Z., Sullivan, D., & Atchley, R. (2011). Embodied metaphor and the "true" self: Priming entity expansion and protection influences intrinsic self-expressions in self-perceptions and interpersonal behavior. *Journal of Experimental Social Psychology, 47,* 79–87.

Lee, S. W. S., Chen, K., Ma, C., & Hoang, J. (2024). Wipe it off: A meta-analytic review of the psychological consequences and antecedents of physical cleansing. *Psychological Bulletin, 150*(4), 355–398.

Maslow, A. (1968). Existential psychology—what's in it for us? In R. May (Ed.), *Existential psychology* (pp. 52–60). Random House.

May, R. (1968). The emergence of existential psychology. In R. May (Ed.) *Existential psychology* (pp. 11–51). Random House.

McAdams, D. (2001). The psychology of life stories. *Review of General Psychology, 5,* 100–122.

McMullen, L., & Conway, J. (2002). Conventional metaphors for depression. In S. Fussel (Ed.), *The verbal communication of emotions: Interdisciplinary perspectives* (pp. 167–181). Erlbaum.

Michotte, A. (1963). *The perception of causality* (T. Miles, Trans.). Methuen. (Original work published 1946)

Morris, M., Sheldon, O., Ames, D., & Young, M. (2007). Metaphors and the market: Consequences and preconditions of agent and object metaphors in stock market commentary. *Organizational Behavior and Human Decision Processes, 102,* 174–192.

Moser, K. (2007). Metaphors as symbolic environment of the self: How self-knowledge is expressed verbally. *Current Research in Social Psychology, 12,* 151–178.

Rothschild, Z., Landau, M. J., & Sullivan, D. (2011). By the numbers: Structure-seeking individuals prefer quantitative over qualitative representations of personal value to compensate for the threat of unclear performance contingencies. *Personality and Social Psychology Bulletin, 37,* 1508–1521.

Sani, F. (2008). *Self-continuity.* Psychology Press.

Schlegel, R., Hicks, J., Arndt, J., & King, L. (2009). Thine own self: true self accessibility and meaning in life. *Journal of Personality and Social Psychology, 96,* 473–490.

Sedikides, C., Slabu, L., Lenton, A. P., & Thomaes, S. (2017). State authenticity. *Current Directions in Psychological Science, 26,* 521–525.

Shaver, P., & Mikulincer, M. (Eds.) (2012). *Meaning, mortality, and choice: The social psychology of existential concerns.* American Psychological Association.

Steger, M. F., Frazier, P., Oishi, S., & Kaler, M. (2006). The meaning in life questionnaire: Assessing the presence of and search for meaning in life. *Journal of Counseling Psychology, 53,* 80–93.

Stevens, W. (1967). *Opus posthumous* (S. F. Morse, Ed.). Knopf.

Stookey, L. (2004). *Thematic guide to world mythology.* Greenwood Press.

Sullivan, D., Landau, M. J., Young, I., & Stewart, S. (2014). The dramaturgical perspective in relation to self and culture. *Journal of Personality and Social Psychology, 107,* 767–790.

Trope, Y., & Liberman, N. (2010). Construal-level theory of psychological distance. *Psychological Review, 117,* 440–463.

von Winterfeldt, D., & Edwards, W. (1986). *Decision analysis and behavioral research.* Cambridge University Press.

Zestcott, C., Stone, J., & Landau, M. J. (2017). The role of conscious attention in how weight serves as an embodiment of importance. *Personality and Social Psychology Bulletin, 43,* 1712–1723.

CHAPTER 36

Cultural–Existential Psychology

The Societal Roots of Threat and Defense

Daniel Sullivan, Alexis N. Goad, Roman Palitsky, Harrison J. Schmitt, *and* Isaac F. Young

Cultural–existential psychology refers to any study or theory that combines the perspectives and methods of two areas of social psychology, namely existential social psychology and cultural psychology.

EXISTENTIAL SOCIAL PSYCHOLOGY

Existential psychology shares three foundational ideas with existential philosophy (Sullivan & Palitsky, 2017): (1) the uniqueness of the human species (stemming from symbolic consciousness) and the human individual (stemming from temporal finitude); (2) the indissolubility of the person's body, mind, and the concrete, historical situation in which they are located; and (3) the ubiquity of freedom and threat in human experience. In social psychology, existential psychology was inaugurated as a subfield almost four decades ago with the creation of terror management theory (TMT; Greenberg et al., 1986), which proposes that people are motivated to maintain the symbolic resources of self-esteem and a meaningful cultural worldview in order to protect themselves from the awareness of inevitable death. Hundreds of studies carried out in dozens of countries have shown that reminding people of their mortality prompts compensatory investment in cultural beliefs or markers of self-worth, even to the point of aggression against others who endorse opposing ideologies (Pyszczynski et al., 2015). These studies demonstrate that humans often rely on symbolic resources to maintain equanimity in the face of symbolic threats to life's meaning.

By bridging existential philosophical insights with empirical methods, TMT inaugurated a broader area of research: existential social psychology. Hart (2014) offered a distillation of three main domains of existential psychological research, which primarily concern threats and defenses that respond to those threats. These domains comprise interpersonal relationships (e.g., Baumeister & Leary, 1995), self-esteem (e.g., Greenberg et al., 1992), and cultural meaning/worldviews (e.g., Heine et al., 2006). Hart (2014) described these domains as functioning like a "security system," in which the domains are linked via fluid compensation: Threats in any of the domains can impact a person's global sense of security, which would affect the other domains. For example, personal relationship threats can undermine security, which also affects self-esteem. However, one can also compensate for a threat in one domain by means of another domain. For example, personal relationships (Mikulincer et al., 2003) and self-esteem (Greenberg et al., 1992) can function as buffers against existential threats in other domains.

CULTURAL PSYCHOLOGY

Cultural psychology examines culture as a psychological phenomenon (i.e., how minds produce culture) and psychology as a cultural phenomenon (i.e., how cultures produce minds). One of the guiding dictums of cultural psychology is the notion of mutual constitution (Markus & Kitayama, 2010): Culture and mind "make each other up" in reciprocal processes. Thus, the products and environments that constitute the "public sphere" are infused with the intentions of individuals. In some cultures, news stories make more dispositional (versus situational) attributions; artworks emphasize individual actors rather than surrounding landscapes; and street corners tend to have more clearly defined and streamlined—rather than ambiguous and cluttered—features (Morling & Lamoreaux, 2008). This intentionality in cultural environments in turn feeds back into the intentionalities of subjects living in those environments. For instance, settings with more residentially mobile individuals become filled with bureaucratic and standardized spaces, which then attract more residentially mobile individuals (Oishi, 2014).

Cultural psychologists have conducted hundreds of studies over the past 35 years documenting psychological variability between (and within) cultural groups. Famously, research has established that cultures vary on a continuum of individualism–collectivism (Triandis, 1995). *Collectivism* is a cultural orientation in which individuals have sociocentric values (e.g., prioritizing group goals), construe themselves as interdependent with others and sharing common identity, and experience embedded relatedness with low residential and relational mobility and thick social ties. *Individualism* is a cultural orientation in which individuals have egocentric values (e.g., prioritizing personal goals), construe themselves as independent and possessing unique identity, and experience abstracted independence with high residential and relational mobility and thin social ties (Adams & Plaut, 2003; Markus & Kitayama, 2010).

Existential and cultural psychology share an understanding of the importance of culture in human existence, which was also a perennial concern of 20th-century philosophy and social science. We therefore begin this chapter with an outline of the antecedents of cultural–existential theory in *philosophical* and *psychological anthropology*, as well as *existential philosophy*. We then overview contemporary theory and research in this area.

THE ORIGINS OF CULTURAL–EXISTENTIAL PSYCHOLOGY

Philosophical and Psychological Anthropology

"Modern" anthropology was influenced by 19th-century German social theory, in particular the work of Nietzsche and Weber (Lindholm, 2001). One throughline of these perspectives is that cultures exist and evolve in large part to convince their members that life is worth living despite material hardship and the human potential to grasp meaninglessness and futility. Conversely, the means by which cultures provide sense and purpose also make individuals vulnerable to existential threat (Sullivan, 2013). For example, belonging to a group can furnish security and meaning while also creating guilt at the prospect of transgressing against the group's norms. This duality was observed in the foundational work of anthropology: Whereas Malinowski emphasized how religious rituals neutralize anxiety, Radcliffe-Brown pointed out that the taboos set by culture actually generate considerable psychological stress (Homans, 1941), an idea that was already influential in psychoanalysis (Freud, 1913/1946).

Building on such notions and the growing foundation of social science, certain 20th-century philosophers attempted to illuminate the nature of the human condition. The key contribution of philosophical anthropology to cultural–existential psychology can be summarized by the observation that the worlds in which we psychologically exist are determined, in large part, by our culturally laden perceptions and motivations. As anthropologist A. I. Hallowell (1954/1967) stated, "Cultures not only share a common function in mediating self-objectification, it is one of their concomitant functions to constitute the self as a primary object of value in a world of other objects" (p. 102). This analysis would be echoed by Ernest Becker (1971) a few years later, when he defined culture as a system constructed "to provide the individual with the conviction that he is *an object of primary value in a world of meaningful action*" (p. 79).

The symbolic consciousness that affords cultural construction emerged as a result of a multifaceted evolutionary process referred to by Susanne Langer (1988) as the "great shift" from other-than-human to human psychology. According to Langer, other-than-human animals exist in an "animal ambient" in which cognition and perception are highly episodic. The evolutionary transition from the animal to the human ambient occurred as a function of the cognitively mediated *symbol*. The ability to think and communicate through symbols allowed humans to cognitively "fix" objects, facilitating the emergence of a social environment consisting of other symbolically conscious beings. Language further facilitated the emergence of long-term, self-referential memory and autobiographical time as a dimension of phenomenological experience. Philosophical anthropologists proposed that this symbolic scaffolding is able to occur largely because humans have an extended period of neoteny or prereproductive development. Human offspring have among the longest periods of dependence on their parents of any animal, an adaptation that has been attributed to the need for building complex social skillsets (Keller & Kärtner, 2013; Konner, 2007). Arnold Gehlen (1980) argued that this fact means that human behavior patterns are largely open-ended and require external guidance. As a result, nearly all cultural practices partly provide the individual with what Gehlen (1980) called institutionalizations—guidelines for behavior that symbolically anchor an extended temporal perspective to meaningful activity in the present.

In tandem with the work of such philosophical anthropologists, many European and North American anthropologists of the early 20th century attempted to understand the psychological experience of people from different cultures (often in the Global South). Some of these efforts eventually coalesced in the subfield known as psychological anthropology, which anticipated the central doctrines of cultural psychology (e.g., mutual constitution). Important for cultural–existential psychology was the fact that certain anthropologists believed cultural patterns were most directly observable when enacted by individuals in response to existential threat. For example, Edward Evans-Pritchard developed his "theory of social accountability" through the insight "that the essential point for [cross-cultural] comparison is that at which people meet misfortune" (Douglas, 1980, p. 3). John Gillin (1967) went so far as to argue that culture itself may be defined as a system that predisposes individuals to perceive certain events and information as threatening, and to employ certain defenses for coping with or repressing those threats.

Existential Philosophy

Due to their cognitive capacities, people are capable of confronting what Camus (1942/2004) called the basic question of life: whether it is worth living in the face of knowledge of death's inevitability. The awareness of finitude is a throughline in existential philosophy and animates one of its central observations: Human lives and human plans are shaped by responses to existential anxiety, which Paul Tillich (1952) defined as "the existential awareness of nonbeing" (p. 35). Awareness of nonbeing not only entails a direct focus on mortality but also includes the fragility of the symbolic modes of being in which humans participate, and which give people a sense of ultimacy or continuity. For example, experiences that call into question one's sense of meaning or personal value can serve as reminders of the state of nonbeing we all approach. The fragility of the culturally mediated world threatens the possibility of nihilism: that life is meaningless and not worth living.

Understanding how individuals and cultures respond to such threats has been a consistent interest for existential philosophers. Several categorical schemes for distinguishing between different common experiences of threat and defense have been articulated, which often take the form of a dialectic, or a dynamic oscillation between two opposing "poles" of threat (Schneider, 1999), also characterized as existentialism's *threat dialectic theory* (Sullivan et al., 2012a). According to Nietzsche, culture must defend against two primary possible forms of nihilism (Reginster, 2006). One is *nihilistic disorientation*—the conviction that our cultural values, beliefs, and goals are not worth upholding or achieving, connoting that our lives lack meaning *regardless* of what we are personally capable of. The other is *nihilistic despair*—the conviction that we personally are not capable of achieving our cultural values, beliefs, and goals, connoting that our lives lack meaning *because* of what we are personally (not) capable of. In order to convince us that life is worth living despite the guarantee of mortality, culture must neutralize the threats of both nihilistic disorientation and despair.

Sartre (1956) later asserted that humans are defined by *facticity* (unchangeable aspects of identity, embodiment, and historical circumstance), but aware of their potential for and motivated toward *transcendence* (altering or overcoming facticity by asserting free will). He proposed that humans cannot tolerate pure facticity or transcendence, and hence often dialectically defend against these realities through two forms of bad faith: flight from transcendence and flight from facticity. When a person experiences the threat of the abstract, of too much ambiguity in a situation, they flee (in dialectical fashion) toward the concrete, toward clear and unambiguous identities, definitions, and objects. On the other hand, when a person experiences inadequacy or guilt, they flee (again dialectically) toward the opposite pole, toward abstraction, away from concrete identities and the facticity of their existence. In one application of Sartre's framework, Palitsky and colleagues (2021) examined social responses to the COVID-19 pandemic as driven either by flight from transcendence (i.e., too much uncertainty), resulting in rigid embrace of rules, safety precautions, and social norms; or by flight from facticity (i.e., too much constraint), resulting in rigid emphases on autonomy, denying rules, and rejecting social norms.

Dialectical systems of threat and defense have been a focus of experimental and observational study in social existential psychology, as they lend themselves to operationalization and empirical manipulation. In such research, participants are often exposed to one pole of the threat dialectic while responses that emphasize the other side of the dialectic are investigated as dependent variables. In turn, these threat-response systems are reflected in social psychological theory, including explanatory frameworks for motives to reduce self-uncertainty through group identification (Hogg, 2007), the experience of discrepancies between one's self-understanding and standards of evaluation (e.g., Higgins, 1989), and emotional responses to one's personal transgressions (e.g., guilt and shame; Tangney & Dearing, 2003).

FIRST MAJOR PREMISE OF CULTURAL–EXISTENTIAL PSYCHOLOGY: A THREAT–CULTURE CYCLE

As formulated by Sullivan (2016) based on the work and scholarly traditions described above, cultural–existential psychology is rooted in two premises. The first is that of the *threat–culture cycle*: how culture and existential threat reciprocally constitute one another as individuals in a culture defensively negotiate threatening situations. The threat–culture cycle has two aspects. First, cultures provide psychological *threat interpretations*, through which they define what kinds of information and events are experienced as threatening. In three different cultures, people may alternatively be extremely anxious about the possibility that their neighbors may use witchcraft against them, or that they may not be able to own as many luxury commodities as their neighbors, or that they have behaved in such a way as to lose God's favor and protection. Moreover, they may worry about one of these possibilities without being in the least bit concerned about the other two. The differential emphasis on these different kinds of threats is driven by cultural threat interpretations. Second, cultures provide *threat responses*—culturally afforded and sanctioned defensive behaviors and attitudes that can grant people psychological solace in the face of culturally interpreted existential threats. In the same three different cultures, people may ritualistically guard themselves against witchcraft, or they may consume mind-altering drugs in order to cope with feelings of status anxiety, or they may engage in rituals of penance—such as reform through punishment—to restore their favor in God's eyes. Oriented toward addressing particular threats (e.g., existential uncertainty or guilt), these responses reinforce the cultural frameworks in which individuals operate while providing sanctioned responses that temporarily mitigate core anxieties.

The study of threat interpretations and responses has increasingly been delegated to the subfields of cultural psychology and existential social psychology, respectively. The concept of the threat–culture cycle helps unite these fields by emphasizing that one of the ways culture shapes individual psychology is through the symbolic coding of (non-)threatening situations. At the same time, people's psychological resistance to existential threat—their enactment of worldview defense when they are confronted by thoughts of mortality or meaninglessness, for example—are a primary motivational source of the perpetuation of cultural ideas and practices.

In this way the threat–culture cycle is often conservative. Our culture tends to tell us that we should be anxious about information and events that deviate from locally defined normality and further supplies us with defenses that often involve bolstering cultural norms. A self-sustaining culture is therefore one in which experiences of personal threat psychologically attach individuals even more strongly to the culture. However, it is also possible for the threat–culture cycle to move in more radical patterns of cultural evolution. If existing cultural interpretations and defense mechanisms fail to psychologically assuage the majority of cultural members who are experiencing threat, then their threat responses may eventually lead to cultural change rather than cultural conservation. Cultural leaders or influential groups may engage in cultural *innovation* in the face of threats, which the culture is unable to mitigate. More radically, it is possible for *revolutionary* or *counterrevolutionary* change to occur within a society as its threat responses accumulate and drive the culture in new directions. Under revolutionary circumstances, people confronted by material threat (e.g., low wages; famine) develop a counterculture that offers a new set of values and beliefs by which to live. In a counterrevolution, elites (e.g., politicians and pundits) channel widespread existential threat into scapegoating of deviant or minority groups to bolster the status quo.

REVIEW OF RESEARCH SUPPORTING A THREAT–CULTURE CYCLE

Cultural Variation in Interpretations of and Explanations for Threat

Some cross-cultural research documents that cultures vary in the chronic salience of particular threats. Summarizing a number of studies examining cultural differences in the experience of agency, Gibbs and colleagues (2023) have argued that people in more individualistic contexts are especially susceptible, and defensively respond, to perceived threats to personal control, whereas such threats may be less salient for people from more collectivistic backgrounds.

Other research examines cultural differences in how people interpret the causes and consequences of seemingly similar threat experiences. According to the perspectives that influenced cultural–existential psychology—in particular, psychological anthropology and existential philosophy—one of the most pervasive forms of existential threat is potentially meaningless suffering. Physical or mental illness, sudden natural disaster, and other sources of intense suffering in life would have even more drastic impact if they could not be explained in ways that allow sufferers to uphold or accommodate their existing worldviews. Therefore, one domain of research relevant to culture's role in threat interpretation is the body of studies of cross-cultural variation in explanations for suffering. As an example, in a highly influential chapter, Shweder and colleagues (1997) drew on a wide range of early ethnographic data to identify three major types of causal explanation for suffering around the globe: biomedical causality, which traces suffering to environmental factors outside of direct human control (e.g., understandings of illness as caused by viruses or bacteria); interpersonal causality, which traces suffering to violations and transgressions in the web of human relationships (e.g., understandings of illness as caused by witchcraft, prompted by interpersonal envy); and moral causality, which traces suffering to personal or community failures in an ideological or transcendental realm (e.g., understandings of illness as caused by sinfulness or failure to perform proper rituals). It is possible that such variation in causal explanations for suffering may even extend to different interpretations of extreme forms of psychological threat, such as traumatic stressors or psychopathology. Chentsova-Dutton and Maercker (2019) proposed that there are different "cultural scripts" for trauma, providing distinct expectations for what occurs over time when a person is traumatized, and which can be used to interpret one's own experience when confronted by potentially traumatic events. One of the cultural differences they observed is that "cognitive and emotional changes are foregrounded in scripts about trauma from Western countries, while bodily sensations and spiritual concerns are foregrounded in scripts from non-Western countries" (Chentsova-Dutton & Maercker, 2019, p. 12).

Building on such theoretical frameworks, some of our prior research has investigated the cultural variables associated with two prominent forms of suffering interpretation: *repressive* and *redemptive* suffering construals. A repressive suffering construal is the combination of an etiological account of suffering as caused by deviant or immoral behavior and a teleological account of suffering as having a sociocentric function (i.e., to strengthen social bonds or the moral order by preventing future deviant behavior). A redemptive suffering construal is the combination of a causal account of suffering in which it is organic to existence and unavoidable, and a teleological account of suffering as having an egocentric function (i.e., to strengthen processes of individuation and growth). These two suffering interpretations correspond with cultural variation in individualism–collectivism. Given the emphasis on maintaining harmony and relationships, cultural collectivism may afford a greater tendency toward repressive construals, whereas individualism may afford a greater tendency toward redemptive construals.

A correlational study of U.S. participants indeed found that dispositional collectivism predicted greater endorsement of repressive construals, a relationship statistically mediated by higher expressed social morality (endorsing the notion that morality is a social, rather than personal, construct; Sullivan et al., 2012b). Converging experimental evidence from U.S. samples showed that primed collectivist orientation increased repressive construals of both abstract (i.e., "suffering in general") and specific forms of suffering (e.g., the experience of AIDS; Sullivan et al., 2012b). Another investigation documented that Chinese citizens showed higher levels of teleological, but not causal, repressive construal compared to U.S. citizens (Sullivan et al., 2016). In other words, Chinese and North American participants were equally likely to make moralistic attributions for suffering, but Chinese individuals were more likely to endorse a prosocial function of suffering. That Chinese people associated more prosocial outcomes with suffering may be one reason why, overall, Chinese (compared to North American) participants have reported stressful experiences to have more elements of positivity and meaningfulness (Ji et al., 2022).

On the other hand, studies from narrative psychology suggest that redemptive narratives of suffering—which imply that the individual should experience personal growth as a result of negative life events—represent a "master narrative" in U.S. culture (McAdams, 2006). In the context of interpreting suffering caused by depression, Palitsky and colleagues (2019) found an association between more redemptive construals and belief in a humanist worldview (which blends elements of individualist and secular ideology). A study experimentally raised or lowered participants' beliefs that they were likely to experience depression in the future. Participants who subscribed to a humanist worldview were more prone to endorse redemptive construals of depression-related suffering when they believed themselves to be at greater risk, demonstrating the defensive function of redemptive construals.

Cultural Variation in Threat Responses

The studies just reviewed offer a window on cultural variability in threat interpretation by documenting how different societies make sense of potentially meaningless suffering in culture-consistent ways. Other studies have examined the influence of culture on patterns of defensive response to threats. For example, although TMT research has shown that people in various cultures who have been reminded of their mortality compensatorily respond by investing in worldview defense or self-enhancement, some studies attest to cultural nuance in this process. Building on the observation that Chinese participants saw greater positive and meaningful elements in suffering (Ji et al., 2022), a series of studies demonstrated that Northeast Asian (compared to North American) participants responded to thoughts of death with greater psychological investment in enjoyable aspects of life (Ma-Kellams & Blascovich, 2012). Mortality reminders lead to increased endorsement of individualist values among Australians, but not among Japanese participants (Kashima et al., 2004). On the other hand, such reminders have led to greater nationalism among Chinese but not U.S. participants (Routledge et al., 2013).

Religion is another cultural domain highly relevant to existential psychology. Probably the most extensive cross-cultural examination of death anxiety and associated defensive responses comes from Jong and Halberstadt (2016), who investigated cultural variability in the relationship between mortality concerns and religiosity. Interestingly, they found that when participants were asked to freely report their most prominent fears, about half of U.S. participants reported death among these fears, but only about a quarter of participants in other countries (Brazil, Russia, South Korea, the Philippines) did so. Furthermore, in their review of relevant studies, Jong and Halberstadt found evidence for a curvilinear relationship in the association between death anxiety and religiosity—in other words, self-reported death anxiety is relatively low for religious individuals who have relatively strong religious beliefs *and also* for secular individuals who may have other ways of managing death anxiety. This pattern is consistent with TMT's worldview defense hypothesis: People who feel relatively secure in their worldview (religious or secular) are comparatively buffered against thoughts of death. Having developed culturally translatable measures of death fear and religiosity, Jong and Halberstadt found that the curvilinear relationship between strength of religious belief and death anxiety was replicated in South Korea, which was similar to U.S. samples with Christianity being the most common religious affiliation and with relatively even representation of religious and secular individuals. However, among Japanese participants—where Buddhism (rather than Christianity) was the most common affiliation—there was no observed relationship between level of religious belief and reported fear of death. This is at least tentative evidence for cultural nuance in the relationship between religion and existential concerns; for instance, different patterns in Japan may reflect the representation of mortality in Buddhism versus Christianity, or the different historical developments of societal religiosity across cultures.

Examining a different form of threat response moderated by religion, Cohen and colleagues (2014) conducted several studies on the defensive process of sublimation—channeling repressed motivation connected with socially taboo experiences of sexuality and aggression into socially approved, creative productivity. They identified religious affiliation as a crucial cultural component of sublimation behavior. In experiments, some religious participants were induced to suppress feelings of anger or contemplate incestuous thoughts, while others were not. Protestants who experienced the induction (compared to Protestants who did not, and members of other religious communities—Catholics and Jews—who did) were more likely to expend effort on creative tasks (Kim et al., 2013). In a survey of representative U.S. residents, Hudson and Cohen

(2016) even found that Protestants who reported feelings of sexual conflict were more likely to have professions that require greater creativity (an effect not observed among Catholics and Jews in the sample).

SECOND MAJOR PREMISE OF CULTURAL–EXISTENTIAL PSYCHOLOGY: A TYPOLOGY OF THREAT ORIENTATIONS

Building from the concept of the threat–culture cycle, Sullivan (2013, 2016) proposed a typology of two major *threat orientations*, which characterize the patterns of threat and defense most often observed across diverse cultures. As described earlier, Nietzsche argued nihilism can take the form of disorientation—an ultimate threat to cultural worldview—or despair—an ultimate threat to self-esteem. Correspondingly, cultures can be classified on the basis of the type of nihilism against which they primarily protect their members. According to threat-dialectic theories, the choice of defense against threat is always one-sided and involves a tradeoff: A cultural system tends to shelter individuals from one form of nihilism by orienting them toward lower-level experiences of the opposite pole of existential threat.

Accordingly, some cultures may be called *disorientation-avoidant* (DISA), and therefore "guilt-oriented," meaning that cultural beliefs and socialization operate to neutralize the threat of meaninglessness; as a tradeoff, they orient individuals toward experiences of guilt. In DISA cultures, the primary concern is to protect the sacred nature of cultural values against their potential disconfirmation through relativism, skepticism, and so on. DISA cultures position their members to prevent the emergence of nihilistic disorientation and equip them with interpretations that involve tracing these threats to the inadequacy and immorality of the self or the community. At the same time, these cultures further equip their members with defenses that involve reasserting what Rothbaum and colleagues (1982) called *secondary control*: the perception that broader forces, which are outside the self but nonrandom and generally benevolent (e.g., God, ancestors, government leaders) are in control of events and the environment. Although DISA cultures may be effective at preventing disorientation, they potentially expose their members to nihilistic despair by encouraging them to critically reflect on whether they are meeting the strict standards of value upheld by their society.

By contrast, other cultures are *despair-avoidant* (DESA), and hence "uncertainty-oriented," meaning that attributional patterns acquired through socialization operate to neutralize the threat of personal guilt by strategically delegitimizing cultural standards of self-evaluation or judgment. DESA cultures focus on the avoidance of personalized feelings of despair that can arise from low self-esteem, inadequacy, or alienation among members of the culture. They equip their members with threat interpretations and defenses that take such forms as self-serving biases, greater relational mobility, and cultural relativism. Many defenses in DESA culture involve maintaining *primary control* in the face of threat (Rothbaum et al., 1982), that is, maintaining the conviction that one can personally control life outcomes when confronted with seemingly contradictory evidence. Although DESA cultures can effectively protect individuals from the despair of personal condemnation, they potentially expose their members to nihilistic disorientation by undermining commitment to any particular cultural value system.

These threat orientations are overviewed in Table 36.1, which also lists a series of cultural forms (i.e., culturally variable factors, worldviews, or systems) that tend to be associated with them. A primary cultural variable that influences the development of these threat orientations is *reflexivity*. In general, reflexivity refers to the capacity of a person, group, or human-created system to critically reflect on the sources and causes of their knowledge and behavior; cultural reflexivity specifically describes the extent to which a culture has widely available and cumulative data about its history and practices (Archer, 2012; Giddens, 1991; Hsu & Elliott, 2015). Widespread affordance of reflexivity in a culture has important implications for threat interpretation and response. If people in a culture have less awareness of the human origins of their values and beliefs, they are less likely to question the legitimacy of those

TABLE 36.1. DISA and DESA Threat Orientations: Typical Existential Components and Associated Cultural Forms

	DISA ("guilt-oriented")	DESA ("uncertainty-oriented")
Typical existential threat	Guilt	Anxiety
Typical existential defense	Worldview defense/secondary control	Self-enhancement/primary control
Degree of reflexivity	Low	High
Worldview	Religious	Secular
Social orientation	Collectivist	Individualist
Social control	Tight	Loose

values and beliefs; hence, lower-reflexivity cultures tend to have a DISA threat orientation. If people in a culture are socialized to reflect on and question the human origins of their values and beliefs, they are more likely to modify those values and beliefs in pursuit of their personal goals; hence, higher-reflexivity cultures tend to have a DESA orientation.

Reflexivity is thus a cultural form that proximally influences the development of threat orientations. However, there is also a constellation of cultural forms that in turn tend to be associated with the emergence and maintenance of reflexivity. Specifically, reflexive cultures generally tend to be lower in (orthodox) religiosity, more individualist, and less tightly controlled. Religion has often been psychologically defined as a pattern of cultural belief and behavior on which individuals rely to cope with existential threat (Batson et al., 1993). Religiosity relates to threat orientation particularly when conceptualized along a dimension from religious fundamentalism to secularism. Drawing on a dataset of large samples from 14 countries representing major religious traditions (multiple branches of Christianity, as well as Judaism, Islam, and Buddhism), Saroglou and colleagues (2022) recently defined *fundamentalism* as "cognitive and moral rigidity, a combination of dogmatic, inflexible, belief . . . with moral rigorism and conservatism through conformity to religious norms" (p. 568). Fundamentalism can be seen as an extreme form of religiosity to be contrasted with *secularism,* sociologically defined as participation in a (sub-)culture in which religion appears to be a lifestyle or choice that may be invalid, rather than an inherently given mode of being (Casanova, 2012; Taylor, 2007). At the individual level, secularism can be understood as a questing and uncertain or open-ended mindset toward spiritual matters (van Pachterbeke et al., 2012). Van Mulukom and colleagues (2023) have recently identified a secular worldview among people who identify as atheist or nonreligious in 10 (generally higher-income) countries around the globe, consisting of primary components such as a belief in the power and potential of science as well as a humanist value system (emphasizing the special nature and rights of humans as well as the potential for human progress).

Such recent large datasets provide evidence that whereas religious fundamentalism is more associated with group belongingness (Saroglou et al., 2022), secularism is more associated with an emphasis on individual agency and freedom (van Mulukom et al., 2023). The religious–secular dimension is therefore correlated with another cultural form, that of individualism and collectivism. A great deal of theory and evidence indicates that, historically, devout religiosity and collectivist social orientation were normative in most human societies, and the rise of individualism tends to be associated with a move toward secularity or away from more devout, all-encompassing, or fundamentalist forms of religiosity (e.g., Bellah, 1964; Durkheim, 1972; Gauchet, 1997; Norris & Inglehart, 2012).

A final cultural factor that, along with religiosity and collectivism, influences both reflexivity and threat orientation is the emphasis on social control exerted in the society—in other words, the way in which social behavior is regulated. Gelfand and colleagues (2011) described a continuum of social control that ranges from tight to loose. Cultures with *tight* social control exhibit a DISA orientation; they are characterized by strong situational norms for behavior across environments and tough sanctions for behavioral deviation, whereas those with *loose* control have a more DESA orientation; they possess less clear or rigid situational norms and fewer or weaker sanctions for deviance (Gelfand et al., 2011). In tight cultures, exposure to threat tends to evoke more conservative reactions of bolstering group norms and identity (Gelfand, 2021). In loose cultures, individuals respond to threat in more idiosyncratic ways and by bolstering personal control or agency; furthermore, freer flow of information and greater tolerance of deviance encourage critical reflection on self and culture.

Importantly, cultural tendencies toward DISA/DESA orientations are not monolithic or static, as socioecological factors afford variation within cultures and shifts in cultural values and lifeways over time (Greenfield, 2018; Weinstock, 2015). For instance, although secularism is generally associated with cultural reflexivity and looseness, and thus theoretically should afford a DESA orientation, it is also not historically uncommon for DISA movements or subcultures to arise within or directly in response to secular culture, as has occurred in some instances of state-sanctioned fascism or communism. Accordingly, it should also be borne in mind that the threat orientations are ideal types and although they may be generally afforded by the cultural forms listed in Table 36.1, they can manifest in different ways in particular historical and geographical contexts. Such historical nuance notwithstanding, summarizing across the cultural forms from Table 36.1, collectivist, tightly controlled, and fundamentalist-religious cultures are likely to have a DISA threat orientation in which their members are more disposed toward guilt than anxiety, and typically defend against threats by relying on their cultural worldview or the secondary control of external agents (e.g., God or group leaders). By contrast, individualist, loosely controlled, and secular cultures are likely to have a DESA threat orientation in which their members are more disposed toward anxiety than guilt and typically defend against threats through self-enhancement or reassertion of personal, primary control.

Research Supporting Threat Orientation Theory

Several recent studies have investigated the threat dialectic theory from existentialism, which proposes that anxiety and guilt are major categories of existential threat and that they are accompanied by characteristic defensive reactions. Young and colleagues (2018) found evidence that anxiety is a "separating" emotion (i.e., it accompanies feelings of disconnection from one's environment) associated with the threat of abstraction and uncertainty, whereas guilt is a "binding" emotion (i.e., it accompanies strong ties to one's environment), which prompts individuals to restore bonds between the self and others or the self and environment (cf. Rank, 1945). Young and colleagues observed, first, that individuals who experienced more dispositional disconnection (vs. connection) from their daily environments were more prone to anxiety (vs. guilt) feelings. In a subsequent study they experimentally manipulated feelings of connection or disconnection to the environment. The former experience led to elevated guilt, and the latter to elevated anxiety. Other work has examined how the same negative event may be construed as either a threat to control and uncertainty—hence, an experience of anxiety—or as a threat to the self's moral value and worth—hence, an experience of guilt. A study by Rothschild and colleagues (2012) showed that global climate change can be experienced either as anxiety-inducing—when understood as an overwhelming catastrophe that humans cannot fully understand or intervene upon—or guilt-inducing—when understood as the direct result of human actions, including those of the study participants. Those participants who were induced to consider climate change as a moral threat showed motivation to engage in future reparative behavior to reduce climate change, unless they could alleviate their guilt by blaming a scapegoat group (oil companies). Those participants induced to consider climate change as an uncertainty threat, by contrast, were solely motivated to blame a scapegoat group for the threat and did not report the same reparative intentions.

Individual-level variation in the construal of negative events as either anxiety- or guilt-inducing can entail distinct behavioral patterns of response. Further research on the psychology of climate change (Rothschild & Keefer, 2023) demonstrated that different individuals are motivated to respond to distinctive threat framings with defensive scapegoating. Among U.S. participants, those high in the psychological need for closure (who are less tolerant of uncertainty) were especially likely to blame a scapegoat group (China) for climate change when it was framed as an ambiguous and indeterminate threat. However, those who identified more strongly with their national ingroup were especially likely to blame China for climate change when it was framed as the consequence of immoral U.S. actions. In a more applied examination, Gao and colleagues (2024) examined how people respond to negative social interactions in the workplace in China. Specifically, they examined emotional reactions to participating in workplace gossip and found that individuals who felt more anxious after such events engaged in defensive behaviors designed to bolster their personal identity at the expense of their organizational identity. By contrast, individuals who felt more guilty after participating in gossip were more likely to subsequently attempt to make amends by ingratiating themselves with their supervisors.

Such research is consistent with threat orientation theory's proposition that different cultural factors are associated with distinct patterns of threat interpretation, but these particular studies do not connect people's dispositional threat interpretations to elements of their cultural background. However, in one relevant study, Young and colleagues (2021a) examined experiences of guilt and shame across five nations (United States, China, India, Iran, and Spain). They found that, among all participants, those individuals higher in a form of collectivism that emphasizes interpersonal relationships reported being more prone to engage in reparative behavior after experiencing guilt; whereas those individuals higher in a form of individualism that emphasizes competition and status reported being more likely to withdraw from uncomfortable interpersonal situations. Unlike guilt, shame prompts individuals to avoid social engagement, and meta-analytic research has shown that shame (but not guilt) and anxiety feelings are strongly related (Cândea & Szentagotai-Tătar, 2018). Thus, Young and colleagues' cross-cultural study may be taken as indirect but compelling evidence that collectivism predisposes individuals to guilt reactions, whereas individualism predisposes individuals to shame and anxiety reactions. Indeed, an analysis of 25 countries found that prevalence of anxiety disorders was positively related to a more individualistic profile of cultural values (high egalitarian values and lower values of hierarchy; Heim et al., 2017).

A few additional studies have examined in greater detail the proposal that there are distinct cultural patterns that orient individuals either toward guilt or toward anxious uncertainty. In the original explication of cultural–existential psychology, Sullivan (2016) reported a cross-cultural investigation that compared a standard psychology research sample—U.S. undergraduates—to two subcultural groups representing fundamentalist-religious and secular tendencies. The fundamentalist-religious group was a sample drawn from a traditionalist Mennonite community (for a detailed description of this group and their worldview, see Jantz, 2020). These Mennonites maintain a collectivist subculture emphasizing separation from the temptations and sins of mainstream capitalist "secular" society. They place great importance on living together in harmony and mutual support with their family and other members of their local church community. Congregations negotiate local normative practices, which typically involve unspoken rules for plain attire (especially for women) and the avoidance of any objects, entertainments, or activities that might be construed as selfish or materialistic. Members of this community were compared to a secular group represented by Unitarian Universalists (for a description of this tradition and community, see McKanan, 2013). Unitarian Universalism is a liberal religion that centers on ethics rather than creed: Its members emphasize the solidarity and commitment to social reform that can attend religious participation, rather than particular elements of doctrine. They follow a set of seven principles that share some similarities with the secular worldview identified by van Mulukom and colleagues (2023; e.g., individual dignity).

When comparing samples from these three subcultural groups, Sullivan (2016) found evidence for the DISA/DESA patterns of threat orientation. The traditionalist Mennonites—who scored higher on measures of fundamentalist religiosity and collectivism—were relatively more prone to guilt feelings compared to the other groups. The undergraduates and Unitarian Universalists—who scored higher on measures of secularity, humanism, and individualism—were relatively more prone to anxiety feelings compared to the Mennonites. Beyond threat interpretation, the groups also showed culturally distinct patterns of threat response: For example, among the undergraduates, self-esteem was negatively correlated with feelings of death anxiety, a relationship not observed in the Mennonite sample; whereas among the Mennonites, belief in God's power and control was negatively correlated with death anxiety, a relationship not observed in the undergraduate sample. A further qualitative study with these groups found evidence of different patterns of response when participants imagined coping with the threat of natural disaster (Sullivan et al., 2022). Traditionalist Mennonites discussed themes of transcendence and nonattachment in the context of disaster, meaning they cope with such events by relying on secondary control mechanisms—belief in God's protection and adjustment to the environment by relinquishing worldly goods. By contrast, Unitarian Universalists tended to mention relying on a sense of inner strength to cope with disaster, while also emphasizing that the loss of personally significant possessions and property would represent a major psychological threat.

Drawing on much larger samples of U.S. residents, Young and colleagues (2021b) utilized a person-centered and cluster-analytic approach to identify characteristic patterns of threat orientation and their cultural associations. Participants completed a variety of survey items assessing their level of concern about different potential sources of psychological insecurity. Data patterns revealed that people tended to cluster in groups of (1) *socially concerned* participants (corresponding to the DISA/guilt orientation) who were secure in their sense of meaningfulness but relatively sensitive to threats that they were exhibiting deviant behavior or breaking social relationships and (2) *meaning-concerned* participants (corresponding to the DESA/uncertainty orientation) who were secure in their sense of self but relatively sensitive to the possibility of meaninglessness in their lives. Supporting threat orientation theory, the socially concerned/DISA participants scored higher in religiosity and collectivism, whereas the meaning-concerned/DESA participants scored higher in secularity and individualism.

Closely related research highlights another aspect of existential theory, namely that there are varying levels of threat experience. Lower-level, everyday experiences of anxiety and guilt can trigger dialectical defenses. If these are unsuccessful or the negative emotions are sustained over time, higher-level, more severe threat experiences may result, possibly leading to the experience of nihilism and withdrawal from life (Sullivan et al., 2012a). Reiss and colleagues (2021) recently asked a sample of Austrian participants to describe in detail their emotional and motivational experience when they are confronted by different types of existential threats. Using cluster analysis, they found three patterns in the phenomenological experience of threat. Supporting Tillich's analysis, death anxiety emerged as a unique cluster. A second cluster seemed to represent concrete threat experiences involving vigilance and arousal in social environments. Finally, a third cluster represented more abstract and severe threat experiences more closely connected to potential nihilism. In their own cluster analysis of threat orientations, Young and colleagues (2021b) found that meaning-concerned (i.e., DESA) individuals were more prone to report higher-level and diffuse distress. In contrast, those who were greater in social concern (i.e., DISA) reported more concern regarding their social and physical surroundings, reflecting more vigilance and attentiveness to their immediate surroundings. Also attesting to variation in the severity of existential threats, Hayes and Hubley (2017) have proposed a model of death awareness and psychopathology. Their work shows that if individuals possess a meaningful goal when they are confronted with death awareness, they will defensively invest in the goal, reducing their feelings of distress but increasing their susceptibility to concern regarding their ability to achieve the goal. On the other hand, if individuals do not have a clear goal to pursue, confrontation by thoughts of mortality will increase feelings of distress and tendencies to withdraw, decreasing direct self-evaluative concerns but potentially leading to nihilistic despair.

Although work on variation in the severity of existential threat experience is relatively new, it represents one possible avenue among others for the development of existential social psychology broadly and cultural–existential psychology in particular. One suggestive but underdeveloped implication of the studies just discussed is that DESA/uncertainty orientation may lead to higher incidence of behavioral disorders compared to other threat orientations, especially if individualist and secular tendencies are taken to extremes. The data thus far suggest (in U.S. and European samples) that strongly individualist participants are less likely to have a strong sense of meaning in their lives, which could open a psychological gateway to nihilism.

FUTURE DIRECTIONS IN CULTURAL–EXISTENTIAL PSYCHOLOGY

The subfields of cultural and experimental existential psychology are only approximately 40 years old in their current incarnations. Systematic efforts to unite them are even more recent. And yet, as discussed, the theoretical background of these contemporary research efforts effectively coincides with the inception of modern social science in the Global North. There is ample research documenting the diverse ways in which culture interprets and filters the experiences of existential threat and response, as well as a growing body of work that suggests one major way in which these interpretations are patterned. Specifically, some cultures characterized by lower reflexivity, collectivism, and tightness afford interpretations of threat as stemming from failures to uphold cultural standards, while protecting the sense that there are sacred values and meaning that transcend individual experience. On the other hand, cultures characterized by greater reflexivity, individualism, and looseness defend the sacrosanct nature of the individual's self-worth and inalienable rights, while interpreting threat as stemming from a hostile, chaotic, and perhaps meaningless world.

Moving forward, it will be important for research on the intersection of culture and existential threat to employ dynamic methods, as well as flexible theoretical interpretations rooted in historical understanding, to avoid the tendency for research to reify culture. The DISA and DESA threat orientations are patterns and possibilities that recur throughout history in a variety of forms and combinations. It is possible for subcultural groups in a society to experience either or both of these tendencies in different situations, and historical circumstances may move entire cultures rapidly in one direction or the other. It is also likely that individual patterns of orientation and threat response vacillate and change over time. However, temporal trajectories of individual existential orientations remain largely unexamined (Palitsky et al., 2020). Like other binaries in the history of psychology and social science, the threat orientation theory is one way of making sense of the diversity of human experience, drawing on seemingly universal existential themes. Yet if a lesson is to be learned from existentialism, it is that all humans have responsibility for their lives, and for the way they meet threats with dignity and frailty (Jackson, 2005). And, indeed, individuals and groups slowly change the course of cultural history in the creative and desperate ways they fight against threats.

Probably the most comprehensive vision of cultural–existential psychology yet developed can be found in Jean-Paul Sartre's late work *Critique of Dialectical Reason*, which represented his attempt to interweave existentialism and Marxism (for a summary, see Sullivan, 2021). That work attempted nothing less than an understanding of human history as the cumulative result of the countless acts of successive generations of self-responsible and radically free individuals. Two premises can be drawn from that work that may profitably guide future research on culture and existential threat.

The first is that threats do not merely arise naturally as "existential givens" of human experience with which all individuals are confronted in the same way but, rather, they are actively produced and shaped by human culture. Humans create history, yes; but in doing so they create the history of others (and thus are also the recipients of history created by others). The acts of transcendence and freedom of some individuals are *simultaneously* the conditions of constraint and facticity for others, and this is true both intergenerationally (e.g., the productive capacity and energy consumption of today is the environmental catastrophe of tomorrow) and between cultural groups at any moment in history (hence Ruth Wilson Gilmore's, 2022, definition of racism as the systematic distribution between people of premature death). The COVID-19 pandemic confronted all people with a glaring indication of the extent to which contemporary social interconnection exposes us immediately to geographically distal threats; and yet historic resource disparities ensure that people do not all meet such threats with the same defensive capacities (see Palitsky et al., 2021). We can also consider how economic growth and the experience of luxury for some in the United States has been partly fueled in the last five decades by the proliferation of debt mechanisms that have disenfranchised much of the lower and working classes, leading in many instances to their criminalization and imprisonment (Goad et al., 2025). These examples suggest the importance of theorizing the distribution of existential threat, and disparities of response, within and across (as well as between) cultures and generations.

Another premise from Sartre's framework crucial for future work is that existential threat response can be generative of cultural change. According to Sartre, people undergo the most profound forms of social identity and collective consciousness when they experience the threat of mortality as a collective, rather than merely individual, phenomenon. When individuals recognize that their entire cultural group is equally threatened by the possibility of premature or violent death, they cease to live as isolates and engage in collective action to fight back against the source of the threat. This premise should be kept in mind when researching contemporary forms of cultural change and social resistance, whether this be the responses of racialized group members to police violence or military oppression (Burson & Godfrey, 2020) or the efforts of activists to recognize and halt the effects of global climate change (Van Stekelenburg & Klandermans, 2023). Existential threat defines not only the boundaries of our individual lives, but the contours of our responsibility toward, and shared fate with, others. Cultural history represents an expanding repertoire of ways in which people have come to terms with human reality, a repertoire on which we can draw when we understand death as a font of both division and communion.

REFERENCES

Adams, G., & Plaut, V. C. (2003). The cultural grounding of personal relationship: Friendship in North American and West African worlds. *Personal Relationships, 10*(3), 333–347.

Archer, M. S. (2012). *The reflexive imperative in late modernity.* Cambridge University Press.

Batson, C. D., Schoenrade, P., & Ventis, W. L. (1993). *Religion and the individual.* Oxford University Press.

Baumeister, R. F., & Leary, M. R. (1995). The need to belong: Desire for interpersonal attachments as a fundamental human motivation. *Psychological Bulletin, 117*(3), 497–529.

Becker, E. (1971). *The birth and death of meaning* (2nd ed.). The Free Press.

Bellah, R. N. (1964). Religious evolution. *American Sociological Review, 29*(3), 358–374.

Burson, E., & Godfrey, E. B. (2020). Intraminority solidarity: The role of critical consciousness. *European Journal of Social Psychology, 50,* 1362–1377.

Camus, A. (2004). The myth of Sisyphus. In G. Marino (Ed.), *The basic writings of existentialism* (pp. 441–494). Modern Library. (Original work published 1942)

Cândea, D.-M., & Szentagotai-Tătar, A. (2018). Shame-proneness, guilt-proneness and anxiety symptoms: A meta-analysis. *Journal of Anxiety Disorders, 58,* 78–106.

Casanova, J. (2012). Religion, the Axial Age,

and secular modernity in Bellah's theory of religious evolution. In R. N. Bellah & H. Joas (Eds.), *The Axial Age and its consequences* (pp. 191–221). Harvard University Press.

Chentsova-Dutton, Y., & Maercker, A. (2019). Cultural scripts of traumatic stress: Outline, illustrations, and research opportunities. *Frontiers in Psychology.*

Cohen, D., Kim, E., & Hudson, N. W. (2014). Religion, the forbidden, and sublimation. *Current Directions in Psychological Science, 23,* 208–214.

Douglas, M. (1980). *Edward Evans-Pritchard.* Viking Press.

Durkheim, E. (1972). *Emile Durkheim: Selected writings* (A. Giddens, Ed.). Cambridge University Press.

Freud, S. (1946). *Totem and taboo* (A. Brill, Trans.). Vintage Books. (Original work published 1913)

Gao, Q., Zhang, K., Cao, Y., Li, J., Bian, R., & Wang, X.-H. (2024). The effect of negative workplace gossip about supervisor on workplace deviance and impression management: The mediating roles of anxiety and guilt. *Journal of Business Psychology, 39,* 435–454.

Gauchet, M. (1997). *The disenchantment of the world: A political history of religion.* Princeton University Press.

Gehlen, A. (1980). *Man in the age of technology.* Columbia University Press.

Gelfand, M. J. (2021). Cultural evolutionary mismatches in response to collective threat. *Current Directions in Psychological Science, 30,* 401–409.

Gelfand, M. J., Raver, J. L., Nishii, L., Leslie, L. M., Lun, J., Lim, B. C., . . . Yamaguchi, S. (2011). Differences between tight and loose cultures: A 33-nation study. *Science, 332*(6033), 1100–1104.

Gibbs, W. C., Kim, H. S., Kay, A. C., & Sherman, D. K. (2023). Who needs control?: A cultural perspective on the process of compensatory control. *Social and Personality Psychology Compass, 17.*

Giddens, A. (1991). *Modernity and self-identity.* Stanford University Press.

Gillin, J. (1967). The balance of threat and security in Mesoamerica: San Carlos. In R. Hunt (Ed.), *Personalities and cultures: Readings in psychological anthropology* (pp. 139–149). Natural History Press.

Gilmore, R. W. (2022). *Abolition geography* (B. Bhandar & A. Toscano, Eds.). Verso.

Goad, A. N., Jimenez, T., Jones, T. K., Schmitt, H. S., Sedivy, L., & Sullivan, D. (2025). *Credit, cops, and cages: A theory of capitalist individualism.* Bloomsbury.

Greenberg, J., Pyszczynski, T., & Solomon, S. (1986). The causes and consequences of a need for self-esteem: A terror management theory. In R. F. Baumeister (Ed.), *Public self and private self* (pp. 189–212). Springer.

Greenberg, J., Solomon, S., Pyszczynski, T., Rosenblatt, A., Burling, J., Lyon, D., . . . Pinel, E. (1992). Why do people need self-esteem?: Converging evidence that self-esteem serves an anxiety-buffering function. *Journal of Personality and Social Psychology, 63*(6), 913–922.

Greenfield, P. M. (2018). Studying social change, culture, and human development: A theoretical framework and methodological guidelines. *Developmental Review, 50,* 16–30.

Hallowell, A. I. (1967). The self and its behavioral environment. In *Culture and experience* (pp. 75–110). Schocken Books. (Original work published 1954)

Hart, J. (2014). Toward an integrative theory of psychological defense. *Perspectives on Psychological Science, 9,* 19–39.

Hayes, J., & Hubley, C. (2017). Between a rock and a hard place: When affirming life reduces depression, but increases anxiety. *Journal of Social and Clinical Psychology, 36,* 860–882.

Heim, E., Wegmann, I., & Maercker, A. (2017). Cultural values and the prevalence of mental disorders in 25 countries: A secondary data analysis. *Social Science and Medicine, 189,* 96–104.

Heine, S. J., Proulx, T., & Vohs, K. D. (2006). The meaning maintenance model: On the coherence of social motivations. *Personality and Social Psychology Review, 10,* 88–110.

Higgins, E. T. (1989). Self-discrepancy theory: What patterns of self-beliefs cause people to suffer? In L. Berkowitz (Ed.), *Advances in experimental social psychology* (Vol. 22, pp. 93–136). Academic Press.

Hogg, M. A. (2007). Uncertainty-identity theory. In M. P. Zanna (Ed.), *Advances in experimental social psychology* (Vol. 39, pp. 69–126). Academic Press.

Homans, G. C. (1941). Anxiety and ritual: The theories of Malinowski and Radcliffe-Brown. *American Anthropologist, 43*(2), 164–172.

Hsu, E. L., & Elliott, A. (2015). Social acceleration theory and the self. *Journal for the Theory of Social Behaviour, 45,* 397–418.

Hudson, N. W., & Cohen, D. (2016). Taboo desires, creativity, and career choice. *Motivation and Emotion, 40,* 404–421.

Jackson, M. (2005). *Existential anthropology.* Berghahn Books.

Jantz, R. C. (2020). *Living in the world.* Wipf & Stock.

Ji, L.-J., Yap, S., Khei, Z. A. M., Wang, X., Chang, B., Shang, S. X., & Cai, H. (2022). Meaning in stressful experiences and coping across cultures. *Journal of Cross-Cultural Psychology, 53,* 1015–1032.

Jong, J., & Halberstadt, J. (2016). *Death anxiety and religious belief: An existential psychology of religion.* Bloomsbury.

Kashima, E. S., Halloran, M., Yuki, M., & Kashima, Y. (2004). The effects of personal and collective mortality salience on individualism: Comparing Australians and Japanese with higher and lower self-esteem. *Journal of Experimental Social Psychology, 40,* 384–392.

Keller, H., & Kärtner, J. (2013). Development—The culture-specific solution of universal developmental tasks. In M. L. Gelfand, C.-Y., Chiu, & Hong, Y. Y. (Eds.), *Advances in culture and psychology* (Vol. 3, pp. 63–116). Oxford University Press.

Kim, E., Zeppenfeld, V., & Cohen, D. (2013). Sublimation, culture, and creativity. *Journal of Personality and Social Psychology, 105,* 639–666.

Konner, M. (2007). Evolutionary foundations of cultural psychology. In S. Kitayama & D. Cohen (Eds.), *Handbook of cultural psychology* (pp. 77–105). Guilford Press.

Langer, S. K. (1988). *Mind: An essay on human* feeling (abridged ed.). Johns Hopkins University Press.

Lindholm, C. (2001). *Culture and identity: The history, theory, and practice of psychological anthropology.* McGraw-Hill.

Ma-Kellams, C., & Blascovich, J. (2012). Enjoying life in the face of death: East–West differences in responses to mortality salience. *Journal of Personality and Social Psychology, 103,* 773–786.

Markus, H. R., & Kitayama, S. (2010). Cultures and selves: A cycle of mutual constitution. *Perspectives on Psychological Science, 5,* 420–430.

McAdams, D. P. (2006). *The redemptive self: Stories Americans live by.* Oxford University Press.

McKanan, D. (2013). Unitarianism, Universalism, and Unitarian Universalism. *Religion Compass, 7,* 15–24.

Mikulincer, M., Florian, V., & Hirschberger, G. (2003). The existential function of close relationships: Introducing death into the science of love. *Personality and Social Psychology Review, 7*(1), 20–40.

Morling, B., & Lamoreaux, M. (2008). Measuring culture outside the head: A meta-analysis of individualism–collectivism in cultural products. *Personality and Social Psychology Review, 12,* 199–221.

Norris, P., & Inglehart, R. (2012). *Sacred and secular: Religion and politics worldwide.* Cambridge University Press.

Oishi, S. (2014). Socioecological psychology. *Annual Reviews of Psychology, 65,* 581–609.

Palitsky, R., Schmitt, H., Sullivan, D., & Young, I. F. (2021). An existential analysis of responses to the 2020 coronavirus outbreak. *Journal of Humanistic Psychology, 61,* 231–243.

Palitsky, R., Sullivan, D., Young, I. F., & Dong, S. (2019). Worldviews and the construal of suffering from depression. *Journal of Theoretical Social Psychology, 3,* 191–208.

Palitsky, R., Sullivan, D., Young, I. F., & Schmitt, H. J. (2020). Religion and the construction of identity. In K. E. Vail & C. Routledge (Eds.), *The science of religion, spirituality, and existentialism* (pp. 207–222). Academic Press.

Pyszczynski, T., Solomon, S., & Greenberg, J. (2015). Thirty years of terror management theory: From genesis to revelation. *Advances in Experimental Social Psychology, 52,* 1–70.

Rank, O. (1945). *Will therapy* and *Truth and reality* (J. Taft, Trans.). Knopf (Original works published 1929–1931)

Reginster, B. (2006). *The affirmation of life: Nietzsche on overcoming nihilism.* Harvard University Press.

Reiss, S., Leen-Thomele, E., Klackl, J., & Jonas, E. (2021). Exploring the landscape of psychological threat: A cartography of threats and threat responses. *Social and Personality Psychology Compass, 15*(4), e12588.

Rothbaum, F., Weisz, J. R., & Snyder, S. S. (1982). Changing the world and changing the self: A two-process model of perceived control. *Journal of Personality and Social Psychology, 42,* 5–37.

Rothschild, Z. K., & Keefer, L. A. (2023). Who scapegoats?: Individual differences moderate the dual-motive model of scapegoating. *Journal of Research in Personality, 105.*

Rothschild, Z. K., Landau, M. J., Sullivan, D., & Keefer, L. A. (2012). A dual-motive model of the motives underlying scapegoating: Displacing blame to reduce guilt or increase control. *Journal of Personality and Social Psychology, 102,* 1148–1163.

Routledge, C., Juhl, J., Vess, M., Cathey, C., & Liao, J. (2013). Who uses groups to transcend the limits of the individual self? Exploring the effects of interdependent self-construal and mortality salience on investment in social groups. *Social Psychological and Personality Science, 4,* 483–491.

Saroglou, V., Clobert, M., Cohen, A. B., Johnson, K. A., Ladd, K. L., Brandt, P.-Y., . . . Valladares, J. T. (2022). Fundamentalism as dogmatic belief, moral rigorism, and strong groupness across cultures: Dimensionality, underlying components, and related interreligious prejudice. *Psychology of Religion and Spirituality, 14,* 558–571.

Sartre, J.-P. (1956). *Being and nothingness: An essay in phenomenological ontology* (H. Barnes, Trans.). Philosophical Library.

Schneider, K. J. (1999). *The paradoxical self: Toward an understanding of our contradictory nature.* Humanity Books.

Shweder, R. A., Much, N. C., Mahapatra, M., & Park, L. (1997). The "big three" of morality (autonomy, community, divinity) and the "big three" explanations of suffering. In A. Brandt & P. Rozin (Eds.), *Morality and health* (pp. 119–169). Routledge.

Sullivan, D. (2013). From guilt-oriented to uncertainty-oriented culture: Nietzsche and Weber on the history of theodicy. *Journal of Theoretical and Philosophical Psychology, 33*(2), 107–124.

Sullivan, D. (2016). *Cultural-existential psychology: The role of culture in suffering and threat.* Cambridge University Press.

Sullivan, D. (2021). Sartre's *Critique of Dialectical Reason* and new materialism. *ANGELAKI, 26,* 31–48.

Sullivan, D., Landau, M. J., & Kay, A. C. (2012a). Toward a comprehensive understanding of existential threat: Insights from Paul Tillich. *Social Cognition, 30*(6), 734–757.

Sullivan, D., Landau, M. J., Kay, A. C., & Rothschild, Z. K. (2012b). Collectivism and the meaning of suffering. *Journal of Personality and Social Psychology, 103*(6), 1023–1039.

Sullivan, D., & Palitsky, R. (2017). An existential-psychological perspective on the human essence. In M. van Zomeren & J. Dovidio (Eds.), *The handbook of the human essence* (pp. 21–34). Oxford University Press.

Sullivan, D., Schmitt, H. J., & Goad, A. N. (2022). The socio-material force theory of identity. *Theory and Psychology, 32,* 353–374.

Sullivan, D., Stewart, S. A., Landau, M. J., Liu, S., Yang, Q., & Diefendorf, J. (2016). Exploring repressive suffering construal as a function of collectivism and social morality. *Journal of Cross-Cultural Psychology, 47,* 903–917.

Tangney, J. P., & Dearing, R. L. (2003). *Shame and guilt.* Guilford Press.

Taylor, C. (2007). *A secular age.* Belknap Press.

Tillich, P. (1952). *The courage to be.* Yale University Press.

Triandis, H. C. (1995). *Individualism and collectivism.* Westview Press.

van Mulukom, V., Turpin, H., Haimila, R., Purzycki, B. G., Bendixen, T., Kundtová Klocová, E., . . . Farias, M. (2023). What do nonreligious nonbelievers believe in?: Secular worldviews around the world. *Psychology of Religion and Spirituality, 15,* 143–156.

Van Pacterbeke, M., Keller, J., & Saroglou, V. (2012). Flexibility in existential beliefs and worldviews: Introducing and measuring existential quest. *Journal of Individual Differences, 33,* 2–16.

Van Stekelenburg, J., & Klandermans, B. (2023). *A social psychology of protest.* Cambridge University Press.

Weinstock, M. (2015). Changing epistemologies under conditions of social change in two Arab communities in Israel. *International Journal of Psychology, 50*(1), 29–36.

Young, I. F., Razavi, P., Cohen, T. R., Yang, Q., Alabèrnia-Segura, M., & Sullivan, D. (2021a). A multidimensional approach to the relationship between individualism-collectivism and guilt and shame. *Emotion, 21*(1), 108–122.

Young, I. F., Sullivan, D., Hart, J., & Palitsky, R. (2021b). Insecurity orientations: A person-centered approach to existential concerns. *Personality and Individual Differences, 168.*

Young, I. F., Sullivan, D., Stewart, S. A., & Palitsky, R. (2018). The existential approach to place: Consequences for emotional experience. *Journal of Environmental Psychology, 60,* 100–109.

CHAPTER 37

A Hero's Wrath

Taming the Sense of Chaos and Cultivating a Meaningful Sense of Self through Moral Outrage

Zachary K. Rothschild *and* Lucas A. Keefer

On January 6, 2021, in the middle of a global pandemic, an estimated 120,000 people came to Washington, DC, to protest the results of the U.S. presidential election (Arkon, 2021). In the end, over 1,000 people were charged with various acts of violence or trespassing on the Capitol building. Interviews and court proceedings reveal that many of the perpetrators came to express anger at what they believed was a grave injustice: an attempt by corrupt politicians and "Deep State" actors to steal the election (January 6 Committee Final Report). They saw themselves not as villains, but as heroes putting themselves at risk to save democracy and freedom from evil forces.

While some may be shocked at the protestors' anger and moral grandiosity, Becker (1973) proposed that people all share a similar ache for heroism, driven by the need to believe in our own enduring value and significance. Taking Becker's claims seriously, we consider the possibility that righteous anger may sometimes serve as a means of heroizing ourselves in service to deeper existential concerns. Narrowly, this pursuit of heroism refers to the need to perceive oneself as a moral agent acting in a rigid framework in which the lines between good and evil are drawn in stark relief. In a psychological sense, this entails an unshakeable faith in two "truths": (1) that the world allows for meaningful action against irredeemable foes and (2) a basic certitude in one's moral righteousness. We start this chapter by examining what it means to be a hero, and the existential concerns that might motivate people to pursue a heroic identity. We then draw on Becker's theorizing, and recent empirical evidence, to consider how identifying clear villains and expressing outrage in the name of justice can serve to cultivate a heroic self-image in a chaotic world where one's own goodness and significance are uncertain.

HEROES: MORAL AGENTS STANDING AGAINST EVIL ON BEHALF OF OTHERS

The idea of a heroic figure seems as old as literature itself. Although the substance has evolved over time, ancient literature such as the Homeric epics or the *Epic of Gilgamesh* tell stories of moral avatars overcoming challenges in righteous pursuit of a greater good.

The enduring appeal of the noble hero across cultures and histories encouraged theorists to propose that the hero is more than just a garden-variety concept; rather, it has a unique psychological importance. Most directly, Jung (e.g., 1959) proposed that the hero's universality was a manifestation of its central importance in human nature.

The hero archetype is an intuitive persona representing humanity's need for both moral exemplars and reassurance that morality's rewards await the virtuous, no matter what slings and arrows come in the short term. Analysts have embraced this view (most famously Joseph Campbell, 1949) seeking a psychological explanation for the recurrent appeal of the hero's journey through adversity and growth.

More recent psychological analysis sought to establish thematic coherence underlying hero concepts (Kinsella et al., 2015b). This prototype analysis indicated that heroes tend to embody core personality attributes. Heroes are seen centrally as *morally virtuous*; their conviction, integrity, self-sacrifice, and altruism are critical elements in their inspirational role. Additionally, the heroic prototype subsumes *action-oriented* personality traits such as bravery, courage, and determination. In one study, when participants were asked what heroes (vs. leaders or role models) are like and what they do, heroes were distinguished by their tendency to act against evil as a means of saving or protecting others (Kinsella et al., 2015a).

Setting aside questions about variation in hero myths and concepts, a couple of key themes are worth noting. First, heroes are moral agents whose role is to directly achieve some moral end. Comic books, mythology, Hollywood films, poems, and plays provide daily examples of moral heroes reflecting an idealized moral image to which audiences can aspire. These narratives tell us that a hero's virtue manifests in their selfless opposition to malevolent actors and injustices on behalf of others. This long-standing archetype, with seemingly endless appeal, has encouraged theorists like those above to consider that heroes have some fundamental psychological importance. We turn next to perspectives that suggest heroism likely serves a variety of existential psychological functions.

EXISTENTIAL ROOTS OF HEROIC PURSUITS

One reason why heroes have captured the imaginations of generations may be because they confront existential challenges that all individuals face. Every hero provides a slate of idealized moral traits that offer individuals a framework for thinking about their own ideal selves. Below, we explore two existential perspectives that help explain why people tend to be profoundly and universally captivated by heroism.

Death Transcendence

Ernest Becker (1973) believed that human pursuits are profoundly shaped by the desire to escape an honest reckoning with our mortality. In his view, human striving commonly attempts to symbolically transcend one's brief life by seeing oneself as a valuable and lauded part of a larger and more enduring cultural worldview. Symbolic immortality offers a palliative against anxieties about death. Work in terror management theory (Solomon et al., Chapter 6, this volume) offers some empirical support for Becker's view.

While there are many ways to be remembered (and thus achieve symbolic immortality), heroes offer a clear prototype for a successful path into a culture's long-term memory. As noted above, cultures routinely tell and retell hero myths, carve statues to celebrate their heroes, mark off holidays to commemorate their lives, and so on. And thus, for Becker, people strive to see themselves as heroes in the hope that they will "transcend the limitations of the human condition and achieve victory over impotence and finitude" (1975, p. 31). So central is this need, that Becker believed every society is in essence a "hero system" that offers routes for "heroic victory over evil and death" (p. 124).

McCabe and colleagues (2015) have conducted some of the only empirical research testing Becker's claim that concerns about one's mortality can fuel the pursuit of a heroic self-image. In one subtle study, individuals reminded of their mortality (vs. exam failure) reported less pain during a physically painful situation (having a hand in a bucket of ice water) if they were also primed to think of endurance as a heroic (vs. generally positive) trait. Reminders of death elicited a motivation to prove oneself as possessing heroic (and not merely positive) traits. This comparison is critical: Death salience did not encourage pain endurance for the sake of being a *better* person but did do so for the sake of being a more *heroic* person.

Additionally, experimental studies show that individuals who were randomly assigned to receive feedback confirming (vs. disconfirming) their heroism showed reduced salience of thoughts related to death in a behavioral assessment (word-stem completion; Greenberg et al., 1994). In other words, the feeling that one is heroic helps keep thoughts about mortality further from conscious awareness, demonstrating the protective benefits of heroism that Becker theorized.

McCabe and colleagues (2016) also investigated whether the death-denying desire for heroic transcendence can motivate individuals to identify with other heroic individuals. In their initial study, participants were asked to think of a hero and rate the extent to which they included that individual in their sense of self. They found that self-focused participants reminded of death (vs. uncertainty) tended to see greater overlap between themselves and a hero. Heightening thoughts of one's finite existence motivated stronger identification with a hero.

In a final study, McCabe and colleagues (2016) assessed whether hero identification could attenuate thoughts of death. They found that following a reminder of death (vs. pain), participants induced to identify with a hero showed reduced salience of death-related words, but only when the hero's legacy and sacrifice were emphasized. This suggests that the potency of heroic identification is closely tied to the symbolic immortality afforded to heroes.

Meaning in Life

Viktor Frankl (1969/1981) proposed that "the will to meaning" is a separate but equally fundamental motivation. Consistent with Frankl's theorizing, research has found that people tend to see their lives as meaningful and seek to restore meaningful self-views when threatened (Baumeister, 1991). Insofar as heroes are seen to "personify what it means to live a meaningful life," the desire to be heroic may reflect a deeper need for personal meaning (Kinsella et al., 2019, p. 475).

Converging tripartite models (e.g., George & Park, 2016; Martela & Steger, 2016) suggest that personal meaning emerges from experiences of coherence, purpose, and significance in one's life. Below we review evidence suggesting that a heroic sense of self can satisfy each interlocking but distinct component.

Coherence

Meaning as coherence refers to the ability to make sense of oneself and one's experiences (Martela & Steger, 2016). Personal meaning relies on a self-concept that provides a coherent (clear, stable, and consistent) sense of identity (Campbell et al., 1996). Shin and colleagues (2016) found that participants who felt their lives were more meaningful tended to be those who had a more clearly defined and internally consistent self-concept (Shin et al., 2016).

Waterman (1993) proposed that personal meaning depends on the perceived coherence between one's avowed true self-concept (a cognitive schema representing one's perceived essential nature) and one's expressed values, goals, and actions. Consistent with this premise, research has shown that people who rate themselves as more authentic (true to themselves) report feeling that their lives are more meaningful (Guenther et al., 2023). In other words, we see our lives as meaningful to the extent that they appear aligned with what we perceive to be our essential nature (Schlegel et al., 2009).

Theorists have proposed that heroes directly satisfy the need for a coherent understanding of the avowed or ideal self. Specifically, Allison and Goethals (2015) proposed a framework suggesting that heroes fulfill two critical needs: *epistemic* and *energizing.* In other words, heroes allow individuals to understand how to live and, through identification, motivate the pursuit of those clear exemplars. Research has also shown that people view their true self to be fundamentally moral and good (Strohminger et al., 2017). As such, a heroic self-narrative offers a framework for understanding the self and interacting with the world that people are likely to perceive as authentic, and thus meaningful.

Purpose

Frankl (1969/1981) claimed that seeing one's life as purposeful, oriented toward something greater than oneself, is a central feature of experiencing life as meaningful. Purpose has been described as the essence of heroic action (Bronk & Riches, 2017). Heroes have a clear and morally compelling purpose, to selflessly help others and uphold core moral principles like justice.

This suggests that adopting a heroic purpose may foster personal meaning. Consistent with this idea, Smaliukienė and colleagues (2023) found that military personnel viewed their service as more meaningful to the extent that they also viewed it as having a more prosocial purpose. Other research has shown that acting for the benefit of others is associated with greater personal meaning (Klein, 2017), and that threats to meaning motivate efforts to see one's actions as more virtuous and prosocial (Van Tongeren et al., 2016).

Significance

The last component of personal meaning is the sense that one's life matters and is worth living (Martela & Steger, 2016). Significance, sometimes referred to as existential mattering (George & Park, 2014), connects with Becker's theorizing that people strive to see their lives as making an enduring positive mark on the world. If meaning as purpose is about the *goal* of making a valuable contribution to humanity, meaning as significance is about believing that one *is making* a valuable contribution.

Value and impact are part and parcel of our understanding of heroism. As previously discussed, heroes are lauded as moral exemplars that make the world a better place. The scope of the hero's impact and tendency to prioritize the well-being of others imbues their actions with greater significance. As such, possessing a heroic sense of self may bolster personal meaning by affirming that one's actions and sacrifices matter in the lives of others. This is consistent with the finding that perceiving one's life as having a positive impact on others is strongly associated with seeing one's life as meaningful (Fuhrer & Cova, 2023).

Most existing research on meaning and heroism has focused on how personal and cultural heroes may be a source of meaning for other people (see Green et al., 2017; Kinsella et al., 2019). However, the aforementioned analysis suggests that acting or even just imagining oneself to be heroic should also be an appealing route for those seeking to bolster or maintain a sense of personal meaning. Supporting this claim, Dakin and colleagues (2021) found that individuals reporting a greater search for meaning (e.g., "I am looking for something that makes my life meaningful") also reported a greater willingness to engage in heroic actions like donating a kidney to someone in need or sacrificing one's life to save others (including people from their hometown, people from Africa, chimpanzees, and redwood trees).

Igou and colleagues (2018) examined whether perceiving threats to one's personal meaning may motivate people to cultivate a heroic self-image. In one experiment, participants were randomized to experience a threat to their personal meaning (by focusing on their biggest regret in life) or not. The study's primary outcome was an assessment of participants' heroism motivation (e.g., "It is significant to my life to be seen as someone who has the qualities of a hero"; "It is important to me to be seen as someone who can act heroically"). Thinking about personal regret spurred an increased desire to be heroic and this effect was driven in part by a threat-induced increase in participants' search for meaning. Interestingly, independent of meaning-seeking, general self-enhancement concerns also predicted heroism motivation. This suggests that needs for meaning and value may represent distinct reasons for pursuing a heroic self-concept.

Summary

People must address the awareness of their mortality and have a need for meaning reflected in subordinate needs for coherence, purpose, and significance. Both needs seem to be addressed by becoming and being heroic. Heroes are memorialized in ways that make heroism a compelling response to death awareness. Additionally, heroes provide clear guidance on how to live meaningfully (coherence), provide a blueprint for living purposefully (purpose), and impact the world in ways that create positive moral change (significance).

But how can a person come to see themselves as a hero in a chaotic world of haphazard threats and diverse moral values? Below we summarize two lines of research that explore two psychological processes underpinning the hero's quest: namely, those by which a villain is discovered/created in the social environment and, in tandem, those by which the self is perceived as capable of moral heroism. In both cases, we highlight the unique role that moral outrage against a focal enemy plays in promoting these outward and inward facing perceptions, respectively.

IN SEARCH OF VILLAINS: FETISHIZING EVIL TO CREATE A WORLD FOR HEROIC ACTION

Although heroism seems at first glance to reflect the hero's personal virtue and drive, heroism requires a particular socioecological context. A world where suffering and injustice are the result of impersonal, random misfortune, precludes the possibility of a heroic triumph over evil. Therefore, at minimum, a sense of heroism often relies on the perception that *evil exists* and that some *adversary clearly embodies it* to create conditions that allow heroes to address a moral challenge.

To unpack how people identify moral enemies, researchers have looked to diverse phenomena, including the viral video campaign "Stop Kony" (Sullivan et al., 2016). This online campaign, spearheaded by the group Invisible Children, sought to publicize the mistreatment and violence experienced by citizens in central Africa at the hands of Joseph Kony and his militia, the Lord's Resistance Army. Sullivan and colleagues (2016) conducted two studies demonstrating that while a simple depiction of Kony as directly responsible for the suffering of 30,000 children elicited moral outrage, outrage was diminished when individuals learned about the true complexity of the situation. In other words, moral outrage was strongest in a low-information environment in which Kony's actions could clearly be identified as evil and in which no external attributions were available to explain them beyond his inherent viciousness. Unlike the more complex description of events, the simple framing of Kony as a singularly important villain provided a simple solution for improving life in Uganda: killing or capturing Kony.

The social-cognitive processes that individuals enact to identify sources of evil serve directly as a means of addressing existential psychological threats (e.g., Rothschild et al., 2020; Sullivan et al., 2010). In Becker's (1975) view, enemies fulfill a vital function by allowing individuals to localize and explain evil; believing that nefarious agents bear ill will can help reduce the more threatening perception that reality is chaotic. Unlike random misfortune, a clear enemy provides an adversary, who is evil and can be potentially defeated, or at least understood.

In a series of experimental studies, Sullivan and colleagues (2010) found that when individuals were reminded of chaotic hazards in the environment, they were more likely to believe that powerful enemy figures were working against them. For example, when individuals were reminded of uncontrollable (vs. controllable) hazards, they were more likely to believe political conspiracy theories proposing that elections were rigged by the opposing political party's leaders. Participants also showed an increased tendency to attribute myriad negative events to a personal enemy when institutions normally tasked with mitigating harms (i.e., the government) were portrayed as impotent.

This and other research have gone further by showing that this perception of powerful and ill-intentioned enemies ironically boosts perceptions of personal control. In one study, Sullivan and colleagues (2010) found that, following a control threat, participants who read an article attributing vague powers to the terrorist organization Al Qaeda adopted a more internal locus of control. This effect was partially explained by *reduced* concern about the risk of encountering future misfortunes in a mediational analysis.

These findings highlight a somewhat ironic benefit of identifying a clear enemy. On the one hand, knowing that the universe is not fully benevolent and that there are in fact people actively threatening the individual might seem like a source of unease. However, this unease seems somewhat less aversive than the alternative in which threats are completely random and without intention. The work on enemyship shows that individuals prefer the smaller cost in concern over specific threats, compared to the more global anxieties that might result from confrontation with the broader chaos and meaninglessness of the universe.

Research has even found a similar tradeoff with enemies who are not human at all. After being reminded of random hazards in the environment, individuals with a greater fear of spiders perceived a greater sense of personal control after having the opportunity to focus on images of spiders (vs. grass) (Rothschild et al., 2020). This pattern is doubly ironic: These individuals both were reminded of chaotic hazards and reported high fear of the very thing they encountered in the task. Nevertheless, in two studies (including one preregistered replication) Rothschild and colleagues found the same result—namely, that reminders of a particular focal enemy helped reduce anxieties about chaos in the world writ large. These findings support Becker's (1975) contention that uncontrollable hazards become subsumed by a focal enemy, creating a simpler, safer, and more controllable conception of reality.

Relatedly, Rothschild and colleagues (2012) found that when people encountered a complex negative event without a clear cause (e.g., global climate change), they were motivated to attribute blame for that event to a target outgroup (e.g., oil companies), so long as the target was seen as powerful and malicious enough to serve as a scapegoat. Blaming a scapegoat under such conditions was found to bolster participants' feelings of personal control. Rothschild and Keefer (2023) replicated this pattern and further found that this kind of scapegoating was driven by concern that the harmful effects of climate change were beyond one's control.

The aforementioned research provides converging evidence that the tendency to focalize, or as Becker would say, fetishize, evil appears to serve an underlying desire to see the world as a place where one can effectively assert one's will. While there are a litany of ways to bolster perceptions of control (Landau et al., 2015), we propose that fetishizing evil is unique insofar as it helps create a world for heroic action. However, the process of enemyship appeals to the would-be hero only insofar as it creates an embodiment of evil that can be heroically opposed. Consistent with this premise, Schöpfer and colleagues (2023) found that meaning-seeking participants were more likely to believe in nefarious conspiracies if they thought they could personally or collectively take action against the conspirators. Furthermore, belief in these conspiracies predicted a greater sense that one's own life mattered. In other words, people endorsed conspiracy theories because they offered a sense of moral agency, a means of opposing evil, and potential to have a positive impact on the world.

This illustrates that focalizing evil may be necessary but not sufficient to heroize the self; one must also have the opportunity to oppose that evil. This may occur through action or through sentiment implying a desire to move against an enemy. Motro and Sullivan (2017) sought to examine the role that anger plays in the process of enemyship. As an approach-oriented emotion associated with perceptions of high certainty and control (Ellsworth & Scherer, 2003), anger motivates action to confront or punish the perceived source of a moral violation (Carver & Harmon-Jones, 2009).

Motro and Sullivan (2017) exposed individuals to a control threat (or not) then assigned participants to focus on either the anger they experienced while thinking about an enemy (enemy-directed anger condition), an enemy without considering their anger (enemy-only condition), the experience of anger without an enemy (anger-only condition), or neither an enemy nor the experience of anger (absent condition). A series of experimental tests found that relative to the other conditions, enemy-directed anger bolstered feelings of personal control and certainty, which in turn increased participants' general motivation. This suggests that anger is a motivating and clarifying emotion that amplifies the psychological functionality of enemyship.

This research provides evidence that fetishizing evil in a villain, against whom one can direct feelings of anger, attenuates anxieties about chaotic risks while bolstering feelings of personal control and motivation. While this process may set the stage for heroic action, one must still prove their status as a moral agent with a righteous mission. In the next section we consider the idea that moral outrage, or anger at the perceived violation of a moral principle, like justice or fairness (Batson et al., 2007), may serve this function when directed at a third-party harmdoer.

HEROIC ANGER: MORAL OUTRAGE FOSTERS A MORAL AND MEANINGFUL SENSE OF SELF

To be a hero, individuals must not only be *capable* of virtue; they must *embody* it. What makes a hero is, in part, their absolute moral correctness. Without that, their actions do not rise to a level worthy of remembrance that Becker's analysis would require for symbolic immortality.

But how can the individual, a flesh-and-blood human with moral failings, be assured that they are up to that high bar? One way people may seek assurances about their moral character is by observing their responses to moral violations. People tend to view their emotional responses as particularly insightful because they are perceived to offer an involuntary and unfiltered expression of who they are and what they value (Solomon, 2007). For instance, feeling moral outrage at a third-party perpetrator for harming an innocent victim, signals that one is both concerned about the welfare of others, and motivated to uphold moral principles like justice, even when one is not directly affected. Thus, the experience and expression of outrage would seem to signal one's own moral righteousness. Indeed, a line of research demonstrates that moral outrage has the unique effect of clarifying moral self-perceptions, enhancing the individuals' sense of their moral worth and personal meaning.

Moral Threat Elicits Outrage

While terror management theorists have long argued that self-esteem is a psychological need because of its death-buffering effects (e.g., Pyszczynski et al., 2004), some have suggested an additional need for a moral self-image. Specifically, in an attempt to distinguish the unique benefits of a moral sense of self-worth, Prentice and colleagues (2019) found that feeling moral had unique contributions to well-being over and above autonomy, competence, relatedness, and general self-esteem.

At the group level, studies find that the ingroup's perceived moral status is rated as more important than competence or warmth (Leach et al., 2007). This finding is notable given the fact that those two dimensions make up the core of most social-cognitive research on group perceptions (e.g., Fiske, Cuddy, Glick, & Xu, 2018).

Other evidence suggests that the need for a moral self-image is reflected in defensive responses to distinctly moral threats. Individuals who experience a threat to the moral value of an ingroup have been shown to respond with outrage (e.g., Tauber & van Zomeren, 2013), unless given an opportunity to affirm the group's moral value first (van der Toorn et al., 2015). These studies suggest that anger at an outgroup is driven by a distinctly moral threat and that addressing that threat can diminish the defensive reactions.

In one line of studies, Rothschild and colleagues (2021) found that awareness of a threat to the moral value of an ingroup led to greater derogation of a rival outgroup. Specifically, the researchers used a naturalistic experimental design whereby U.S. partisans' self-identified political party (Republican, Democrat) was crossed with random assignment to articles describing moral failings by either Republican or Democratic politicians. Despite the fact that the ingroup condition described members of one's own party acting immorally, this condition elicited increased derogation of outgroup partisans. This included an increased tendency to express outrage at false statements by outgroup leaders (Study 1), judge an outgroup politician as morally corrupt (Study 2), and view opposing partisans as hateful and malicious (Study 3).

However, although these studies focused on moral threats to personally valued groups, they might be alternatively explained as the result of other non-moral processes. For example, social groups generally support feelings of self-worth and provide a sense of certainty about one's identity (e.g., Luhtanen & Crocker, 1992). So, to check whether moral image threat, specifically, drives moral outrage against target perpetrators, researchers conducted experimental studies that directly examined the role of feelings of personal moral culpability. For example, Rothschild and Keefer (2017) found that individuals with greater guilt about their contributions to sweatshop labor or environmental destruction were more outraged by corporations who could plausibly be viewed as contributing to those issues. In two studies a linear association was found between the amount of guilt individuals felt, and how incensed they were over corporations perpetrating the same misdeeds.

Outrage and Moral Image Maintenance

Outrage is more than just a consequence of moral threat; it is also an effective treatment. In the same article (Rothschild & Keefer, 2017), researchers found that when individuals expressed outrage following a moral value threat, they subsequently evaluated themselves as more virtuous. Yet this effect is not a blanket positive shift in esteem. Green and colleagues (2019) found that individuals who expressed moral outrage viewed themselves as more moral but not higher in other positive (agentic) traits.

Other evidence that moral outrage serves in part to restore a moral self-image comes from studies showing that affirmation of the individual's sense of personal moral value can reduce threat-induced expressions of outrage. This was initially tested by Rothschild and Keefer (2017); individuals first expressed their levels of guilt for contributing to sweatshop labor and learned about a blameworthy target: an international cell-phone manufacturer. Then half the participants (randomly assigned) were asked to write about what makes them a good person versus a matched non-moral affirmation. While guilt was associated with subsequent outrage among those exposed to a non-moral affirmation, the relationship between guilt and outrage at the sweatshop-supporting corporation was eliminated after individuals were made to feel like a morally good person. The fact that this affirmation was effective even in a completely irrelevant context suggests that for some, moral outrage stems more from nonspecific concerns about moral self-image than domain-specific concerns about a particular issue.

Further research on scapegoating as a means of moral image maintenance demonstrated that righteous anger can "purify" one's moral self-image. In one such investigation Rothschild and colleagues (2012) found that individuals who were reminded of their own negative impact on the environment ascribed greater blame to oil companies for environmental hazards and that this effect was driven by state feelings of guilt. Supporting a moral image maintenance explanation, research found that scapegoating after a value threat was eliminated if individuals were given a nonspecific moral affirmation. Another project Rothschild and colleagues (2013) found that self-identified middle-class Americans reminded of their group's negative impact on the working-class felt greater collective guilt, unless they were given the opportunity to scapegoat illegal immigrants as an alternative source of blame. Those who were able to displace blame onto illegal immigrants expressed greater outrage at immigrants on behalf of working-class Americans.

The fact that moral anger in part addresses concerns with moral image was further examined by investigations of who is likely to deploy scapegoating as a moral image defense (Rothschild & Keefer, 2023). In this work, researchers found that individuals given a value threat did not universally blame a candidate outgroup (China) for their own group's harmful environmental impact; rather, the effects observed in the previous studies varied strongly as a function of individuals' collective narcissism. Those who had a strong preexisting commitment to the superiority of their group were ostensibly more threatened by an ingroup moral culpability manipulation and thus more motivated to lash out at a target scapegoat to defend the value of their group. In contrast, a collective moral image threat failed to elicit defensiveness among individuals with no moral commitment to the ingroup.

In a separate series of studies (Rothschild & Keefer, 2018), researchers found that the guilt-driven increases in outrage at third-party perpetrated injustice was only found among those dispositionally low in the trait of justice sensitivity. In other words, the individuals who expressed elevated outrage at third-party perpetrated injustices when their own moral standing was threatened, tended not to be bothered by justice violations in general (low in justice sensitivity). This provides additional evidence that the threat-induced increase in outrage found in the previous studies was not about concerns with justice per se, but about concern with individuals' own moral status.

These results suggest that people are motivated to maintain a sense of their moral worth and may attempt to do so by derogating outgroups when their own morality is in question. In such cases, perceiving an outgroup as malevolent and expressing anger at their misdeeds on behalf of others may reassure the individual that they are morally righteous. In such instances, outrage appears to replace concerns about one's own moral inadequacies with a sense of heroic morality.

Outrage and Meaning Maintenance

While less focus has been given to moral outrage as a source of meaning, initial research demonstrates a clear role. In an initial investigation (Rothschild & Keefer, 2022), researchers asked individuals to provide reports for 1 week on the outrage they experienced after reading news on social media each day as well as daily feelings of meaning in life. We found that levels of moral outrage about injustice were associated with stronger feelings of daily meaning but only among individuals highly committed to justice as a personal value.

But does outrage actually satisfy needs for meaning? To test this, researchers conducted an experiment manipulating both a meaning threat and the order in which participants reported on their feelings of outrage and meaning in life. Among those with a strong commitment to justice, expressing anger about the mistreatment of workers eliminated the effect of the meaning threat. Notably, participants who reported on their personal meaning before assessing outrage showed the threat effect—meaning was effectively reduced by the threat manipulation among our highly justice sensitive participants initially—but outrage effectively buffered this threat.

Finally, researchers tested the possibility that meaning affirmation might reduce moral outrage among those individuals highly committed to justice. Using a large, preregistered experimental design, researchers measured dispositional concern with justice, then asked all participants to complete a task shown in past research to threaten meaning in life. Participants were then randomly assigned to write about something that made their lives meaningful (self-meaning affirmation), that made a close friend or family member's life meaningful (other-meaning affirmation), or their morning routine (control). The research found that outrage over sweatshop labor was diminished after completing the self- but not the other-meaning affirmation, and that this effect again held only among those individuals with a strong commitment to justice.

Interestingly, participants' reported sense of coherence, purpose, and significance/mattering all mirrored the primary effects for their overall perceived meaning in life. These findings are consistent with previous theory and research on why a heroic sense of self may serve as a source of meaning. The fact that outrage at injustice only bolstered meaning among justice-sensitive participants is consistent with the notion that personal meaning can emerge from the perceived congruence between one's outwardly expressed, and one's inwardly held core values.

FUTURE DIRECTIONS

Above we have discussed the ways that moral outrage uniquely props up a sense of personal heroism. However, this work is relatively novel and bears development. Below we highlight recommendations for integrating this work into broader literature in existential and social psychology and point toward avenues for further considering the unique ways that heroism integrates concepts of self, morality, and evil in the lives of everyday social agents.

Outrage and Existential Concerns

First, we initiated our discussion of heroism by introducing Becker's view that individuals have a need for heroism to address concerns about mortality. By that view, death concerns are ameliorated by a sense of symbolic immortality. Personal status as a hero provides a powerful dose of symbolic immortality ostensibly able to cement the individual's status as a culturally enduring figure. Nevertheless, the studies viewed above test only a small portion of that larger account. Specifically, the work reviewed above demonstrates only that outrage provides a sense of personal heroism and sharpens the lines around moral outgroups to reaffirm personal (and collective) value and meaning. In none of the studies above have researchers yet moved to the next step of assessing whether or how this affirmed sense of moral value contributes to larger existential concerns around mortality. However, one possible link to that broader existential concern comes from the studies demonstrating that moral outrage bolsters a sense of personal meaning among justice-sensitive individuals (Rothschild & Keefer, 2022). To the extent that a sense of meaning in life serves as a fundamental buffer against larger existential anxieties (Greenberg et al., 2014), outrage seems to be a path that could promote existential security by way of clarified purpose, significance, or coherence (all three were enhanced by moral outrage; Rothschild & Keefer, 2022).

Admittedly this is not quite what Becker proposed, but the fact that moral outrage also affirms a sense of personal value (e.g., Rothschild & Keefer, 2017) suggests that moral outrage may buffer death anxiety through self-esteem-related mechanisms, such as those outlined by terror management theory. Specifically, terror management theory has long endorsed the view that self-esteem buffers death anxiety because it conveys to individuals that they have successfully achieved cultural benchmarks for symbolic immortality (e.g., Greenberg et al., 1992). So, in addition to the meaning afforded by moral outrage, future work may also benefit from considering how the affirmed value provided by moral outrage may achieve some of the same processes ascribed to self-esteem. For example, to the extent that outrage mitigates moral threats, it may also affirm a sense of moral virtue and corresponding sense of symbolic immortality.

Routes to Heroism

While we set out this discussion highlighting the importance of heroism as a construct, we have not yet discussed how outrage may compare to other more direct routes to achieving heroism. After all, most hero myths speak of more than angry tweets. For most heroes, heroism is earned through prosocial works, sacrifice, and victory over a moral adversary. This simple fact suggests that outrage may be little more than a quick (and largely effortless) way of *feeling* heroic without the struggles that actual heroes typically endure. Accordingly, individuals who have a sense of their own heroism affirmed in other ways (e.g., reminders of their sacrifices or prosociality) may be less motivated to lash out with moral outrage following a threat to their moral self-image (initial evidence suggests so; Rothschild & Keefer, 2017).

Doing heroic things may then subvert the need to *feel* heroic by way of moral outrage. Studies have shown that prosocial behavior can reduce guilt (e.g., Estrada-Hollenbeck & Heatherton, 1998) and that reminders of guilt (e.g., Catholics reminded of their last confession) elicit more prosocial behavior (e.g., McKay et al., 2013). Self-sacrifice directly attests to the individual's moral character without reliance on an external adversary or the negative consequences that follow. Accordingly, interventions based around heroic action may provide a way to supplant some of the more detrimental consequences of heroic thinking observed in our work on moral outrage.

On a more cautionary note, relatively easy expressions of outrage that amount to mere hand wringing may sometimes undermine more effortful and costly actions to address injustices. Initial evidence lends credence to this possibility. In one set of studies, Rothschild and colleagues (2025) found when White U.S. participants were reminded of their racial privileges, having the opportunity to express outrage at another individual's racist behavior attenuated participants' own willingness to donate time and money to address systemic racism.

Outrage in Context

Moral outrage elicits intense motivation to punish perceived moral transgressions. Based on our research, this desire to punish can stem in part from personal moral image concerns. In essence, the greater the feeling of personal guilt, the stronger the desire to enforce moral norms (e.g., Rothschild & Keefer, 2017, Study 1). But despite their claims to absolutism, moral norms are deployed in surprisingly flexible ways. For example, research on construal level demonstrates that individuals taking a more distant, abstract stance toward an issue tend to employ more rigid moral rules, while those closer to a situation may be more likely to consider exemptions (Eyal & Liberman, 2012; Eyal et al., 2008). Indeed, studies show that a more abstract mindset yields greater consistency of moral responses (Alper, 2018), suggesting more rigid obedience to individuals' core moral convictions.

To the extent that heroism entails a clear cognitive demarcation between good and evil, it seems that heroic thought may be more effective among individuals taking a more abstract or otherwise rule-based approach to moral reasoning in a given context. In other words, individual variation in core values (e.g., Alper, 2020) may suggest differences not only in targets of moral outrage but also more fundamentally in whether outrage is useful as a strategy at all. Minimally, an agent must have internalized moral values germane to a target for outrage to afford feelings of heroism (and see the work described previously, establishing intrinsic commitment to justice as a moderator of the link between moral outrage and meaning; Rothschild & Keefer, 2022).

Additionally, diversity in patterns of moral cognition may explain why moral outrage often fails to generate sustained political or social change. To the extent that moral outrage is driven by principled moral rules, the presence of concrete barriers to action may undermine the abstract values that could otherwise call individuals to heroic action. It is clear that anger can drive actions like protest (e.g., Jost et al., 2012), but in the digital age outrage is often expressed in less disruptive ways, like posting on a private feed (Brady & Crockett, 2019). More substantively, this perspective suggests that a more concrete mindset or other disruption to the abstract principles that undergird moral outrage may reduce its impact as a means of securing a moral self-image. For example, consideration of the villain's motives or extenuating factors may force individuals to adopt less morally rigid perceptions that undermine both outrage and its impacts described above.

Heroes, Villains, Sidekicks, and Audiences

Although we have focused on moral outrage's intraindividual effects on existential needs, it is ultimately a social emotion that can be felt only within dyadic (or larger) relational contexts. Our research has had little to say about outrage's place in the social environment beyond noting that context affords targets able to serve as outlets for self-serving outrage. Larger questions about moral outrage's place in politics, social media, education, or other social contexts could draw critical lessons from an existential perspective. The research reviewed previously explored how moral outrage props up both anxiety-reducing perceptions of enemies and affirming perspectives of the self. The inevitability of existential concerns may help explain both the enduring presence of moral outrage in society and variations across groups, contexts, and eras. For example, the analysis reviewed above suggests that moral outrage may be a particularly alluring psychological defense among those who experience less control or have higher proneness to guilt (e.g., Quiles & Bybee, 1997).

Social media bears particular mention given the importance of having a viable enemy who could plausibly bear responsibility for evil (e.g., Rothschild et al., 2012). In a more restricted information environment, individuals may not have many known enemies capable of serving as viable targets for moral outrage. In contrast, social media provides an almost unlimited pool of outrage candidates (e.g., Crockett, 2017). While proposing a link between social media and outrage is hardly a novel insight, an existential perspective can shed light on why people devote so much time and energy to reading about unpleasant things and people online. After all, it is counterintuitive that people would choose to spend time watching videos of police killings or reading about despised public figures. The work in this chapter suggests that all this unpleasantness addresses vital existential needs for a positive self-image and sense of meaning that may ultimately diminish mortality concerns. As Green and colleagues (2019) observed, individuals who bolstered their moral self-perceptions through outrage also tended to seek out information to sustain feelings of outrage. What draws people to unpleasant information is, in part, a need to feel heroic in a digital age that is increasingly isolating individuals behind screens and abstract systems for interaction (e.g., reactions, ratings; Turkle, 2012).

One of the things that makes heroism valuable from a Beckerian perspective is that it can be a route to symbolic immortality; but the hidden requirement is that heroism be public enough that individuals can establish their memory in the minds of others. In other words, heroism's worth to the individual is derived in part from its social validity in the eyes of others. In our experimental research thus far, we have focused on either universally despised targets (e.g., sweatshop labor; Rothschild et al., 2017) or relied on naturally occurring groups that carry at least some social validity for the individual (e.g., political parties; Rothschild et al., 2021). Much more work remains to be done in unpacking senses of moral outrage in more pluralistic or extreme contexts. For instance, research on perpetrators of mass violence consistently observes a common desire for personal significance and/or a wish to be remembered as a martyr or hero (Knoll, 2010; Kruglanski et al., 2013; Langman, 2020). These perceptions are commonly propped up by grandiose beliefs that others would come to see the killer's perspective eventually, even if they could not at the time of the violence. For example, Dylan Roof believed that after killing nine people, his actions in defense of White supremacy would be widely lauded and that he would be pardoned and appointed to governor of the state of South Carolina (*United States of America v. Dylan Storm Roof*, 2016, cited in Langman, 2020). Even in extreme cases like these, heroism is not merely in the eye of the beholder; perception of a heroic legacy requires acceptance and social validation by a real or imagined audience.

CONCLUSION

In this chapter we explored how moral outrage plays a critical role in addressing existential concerns through the vehicle of heroism. Following Becker's notion that individuals have a drive toward heroism to address death anxiety, we focused on the ways that enemies—and anger toward those enemies—support the individual's sense of their own heroism. The evidence reviewed above suggests that this drive to achieve a heroic self-image may lead us to seek out villains, against whom our outrage may serve as a testament to our own righteousness and provide us with the purpose, certainty, direction, and control necessary to don a mantle of heroism that elevates everyday action to the moral and transcendental.

Experimental evidence clearly establishes that needs for external control and meaning are addressed by anger toward focal enemies and further that individuals can maintain a sense of their own moral value through opposition to perceived sources of evil. Despite how commonplace outrage about perceived injustice may be in daily life, its use may, in many cases, be addressing fundamental human concerns about meaning, self-esteem, control, and perhaps in a more abstract way, death. Existential psychology could benefit from greater consideration of the ways that everyday efforts at personal heroism reflect ongoing projects to live lives free of the deluge of anxieties that accompany self-awareness.

For those who are concerned about outrage, the research in this chapter speaks to the importance of existential security as a means of defusing its worst excesses. To the extent that people rage against others to address existential concerns, alternative routes to meaning, control, and value may all help in various contexts to turn down the temperature in various situations. With that being said, the fact that outrage and heroism address so many existential needs may mean that applying this knowledge requires sensitivity to the motives behind specific expressions. Enhancing individuals' sense of meaning in life may do little to reduce polarization among those seeking control or personal moral value through an enemy (see Rothschild & Keefer, 2023).

At this stage, the research on moral outrage points toward its many roles but raises many questions about why people may opt to rely on moral outrage over other strategies for addressing existential concerns. Because moral outrage is expressed in interpersonal contexts, often to those sharing the self's views, it may be that the ultimate causes lie outside the individual in cultural norms about the acceptability of outrage as a psychological strategy. Nevertheless, the role of deep personal concerns has been grounded in several compelling lines of research that point toward the need for much greater attention in future work.

REFERENCES

Allison, S. T., & Goethals, G. R. (2015). Hero worship: The elevation of the human spirit. *Journal for the Theory of Social Behavior, 46*(2), 187–210.

Alper, S. (2018). An abstract mind is a principled one: Abstract mindset increases consistency in responses to political attitude scales. *Journal of Experimental Social Psychology, 77,* 89–101.

Alper, S. (2020). Explaining the complex effect of construal level on moral and political attitudes. *Current Directions in Psychological Science, 29*(2), 115–120.

Arkon, W. M. (2021, December 23). Exclusive: Classified documents reveal the number of January 6 protestors. *Newsweek.* www.newsweek.com/exclusive-classified-documents-reveal-number-january-6-protestors-1661296.

Batson, C. D., Kennedy, C. L., Nord, L. A., Stocks, E. L., Fleming, D. Y. A., Marzette, C. M., . . . Zerger, T. (2007). Anger at unfairness: Is it moral outrage? *European Journal of Social Psychology, 37*(6), 1272–1285.

Baumeister, R. F. (1991). *Meanings of life.* Guilford Press.

Brady, W. J., & Crockett, M. J. (2019). How effective is online outrage? *Trends in Cognitive Sciences, 23*(2), 79–80.

Bronk, K. C., & Riches, B. R. (2017). The intersection of purpose and heroism. In S. T. Allison, R. Kramer, & G. Goethals (Eds.), *Handbook of heroism and heroic leadership* (pp. 495–506). Routledge.

Becker, E. (1973). *Denial of death.* Free Press.

Becker, E. (1975). *Escape from evil.* Free Press.

Campbell, J. (1949). *The hero with a thousand faces.* Princeton University Press.

Campbell, J. D., Trapnell, P. D., Heine, S. J., Katz, I. M., Lavallee, L. F., & Lehman, D. R. (1996). Self-concept clarity: Measurement, personality correlates, and cultural boundaries. *Journal of Personality and Social Psychology, 70*(1), 141–156.

Carver, C. S., & Harmon-Jones, E. (2009). Anger is an approach-related affect: Evidence and implications. *Psychological Bulletin, 135*(2), 183–204.

Crockett, M. J. (2017). Moral outrage in the digital age. *Nature Human Behavior, 1,* 769–771.

Dakin, B. C., Laham, S. M., Tan, N. P. J., & Bastian, B. (2021). Searching for meaning is associated with costly prosociality. *PLOS One, 16*(10), 1–25.

Ellsworth, P. C., & Scherer, K. R. (2003). Appraisal processes in emotion. In R. J. Davidson, K. R. Scherer, & H. H. Goldsmith (Eds.), *Handbook of affective sciences* (pp. 572–595). Oxford University Press.

Estrada-Hollenbeck, M., & Heatherton, T. F. (1998). Avoiding and alleviating guilt through prosocial behavior. In J. Bybee (Ed.), *Guilt and children* (pp. 215–231). Academic Press.

Eyal, T., & Liberman, N. (2012). Morality and psychological distance: A construal level theory perspective. In M. Mikulincer & P. R. Shaver (Eds.), *The social psychology of morality: Exploring the causes of good and evil* (pp. 185–202). American Psychological Association.

Eyal, T., Liberman, N., & Trope, Y. (2008). Judging near and distant virtue and vice. *Journal of Experimental Social Psychology, 44*(4), 1204–1209.

Fiske, S. T., Cuddy, A. J., Glick, P., & Xu, J. (2018). A model of (often mixed) stereotype content: Competence and warmth respectively follow from perceived status and competition. In S. T. Fiske (Ed.), *Social cognition* (pp. 162–214). Routledge.

Frankl, V. E. (1981). *The will to meaning: Foundations and applications of logotherapy.* New American Library. (Original work published 1969)

Fuhrer, J., & Cova, F. (2023). What makes a life meaningful?: Folk intuitions about the content and shape of meaningful lives. *Philosophical Psychology, 36*(3), 477–509.

George, L. S., & Park, C. L. (2014). Existential mattering: bringing attention to a neglected but central aspect of meaning? In A. Batthyany & P. Russo-Netzer (Eds.) *Meaning in positive and existential psychology* (pp. 39–51). Springer.

George, L. S., & Park, C. L. (2016). Meaning in life as comprehension, purpose, and mattering: the promise of a tripartite conceptual model. *Review of General Psychology, 20,* 205–220.

Green, J. D., Sedikides, C., Van Tongeren, D. R., Behler, A. M., & Barber, J. M. (2019). Self-enhancement, righteous anger, and moral grandiosity. *Self and Identity, 18*(2), 201–216.

Green, J. D., Van Tongeren, D. R., Cairo, A. H.,

& Hagiwara, N. (2017). Heroism and the pursuit of meaning. In S. T. Allison, G. R. Goethals, & R. M. Kramer (Eds.) *Handbook of heroism and heroic leadership* (pp. 529–546). Routledge.

Greenberg, J., Pyszczynski, T., Solomon, S., Simon, L., & Breus, M. (1994). The role of consciousness and accessibility of death-related thoughts in mortality salience effects. *Journal of Personality and Social Psychology, 67,* 627–637.

Greenberg, J., Solomon, S., Pyszczynski, T., Rosenblatt, A., Burling, J., Lyon, D., . . . Pinel, E. (1992). Why do people need self-esteem?: Converging evidence that self-esteem serves an anxiety-buffering function. *Journal of Personality and Social Psychology, 63,* 913–922.

Greenberg, J., Vail, K., & Pyszczynski, T. (2014). Terror management theory and research: How the desire for death transcendence drives our strivings for meaning and significance. *Advances in Motivation Science, 1,* 85–134.

Guenther, C. L., Zhang, Y., & Sedikides, C. (2023). The authentic self is the self-enhancing self: A self-enhancement framework of authenticity. *Personality and Social Psychology Bulletin,* 1–15.

Igou, E. R., Van Tilburg, W. A., Kinsella, E. L., & Buckley, L. K. (2018). On the existential road from regret to heroism: Searching for meaning in life. *Frontiers in Psychology, 9,* 1–10.

Jost, J. T., Chaikalis-Petritsis, V., Abrams, D., Sidanius, J., van der Toorn, J., & Bratt, C. (2012). Why men (and women) do and don't rebel: Effects of system justification on willingness to protest. *Personality and Social Psychology Bulletin, 38*(2), 197–208.

Jung, C. G. (1959). *The archetypes and the collective unconscious.* Princeton University Press.

Kinsella, E. L., Ritchie, T. D., & Igou, E. R. (2015a). Lay perspectives on the social and psychological functions of heroes. *Frontiers in Psychology, 6,* 1–12.

Kinsella, E. L., Ritchie, T. D., & Igou, E. R. (2015b). Zeroing in on heroes: A prototype analysis of hero features. *Journal of Personality and Social Psychology, 108*(1), 114–127.

Kinsella, E. L., Igou, E. R., & Ritchie, T. D. (2019). Heroism and the pursuit of a meaningful life. *Journal of Humanistic Psychology, 59*(4), 474–498.

Klein, N. (2017). Prosocial behavior increases perceptions of meaning in life. *Journal of Positive Psychology, 12*(4), 354–361.

Knoll, J. L. (2010). The "pseudocommando" mass murder: Part I, the psychology of revenge and obliteration. *Journal of the American Academy of Psychiatry and the Law, 38*(1), 87–94.

Kruglanski, A. W., Bélanger, J. J., Gelfand, M., Gunaratna, R., Hettiarachchi, M., Reinares, F., . . . Sharvit, K. (2013). Terrorism—A (self) love story: Redirecting the significance quest can end violence. *American Psychologist, 68*(7), 559–575.

Landau, M. J., Kay, A. C., & Whitson, J. A. (2015). Compensatory control and the appeal of a structured world. *Psychological Bulletin, 141*(3), 694–722.

Langman, P. (2020). Desperate identities: A bio-psycho-social analysis of perpetrators of mass violence. *Criminology and Public Policy, 19*(1), 61–84.

Leach, C. W., Ellemers, N., & Barreto, M. (2007). Group virtue: The importance of morality (vs. competence and sociability) in the positive evaluation of in-groups. *Journal of Personality and Social Psychology, 93*(2), 234.

Luhtanen, R., & Crocker, J. (1992). A collective self-esteem scale: Self-evaluation of one's social identity. *Personality and Social Psychology Bulletin, 18*(3), 302–318.

Martela, F., & Steger, M. F. (2016). The three meanings of meaning in life: Distinguishing coherence, purpose, and significance. *Journal of Positive Psychology, 11*(5), 531–545.

McCabe, S., Carpenter, R. W., & Arndt, J. (2015). The role of mortality awareness in heroic enactment. *Journal of Experimental Social Psychology, 61,* 104–109.

McCabe, S., Carpenter, R. W., & Arndt, J. (2016). The role of mortality awareness in hero identification. *Self and Identity, 15*(6), 707–726.

McKay, R., Herold, J., & Whitehouse, H. (2013). Catholic guilt?: Recall of confession promotes prosocial behavior. *Religion, Brain and Behavior, 3*(3), 201–209.

Motro, D., & Sullivan, D. (2017). Could two negative emotions be a positive?: The effects of anger and anxiety in enemyship. *Journal of Experimental Social Psychology, 69,* 130–143.

Prentice, M., Jayawickreme, E., Hawkins, A., Hartley, A., Furr, R. M., & Fleeson, W. (2019). Morality as a basic psychological need. *Social Psychological and Personality Science, 10*(4), 449–460.

Pyszczynski, T., Greenberg, J., Solomon, S., Arndt, J., & Schimel, J. (2004). Why do people need self-esteem?: A theoretical and empirical review. *Psychological Bulletin, 130*(3), 435–468.

Quiles, Z. N., & Bybee, J. (1997). Chronic and predispositional guilt: Relations to mental health, prosocial behavior, and religiosity. *Journal of Personality Assessment, 69*(1), 104–126.

Rothschild, Z. K., Hauri, J., & Keefer, L. A. (2020). Specific phobias: Maintaining control in the face of chaotic threats. *Journal of Social and Clinical Psychology, 39*(5), 383–418.

Rothschild, Z. K., & Hugee, M. (2025). Demotivating justice: White Americans' outrage at individual bigotry may reduce action to address systematic racial inequity. *Personality and Social Psychology Bulletin.*

Rothschild, Z. K., & Keefer, L. A. (2017). A cleansing fire: Moral outrage alleviates guilt and buffers threats to one's moral identity. *Motivation and Emotion, 41*(2), 209–229.

Rothschild, Z. K., & Keefer, L. A. (2018). Righteous or self-righteous anger?: Justice sensitivity moderates defensive outrage at a third-party harmdoer. *European Journal of Social Psychology, 48*(4), 507–522.

Rothschild, Z. K., & Keefer, L. A. (2022). Meaningful outrage: Anger at injustice bolsters meaning for justice sensitive individuals. *European Journal of Social Psychology, 52,* 124–146.

Rothschild, Z. K., & Keefer, L. A. (2023). Who scapegoats?: Individual differences moderate the dual-motive model of scapegoating. *Journal of Research in Personality, 105*, 104400

Rothschild, Z. K., Keefer, L. A., & Hauri, J. (2021) Defensive partisanship?: Evidence that in-party scandals increase out-group hostility. *Political Psychology, 42*(1), 3–21.

Rothschild, Z. K., Landau, M. J., Molina, L. E., Branscombe, N. R., & Sullivan, D. (2013). Displacing blame over the ingroup's harming of a disadvantaged group can fuel moral outrage at a third-party scapegoat. *Journal of Experimental Social Psychology, 49*(5), 898–906.

Rothschild, Z. K., Landau, M. J., Sullivan, D., & Keefer, L. A. (2012). A dual-motive model of scapegoating: Displacing blame to reduce guilt or increase control. *Journal of Personality and Social Psychology, 102,* 1148–1163.

Schlegel, R. J., Hicks, J. A., Arndt, J., & King, L. A. (2009). Thine own self: true self-concept accessibility and meaning in life. *Journal of Personality and Social Psychology, 96*(2), 473–490.

Schöpfer, C., Abatista, A. G. F., Fuhrer, J., & Cova, F. (2023). "Where there are villains, there will be heroes": Belief in conspiracy theories as an existential tool to fulfill need for meaning. *Personality and Individual Differences, 200.*

Shin, J. Y., Steger, M. F., & Henry, K. L. (2016). Self-concept clarity's role in meaning in life among American college students: A latent growth approach. *Self and Identity, 15*(2), 206–223.

Smaliukienė, R., Bekesiene, S., Kanapeckaitė, R., & Meidutė-Kavaliauskienė, I. (2023). Meaning in military service among reservists: Measuring the effect of prosocial motivation in a moderated-mediation model. *Frontiers in Psychology, 14.*

Solomon, R. C. (2007). *True to our feelings: What our emotions are really telling us.* Oxford University Press.

Strohminger, N., Knobe, J., & Newman, G. (2017). The true self: A psychological concept distinct from the self. *Perspectives on Psychological Science, 12*(4), 551–560.

Sullivan, D., Landau, M. J., & Kay, A. C. (2016). When enemies go viral (or not)—A real-time experiment during the "Stop Kony" campaign. *Psychology of Popular Media Culture, 5*(1), 15–26.

Sullivan, D., Landau, M. J., & Rothschild, Z. K. (2010). An existential function of enemyship: Evidence that people attribute influence to personal and political enemies to compensate for threats to control. *Journal of Personality and Social Psychology, 98,* 434–449.

Täuber, S., & van Zomeren, M. (2013). Outrage towards whom?: Threats to moral group status impede striving to improve via out-group-directed outrage. *European Journal of Social Psychology, 43*(2), 149–159.

Turkle, S. (2012). *Alone together: Why we expect more from technology and less from each other.* Basic Books.

Van der Toorn, J., Ellemers, N., & Doosje, B. (2015). The threat of moral transgression: The impact of group membership and moral opportunity. *European Journal of Social Psychology, 45*(5), 609–622.

Van Tongeren, D. R., Green, J. D., Davis, D. E., Hook, J. N., & Hulsey, T. L. (2016). Prosociality enhances meaning in life. *Journal of Positive Psychology, 11*(3), 225–236.

Waterman, A. S. (1993). Two conceptions of happiness: Contrasts of personal expressiveness (eudaimonia) and hedonic enjoyment. *Journal of Personality and Social Psychology, 64*(4), 678–691.

CHAPTER 38

Life in Plastic, Not So Fantastic

A Barbie-Informed Feminist Existential Perspective on the Objectification of Women

Jamie L. Goldenberg, Tomi-Ann Roberts, *and* Roxanne N. Felig

In the film *Barbie*, directed by Greta Gerwig (2023), life in plastic is fantastic—that is, until midway through a euphoric dance number, when Barbie blurts out "Do you guys ever think about dying?" The music screeches to a halt and the next morning Barbie's natural body asserts itself, with bad breath, flat feet, and even cellulite. Death awareness and imperfect bodies have no place in Barbieland, and so, Barbie embarks on a journey to restore her perfectly arched feet and abandon her irrepressible thoughts of death. In a recent commentary in the feminist magazine *Ms.*, Roberts and Goldenberg (2024) suggested that this film can be viewed as a cinematic depiction of feminist existential theory on the objectification of women.

Feminist scholars (e.g., de Beauvoir, 1949/1989) have pointed the finger at the patriarchy as an underlying cause of women's objectification. We agree, but with an added existential twist. As highlighted in this volume, and in research on terror management theory (Greenberg et al., 1986; Solomon et al., 2015), investment in sociocultural beliefs systems, including patriarchy, can be understood as serving an important psychological function—death denial. We maintain that this is true especially with respect to the treatment of women and their bodies (Goldenberg & Roberts, 2004, 2010). Objectification dehumanizes women and strips them of their autonomy (Nussbaum, 2001), but in doing so, it also provides an existential perk: Objects, like Barbies, cannot die (Goldenberg, 2013). In this chapter we examine objectification through this feminist existential lens, suggesting that patriarchal control of women's bodies works in tandem with existential concerns rooted in the awareness of death. We conclude by considering some recent work suggesting that, perhaps, women can turn the tides of patriarchy, and the consequences of objectification, through autonomous, self-determined motivation (Felig & Goldenberg, 2024).

THE BODY AS AN EXISTENTIAL THREAT

In contrast to Barbie dolls, for whom death and genitals do not exist, in the real world, and for real women, they do. We suggest this as a starting point for our feminist existential perspective on the objectification of women. The management of existential concerns, from the perspective of terror management theory, involves embedding oneself into a meaningful, and symbolic, cultural existence, in a sense severing the connection to the natural, animal world. In the words of Ernest Becker (1973), whose *Denial of Death* laid the theoretical groundwork for terror management theory, human beings are "out of nature and hopelessly in it" "up in the stars and yet housed in a heart-pumping, breath-gasping body . . . material fleshy casing that is alien to *him* in many ways—the strangest and most repugnant way being that it aches and bleeds and will decay and die" (p. 26). To the extent that human beings grapple with concerns about their mortality, the physical body, in all its frailty, poses a problem. Not only does the body die, but if one is fortunate enough to live for 80 or so years, it dies slowly, oozing life and bodily fluids along the way.

Empirical research derived from terror management theory provides evidence that most of us are deeply unsettled by the physical aspects of the body, and that existential concerns fuel this discomfort (Goldenberg, 2012; Goldenberg et al., 2000). Using a terror management paradigm, where people are reminded of their mortality (mortality salience) and reactions are observed, one sees an increase in how disgusting people find natural bodily functions, such as using the toilet (Goldenberg et al., 2001). And this applies not just to potty behavior, but to more agreeable physical acts as well. Priming mortality salience leads people to report less interest in the physical aspects of sex (Goldenberg et al., 1999) and other pleasurable physical sensations (e.g., a foot massage, Goldenberg et al., 2006). Demonstrating that this existential threat is associated with concerns about being a physical creature, a number of experiments incorporate a human creatureliness manipulation (an essay describing the similarities between humans and other animals) and find that this, alone or in combination with mortality salience, increases these negative reactions to the body (Cox et al., 2007b; Goldenberg et al., 2002). Research also supports bidirectionality in this relationship between our embodied lives and existential threat, revealing that thoughts of death become more accessible when people are reminded of the body and sex (Cox et al., 2007b; Goldenberg et al., 1999, 2002).

Our feminist existential perspective posits that while all bodies are existentially troubling, women's bodies, and their unique bodily functions, are especially problematic. As Camille Paglia (1990, p. 9) noted, "nature's burden falls more heavily on one sex." Evolutionary psychologists have observed this same imbalance with respect to women's and men's unequal contribution to the reproduction of the species: years of menstruation, 9 months of pregnancy, and weeks, months or even years of lactating breasts, for women, compared to an obligatory bodily contribution that can be measured in minutes for men. This, in the context of the patriarchy, where men have the power to decide which aspects of humanity are celebrated and which are condemned, creates the perfect recipe for the stigmatization of women's reproductive functions.

In our research examining reactions to women's menstruation (Roberts et al., 2002), both men and women viewed a woman as less competent and less likable when she appeared to inadvertently drop a wrapped tampon out of her backpack, compared to an equally feminine but less offensive hair barrette, and the presence of the tampon led participants to distance themselves physically from the woman, sitting further away from her. Similarly, customers portrayed as pregnant (wearing a pregnancy prosthesis) faced more hostile behavior by store employees than did women portrayed as not pregnant (Hebl et al., 2007). Additionally, women depicted as posing with their bare pregnant belly on display, compared to their pregnant belly covered, were perceived as lower in humanness, and this in turn contributed to the belief that these women would be unfit mothers and should be denied financial support (Ligman et al., 2025). Moreover, supporting not just our feminist position, but also the existential position, reminders of mortality have exacerbated negative reactions to women's reproductive functions, such as in response to a scenario depicting a woman breastfeeding her infant in public (Cox et al., 2007a). Mortality reminders also decreased how much participants reported liking, and how close they positioned their chairs in anticipation of meeting, a task partner described as breastfeeding (versus bottle feeding) in another room (Cox et al., 2007a). Mortality salience in conjunction with a breastfeeding prime also served to increase cognitions associated with human creatureliness (Cox et al., 2007a), and priming human creatureliness increased disapproval of pregnant, compared to nonpregnant, images of actresses Demi Moore and Gwyneth Paltrow (Goldenberg et al., 2007).

Given this research, it is not surprising that Barbie dolls, despite being adult women with breasts and hips, lack identifiable genitalia and nipples. As well, among the myriad "specialty" Barbie dolls to hit the market, Midge, the pregnant Barbie, and Growing Up Skipper, whose breasts developed by pumping her arm, did not sell well and were discontinued. Menstruating Barbie would be, of course, out of the question. Such poor-selling and even inconceivable Barbies are Mattel's illustration of our existential, feminist claim that women's bodies pose a particular problem that is fueled by mortality concerns, which may be alleviated through objectification.

AN EXISTENTIAL FUNCTION OF THE OBJECTIFICATION OF WOMEN

Building on the terror management framework, Goldenberg and Roberts (2004, 2010) argued that in the same way concerns surrounding physical death are managed symbolically, though investment in meaningful cultural worldviews, the threat associated with women's bodies is managed by transforming the physical body into a cultural symbol. Women's bodies are stripped of the threatening association with reproduction and held to high standards of beauty and perfection. Consider the frequency with which viewers are ever shown an ad for a menstrual product that depicts a woman experiencing premenstrual symptoms, or which uses real or any fluid resembling menstrual blood to demonstrate product effectiveness. Mostly viewers are regaled with mysterious blue liquid poured onto panty liners and smiling, active young women wearing white clothing. In fact, a content analysis of menstrual product advertisements found that idealized, but not overly sexualized, depictions of women in menstrual product advertisements were common, offering support that the threat of women's bodies may be quelled through objectification (Erchull, 2013).

In the previously described tampon-drop study (Roberts et al., 2002), the woman who dropped the tampon was not only viewed more negatively, but participants in the tampon condition reported that they thought it was more important for a woman to be beautiful than competent relative to participants who witnessed the dropping of a hair barrette. In other research, mortality primes have been shown to increase how important appearance is for other women (Grabe et al., 2005). It is no surprise, from this perspective, that one sees gendered cultural expectations of body hair removal, perfectly applied makeup, and restrictive clothing meant to look good, rather than feel good, such that media depictions of women's bodies are curated and controlled so as to not be existentially problematic. The increased interest in plastic surgery during the pandemic is perhaps also consistent with this position (Lem et al., 2023; Liu et al., 2021). Evidence that women's appearance becomes more important in the light of existential concerns supports the premise that the objectification of women can be a response to existential concerns; but, we suggest, it does not stop there.

Objectification involves not just a focus on appearance over other aspects of human bodies, but philosophical treatises on objectification (Kant, 1963; Langton, 2009; Nussbaum, 1995) argue that this way of viewing and treating others goes beyond the figurative, transforming them into *things* that assume qualities of objects in a literal sense. Consistent with this, when observers focus on a woman's appearance, they tend to perceive her as less characteristic of what it means to be human. Heflick and Goldenberg (2009) instructed male and female participants to focus on the appearance of a famous woman (Sarah Palin or Angelina Jolie), compared to focusing on the person herself, and found that this led participants to perceive the target as lower in the characteristics that they associated with human nature (cf. Haslam, 2006) and as less competent. In the 2008 election, a focus on vice presidential candidate Sarah Palin's appearance reduced intentions to vote for the

McCain-Palin ticket, and this effect was mediated by perceptions of her competence and human nature (Helfick & Goldenberg, 2009). Notably, these same results do not occur when men are the targets. In another series of studies (Heflick et al., 2011), female targets, including Michelle Obama, but not male targets, including Barack Obama, were perceived as less competent, warm, and moral (traits associated with perceptions of humanness, Gray et al., 2007; Harris & Fiske, 2009; Haslam, 2006) when participants were instructed to focus on their appearance.

Other research converges with this idea that objectification of others results in increased attributions of *thing*-ness (Bernard et al., 2012; Fiske et al., 2007), which, with a few exceptions (Loughnan et al., 2010), is found to be especially true when the targets are women. Cognitively, sexualized women—but not men—are processed in a manner more similar to objects than to humans (e.g., recognized equally well upside down as right-side-up; see Bernard et al., 2012; Gervais et al., 2012). Other research investigating neural patterns finds that objectified women, more so than objectified men, are perceived more similarly to doll-like objects (Vaes et al., 2019). This research converges to support the position that when objectified, women are literally perceived as things, much like Barbie dolls.

As objects cannot suffer, feel pain, or have subjective experiences, people may make the same inferences when objectifying women. Morris and colleagues (2018) tested this empirically, finding that in response to a social media profile in which a woman's appearance was prominent, with a focus on beauty and fashion, participants objectified her—that is, they attributed to her fewer of the qualities associated with human nature. This, in turn, promoted a perception of the woman as less able to feel pain, with participants reporting that they thought the woman would feel less pain in response to such experiences as a root canal or burning her hand on a hot stove. It follows that if objectified women are perceived as less able to feel the pain of a root canal, then this might set the stage for a willingness to harm them, or to be less concerned when they are harmed. Consistent with this, correlational evidence has documented an association between objectification of women and violence against them (Johnson et al., 2018). Loughnan and colleagues (2010) found that participants self-reported more willingness to give "pain-causing pills" to an objectified target, and subsequently reported less concern for the target when she was harmed, and going beyond a hypothetical scenario, Vasquez and colleagues (2017) found that participants subjected an objectified woman to more pain by determining longer amounts of time for her to submerge her hand in ice cold water.

A number of experiments have demonstrated that the perception of humanness, or rather, a lack of it, is instrumental in these outcomes. In an investigation of online harassment (Ligman et al., 2025), participants viewed mock social media profiles of the same woman shown in either an objectified or a nonobjectified way and later learned she had experienced online sexual aggression. Participants were more tolerant of aggression depicted against a woman and were more likely to engage in a hostile behavior toward her (sending her a harassing message), when her Instagram profile was highly sexualized. Critically, participants' denial of the woman's human-like qualities, such as the ability to think analytically, explained these tendencies. In the context of a physical domestic violence incident, participants rated an objectified women as experiencing less physical and emotional pain and suffering, despite learning that she had been thrown against a wall and showed visible bruising (Felig et al., 2023). These perceptions were explained by participants' association of the woman with literal objects, not with animals, which is consistent with theorizing, and other research (Morris et al., 2018) demonstrating that if objects cannot suffer, neither can objectified women.

Sexually objectifying teenage and very young preteen girls can carry the same consequences in terms of denial of their personhood and hence poor regard for their well-being. In a study of adolescents, Vasquez and colleagues (2016) found that higher scores on a measure of sexual objectification (e.g., "Girls are only good for their body") predicted greater aggression toward girls as well as gang affiliation. In an experimental study, Holland and Haslam (2016) compared adults' views of girls depicted in clothing advertisements in a two-piece swimsuit, compared with a track suit, and found that when asked to consider the target girl's experience of bullying, adults rated the scantily clad girl as more responsible for the behavior that harmed her, and less in need of adult intervention or sympathy. Similarly, Pacilli and colleagues (2019) found that when a girl was the victim of bullying and portrayed as sexualized, compared to nonsexualized, helping intentions were reduced as a function of her dehumanization.

Notably, from the perspective of our feminist existential theorizing, men are not merely innocent bystanders, recipients of objectifying media and influenced by it. Rather, their own existential concerns compel them to seek out objectifying content. Building on research by Landau and colleagues (2006) showing that reminders of mortality reduce men's reported attraction to a sexually seductive woman, Morris and Goldenberg (2015) examined whether the literal objectification of a woman's body might remediate this threat and make for an existentially safer attraction to women. Men were primed with mortality salience and presented with a product advertisement featuring a sexualized woman (e.g., a Budweiser beer model) either merged with a literal object (i.e., as if she were the label on the beer bottle), or separate from the object (i.e., the same woman next to the beer bottle). Replicating the results of Landau and colleagues (2006), when heterosexual men were primed with death, they reported finding the sexualized woman less attractive when she was presented as separate from the object. Moreover, literal objectification not only reduced this effect, but completely reversed it: In response to a mortality prime, men reported that the same woman merged with the beer bottle was *more* attractive, compared to men in the control condition. In other research, mortality reminders increased men's attractiveness ratings, not of real women, but of female mannequins (Goldenberg & Morris, 2016), similar to Barbie dolls. Additionally, men who objectify women attribute reduced humanness toward their own female partners, which then predicted a greater likelihood of enacting intimate partner violence against them (Sáez et al., 2020).

These findings converge to suggest a chilling conclusion: Objectified women and girls are not simply valued for their appearance; rather, they are perceived and treated as lacking the very qualities that make them human and alive. They are reduced to *things* to be instrumentalized and toyed with, like Barbie dolls, or even harmed. In the Barbie film, Barbieland is a place of blissful eternal recurrence, where Barbies hold the power, serving as president, doctors, and supreme court justices, and Kens are "just Ken." But after death awareness sets in, and a foray to the real world introduces Kens to patriarchy in the form of the all-male executive board of Mattel, and horses, Barbieland's Kens subvert the gendered power to their benefit, now objectifying Barbies as those with existential knowledge of death are motivated to do.

WOMEN'S SELF-OBJECTIFICATION THROUGH A FEMINIST EXISTENTIAL LENS

In a stark contrast to Barbieland, where women hold power and are valued for their intellect and capabilities, reality thrusts Barbie into the world of the male gaze and patriarchy, where she suddenly experiences what it's like to be looked at and treated as a body meant for visual consumption. "Why are these men looking at me?" she remarks as catcalls, whistles, and comments about her appearance are hurled her way. "I feel kind of ill at ease. I don't know the word for it, but I'm conscious, but it's myself that I'm conscious of." The word that Barbie is looking for is *self-objectification.*

Objectification theory (Fredrickson & Roberts, 1997) posits that objectifying treatment and exposure to chronic cultural depictions of objectified women leads many women and girls to internalize an objectifying perspective on their bodies, becoming preoccupied with their physical appearance as a way of anticipating their treatment in a sexualizing and objectifying world. Cognitive developmental theories of gender development (e.g., Warin, 2000) argue that once children understand their membership in a gender category, they value the behaviors, appearance norms, attitudes, and objects associated with their gender, and align themselves accordingly. Sexually objectified, genital-less and nipple-less Barbie dolls serve as aspirational models of femininity for girls, and playing with them surely solidifies self-objectification as an essential component of "succeeding" in a feminine gender (Roberts, 2013). Consistently, Starr and Ferguson (2012) found that when presented with sexualized, adult dolls like Barbie or Bratz, versus nonsexualized paper dolls, 6- to 9-year-old girls indicated that they wished they looked like the sexy doll and thought that this doll would be more popular at school and have more friends and more kids wishing to sit next to her at the lunch table than the nonsexualized paper doll would.

After Barbies are no longer fun to play with, much research supports that the more teen girls and young adult women consume sexually objectifying cultural content like fashion magazines, blogs, or social media, the more they endorse sexiness as of primary importance in judging women's value, and the more they self-objectify (e.g., Ward, 2002, 2016). But self-objectification and its associated "body projects" of disciplining the body and mind to align with cultural standards of Barbie-style appearance carries a host of behavioral, cognitive, and emotional consequences, from feelings of shame, anxiety, and depression to sexual dysfunction and disordered eating, which has been demonstrated over decades of research (Moradi & Huang, 2008; Roberts et al., 2018).

Our feminist existential perspective suggests that self-objectification serves the function for women themselves of psychic distancing from their own creaturely nature, and several studies have found that indeed the more women self-objectify, the more they feel emotions such as disgust and shame toward their bodies' reproductive functioning, including menstruation, and the more they tend to opt for menstrual suppression to eliminate their periods altogether (e.g., Johnston-Robledo et al., 2003, 2007; Roberts, 2004). Young women higher in self-objectification are less likely to seek preventative sexual and reproductive health care (Holland et al., 2020). Pregnant and postpartum women higher in self-objectification show more body shame, more concerns about the negative impact of breastfeeding on their bodies and sexuality, barriers to breastfeeding, and fear of childbirth (Beech et al., 2020).

Although the focus on women's appearance is the hallmark of objectification and objectification theory, classical theorizing about objectification (Kant, 1963; Nussbaum, 1995) suggests that objectification, quite literally, refers to viewing a person as more like an object and less like a human being. The same reasoning applies to the self, when women self-objectify. Just as women who are objectified by others are perceived as less capable of feeling emotional distress and experiencing physical pain (Felig et al., 2023), women who tend to objectify themselves feel less connected to their body (Piran et al., 2020) and have muted awareness of their emotions (Myers & Crowther, 2008). This disconnect from the self manifests in lab situations, where women high in self-objectification show difficulty accurately detecting their heartbeat (Ainley & Tsakiris, 2013), and in real-world settings, where unlike women low in self-objectification, women higher in self-objectification do not report feeling cold in relation to how much skin they have exposed (Felig et al., 2022). Just as objects do not feel physical or physiological sensations, it seems that self-objectification provides women with a respite from the sensation of being, which may serve an existential purpose, as objects cannot feel and do not die.

Morris and colleagues (2014) directly tested this feminist existential explanation of self-objectification, examining the tendency to perceive the self as an object in response to being primed with existential concerns and female reproduction. In a first study, when a mortality prime was coupled with an image of a pregnant (vs. nonpregnant) woman whose belly was exposed, female participants responded by placing more value on their own body's appearance, relative to its competence—that is, they self-objectified, as it is typically operationalized. Additionally, these women denied themselves of traits considered essential to human nature, effectively viewing themselves in terms more consistent with how one views objects (cf. Haslam, 2006). These responses were not observed among participants who were men. In a second study, women participants were asked by a female experimenter if they had a tampon (vs. a pencil). This, in conjunction with a mortality salience manipulation, did not increase the appearance emphasis; it did, however, lead participants to deny themselves traits essential to human nature, again replicating the "literal objectification" effect. These results suggest that although appearance striving might be an effective means to manage the threat of death in some circumstances (perhaps in response to pregnancy, a more appearance-relevant behavior than menstruation), literal (self) objectification offers a broader psychological protective function. Providing further evidence for literal self-objectification as an existential defense, women, but not men, responded to mortality salience and women's reproduction primes by implicitly and explicitly associating themselves with objects, and an explicit association of the self with objects functioned to reduce the amount of time participants spent writing about death.

While a disconnect from the physical body can, at times, prove existentially soothing, like any other psychological defense, including defenses against existential concerns, self-objectification comes at a cost. Women take a number of hits to their self-esteem, and their overall well-being (Breines et al., 2008), but with ever-changing appearance standards telling women what they should look like, women may constantly be changing themselves in response. Women high in self-objectification rely more heavily on external and sociocultural standards to define who they are (Fredrickson & Roberts, 1997; Vartanian, 2009), and also report a less stable, less well-defined sense of self (Cui & Fang, 2022). Recent empirical evidence confirms this relationship with an unclear sense of self, finding that high trait self-objectification (Felig & Goldenberg, 2024) as well as engaging in momentary objectifying behaviors (i.e., editing a selfie; Felig, 2020) is associated with lower self-concept clarity, whereby women know themselves less well. This suggests that self-objectification extends beyond internalizing an observer's perspective of the body and valuing one's appearance and involves a fundamental denial of self. When considered in line with our previous discussion of literal objectification, it appears that self-objectification can be literal, too, distancing women not just from their physical sensations, but from who they are as human beings.

Perhaps this is why Calogero (2013) found that woman who are high in self-objectification are less likely to question gender inequality—"objects don't object"—and why, when Ken brings the patriarchy to Barbieland, establishing Kendom, Barbies find relief in "giving their brains a break," by giving up their careers as doctors and supreme court members to wear bikinis and cheerleader's and maid's uniforms, serving their Kens brewskie beers and being a "helpful decoration."

TAKING BACK THE BODY AND SELF: SELF-DETERMINED APPEARANCE STRIVING

That women should renounce the patriarchal notion of feminine beauty is a central mantra of feminism (e.g., Bartky, 1988; Orbach, 2019; Wolf, 1991), and objectification theory and the surrounding research has come to the same conclusion, amassing a large literature to support that women are harmed by self-objectification and its relentless focus on physical appearance as one's primary pathway for personal esteem (cf. Roberts et al., 2018). But, at the risk of carrying our Barbie analysis too far, we do not think it coincidental that in Barbieland, before exposure to patriarchy, and death, the Barbies joyfully and autonomously decided not only what they wanted to do and be, but also how they wanted to look.

The importance of autonomy and "choice" is central in both feminist (Hirshman, 2006; see also Budgeon, 2015) and existential dialogue (e.g., Yalom, 1980). Whereas second wave feminism focused on the limitation in women's choices (e.g., Friedan, 1963), third wave feminists shifted the focus on the act of choosing, with the position of "choice feminism" (Hirshman, 2006) arguing that feminism should aim to validate not the contents of women's choices, but the act of choosing (see Budgeon, 2015, for a critique of this perspective). Likewise, the importance of choice and self-determination has been considered from the perspective of terror management theory (Pyszczynski et al., 2003), with research demonstrating that people are less defensive against the terror of death when the contents of their self-esteem are more intrinsic and self-determined (e.g., Vail et al., 2020).

Some suggestive work exists to support a connection between intrinsically motivated appearance striving and greater well-being.

For example, Pellizzer and colleagues (2016) found that recreational pole dancers scored lower in self-objectification than a comparison sample of university women. Further, for these recreational pole dancers, their enjoyment of sexualization directly and positively predicted greater embodiment, or awareness of and sense of connectedness with one's body. When this is contrasted with other research showing that professional exotic dancers have higher self-objectification and poorer self-esteem than nondancers (Downs et al., 2006), it points to the potential for intrinsically motivated pathways of sexualized body appreciation and well-being, where self-sexualizing "for fun" may yield better outcomes than doing so for extrinsic rewards such as pay. Another study examining the role of close relationships in young adult women's positive body image found that autonomous self-determined motivation messages around one's body, especially from mothers (e.g. "My mother encourages me to be healthy because it's fun"), significantly predicted body appreciation, whereas controlled motivation messages from mothers (e.g., "My mother encourages me to be healthy because then I will receive compliments") predicted body dissatisfaction (Arroyo et al., 2020).

Along these lines, Felig and Goldenberg (2025) recently turned to self-determination theory (Ryan & Deci, 2000) to examine the role of perceived autonomy in determining whether and under what conditions the pursuit of beauty and desirability harms women. This work offers preliminary evidence that perceptions of autonomy moderate the impact of self-objectifying behaviors on body shame and also clarity of the self-concept. In other research, feminist women, who report engaging in "beauty work" as much as women who do not identify as feminists (Siegel & Calogero, 2019), indicated a willingness to pay greater sums of money for premium beauty products because they view their decision to invest in their appearance as their own choice (Harrold et al., 2023). From the perspective of feminism and existentialism, "choice" is critical to well-being, and we suggest this is no less true when it comes to the behaviors that real women engage in to enhance their appearance.

Acknowledging that today's world affords women a universe of options for appearance enhancement, from cosmetics to surgery, feminist legal scholar Deborah Rhode (2016) has argued that, if "appearance is a feminist issue . . . then the women's movement must develop a concept of beauty that is a source of pleasure rather than shame, and that enhances, rather than dictates self-worth" (p. 697). We could not agree more. However, for such a dream of self-determined appearance striving to be realized, we must recognize that the contexts of such choices in the real world (unlike in Barbieland) are still sexist (Pollitt, 2007), and the standards are still overwhelmingly White, slender, smooth-skinned, and youthful (like Barbie). Schools, the workplace, and the court of public opinion raging on social media inequitably punish girls and women for the appearance choices they make, from sending African American girls home from school for their "natural" hair to Donald Trump demeaning the faces and bodies of his women rivals. Our job in exploring the benefits to well-being of girls' and women's self-determined pursuit of beauty must go hand in hand with critiquing the culture that dictates what constitutes "beautiful" and that inequitably ties one's gender's worth so tightly to it.

CONCLUSION

In seeking answers to why women are often objectified and why women objectify themselves, we turn to a position informed by both feminist and existential perspectives. This combined perspective offers explanations rooted in not only the patriarchal control of women's bodies but also the psychological protection it affords all of us humans, who find our creatureliness, and hence our mortality, concerning. The body of work using the empirical methods derived for psychological science from both terror management theory and objectification theory provides evidence that existential concerns make people uncomfortable with the physicality of the body, and this is especially true when it comes to the things that women's bodies do in the service of reproduction. In this threat, and the need to defend against it, we find an impetus for objectification, both of women by others and of women themselves. The focus on the external appearance of women's bodies leads to a view of women as *things*, literal objects like Barbie dolls. This harms them, but it also protects them, as it protects men. In this dynamic, quite cleverly illustrated by the *Barbie* movie, the roots of objectification can perhaps be better understood.

In moving beyond the terror, we suggest a solution rooted in both existentialism and feminism, where *choice* is the crux of the matter. We suggest that, along with feminist work on the collective level to fight for women's rights to their own bodily autonomy and choice (legal protections for reproductive rights and against sexual misconduct in the workplace and at school), a sense of personal autonomy for girls and women to dress and move their bodies as they wish may go a long way in protecting against the harms of objectification. Though we have no choice but to die, and, perhaps, no choice but to be threatened by this fact, we do have a choice as to how we respond to that threat.

The conclusion of the *Barbie* movie is an ideal place to end our chapter, where Barbie, holding hands with Ruth Handler, her creator, sees a vision of the ordinary lives of ordinary girls and women, making their own choices; some are wearing "a flattering top," some are fat and some are thin, some are old with wrinkled faces, who likely would respond, "I know it!" when told they're beautiful. Seeing this, Barbie says, "I want to be part of the people that make meaning, not the thing that's made. I want to do the imagining. I don't want to be the idea." Barbie makes her choice, no longer a doll, but a real woman. And her first stop? Obviously, the gynecologist.

REFERENCES

Ainley, V., & Tsakiris, M. (2013). Body conscious?: Interoceptive awareness, measured by heartbeat perception, is negatively correlated with self-objectification. *PLOS One, 8*, e55568.

Arroyo, A., Burke, T. J., & Young, V. J. (2020). The role of close relationships in promoting weight management and body image outcomes: An application of confirmation, self-determination, social control and social support. *Journal of Social and Personal Relationships, 37*, 1030–1050.

Bartky, S. L. (1988). Foucault, femininity, and the modernization of patriarchal power. In I. Diamond & L. Quinby (Eds.), *Feminism and Foucault: Reflections on resistance* (pp. 61–86). Northeastern University Press.

Becker, E. (1973). *The denial of death*. Free Press.

Beech, O. D., Kaufmann, L., & Anderson, J. (2020). A systematic literature review exploring objectification and motherhood. *Psychology of Women Quarterly, 44*(4), 521–538.

Bernard, P., Gervais, S., Allen, J., Campomizzi, S., & Klein, O. (2012). Integrating sexual objectification with object versus person recognition: The sexualized body-inversion hypothesis. *Psychological Science, 23*(5), 469–471.

Breines, J. G., Crocker, J., & Garcia, J. A. (2008). Self-objectification and well-being in women's daily lives. *Personality and Social Psychology Bulletin, 34*(5), 583–598.

Budgeon, S. (2015). Individualized femininity and feminist politics of choice. *European Journal of Women's Studies, 22*(3), 303–318.

Calogero, R. M. (2013). Objects don't object: Evidence that self-objectification disrupts women's social activism. *Psychological Science, 24*(3), 312–318.

Cox, C. R., Goldenberg, J. L., Arndt, J., & Pyszczynski, T. (2007). Mother's milk: An existential perspective on negative reactions to breast-feeding. *Personality and Social Psychology Bulletin, 33*(1), 110–122.

Cox, C. R., Goldenberg, J. L., Pyszczynski, T., & Weise, D. (2007). Disgust, creatureliness and the accessibility of death-related thoughts. *European Journal of Social Psychology, 37*(3), 494–507.

Cui, J., & Fang, Y. (2022). Mediating effects of self-concept clarity and self-objectification on the relationship between celebrity worship and the process of considering cosmetic surgery among Chinese undergraduates. *BMC Psychology, 10*(1), 259.

de Beauvoir, S. (1989). *The second sex* (H. M. Parshley, Trans.). Vintage Books (Original work published 1949)

Downs, D., James, S., & Cowan, G. (2006). Body objectification, self- esteem, and relationship satisfaction: A comparison of exotic dancers and college women. *Sex Roles, 54*, 745–752.

Erchull, M. J. (2013). Distancing through objectification?: Depictions of women's bodies in menstrual product advertisements. *Sex Roles, 68*, 32–40.

Felig, R. N. (2020). *Editing the self away: The effects of photo manipulation on perceptions of the self*. USF Tampa Graduate Theses and Dissertations. https://digitalcommons.usf.edu/etd/8195.

Felig, R. N., Courtney, E. P., Lee, K. J., Ligman, K. M., & Goldenberg, J. L. (2023). Objects do not suffer: An impact of mechanistic de-

humanization on perceptions of women's suffering and lack of justice in domestic assault. *Journal of Interpersonal Violence.*
Felig, R. N., & Goldenberg, J. L. (2024). *Women undefined: A longitudinal investigation of sexual harassment on self-objectification and self-concept clarity.* Manuscript under review.
Felig, R. N., & Goldenberg, J. L. (2025). *Self-determined self-objectification: Autonomy as a moderator of the harms of self-objectification.* Manuscript in preparation.
Felig, R. N., Jordan, J. A., Shepard, S. L., Courtney, E. P., Goldenberg, J. L., & Roberts, T. A. (2022). When looking "hot" means not feeling cold: Evidence that self-objectification inhibits feelings of being cold. *British Journal of Social Psychology, 61(2),* 455–470.
Fiske, S. T., Cuddy, A. J., & Glick, P. (2007). Universal dimensions of social cognition: Warmth and competence. *Trends in Cognitive Sciences, 11*(2), 77–83.
Fredrickson, B. L., & Roberts, T. A. (1997). Objectification theory: Toward understanding women's lived experiences and mental health risks. *Psychology of Women Quarterly, 21*(2), 173–206.
Friedan, B. (1963). *The feminine mystique.* Norton.
Gervais, S. J., Vescio, T. K., Förster, J., Maass, A., & Suitner, C. (2012). Seeing women as objects: The sexual body part recognition bias. *European Journal of Social Psychology, 42*(6), 743–753.
Gerwig, G. (Director). (2023). *Barbie* [film]. Warner Bros.
Goldenberg, J. L. (2012). A body of terror: Denial of death and the creaturely body. In P. R. Shaver & M. Mikulincer (Eds.), *Meaning, mortality, and choice: The social psychology of existential concerns* (pp. 93–110). American Psychological Association.
Goldenberg, J. L. (2013). Immortal objects: The objectification of women as terror management. In S. J. Gervais & S. J. Gervais (Eds.), *Objectification and (de)humanization: 60th Nebraska Symposium on Motivation* (pp. 73–95). Springer Science + Business Media.
Goldenberg, J. L., Cox, C. R., Pyszczynski, T., Greenberg, J., & Solomon, S. (2002). Understanding human ambivalence about sex: The effects of stripping sex of meaning. *Journal of Sex Research, 39*(4), 310–320.
Goldenberg, J. L., Goplen, J., Cox, C. R., & Arndt, J. (2007). "Viewing" pregnancy as an existential threat: The effects of creatureliness on reactions to media depictions of the pregnant body. *Media Psychology, 10*(2), 211–230.
Goldenberg, J. L., Hart, J., Pyszczynski, T., Warnica, G. M., Landau, M., & Thomas, L. (2006). Ambivalence toward the body: Death, neuroticism, and the flight from physical sensation. *Personality and Social Psychology Bulletin, 32*(9), 1264–1277.
Goldenberg, J. L., & Morris, K. L. (2016). Death and the real girl: The role of existential concerns in men's attraction to women as objects. In T.-A. Roberts, N. Curtin, L. Cotina, & L. E. Duncan (Eds.), *Gender beyond difference: Best practices in feminist psychological science* (pp. 29–42). Springer.
Goldenberg, J. L., Pyszczynski, T., Greenberg, J., & Solomon, S. (2000). Fleeing the body: A terror management perspective on the problem of human corporeality. *Personality and Social Psychology Review, 4,* 200–218.
Goldenberg, J. L., Pyszczynski, T., Greenberg, J., Solomon, S., Kluck, B., & Cornwell, R. (2001). I am NOT an animal: Mortality salience, disgust, and the denial of human creatureliness. *Journal of Experimental Psychology: General, 130,* 427–435.
Goldenberg, J. L., Pyszczynski, T., McCoy, S. K., Greenberg, J., & Solomon, S. (1999). Death, sex, love, and neuroticism: Why is sex such a problem? *Journal of Personality and Social Psychology, 77,* 1173–1187.
Goldenberg, J. L., & Roberts, T. A. (2004). The beast within the beauty: An existential perspective on the objectification and condemnation of women. In J. Greenberg, S. L., Koole, & T. Pyszczynski (Eds.), *Handbook of experimental existential psychology* (pp. 71–85). Guilford Press.
Goldenberg, J. L., & Roberts, T. A. (2010). The birthmark: An existential account of why women are objectified. In R. Calogero, S. Tantleff-Dunn, & J. K. Thompson (Eds.), *The objectification of women: Innovative directions in research and practice* (pp. 77–100). American Psychological Association.
Grabe, S., Routledge, C., Cook, A., Andersen, C., & Arndt, J. (2005). In defense of the body: The effect of mortality salience on female body objectification. *Psychology of Women Quarterly, 29*(1), 33–37.
Gray, H., Gray, K., & Wegner, D. M. (2007). Dimensions of mind perception. *Science, 315,* 619.
Greenberg J., Pyszczynski T., & Solomon S. (1986). The causes and consequences of a need for self-esteem: A terror management theory. In Baumeister, R. F. (Eds.), *Public self and private self* (pp. 189–212). Springer.
Harris, L. T., & Fiske, S. T. (2009). Social neuroscience evidence for dehumanised perception. *European Review of Social Psychology, 20*(1), 192–231.
Harrold, M. L., Miller, C. J., & Perkins, A. W.

(2023). Pink tasks: Feminists and their preferences for premium beauty products. *Psychology and Marketing, 40*(8), 1658–1671.
Haslam, N. (2006). Dehumanization: An integrative review. *Personality and Social Psychology Review, 10*(3), 252–264.
Hebl, M. R., King, E. B., Glick, P., Singletary, S. L., & Kazama, S. (2007). Hostile and benevolent reactions toward pregnant women: Complementary interpersonal punishments and rewards that maintain traditional roles. *Journal of Applied Psychology, 92*(6), 1499–1511.
Heflick, N. A., & Goldenberg, J. L. (2009). Objectifying Sarah Palin: Evidence that objectification causes women to be perceived as less competent and less fully human. *Journal of Experimental Social Psychology, 45,* 598–601.
Heflick, N. A., Goldenberg, J. L., Cooper, D. P., & Puvia, E. (2011). From women to objects: Appearance focus, target gender, and perceptions of warmth, morality and competence. *Journal of Experimental Social Psychology, 47,* 572–581.
Hirshman, L. R. (2006). *Get to work: A manifesto for women of the world.* Viking.
Holland, E., & Haslam, N. (2016). Cute little things: The objectification of prepubescent girls. *Psychology of Women Quarterly, 40*(1), 108–119.
Holland, K. J., Silver, K. E., Cipriano, A. E., & Brock, R. L. (2020). Internalized body stigma as a barrier to accessing preventative healthcare for young women. *Body Image, 35,* 217–224.
Jonnson, M. R., Langille, J. I., & Walsh, Z. (2018). The role of objectification in the victimization and perpetration of intimate partner violence. *Violence and Victims, 33*(1), 23–39.
Johnston-Robledo, I., Ball, M., Lauta, K., & Zekoll, A. (2003). To bleed or not to bleed: Young women's attitudes toward menstrual suppression. *Women and Health, 38*(3), 59–75.
Johnston-Robledo, I., Voigt, J., Sheffield, K., & Wilcox-Constantine, J. (2007). Reproductive shame: Self-objectification and women's attitudes toward their reproductive functioning. *Women and Health, 46*(1), 25–39.
Kant, I. (1963). *Lectures on ethics* (L. Infield, Trans.). Harper & Row. (Original work published 1780–1781)
Landau, M. J., Goldenberg, J. L., Greenberg, J., Gillath, O., Solomon, S., Cox, C., & Pyszczynski, T. (2006). The siren's call: Terror management and the threat of men's sexual attraction to women. *Journal of Personality and Social Psychology, 90*(1), 129–146.
Langton, R. (2009). *Sexual solipsism: Philosophical essays on pornography objectification.* Oxford University Press.
Lem, M., Kim, J. K., Pham, J. T., & Tang, C. J. (2023). Effect of the COVID-19 pandemic on global interest in plastic surgery. *JPRAS Open, 37,* 63–71.
Ligman, K. M., Courtney, E. P., Roberts T-A., & Goldenberg, J. (2025). Cover up that "baby bump": Displaying the pregnant body undermines women's perceived humanness. *Sex Roles, 91*(8), 1–18.
Ligman, K. M., Felig, R. N., & Goldenberg, J. L. (2024). An unsafe space: Sexualization, dehumanization, and the harassment of women on social media. *Psychology of Popular Media, 14*(1), 42–53.
Liu, W., Wei, Z., Cheng, X., Pang, R., Zhang, H., & Li, G. (2021). Public interest in cosmetic surgical and minimally invasive plastic procedures during the COVID-19 pandemic: Infodemiology study of Twitter data. *Journal of Medical Internet Research, 23*(3).
Loughnan, S., Haslam, N., Murnane, T., Vaes, J., Reynolds, C., & Suitner, C. (2010). Objectification leads to depersonalization: The denial of mind and moral concern to objectified others. *European Journal of Social Psychology, 40*(5), 709–717.
Moradi, B., & Huang, Y. P. (2008). Objectification theory and the psychology of women: A decade of advances and future directions. *Psychology of Women Quarterly, 32,* 377–398.
Morris, K. L., & Goldenberg, J. L. (2015). Objects become her: The role of mortality salience on men's attraction to literally objectified women. *Journal of Experimental Social Psychology, 56,* 69–72.
Morris, K. L., Goldenberg, J. L., & Boyd, P. (2018). Women as animals, women as objects: Evidence for two forms of objectification. *Personality and Social Psychology Bulletin, 44,* 1302–1314.
Morris, K. L., Goldenberg, J. L., & Heflick, N. A. (2014). Trio of terror (pregnancy, menstruation, and breastfeeding): An existential function of literal self-objectification among women. *Journal of Personality and Social Psychology, 107,* 181–198.
Myers, T. A., & Crowther, J. H. (2008). Is self-objectification related to interoceptive awareness?: An examination of potential mediating pathways to disordered eating attitudes. *Psychology of Women Quarterly, 32,* 172–180.
Nussbaum, M. (1995). Objectification. *Philosophy and Public Affairs, 24,* 249–291.
Orbach, S. (2019). *Bodies.* Profile Books.
Pacilli, M. G., Spaccatini, F., Barresi, C., & Tomasetto, C. (2019). Less human and help-worthy: Sexualization affects children's percep-

tions of and intentions toward bullied peers. *International Journal of Behavioral Development, 43,* 481–491.
Paglia, C. (1990). *Sexual personae: Art and decadence from Nefertiti to Emily Dickinson.* Random House.
Pellizzer, M., Tiggemann, M., & Clark, L. (2016). Enjoyment of sexualization and positive body image in recreational pole dancers and university students. *Sex Roles, 74,* 35–45.
Piran, N., Teall, T., & Counsell, A. (2020). The experience of embodiment scale: Development and psychometric evaluation. *Body Image, 34,* 117–134.
Pollitt, K. (2007). *Learning to drive, and other life stories.* Random House.
Pyszczynski, T., Greenberg, J., & Goldenberg, J. L. (2003). Freedom versus fear: On the defense, growth, and expansion of the self. In M. R. Leary & J. P. Tangney (Eds.), *Handbook of self and identity* (pp. 314–343). Guilford Press.
Rhode, D. L. (2016). Appearance as a feminist issue. *SMU Law Review, 69,* 697–710.
Roberts, T. A. (2004). Female trouble: The menstrual self-evaluation scale and women's self-objectification. *Psychology of Women Quarterly, 28*(1), 22–26.
Roberts, T.-A. (2013). She's so pretty, she looks just like a Bratz doll!: Theoretical foundations for understanding girls' and women's self-objectification. In E. Zurbriggen & T.-A. Roberts (Eds.), *The sexualization of girls and girlhood: Causes, consequences, and resistance* (pp. 22–35). Oxford University Press.
Roberts, T.-A., Calogero, R. M. & Gervais, S. J. (2018). Objectification theory's continuing contribution to feminist psychology. In J. White & C. Travis (Eds.), *APA handbook of the psychology of women* (pp. 249–271). American Psychological Association.
Roberts, T. A., & Goldenberg, J. L. (2024, January 11). Barbie's existential crisis and the fight for reproductive justice. *Ms. Magazine.* https://msmagazine.com/2024/01/11/death-barbie-abortion-supreme-court/.
Roberts, T., Goldenberg, J. L., Power, C., & Pyszczynski, T. (2002). "Feminine protection": The effects of menstruation on attitudes towards women. *Psychology of Women Quarterly, 26*(2), 131–139.
Ryan, R. M., & Deci, E. L. (2000). Self-determination theory and the facilitation of intrinsic motivation, social development, and well-being. *American Psychologist, 55*(1), 68–78.
Sáez, G., Riemer, A. R., Brock, R. L., & Gervais, S. J. (2020). The role of interpersonal sexual objectification in heterosexual intimate partner violence from perspectives of perceivers and targets. *Journal of Interpersonal Violence, 37*(3-4), 1430–1455.
Siegel, J. A., & Calogero, R. M. (2019). Conformity to feminine norms and self-objectification in self-identified feminist and non-feminist women. *Body Image, 28,* 115–118.
Solomon S., Greenberg J., & Pyszczynski T. (2015). *The worm at the core: On the role of death in life.* Random House.
Starr, C. R., & Ferguson, G. M. (2012). Sexy dolls, sexy grade-schoolers?: Media and maternal influences on young girls' self-sexualization. *Sex Roles, 67,* 463–476.
Vail, K. E. III, Conti, J. P., Goad, A. N., & Horner, D. E. (2020). Existential threat fuels worldview defense, but not after priming autonomy orientation. *Basic and Applied Social Psychology, 42*(3), 150–166.
Vaes, J., Cristoforetti, G., Ruzzante, D., Cogoni, C., & Mazza, V. (2019). Assessing neural responses towards objectified human targets and objects to identify processes of sexual objectification that go beyond the metaphor. *Scientific Reports, 9*(1), 6699.
Vartanian, L. R. (2009). When the body defines the self: Self-concept clarity, internalization, and body image. *Journal of Social and Clinical Psychology, 28*(1), 94–126
Vasquez, E., Ball, L., Loughnan, S., & Pina, A. (2017). The object of my aggression: Sexual objectification increases physical aggression towards women. *Aggressive Behavior, 44*(1), 5–17.
Vasquez, E., Osinnowo, K., Pina, A., Ball, L., & Bell, C. (2016). The sexual objectification of girls and aggression towards them in gang and non-gang affiliated youth. *Psychology, Crime, and Law, 23,* 459–471.
Ward, L. M. (2002). Does television exposure affect emerging adults' attitudes and assumptions about sexual relationships?: Correlational and experimental confirmation. *Journal of Youth and Adolescence, 31,* 1–15.
Ward, L. M. (2016). Media and sexualization: State of empirical research, 1995–2015. *Journal of Sex Research, 53,* 560–577.
Warin, J. (2000). The attainment of self-consistency through gender in young children. *Sex Roles, 42,* 209–231.
Wolf, N. (1991). *The beauty myth: How images of beauty are used against women.* Vintage.
Yalom, I. D. (1980). *Existential psychotherapy.* Basic Books.

CHAPTER 39

State Authenticity as Identity-Based Fit to Environment

The SAFE Model

Constantine Sedikides *and* Toni Schmader

People's sense of who they are can be reflected by (or feel at odds with) the environments they are in. In such a way, person–environment fit can have consequences for state authenticity and ensuing behavior. Guided by the state authenticity as fit to the environment (SAFE) model (Schmader & Sedikides, 2018), we describe three types of person–environment fit: self-concept, goal, and social. Situations can explicitly or subtly cue each of these types of fit to one's identity, triggering state authenticity. In turn, people are motivated to seek out or remain in situations that afford authenticity and avoid or leave those that do not. When situational cues systematically cue a sense of identity misfit for a group of people, these tendencies can lead to self-segregation. We review emerging evidence for the SAFE model, consider implications, and discuss unresolved issues.

AUTHENTICITY

The human pursuit of meaning often involves navigating a rocky terrain. Humanistic psychologists argued that the advanced territory of that terrain is signposted by self-growth and self-actualization, ending at self-transcendence (Maslow, 1943; Rogers, 1961). Reaching the destination, one could enjoy peak experiences of being-cognition where "the person can then become relatively egoless" (Maslow, 1961/1999, p. 117), "leaving behind self-consciousness and self-observation . . . [and becoming] a strong real self" (Maslow, 1961/1999, p. 125). Becoming "a strong real self," then, was considered a primary human need. Humanistic psychologists took their cue from existential philosophers (e.g., Albert Camus, Simone de Beauvoir, Martin Heidegger, Søren Kierkegaard, Jean-Paul Sartre), who championed the value of realizing one's true self. The pertinent concept is authenticity, "the reduction of phoniness toward the zero point" (Maslow, 1971, p. 183) or "the unobstructed operation of one's true self in one's daily enterprise" (Goldman & Kernis, 2002, p. 293).

From an empirical standpoint, authenticity was first conceptualized as a personality trait. According to the multicomponent authentic functioning model (Kernis & Goldman, 2006), the trait has four constituents: (1) awareness: understanding one's strengths and weaknesses; (2) unbiased processing: accepting both positive and negative feedback; (3) behavior: acting consistently with one's values, preferences, and needs; and (4) relational orientation: having trusting, veritable social bonds. Those four constituents were condensed into three by the authentic personality model (Wood et al., 2008): (1) authentic living: acting congruently with one's values, preferences, and needs; (2) (non)accepting external influence: rebuffing social pressure; and (3) (absence of) self-alienation: being in touch with one's internal world. Trait authenticity is positively associated with approach orientation such as promotion focus (Kim et al., 2019) or problem-focused coping (e.g., planning, active coping; Kernis & Goldman, 2006), employee engagement (Sutton, 2020), and psychological well-being (Rivera et al., 2019; Sutton, 2020).

Although authenticity varies between persons (consistent with this trait approach), it also varies within persons. That is, authenticity fluctuates momentarily or as a function of situations (Lenton et al., 2013; Lenton et al., 2016). In fact, state or felt authenticity varies to a greater extent within persons than it does between persons (Fleeson & Wilt, 2010; Landa & English, 2022). Consequently, authenticity can also be conceptualized as a psychological state, "the sense or feeling that one is currently in alignment with one's true or genuine self, that one is being his or her real self" (Sedikides et al., 2017, p. 521). State authenticity is formed by two constituents, authentic living and absence of self-alienation (Lenton et al., 2014). Finally, like trait authenticity, state authenticity is related to approach orientation such as likelihood of pro-environmental action (i.e., monetary donations; Yang et al., 2021), is linked to engagement in moral behaviors at the workplace (Zhang et al., 2019), and is associated with or increases psychological well-being (Bailey et al., 2020; Kelley et al., 2022; Thomaes et al., 2017).

State authenticity has been gaining traction in the literature (Chen, 2019; Sedikides et al., 2019; Vess, 2019). People aspire to "be themselves," as authenticity is frequent in daily life and more so than inauthenticity (Huber et al., 2022; Lenton et al., 2013). But, if authenticity varies within person from one situation to the next, what quality of those situations predicts state authenticity? Also, what are the consequences of felt authenticity, and do these consequences differ among social groups? These are questions that the SAFE model addresses.

THE SAFE MODEL

The SAFE model (Schmader & Sedikides, 2018) seeks to identify the processes through which people self-segregate by identity into different situations. According to the model, state authenticity is experienced when aspects of one's identity seem to fit or be matched by the environment. Whereas fit engenders the experience of fluency, a lack of fit creates friction. The subjective experience of fluency or friction is perhaps what is coded as state authenticity. In turn, state authenticity entails motivational and behavioral consequences. We describe below in more detail the key tenets of the model.

Fit and Fluency

Person–environment fit occurs when personality and environmental attributes are well matched (Kristof-Brown & Guay, 2011). Fit is a fulcrum construct in psychology, presumed to underlie, in part, attitudes, motivation, and behavior (Su et al., 2015; Van Vianen, 2018; Walsh et al., 2000). The SAFE model distinguishes among three forms of fit that constitute separate pathways to authenticity. Self-concept fit cues the cognitive component of authenticity, goal fit cues the motivational component, and social fit cues the interpersonal component.

Self-concept fit refers to the match between static cues in an environment and valued characteristics of the self. It occurs, for example, when a scientist is at a science museum or a gardener is at a gardening show. In such cases, the environment activates central and default (i.e., chronically available) self-facets (Schmader et al., 2014), that is, traits, memories, and values tethered with being a "scientist" or "gardener." The environment matches one's working self-concept (Markus & Wurf, 1987) and feels familiar. For this reason, the individual experiences perceptual fluency. Put otherwise, frequent exposure to the same working self-concept in identical or similar situations (Montoya et al., 2017) aids fluent processing of self-relevant information. Perceptual fluency leads to considering the relevant message as truer (Reber & Unkelbach, 2010). Hence, the cognitive outcome of perceptual fluency is a sense of the self as true (i.e., state authenticity). Alternatively, the cognitive outcome of perceptual disfluency (e.g., an atheist in a religious service or a tone-deaf person at the symphony) evokes inauthenticity.

Goal fit refers to the match between institutional structures or norms in the environment and one's own valued goals. It occurs, for example, when a high achiever works for an ambitious organization or a person high on openness to experience learns about a new culture. In such cases, the environment activates internalized or valued goals, heightening interest in them (Higgins, 2005) and rendering them more subjectively affordable (Diekman et al., 2017). When the environment matches one's goals, the person experiences motivational fluency. This fluency can be experienced as a sense of one's actions having value (Avnet & Higgins, 2003) or being autonomous (Heppner et al., 2008) or of one's judgments being correct (Camacho et al., 2003). Such experiences of self-determination are often regarded as overlapping with authenticity (Ryan & Deci, 2017). Alternatively, the outcome of motivational disfluency (e.g., an extraverted student completing a class assignment individually rather than as part of a working group) elicits inauthenticity and more hesitation toward goals.

Social fit refers to the match between the social environment and the self, or the extent to which others validate who one is. It occurs when a person feels comfortable to self-disclose among friends or when an employee is regularly invited to lunch and after-work drinks by their colleagues. In such cases, the person has the opportunity to express themselves relatively unencumbered by social expectations or constraints. The person feels that they are not judged by others and are accepted by them. For this reason, the person experiences interpersonal fluency. Indeed, hanging out with friends is positively associated with authenticity (Lenton et al., 2013), supportive relationships promote authenticity (DiDonato & Krueger, 2010), and an audience that has a favorable (vs. unfavorable) attitude toward the topic of a communicators' autobiographical memory increases communicator felt authenticity (Boytos et al., 2023). Alternatively, interpersonal disfluency (i.e., a student sensing avoidance from their classmates), can lead to inauthenticity.

Consequences of Fit and Fluency

The SAFE model posits that self-concept, goal, and social fit conduce to state authenticity via cognitive, motivational, and interpersonal fluency, respectively. Authenticity, in turn, drives one's selection of situations. But what are the consequences of the fit–fluency–authenticity chain?

Authenticity is approach-oriented (Kernis & Goldman, 2006; Kim et al., 2019; Yang et al., 2021). In the case of self-concept fit, people are likely to approach situations that facilitate further processing fluency or avoid situations that impede it (Song & Schwarz, 2009). Perceptual fluency will shape self and social perception (Claypool et al., 2012). As such, people will favor situations that reinforce the default self-concept or disfavor situations that undermine it. For example, a pilot traveling to Washington, DC, for the first time might be more likely to visit the Smithsonian Air and Space Museum, whereas a high school history teacher might prefer to check out the National Archives to see the Declaration of Independence. Even though each might have more to learn by visiting the other site, the tendency to select a situation that activates core aspects of the self-concept will likely aid psychological well-being (Dufner et al., 2019).

Authenticity is also linked to stronger engagement (Sutton, 2020; Zhang et al., 2019). In the case of goal fit, people are likely to prefer situations that sustain motivational fit and disapprove of those that disrupt it (Milyavskaya et al., 2015). Motivational fluency has an impact on engagement (Diekman et al., 2017), in that people embrace situations that enhance engagement and shy away from those that diminish it. For instance, a highly competitive person might prefer to join and perform better on a sports team that rewards individual accomplishment and emphasizes winning games over enjoyment. A more cooperative person might join and perform better on a sports team that rewards team success and emphasizes cohesion. Again, the experience of goal fit in the environment will likely aid psychological well-being (Vainio & Daukantaitė, 2016).

Authenticity can also have implications for retention. Often one's initial attraction to a situation is guided by either self-concept or goal fit. People choose degree programs or jobs, for example, because they see them as being a good fit to their abilities, interests, and values. Once there, however, the social environment of that setting often becomes a more powerful predictor of experience. As such, people will persist longer in academic programs and jobs where they experience interpersonal fluency evincing lower turnover (Walton et al., 2012). Such situation selection will likely engender psychological well-being (Baumeister & Leary, 1995). But people might also self-select out of environments that otherwise fit who they are (high self-concept fit) and what they want to do (high goal fit), if the people in that environment do not allow them to be authentic (low social fit). For instance, a communal person who was originally attracted to a career in early childhood education might eventually change their career path if they continually find that their coworkers question this commitment.

On the Distinctiveness versus Interrelation of the Three Types of Fit

The three types of fit, and corresponding routes to authenticity, are theoretically and empirically distinct. Yet they are often interrelated. That is, a particular environment might cue more than one form of fit. As an example, being accepted by one's colleagues and feeling securely embedded in social context (social fit) might energize an employee to strive harder in attaining personal or organizational goals (motivational fit). Likewise, attaining such goals (motivational fit) might validate one's self-view as competent and effective in that setting (self-concept fit). To measure distinctions and interrelationships among these three types of fit, recent research has aimed to validate measures to assess each type of fit independently. Such measures then pave the way for ongoing and future research assessing common and distinct consequences of each type of fit. Two studies, described next, took this step.

SUPPORT FOR THE SAFE MODEL

One approach to measuring fit and its relation with state authenticity is to assess participants' subjective sense of fit with a given context and whether between-person variation in each type of fit uniquely predicts state authenticity. Aday and colleagues (2024, Study 1) began by developing a self-report scale that assessed self-concept, goal, and social fit as unique predictors of state authenticity among samples of undergraduate students at their university. The scale consists of 12 items. Four items refer to self-concept fit (e.g., "Even when I'm alone and doing nothing, simply being at [university name] makes me feel like myself"; "I feel 'at home' when I'm at [university name]"), four items refer to goal fit (e.g., "[University name] is a place where I feel intrinsically motivated by my own goals"; "I feel that [university name] is a place that allows me to realize my own goals"), and four items refer to social fit (e.g., "When I'm around [other students] on campus, I feel like I can act natural"; "Other students at [university name] do NOT judge me for being myself"). Although the scale was validated among university students, an additional sample of organizational employees produced similar results. The scale evinced good factor structure and good convergent validity (with belonging) and discriminant validity from other constructs (i.e., autonomy, relatedness, competence, strength of self, goal motivation, social belonging). Although the three types of fit were positively intercorrelated, they were also distinct constructs.

Participants in Study 1 of Aday and colleagues (2024) also completed a face valid measure of state authenticity ("At [University], I feel . . ." 1 = *inauthentic*, 7 = *authentic*) and dropout intentions (e.g., "I often think about dropping out"; "I will likely actively look to transfer out of [University] in the next year"). All three forms of fit significantly and uniquely predicted state authenticity. Moreover, self-concept and goal fit significantly and uniquely predicted dropout intentions, although social fit did not. Alternative constructs (i.e., positive affect, negative affect, social desirability) did not explain better the association between fit and state authenticity.

This cross-sectional study validated a new SAFE scale that can be used to measure between-person variation in fit and authenticity as situated within a certain context. To examine state-level experiences and fit and authenticity in Study 2, Aday and colleagues (2024) implemented ecological momentary assessment aiming to find out how these variables fluctuate from one situation to the next within persons. At baseline, university students completed a 12-item trait authenticity scale (Wood et al., 2008; "I live in accordance with my values and beliefs"; "I always stand by what I believe in"). Approximately a month later, they began a 2-week experience-sampling phase. They received daily prompts to complete a 3-minute survey via smartphone, tablet, or laptop. The survey started with questions about participants' current context (e.g., "What are you doing right now?"). Then, it assessed transient fit measured via the highest-loading item from their corresponding subscale of the SAFE model scale: "Just being here in this space suits the way I see myself" (*self-concept fit*), "This is a place where I feel intrinsically motivated by my own goals" (*goal fit*), "I can act natural around the people who are here" (*social fit*). The assessment of state authenticity, as in Study 1, followed. Finally, participants responded to items measuring—at the state level—willingness to return ("Are you likely to return to this setting?"), university attachment (1 = *completely emotionally disengaged from [University]*, 7 = *strongly emotionally attached to [University]*), and burnout ("Right now, I feel emotionally drained"). On half of the trials, participants also completed a working-memory capacity task as a performance-based index of cognitive fluency (Riediger et al., 2011). This task is a memory-updating task in which participants memorize four displayed numbers, which subsequently disappear. A single-digit addition or subtraction updating operation (e.g., +6) appears next. Participants update the original number according to the operation and hold that new number in working memory. After 3.5 seconds, the updating operation disappears and a new operation comes into view. In all, participants in this study remembered and inputted four updated numbers.

The between-person results from Study 1 were replicated in Study 2. Participants who on average across situations reported greater state authenticity also on average reported greater self-concept, goal, and social fit. The within-person effects were revealing: Each outcome was uniquely predicted by one or more forms of fit. In particular, all three forms of fit significantly predicted state authenticity; that is, when participants reported higher fit on campus, they also relayed feeling more authentic. Moreover, when participants felt more self-concept, goal, and/or social fit, they were also more willing to return to that situation. Further, each of self-concept, goal, and social fit felt on campus significantly and uniquely predicted attachment to the university. These findings provide evidence that each type of fit might underlie situation selection. In addition, participants reported more burnout in situations in which they experienced less self-concept fit, while their working-memory capacity was higher in situations in which they experienced greater self-concept fit, consistent with the SAFE model's tenet that self-concept fit cues cognitive fluency.

Aday and colleagues (2024) proceeded to test whether momentary variation in authenticity predicts momentary outcomes. They found that for the most part, it does. In situations in which participants felt more authentic, they reported stronger willingness to return, greater attachment to the university, and weaker burnout. Authenticity did not predict momentary variation in working-memory capacity. Lastly, variation in state authenticity mediated the effects of all forms of fit on attachment to the university and the effect of self-concept fit on burnout, but it did not mediate effects on willingness to return to the situation.

Finally, this study also provided evidence that each type of fit is cued by distinct features of the environment. Self-concept fit was elevated in situations that were highly familiar and freely chosen, goal fit was higher when people were engaged in active (vs. passive) tasks, and social fit was higher in situations involving close others (vs. alone) and social (vs. solitary) tasks. Taken together, Study 2 offered insight into how fit and authenticity varies across situations within persons in support of the SAFE model.

IMPLICATIONS OF THE SAFE MODEL

Cultural Defaults and the Experience of Fit

The SAFE model has implications for how environments can systematically cue varying levels of fit and authenticity for different identity groups. Given that many environments are designed by and for members of advantaged groups (e.g., in regard to race/ethnicity, gender, or social class), they often constitute the cognitive and social default (Cheryan & Markus, 2020). For instance, in the United States, the racial category "White" is implicitly associated with the concept "American," U.S.-born ethnic minorities are rated as less American than White Europeans (Devos & Banaji, 2005), and valued cultural traits are assumed to characterize men more than women (Cuddy et al., 2015). As a result, cultural cues, institutional structures, and social context more readily signal self-concept fit, goal fit, and social fit for advantaged group members. In contrast, the same environmental features might cue a lack of fit and inauthenticity for members of disadvantaged groups.

Self-Concept Fit

Those who are the cultural default more often encounter environmental cues that feel familiar, elevating the cognitive benefits of self-concept fit. When self-concept fit and processing fluency are strengthened, resources are freed for being-cognition and authenticity. Therefore, advantaged group members should more often experience reduced self-consciousness and increased flow states (Csikszentmihalyi, 1975). For example, leaders are less likely to be aware of themselves as shown by their lower likelihood of first-person pronoun ("I") use (Pennebaker, 2011). Authenticity, in turn, will facilitate task engagement or persistence, increasing the probability of success (Schmader et al., 2001).

Those from disadvantaged groups often find themselves needing to adjust and adapt to advantaged group contexts that might not feel familiar or match their identity. As a result, they might more often experience lower self-concept fit and processing disfluency. The same context that feels fluent for the advantaged group might elicit uncertainty for those who encounter negative group stereotypes that are at odds with their own self-view (Schmader et al., 2014). To resolve uncertainty, members of disadvantaged groups might direct conscious attention to the self or social identity, monitoring and analyzing their behavior or performance (Schmader et al., 2008, 2009), becoming more susceptible to errors (Forbes et al., 2008). This deliberate focus on the self will disrupt fluency and being-cognition, making the individual feel less true to themselves. The ensuing inauthenticity will culminate in obstruction of task engagement or persistence, decreasing the probability of success (Schmader et al., 2001).

Goal Fit

Those from culturally advantaged groups more frequently encounter institutional structures that align with and afford their valued goals. As a result, goal fit and motivational fluency will be enhanced, strengthening internalized or autonomous goals. This alignment between one's own goals and the way society and its institutions are structured increases the perceived value of one's actions and state authenticity.

In contrast, being the disadvantaged group in a world of institutions that have been created by those who are advantaged can have motivational liabilities. These include goal misfit and motivational disfluency, which will increase goal coercion and restrict goal internalization. When one's own goals feel at odds with the actions that are valued in a setting, people feel inauthentic. For instance, a university student from a lower social class background might feel dissonance for having to behave similarly to middle-class students at the university in order to fit in (Brummelman & Sedikides, 2023) and might perform more poorly as a result (Phillips et al., 2020). As another example, disadvantaged group members might spurn the values of their own group in order to conform to advantaged group norms (Henrich & Gil-White, 2001). An Asian student, for example, who is competent in math may decide to take literature classes instead to escape prevalent stereotypes about his group, or a woman might purposely downplay aspects of her feminine identity in order to conform to male default culture in her STEM classes (Pronin et al., 2004).

Social Fit

Finally, as a member of a culturally advantaged group, many environments will include others who share their same identity.

As a result, one can often enter into contexts assuming that other people in that setting will accept them as they are and value their contributions. These social benefits enhance social fit and interpersonal fluency, which lifts authenticity. Those same situations, however, can imply social misfit and interpersonal disfluency for those from disadvantaged groups who are often negatively stereotyped. As such, members of disadvantaged groups can come to chronically expect social rejection, inhibiting feelings of authenticity.

For example, disadvantaged group members experience social misfit in domains where they are negatively stereotyped (Walton & Cohen, 2007), cuing avoidance behavior. For example, social misfit in a STEM topic fuels greater anxiety and lower interest among women (Cheryan et al., 2009). Avoidance behavior at the group level leads to self-segregation. For instance, older adults prefer to exercise alongside similar others rather than with younger adults (Dunlop & Schmader, 2014). In addition, disadvantaged group members may attempt to reduce social misfit by engaging in compensatory behaviors likely to curtail stereotyping of their group. As a case in point, overweight persons may be hyperfriendly (Miller et al., 1995) and Black persons may be hyperengaging in social interactions with a White person, seeking to put their conversational partner at ease (Shelton et al., 2005). These strategies will compound inauthenticity due to a lack of social fit (English et al., 2012). However, those in the majority can also signal social fit by creating supportive social connections with members of marginalized groups (Cyr et al., 2021; Hall et al., 2019).

Preliminary Findings

There is emerging evidence that those who are marginalized often feel less authentic in environments where they are not the cultural default. For example, in Aday and colleagues research (2024, Study 1, supplemental analyses), students of color, compared to their White peers, reported feeling less authentic at their university, an effect that was related to experiencing less self-concept and goal (but not social) fit. In a momentary ecological assessment study, university students with more experiences of marginalization in the classroom reported lower authenticity in conjunction with lower self-concept and social (but not goal) fit (Guo & Schmader, 2024). Finally, within engineering majors women reported lower state authenticity than men did, and this gender difference was mediated by lower levels of each type of fit independently (Guo & Schmader, 2024). The SAFE model thus offers promise for identifying the distinct types of fit that might undermine state authenticity for different marginalized groups in distinct contexts. Such findings can help organizations target interventions for fostering greater inclusion.

Self-Segregation

The SAFE model also has implications for self-segregation, that is, the tendency for people to prefer environments that cue and bolster their identity (above and beyond the direct influence of prejudice and discrimination that create realistic barriers to integration). Patterns of self-segregation can result from each form of fit. For example, people are attracted to situations that elicit greater self-concept fit, as when people move to places where others share their same personality, ideology, race, and ethnicity (Ihlanfeldt & Scafidi, 2002; Motyl, 2016; Rentfrow et al., 2008). People also self-select into educational and occupational opportunities that enhance goal fit. Examples include career choices based on gender (e.g., girls opting out of STEM subjects), core values (Diekman et al., 2017), or ideological conviction (Peterson & Morgan, 1995). Lastly, people readily seek out friendships and relationships that foster social fit and acceptance. Examples are friendship networks clustered in terms of immigrant status, social class, or race and ethnicity (Charles, 2000; Kye, 2023; Musterd & Ostendorf, 1998).

Self-segregation, as per the SAFE model, is partly motivated by the desire for authenticity. The selected environments activate the default self, allow completion of valued goals, or validate the self. Self-segregation is also motivated by the desire to avoid inauthenticity, that is, to escape environments that feel disfluent with the default self, obstruct one's important goals, and invalidate the self. Such environments may induce stress, lower performance, and increase intergroup alienation if not outright hostility.

Self-segregation can have salutary effects, alleviating some of the negative psychological ramifications of inauthenticity. However, it can also propagate social inequality and hinder social mobility (Cutler & Glaeser, 1997; Ihlanfeldt & Scafidi, 2002). Yet these presumed outcomes of self-segregation can be overridden by various experiences, interventions, or norms. These include having role models, acquiring access to positions of status and power, embracing the value of diversity (Smith, 1990), promoting diversity in the workplace (Bond, 2008), and interacting with an outgroup member or fostering intergroup contact (Pettigrew & Tropp, 2006). Counteracting strong tendencies toward self-segregation often requires active efforts to embrace or reframe experiences of misfit in a more positive light, as something to approach rather than avoid. For example, people high in openness to new experiences, those who value diversity and inclusion, and individuals from cultures that value harmony might experience situations of identity misfit in more favorable ways, allowing them to grow and adapt through self-uncertainty rather than feel inauthentic (Guo & Schmader, 2025).

UNRESOLVED ISSUES

Having outlined the model, described support for it, and considered implications, we now turn to a discussion of a selection of unresolved issues (see also Schmader & Sedikides, 2018).

Is Self-Segregation a Choice?

Some scholars have considered the possibility that self-segregation is a choice that members of disadvantaged groups make (Block et al., 2018; Ceci et al., 2014; Lippa, 1998). That is, when members of disadvantaged groups settle into the identity safety afforded by self-concept, goal, and social fit, they are electing to avoid other opportunities for where to live, what careers to pursue, or what people to befriend. For example, Ceci and colleagues (2014) have suggested that gender disparities in STEM reflect women's and men's different choices, not discrimination.

To some extent, self-segregation is a choice. However, such choices are not free of social constraints. The SAFE model outlines the various ways in which the same environment can cue fit and fluency for those who are advantaged, and misfit and friction for those who are disadvantaged. The equality of opportunity in the context can mask the ways in which inequities of fit still persist (Purdie-Vaughns et al., 2008). As a result of these more subtle forces, patterns of self-segregation result from implicit or automatic processing, rather than controlled or deliberate processing, habituated over time by environmental influences and strong social norms (Aday & Schmader, 2019). Also, the identity congruent choices that people make may be rationalized after the fact as being more autonomous than they actually are (Kay et al., 2002; Nisbett & Wilson, 1977; see also Aday & Schmader, 2019). Finally, such choices can be met with social support from ingroup members (Schopler et al., 1993), solidifying the choices as normative behavior.

When Is Inauthenticity Tolerable?

Some disadvantaged group members may shy away from self-segregation. Instead, they may seemingly tolerate, or even seek out, inauthenticity. How can their behavior be explained?

What appears to be inauthenticity tolerance may, in part, be uncertainty coping (Guo & Schmader, 2025). That is, individuals encountering self-concept, goal, or social misfit may feel uncertain about themselves, their goals, or their social efficacy (Campbell, 1990; Choi & Hogg, 2020; Ntoumanis & Sedikides, 2018). Their uncertainty will be higher if they appraise the self as malleable (rather than stable; Dweck, 2006), are high (rather than low) on openness to experience (McCrae & Costa, 1987), value diversity and inclusion (Green et al., 2021; Page-Gould et al., 2008), and come from cultures that emphasize harmony (Zhang et al., 2005). That is, for some individuals, situations of person–environment misfit are opportunities to learn and grow.

Does High Authenticity Deter Self-Segregation?

At the core of the SAFE model is the tenet that situation selection, including self-segregation, is at the service of attaining authenticity. But what if one feels authentic in the first place? Put otherwise, what if one already enjoys an environment that is low on authenticity variability or that affords stable levels of authenticity?

On the one hand, several theoretical statements predict that authenticity would act as a balancing feedback mechanism, counteracting threats to one's identity and sustaining psychological equilibrium (Reed et al., 2021). These statements include self-affirmation theory (Steele, 1988), the mnemic neglect model (Sedikides et al., 2016), attachment theory (Shaver & Mikulincer, 2008), and terror management theory (Pyszczynski et al., 2004). On the other hand, the individual does not act alone. As a group member, the individual is influenced by social context and so is prone to making contextual decisions. Although one may feel fairly authentic, fellow ingroup members may not feel so. The ingroup, then, may exert social pressure in favor of self-segregation. An interesting dynamic refers to the extent to which a person who experiences high levels of authenticity belongs to, and interacts with, a group low on collective authenticity, and vice versa (cf. Sedikides et al., 2013).

Is Authenticity Good for Stigmatized Individuals?

The SAFE model posits not only that all forms of fit are linked with higher authenticity, but also that the expression of authenticity is associated with desirable consequences for the disadvantaged group. This may not be the case for all groups in all contexts. In particular, gender- and sexuality-diverse (LGBTQIAP+) individuals and other disadvantaged groups with concealable stigmas often face a unique dilemma of when, where, and with whom they can be authentic.

In many cultures, the expression of authenticity on the part of LGBTQIAP+ individuals is problematic, if not illegal, leading to concealment of one's identity. Such concealment may undermine approach orientation, engagement, and psychological health (Hatzenbuehler, 2009; Meyer, 2003; Stonewall, 2018). Although the ability to live authentically might be possible in more progressive nations, those in sexually restrictive cultures are often not afforded the ability to live authentically. In those situations, self-segregation might be more extreme. Alternatively, the peril of stigma might lead people to pursue assimilation when it is possible, even though this meant forgoing authentic living.

Patterns of Self-Segregation by the Advantaged Group

Although the SAFE model emphasizes understanding situations where members of marginalized groups self-segregate from those who are advantaged, the same processes can be applied to understand the experience of advantaged group members who feel that their identity is marginalized in conversations about diversity, equity, and inclusion (DEI), and are threatened by their own group becoming a numerical minority (Craig et al., 2018). Members of the majority group in a society often assume that messaging around diversity and inclusion does not include them (Dover et al., 2016). Thus, they may experience progressive efforts to support DEI initiatives in increasingly diverse societies as a threat. This form of identity threat contributes to rising support for authoritarian leaders who promote protectionist agendas (Major et al., 2018).

Such threats can be couched in the SAFE model. Members of the advantaged group who long enjoyed the benefits of being-cognition now find themselves more aware of their social identities (Rios & Mackey, 2022), likely resulting in less self-concept fit. Additionally, institutional discussions of equity often encourage leaders to rethink and expand their views of success and merit, which can cue lower goal fit for those who prefer the cultural default definitions of success (Folberg et al., 2024). Finally, efforts to diversify and integrate society can lead to lower social fit as members of the advantaged group find they need to adjust their behaviors to be more inclusive of others with different perspectives and/or fear being perceived as prejudiced (Kaiser et al.,

2022). In each case, weaker feelings of fit and authenticity are likely to drive the same tendency to self-segregate and reject policies and initiatives aimed at increasing DEI. Consequently, members of both advantaged and disadvantaged groups can feel polarized from one another by these processes. Efforts at bridging these groups are needed to break down self-segregation tendencies and achieve integration.

CONCLUDING COMMENTS

The pursuit of meaning is at the core of existential concerns (Becker, 1973; Frankl, 1959/2006; Hicks & Routledge, 2013). This pursuit can be partially satisfied by attaining authenticity, as per the SAFE model. Authenticity is attainable via fit of identity characteristics (self-concept, goals, sociality) with the environment. These basic tenets of the SAFE model have received empirical backing, paving the way for future work on how environments constructed for and by advantaged groups signal misfit and inauthenticity for those who are disadvantaged. If systemic disadvantages in the ability to feel authentic are found to be a core driver of self-segregation, future research might seek to identify meaningful ways to increase fit and authenticity for diverse groups.

REFERENCES

Aday, A., Guo, Y., Mehta, S., Chen, S., Hall, W., Götz, F., . . . Schmader, T. (2024). The SAFE model: State authenticity as a function of three types of fit. *Personality and Social Psychology Bulletin, 51*(8), 1472–1489.

Aday, A., & Schmader, T. (2019). Seeking authenticity in diverse contexts: How identities and environments constrain "free" choice. *Social and Personality Psychology Compass, 13*(6), Article e12450.

Avnet, T., & Higgins, E. T. (2003). Locomotion, assessment, and regulatory fit: Value transfer from "how" to "what." *Journal of Experimental Social Psychology, 39*(5), 525–530.

Bailey, E. R., Matz, S. C., Youyou, W., & Iyengar, S. S. (2020). Authentic self-expression on social media is associated with greater subjective well-being. *Nature Communications, 11*, Article 4889.

Baumeister, R. F., & Leary, M. R. (1995). The need to belong: Desire for interpersonal attachments as a fundamental human motivation. *Psychological Bulletin, 117*(3), 497–529.

Becker, E. (1973). *The denial of death.* Free Press.

Block, K., Croft, A., De Souza, L., & Schmader, T. (2018). Do people care if men don't care about caring? The asymmetry in support for changing gender roles. *Journal of Experimental Social Psychology, 83*(3), 112–131.

Bond, M. A. (2008). *Workplace chemistry: promoting diversity through organizational change.* University Press of New England.

Boytos, A. S., Costabile, K. A., & Logan, T. R. (2023). Describing autobiographical memories: Effects of shared reality and audience attitude valence on perceived authenticity and self-esteem. *Self and Identity, 22*(1), 77–101.

Brummelman, E., & Sedikides, C. (2023). Unequal selves in the classroom: Nature, origins, and consequences of socioeconomic disparities in children's self-views. *Developmental Psychology, 59*(1), 1962–1987.

Camacho, C. J., Higgins, E. T., & Luger, L. (2003). Moral value transfer from regulatory fit: What feels right is right and what feels wrong is wrong. *Journal of Personality and Social Psychology, 84*(3), 498–510.

Campbell, J. D. (1990). Self-esteem and clarity of the self-concept. *Journal of Personality and Social Psychology, 59*(3), 538–549.

Ceci, S. J., Ginther, D. K., Kahn, S., & Williams, W. M. (2014). Women in academic science: A changing landscape. *Psychological Science in the Public Interest, 15*(3), 75–141.

Charles, C. Z. (2000). Neighborhood racial composition preferences: Evidence from a multiethnic metropolis. *Social Problems, 47*(3), 379–407.

Chen, S. (2019). Authenticity in context: Being true to working selves. *Review of General Psychology, 23*(1), 60–72.

Cheryan, S., & Markus, H. R. (2020). Masculine defaults: Identifying and mitigating hidden cultural biases. *Psychological Review, 127*(6), 1022–1052.

Cheryan, S., Plaut, V. C., Davies, P. G., & Steele, C. M. (2009). Ambient belonging: How stereotypical cues impact gender participation in computer science. *Journal of Personality and Social Psychology, 97*(6), 1045–1060.

Choi, E. U., & Hogg, M. A. (2020). Self-uncertainty and group identification: A meta-analysis. *Group Processes and Intergroup Relations, 23*(4), 483–501.

Claypool, H. M., Housley, M. K., Hugenberg, K., Bernstein, M. J., & Mackie, D. M. (2012). Easing in: Fluent processing bring others into the ingroup. *Group Processes and Intergroup Relations, 15*(4), 441–455.

Craig, M. A., Rucker, J. M., & Richeson, J. A. (2018). The pitfalls and promise of increasing racial diversity: Threat, contact, and race relations in the 21st century. *Current Directions in Psychological Science, 27*(3), 188–193.

Csikszentmihalyi, M. (1975). *Beyond boredom and anxiety: Experiencing flow in work and play*. Jossey-Bass.

Cuddy, A. J. C., Wolf, E. B., Glick, P., Crotty, S., Chong, J., & Norton, M. I. (2015). Men as cultural ideals: Cultural values moderate gender stereotype content. *Journal of Personality and Social Psychology, 109*(4), 622–635.

Cutler, D. M., & Glaeser, E. L. (1997). Are ghettos good or bad? *Quarterly Journal of Economics, 1112*(3), 827–872.

Cyr, E. N., Bergsieker, H. B., Dennehy, T. C., & Schmader, T. (2021). Mapping social exclusion in STEM to men's implicit bias and women's career costs. *Proceedings of the National Academy of Sciences, 118*(40).

Devos, T., & Banaji, M. R. (2005). American = White? *Journal of Personality and Social Psychology, 88*(3), 447–466.

DiDonato, T. E., & Krueger, J. I. (2010). Interpersonal affirmation and self-authenticity: A test of Rogers's self-growth hypothesis. *Self and Identity, 9*(3), 322–336.

Diekman, A. B., Steinberg, M., Brown, E. R., Belanger, A. L., & Clark, E. K. (2017). A goal congruity model of role entry, engagement, and exit: Understanding communal goal processes in STEM gender gaps. *Personality and Social Psychology Review, 21*(2), 142–175.

Dover T. L., Major B., & Kaiser C. R. (2016). Members of high-status groups are threatened by pro-diversity organizational messages. *Journal of Experimental Social Psychology, 62*, 58–67.

Dufner, M., Gebauer, J. E., Sedikides, C., & Denissen, J. J. A. (2019). Self-enhancement and psychological adjustment: A meta-analytic review. *Personality and Social Psychology Review, 23*(1), 48–72.

Dunlop, W. L., & Schmader, T. (2014). For the overweight, is proximity to in-shape, normal-weight exercisers a deterrent or an attractor?: An examination of contextual preferences. *International Journal of Behavioral Medicine, 21*(1), 139–143.

Dweck, C. S. (2006). *Mindset: The new psychology of success*. Random House.

English, T., John, O. P., Srivastava, S., & Gross, J. J. (2012). Emotion regulation and peer-rated social functioning: A four-year longitudinal study. *Journal of Research in Personality, 46*(6), 780–784.

Fleeson, W., & Wilt, J. (2010). The relevance of Big Five trait content in behavior to subjective authenticity: Do high levels of within-person behavioral variability undermine or enable authenticity achievement? *Journal of Personality, 78*(4), 1353–1382.

Folberg, A. M., Dueland, L. B., Swanson, M., Stepanek, S., Hebl, M., & Ryan, C. S. (2024). Racism underlies seemingly race-neutral conservative criticisms of DEI statements among Black and White people in the United States. *Journal of Occupational and Organizational Psychology*.

Forbes, C. E., Schmader, T., & Allen, J. J. B. (2008). Error monitoring in an intellectually threatening environment. *Social Cognitive Affective Neuroscience, 3*(5), 253–261.

Frankl, V. (2006). *Man's search for meaning*. Beacon Press. (Original work published 1959)

Goldman, B. M., & Kernis, M. H. (2002). The role of authenticity in healthy psychological functioning and subjective well-being. *Annals of the American Psychotherapy Association, 5*(6), 18–20.

Green, P. A., Briffa, M., & Cant, M. A. (2021). Assessment during intergroup contests. *Trends in Ecology and Evolution, 36*(2), 139–150.

Guo, Y., & Schmader, T. (2024). *Does marginalization undermine fit and state authenticity?* Unpublished data, University of British Columbia.

Guo, Y., & Schmader, T. (2025). Inauthentic or merely uncertain: When do people tolerate situations of identity misfit? In P. Carroll, K. Rios, & K. Oleson (Eds.), *Handbook of the uncertain self* (2nd ed., pp. 132–146). Routledge.

Hall, W., Schmader, T., Aday, A., & Croft, E. (2019). Decoding the dynamics of social identity threat in the workplace: A within-person analysis of women's and men's interactions in STEM. *Social Psychological and Personality Science, 10*(4), 542–552.

Hatzenbuehler, M. L. (2009). How does sexual minority stigma "get under the skin"?: A psychological mediation framework. *Psychological Bulletin, 135*(5), 707–730.

Henrich, J., & Gil-White, F. (2001). The evolution of prestige: Freely conferred status as a mechanism for enhancing the benefits of cultural transmission. *Evolution and Human Behavior, 22*(3), 165–196.

Heppner, W. L., Kernis, M. H., Nezlek, J. B., Foster, J., Lakey, C. E., & Goldman, B. M. (2008). Within-person relationships among daily self-esteem, need satisfaction, and authenticity. *Psychological Science, 19*(11), 1140–1145.

Hicks, J. A., & Routledge, C. (Eds.). (2013). *The experience of meaning in life: Classical perspectives, emerging themes, and controversies*. Springer Science + Business Media.

Higgins, E. T. (2005). Value from regulatory fit. *Current Directions in Psychological Science, 14*(4), 209–213.

Huber, C., Germar, M., & Mojzisch, A. (2022). Authenticity occurs more often than inauthenticity in everyday life: Evidence from retrospective reports. *Social Psychology, 53*(2), 63–72.

Ihlanfeldt, K. R., & Scafidi, B. (2002). Black self-segregation as a cause of housing segregation: Evidence from the multi-city study of urban inequality. *Journal of Urban Economics, 51*(2), 366–390.

Kaiser, C. R., Dover, T. L., Small, P., Xia, G., Brady, L. M., & Major, B. (2022). Diversity initiatives and white Americans' perceptions of racial victimhood. *Personality and Social Psychology Bulletin, 48*(6), 968–984.

Kay, A. C., Jimenez, M. C., & Jost, J. T. (2002). Sour grapes, sweet lemons, and the anticipatory rationalization of the status quo. *Personality and Social Psychology Bulletin, 28*(9), 1300–1312.

Kelley, N. J., Davis, W. E., Dang, J., Liu, L., Wildschut, T., & Sedikides, C. (2022). Nostalgia confers psychological wellbeing by increasing authenticity. *Journal of Experimental Social Psychology, 102,* Article 104379.

Kernis, M. H., & Goldman, B. M. (2006). A multicomponent conceptualization of authenticity: Theory and research. *Advances in Experimental Social Psychology, 38,* 284–357.

Kim, J., Chen, K., Davis, W. E., Hicks, J. A., & Schlegel, R. J. (2019). Approaching the true self: Promotion focus predicts the experience of authenticity. *Journal of Research in Personality, 78,* 165–176.

Kristof-Brown, A., & Guay, R. P. (2011). Person–environment fit. In S. Zedeck (Ed.), *APA handbook of industrial and organizational psychology: Vol. 3. Maintaining, expanding, and contracting the organization* (pp. 3–50). American Psychological Association.

Kye, S. (2023). The rise of Asian ethnoburbs: A case of self-segregation? *Sociology of Race and Ethnicity, 9*(3), 377–394.

Landa, I., & English, T. (2022). Variability in state authenticity predicts daily affect and emotion regulation. *Emotion, 22*(8), 1995–1999.

Lenton, A. P., Bruder, M., Slabu, L., & Sedikides, C. (2013). How does "being real" feel?: The experience of state authenticity. *Journal of Personality, 81*(3), 276–289.

Lenton, A. P., Slabu, L., Bruder, M., & Sedikides, C. (2014). Identifying differences in the experience of (in)authenticity: A latent class analysis approach. *Frontiers in Psychology: Personality Science and Individual Differences, 5,* Article 770.

Lenton, A. P., Slabu, L., & Sedikides, C. (2016). State authenticity in everyday life. *European Journal of Personality, 30*(1), 64–82.

Lippa, R. (1998). Gender-related individual differences and the structure of vocational interests: The importance of the people–things dimension. *Journal of Personality and Social Psychology, 74*(4), 996–1009.

Major, B., Blodorn, A., & Major Blascovich, G. (2018). The threat of increasing diversity: Why many White Americans support Trump in the 2016 presidential election. *Group Processes & Intergroup Relations, 21*(6), 931–940.

Markus, H., & Wurf, E. (1987). The dynamic self-concept: A social psychological perspective. *Annual Review of Psychology, 38,* 299–337.

Maslow, A. H. (1943). A theory of human motivation. *Psychological Review, 50*(4), 370–396.

Maslow, A. H. (1971). *The farther reaches of human nature.* Viking.

Maslow, A. H. (1999). Peak-experiences as acute identity experiences. In *Toward a psychology of being* (3rd ed., pp. 113–125). Wiley. (Reprinted from 1961, *American Journal of Psychoanalysis, 21,* 254–260)

McCrae, R. R., & Costa, P. T. (1987). Validation of the five-factor model of personality across instruments and observers. *Journal of Personality and Social Psychology, 52*(1), 81–90.

Meyer, I. H. (2003). Prejudice, social stress, and mental health in lesbian, gay, and bisexual populations: Conceptual issues and research evidence. *Psychological Bulletin, 129*(5), 674–697.

Miller, C. T., Rothblum, E. D., Felicio, D., & Brand, P. (1995). Compensating for stigma: Obese and nonobese women's reactions to being visible. *Personality and Social Psychology Bulletin, 21*(10), 1093–1106.

Milyavskaya, M., Nadolny, D., & Koestner, R. (2015). Why do people set more self-concordant goals in need satisfying domains?: Testing authenticity as a mediator. *Personality and Individual Differences, 77,* 131–136.

Montoya, R. M., Horton, R. S., Vevea, J. L., Citkowicz, M., & Lauber, E. A. (2017). A reexamination of the mere exposure effect: The influence of repeated exposure on recognition, familiarity, and liking. *Psychological Bulletin, 143*(5), 459–498.

Motyl, M. (2016). Liberals and conservatives are (geographically) dividing. In P. Valdesolo & J. Graham (Eds.), *Social psychology of political polarization* (pp. 7–37). Routledge/Taylor & Francis Group.

Musterd, S., & Ostendorf, W. (Eds.). (1998). *Urban segregation and the welfare state: Inequality and exclusion in Western cities.* Routledge.

Nisbett, R. E., & Wilson, T. D. (1977). Telling more than we can know: Verbal reports on mental processes. *Psychological Review, 84*(3), 231–259.

Ntoumanis, N., & Sedikides, C. (2018). Holding on (to the goal) or letting it go and move on?: A tripartite model of goal striving. *Current Directions in Psychological Science, 27*(5), 363–368.

Page-Gould, E., Mendoza-Denton, R., & Tropp, L. R. (2008). With a little help from my cross-group friend: Reducing anxiety in intergroup contexts through cross-group friendship. *Journal of Personality and Social Psychology, 95*(5), 1080–1094.

Pennebaker, J. W. (2011). *The secret life of pronouns: What our words say about us.* Bloomsbury Press.

Peterson, T., & Morgan, L. A. (1995). Separate and unequal: Occupation-establishment sex segregation and the gender wage gap. *American Journal of Sociology, 101*(2), 329–365.

Pettigrew, T. F., & Tropp, L. R. (2006). A meta-analytic test of intergroup contact theory. *Journal of Personality and Social Psychology, 90*(5), 751–783.

Phillips, L. T., Stephens, N. M., Townsend, S. S. M., & Goudeau, S. (2020). Access is not enough: Cultural mismatch persists to limit first-generation students' opportunities for achievement throughout college. *Journal of Personality and Social Psychology, 119*(5), 1112–1131.

Pronin, E., Steele, C. M., & Ross, L. (2004). Identity bifurcation in response to stereotype threat: Women and mathematics. *Journal of Experimental Social Psychology, 40*(2), 152–168.

Purdie-Vaughns, V., Steele, C. M., Davies, P. G., Ditlmann, R., & Crosby, J. R. (2008). Social identity contingencies: How diversity cues signal threat or safety for African Americans in mainstream institutions. *Journal of Personality and Social Psychology, 94*(4), 615–630.

Pyszczynski, T., Greenberg, J., Solomon, S., Arndt, J., & Schimel, J. (2004). Why do people need self-esteem?: A theoretical and empirical review. *Psychological Bulletin, 130*(3), 435–468.

Reber, R., & Unkelbach, C. (2010). The epistemic status of processing fluency as source for judgments of truth. *Review of Philosophy and Psychology, 1*(4), 563–581.

Reed, D. E., Lehinger, E., Cobos, B., Vail, K. E., Nabity, P., Helm, P. J., . . . McGeary, D. D. (2021). Authenticity as a resilience factor against CV-19 threat among those with chronic pain and posttraumatic stress disorder. *Frontiers in Psychology, 12,* Article 643869.

Rentfrow, P. J., Gosling, S. D., & Potter, J. (2008). A theory of the emergence, persistence, and expression of geographic variation in psychological characteristics. *Perspectives on Psychological Science, 3*(5), 339–369.

Riediger, M., Wrzus, C., Schmiedek, F., Wagner, G. G., & Lindenberger, U. (2011). Is seeking bad mood cognitively demanding?: Contra-hedonic orientation and working-memory capacity in everyday life. *Emotion, 11*(3), 656–665.

Rios, K., & Mackey, C. D. (2022). "White" self-identification: A source of uniqueness threat. *Social Psychological and Personality Science, 13*(2), 416–424.

Rivera, G. N., Christy, A. G., Kim, J., Vess, M., Hicks, J. A., & Schlegel, R. J. (2019). Understanding the relationship between perceived authenticity and well-being. *Review of General Psychology, 23*(1), 113–126.

Rogers, C. R. (1961). *On becoming a person: A therapist's view of psychotherapy.* Houghton Mifflin.

Ryan, R. M., & Deci, E. L. (2017). *Self-determination theory: Basic psychological needs in motivation, development, and wellness.* Guilford Press.

Schmader, T., Croft, A., & Whitehead, J. (2014). Why can't I just be myself?: A social cognitive analysis of the working self-concept under stereotype threat. *Social Psychological and Personality Science, 5*(1), 4–11.

Schmader, T., Forbes, C. E., Zhang, S., & Mendes, W. B. (2009). A metacognitive perspective on the cognitive deficits experienced in intellectually threatening environments. *Personality and Social Psychology Bulletin, 35*(5), 584–596.

Schmader, T., Johns, M., & Forbes, C. (2008). An integrated process model of stereotype threat effects on performance. *Psychological Review, 115*(2), 336–356.

Schmader, T., Major, B., & Gramzow, R. H. (2001). Coping with ethnic stereotypes in the academic domain: Perceived injustice and psychological disengagement. *Journal of Social Issues, 57*(1), 93–111.

Schmader, T., & Sedikides, C. (2018). State authenticity as fit to environment (SAFE): The implications of social identity for fit, authenticity, and self-segregation. *Personality and Social Psychology Review, 22*(3), 228–259.

Schopler, J., Insko, C. A., Graetz, K. A., Drigotas, S., Smith, V. A., & Dahl, K. (1993). Individual-group discontinuity: Further evidence for mediation by fear and greed. *Personality and Social Psychology Bulletin, 19*(4), 419–431.

Sedikides, C., Gaertner, L., Luke, M. A., O'Mara, E. M., & Gebauer, J. (2013). A three-tier hierarchy of motivational self-potency: Individual self, relational self, collective self. *Advances in Experimental Social Psychology, 48*, 235–295.

Sedikides, C., Green, J. D., Saunders, J., Skowronski, J. J., & Zengel, B. (2016). Mnemic neglect: Selective amnesia of one's faults. *European Review of Social Psychology, 27*(1), 1–62.

Sedikides, C., Lenton, A. P., Slabu, L., & Thomaes, S. (2019). Sketching the contours of state authenticity. *Review of General Psychology, 23*(1), 73–88.

Sedikides, C., Slabu, L., Lenton, A. P., & Thomaes, S. (2017). State authenticity. *Current Directions in Psychological Science, 26*(1), 515–520.

Shaver, P. R., & Mikulincer, M. (2008). Adult attachment and cognitive and affective reactions to positive and negative events. *Social and Personality Psychology Compass, 2*(5), 1844–1865.

Shelton, J. N., Richeson, J. A., & Salvatore, J. (2005). Expecting to be the target of prejudice: Implications for interethnic interactions. *Personality and Social Psychology Bulletin, 31*(9), 1189–1202.

Smith, D. G. (1990). Embracing diversity as a central campus goal. *Academe, 76*(6), 29–33.

Song, H., & Schwarz, N. (2009). If it's difficult to pronounce, it must be risky: Fluency, familiarity, and risk perception. *Psychological Science, 20*(2), 135–138.

Steele, C. M. (1988). The psychology of self-affirmation: Sustaining the integrity of the self. *Advances in Experimental Social Psychology, 21*, 261–302.

Stonewall. (2018). *LGBT health in Britain* (p. 21). Stonewall. www.stonewall.org.uk/lgbt-britain-health.

Su, R., Murdock, C., & Rounds, J. (2015). Person-environment fit. In P. J. Hartung, M. L. Savickas, & W. B. Walsh (Eds.), *APA handbook of career intervention: Vol. 1. Foundations* (pp. 81–98). American Psychological Association.

Sutton, A. (2020). Living the good life: A meta-analysis of authenticity, well-being and engagement. *Personality and Individual Differences, 153*, Article 109645.

Thomaes, S., Sedikides, C., Van den Bos, N., Hutteman, R., & Reijntjes, A. (2017). Happy to be "me"? Authenticity, psychological need satisfaction, and subjective well-being in adolescence. *Child Development, 88*(4), 1045–1056.

Van Vianen, A. E. M. (2018). Person–environment fit: A review of its basic tenets. *Annual Review of Organizational Psychology and Organizational Behavior, 5*, 75–101.

Vainio, M. M., & Daukantaitė, D. (2016). Grit and different aspects of well-being: Direct and indirect relationships via sense of coherence and authenticity. *Journal of Happiness Studies: An Interdisciplinary Forum on Subjective Well-Being, 17*(5), 2119–2147.

Vess, M. (2019). Varieties of conscious experience and the subjective awareness of one's "true" self. *Review of General Psychology, 23*(1), 89–98.

Walsh, W. B., Craik, K., & Price, R. H. (2000). *Person–environment psychology* (2nd ed.). Erlbaum.

Walton, G. M., & Cohen, G. L. (2007). A question of belonging: Race, social fit, and achievement. *Journal of Personality and Social Psychology, 92*(1), 82–96.

Walton, G. M., Cohen, G. L., Cwir, D., & Spencer, S. J. (2012). Mere belonging: The power of social connections. *Journal of Personality and Social Psychology, 102*(3), 513–532.

Wood, A. M., Linley, P. A., Maltby, J., Baliousis, M., & Joseph, S. (2008). The authentic personality: A theoretical and empirical conceptualization and the development of the Authenticity Scale. *Journal of Counseling Psychology, 55*(3), 385–399.

Yang, Y., Zhu, S., Gan, Y., & Dang, J. (2021). To be authentic, to be eco: Exploring the link between authenticity and pro-environmental behavior. *Frontiers in Psychology, 12*, Article 755860.

Zhang, H., Chen, K., Schlegel, R., Hicks, J., & Chen, C. (2019). The authentic moral self: Dynamic interplay between perceived authenticity and moral behaviors in the workplace. *Collabra: Psychology, 5*(1), Article 48.

Zhang, Y. B., Lin, M.-C., Nonaka, A., & Beom, K. (2005). Harmony, hierarchy and conservatism: A cross-cultural comparison of Confucian values in China, Korea, Japan, and Taiwan. *Communication Research Reports, 22*(2), 107–115.

CHAPTER 40

Narrative Identity

Dan P. McAdams *and* Sebnem Ture

Narrative identity is the story that evolves in the mind of a person to depict who they are and how they have come to be the person they are becoming (McAdams, 2021; McAdams & McLean, 2013). Rather than providing a veridical rendering of past events, narrative identity reconstructs the autobiographical past and imagines the future, functioning as a personal myth that affirms a sense of temporal coherence, integration, and purpose in life. It is through our life stories that we find meaning in our lives, as both authors of those stories and protagonists who push the plotlines forward (Bruner, 1990; Freeman, 1993; Josselson, 2009). Narrative identity functions as an important psychological resource for adapting to the daunting demands of modern life (Giddens, 1991; Taylor, 1989), as it shapes self-understanding, influences the choices we make, and partly determines the psychological quality of the lives we live.

In first proposing a life-story model of identity, McAdams (1985) situated the concept of narrative identity within the fields of personality and lifespan developmental psychology. The original theory was framed within the context of Henry Murray's (1938) personological tradition and the psychodynamic writings of Erik Erikson (1958, 1963). McAdams (1985, 1996) aimed to reformulate Erikson's concept of identity in narrative terms, as an inner story that a person begins composing in the emerging adulthood years. And he sought to import the empirical study of life stories into the realm of personality research, introducing an experience-rich perspective to a scientific field dominated at the time by the study of decontextualized personality traits.

That said, the original conception of life stories, as it emerged in the late 1980s, was also strongly influenced by existentialist philosophy and the writings of Jean-Paul Sartre (McAdams, 1985, 1993). In the years following, selected research programs generated by the concept of narrative identity (e.g., McAdams, 2013b, 2019b; McAdams & de St. Aubin, 1992; McAdams & Guo, 2015; McAdams et al., 2022) owed their inspiration, in part, to the writings of other existentialist scholars and thinkers, like Ernest Becker and Albert Camus. Moreover, the study of narrative identity focused from the outset on classic themes in existential psychology, such as meaning, identity, freedom, and the anticipation of death (Koole et al., 2006). With all this in mind, the purpose of this chapter is to present a broad overview of the scientific study of narrative identity within an existentialist frame. We aim to reveal connections between existential psychology and the study of narrative identity—a concept that itself was partly inspired by existentialism, and that has, over the subsequent couple decades, generated many different lines of research in a range of domains in psychological science.

LIFE STORIES (AND THE LEGACY OF JEAN-PAUL SARTRE)

In his eight-stage model of psychosocial development, Erikson (1963) identified identity versus role confusion to be the central dynamic for the adolescent and emerging adulthood years. At this time in the life course, the young person may be preoccupied with identity questions such as "Who am I?" and "How do I fit into the adult world?" According to Erikson, the young person may eventually resolve these questions by developing a new self-conception that provides a sense of inner sameness, even as they move across many different roles, and a sense of personal continuity, even as they continue to change over time. As Erikson saw it, identity formation involves arranging the self in such a way as to integrate a life in time and in social space while situating the young person within a meaningful societal niche.

But what explicit form might that self-arrangement take? If one could literally "see" an identity, what might it look like? McAdams (1985) proposed that it might look like a *story*. Constructing an internalized and evolving story of the self, McAdams argued, might do for the young person what Erikson insisted identity itself does. Indeed, stories capture experience as it unfolds over time, structured temporally in terms of beginnings, middles, and endings. As such, a life story might tell us who we were, who we are, and who we may become in the future. With manifold characters and plots, stories convey the richness of lived experience—the different and conflicting selves that make "me" up. Stories organize the diversity of selfhood into a coherent narrative frame. They explain who we are, both to ourselves and to others. They provide our lives with meaning and purpose while helping situate us as actors and agents in the world, who reflect upon it all as authors (McAdams, 2013a). McAdams proposed that we begin working on our life stories, through introspection and social interaction, in the emerging adulthood years. As autobiographical authors, we continue to work on our stories across the adult life course, as identity continues to develop and change.

In a famous quote from *Nausea*, the existentialist philosopher Jean-Paul Sartre (1964) wrote, "This is what fools people: a man is always a teller of tales, he lives surrounded by his stories and the stories of others, he sees everything that happens to him through them; and he tries to live his life as if he were telling a story" (p. 39). Among the most important sources McAdams (1985, 1993) drew upon in formulating the life-story model of identity was Sartre's existentialist idea of the *true novel* (Charme, 1984; Sartre, 1965). In some of his writings, Sartre imagined the self as a retrospective story that creates order out of the chaos of personal experience. Because traditional myths no longer provide meaning for modern adults, Sartre suggested, many people create their own myths about themselves to experience meaning. Ideally, a person's true novel should reflect a central truth or dilemma about their own lives and about the historical moment in which they live.

Sartre may have been ambivalent, however, about the validity and value of the stories people tell about their lives. After all, the next sentence in the *Nausea* quote is this: "But you have to choose: Live or tell." The implication is that the true novel may occlude authentic lived experience. People cannot live and tell at the same time, and telling may, in some sense, get in the way of living—may even constitute "bad faith" when conventional narration strips away the unique phenomenology of an experienced event. Then again, narration may be the prime manner by which modern people, "thrown" into a chaotic world as Heidegger famously contended, try to create order and discern meaning amid it all. Contemporary philosophers continue to debate whether Sartre truly endorsed a narrative approach to understanding the self and identity. But from the standpoint of narrative psychology, he is viewed as a philosophical antecedent, along with Paul Ricouer (1984) and others who have strongly advocated for life-narrative perspectives in philosophy (e.g., Schechtman, 1996). The main idea running through these works is that human beings are storytellers by nature (McAdams, 2019a), as well as by culture (Hammack,

2008), and that people make meaning in life through narrative.

Working within the field of personality science, McAdams (1985, 1996) sought to examine variation in the stories people tell about their lives. He proposed that individual differences in narrative identity distinguish one person from the next, just as do conventional personality traits (the person as social actor) and goals/values (the person as motivated agent). As autobiographical authors, people may differ from each other in terms of the processes involved in life-story construction and in terms of the stories they tell. Focusing mainly on the latter, McAdams (1985) developed a life-story interview for collecting data on narrative identity. The interview asks the person first to think about their life as if it were a novel and to briefly summarize each of the chapters in the novel. Then, the interview poses a series of questions that ask the participant to describe in detail particular scenes in the life story (such as high points, low points, and turning points), to identify key characters and challenges, to anticipate chapters to come in the future, to articulate basic values and beliefs (especially religious and political values and beliefs), and finally to identify key themes or motifs that run through the interview text. Similar procedures have been developed for online data collection, usually focusing on but a few prompts from the longer interview.

After collecting the qualitative life-story data, researchers today typically initiate a quantification process by crafting coding schemes or utilizing preexisting ones. The quantification of the qualitative data is necessary for hypothesis-testing research, as it allows researchers to look at associations between narrative identity and other important metrics that are often quantitative in nature (e.g., self-report data). A recent factor analysis of coding procedures applied to a large number of narrative protocols from different labs revealed three main groupings of coding schemes—those focused on (1) social and emotional functioning of the characters in the story; (2) structural features of the story itself, such as coherence; and (3) the quality of autobiographical reasoning and meaning making displayed by the narrator of the story (McLean et al., 2020).

Determining which segments of the life-story accounts to code and what coding schemes to employ is dependent on the study hypotheses. Researchers may choose to concentrate on one single narrative scene, such as "the most unstable, troubled, or discouraging time in your life" (Pals, 2006), a memory of a yearly life challenge (Lind et al., 2024), or a major historical event the person witnessed (Ture et al., 2025). Alternatively, they may analyze many different narrative scenes and aggregate scores across scenes, which together reflect a participant's overarching narrative identity, or trace how particular themes emerge across different parts of an entire life story (Mayukha et al., 2025). In the latter approach, researchers have, for example, combined data from various key scenes, including low points, biggest failures/regrets, significant religious/spiritual experiences, expected future scenes and chapters, and overall life themes, to assess variation in narrative themes such as self-transcendence (Reischer et al., 2021).

Coding schemes typically involve making ratings ranging from a low score to a high score. For example, the narrative theme of communion (the extent to which a character feels that they experience positive relationships with others) is a socioemotional theme measured through a coding scale that ranges from 0 to 4. A score of 0 indicates that the protagonist feels completely isolated from others, and strong disconnection language is present in the narrative, while a score of 4 indicates that the protagonist feels highly connected to others, and rich connection language is predominant in the narrative. Typically, a pair of research assistants, who are unaware of the study's hypotheses but trained to use the coding manuals, independently read each narrative account and assign a score. They review the same narratives separately until achieving good interrater reliability. Once reliability is attained, coders either divide the remaining data between them to be coded, or they continue coding all the data. For the latter, consensus codes are used for analysis, or respective coder's independent scores are averaged.

As a final step, the quantified narrative data may then be linked to other data from the same participants. For example, prior empirical research has shown that communion in individuals' love narratives—stories about romantic relationships in one's life—correlates positively with self-reported positive outcomes within the relationship domain (Bühler & Dunlop, 2019). For further insights into conventional procedures for conducting empirical research involving narratives, refer to Adler and colleagues (2017).

Developmental research has shown that it is not until adolescence that people develop the cognitive wherewithal to construct narrative identities. While differences in childhood storytelling have implications for narrative identity down the road (Fivush et al., 2019), adolescence typically marks the emergence of autobiographical reasoning, which jump-starts life-narrative processes (Habermas & Bluck, 2000). Through autobiographical reasoning, young people attribute meaning to remembered scenes in their lives. For example, an 18-year-old girl may recall a junior high school incident of online bullying as marking a turning point. As she makes sense of her life in retrospect, she now believes that her days were filled with joy and laughter in grade school, but after she was bullied, she began to distrust people. She makes an authorial decision to see her life in this way. Another teenaged girl, recently graduated from high school, looks back on the last 4 years as a period of social maturation and success. She came into her own during that time, she feels. She now looks to the future with a mix of confidence and uncertainty. She is not sure what will happen next, but her story tells her that she may be able to build on her newfound strengths.

As young people use autobiographical reasoning to make narrative meaning in their lives, they discuss and enact those meanings within important interpersonal relationships. Researchers have documented the ways in which young people begin to share personal stories with each other and how the reactions those stories elicit from interlocuters change the stories themselves (Pasupathi & Billitteri, 2015), accentuating certain ideas and discounting others, as selves create stories, which create new selves, and narrative identity grows and changes over time (Lilgendahl & McLean, 2020; McLean et al., 2007). We become new persons as our stories change, stories that themselves describe the existential process of becoming. Going back to Sartre (1964), people tell as they live, and live as they tell. Narration shapes action, and action, in turn, shapes the narratives we construct to explain our acts.

In his copious writings on identity, Erikson (1958, 1963) frequently highlighted the ideological nature of the adolescent mind. From the beginning, research on narrative identity prioritized the role of religious and political values in life stories. McAdams (1985) proposed that life narratives are structured within an *ideological setting*, which specifies the backdrop of belief and value against which the story's plot unfolds. A strong line of research on narrative identity has examined variation in political and religious values (e.g., Hanek et al., 2011; McAdams et al., 2008). For example, studies have shown that political conservatives in the United States tend to construct stories for their lives that emphasize the challenge of self-control and the value of strong authority to rein in the worst instincts of human beings. Christian conservatives tend to see God as a supreme king who rules with a firm hand. They fear chaos; God and good government ideally protect them from that danger (McAdams & Albaugh, 2008). By contrast, political liberals in the United States tend to construct life stories underscoring self-discovery and the power of nurturance. Christian liberals imagine God as a benevolent provider. They fear emptiness, and they expect God and good government to provide them with the resources they need to grow and flourish (McAdams & Albaugh, 2008).

Variations in the structure and content of narrative identity have been repeatedly linked to self-report assessments of mental health and well-being. Indeed, the predictive efficacy of narrative indices is robust enough to explain additional variance in well-being above and beyond the strong effects exerted by personality traits such as extraversion and neuroticism (Adler et al., 2016). Studies have consistently shown that psychological well-being is positively associated with life narratives exhibiting high levels of (1) *coherence* (accounts are well-structured and easy to follow), (2) *agency* (the protagonist experiences self-efficacy or control), (3) *communion* (the protagonist enjoys positive interpersonal relationships), and (4) *redemption* (accounts track the move from suffering to enhancement or growth) (e.g., Adler et al., 2015; McAdams & Guo, 2015; Waters & Fivush, 2015). Stories suffused with the imagery of *contamination*, wherein an emotionally positive scene turns suddenly negative, have been shown to be strongly associated with depression (Adler et al., 2006).

Recent work has expanded the study of life stories into the realm of psychopathology, with special attention paid to personality disorders (Lind et al., 2022). Studies have shown that people suffering from personality disorders often construct life-narrative accounts that are highly incoherent and suffused with negative emotion, deviate markedly from normative scripts for development, exhibit low levels of agency, and describe a longing for communion that is repeatedly thwarted (Lind et al., 2021; Shiner et al., 2021).

Other researchers have begun to apply narrative-identity concepts to understanding the etiology and course of schizophrenia-spectrum disorders. Cowan, Mittal, and McAdams (2021) have proposed a model that follows the development of narrative identity over the course of psychotic illness. Reviewing 30 studies that examine the intersection of life stories and psychosis, they suggest that (1) a strong focus on suffering in autobiographical memory arises in childhood for individuals afflicted with these severe disorders, (2) disjointed structure of narrative accounts emerges in middle-to-late adolescence, and (3) detached narration begins to appear around the time of the person's first psychotic episode. The decline and disintegration of narrative identity over time marks a severe breakdown in the person's ability to make fundamental meaning out of life, systematically tracking the tragic course of the illness. The model aims to shed light on the existential mysteries of severe psychopathology and suggest new aims for treatment.

GENERATIVITY AND THE REDEMPTIVE SELF (ENTER ERNEST BECKER)

In *The Denial of Death*, Ernest Becker (1973) argued that human beings engage in a range of life projects—from creating art to building institutions—as a way of finding meaning in the face of mortality. Situated between the beasts and the angels, Becker wrote, human beings are painfully aware of their corporeality even as they long for the transcendent. The fear of death is primal. We know that our bodies will deteriorate, die, and decay—from dust to dust, ashes to ashes. Or at least we know it at some level, because we also act in ways that suggest a denial of the reality. The fear of death operates as a prime motivator, Becker suggested, for much of what human beings do in daily life, and it lies behind our greatest achievements in art, government, science, religion, and society. We work hard to create products and achieve outcomes that will outlive the self, aiming to defy death and achieve a kind of symbolic immortality. Through the things we make, the people we care for, and the ideas we promulgate, we aim to create something—anything—that may live on as a legacy of the self. We can never know if what we have to offer for future generations is worthy and good, but we are compelled to push forward anyway, in the face of death.

This profoundly existential sentiment is captured powerfully in the following passage from Becker's seminal text: "Who knows what form the forward movement of life will take in the time ahead or what use it will make of our anguished searching? The most that any of us can seem to do is to *fashion* something—an object or ourselves—and drop it into the confusion, make an *offering* of it, so to speak, to the life force" (Becker, 1973, p. 173, emphasis added).

It is well known that Becker's perspective served as the starting point for terror management theory, one of the most formidable conceptions in social psychology (Greenberg et al., 1990). The core existentialist idea here is that people manage the fear of mortality by finding comfort and security in cultural beliefs that offer lasting meaning and value. Becker's writing, however, has also exerted a strong impact on the study of narrative identity. Life stories incorporate imagined endings, increasingly so as people grow older and the prospect of death becomes more salient. McAdams (1985) argued that in midlife and beyond adults tend to project scripts for the future chapters in their life narratives that aim to leave a positive legacy of the self, as a symbolic immortality project. The creation of such a *generativity script* often makes for the creative blending or juxtaposition of thematic lines of agency and communion in narrative identity (McAdams et al., 1986). The idea that such a script anticipates ways in which the person's life activities and commitments may positively impact future generations recalls Erikson's (1963, 1969) concept of generativity, which he conceived as the midlife adult's concern for and commitment to promoting the well-being of future generations.

While Erikson tended to emphasize the communal virtue of care in his writings on generativity, he also gestured toward agency and the generative person's desire to generate people, things, and ideas that may outlive the self (Kotre, 1984). Following Otto Rank, Becker (1973) used the term *heroism* to describe the generative process of fashioning something out of the self and then offering it up as a gift to the future. Becker's conception foregrounds agency over communion and suggests a more muscular conception of how human beings orient themselves to future generations. Drawing on both Erikson and Becker, McAdams and de St. Aubin (1992) reformulated the concept of generativity to explicitly include both an agentic drive for symbolic immortality and a communal desire to nurture and care for the next generation, and they developed and validated self-report measures to assess individual differences in generativity. They then launched a long-term program of research, employing both quantitative and qualitative methods, to examine the life stories of highly generative adults. Committing oneself to promoting the well-being of future generations and leaving a positive legacy of the self is risky business, many would say. *It is difficult to be a highly generative adult.* The effort often requires significant sacrifice, and there are no guarantees that one's efforts will lead to the desired impact. What kinds of narrative identities, therefore, do caring and productive midlife adults construct to support their generative efforts? How do those life stories compare with the narrative identities constructed by adults lower in generativity?

Research has revealed that highly generative American adults in their midlife years tend, more than their less generative counterparts, to construe their lives as tales of redemption (McAdams, 2013b). Replicated empirical studies and case biographies demonstrate that midlife American adults who score high on well-validated measures of generativity often construct variations on a general story prototype called the *redemptive self* (e.g., Dunlop, 2021; McAdams, 2011; McAdams et al.,1997; McAdams & Guo, 2015; Perlin & Fivush, 2021; Walker & Frimer, 2007). It is a heroic tale of the sort that resonates with Becker's (1973) narrative sensibility and with a long-standing American mythos regarding how to live a good American life. As such, the redemptive self qualifies as a *master cultural narrative* in American society (McLean & Syed, 2015). The story is ever-present in a wide range of characteristically American cultural products, such as Hollywood movies, classic American fiction, presidential speeches, self-help regimens, and personal essays that students write for admission to college (McAdams, 2013b).

In the redemptive self, a gifted (special, chosen, lucky) protagonist journeys forth into a dangerous world (where bad things often happen to other people) and, equipped with moral steadfastness and a sense of personal manifest destiny, overcomes adversity, and turns suffering into enhancement, with the expectation of continuing to exert a positive impact for future generations (McAdams, 2013b). This kind of life story supports generativity in many ways. For example, by juxtaposing the idea that (1) "I am special" and (2) "The world is dangerous" (and, therefore, "it needs me"), the story challenges the main character to commit to prosocial projects of various kinds, as a way of giving back in gratitude. By suggesting that suffering can often be overcome, furthermore, the story gives the generative adult the confidence that the hard work and many setbacks that generativity typically entails and demands will eventually yield dividends. The redemptive-self narrative bears some resemblance to Joseph Campbell's (1949) conception of the myth of the hero, though there are important differences as well. In this regard, it is noteworthy that a recent set of studies showed that when people see their lives as resembling the journey of the hero, as depicted by Campbell, their sense that life has meaning and purpose tends to increase (Rogers et al., 2023).

As a master cultural narrative in American society, the redemptive self exemplifies cardinal values that Americans have historically cherished, such as rugged individualism, self-improvement, resilience, personal growth, and charity. This widely recognized form of narrative identity resonates strongly for many Americans, especially in their midlife years, and it serves to promote prosocial, generative commitments that might otherwise be more difficult to sustain (McAdams, 2013b, 2019b). Like any cultural ideal, however, the redemptive self is not so elastic and accommodating as to capture the lived experience of all highly generative American adults, let alone all Americans. And its applicability to the lives of people living in other societies, perhaps especially non-Western societies and those of the global South, may not be especially strong. Every culture projects its own storehouse of valued images, metaphors, characters, plotlines, and life tropes for living a good and generative life. People living within the orbit of that culture may borrow narrative material from the storehouse to make meaning of their own lives. As autobiographical authors, they experience varying levels of freedom (versus constraint) in their efforts to do so.

The existential issue of freedom proves to be especially fraught in the literature on narrative identity. On the one side, narrative identity features authorial processes that suggest self-determination and the freedom to construct one's life in ways that conform to personal wishes and values. In *Man's Search for Meaning*, Viktor Frankl (1963/1984) wrote that his Nazi captors could control nearly every aspect of his existence in the concentration camp, save his inner attitude about things. The freedom to think about things in your own way, to make self-determined meaning in the privacy of your own mind, may seem to be inviolate. And yet we find that even our innermost thoughts and fantasies may, at minimum, be contoured and colored by external realities. How much freedom do we really have?

Meaning making through life narrative is never an exclusively private affair. For better and for worse, master cultural narratives shape how people living within the parameters of a given culture give meaning to their lived experience (Hammack, 2008; McLean & Syed, 2015; Rogers, 2020). These broad and highly prescriptive stories about how to live a good life in a particular cultural context can constrain as much as they inspire. Furthermore, they typically reinforce existing power dynamics within a given society, affirming the values and perspectives of its most privileged members (Syed & McLean, 2022). Master cultural narratives are often ubiquitous and invisible (McLean & Syed, 2015), like water to a fish. We swim within a sea of narrative, often oblivious to alternative possibilities in living that might arise in different narrative ecologies.

That said, researchers who focus their inquiry on master cultural narratives often speak, as well, of alternative *counter narratives* that people may construct as they aim to defy, or push back against, the rigid strictures of master stories (Bamberg & Andrews, 2004; McLean & Syed, 2015). In a similar vein, narrative therapists speak of *emancipatory discourses* that may arise during therapy, as they encourage their clients to shed the constraints of convention and thereby find new stories that better capture and give meaning to their lived experience (McLeod, 2004; White & Epston, 1990). These perspectives assert again the power of human agency and autonomous authorship, hinting at a complex dialectic between self and society. Even as researchers and scholars, therefore, offer multiple (and sometimes conflicting) points of view, it is clear that the existential issue of freedom (versus constraint) in the construction of selfhood remains a central concern in the scientific literature on narrative identity.

THE THEME OF ACCEPTANCE IN LIFE NARRATIVE (AND THE INFLUENCE OF ALBERT CAMUS)

In the early days of the COVID-19 pandemic, the *New York Times* columnist David Brooks (2020) wrote of the power of redemptive stories to make sense of difficult times. Brooks expressed the hope that Americans might find long-term redemptive meaning in the wake of the virus. He wrote,

"We will look back on this as one of the most meaningful periods in our lives. Our long-term well-being depends on the story we tell about this moment. It's the way we tie our moment of suffering to a larger narrative of redemption. It's the way we then go out and stubbornly live out that story. The plague today is an invisible monster, but it gives birth to a better world" (Brooks, 2020).

In characterizing COVID-19 as "the plague," Brooks (2020) gestured to Albert Camus's (1947) novel of the same name. Considered one of the canonical literary works in the existentialist tradition, *The Plague* tells the fictional story of a virus spreading uncontrollably through a small city on the Algerian coast. For a year, the citizens are locked down and cut off from the rest of the world, as the epidemic claims tens of thousands of lives. And then one day, the dying ends, for no apparent reason. The afflicted begin to recover. The survivors rejoice. It seems like a happy ending. But the novel's protagonist, Dr. Rieux, cautions against a redemptive interpretation: "The tale could not be one of final victory. It could be only the record of what had had to be done, and what assuredly would have to be done again in the never ending fight against terror and its relentless onslaughts, despite their personal afflictions, by all who, while unable to be saints but refusing to bow down to pestilence, strive their utmost to be healers" (Camus, 1947, p. 278).

As the protagonist of the novel, Dr. Rieux works tirelessly to be a "healer." But here is the irony: *He never heals anybody.* Despite his best efforts and up until the moment the virus suddenly abates, every one of his patients dies. *The Plague* is not a heroic story about overcoming adversity. "There's no heroism in this," Rieux says. "It's a matter of common decency" (p. 150). *The Plague* is instead a more sober story of *managing* adversity in a world that invokes random acts of suffering while sorely testing the limits of human agency. As the *protagonist* of the story, Dr. Rieux's role is to comfort people and validate their suffering. But as the novel's *narrator*, Dr. Rieux's role is to *bear witness* to the suffering and the death he has seen—to *tell the story*, so that we never forget the suffering.

Reprising themes that run through the social gerontology literature and that feature prominently in Erikson's (1982) writings on ego integrity, *The Plague* suggests a broad cultural narrative that runs counter to the redemptive self. It is a narrative of *radical acceptance* wherein protagonists who are unable to overcome adversity need, instead, to come to terms with it, and to accept certain inevitabilities in life, including its tragic features (Alon & Omer, 2004; McAdams, 2023; McAdams et al., 2022). In this kind of story, the setting is a world of uncertainty, unpredictable change, and serendipity—akin to life in the time of a plague, as the world experienced it with COVID-19. The idealized goal in the story is to come to terms with life, reconcile conflict to minimize regret, to manage adversity (because adversity cannot always be overcome), and to sustain bonds of intimacy and warmth. With personal qualities like grace, humility, common decency, flexibility, and relentless compassion, Dr. Rieux is one model of the kind of protagonist who flourishes in this kind of postredemptive narrative. As both Camus and Becker knew, the plague—in one form or another—will always be with us. We need to be aware of our constraints. We need to be clear-eyed in the face of our limitations. We need to learn how to live with adversity when we cannot fully defeat it. And like Dr. Rieux, we need to bear witness.

Stories of radical acceptance may become especially relevant for narrative identity as people move through midlife and into their later years (Kenyon et al., 2010). As older adults experience the physical decline and interpersonal losses that invariably accompany aging, life stories that champion triumph over adversity may no longer capture lived experience, nor affirm health and well-being. Some forms of adversity cannot be overcome, increasingly so perhaps in later life. Instead, one may seek to come to terms with adversity, to manage it, to find new ways of living with limitations and constraint. As narratives of acceptance bring into bold relief the protagonist's vulnerabilities, they also prioritize interpersonal contexts that reinforce common decency, compassion, and intimate bonds, as we see with Dr. Rieux in *The Plague*.

Erikson (1963, 1982) identified ego integrity versus despair as the psychosocial centerpiece for the last stage in his developmental model, associated with late life. As Erikson saw it, achieving ego integrity involves an *acceptance* of one's life as something good and worthwhile, as if it were a good *gift* gracefully received. In a study of narrative identity in late midlife, Hollen Reischer and her colleagues found that scores on a self-report measure of ego integrity were negatively associated with regret, even as older adults' stories acknowledged shortcomings, constraints, and disappointments (Reischer et al., 2021). In their life-narrative accounts, the late midlife adults high in ego integrity underscored a deep appreciation for, and acceptance of, their lives as having unfolded in ways that seemed, in retrospect, right and good.

Narratives of acceptance are increasingly featured in the growing literatures on narrative medicine (Garden, 2010), the recovery movement (Altmaeir, 2017), and disability studies (Adler, 2018). With respect to disability, heartwarming (and sometimes miraculous) stories wherein disabled people, in the harsh face of their limitations, achieve heroic feats, provide an inspiring discourse in the popular press and on social media. But these remarkably redemptive accounts are, by definition, the awe-inspiring exceptions to the rule. The promulgation of these kinds of stories—derisively termed "crip-porn" by some critics—belie the clear-eyed reality of most disabled people's lives (Adler, 2018). They set a standard for achievement that is nearly impossible to reach.

For many afflicted with physical or mental disabilities, by contrast, the prime challenges in life revolve around coming to terms with limitations rather than heroically overcoming them. Research in this area tends to deemphasize the idea of overcoming one's disability in favor of acceptance (Adler et al., 2021). For example, Siebers (2017) has written that "in almost every case . . . people with disabilities have a better chance of future happiness and health if they accept their disability as a positive identity and benefit from the knowledge embodied in it" (p. 326). Adler (2018) has suggested that acceptance of one's disability (1) helps a person integrate discordant aspects of the self, bringing mind and body into closer alignment and (2) enables one to take "a sense of pride in one's difference" (p. 814). Moreover, acceptance paves the way for developing meaningful relationships with other members of the disability community.

Stories of radical acceptance offer a template for narrative identity that diverges sharply from the heroic, redemptive stories that so many Americans love. Despite their sharp differences, nonetheless, both forms hold value for conferring meaning and purpose in human lives. And there are surely many more, countless stories perhaps, that autobiographical authors may appropriate to make positive meaning in their lives. The science of narrative identity looks out upon a wide vista for the future. We have just begun to understand the stories people live by. There are still so many questions to ask and problems to confront.

CONCLUSION

Narrative identity is the person's story of who they have been, who they are now, and who they believe they are becoming in the future. As an internalized and evolving saga of the self, narrative identity is a psychological concept with a strong existentialist sensibility. Over the past three decades, the existentialist writings of Jean-Paul Sartre, Ernest Becker, and Albert Camus have had an abiding, and heretofore underappreciated, effect on theory and research in the study of narrative identity. Sartre's ideas regarding the dialectic between narrating life and living life, captured in his concept of the true novel, foreshadowed the emergence of narrative identity as a scientific concept in the 1980s. Becker's profound musings on the meaning of heroism in life (and in the face of death) and the primal drive to fashion an offering of the self to posterity has informed contemporary perspectives on generativity, which, in turn, feature prominently in life-narrative studies. The ramifying empirical literature on the redemptive self—a form of narrative identity so favored by highly generative American adults—owes a debt to Ernest Becker's *The Denial of Death*. And recent research and theorizing on narratives of acceptance owe as much, if not more, to

Albert Camus and his existentialist masterpiece *The Plague*.

Research on narrative identity has repeatedly shown that the stories people construct to make sense of their lives speak directly to the classic existentialist issues of meaning, identity, freedom, and the anticipation of death. Life-narrative studies are flourishing in the fields of personality, developmental, social, cognitive, cultural, and political psychology today, and in other social-science disciplines. The concept of narrative identity holds tremendous interdisciplinary appeal, informing intellectual projects that run the gamut from philosophy (e.g., Binder, 2022) to cognitive neuroscience (e.g., D'Argembeau et al., 2014). Part of that appeal surely derives from its exploration of some of the same issues that the science of existential psychology has perennially focused on. With that fortuitous overlap in mind, future research can benefit greatly from a more concerted effort to develop meaningful linkages between existential psychology and the empirical study of narrative identity.

REFERENCES

Adler, J. M. (2018). Bringing the (disabled) body to personality psychology: A case study of Samantha. *Journal of Personality, 86,* 803–824.

Adler, J. M., Dunlop, W. L., Fivush, R., Lilgendahl, J. P., Lodi-Smith, J., McAdams, D. P., . . . Syed, M. (2017). Research methods for studying narrative identity: A primer. *Social Psychological and Personality Science, 8,* 519–527.

Adler, J. M., Kissel, E., & McAdams, D. P. (2006). Emerging from the CAVE: Attributional style and the narrative study of identity in midlife adults. *Cognitive Therapy and Research, 30,* 39–51.

Adler, J. M., Lakmazaheri, A., O'Brien, E., Palmer, A., Ried, M., & Tawes, E. (2021). Identity integration in people with acquired disabilities: A qualitative study. *Journal of Personality, 89,* 84–112.

Adler, J. M., Lodi-Smith, J., Philippe, F., & Houle, I. (2016). The incremental validity of narrative identity in predicting well-being: A review of the field and recommendations for the future. *Personality and Social Psychology Review, 20,* 142–175.

Adler, J. M., Turner, A., Brookshier, K. M., Monahan, C., Walder-Biesanz, I., Harmeling, J. H., . . . Oltmanns, T. F. (2015). Variation in narrative identity is associated with trajectories of mental health over several years. *Journal of Personality and Social Psychology, 108,* 476–496.

Alon, N., & Omer, H. (2004). Demonic and tragic narratives in psychotherapy. In A. Lieblich, D. P. McAdams, & R. Josselson (Eds.), *Healing plots: The narrative basis of psychotherapy* (pp. 29–48). APA Books.

Altmaeir, B. (Ed.). (2017). *Meaning reconstruction after trauma.* Elsevier.

Bamberg, M., & Andrews, M. (Eds.). (2004). *Considering counter narratives: Narrating resistance, making sense.* Benjamins.

Becker, E. (1973). *The denial of death.* Free Press.

Binder, P.-E. (2022). Facing the uncertainties of being a person: On the role of existential vulnerability in personal identity. *Philosophical Psychology, 37*(8), 2220–2243.

Brooks, D. (2020, March 26). The moral meaning of the plague. *New York Times.* www.nytimes.com/2020/03/26/opinion/coronavirus-meaning.html.

Bruner, J. S. (1990). *Acts of meaning.* Harvard University Press.

Bühler, J. L., & Dunlop, W. L. (2019). The narrative identity approach and romantic relationships. *Social and Personality Psychology Compass, 13*(4), e12447.

Campbell, J. (1949). *The hero with a thousand faces.* Bollingen Foundation

Camus, A. (1947). *The plague.* Knopf.

Charme, S. T. (1984). *Meaning and myth in the study of lives: A Sartrean perspective.* University of Pennsylvania Press.

Cowan, H. R., Mittal, V. A., & McAdams, D. P. (2021). Narrative identity in the psychosis spectrum: A systematic review and developmental model. *Clinical Psychology Review, 88,* 102067.

D'Argembeau, A., Cassol, H., Phillips, C., Balteau, B., Salmon, E., & Van de Londen, M. (2014). Brains creating stories of selves: The neural basis of autobiographical reasoning. *Social Cognitive Affective Neuroscience, 9*(5), 646–652.

Dunlop, W. L. (2021). Everything you wanted to know about redemptive stories* (*but were afraid to ask). *Journal of Research in Personality, 92,* 104078.

Erikson, E. H. (1958). *Young man Luther: A study in psychoanalysis and history.* Norton.

Erikson, E. H. (1963). *Childhood and society* (2nd ed.). Norton.

Erikson, E. H. (1969). *Gandhi's truth.* Norton.

Erikson, E. H. (1982). *The life cycle completed.* Norton.

Fivush, R., Reese, E., & Booker, J. (2019). Developmental foundations for the narrative author in early mother–child reminiscing. In D. P. McAdams, R. L. Shiner, & J. L. Tackett (Eds.), *Handbook of personality development* (pp. 399–417). Guilford Press.

Frankl, V. (1984). *Man's search for meaning* (3rd ed.). Washington Square Press. (Original work published 1963)

Freeman, M. (1993). *Rewriting the self: History, memory, narrative.* Routledge.

Garden, R. (2010). Telling stories about illness and disability: The limits and lessons of narrative. *Perspectives in Biology and Medicine, 53,* 121–135.

Giddens, A. (1991). *Modernity and self-identity: Self and society in the late modern age.* Stanford University Press.

Greenberg, J., Pyszczynski, T., Solomon, S., Rosenblatt, A., Veeder, M., Kirkland, S, & Lyon, D. (1990). Evidence for terror management theory II: The effects of mortality salience on reactions to those who threaten or bolster the cultural worldview. *Journal of Personality and Social Psychology, 58,* 308–318.

Habermas, T., & Bluck, S. (2000). Getting a life: The emergence of the life story in adolescence. *Psychological Bulletin, 128,* 748–769.

Hammack, P. L. (2008). Narrative and the cultural psychology of identity. *Personality and Social Psychology Review, 12,* 222–247.

Hanek, K. J., Olson, B., & McAdams, D. P. (2011). Political orientation and the psychology of Christian prayer: How conservatives and liberals pray. *International Journal for the Psychology of Religion, 21,* 30–42.

Josselson, R. (2009). The present of the past: Dialogues with memory over time. *Journal of Personality, 77,* 647–668.

Kenyon, G., Bohlmeijer, E., & Randall, W. L. (Eds.). (2010). *Storying later life: Issues, investigations, and interventions in narrative gerontology.* Oxford University Press.

Koole, S. L., Greenberg, J., & Pyszczynski, T. (2006). Introducing science to the psychology of the soul: Experimental existential psychology. *Current Directions in Psychological Science, 15,* 212–216.

Kotre, J. (1984). *Outliving the self: Generativity and the interpretation of lives.* Johns Hopkins University Press.

Lilgendahl, J. P., & McLean, K. C. (2020). Narrative identity processes and patterns of adjustment across the transition to college: A developmentally contextualized approach. *Journal of Personality and Social Psychology, 119,* 960–977.

Lind, M., Adler, J. M., & Clark, L. (2021). Narrative identity and personality disorder: An empirical and conceptual review. *Current Psychiatry Reports, 22,* 67.

Lind, M., Sharp, K., & Dunlop, W. L. (2022). Why, how, and when to integrate narrative identity within dimensional approaches to personality disorders. *Journal of Personality Disorders, 36,* 377–398.

Lind, M., Ture, S., McAdams, D. P., & Cowan, H. R. (2024). Narrative identity, traits, and trajectories of depression and well-being: A 9-year longitudinal study. *Psychological Science, 35*(12), 1325–1339.

Mayukha, A., Guzman, A., Jitklongsub, S., & McAdams, D. P. (2025). "I want to lift my people up": Exploring the psychological correlates of racial themes within the life stories of midlife Black Americans. *Journal of Personality, 93*(2), 320–340.

McAdams, D. P. (1985). *Power, intimacy, and the life story: Personological inquiries into identity.* Dorsey Press.

McAdams, D. P. (1993). *The stories we live by: Personal myths and the making of the self.* William Morrow.

McAdams, D. P. (1996). Personality, modernity, and the storied self: A contemporary framework for studying persons. *Psychological Inquiry, 7,* 295–321.

McAdams, D. P. (2011). *George W. Bush and the redemptive dream: A psychological portrait.* Oxford University Press.

McAdams, D. P. (2013a). The psychological self as actor, agent, and author. *Perspectives on Psychological Science, 8,* 272–295.

McAdams, D. P. (2013b). *The redemptive self: Stories Americans live by* (revised and expanded edition). Oxford University Press.

McAdams, D. P. (2019a). First we invented stories, then they changed us: The evolution of narrative identity. *Evolutionary Studies in Imaginative Culture, 3,* 1–18.

McAdams, D. P. (2019b). "I am what survives me": Generativity and the self. In J. A. Frey & C. Vogler (Eds.), *Self-transcendence and virtue: Perspectives from philosophy, psychology, and theology* (pp. 251–273). Routledge.

McAdams, D. P. (2021). Narrative identity and the life story. In O. P. John & R. W. Robins (Eds.), *Handbook of personality: Theory and research* (4th ed., pp. 122–141). Guilford Press.

McAdams, D. P. (2023). Stories of crisis: Denial, redemption, and radical acceptance in the time of COVID-19. In M. Dege & I. Strasser (Eds.), *Narrative in crisis: Reflections on the limits of storytelling* (pp. 35–48). Oxford University Press.

McAdams, D. P., & Albaugh, M. (2008). What if there were no God?: Politically conservative and liberal Christians imagine their lives without faith. *Journal of Research in Personality, 42,* 1668–1672.

McAdams, D. P., Albaugh, M., Farber, E., Daniels, J., Logan, R. L., & Olson, B. (2008). Family metaphors and moral intuitions: How conservatives and liberals narrate their lives. *Journal of Personality and Social Psychology, 95,* 978–990.

McAdams, D. P., & de St. Aubin, E. (1992). A theory of generativity and its assessment through self-report, behavioral acts, and narrative themes in autobiography. *Journal of Personality and Social Psychology, 62,* 1003–1015.

McAdams, D. P., Diamond, A., de St. Aubin, E., & Mansfield, E. (1997). Stories of commitment: The psychosocial construction of generative lives. *Journal of Personality and Social Psychology, 72,* 678–694.

McAdams, D. P., & Guo, J. (2015). Narrating the generative life. *Psychological Science, 26,* 475–483.

McAdams, D. P., Logan, R. L., & Reischer, H. N. (2022). Beyond the redemptive self: Narratives of acceptance in later life (and other contexts). *Journal of Research in Personality, 100,* 104286.

McAdams, D. P., & McLean, K. C. (2013). Narrative identity. *Current Directions in Psychological Science, 22,* 233–238.

McAdams, D. P., Ruetzel, K., & Foley, J. (1986). Complexity and generativity at midlife: A study of biographical scripts for the future. *Journal of Personality and Social Psychology, 50,* 800–807.

McLean, K. C., Pasupathi, M., & Pals, J. L. (2007). Selves creating stories creating selves: A process model of self-development. *Personality and Social Psychology Review, 11,* 262–278.

McLean, K. C., & Syed, M. (2015). Personal, master, and alternative narratives: An integrative framework for understanding identity development in context. *Human Development, 58,* 318–349.

McLean, K. C., Syed, M., Pasupathi, M., Adler, J. M., Dunlop, W. L., Drustrup, D., . . . McCoy, T. (2020). The empirical structure of narrative identity: The initial Big Three. *Journal of Personality and Social Psychology, 119,* 920–944.

McLeod, J. (2004). The significance of narrative and storytelling in post-psychological counseling and psychotherapy. In A. Lieblich, D. P. McAdams, & R. Josselson (Eds.), *Healing plots: The narrative basis of psychotherapy* (pp. 11–27). American Psychological Association.

Murray, H. A. (1938). *Explorations in personality.* Oxford University Press.

Pals, J. L. (2006). Narrative identity processing of difficult life experiences: Pathways of personality development and positive self-transformation in adulthood. *Journal of Personality, 74*(4), 1079–1110.

Pasupathi, M., & Billitteri, J. (2015). Being and becoming through being heard: Listener effects on stories and selves. *International Journal of Listening, 29,* 67–84.

Perlin, J. D., & Fivush, R. (2021). Revisiting redemption: A life-span developmental account of the functions of narrative redemption. *Human Development, 65,* 23–42.

Reischer, H. N., Roth, L. J., Villarreal, J. A., & McAdams, D. P. (2021). Self-transcendence and life stories of humanistic growth among late-midlife adults. *Journal of Personality, 89,* 305–324.

Ricoeur, P. (1984). *Time and narrative* (Vol. 1) (K. McGlaughlin & D. Pellauer, Trans.). University of Chicago Press.

Rogers, B. A., Chicas, H., Kelly, J. M., Kubin, E., Christian, M. S., Kachanoff, F. J., . . . Gray, K. (2023). Seeing your life as a hero's journey increases meaning in life. *Journal of Personality and Social Psychology, 125,* 752–778.

Rogers, L. O. (2020). "I'm kind of a feminist": Using master narratives to understand gender identity in middle childhood. *Child Development, 91,* 179–196.

Sartre, J.-P. (1964). *Nausea* (L. Alexander, Trans.). New Directions.

Sartre, J.-P. (1965). *Essays on existentialism.* Citadel Press.

Schechtman, M. (1996). *The constitution of selves.* Cornell University Press.

Shiner, R. L., Klimstra, T. A., Denissen, J. J. A., & See, A. Y. (2021). The development of narrative identity and the emergence of personality disorders in adolescence. *Current Opinion in Psychology, 37,* 1–5.

Siebers, T. (2017). Disability and the theory of a complex embodiment: For identity politics in a new register. In L. J. Davis (Ed.), *The disability reader* (5th ed., pp. 272–291). Routledge.

Syed, M., & McLean, K. C. (2022). Who gets to live a good life? Master narratives, identity, and well-being within a marginalizing society. *Journal of Research in Personality, 100,* 104285.

Taylor, C. (1989). *Sources of the self: The making of the modern identity.* Harvard University Press.

Ture, S., Bonner, C. V., Yuan, M., & McAdams, D. P. (2025). Historical consciousness: Recollections of major historical events in the personal life story. *Personality and Social Psychology Bulletin, 51*(3), 1–16.

Walker, L., & Frimer, J. (2007). Moral personality of brave and caring exemplars. *Journal of Personality and Social Psychology, 78,* 907–942.

Waters, T. E. A., & Fivush, R. (2015). Relations between narrative coherence, identity, and psychological well-being in emerging adulthood. *Journal of Personality, 83,* 441–451.

White, M., & Epston, M. (1990). *Narrative means to therapeutic ends.* Norton.

CHAPTER 41

How and Why Does Personality Change across the Lifespan?

Muchen Xi *and* Joshua J. Jackson

Personality is consistent yet changeable. For many, this duality is challenging to comprehend, much like in quantum physics, where two seemingly separate processes are valid at the same time. From an existential perspective, personality can be seen as a person's "way of being" in the world—an ongoing process shaped by choices, experiences, and the search for meaning. Existential psychology, with its focus on "being" and "becoming," invites us to consider how personality reflects both the continuity of one's core self and the potential for transformation. If we frame personality development as a process of navigating existential questions—such as what to do, who to be, how to live, and why—we see that the apparent contradiction between consistency and change is a reflection of our existential struggle to forge and refine our identity over time.

Within personality development, this seeming contradiction occurs because of three primary factors: First, there are many types of change, so when we say someone's personality has changed, it can have different meanings. Second, people are poor at comprehending different time scales; for example, height is very consistent from day to day, but from the cradle to the grave, it changes substantively. Third, change and consistency are much like the proverbial half-empty, half-filled glass of water, which one might interpret differently depending on one's perspective. Rather than viewing personality as consistent or changing, it is best to think of these along a continuum such that personality can be somewhat consistent but is also changing.

Below, we describe the different types of personality change and review evidence for the change and consistency across these types. We then describe the processes that result in various types of change and consistency. Aligning with the suggestions of existential psychological perspectives, research shows that these changes can occur both unintentionally as a response to life events (Bleidorn et al., 2018; Bühler et al., 2024) or existential crises and intentionally as people seek to align their "way of being" with their evolving sense of purpose and authenticity. For example, Nietzsche's idea of "becoming who one is" suggests that individuals are not fixed beings but are constantly in the process of self-creation, guided by their values, desires, and the courage to break free from societal norms or self-imposed limitations. Research indicates that intentional personality change requires certain preconditions, such as awareness, motivation, and sustained effort (Caspi & Roberts, 1999)—mirroring existential themes of taking responsibility for one's existence and embracing the discomfort of growth.

TYPES OF CONSISTENCY AND CHANGE

In this section, we review six different types of personality change (or the opposite of change: consistency). We first describe the widely studied rank-order consistency, mean-level change, and individual differences in mean-level change. Then, we highlight the findings in three underappreciated metrics of within-person consistency and change (ipsative consistency, structural consistency, and idiographic consistency). Importantly, these types of changes are primarily orthogonal to one another, meaning there could be changes occurring for one type of change, while there may or may not be changes occurring in other metrics.

Rank-Order Consistency

Rank-order consistency (or differential consistency) examines whether someone high on a trait relative to a group will still be high on that trait relative to the group at a different time period. The test of this is the simple correlation of personality scores across two time points. Meta-analytic reports drawing on diverse longitudinal studies (e.g., Anusic & Schimmack, 2016; Ardelt, 2000; Bazana & Stelmack, 2004; Bleidorn et al., 2022; Ferguson, 2010) have consistently demonstrated that personality traits exhibit moderate to high rank-order consistency, with correlations typically situated between 0.40 and 0.60 over intervals of 4 to 10 years. This evidence underlines a fundamental aspect of personality traits: Despite fluctuations over time, a significant degree of stability is maintained, suggesting an inherent resilience of personality traits across decades regardless of the slings and arrows life may throw at someone. But this also means that people are not entirely consistent, and changing is possible.

Research shows a marked increase in the rank-order stability of personality traits from adolescence to mid-adulthood, reflecting a consolidation phase coinciding with life transitions such as completing education, entering the workforce, and starting families (Bleidorn et al., 2022). Adolescence and early adulthood thus represent a period of heightened personality malleability, during which individuals are more likely to explore their identities and confront existential questions about who they want to be. By mid-adulthood, personality stability plateaus, reaching its peak in middle age (Bleidorn et al., 2022; Fraley & Roberts, 2005). Empirical estimates show stability rising from $r = 0.40$ in youth to $r = 0.62$ by age 30, and peaking at $r = 0.75$ around age 50 (Bleidorn et al., 2022). This pattern holds across the Big Five traits, regardless of assessment method or gender (Caspi et al., 2005), suggesting that middle age tends to be less existentially volatile. In later life, the trajectory of personality stability becomes more complex. Some studies report declines in trait stability among older adults (Ardelt, 2000; Lucas & Donnellan, 2011; Specht et al., 2011; Terracciano et al., 2006; Wortman et al., 2012), whereas others find relatively high stability beyond age 70, with correlations ranging from $r = 0.50$ to $r = 0.80$ (Ferguson, 2010; Kandler et al., 2015). This inconsistency points to a more nuanced view of personality development in later adulthood, likely shaped by health, life transitions, and cognitive changes.

Findings on rank-order consistency in personality development align with existential psychology's view of life as a journey of exploration, choice, and self-definition. The lower consistency observed in adolescence reflects a phase of identity exploration, as individuals navigate diverse roles and values (Erikson, 1968). From an existential perspective, this stage involves the challenge of self-definition and the pursuit of authenticity, echoing Sartre's (1943) notion that existence precedes essence. In middle adulthood, peak personality stability corresponds with a consolidation of self through established roles in work, family, and community—roles that reflect committed, value-aligned choices. This pattern resonates with Kierkegaard's (1849) and Heidegger's (1927) emphases on authentic existence shaped by deliberate commitment. In late adulthood, the variability in consistency mirrors existential themes of reevaluating purpose and confronting mortality. Health changes, loss, or retirement can prompt a reassessment of identity, with some maintaining stability and others adapting to new existential concerns (Frankl, 1959; Nietzsche, 1886). This underscores the lifelong process of meaning making in response to life's ultimate questions (Heidegger, 1927; Sartre, 1943).

Mean-Level Change

While the findings in rank-order stability indicate moderately stable patterns of personality changes relative to other people, they do not reveal how personality traits, on average in a population, change in magnitude. Mean-level changes in personality are demonstrated by the absolute increment or drop in the expression of personality traits over time. Unlike the patterns of rank-order stabilities, where estimates of consistency were similar in magnitude across different dimensions of personality, there are more nuances in the mean-level changes in personality traits.

During childhood and adolescence, individuals often experiment with various identities, resulting in diverse social contexts and minimal normative mean-level changes in personality traits (Borghuis et al., 2017; Göllner et al., 2017; Roberts et al., 2006). In early adulthood, personality becomes more integrated and stable, marked by increases in conscientiousness, emotional stability (i.e., lower neuroticism), and agreeableness—an established pattern known as the maturity principle (Bleidorn et al., 2022; Roberts et al., 2005). This trend has been consistently observed across cross-sectional (Soto et al., 2011), longitudinal (e.g., Lucas & Donnellan, 2011; Oltmanns et al., 2020), and cross-cultural studies (Bleidorn et al., 2013), with mean-level changes approaching nearly a full standard deviation across the lifespan.

In contrast, developmental patterns for extraversion and openness are less consistent. Both traits tend to increase gradually from adolescence into early adulthood and peak in midlife (Bleidorn et al., 2022; Lüdtke et al., 2011), though some studies report gradual declines across the lifespan (Lucas & Donnellan, 2011). Facet-level analyses offer more nuance: For example, increases in dominance (a facet of extraversion) are more pronounced than changes in social vitality (Roberts et al., 2006), and openness facets follow different trajectories—intellectual interests correlate with educational attainment, while aesthetic interests relate more to unconventional career pursuits (Schwaba et al., 2019).

In contrast to the well-established effort studying changes in personality in early life, the development of personality traits in later life only received its deserved attention in recent years. While several longitudinal studies show a drop in mean-level conscientiousness and emotional stability in older adulthood and late life (Kandler et al., 2015; Mueller et al., 2016), other studies show both traits remain at the higher level reached in early adulthood without a decline (Kuzma et al., 2011; Mõttus et al., 2012). In a recent meta-analysis, Bleidorn and colleagues (2022) analyzed findings from 276 longitudinal studies showing a gradual decline in agreeableness after late adulthood and a more pronounced drop in conscientiousness in similar periods but cumulative gains in emotional stability (the opposite of neuroticism) across the lifespan. The trajectories regarding extraversion and openness in later life have similar nuances (Brandt et al., 2023), with some evidence showing perpetual increases (Mueller et al., 2016) and others showing prominent drops in late life (Schwaba et al., 2018). More work is needed to help understand the patterns of development in later life, especially given that this time period involves many difficulties, such as selection bias (people who have certain traits are more likely to pass away younger), as well as assessment challenges (e.g., conscientiousness measures were developed with younger individuals in mind—how do people fill out personality items that specifically reference work when they are retired?).

Mean-level changes in personality traits across the lifespan align with existential psychology's view of human development as an ongoing process of becoming, adaptation, and meaning making. The relative stability in traits during childhood and adolescence reflects a phase of identity exploration, consistent with Kierkegaard's (1843) "aesthetic stage," where individuals pursue possibilities without committing to a fixed self-concept. In early adulthood, increases in conscientiousness, emotional stability, and agreeableness—commonly known as the maturity principle—mark a period of existential consolidation. This phase involves committing to careers, relationships, and social roles, requiring heightened responsibility and emotional regulation, echoing Heidegger's (1927) notion of confronting freedom through meaningful choice. A sense of purpose during this time supports identity stabilization and trait development (Hill & Burrow, 2012; Hill et al., 2016).

In middle adulthood, personality traits typically plateau as individuals deepen existing commitments, refining their identities in line with core values and long-term goals. This process aligns with existential themes of authenticity and Nietzsche's (1886) concept of the "will to power" as a drive toward self-overcoming and self-definition. Purpose in life has been linked to psychological resilience and well-being, serving as a buffer against midlife stress and existential anxiety (Hill & Turiano, 2014). In later adulthood, nuanced changes—such as declines in conscientiousness and agreeableness and variability in emotional stability and openness—reflect existential challenges like confronting mortality, adapting to loss, and reassessing meaning (Frankl, 1959; Sartre, 1943).

Individual Differences in Mean-Level Change

The mean-level changes in personality reveal the average or normative pattern of personality trait change over time. Suppose all individuals follow this universal pattern of change. In that case, the rank-order stability of personality traits should be perfect, such that the most agreeable person at age 20 will still be the most agreeable person at age 40, as everyone changes in the same direction at the same rate. However, the findings regarding rank-order stability tend to hover between moderate to high but will never reach perfect, indicating individual differences in how one's personality would change. Individual differences in mean-level change reflect absolute changes for a single individual, regardless of the normative pattern of change. For example, some people may decrease in conscientiousness over time despite the average tendency to increase in conscientiousness over the lifespan.

Individual differences in change are found across the entire lifespan, occurring in childhood and adolescence (De Fruyt et al., 2006) as well as in late life (Graham et al., 2020; Schwaba & Bleidorn, 2018). For example, although people, in general, tend to increase their emotional stability as they mature through age, some people remain at the same level of neuroticism, the counterpart of emotional stability, without any drop (Mroczek et al., 2021; Mroczek & Spiro, 2003). These patterns indicate that while there is a tendency to change in normative directions, it is not guaranteed to occur for every person.

The idiosyncratic trajectory of personality development reflects the idea that people encounter different experiences and that these experiences shape who they are. If people are differently exposed to unique life experiences, then we would expect individual differences in mean-level change (see more below about what drives personality changes). For example, effort investment and commitment in education and the workplace have been found to predict increases in conscientiousness (Göllner et al., 2017; Hudson et al., 2012). Moreover, promotion and status attainment in professional development have been associated with gaining in extraversion and conscientiousness (Roberts et al., 2003; Wille et al., 2012). Moreover, positive relationship experiences with committed partners were found to be associated with an increment in emotional stability and conscientiousness (Lehnart et al., 2010; Robins et al., 2002; Scollon & Diener, 2006). Hence, although there exist general trends in the development of personality traits through aging (e.g., the maturity principle), individuals' unique trajectories can largely deviate from the typical pattern adapting to their unique life experiences.

Profile or Ipsative Consistency

While rank-order consistency—stability in individuals' relative positions on a single trait over time—is often used to demonstrate personality stability across the lifespan (Roberts & DelVecchio, 2000), two less frequently examined but equally important forms of stability are *profile consistency* and *structural consistency* focusing on the intraindividual variability of personality. These approaches focus on how personality is organized within individuals rather than between them, providing a more person-centered understanding of stability and change.

Profile consistency (or *ipsative consistency*) reflects the stability of the relative configuration of multiple traits within a person over time. Unlike rank-order stability, which compares individuals to one another on a single trait, profile consistency compares the internal ordering of a person's traits across time. For example, if someone increases in extraversion but also increases equally in other traits, no change in profile would be detected because the relative rank ordering remains the same. Thus, profile consistency captures intraindividual personality structure, with change defined by shifts in the relative importance of traits over time.

Empirical work demonstrates that profile consistency is generally lower in adolescence, increases into early and mid-adulthood, and plateaus from adulthood into later life (McCrae & Costa, 2003; Poier, 2022). This developmental pattern mirrors identity consolidation processes, where young people experiment with various roles and values, and adults settle into more stable configurations. For example, one longitudinal study found that individuals' trait profiles were remarkably consistent over a 4-year period (Mõttus et al., 2012), a finding replicated across other time spans and developmental stages (Block, 1971; Gilbert et al., 2021; Ibáñez et al., 2016; Jackson & Beck, 2021; Klimstra et al., 2009; Terracciano et al., 2010).

Importantly, individual differences in profile consistency have also been observed. Wright and Jackson (2023) examined longitudinal data across multiple waves spanning more than a decade and found high overall profile stability, but also substantial variability in the degree of consistency between individuals. These differences remained even after controlling for age, education, and maturity. Some individuals were consistently more stable across time, while others showed more variability—suggesting that consistency itself may be a personality characteristic. People who frequently change their internal configuration of traits may be those who are more open, flexible, or constantly renegotiating their identities. For instance, someone who seems to "reinvent" themselves annually may persistently grapple with existential questions about who they are, whereas others may have reached a stage of commitment and stability that endures for decades.

Of course, temporary disruptions to profile consistency can also result from external events. For example, life transitions—like becoming a parent—may temporarily alter trait salience, increasing conscientiousness and neuroticism in response to new demands. These shifts may reduce profile stability in the short term but reflect adaptive reordering rather than deep instability. To test whether such inconsistency was due to environmental disruptions or intrinsic individual differences, Wright and Jackson (2023) analyzed long-term patterns across many waves. They found that environmental effects alone could not account for the variability—suggesting that the tendency to change or stay stable is a persistent individual difference in itself.

Structural Change

Complementing *profile consistency* is *structural consistency*, which refers to whether the organization of traits (e.g., the coherence of the Big Five model) remains stable across time and age. While the Big Five is often assumed to be a stable and universal structure, most personality assessments and factor analyses have focused on younger adults. Tests in other populations often aim to replicate the Big Five rather than investigate whether it remains the best-fitting model across different life stages (Caspi & Roberts, 2001). However, some findings challenge this structural assumption.

A few studies examine the factor structure of personality specifically, with most only ensuring that the factor structure reasonably works across different ages rather than identifying the best factor structure for any particular age. For instance, Beck, Condon, and Jackson (2023) found that while younger adults' responses clustered neatly into the Big Five structure, older adults showed a more complex and less differentiated pattern. Items did not load cleanly onto five distinct factors, suggesting that aging may bring a reorganization of how traits are structured. This may result from changing roles and experiences that alter the salience and integration of certain traits. For example, conscientiousness items referencing work behavior may be less relevant to retirees and thus may no longer cluster meaningfully. Such differences in structure only appear over extended time frames. Despite age and social role changes that occur across the lifespan, the structure of personality appears very robust over modest timeframes of a decade or less. For example, life events that are thought to lead to personality change (e.g., retirement, parenthood) do not change the structure of personality comparing pre- and post-event (Jackson & Beck, 2021). That is, how personality is configured within a person is robust to these life events. In general, these two seemingly contradictory results reflect the field in that some studies find that the Big Five factors show consistency across time (Allemand et al., 2007; Brandt et al., 2023; Jackson et al., 2009; Mõttus et al., 2012; Schwaba & Bleidorn, 2018), whereas others identify some potential misfit (Marsh et al., 2013; Nye et al., 2016; Olaru et al., 2018; Tackett et al., 2009).

These two frameworks—profile and structural consistency—reveal both robustness and plasticity in personality development. Over shorter periods, both profile and structure tend to be stable, even in the face of life transitions. Yet over longer timescales, subtle reorganizations can occur, reflecting both developmental and existential processes. From an existential psychology perspective, these patterns underscore personality development as a dynamic interplay between stability and the ongoing construction of meaning. During adolescence, lower profile and structural consistency align with themes of identity exploration and self-definition. This is a stage marked by the freedom to explore different possibilities and values, resonating with Sartre's (1943) concept that existence precedes essence, and Kierkegaard's (1843) notion of the aesthetic stage—where individuals pursue diverse roles without firm commitments.

As individuals transition into early and mid-adulthood, rising profile consistency and relative structural stability reflect a process of existential consolidation. Commitments to relationships, careers, and worldviews often bring coherence to identity, leading to a more stable self-configuration (Heidegger, 1927; Sarbin, 1967). This midlife phase reflects Nietzsche's (1886) idea of the "will to power," where individuals strive for authenticity through the alignment of their values and actions. Consistency during this phase implies not rigidity but rather the integration of values into a coherent and lived identity across roles.

In later adulthood, observed variability in both profile and structural consistency can be understood as part of the existential work of aging. Individuals may reevaluate priorities, experience shifts in roles or health, and confront questions of legacy and mortality. Some show remarkable stability; others undergo meaningful reorganization of traits. These changes are not regressions but reflect a continued search for coherence and significance in later life (Frankl, 1959; Yalom, 1980). The fluidity observed in aging personalities reinforces the view that personality is not fixed but evolves in dialogue with life's changing demands—an ongoing project of becoming, situated in both structure and self-understanding.

Idiographic Change

The types of change described above make assumptions about how best to describe personality in terms of the content and the structure. Change, in the above manner, is constrained by the set of variables or traits measured by the researchers. That is, the choice of which personality questionnaire to give to a person assumes that this questionnaire is not only the best description of personality (e.g., Big Five) but also applicable to that person. Similarly, the associations between variables are often assumed to be universally generalizable to the broader population. However, there is accumulating evidence that people are unique in the content and structure of personality (Beck & Jackson, 2020, 2022a, 2022b). For example, the processes that lead an individual to procrastinate, a marker of conscientiousness (Jackson et al., 2009), differ from one person to the next (Beck & Jackson, 2022a, 2022b). This means that we may potentially miss the aspects of change that are important to an individual when we examine change at the population or sample level.

In contrast, idiographic models are built on a single individual and thus personalized, thereby allowing people to differ among many dimensions and associations between dimensions (Beck & Jackson, 2022c; Mischel 2004). Rather than starting with the assumption that people are similar and only differ in degree (e.g., some people increase whereas others decrease on a trait), the idiographic change allows the loosening of many of the assumptions of how variables relate to one another. This type of change is analyzed at the $N = 1$ level, making no assumptions that people are similar in their personality. These types of models are just starting to be tested within personality development, but two examples show interesting results.

Beck and Jackson (2020) asked whether the structure of personality may differ between people. Rather than assume the Big Five is the best for everyone, they looked at the interrelationships among variables to see how they relate to one another. This is similar to the profile or ipsative type of change but differs in that while the profile or ipsative type characterizes change as a single metric that captures, in general, the relative rank ordering of variables within a person, the idiographic models focus on the specific associations among variables to see how they are related across time. Notably, they found that people differed in the association between variables: For example, being extraverted may not coincide with neuroticism for some people but does coincide for others. Interestingly, these associations were quite consistent across a 2-year period. Importantly, however, they found that some people were very consistent, whereas others were very inconsistent. These findings were replicated in another sample of individuals tested across the onset of the COVID-19 pandemic; again, some people were consistent, especially in the face of an ongoing pandemic, whereas others were relatively inconsistent in their idiographic personality structures (Beck & Jackson, 2022b).

A second example of testing idiographic personality development looked at the associations between variables weekly across a year (Beck & Jackson, 2022a). Again, personality was investigated as the association between variables analyzed at the individual level where everyone could have different associations between variables such as extraversion and neuroticism. Rather than look at consistency, they asked whether there were notable deviations in the person-typical associations between variables—and if these deviations lasted, indicating a shift in one's personality. For over a quarter of participants, deviations from the expected associations between variables occurred. These findings suggest that personality changed quickly, over the timeframe of a week or two, while much of the literature suggests that personality change happens slowly and gradually across time. These changes would have been dismissed as noise if not treated idiographically; thus, the extant literature likely undercounts how much personality development occurs.

The existence of individual differences in mean-level and idiographic changes in personality highlights the uniquely personal nature of human development, reflecting the existential journey of "being and becoming." From an existential perspective, these differences emphasize that each person's developmental trajectory is shaped by personal choices, experiences, and the meanings they derive from them, resonating with Sartre's (1943) notion that existence precedes essence, where individuals define themselves through their actions. Unlike a uniform path, this variability reflects the freedom and responsibility individuals have in crafting their identities, aligning with Heidegger's (1927) concept of authenticity—living following one's own values rather than conforming to external norms.

The idiosyncratic paths people take—shaped by unique encounters like career achievements or personal relationships—demonstrate that identity is not a fixed set of traits but a dynamic, evolving project. This view aligns with Nietzsche's (1886) idea of self-overcoming, where individuals continuously strive to redefine themselves in the face of life's challenges. Such differences underscore the existential psychological perspective that identity is perpetually in flux, a continuous process of self-definition as individuals respond to the demands and uncertainties of life, including the fundamental questions of what to do, who to be, how to live, and why (Frankl, 1959; Yalom, 1980). Understanding these individual differences in personality development not only acknowledges the diversity of human experience but also celebrates the existential reality that each person's journey is deeply personal, shaped by the freedom to choose and the courage to live authentically.

DEVELOPMENTAL MECHANISMS LEADING TO TRAIT-LEVEL PERSONALITY CHANGE

Despite long-term consistency, personality remains only partially solidified and can change across the lifespan. Understanding how personality changes requires considering multiple levels of analysis (Rosenberg, 1998). At the broadest level are latent traits (e.g., the Big Five); at the midlevel, habits—stable behavioral patterns like punctuality; and at the lowest level, momentary manifestations of affect, behavior, cognition, and desires. Change typically follows a bottom-up process, beginning with immediate state-level shifts and, over time, influencing habits and eventually traits. Direct trait change is rare without biological intervention (Caselli et al., 2018; Quilty et al., 2008; Roberts & Jackson, 2008; Terracciano et al., 2018; Jackson et al., 2021), and simply understanding a trait's value (e.g., conscientiousness) is rarely sufficient for transformation.

Therapeutic approaches often reflect this complexity by targeting more malleable, short-term behaviors rather than attempting to directly alter traits (Chapman et al., 2014; Magidson et al., 2014; Sander et al., 2017). Lasting personality change requires consistent shifts in state-level behaviors that evolve into habits and, eventually, traits (Geukes et al., 2018; Wrzus & Roberts, 2017). Yet deviating from trait-typical behaviors alone is not enough (Sauer-Zavala et al., 2017). No single mechanism is sufficient for change; rather, change arises from the interplay of multiple factors.

A comprehensive review of empirical and theoretical works (Allemand & Flückiger, 2017; Hampson, 2012; Roberts & Caspi, 2003; Specht et al., 2014; Wrzus & Roberts, 2017) helps identify four key mechanisms: preconditions (readiness to change), triggers (events prompting state shifts), reinforcers (sustaining new behaviors), and integrators (embedding changes into identity) (Jackson & Wright, 2024). These mechanisms map a pathway from state changes to lasting trait change. However, disruption at any stage can halt the process, and none of these mechanisms alone can produce enduring change—highlighting the need for a multifaceted, sustained approach.

Preconditions

Preconditions refer to the specific circumstances or settings that facilitate the possibility of personality change (Hennecke et al., 2014). In therapeutic contexts, for example, the success of the process can be influenced by the patient's receptiveness or resistance to treatment. Similarly, in everyday life, individuals may either open themselves to change or block it, whether intentionally or not. A key aspect of initiating personality change is the individual's genuine desire or motivation to alter aspects of their personality, whether for personal growth or to achieve other objectives (Hennecke et al., 2014; Hudson & Fraley, 2015). Superficial changes in behavior or actions, done without genuine desire or merely for external validation, seldom lead to meaningful or enduring changes in personality traits (Hudson et al., 2019). Consider a student who studies hard to achieve good grades, driven by the desire to please their parents or secure a spot in a good college. Although this behavior might seem like a shift toward diligence, it will not lead to an actual change in the student's personality unless they develop a genuine motivation to learn for the sake of learning itself. However, if they embrace learning beyond external rewards, this shift in values can lead to lasting changes in their personality.

To achieve lasting change, it must be realistic and within one's reach. (Hennecke et al., 2014; Lücke et al., 2021). For example, a person may want to reduce their anxiety. However, their life (and society) might be too stressful for them to make much progress. The capacity for change depends on the individual's ability to adopt new behaviors or mindsets, which may be limited by cognitive or emotional resources (Gallagher et al., 2011), such as if they are exhausted by their daily responsibilities. Effective personality change requires not just the intention but also the practical means to act differently in various situations, underscoring the complexity (and potential inequalities) of transforming one's personality.

Triggers

Triggers are specific experiences that prompt state-level changes in feelings, behaviors, thoughts, or desires (Magidson et al., 2014; Wrzus & Roberts, 2017). These can arise from external factors such as situations or tasks, as well as internal states like emotional or physical reactions (Borghuis et al., 2020; Quintus et al., 2021; Wrzus et al., 2021). A single triggered state rarely produces lasting personality change—for instance, an introvert might temporarily act outgoing at a party without fundamentally altering their trait-level introversion. However, repeated exposure to consistent triggers may lead to more enduring trait change.

Triggers can include major life events, social role transitions, developmental milestones, therapeutic and educational experiences, emotion regulation strategies, or cognitive shifts (Denissen et al., 2019; Helson et al., 2002; Hudson & Roberts, 2016; Hutteman et al., 2014; Koval et al., 2023; Roberts et al., 2017; Specht et al., 2011). These influences affect not only the immediate situation but also how individuals interpret and engage with their environments (Kuper et al., 2022; Rauthmann et al., 2015).

Ideally, there is a clear link between a trigger and its behavioral consequences. Thus, personality change often requires more than exposure to new situations; it involves cognitive strategies that reframe familiar experiences. This reframing alters not just behaviors, but also interpretations and expectations. Returning to the student example, a shift from viewing assignments as grade requirements to seeing them as opportunities for growth may foster sustained curiosity and engagement. Such mindset shifts, akin to therapeutic practices, promote lasting personality change through the interplay of triggers and intentional cognitive adjustments.

Reinforcers

While triggers initiate changes in how we feel, think, behave, and desire, for these changes to become lasting, they need to be consistently repeated (Danner et al., 2008; Roberts & Jackson, 2008; Verplanken & Orbell, 2022; Wrzus & Roberts, 2017). Altering behavior momentarily is relatively straightforward, yet embedding these changes into our routine, making them automatic and habitual, proves more challenging. Often, we might resist triggers due to their discomfort or the effort they demand. Therefore, reinforcement, whether internal or external, plays a crucial role in ensuring continued exposure to triggers, facilitating the development of habits and enduring change (Aarts & Dijksterhuis, 2000; Bleidorn & Hopwood, 2024; Chapman et al., 2014; Lally et al., 2010; Magidson et al., 2014).

Reinforcement also occurs at a social level, where social expectations, contingent outcomes, and consequences for not meeting these expectations guide behavior (Bicchieri, 2006; Fehr & Schurtenberger, 2018). New jobs, for instance, come with understood behaviors considered acceptable (like punctuality) and unacceptable (such as theft) (Hoff et al., 2021; Sutin et al., 2009). Adhering to these norms has significant implications for one's professional relationships and income, providing strong motivation to conform to societal expectations. These reinforcers (paired with preconditions and triggers) have the potential to shift one's behavior long term. However, those shifts in behavior might not lead to personality change without integration processes at play.

Integrators

To solidify new habits and foster lasting personality change, reinforcers must sustain state-level changes over time. Behavior becomes routine through repeated reinforcement—such as reminders or investments like a gym membership—but for these habits to translate into personality change, they must generalize across multiple life domains. Drawing from cognitive training research, this transition requires skill transference across contexts (Sala et al., 2019). True personality change involves broad, multidomain adaptations rather than isolated behavioral tweaks (Olaru et al., 2024). This transformation is facilitated by introspective processes that integrate new behaviors into one's self-concept (Roberts & Caspi, 2003).

For instance, an individual may recognize that discipline developed at the gym reflects a broader conscientious identity, which can inform behaviors in other settings.

External validation also plays a key role. When changes are recognized by close others—friends, family, or partners—these others reinforce the authenticity and social acceptance of the evolving personality (Jackson et al., 2015; Smith et al., 2008; Wright et al., 2022). Alignment between self-perception and external feedback signals that personality adjustments are becoming embedded in one's identity.

Additionally, personality change can unfold through more implicit, associative processes. Reinforcement and feedback gradually reshape self-perception, even without deliberate reflection (Caspi & Roberts, 2001; Seger, 1994; Wrzus & Roberts, 2017). For example, a teenager gaining responsibility through a job may develop time management and self-discipline, and positive feedback can reinforce a new identity as capable and responsible. Together, these reflective and associative mechanisms highlight that enduring personality change is a multifaceted process, shaped by conscious integration, social reinforcement, and subtle shifts in self-understanding.

Summary

The journey to trait-level personality change can be captured by the phrase "Fake it till you make it—and believe it—across multiple aspects of life." This process unfolds through four core mechanisms: preconditions (readiness and openness to change), triggers (experiences that prompt state-level shifts), reinforcers (sustained repetition and validation of new behaviors), and integrators (the assimilation of changes into one's identity across contexts).

Viewed through an existential lens, these mechanisms reflect the ongoing negotiation of identity and the pursuit of meaning. *Preconditions* such as the desire for growth exemplify authentic living, where individuals exercise existential freedom and responsibility by making deliberate, value-aligned choices (May, 1958; Sartre, 1943). When pursued intentionally—such as cultivating conscientiousness—personality change becomes an act of self-creation, resonating with existential themes of purpose and commitment (Heidegger, 1927). *Triggers*, whether self-directed or externally imposed, initiate immediate shifts in emotion, cognition, or behavior that may accumulate into broader trait changes. When *reinforced* through positive feedback and congruent life experiences, these changes can be *integrated* into one's self-concept, aligning with Nietzsche's (1886) notion of self-overcoming as a path to authenticity. This process reflects the existential task of maintaining coherence and authenticity amid life's inherent flux (Heidegger, 1927). Ultimately, personality change—intentional or not—is a central feature of the human condition: a continual shaping of the self in response to uncertainty, experience, and the quest for meaning (Sartre, 1943; Yalom, 1980).

DEVELOPMENTAL MECHANISMS PREVENTING TRAIT-LEVEL CHANGE

Nevertheless, personality is an inherently stable system (Anusic & Schimmack, 2016; Terracciano et al., 2010; Wright & Jackson, 2023). For example, people generally do not show lasting changes in their traits or satisfaction after major life events; instead, they often revert to their previous levels within months or a few years after changes due to the events (Denissen et al., 2019; Schwaba & Bleidorn, 2018; Specht et al., 2011). Events like becoming a parent or losing a job typically do not lead to long-term personality shifts, emphasizing the resilience of personality against change (Asselmann & Specht, 2021; Denissen et al., 2019; van Scheppingen et al., 2016). To complement the previous discussion on the mechanism of change, in this section, we discuss the mechanisms preventing change (Jackson & Wright, 2024).

Comfort Zone

First, acting outside one's usual behavior range is strenuous and can feel unnatural (Gallagher et al., 2011), leading individuals to gravitate toward or shape environments that reinforce their original personality traits. People often engage in self-selection of familiar experiences (Denissen et al., 2014; Roberts & Nickel, 2021) or manipulate their surroundings to ensure consistency with their personality (Roberts & Nickel, 2021; Scarr & McCartney, 1983), avoiding situations that feel discordant. Additionally, other people often play a role in reinforcing one's personality by selecting one into environments that match one's existing traits, thus acting as gatekeepers preventing personality change (Schneider et al., 1998). The cycle of selection and self-segregation illustrates how both internal preferences and external influences work together to maintain personality stability.

Effort

Second, temporary shifts in a person's emotions, behavior, thoughts, and desires may not last long enough to become permanent due to the effort required to maintain them, which can deplete one's self-regulation abilities. Consequently, individuals often revert to their original dispositions and habits. The duration necessary for state changes to become stable trait changes varies, with habit formation typically requiring weeks to months and changes from interventions or therapy occurring over weeks.

Underdoing It, Overdoing It

Third, for personality changes to be effective and lasting, they need to be realistically aligned with what an individual can handle. Too ambitious changes can lead to discomfort and avoidance, while minimal changes might not be sufficient to engage reinforcing mechanisms. Successful changes should build on existing capabilities within the individual's "zone of proximal development," as seen in methods like exposure therapy, which uses progressively challenging exposures to facilitate change.

Inattentiveness

Last but not least, even if individuals develop new habits or behaviors, they may not recognize these changes or relate them to their self-concept, which can hinder lasting personality change. The lack of self-perception of change can be a significant obstacle, though it can sometimes be mitigated by external validation, which helps affirm and solidify the new behaviors as part of one's identity.

Summary

Just as some factors promote personality change, there are also mechanisms that encourage stability and resist change. People often prefer consistency, seeking to maintain a familiar environment and a stable self-image. Everyday challenges that disrupt successful and lasting behavioral changes also impose limits on the extent and possibility of such changes (Caspi et al., 2005; Roberts, 2006; Scarr & McCartney, 1983; Swann et al., 2003). Resistance to personality change aligns with the existential need for stability, coherence, and authenticity. People often avoid changes that disrupt their established self-concept, seeking consistency with their core values (Kierkegaard, 1849; May, 1958). Familiar environments reinforce this comfort zone, serving as a buffer against the anxiety of confronting unfamiliar aspects of the self (Heidegger, 1927).

Even when individuals attempt change, sustained effort can be exhausting, especially if changes lack alignment with personal meaning or exceed one's "zone of proximal development" (Frankl, 1959). Without conscious reflection, even meaningful behaviors may fail to integrate into the self-concept, rendering change superficial. Existential psychology emphasizes that genuine transformation requires self-awareness, intentionality, and alignment with one's evolving identity (Nietzsche, 1886; Sartre, 1943).

Ultimately, existential psychology frames resistance to personality change as part of the broader human inclination toward psychological coherence. Balancing this desire for stability with the courage to pursue meaningful, authentic transformation represents a central existential challenge—one that calls for conscious, deliberate engagement in personal growth.

CONCLUSION

This exploration of personality development and change through the lens of existential psychology provides a profound understanding of human life as an ongoing journey of "being and becoming." This perspective invites us to view personality developments as objective outcomes but as a fluid and evolving construct shaped by intentional actions and existential challenges.

Throughout this chapter, we have considered personality as a person's particular way of being—a unique manifestation of one's existence that can take various forms and structures and may change (or remain stable) over time. The research on personality development reveals that change is not only possible but can occur in diverse ways—through shifts in rank order, mean levels, individual profiles, or structural organization. These findings challenge the notion of personality as fixed, instead highlighting its adaptability in response to life's existential challenges. They underscore the essential role of personal agency and individuals' choices in shaping their identities while acknowledging the impact of external circumstances beyond one's control. The balance between stability and change reflects the broader human struggle to create a coherent self amid the unpredictability of existence.

Drawing from existential insights, we see that intentional personality changes—rooted in conscious, value-driven decisions—reflect a profound commitment to authenticity and self-definition. This intentional engagement aligns with the existential call to become who one is, illustrating that personal growth is an actively ongoing process. The mechanisms that facilitate or hinder personality change, such as preconditions, triggers, reinforcers, and integrators, further illustrate the dynamic interplay between agency and circumstance. They suggest that change is most enduring when it is both intentional and supported by consistent reinforcement, aligning actions with one's broader life narrative. At the same time, the factors that prevent change, like comfort zones or resistance to unfamiliar experiences, reflect the existential tension between the desire for growth and the comfort of stability. This tension speaks to the fundamental human challenge of navigating between the known and the unknown, the secure and the transformative. By doing so, we are reminded that our identities are not static endpoints but dynamic and evolving responses to the profound questions that define human existence.

REFERENCES

Aarts, H., & Dijksterhuis, A. (2000). Habits as knowledge structures: Automaticity in goal-directed behavior. *Journal of Personality and Social Psychology, 78,* 53–63.

Allemand, M., & Flückiger, C. (2017). Changing personality traits: Some considerations from psychotherapy process-outcome research for intervention efforts on intentional personality change. *Journal of Psychotherapy Integration, 27,* 476–494.

Allemand, M., Zimprich, D., & Hertzog, C. (2007). Cross-sectional age differences and longitudinal age changes of personality in middle adulthood and old age. *Journal of Personality, 75*(2), 323–358.

Anusic, I., & Schimmack, U. (2016). Stability and change of personality traits, self-esteem, and well-being: Introducing the meta-analytic stability and change model of retest correlations. *Journal of Personality and Social Psychology, 110,* 766–781.

Ardelt, M. (2000). Still stable after all these years: Personality stability theory revisited. *Social Psychology Quarterly,* 392–405.

Asselmann, E., & Specht, J. (2021). Testing the social investment principle around childbirth: Little evidence for personality maturation before and after becoming a parent. *European Journal of Personality, 35*(1), 85–102.

Bazana, P. G., & Stelmack, R. M. (2004). Stability of personality across the life span: A meta-analysis. In *On the psychobiology of personality: Essays in honor of Marvin Zuckerman* (pp. 113–144). Elsevier.

Beck, E. D., Condon, D., & Jackson, J. (2023). Interindividual age differences in personality structure. *European Journal of Personality, 37*(3), 257–275.

Beck, E. D., & Jackson, J. J. (2020). Consistency and change in idiographic personality: A longitudinal ESM network study. *Journal of Personality and Social Psychology, 118*(5), 1080.

Beck, E. D., & Jackson, J. J. (2022a). Detecting idiographic personality change. *Journal of Personality Assessment, 104,* 467–483.

Beck, E. D., & Jackson, J. J. (2022b). Idiographic personality coherence: A quasi-experimental longitudinal ESM study. *European Journal of Personality, 36,* 391–412.

Beck, E. D., & Jackson, J. J. (2022). Personalized prediction of behaviors and experiences: An idiographic person–situation test. *Psychological Science, 33*(10), 1767–1782.

Bicchieri, C. (2006). *The grammar of society: The nature and dynamics of social norms.* Cambridge University Press.

Bleidorn, W., & Hopwood, C. J. (2024). A motivational framework of personality development in late adulthood. *Current Opinion in Psychology, 55,* 101731.

Bleidorn, W., Hopwood, C. J., & Lucas, R. E. (2018). Life events and personality trait change. *Journal of Personality, 86,* 83–96.

Bleidorn, W., Klimstra, T. A., Denissen, J. J., Rentfrow, P. J., Potter, J., & Gosling, S. D. (2013). Personality maturation around the world: A cross-cultural examination of social-investment theory. *Psychological Science, 24*(12), 2530–2540.

Bleidorn, W., Schwaba, T., Zheng, A., Hopwood, C. J., Sosa, S. S., Roberts, B. W., & Briley, D. A. (2022). Personality stability and change: A meta-analysis of longitudinal studies. *Psychological Bulletin, 148*(7–8), 588.

Block, J. (1971). *Lives through time.* Bancroft Books.

Borghuis, J., Denissen, J. J., Oberski, D., Sijtsma, K., Meeus, W. H., Branje, S., . . . Bleidorn, W. (2017). Big Five personality stability, change, and codevelopment across adolescence and early adulthood. *Journal of Personality and Social Psychology, 113*(4), 641.

Borghuis, J., Bleidorn, W., Sijtsma, K., Branje, S., Meeus, W. H., & Denissen, J. J. (2020). Longitudinal associations between trait neuroticism and negative daily experiences in adolescence. *Journal of Personality and Social Psychology, 118*(2), 348.

Brandt, N. D., Drewelies, J., Willis, S. L., Schaie, K. W., Ram, N., Gerstorf, D., & Wagner, J. (2023). Beyond Big Five trait domains: Stability and change in personality facets across midlife and old age. *Journal of Personality, 91*(5), 1171–1188.

Bühler, J. L., Orth, U., Bleidorn, W., Weber, E., Kretzschmar, A., Scheling, L., & Hopwood, C. J. (2024). Life events and personality change: A systematic review and meta-analysis. *European Journal of Personality, 38*(3), 544–568.

Caselli, R. J., Langlais, B. T., Dueck, A. C., Henslin, B. R., Johnson, T. A., Woodruff, B. K., . . . Locke, D. E. (2018). Personality changes during the transition from cognitive health to mild cognitive impairment. *Journal of the American Geriatrics Society, 66*(4), 671–678.

Caspi, A., & Roberts, B. W. (1999). Personality continuity and change across the life course. In L. A. Pervin & O. P. John (Eds.), *Handbook of personality: Theory and research* (2nd ed., pp. 300–326). Guilford Press.

Caspi, A., & Roberts, B. W. (2001). Personality development across the life course: The argument for change and continuity. *Psychological Inquiry, 12,* 49–66.

Caspi, A., Roberts, B. W., & Shiner, R. L. (2005). Personality development: Stability and change. *Annual Review of Psychology, 56,* 453–484.

Chapman, B. P., Hampson, S., & Clarkin, J. (2014). Personality-informed interventions for healthy aging: Conclusions from a National Institute on Aging workgroup. *Developmental Psychology, 50,* 1426–1441.

Danner, U. N., Aarts, H., & de Vries, N. K. (2008). Habit vs. intention in the prediction of future behaviour: The role of frequency, context stability and mental accessibility of past behaviour. *British Journal of Social Psychology, 47,* 245–265.

De Fruyt, F., Bartels, M., Van Leeuwen, K. G., De Clercq, B., Decuyper, M., & Mervielde, I. (2006). Five types of personality continuity in childhood and adolescence. *Journal of Personality and Social Psychology, 91*(3), 538.

Denissen, J. J. A., Luhmann, M., Chung, J. M., & Bleidorn, W. (2019). Transactions between life events and personality traits across the adult lifespan. *Journal of Personality and Social Psychology, 116,* 612–633.

Denissen, J. J. A., Ulferts, H., Lüdtke, O., Muck, P. M., & Gerstorf, D. (2014). Longitudinal transactions between personality and occupational roles: A large and heterogeneous study of job beginners, stayers, and changers. *Developmental Psychology, 50,* 1931–1942.

Erikson, E. H. (1968). *Identity: Youth and crisis.* Norton.

Fehr, E., & Schurtenberger, I. (2018). Normative foundations of human cooperation. *Nature Human Behaviour, 2,* 458–468.

Ferguson, C. J. (2010). A meta-analysis of normal and disordered personality across the life span. *Journal of Personality and Social Psychology, 98*(4), 659.

Fraley, R. C., & Roberts, B. W. (2005). Patterns of continuity: A dynamic model for conceptualizing the stability of individual differences in psychological constructs across the life course. *Psychological Review, 112*(1), 60.

Frankl, V. E. (1959). The spiritual dimension in existential analysis and logotherapy. *Journal of Individual Psychology, 15,* 157–165.

Gallagher, P., Fleeson, W., & Hoyle, R. (2011). A self-regulatory mechanism for personality trait stability: Contra-trait effort. *Social Psychological and Personality Science, 2,* 333–342.

Geukes, K., Zalk, M., & Back, M. D. (2018). Understanding personality development: An integrative state process model. *International Journal of Behavioral Development, 42,* 43–51.

Gilbert, K., Whalen, D. J., Jackson, J. J., Tillman, R., Barch, D. M., & Luby, J. L. (2021). Thin slice derived personality types predict longitudinal symptom trajectories. *Personality Disorders: Theory, Research, and Treatment, 12*(3), 275.

Göllner, R., Roberts, B. W., Damian, R. I., Lüdtke, O., Jonkmann, K., & Trautwein, U. (2017). Whose "storm and stress" is it?: Parent and child reports of personality development in the transition to early adolescence. *Journal of Personality, 85*(3), 376–387.

Graham, E. K., Weston, S. J., Gerstorf, D., Yoneda, T. B., Booth, T. O. M., Beam, C. R., . . . Mroczek, D. K. (2020). Trajectories of Big Five personality traits: A coordinated analysis of 16 longitudinal samples. *European Journal of Personality, 34*(3), 301–321.

Hampson, S. E. (2012). Personality processes: Mechanisms by which personality traits "get outside the skin." *Annual Review of Psychology, 63,* 315–339.

Heidegger, M. (1927). *Being and time.* SCM Press.

Helson, R., Kwan, V. S. Y., John, O. P., & Jones, C. (2002). The growing evidence for personality change in adulthood: Findings from research with personality inventories. *Journal of Research in Personality, 36,* 287–306.

Hennecke, M., Bleidorn, W., Denissen, J. J. A., & Wood, D. (2014). A three-part framework for self-regulated personality development across adulthood. *European Journal of Personality, 28,* 289–299.

Hill, P. L., & Burrow, A. L. (2012). Viewing purpose through an Eriksonian lens. *Identity: An International Journal of Theory and Research, 12*(1), 74–91.

Hill, P. L., Edmonds, G. W., Peterson, M., Luyckx, K., & Andrews, J. A. (2016). Purpose in life in emerging adulthood: Development and validation of a new brief measure. *Journal of Positive Psychology, 11*(3), 237–245.

Hill, P. L., & Turiano, N. A. (2014). Purpose in life as a predictor of mortality across adulthood. *Psychological Science, 25*(7), 1482–1486.

Hoff, K. A., Einarsdóttir, S., Chu, C., Briley, D. A., & Rounds, J. (2021). Personality changes predict early career outcomes: Discovery and replication in 12-year longitudinal studies. *Psychological Science, 32,* 64–79.

Hudson, N. W., & Fraley, R. C. (2015). Volitional personality trait change: Can people choose to change their personality traits? *Journal of Personality and Social Psychology, 109*(3), 490–507.

Hudson, N. W., & Roberts, B. W. (2016). Social investment in work reliably predicts change in conscientiousness and agreeableness: A direct replication and extension of Hudson, Roberts, and Lodi-Smith (2012). *Journal of Research in Personality, 60,* 12–23.

Hudson, N. W., Roberts, B. W., & Lodi-Smith, J. (2012). Personality trait development and social investment in work. *Journal of Research in Personality, 46*(3), 334–344.

Hudson, N. W., Briley, D. A., Chopik, W. J., & Derringer, J. (2019). You have to follow through: Attaining behavioral change goals predicts volitional personality change. *Journal of Personality and Social Psychology, 117*(4), 839.

Hutteman, R., Hennecke, M., Orth, U., Reitz, A. K., & Specht, J. (2014). Developmental tasks as a framework to study personality development in adulthood and old age. *European Journal of Personality, 28,* 267–278.

Ibáñez, M. I., Viruela, A. M., Mezquita, L., Moya, J., Villa, H., Camacho, L., & Ortet, G. (2016). An investigation of five types of personality trait continuity: A two-wave longitudinal study of Spanish adolescents from age 12 to age 15. *Frontiers in Psychology, 7,* 163412.

Jackson, J. J., & Beck, E. D. (2021). Personality development beyond the mean: Do life events shape personality variability, structure, and ipsative continuity? *Journals of Gerontology: Series B, 76*(1), 20–30.

Jackson, J. J., Bogg, T., Walton, K. E., Wood, D., Harms, P. D., Lodi-Smith, J., . . . Roberts, B. W. (2009). Not all conscientiousness scales change alike: a multimethod, multisample study of age differences in the facets of conscientiousness. *Journal of Personality and Social Psychology, 96*(2), 446.

Jackson, J. J., Beck, E. D., & Mike, A. (2021). Personality interventions. In O. P. John & R. W. Robins (Eds.), *Handbook of personality: Theory and research* (4th ed., pp. 793–805). Guilford Press.

Jackson, J. J., Connolly, J. J., Garrison, S. M., Leveille, M. M., & Connolly, S. L. (2015). Your friends know how long you will live: A 75-year study of peer-rated personality traits. *Psychological Science, 26,* 335–340.

Jackson, J. J., & Wright, A. J. (2024). The process and mechanisms of personality change. *Nature Reviews Psychology, 3*(5), 305–318.

Kandler, C., Kornadt, A. E., Hagemeyer, B., & Neyer, F. J. (2015). Patterns and sources of personality development in old age. *Journal of Personality and Social Psychology, 109*(1), 175.

Kierkegaard, S. (1843). Either/or. In R. Solomon (Ed.), *Existentialism* (2nd ed., pp. 8–14; D. Swenson & L. Swenson, Trans.). Oxford University Press.

Kierkegaard, S. (1849). *The sickness unto death.* Princeton University Press.

Klimstra, T. A., Hale, W. W. III, Raaijmakers, Q. A., Branje, S. J., & Meeus, W. H. (2009). Maturation of personality in adolescence. *Journal of Personality and Social Psychology, 96*(4), 898.

Koval, P., Kalokerinos, E. K., Greenaway, K. H., Medland, H., Kuppens, P., Nezlek, J. B.,

. . . Gross, J. J. (2023). Emotion regulation in everyday life: Mapping global self-reports to daily processes. *Emotion, 23*(2), 357.

Kuper, N., Breil, S. M., Horstmann, K. T., Roemer, L., Lischetzke, T., Sherman, R. A., . . . Rauthmann, J. F. (2022). Individual differences in contingencies between situation characteristics and personality states. *Journal of Personality and Social Psychology, 123*(5), 1166.

Kuzma, E., Sattler, C., Toro, P., Schönknecht, P., & Schröder, J. (2011). Premorbid personality traits and their course in mild cognitive impairment: Results from a prospective population-based study in Germany. *Dementia and Geriatric Cognitive Disorders, 32*(3), 171–177.

Lally, P., van Jaarsveld, C. H. M., Potts, H. W. W., & Wardle, J. (2010). How are habits formed: Modelling habit formation in the real world. *European Journal of Social Psychology, 40,* 998–1009.

Lehnart, J., Neyer, F. J., & Eccles, J. (2010). Long-term effects of social investment: The case of partnering in young adulthood. *Journal of Personality, 78*(2), 639–670.

Lucas, R. E., & Donnellan, M. B. (2011). Personality development across the life span: longitudinal analyses with a national sample from Germany. *Journal of Personality and Social Psychology, 101*(4), 847.

Lücke, A. J., Quintus, M., Egloff, B., & Wrzus, C. (2021). You can't always get what you want: The role of change goal importance, goal feasibility and momentary experiences for volitional personality development. *European Journal of Personality, 35,* 690–709.

Lüdtke, O., Roberts, B. W., Trautwein, U., & Nagy, G. (2011). A random walk down university avenue: life paths, life events, and personality trait change at the transition to university life. *Journal of Personality and Social Psychology, 101*(3), 620.

Magidson, J. F., Roberts, B. W., Collado-Rodriguez, A., & Lejuez, C. W. (2014). Theory-driven intervention for changing personality: expectancy value theory, behavioral activation, and conscientiousness. *Developmental Psychology, 50,* 1442.

Marsh, H. W., Nagengast, B., & Morin, A. J. (2013). Measurement invariance of big-five factors over the life span: ESEM tests of gender, age, plasticity, maturity, and la dolce vita effects. *Developmental Psychology, 49*(6), 1194.

May, R. (1958). The origins and significance of the existential movement in psychology. In R. May, E. Angel, & H. F. Ellenberger (Eds.), *Existence: A new dimension in psychiatry and psychology* (pp. 3–36). Basic Books.

McCrae, R. R., & Costa, P. T. (2003). *Personality in adulthood: A five-factor theory perspective.* Guilford Press.

Mischel, W. (2004). Toward an integrative science of the person. *Annual Review of Psychology, 55,* 1–22.

Mõttus, R., Johnson, W., & Deary, I. J. (2012). Personality traits in old age: measurement and rank-order stability and some mean-level change. *Psychology and Aging, 27*(1), 243.

Mroczek, D. K., Graham, E. K., Turiano, N. A., & Aro-Lambo, M. O. (2021). Personality development in adulthood and later life. In O. P. John & R. W. Robins (Eds.), *Handbook of personality: Theory and research* (4th ed., pp. 336–351). Guilford Press.

Mroczek, D. K., & Spiro, A. III. (2003). Modeling intraindividual change in personality traits: Findings from the Normative Aging Study. *Journals of Gerontology Series B: Psychological Sciences and Social Sciences, 58*(3), P153–P165.

Mueller, S., Wagner, J., Drewelies, J., Duezel, S., Eibich, P., Specht, J., . . . Gerstorf, D. (2016). Personality development in old age relates to physical health and cognitive performance: Evidence from the Berlin Aging Study II. *Journal of Research in Personality, 65,* 94–108.

Nietzsche, F. (1886). *Beyond good and evil.* Dover.

Nye, C. D., Allemand, M., Gosling, S. D., Potter, J., & Roberts, B. W. (2016). Personality trait differences between young and middle-aged adults: Measurement artifacts or actual trends? *Journal of Personality, 84*(4), 473–492.

Olaru, G., Schroeders, U., Wilhelm, O., & Ostendorf, F. (2018). A confirmatory examination of age-associated personality differences: Deriving age-related measurement-invariant solutions using ant colony optimization. *Journal of Personality, 86*(6), 1037–1049.

Olaru, G., Stieger, M., Rüegger, D., Kowatsch, T., Flückiger, C., Roberts, B. W., & Allemand, M. (2024). Personality change through a digital-coaching intervention: Using measurement invariance testing to distinguish between trait domain, facet, and nuance change. *European Journal of Personality, 38*(2), 141–157.

Oltmanns, J. R., Jackson, J. J., & Oltmanns, T. F. (2020). Personality change: Longitudinal self-other agreement and convergence with retrospective-reports. *Journal of Personality and Social Psychology, 118,* 1065–1079.

Poier, S. (2022). How stable is your customer?: Individual and ipsative consistency of consumers' Big Five personality traits. *Contemporary Economics, 16*(3), 297–316.

Quilty, L. C., Meusel, L. A. C., & Bagby, R. M.

(2008). Neuroticism as a mediator of treatment response to SSRIs in major depressive disorder. *Journal of Affective Disorders, 111*(1), 67–73.

Quintus, M., Egloff, B., & Wrzus, C. (2021). Daily life processes predict long-term development in explicit and implicit representations of Big Five traits: Testing predictions from the TESSERA framework. *Journal of Personality and Social Psychology, 120,* 1049–1073.

Rauthmann, J. F., Sherman, R. A., & Funder, D. C. (2015). Principles of situation research: Towards a better understanding of psychological situations. *European Journal of Personality, 29,* 363–381.

Roberts, B. W. (2006). Personality development and organizational behavior. *Research in Organizational Behavior, 27,* 1–40.

Roberts, B. W., Walton, K. E., & Viechtbauer, W. (2006). Patterns of mean-level change in personality traits across the life course: A meta-analysis of longitudinal studies. *Psychological Bulletin, 132*(1), 1.

Roberts, B. W., & Caspi, A. (2003). The cumulative continuity model of personality development: Striking a balance between continuity and change in personality traits across the life course. In U. M. Staudinger & U. Lindenberger (Eds.), *Understanding human development* (pp. 183–214). Springer.

Roberts, B. W., Caspi, A., & Moffitt, T. E. (2003). Work experiences and personality development in young adulthood. *Journal of Personality and Social Psychology, 84,* 582–593.

Roberts, B. W., & DelVecchio, W. F. (2000). The rank-order consistency of personality traits from childhood to old age: A quantitative review of longitudinal studies. *Psychological Bulletin, 126*(1), 3.

Roberts, B. W., & Jackson, J. J. (2008). Sociogenomic personality psychology. *Journal of Personality, 76,* 1523–1544.

Roberts, B. W., Luo, J., Briley, D. A., Chow, P. I., Su, R., & Hill, P. L. (2017). A systematic review of personality trait change through intervention. *Psychological Bulletin, 143*(2), 117.

Roberts, B. W., & Nickel, L. B. (2021). Personality development across the life course: A neo socioanalytic perspective. In O. P. John & R. W. Robins (Eds.), *Handbook of personality: Theory and research* (4th ed., pp. 259–283). Guilford Press.

Roberts, B. W., Wood, D., & Smith, J. L. (2005). Evaluating five factor theory and social investment perspectives on personality trait development. *Journal of Research in Personality, 39,* 166–184.

Robins, R. W., Caspi, A., & Moffitt, T. E. (2002). It's not just who you're with, it's who you are: Personality and relationship experiences across multiple relationships. *Journal of Personality, 70*(6), 925–964.

Rosenberg, E. L. (1998). Levels of analysis and the organization of affect. *Review of General Psychology, 2,* 247–270.

Sala, G., Aksayli, N. D., Tatlidil, K. S., Tatsumi, T., Gondo, Y., & Gobet, F. (2019). Near and far transfer in cognitive training: A second-order meta-analysis. *Collabra: Psychology, 5*(1), Article 18.

Sander, J., Schmiedek, F., Brose, A., Wagner, G. G., & Specht, J. (2017). Long-term effects of an extensive cognitive training on personality development. *Journal of Personality, 85*(4), 454–463.

Sarbin, T. R. (1967). The dangerous individual: An outcome of social identity transformations. *British Journal of Criminology, 7,* 285–295.

Sartre, J.-P. (1943). *Being and nothingness.* Washington Square Press.

Sauer-Zavala, S., Wilner, J. G., & Barlow, D. H. (2017). Addressing neuroticism in psychological treatment. *Personality Disorders: Theory, Research, and Treatment, 8*(3), 191–198.

Scarr, S., & McCartney, K. (1983). How people make their own environments: A theory of genotype-environment effects. *Child Development, 54,* 424–435.

Schneider, B., Smith, D. B., Taylor, S., & Fleenor, J. (1998). Personality and organizations: A test of the homogeneity of personality hypothesis. *Journal of Applied Psychology, 83,* 462–470.

Schwaba, T., & Bleidorn, W. (2018). Individual differences in personality change across the adult life span. *Journal of Personality, 86*(3), 450–464.

Schwaba, T., & Bleidorn, W. (2019). Personality trait development across the transition to retirement. *Journal of Personality and Social Psychology, 116,* 651–665.

Schwaba, T., Luhmann, M., Denissen, J. J., Chung, J. M., & Bleidorn, W. (2018). Openness to experience and culture-openness transactions across the lifespan. *Journal of Personality and Social Psychology, 115*(1), 118.

Schwaba, T., Robins, R. W., Grijalva, E., & Bleidorn, W. (2019). Does openness to experience matter in love and work?: Domain, facet, and developmental evidence from a 24-year longitudinal study. *Journal of Personality, 87*(5), 1074–1092.

Scollon, C. N., & Diener, E. (2006). Love, work, and changes in extraversion and neuroticism over time. *Journal of Personality and Social Psychology, 91,* 1152–1165.

Seger, C. A. (1994). Implicit learning. *Psychological Bulletin, 115,* 163–196.

Smith, T. W., Uchino, B. N., Berg, C. A., Florsheim, P., Pearce, G., Hawkins, M., . . . Yoon, H. C. (2008). Associations of self-reports versus spouse ratings of negative affectivity, dominance, and affiliation with coronary artery disease: Where should we look and who should we ask when studying personality and health? *Health Psychology, 27*(6), 676.

Soto, C. J., John, O. P., Gosling, S. D., & Potter, J. (2011). Age differences in personality traits from 10 to 65: Big Five domains and facets in a large cross-sectional sample. *Journal of Personality and Social Psychology, 100*(2), 330.

Specht, J., Bleidorn, W., Denissen, J. J., Hennecke, M., Hutteman, R., Kandler, C., . . . Zimmermann, J. (2014). What drives adult personality development: A comparison of theoretical perspectives and empirical evidence. *European Journal of Personality, 28*(3), 216–230.

Specht, J., Egloff, B., & Schmukle, S. C. (2011). Stability and change of personality across the life course: The impact of age and major life events on mean-level and rank-order stability of the Big Five. *Journal of Personality and Social Psychology, 101,* 862–882.

Sutin, A. R., Costa, P. T., Miech, R., & Eaton, W. W. (2009). Personality and career success: Concurrent and longitudinal relations. *European Journal of Personality, 23,* 71–84.

Swann, W. B. Jr., Rentfrow, P. J., & Guinn, J. S. (2003). Self-verification: The search for coherence. In M. R. Leary & J. P. Tangney (Eds.), *Handbook of self and identity* (pp. 367–383). Guilford Press.

Tackett, J. L., Balsis, S., Oltmanns, T. F., & Krueger, R. F. (2009). A unifying perspective on personality pathology across the life span: Developmental considerations for the fifth edition of the Diagnostic and Statistical Manual of Mental Disorders. *Development and Psychopathology, 21*(3), 687–713.

Terracciano, A., Costa, P. T. Jr., & McCrae, R. R. (2006). Personality plasticity after age 30. *Personality and Social Psychology Bulletin, 32*(8), 999–1009.

Terracciano, A., McCrae, R. R., & Costa, P. T., Jr. (2010). Intra-individual change in personality stability and age. *Journal of Research in Personality, 44*(1), 31–37.

Terracciano, A., Stephan, Y., Luchetti, M., & Sutin, A. R. (2018). Cognitive impairment, dementia, and personality stability among older adults. *Assessment, 25,* 336–347.

van Scheppingen, M. A., Jackson, J. J., Specht, J., Hutteman, R., Denissen, J. J., & Bleidorn, W. (2016). Personality trait development during the transition to parenthood: A test of social investment theory. *Social Psychological and Personality Science, 7*(5), 452–462.

Verplanken, B., & Orbell, S. (2022). Attitudes, habits, and behavior change. *Annual Review of Psychology, 73,* 327–352.

Wille, B., Beyers, W., & De Fruyt, F. (2012). A transactional approach to person-environment fit: Reciprocal relations between personality development and career role growth across young to middle adulthood. *Journal of Vocational Behavior, 81*(3), 307–321.

Wortman, J., Lucas, R. E., & Donnellan, M. B. (2012). Stability and change in the Big Five personality domains: evidence from a longitudinal study of Australians. *Psychology and Aging, 27*(4), 867.

Wright, A. J., & Jackson, J. J. (2023). Are some people more consistent? Examining the stability and underlying processes of personality profile consistency. *Journal of Personality and Social Psychology, 124,* 1314–1337.

Wright, A. J., Weston, S. J., Norton, S., Voss, M., Bogdan, R., Oltmanns, T. F., & Jackson, J. J. (2022). Prospective self-and informant-personality associations with inflammation, health behaviors, and health indicators. *Health Psychology, 41*(2), 121.

Wrzus, C., Luong, G., Wagner, G. G., & Riediger, M. (2021). Longitudinal coupling of momentary stress reactivity and trait neuroticism: Specificity of states, traits, and age period. *Journal of Personality and Social Psychology, 121,* 691–706.

Wrzus, C., & Roberts, B. W. (2017). Processes of personality development in adulthood: The TESSERA framework. *Personality and Social Psychology Review, 21,* 253–277.

Yalom, I. D. (1980). *Existential psychotherapy.* Basic Books.

SECTION VI
MEANING AND PURPOSE

CHAPTER 42

Commonplace Meaning in Life

Erica A. Holberg *and* Laura A. King

To commemorate its 350th anniversary in 2010, the Royal Society released digital scans of a number of documents online, providing widespread public access to a treasure trove in the history of science. Among the documents was a biography of Sir Isaac Newton, by William Stukeley. Based on his interview with Newton, Stukeley shared Newton's description of the origins of the law of gravity (Stukeley, 1752, p. 11, emphasis added): "*Why* should that apple always descend perpendicularly to the ground, thought he to himself; occasion'd by the fall of an apple as he sat in a contemplative mood. *Why* should it not go sideways or upward?"

Looking at the world around him, Newton asked, "Why?" In many ways, "Why" questions are the central questions of meaning, both globally ("Why am I here?"; "Why do I live?") and situationally ("Why did that happen?"; "Why did that happen *to me*?"). Newton's experience exemplifies an important truth: Sometimes answers to the "Why" questions of life—those questions asked when meaning is most at stake—are not effortful constructions or creations of the mind. Rather, sometimes, answers to such questions can be found in the natural laws of the world in which we live.

Perhaps the prominence of Viktor Frankl's seminal volume in the inception of the psychology of existential concerns led to psychologists' preoccupation with understanding meaning in its absence—when it is an experience we search for and actively construct. This emphasis is perhaps ironic as Frankl (1956/1992, p. 122) asserted, "What is demanded of [us)] is not, as some existential philosophers teach, to endure the meaninglessness of life, but rather to bear (our) incapacity to grasp its unconditional meaningfulness in rational terms." Frankl viewed life as unconditionally meaningful and suggested that meaning, somewhat like gravity, is discovered (not created). Indeed, Isaac Newton did not search for or construct gravity. He *noticed* it. Newton's eureka moment and the foundation of our understanding of gravity came as a result of gravity doing what gravity does—from an observation of the presence and action of gravity, not its absence. While all of humanity had witnessed objects falling down, Newton attended to the phenomenon and documented its lawfulness. A comprehensive science of meaning in life requires consideration of meaning when, like gravity, it is present, when it is a product of not only searching and constructing but attention, perception, and recognition. Attending to moments when meaning is lacking is undoubtedly important to understanding coping and resilience. However, such attention should not be so selective as to miss meaning when it is readily apparent. Focusing on the presence of meaning requires us not only to confront the fact that life is typically experienced as meaningful, but also to deeply probe all the things in life that may support this perhaps surprisingly commonplace experience.

We begin this chapter by defining *meaning in life* and its facets (coherence, significance, and purpose). Then, we review the commonplace nature of meaning in life and the ways each facet of meaning is supported by common experiences. We then consider the interrelations among the various experiences that make life meaningful and consider their potentially interchangeable nature. Finally, we turn to potential threats to the commonplace experience of meaning in modern life.

DEFINING *MEANING IN LIFE*

As likely noted by many authors in this volume, a sense of inadequacy haunts attempts to characterize the meaning of meaning. Meaning has an ineffable richness, exceeding definitive articulation. Even setting aside the grander concern of the Meaning *of* Life, defining the experience of meaning *in* life has been challenging. As is common in the science of well-being, meaning in life is typically studied as a subjective experience that is available to awareness. Essentially, from this perspective, the best person to tell us if a person's life is meaningful, is the person themselves. Using self-report questionnaires with face-valid items addressing meaning in life (e.g., "My life is meaningful"), research has demonstrated that people who evaluate their lives as meaningful, whatever they think that means, show a broad range of benefits compared to those who view their lives as less meaningful, across diverse outcomes (King & Hicks, 2021; Sutin et al., 2021; Wade et al., 2023; Ward et al., 2023).

A consensus has emerged about at least three experiences that promote the sense that life is meaningful. These themes, or facets, of meaning appear in scholarly conceptual definitions of meaning in life (King et al., 2006) and have garnered empirical support (e.g., Costin & Vignoles, 2020; George & Park, 2016; Martela & Steger, 2023) as approximating a reasonable sense of what makes life meaningful. Specifically, the three facets of meaning include coherence, significance, and purpose. *Coherence* or *comprehensibility* refers to experiencing life as a unified whole, where things fit together and make sense. *Significance* or *existential mattering* refers to the sense that one has had lasting impact on others and the world. Finally, *purpose* refers to dedication to goals and aims, the sense that behavior is directed toward personally desired ends. These three facets may not fully capture all the activities and experiences that make life meaningful, and there may always be a sense that something is missing from our attempts to define meaning in life. Nevertheless, they provide a workable framework for understanding this vital human experience.

Although these three elements have been understood to contribute to meaning in life, globally, their relevance to even more circumscribed contexts is clear. Consider writing a chapter for a handbook. If we wish that chapter to have meaning for readers, we strive toward logic and organization (coherence), a memorable message that will have resonance and impact (significance), and finally, to achieve the goal of persuading readers to a point (purpose).

THE PRESENCE OF MEANING IN EVERYDAY LIFE

Do people experience their lives as coherent, significant, and purposeful? Heintzelman and King (2014b) summarized research using representative samples as well as research samples in which meaning in life self-reports were collected. They found that most people experience life as pretty meaningful. For example, in a survey spanning 132 nations ($N > 100{,}000$; Oishi & Diener, 2014), in answer to the question "Do you feel your life has an important purpose or meaning?," averaged over nations, 91% of participants responded, "Yes." Similarly, in research samples using Likert rating scales, sample means were almost always above the scale midpoint. Life is evaluated as pretty meaningful in samples including undergraduates (including those assigned to "meaning threat" conditions in experiments) and community adults (including those undergoing treatment for cancer, other health concerns, and psychiatric conditions; Heintzelman &

King, 2014b). Surveys of folk beliefs about meaning in life concord with the conclusion that meaning in life is commonplace. Everyday people view meaning in life as a common (and not rare) experience (Heintzelman et al., 2020). While sustained struggle and conscious exertion may be part of the story of meaning in life, struggle and exertion should not be cast in the lead role of the experience of meaning in life. Rather than troublesome and rare, the subjective experience of meaning in life is often effortless and ubiquitous (King, 2012).

What explains the ready availability of meaning in life? One way to think about this question is to consider all the things that might promote the three facets of meaning—resources that might help life make sense and facilitate mattering to the social world and goal pursuit. Indeed, although the meaningful life is sometimes considered a rare achievement or esoteric concern (Baumeister, 1991), decidedly worldly experiences promote the sense that life is meaningful. For example, financial resources predict meaning in life and function similarly to other putative sources of meaning, like religious faith and social relatedness (Ward & King, 2016, 2019). Additionally, both observer ratings and self-reports of physical attractiveness relate positively to self-reported meaning in life (Sanders et al., 2023). It is not difficult to imagine how wealth and attractiveness may contribute to an existence that is less chaotic (coherent) and more memorable (significant) and in which goal pursuits are facilitated (purposeful). However, it is worth noting that financial resources and attractiveness are goods of fortune, largely the products of luck. We see here the interplay of activity and passivity key to an account of meaning's plentiful presence in our lives. That is, not all the meaning we experience is earned or worked for. Meaning can be promoted by experiences that simply happen to us.

The experience of meaning need not always be viewed as the willful imposition of created meaning upon chaos or some blank slate. Rather, we encounter the world as plentiful in meaning: ordered so as to be coherent, full of purpose, and rich with significance. Our world, the people in it, and our own agency afford us plenty with regard to meaning, constraining and guiding our meaning-making activity, and we are sensitive to its plentitude. Made meanings may be most likely to lead to positive resolution when they approximate the feelings of meaning that emerge in daily life from commonplace sources—the feelings that tell us life is meaningful when it is. Next, we review the nuances of commonplace meaning in life with reference to each of its facets—coherence, significance, and purpose—and then turn to the role of positive feelings in commonplace meaning in life.

The World Affords Coherence: Invariants—Natural and Constructed

Coherence—the experience of experience making sense—implies that life events are connected, constituting a unified whole. Some scholars have argued that meaning is, at base, the same as connection, like the link between a word and its meaning (Baumeister & Hippel, 2020). The connections that exist in the world present us with invariants and other steadying regularities, undergirding and supporting reason's work of making, but also perhaps just feeling, coherence. We live in a lawful natural world characterized by constancies, stabilities, and regularities—sunrises and sunsets, winters followed by springs, and objects that fall "perpendicularly to the ground . . . not upward or sideways." Thus, one source for the experience of meaning might be a world that very often makes sense. Still, we might ask, "Does the world often make sense?" Aspects of perception and learning in nonhuman animals and humans point to the conclusion that it does.

Arguably, the general assumption that the world makes sense is an old one for our species. Research on intuitive physics suggests that nonhuman primates possess expectations about the world that are consistent with the laws of physics that operate in the world in which they live (Marciniak et al., 2022). Similarly, research from the nativist perspective on infant cognition suggests human infants come into the world with a nascent cognitive architecture, prepared for understanding physics and mathematics (Spelke, 2022). Infants are ready for and expect a world that conforms to natural laws. Such readiness and expectancies would be profoundly maladaptive for life in a world that did not generally conform to them. Such expectancies exist and persist because they facilitate the survival of organisms navigating a natural world. Such physical invariants are not mere fodder for reason's coherence-making activities but the conditions that make such coherence-making activity possible.

In the "(feeling of) meaning-as-information" approach, Heintzelman and King (2014a) drew links from the Gibsonian view of perception to encounters with objective coherence and subjective meaning. Opposing constructivist views of perception, Gibson argued that organisms are adapted to the environments in which their perceptual organs evolved, such that if invariants are available, an organism can perceive them without the need for construction (e.g., Gibson, 1973, 1979/1986). In conceiving of perception as a direct process that does not require experience or inference, Gibson's account not only makes a claim about how perception works but also locates perception within a natural world flush with sensory data sufficient for accurate judgment. Sensory organs are adapted to function in a particular environment, a world that makes sense. Not simply objects but their relations to each other are detected automatically. The perception of covariation—the perception of connection—occurs without effort, even when such perception is irrelevant to a task (Turk-Browne et al., 2008).

Similarly, Heintzelman and King (2014a) drew a connection between the subjective feeling of meaning and the automatic processes of associative learning. Associative learning is clearly an adaptive trait for all creatures. Like expectancies undergirded by intuitive physics, the capacity to learn from reliable associations would be disastrous for organisms if the world were essentially chaotic. If the capacity to automatically learn associations in the environment is adaptive, then the natural environment must contain such associations (Domjan, 2005). In their behavior, then, all creatures that demonstrate the capacity to extract reliable associations in the environment collectively tell us that they live in a world that contains such associations, a world that often makes sense.

Clearly, meaning is not only objective connection, whether perceived or learned. Meaningfulness is subjectively felt (Rose & King, 2020). Varied evidence supports the potential role of perceived connection in the subjective experience of meaning. In experiments, participants exposed to stimuli that follow patterns (e.g., photos of trees in seasonal order) reported higher meaning in life than did those who saw the same stimuli without such pattern (Heintzelman et al., 2013b). Additionally, the intuitive information-processing system (system 1) is considered the source of the capacity to extract reliable connections in the environment (e.g., Morewedge & Kahneman, 2010). Reliance on intuition (not analytical processing) relates positively to meaning in life (Heintzelman & King, 2016). Intuition is susceptible to subtle cues of accuracy and truth, such as processing fluency (Thompson et al., 2011). When meaning in life items are presented in easy (versus hard) to read fonts, life is rated as more meaningful (Trent et al., 2013). Intuitive knowledge is often described as knowing without knowing why. With regard to the kind of meaning that emerges out of intuitive processes, we might say it represents meaning without *asking* why (Heintzelman & King, 2013a; King, 2012). Meaningfulness can be, at least in part, a deliverance of perception and associative learning, in the absence of conscious effort. Meaning-as-connection is there for the having, integral to how sense-making perceivers move through the world.

Connection emerges not only as a product of natural (or experimentally imposed) predictability or pattern. Human constructions, what we might call invariants of human creation, also serve as sources of the effortless sense of existence fitting together into a coherent, meaningful whole. Large-scale constructed meaning systems, for example as conveyed in culture and religion, may undergird a sense of coherence. Certainly, investment in religious and secular worldviews relates positively to meaning in life (King & Hicks, 2021). Such worldviews provide overarching frameworks that dictate norms and conventions—providing the reliable samenesses we encounter in our lives.

The relevance of worldviews to meaning has long been recognized, and these frameworks likely exist in part to facilitate making sense of existence. Yet, numerous related experiences also likely support meaning via their contribution to coherence. Culturally embedded constancies, such as language, the calendar, and days of the week, likely support a sense of meaning. Rituals—socially shared ceremonies with a dictated order—are also likely a key source of meaning. Research suggests ritual adds meaning to negative events (Norton & Gino, 2014) and to work (Kim et al., 2021). Research also suggests that, spurred by nostalgia, rituals, passed down across generations, support a sense of meaning (Yin et al., 2024). Nostalgia attaches the present self to not only a personal history, but a shared one.

Not only shared rituals but also idiosyncratic habits and routines support the sense of meaning in life. In cross-sectional studies, routinization (the tendency to do the same things every day) predicts higher meaning in life (Heintzelman & King, 2019). In experience-sampling studies, engaging in habitual behavior predicts higher momentary meaning in life (Heintzelman & King, 2019), regardless of the content or goal-relevance of routine activity (Mohideen & Heintzelman, 2023).

Considering the contextual layers in which human life is embedded, from a natural world rich with regularities and connections, to constructed conventions, norms, and worldviews, to shared rituals and idiosyncratic routines and habits, it is not surprising that generally life is felt to be meaningful. All the things that characterize the relatively stable aspects of life, our physical bodies, personality characteristics, identity, autobiographical memories, our social circles—although surely less invariant than gravity—provide a background for meaningfulness through familiarity, predictability, and constancy. A stable sense of self has been shown to enable the experience of meaning in life (Chu & Lowery, 2024). Emotions, like nostalgia, that promote meaning in life also contribute to a sense of self-continuity (Hong et al., 2022). Cross-sectional evidence suggests that cognitive capacities likely to facilitate a sense of continuity, such as episodic memory, relate positively to meaning in life (Sutin et al., 2022). Although such findings are often interpreted as indicating the benefits of meaning for cognitive aging, such capacities may facilitate the experience of one's life as a coherent narrative.

Surely experiences like the regularity of sunrises and sunsets, the days of the week, or the turning of the seasons, may be subtle supports for the experience of meaning. A person might have such experiences and they may contribute to meaning, but the direct connection between such experiences and meaning in life may never be noticed. Are there moments when meaning-as-connection is more vividly present, when meaning *happens* to us, drops vividly upon us, like an apple falling from a tree? Psychologists have long acknowledged that coincidences can sometimes be felt to possess such inescapable, fateful meaning (Freud, 1919/1953; Jung, 1950/1997). Sometimes purely random experiences feel innately and inescapably meaningful—without searching or effortful making. A study of parents of children with Down syndrome, in which they shared narratives about finding out their child had Down syndrome, showed that parents who mentioned a portentous event (e.g., a dream or random experience) experienced higher meaning in parenting a child with Down syndrome (King et al., 2000). Such dramatic, goosebump-inducing experiences may be relatively rare occurrences, but the effects of counterfactual thinking, frequently performed to evaluate alternative possible outcomes, past, present, and future, may function as a smaller-scale reflection of the role of coincidences in meaning.

Counterfactual thinking enhances the subjective meaning experienced in an event (Kray et al., 2010) and in life (Heintzelman et al., 2013a). Counterfactual thinking transforms the reality of life into a series of unlikely events—changing what happened into what was "meant to be." Notably, counterfactual thinking instills an "associative mindset" (McCulloch & Smallman, 2014), suggesting that unlikely coincidences inspire a process of connection seeking. Once again, such connection seeking implicates intuitive processing—to knowing without asking why—which may help explain the sometimes ineffable, even magical quality that characterizes the experience of meaning (Heintzelman & King, 2013a, 2013b).

Existential Mattering: Personal Meaning in a Social World

Existential mattering (or significance) is the experience of meaning through the social world in which we exist. Profound life events, such as the birth of a child or the death of a loved one, stand as strong evidence for the importance of social experience in defining what matters to us and how we matter to each other. Perhaps more than either coherence or purpose, low levels of personal significance have been implicated in particularly dire outcomes. For example, the interpersonal theory of suicide (e.g., Robison et al., 2024) suggests that feeling like a burden (rather than a contributor) and thwarted belongingness are important factors in the prediction of suicide. These aspects of the theory have found consistent empirical support in research (e.g., Okan et al., 2023) and social ostracism predicts suicidal ideation (Chen et al., 2020). Significance quest theory links low levels of personal significance to suicidal terror attacks and radicalization (Kruglanski et al., 2013; Pfundmair et al., 2024). That these extraordinary acts are also fortunately rare suggests that most people do experience a modicum of existential significance. Costin and Vignoles (2020) identified existential mattering as the key to global feelings of meaning in life. If meaning in life is primarily about significance, the commonplace nature of global meaning in life suggests significance, too, must be subjectively bountiful. What might explain the commonplace feeling of mattering?

In contemplating this question, it may be helpful to distinguish "capital-*M*" Mattering from "lowercase-*m*" mattering. When faced with the question of how the individual can transcend the spatial and temporal limitations of their physical existence and Matter in the grand scheme of the universe, our answers may be limited to profound, even historical achievements (e.g., becoming the leader of a nation, discovering a cure for cancer). Significance might seem to require, at the very least, "making it big" in whatever context one occupies. Whether such achievements enhance the experience of personal significance (or meaning in life) is an unanswered empirical question. Foremost, such achievements are not viable options for most people. If, like meaning in life, existential mattering is commonplace, it cannot be reserved for elite achievers. Mattering must be embedded in everyday circumstances.

A key mechanism for commonplace feelings of significance is likely social relationships. Even relatively impersonal social exclusion consistently predicts a lowered sense of one's existence mattering (e.g., Freedman et al., 2024; Williams, 2009). Conversely, romantic relationships (Hadden & Knee, 2018), friendships (O'Rourke et al., 2019), and family (Lambert et al., 2010) contribute to feeling located within a network of social belonging, with these relationships forming coinciding significance-supporting entanglements. Social belonging (Lambert et al., 2013) and relatedness (Hicks & King, 2009b) predict higher meaning in life. This association appears to be reciprocal. Not only does belonging predict greater meaning but meaning, in turn, predicts more belonging (Stavrova & Luhmann, 2016).

Some social relationships appear especially well poised to support existential mattering. While perhaps disruptive to some conceptions of happiness, parenting certainly secures meaning (Corner et al., 2023; Goodman et al., 2019; Nelson et al., 2013). One reason parenting is such a reliable source of significance is because parenting is a generative pursuit. *Generativity*, or concern for leaving a legacy to the next generation, relates positively to meaning in life (Fyffe & Wister, 2016; Hofer et al., 2014). Generative activities, such as mentoring, enhance the experience of meaning in life (Morse et al., 2022), so much so that a history of mentoring can lead to higher generativity long after those activities have ended (Chan & Nakamura, 2016). Directly generative work is one route to a legacy that carries forward in time, but there are more symbolic ways to achieve a sense of mattering, of transcending the threat death poses to individual significance. Activities that benefit society (Huang & Yang, 2023), and dedication to a cause, creative endeavor, or religious or philosophical worldview and larger framework of meaning (Allport, 1961) may provide personal significance and existential mattering.

Other everyday experiences relate positively to significance and meaning. For example, physical attractiveness contributes to meaning in life via significance (Sanders et al., 2023). In everyday life, being remembered (versus forgotten) by others predicts higher meaning in life (King & Geise, 2011; Ray et al., 2019). Everyday significance does not appear to reflect a desire for fame or inaccurate, inflated self-views. Researchers probing posthumous self-verification have asked people how they would like to be remembered in the future, long after they have died (Heintzelman et al., 2016). The vast majority of people preferred to be remembered in ways that constituted genuine reflections of themselves, warts and all. For most people, "lowercase-*m*" mattering may suffice to impart a sense of lasting significance.

Purpose as an All-Purpose Meaning Resource

Historically, feeling that life has goals and aims has been practically synonymous with meaning (King & Hicks, 2021). While purpose does not encompass all of meaning (Park, Chapter 50, this volume), of the three facets of meaning, purpose may serve as a particularly resilient source of meaning in life (Burrow et al., 2024). Certainly, external factors (demands, opportunities) may inform purpose. But, importantly, purpose can also be internally generated—a product of personal agency. In this sense, every problem to be solved in whatever circumstance is a potential purpose and, therefore, a likely source of meaning (Burrow & Hill, 2020).

The resilience of purpose is suggested by research showing its independence from negative experiences. Research suggests that traumatic life experiences in adolescence (when purposes are likely to emerge) are *unrelated* to later adult purpose in life (Pfund et al., 2020). Similarly, Rose and colleagues (2023) argued that significance and coherence resonate with fundamental developmental tasks of childhood, linking significance and coherence to working models of the self and world, respectively. Because of this relevance, they reasoned, adverse childhood experiences (e.g., neglect, abuse) should relate negatively to significance and coherence, but not purpose. Indeed, in adults, a history of adverse childhood experiences predicted lower significance and coherence, but was unrelated to purpose, with results strongly supporting the null hypothesis (Rose et al., 2023).

Although we might think of meaning in life as emerging from a grand life mission, everyday goal pursuit and progress predicts daily meaning in life (King et al., 2006). Thus, even checking off items on our everyday "to do" lists may contribute to commonplace meaning in life. Moreover, the capacity for everyday goals to enhance meaning suggests the potential relevance of smaller, circumscribed goals to the experience of meaning in difficult circumstances. During distressing times, the simple goal of engaging in routine—having dinner with family or enjoying a regular weekend activity—may enhance meaning. The goal of putting one foot in front of the other during times of intense grief may enhance purpose. The goal of a pain-free day for a person in hospice may enhance purpose.

Happiness

Alongside the three facets of meaning, a fourth factor, feeling happy, supports the commonplace experience of meaning in life. Positive affect (feeling happy, cheerful, content) correlates positively with meaning in life, cross-sectionally (King et al., 2006) and in daily reports (Tov & Lee, 2016). Experimentally induced positive mood leads to higher meaning in life (King & Hicks, 2021). In research on folk views of meaning in life, participants high in positive affect and life satisfaction were more likely to view meaning in life as commonplace (Heintzelman et al., 2020). Life satisfaction was negatively related to viewing meaning in life as requiring effort (Heintzelman et al., 2020). When we are happy and satisfied, life feels meaningful.

The notion that simple pleasure plays a role in existential concerns is reflected in socioemotional selectivity theory (Carstensen, 2021), which suggests that, with limited time, positive meaning occupies a central place in human priorities. In keeping with the theory, with age and perceived limited time, positive affect becomes increasingly associated with meaning in life (Hicks et al., 2012). In contexts in which the existential stakes are high, feeling happy may become a central indicator of life's meaning.

The relation between positive affect and meaning in life certainly centers the experience of meaning in the potentially trivial and quotidian. It may seem counterintuitive that meaning in life springs from such a source. However, no evidence suggests that this association is somehow harmful or maladaptive. Rather, the ready availability of positive feelings (Diener et al., 2015), inspired by simple experiences such as listening to music, taking a walk on a sunny day, or connecting with friends, surely supports the commonplace experience of meaning.

Happiness and meaning are both cherished human experiences, and each predicts the other. They both have roles to play in the good life. Yet dedication to meaning may sometimes require a person to disregard personal happiness. The preservation of meaning at the expense of happiness may constitute noble sacrifice, as when a person who sacrifices happiness in the service of duties, such as caring for a loved one. However, the prioritization of meaning may be harmful. For example, people with minoritized gender identities and sexualities may struggle with the conflict between societally and religiously sanctioned meaning and pathways that promise the most personal happiness and fulfillment. The pursuit of meaning and pursuit of happiness can conflict. Although personal happiness may seem like small potatoes relative to the vaunted experience of meaning in life, personal happiness should not always be viewed as the lesser of these experiences.

Intertwined and Interchangeable Aspects of Commonplace Meaning

The varied contributors to meaning in life are deeply interrelated, and they may be interchangeable. Our daily routines, the paths we habitually walk in life, include the faces of people we encounter each day. These people, in turn, are an opportunity to experience significance. It is through social interactions and relationships (likely promoting significance) that stable self (a source of coherence) is verified and affirmed. Enacting purpose by adopting a goal provides everyday existence with beginnings, middles, and ends, likely promoting coherence. Accomplishing a long-cherished goal (purpose) can promote feelings of significance. Likewise, the experience of positive emotion might facilitate seeing the big picture (coherence), energize goal pursuit (purpose), and allow us to recognize our place in our social network (significance).

Research supports the notion that these meaning-relevant experiences are intertwined. Characteristics and experiences clearly relevant to one aspect of meaning can have unexpected relations to other facets. For example, although subclinical narcissism is most clearly relevant to significance, it predicts all three facets of meaning similarly (Womick et al., 2020). Although belongingness appears most central to significance, it relates to all three facets of meaning in life (Costin & Vignoles, 2020). Similarly, the associative mindset, described in the context of coherence, enhances goal-directed pursuits, a clear aspect of purpose (McCulloch & Smallman, 2014). Habits (a source of coherence) often are subjectively mistaken for goal-directed acts, even when they are verifiably merely stimulus-driven (Wood et al., 2022). Generativity, which seems most related to significance, predicts higher meaning in life through the kinds of purposes people pursue (Hofer et al., 2014). Counterfactual thinking boosts meaning especially for those who believe in free will (Seto et al., 2015), suggesting the potential importance of personal significance to coherence. Although the unified life story is practically definitional to coherence, the experience of *purpose* predicts more vivid and rich autobiographical memories in older adults (Sutin et al., 2021). Finally, worldviews, including political ideology and religion, although perhaps most obviously relevant to coherence, appear to contribute to global meaning in life primarily through their links to feelings of existential significance (Womick et al., 2019, 2022).

Not only are the various contributors to meaning deeply related, they may compensate for each other, allowing a person to experience life as meaningful even in the absence of satisfaction of one or more of the others (Zhang et al., 2019). In the research on adverse childhood experiences noted above, Rose and colleagues (2023) found that after writing about a traumatic experience from childhood, those high in adverse childhood experiences experienced lower significance and coherence but a *higher* sense of purpose. Thus, purpose may become increasingly relevant to personal meaning when experience challenges coherence and significance. Similarly, Burrow and colleagues (2024) argued that a sense of purpose is beneficial because it assists in the maintenance of homeostasis, clearly relevant to coherence. These scholars argued that purpose fosters recentering such that when proximal events, whether stressful or uplifting, threaten to disrupt well-being, purpose limits the magnitude of the disruption on the person's equanimity. Finally, people may rely more heavily on positive mood as a source of meaning in life when other sources of meaning (e.g., religious faith, social relatedness) are threatened or lacking (Hicks & King, 2008, 2009b; Hicks et al., 2010; Yu, 2022). The potentially dynamic, interchangeable nature of these fundamental ingredients of meaning may allow people to maintain relatively high levels of meaning in life amid disruptive events that threaten others.

COMMONPLACE MEANING UNDER THREAT

We have argued that meaning in life is commonplace and the contributors to meaning are similarly likely to emerge from quotidian aspects of existence. Yet, in the modern world, the availability of common sources of meaning may be increasingly uncertain. Modern life is characterized by a profoundly confusing cacophony of misinformation, a lack of shared reality, and a (not wholly unjustifiable) mistrust of institutions. Worldwide, people are lonely, isolated, and alienated (Maese, 2023; Murthy, 2023). Contemporary conditions recall warnings by scholars in the earliest days of existential psychology, including Frankl's (1956/1992) "existential vacuum" and Fromm's (1994) concern over the erosion of institutional sources of meaning. These scholars anticipated some of the horrors of life in the 2020s, including the rise of authoritarianism. And research supports the role, however disturbing, of authoritarianism in enhancing meaning in life (Womick et al., 2021). In this context, even foundational sources of meaning may be in jeopardy. Here, we briefly consider one threat to commonplace meaning: climate change.

The Climate Crisis

Having extolled the role of the natural world in the experience of coherence, we must confront the fact that this foundational contributor to meaning is under threat. Climate change constitutes a looming existential threat to humanity. Large-scale catastrophes are more frequent. Weather is more unpredictable, the locating rhythm of seasonal change altered. Where once an unseasonably warm day might have been enjoyed as a respite, it now evokes anxiety. Climate change has created a more dangerous world for all its inhabitants. We see plants, animals, and humans struggling to adapt to a natural world that is quickly becoming inhospitable to them, evoking anxiety (Clayton, 2020) and grief (Cunsolo & Ellis, 2018). Climate change has altered everyday experiences in ways that challenge meaning. For contemporary humans, even natural sources of meaning are in danger of being stripped of their capacity for existential comfort. Natural invariants that undergird meaning are unmistakably varying. Not surprisingly, perhaps, people who read an article conveying that climate change is hopeless (versus that there is still hope) reported lower meaning in life, across all facets of meaning (Edwards, 2024).

Crucial to how climate change threatens meaning is our own role in it. We feel not only anxiety and grief but guilt and helplessness because we know that humans have failed repeatedly to adequately (acknowledge and) respond to the disaster unfolding around us (Tschakert et al., 2017). The profound inability of humanity to come together to confront this crisis challenges the basis of our trust in others, undermining the basic, organizing understanding of what the world is like and what people are like.

Nurturing Commonplace Meaning

This consideration of the climate crisis reminds us of one way in which meaning is not like gravity. Gravity requires no nurturing. But commonplace sources of everyday meaning require care and cultivation. At the systemic level, the failure of institutions and policies to address climate change represents a failure to support the sense that life is meaningful. As individuals we may feel helpless, facing a Sisyphean challenge, changing our own lives in the ways we can control and hoping for the best. Threats to faith in social institutions and our trust and connection with others are not easily surmounted by individual agents working alone. What are we meaning-needing creatures to do?

Perhaps the way to face this challenge is to draw upon quotidian sources of meaning to do better. From our everyday lives, we can find the comfort to reframe the challenges confronting us in ways that seem still true to the depths of the problem but conquerable (coherence), enough connection to others to work together (significance), the strength and flexibility to persist when problems inevitably arise (purpose), and the recognition that small joys found in the task promote a sense that our actions have meaning. Even in the 2020s, our task is not, as noted by Frankl, to endure the meaninglessness of life. Our task is to fully grasp the unconditional meaningfulness of our lives, even when rationality says otherwise. Because we are meaningful creatures, living meaningful lives, in a meaningful world, we must always have reason to hope.

REFERENCES

Allport, G. W. (1961). *Pattern and growth in personality.* Holt, Rinehart & Winston.

Baumeister, R. F. (1991). *Meanings of life.* Guilford Press.

Baumeister, R. F., & Hippel, W. V. (2020). Meaning and evolution: Why nature selected human minds to use meaning. *Evolutionary Studies in Imaginative Culture, 4*(1), 1–18.

Burrow, A. L., & Hill, P. L. (2020). Purpose by design or disaster: Preserving a sense of purpose amid environmental uncertainty. *Journal of Environmental Psychology, 69,* 101436.

Burrow, A. L., Hill, P. L., Stanley, M., & Sumner, R. (2024). The role of purpose in the stress process: A homeostatic account. *Journal of Research in Personality, 108,* 104444.

Carstensen, L. L. (2021). Socioemotional selectivity theory: The role of perceived endings in human motivation. *The Gerontologist, 61*(8), 1188–1196.

Chan, T. M., & Nakamura, J. (2016). A generativity track to life meaning in retirement: Ego-integrity returns on past academic mentoring investments. *Work, Aging and Retirement, 2*(1), 24–37.

Chen, Z., Poon, K.-T., DeWall, C. N., & Jiang, T. (2020). Life lacks meaning without acceptance: Ostracism triggers suicidal thoughts. *Journal of Personality and Social Psychology, 119*(6), 1423–1443.

Chu, C., & Lowery, B. S. (2024). Perceiving a stable self-concept enables the experience of meaning in life. *Personality and Social Psychology Bulletin, 50*(5), 780–792.

Clayton, S. (2020). Climate anxiety: Psychological responses to climate change. *Journal of Anxiety Disorders, 74,* 102263.

Corner, G. W., Rasmussen, H. F., Khaled, M., Morris, A. R., Khoddam, H., Barbee, N., . . . Saxbe, D. (2023). The birth of a story: Childbirth experiences, meaning-making, and postpartum adjustment. *Journal of Family Psychology, 37*(5), 667–679.

Costin, V., & Vignoles, V. L. (2020). Meaning is about mattering: Evaluating coherence, purpose, and existential mattering as precursors of meaning in life judgments. *Journal of Personality and Social Psychology, 118*(4), 864–884.

Cunsolo, A., & Ellis, N. R. (2018). Ecological grief as a mental health response to climate change-related loss. *Nature Climate Change, 8*(4), 275–281.

Diener, E., Kanazawa, S., Suh, E. M., & Oishi, S. (2015). Why people are in a generally good mood. *Personality and Social Psychology Review, 19*(3), 235–256.

Domjan, M. (2005). Pavlovian conditioning: A functional perspective. *Annual Review of Psychology, 56,* 179–206.

Edwards, M. E. (2024). *Hope in the dark: Hope most improves meaning during difficult life events.* Unpublished dissertation, University of Missouri, Columbia.

Frankl, V. E. (1992). *Man's search for meaning* (4th ed.). Beacon Press. (Original work published 1956)

Freedman, G., Powell, D. N., Le, B., & Williams, K. D. (2024). Emotional experiences of ghosting. *Journal of Social Psychology, 164*(3), 367–386.

Freud, S. (1953). The uncanny. In J. Strachey (Ed. & Trans.), *The standard edition of the complete psychological works of Sigmund Freud, Vol. XVII* (pp. 219–252). Hogarth Press. (Original work published 1919)

Fromm E. (1994). *Escape from Freedom.* Henry Holt.

Fyffe, I., & Wister, A. V. (2016). Age differences in Olympic volunteering experiences: An examination of generativity and meaning in life. *Leisure Studies, 35*(5), 638–651.

George, L. S., & Park, C. L. (2016). The Multidimensional Existential Meaning Scale: A tripartite approach to measuring meaning in life. *Journal of Positive Psychology, 12,* 613–627.

Gibson, J. J. (1973). Direct visual perception: A reply to Gyr. *Psychological Bulletin, 79,* 396–397.

Gibson, J. J. (1986). *The ecological approach to visual perception.* Erlbaum. (Original work published 1979)

Goodman, M. L., Gibson, D. C., Keiser, P. H., Gitari, S., & Raimer-Goodman, L. (2019). Family, belonging and meaning in life among semi-rural Kenyans. *Journal of Happiness Studies, 20,* 1627–1645.

Hadden, B. W., & Knee, C. R. (2018). Finding meaning in us: The role of meaning in life in romantic relationships. *Journal of Positive Psychology, 13,* 226–239.

Heintzelman, S. J., Christopher, J., Trent, J., & King, L. A. (2013a). Counterfactual thinking about one's birth enhances well-being judgments. *Journal of Positive Psychology, 8*(1), 44–49.

Heintzelman, S. J., & King, L. A. (2013a). On knowing more than we can tell: Intuition and the human experience of meaning. *Journal of Positive Psychology, 8,* 471–482.

Heintzelman, S. J., & King, L. A. (2013b). The origins of meaning: Objective reality, the unconscious mind, and awareness. In J. A. Hicks & C. Routledge (Eds.), *The experience of meaning in life: Classical perspectives, emerging themes, and controversies* (pp. 87–99). Springer.

Heintzelman, S. J., & King, L. A. (2014a). (The feeling of) meaning-as-information. *Personality and Social Psychology Review, 18,* 153–167.

Heintzelman, S. J., & King, L. A. (2014b). Life is pretty meaningful. *American Psychologist, 69,* 561–574.

Heintzelman, S. J., & King, L. A. (2016). Meaning in life and intuition. *Journal of Personality and Social Psychology, 110,* 477–492.

Heintzelman, S. J., & King, L. A. (2019). Routines and meaning in life. *Personality and Social Psychology Bulletin. 45*(5), 688–699.

Heintzelman, S. J., Mohideen, F., Choi, H., Oishi, S., & King, L. A. (2020). Lay beliefs about meaning in life: Across targets, time, and countries. *Journal of Research in Personality, 88,* 104003.

Heintzelman, S. J., Trent, J., & King, L. A. (2013b). Encounters with objective coherence and the experience of meaning in life. *Psychological Science, 24,* 991–998.

Heintzelman, S. J., Trent, J., & King, L. A. (2016). How would the self be remembered?: Evidence for posthumous self-verification. *Journal of Research in Personality, 61,* 1–10.

Hicks, J. A., & King, L. A. (2008). Religious commitment and positive mood as information about meaning in life. *Journal of Research in Personality, 42*(1), 43–57.

Hicks, J. A., & King, L. A. (2009a). Meaning in life as a subjective judgment and a lived experience. *Social and Personality Psychology Compass, 3/4,* 638–653.

Hicks, J. A., & King, L. A. (2009b). Positive mood and social relatedness as information about meaning in life. *Journal of Positive Psychology, 4*(6), 471–482.

Hicks, J. A., Schlegel, R. J., & King, L. A. (2010). Social threats, happiness, and the dynamics of meaning in life judgments. *Personality and Social Psychology Bulletin, 36*(10), 1305–1317.

Hicks, J. A., Trent, J., Davis, W., & King, L. A. (2012). Positive affect, meaning in life, and future time perspective: An application of socioemotional selectivity theory. *Psychology and Aging, 27,* 181–189.

Hofer, J., Busch, H., Au, A., Poláčková Šolcová, I., Tavel, P., & Tsien Wong, T. (2014). For the benefit of others: Generativity and meaning in life in the elderly in four cultures. *Psychology and Aging, 29*(4), 764–775.

Hong, E. K., Sedikides, C., & Wildschut, T. (2022). How does nostalgia conduce to global self-continuity? The roles of identity narrative, associative links, and stability. *Personality and Social Psychology Bulletin, 48*(5), 735–749.

Huang, M., & Yang, F. (2023). Self-transcendence or self-enhancement: People's perceptions of meaning and happiness in relation to the self. *Journal of Experimental Psychology: General, 152*(2), 590.

Jung, C. G. (1997). Foreword. In R. Wilhelm & C. F. Baynes (Trans.), *I ching or The book of changes* (pp. xxi–xl). Princeton University Press. (Original work published 1950)

Kim, T., Sezer, O., Schroeder, J., Risen, J., Gino, F., & Norton, M. I. (2021). Work group rituals enhance the meaning of work. *Organizational Behavior and Human Decision Processes, 165,* 197–212.

King, L. A. (2012). Meaning: Effortless and ubiquitous. In M. Mikulincer & P. Shaver (Eds)., *Meaning, mortality, and choice: The social psychology of existential concerns* (pp. 129–144). American Psychological Association.

King, L. A., & Geise, A. C. (2011). Being forgotten: Implications for the experience of meaning in life. *Journal of Social Psychology, 151,* 696–709.

King, L. A., & Hicks, J. A. (2021). The science of meaning in life. *Annual Review of Psychology, 72,* 561–584.

King, L. A., Hicks, J. A., Krull, J. L., & Del Gaiso, A. K. (2006). Positive affect and the experience of meaning in life. *Journal of Personality and Social Psychology, 90*(1), 179–196.

King, L. A., Scollon, C. K., Ramsey, C., & Williams, T. (2000). Stories of life transition: Subjective well-being and ego development in par-

ents of children with Down Syndrome. *Journal of Research in Personality, 34*(4), 509–536.
Kray, L. J., George, L. G., Liljenquist, K. A., Galinsky, A. D., Tetlock, P. E., & Roese, N. J. (2010). From what *might* have been to what *must* have been: Counterfactual thinking creates meaning. *Journal of Personality and Social Psychology, 98*(1), 106–118.
Kruglanski, A. W., Bélanger, J. J., Gelfand, M., Gunaratna, R., Hettiarachchi, M., Reinares, F., . . . Sharvit, K. (2013). Terrorism—A (self) love story: Redirecting the significance quest can end violence. *American Psychologist, 68*(7), 559–575.
Lambert, N. M., Stillman, T. F., Baumeister, R. F., Finchman, F. D., Hicks, J. A., & Graham, S. M. (2010). Family as a salient source of meaning in young adulthood. *Journal of Positive Psychology, 5,* 367–376.
Lambert, N. M., Stillman, T. F., Hicks, J. A., Kamble, S., Baumeister, R. F., & Fincham, F. D. (2013). To belong is to matter: Sense of belonging enhances meaning in life. *Personality and Social Psychology Bulletin, 39*(11), 1418–1427.
Maese, E. (2023, October 24). *Almost a quarter of the world feels lonely.* Gallup. https://news.gallup.com/opinion/gallup/512618/almost-quarter-world-feels-lonely.aspx.
Marciniak, D. G., Agra, K., & Agra, P. (2022). *F = ma.* Is the macaque brain Newtonian? *Cognitive Neuropsychology, 39*(5-8), 376–408.
Martela, F., & Steger, M. F. (2023). The role of significance relative to the other dimensions of meaning in life—An examination utilizing the three dimensional meaning in life scale (3DM). *Journal of Positive Psychology, 18*(4), 606–626.
McCulloch, K. C., & Smallman, R. (2014). The implications of counterfactual mind-sets for the functioning of implementation intentions. *Motivation and Emotion, 38,* 635–644.
Mohideen, F., & Heintzelman, S. J. (2023). Routines and meaning in life: Does activity content or context matter? *Personality and Social Psychology Bulletin, 49*(7), 987–999.
Morewedge, C. K., & Kahneman, D. (2010). Associative processes in intuitive judgment. *Trends in Cognitive Sciences, 14*(10), 435–440.
Morse, J. L., Lee, H., Haddock, S. A., & Henry, K. L. (2022). Meaning in life trajectories among college students: Differential effects of a mentoring program. *Journal of Happiness Studies, 23*(1), 285–302.
Murthy, V. (2023). *Surgeon General's advisory on our epidemic of loneliness and isolation.* Office of the U.S. Surgeon General.
Nelson, S. K., Kushlev, K., English, T., Dunn, E. W., & Lyubomirsky, S. (2013). In defense of parenthood: children are associated with more joy than misery. *Psychological Science, 24,* 3–10.
Norton, M. I., & Gino, F. (2014). Rituals alleviate grieving for loved ones, lovers, and lotteries. *Journal of Experimental Psychology: General, 143*(1), 266–272.
Oishi, S., & Diener, E. (2014). Residents of poor nations have a greater sense of meaning in life than residents of wealthy nations. *Psychological Science, 25*(2), 422–430.
Okan, C., Bilson, L., Zhong, D., Weidemann, G., & Bailey, P. E. (2023). Validating the interpersonal theory of suicide among older adults pre-and peri-COVID-19 pandemic. *Aging and Mental Health, 27*(8), 1552–1558.
O'Rourke, J., Harms, C., & Cohen, L. (2019). They're always there for me! Friendship and meaning in young people's lives? *Scandinavian Journal of Psychology, 60*(6), 596–608.
Pfund, G. N., Edmonds, G. W., & Hill, P. L. (2020). Associations between trauma during adolescence and sense of purpose in middle-to-late adulthood. *International Journal of Behavioral Development, 44*(5), 441–446.
Pfundmair, M., Wood, N. R., Hales, A., & Wesselmann, E. D. (2024). How social exclusion makes radicalism flourish: A review of empirical evidence. *Journal of Social Issues, 80*(1), 341–359.
Ray, D. G., Gomillion, S., Pintea, A. I., & Hamlin, I. (2019). On being forgotten: Memory and forgetting serve as signals of interpersonal importance. *Journal of Personality and Social Psychology, 116*(2), 259–276.
Robison, M., Udupa, N. S., Rice, T. B., Wilson-Lemoine, E., Joiner, T. E., & Rogers, M. L. (2024). The interpersonal theory of suicide: State of the science. *Behavior Therapy, 55*(6), 1158–1171.
Rose, H., & King, L. A. (2020). The detection of connections, the *experience* of meaning, and adaptation. *Evolutionary Studies in Imaginative Culture, 4,* 47–50.
Rose, H., Womick, J., & King, L. A. (2023). Purpose maintained: Adverse childhood experiences and meaning in life. *Journal of Personality, 91*(6), 1425–1441.
Sanders, C. A., Jenkins, A. T., & King, L. A. (2023). Pretty, meaningful lives: Physical attractiveness and experienced and perceived meaning in life. *Journal of Positive Psychology, 18*(6), 978–994.
Seto, E., Hicks, J. A., Davis, W. E., & Smallman, R. (2015). Free will, counterfactual reflection, and the meaningfulness of life events. *Social Psychological and Personality Science, 6*(3), 243–250.
Spelke, E. S. (2022). *What babies know: Core*

knowledge and composition (Vol. 1). Oxford University Press.

Stavrova, O., & Luhmann, M. (2016). Social connectedness as a source and consequence of meaning in life. *Journal of Positive Psychology, 11*(5), 470–479.

Stukeley, W. (1752). *Memoirs of Sir Isaac Newton's life.* Royal Society.

Sutin, A. R., Luchetti, M., Aschwanden, D., Stephan, Y., & Terracciano, A. (2021). Sense of purpose in life, cognitive function, and the phenomenology of autobiographical memory. *Memory, 29*(9), 1126–1135.

Sutin, A. R., Luchetti, M., Stephan, Y., Strickhouser, J. E., & Terracciano, A. (2022). The association between purpose/meaning in life and verbal fluency and episodic memory: A meta-analysis of > 140,000 participants from up to 32 countries. *International Psychogeriatrics, 34*(3), 263–273.

Thompson, V. A., Turner, J. A. P., & Pennycook, G. (2011). Intuition, reason, and metacognition. *Cognitive Psychology, 63*(3), 107–140.

Tov, W., & Lee, H. W. (2016). A closer look at the hedonics of everyday meaning and satisfaction. *Journal of Personality and Social Psychology, 111*(4), 585–609.

Trent, J., Lavelock, C., & King, L. A. (2013). Processing fluency, positive affect, and meaning in life. *Journal of Positive Psychology, 8,* 135–139.

Tschakert, P., Barnett, J., Ellis, N., Lawrence, C., Tuana, N., New, M., . . . Pannell, D. (2017). Climate change and loss, as if people mattered: Values, places, and experiences. *Wiley Interdisciplinary Reviews: Climate Change, 8*(5), e476.

Turk-Browne, N. B., Scholl, B. J., Chun, M. M., & Johnson, M. K. (2008). Neural evidence of statistical learning: Efficient detection of visual regularities without awareness. *Journal of Cognitive Neuroscience, 21,* 1934–1945.

Wade, L., Elliott, T. R., Schlegel, R. J., Williamson, M. L., Yoon, M., & Spooner, M. (2023). Resilience and well-being among persons with spinal cord injury/disorders. *Rehabilitation Psychology, 68*(3), 324.

Ward, S. J., & King, L. A. (2016). Poor but happy? Money, mood, and experienced and expected meaning in life. *Social Psychological and Personality Science, 7,* 463–470.

Ward, S. J., & King, L. A. (2019). Exploring the place of financial status in the Good Life: Income and meaning in life. *Journal of Positive Psychology, 14,* 312–323.

Ward, S. J., Womick, J., Titova, M., & King, L. A. (2023). Does meaning in life promote coping? *Personality and Social Psychology Bulletin, 49,* 460–476.

Williams, K. D. (2009). Ostracism: A temporal need-threat model. *Advances in Experimental Social Psychology, 41,* 275–314.

Womick, J., Atherton, B., & King, L. A. (2020). Lives of significance (and purpose and coherence): Narcissism, meaning in life, and subjective well-being. *Heliyon, 6*(5), e03982.

Womick, J., Eckelkamp, J., Luzzo, S., Ward, S. J., Baker, S. G., Salamun, A., & King, L. A. (2021). Exposure to authoritarian values leads to lower positive affect, higher negative affect, and higher meaning in life. *PLOS One, 16*(9), e0256759.

Womick, J., Ward, S. J., Heintzelman, S. J., Woody, B., & King, L. A. (2019). The existential function of right-wing authoritarianism. *Journal of Personality, 87,* 1056–1073.

Womick, J., Woody, B., & King, L. A. (2022). Religious fundamentalism, right-wing authoritarianism, and meaning in life. *Journal of Personality, 90*(2), 277–293.

Wood, W., Mazar, A., & Neal, D. T. (2022). Habits and goals in human behavior: Separate but interacting systems. *Perspectives on Psychological Science, 17*(2), 590–605.

Yin, Y., Jiang, T., Wildschut, T., & Sedikides, C. (2024). Nostalgia, ritual engagement, and meaning in life. *Personality and Social Psychology Bulletin.*

Yu, Y. (2022). Thwarted belongingness hindered successful aging in Chinese older adults: Roles of positive mental health and meaning in life. *Frontiers in Psychology, 13,* 839125.

Zhang, H., Sang, Z., Chan, D. K. S., & Schlegel, R. (2019). Threats to belongingness and meaning in life: A test of the compensation among sources of meaning. *Motivation and Emotion, 43,* 242–254.

CHAPTER 43

Dynamic Variation in Finding Meaning and Purpose in Daily Life

David B. Newman *and* Paul K. Lutz

One of the core concepts of existential psychology is the process through which people find meaning and purpose in their lives. Finding meaning in life often entails the ability to believe your life is coherent, matters, and has a sense of purpose. Though related to hedonic measures of well-being, such as life satisfaction and affect, meaning in life is distinct (Joshanloo, 2016; Steger et al., 2006) and is typically considered to be an important component of eudaimonia and the good life (King & Hicks, 2021). Much of the psychological research on meaning in life has focused on measuring the construct as an individual difference in which people are asked to reflect on their life as a whole. Some people tend to find more meaning in their lives than others. Understanding variation across individuals is important, as many studies have shown that people who find meaning in life report greater well-being (King & Hicks, 2021; Steger et al., 2006), live longer (Boyle et al., 2009), and are healthier (Kim et al., 2013, 2017) than those who report less meaning in life.

Although informative, measuring meaning in life as an individual difference and examining between-person relationships provides no information about within-person relationships and how meaning in life may vary from one time to another (Heintzelman & Mohideen, 2022). People may find their lives to be more or less meaningful at one time than another, depending on the circumstances, situations, and other contextual factors. The fact that the meaning of one's life may change was first proposed by Viktor Frankl, a Holocaust survivor who witnessed the importance of having a sense of meaning and purpose in the direst of circumstances. In his seminal book *Man's Search for Meaning,* he observed that, "The meaning of life differs from man to man, from day to day, from hour to hour. What matters, therefore, is not the meaning of life in general but rather the specific meaning of a person's life at a given moment" (Frankl, 1963). This novel insight was later tested empirically by psychologists who asked people to evaluate how meaningful they found their lives to be on consecutive days (Steger & Frazier, 2005; Steger & Kashdan, 2013). Consistent with Frankl's theory, daily states of meaning varied considerably from one day to the next. The type of method used to measure the fluctuating states of meaning and other relevant constructs is known as ecological momentary assessment (EMA), which includes daily diary and experience-sampling methods (Newman & Stone, 2019; Shiffman et al., 2008; Stone & Shiffman, 1994).

The use of EMA methods in the study of meaning in life can offer several key insights that other methods cannot address. First, EMA methods typically ask participants about their thoughts, feelings, behaviors, and judgments at that particular time or day, thus reducing recall biases and heuristics that often accompany global assessments or long-term recall evaluations. Thus, the judgments that people make in daily life in naturalistic contexts differ markedly from other types of judgments that are utilized in experiments or cross-sectional studies. Second, daily or momentary reports captured from EMA methods can be aggregated to measure individual differences, and these measures are often quite distinct from global assessments. Thus, EMA methods can be used to measure between-person relationships in ways that may differ from single-assessment reports. Third, the use of EMA methods allows researchers to examine within-person processes, which are statistically and psychologically distinct from between-person processes (Affleck et al., 1999; Nezlek, 2001). The examination of within-person relationships opens a wealth of possibilities in helping extend the research on meaning in life.

Before explaining each of these advantages of EMA methods, we first describe daily diary and EMA methods. Then we review studies that touch on each of these advantages. Finally, we end by discussing challenges that accompany the measurement of meaning in daily life and future directions for the field.

OVERVIEW OF EMA METHODS

EMA methods refer to a range of techniques used to capture real-world phenomena by sampling time periods from a person's life. Similar to the way researchers may select a sample of people from the larger population of people, EMA researchers draw on a sample of time points from the larger population of time points of a person's life. There are four attributes or features that define EMA methods. First, participants complete reports in real-world, naturalistic contexts as they live their daily lives. This helps researchers generalize their findings to everyday experiences in contrast to other methods that might elicit responses in artificial settings. This ability to generalize from experiences captured in naturalistic contexts harkens to Brunswik's (1956) term *ecological validity*. Second, participants typically answer questions about their immediate experiences or current states, hence the term *momentary*. This reduces any biases or errors associated with long-term recall reports. Some EMA methods may ask participants to reflect on the past few hours or the present day, but they avoid long-term recall reports. Third, the schedule of assessments in an EMA study reflects a strategic plan. Participants may be prompted to complete a report each time a particular activity occurs (e.g., a social interaction) or they may be prompted to complete reports at randomly selected times throughout the day. Some combination or variation of these schedules could also occur. Fourth, there must be repeated assessments of people's thoughts, feelings, and behaviors over the course of time to provide a sample of time points. Because of this, these methods are sometimes referred to as intensive repeated measures designs. Though most EMA studies will prompt participants to complete multiple assessments each day, end-of-day daily diary studies are often considered a special case of EMA methods. Much of the research on daily experiences of meaning in life comes from daily diary studies, so we include them in this review.

EMA METHODS MINIMIZE RECALL BIASES AND HEURISTICS

The first advantage of EMA methods is that the reports minimize recall biases and heuristics that are inherent in long-term recall (Schwarz, 2012). When people are asked to think about longer time periods, they tend to remember peak moments, recent ones, and frequently occurring occasions (Bradburn et al., 1987; Fredrickson & Kahneman, 1993; Schwarz, 2012). This can be useful when the goal is to capture such memories, but recall reports tend not to provide an accurate picture of average experiences. In studies that have compared aggregated states of affect with recall judgments of the same time period, recall reports tend to be higher than the aggregated states (Broderick et al., 2008; Neubauer et al., 2020; Stone et al., 2010; Wirtz et al., 2003). This demonstrates that feelings and states captured in real time tend to be more mundane and ordinary than people's recollection of the events, feelings, and episodes during the time.

This fact has important implications for the study of meaning in life. By this logic, daily states of meaning in life should not be as extreme as long-term recall reports of meaning in life. Though no study has examined this exact question, Newman and colleagues (2021) compared aggregated daily states of well-being during a typical 2-week period with global evaluations of well-being. Though global evaluations reflect one's life more broadly beyond a 2-week period, the results were consistent with prior research on affective recall. Global evaluations of meaning in life were rated higher than aggregated daily states of meaning in life. The reason for this is presumably because the contexts that influence daily judgments of meaning in life (e.g., working on a paper, eating a typical lunch with friends) differ from the recollections that influence global evaluations of meaning in life (e.g., receiving a promotion at work, enjoying an anniversary dinner). Daily life is much more mundane and ordinary than the peak moments of one's life that come to mind when answering questions about the overall meaning in one's life.

This principle is worth considering when reviewing the literature. For instance, in a thorough review of empirical articles that included a global evaluation of meaning in life, Heintzelman and King (2014) found that the average score was significantly higher than the midpoint of the scale. They concluded that most people tend to think that life is pretty meaningful. Findings about people's experiences of daily meaning in life qualify this conclusion to some degree. Life is certainly quite meaningful when people consider their lives as a whole, but it seems less meaningful in the context of daily life. This discrepancy between global and daily reports of meaning in life is consistent with experimental evidence that found that life seems more meaningful as psychological distance increases (Waytz et al., 2015). According to a construal level theory account (Trope & Liberman, 2010), life seems more meaningful when people think in more abstract, high-level ways as opposed to more concrete, low-level ways. Rare experiences that come to mind in global evaluations may provide more meaning in life than ordinary experiences that come to mind when completing daily questionnaires.

Along these lines, a similar pattern was detected in a study that compared an experimentally induced nostalgic memory with daily nostalgic memories (Newman et al., 2020, Study 5). In this within-subjects experiment with a counterbalanced order, participants wrote about their most nostalgic experience, and they completed a 1-week diary by answering questions about their daily events, states of well-being, and how nostalgic they felt that day. When they felt nostalgic on a particular day, they wrote about the nostalgic feeling. After both tasks, they rated how positive and negative the nostalgic experience was along with their feelings of meaning in life. Meaning in life scores were higher in the long-term recall condition than in the daily life condition. In other words, in this study participants' recollections of their most nostalgic experiences provided more meaning in life than daily, ordinary nostalgic reflections. Once again, this pattern shows that daily experiences differ considerably from long-term recall or global evaluations and highlight the importance of measuring meaning in life in the context of people's daily lives.

These findings lend support to Park's (2010) model that distinguishes global forms of meaning in life from situational forms of meaning. It is important to note that global and situational meaning can influence each other in a reciprocal manner. One's beliefs, goals, and subjective sense of meaning and purpose quite broadly can influence how one interprets situational experiences in daily life. Conversely, the accumulation of daily events and the meaning found in these experiences can influence how people form judgments about their global sense of meaning in life (Newman et al., 2021). The use of daily diary and EMA methods is critical in understanding the dynamic relationships between these different forms of meaning.

EMA METHODS PROVIDE THE MEANS TO EXAMINE INDIVIDUAL DIFFERENCES

Another useful feature of EMA methods is that they allow for the examination of between-person relationships in the study of daily meaning in life. In essence, researchers can calculate an average daily or momentary meaning in life score for each participant across many occasions to form an individual difference measure of meaning in life. Though this type of aggregation score is distinct from a global evaluation, both may be useful, depending on the goals of the research.

This manner of measuring individual differences is similar to an approach known as whole-trait theory (Fleeson, 2001; Fleeson & Jayawickreme, 2015). Instead of relying on global evaluations of personality traits, participants can provide daily reports of their personality states, and these states can be aggregated. Thus, daily and/or situational contexts are accounted for in these assessments used at the individual level, as opposed to trait reports that do not adequately account for multiple contextual factors as they naturally occur.

This technique has been used several times to explain certain attributes about people who find meaning and purpose in their lives. For example, using a 2-week daily diary method, Nezlek and colleagues (2018) found that vegetarians found less meaning in their daily lives relative to semivegetarians and omnivores. In separate EMA and daily diary studies, aggregated momentary states of meaning in life were positively related to everyday routines (Heintzelman & King, 2019), and aggregated daily states of meaning in life were positively related to positive affect (King et al., 2006). That is, people who find meaning and purpose in their daily lives also tend to engage in daily routines and experience high levels of positive affect relative to those who find less meaning and purpose in their daily lives. In other daily diary and EMA studies, conservatives reported greater daily and momentary meaning and purpose in their lives than liberals reported (Newman et al., 2019). These findings were consistent with analyses that examined trait measures or global evaluations of meaning in life. Although aggregated daily states and global reports are distinct types of judgments, they may correlate with other constructs in similar manners.

Finally, in addition to aggregating daily states of meaning in life, researchers can also examine the variation across days for each participant as a measure of instability. For instance, across two daily diary studies, participants who reported unstable levels of daily meaning in life (i.e., high daily variability) had lower global well-being relative to those with higher levels of stability (Steger & Kashdan, 2013). These examples illustrate how EMA methods can be used to examine between-person relationships through some type of aggregation or calculation of daily reports of meaning in life.

EMA METHODS CAN HELP DISTINGUISH WITHIN-PERSON FROM BETWEEN-PERSON RELATIONSHIPS

Though EMA methods can be used to examine between-person relationships, arguably their greatest strength is the means to examine within-person relationships between daily states of meaning in life and other daily events, experiences, feelings, and states. As noted above, between-person relationships and within-person relationships are mathematically orthogonal and represent distinct psychological processes (Affleck et al., 1999; Nezlek, 2001). As an example, consider the relationship between the risk of heart attack and exercise. At a between-person level, they are negatively related; that is, people who exercise frequently have a lower risk of heart attack relative to those who exercise less frequently. In contrast, exercise and risk of heart attack are positively related at a within-person level, that is, people are more likely to have a heart attack while exercising than when not exercising (Curran & Bauer, 2011).

In the research on meaning in life, perhaps the best example of distinguishing between-person from within-person relationships comes from two diary studies on the topic of searching for meaning and presence of meaning in life (Newman et al., 2018). Replicating previous research (Steger et al., 2006), trait measures of searching for and presence of meaning in life were slightly negatively related at a between-person level of analysis. This indicates that people who are searching for meaning in life tend to lack a sense of meaning in life and are generally unhappy with their lives. When the relationship between daily states of searching and presence of meaning in life were examined at a within-person level of analysis, they were positively related. That is, for the average person, on days when they searched for meaning in their lives, they were likely to find more meaning compared to days when they were not searching. This represents a completely different psychological process.

Further, an advantage of examining within-person relationships in a daily diary context is that lagged relationships from one day to the next can provide some insights into the directionality of the relationship. In this particular study, daily states of searching for meaning in life predicted greater levels of presence of meaning in life on the following day, indicating that the process of daily searching for meaning can yield beneficial effects of finding meaning in life (Newman et al., 2018; see also Morse et al., 2021). This type of examination of the directionality of the relationship cannot be conducted in between-person cross-sectional designs, which means we do not know the directionality of the effects at a between-person level of analysis. The distinction of levels of analysis in the relationship between searching for meaning and the presence of meaning highlights distinct processes. At a between-person level, searching for meaning is negatively associated with the presence of meaning in life, presumably because the act of searching for meaning quite broadly indicates one has not been able to find meaning. At a within-person level, the process of searching for meaning in daily life is much more manageable and can lead to the feeling that life is pretty meaningful.

A few other interesting examples that distinguished between-person from within-person variation in the study of meaning in life were captured in an EMA study in which participants reported on their levels of meaning in life during the day while also reporting various activities (Kucinskas et al., 2018). People who frequently listened to the news reported higher average meaning in life than did those who spent less time listening to the news (a positive between-person relationship). In contrast, people reported lower meaning in life during occasions when they listened to the news relative to times when they were not listening to the news (a negative within-person relationship). As yet another example in the opposite direction, people who spent a lot of time eating reported lower meaning in life on average (a negative between-person relationship), whereas people tended to report higher meaning in life during occasions when they were eating compared to moments when they were not (a positive within-person relationship). These examples highlight how different levels of analysis illustrate distinct psychological processes.

With these examples in mind, we now summarize the literature that has examined within-person relationships between meaning in life and other constructs. To help organize this literature, we divide this area of research into three sections. The first considers studies that have examined within-person relationships between meaning in life and other well-being variables. The second reviews how meaning in life is related to outward-focused constructs, such as social relationships, prosociality, and religious/spiritual experiences. The third summarizes how meaning in life is related to inward-focused thoughts, such as thinking about the self, proactive coping, and rumination. Such a categorization may not be perfect, as some variables may fit in multiple groups. Nevertheless, we believe these categories may be useful in helping make sense of studies of within-person relationships.

Meaning in Life and Well-Being

Though meaning in life is usually considered to be a component of well-being, it can be useful to understand how daily meaning in life relates to other aspects of well-being. Not surprisingly, daily states of meaning in life have been positively related to daily life satisfaction, daily positive affect, and daily self-esteem, and negatively related to daily states of negative affect (Newman et al., 2018).

Many of these within-person relationships have been replicated and extended in studies that have found daily meaning in life to be similarly associated with affect, self-esteem, depressive symptoms, and physical symptoms (Hadden & Smith, 2019; Hill, Klaiber, et al., 2022; Jayawickreme et al., 2021). It is worth emphasizing that though the direction of these within-person relationships mirrors those at the between-person level (Steger et al., 2006; Steger et al., 2008b), these within-person relationships represent completely distinct psychological processes. In fact, in separate studies, between-person relationships between aggregated daily states of meaning in life and affect were in the same direction as within-person relationships (Hill et al., 2022a; Jayawickreme et al., 2021). As those studies noted though, understanding the within-person relationships extends the research beyond between-person relationships.

Perhaps more interestingly, several EMA studies have attempted to compare daily meaning in life with other well-being variables. For example, in a series of daily diary studies, Tov and Lee (2016) found that daily meaning in life was more strongly related to daily satisfaction than to daily affect. Moreover, people were able to find some meaning in daily negative events, whereas they generally did not find any satisfaction from daily negative events. In an EMA study that compared momentary states of meaning with momentary states of happiness, Choi and colleagues (2017) found several interesting differences in their associations with various daily activities. Watching TV, playing a game, and attending a staff party were not significantly related to happiness, but they were negatively related to meaning. Participating in a class, visiting a hospital, and working were positively related to momentary states of meaning, but they were negatively related to happiness. Finally, doing housework and studying were positively related to meaning, but they were not significantly (though trending in the negative direction) related to momentary states of happiness. Clearly, daily and momentary states of meaning in life are distinct from other states of well-being. Importantly, these associations differ from studies at between-person levels of analysis that have attempted to compare meaning with other aspects of well-being (Baumeister et al., 2013; Dwyer et al., 2017).

Meaning in Life and Outward Focus

In this section, we review how daily states of meaning relate to experiences that focus one's attention on other individuals or entities that are separate from the self. According to some theoretical accounts, meaning is found when one realizes that the self is part of something bigger than oneself (e.g., Wong, 2014). As an example, social relationships and interactions are some of the key ingredients to a happy life (Diener et al., 2018). The same is true for meaning in life. For example, Machell and colleagues (2015b) found that people found more meaning in their lives on days when they engaged in pleasant social interactions relative to days when they did not experience as many pleasant social interactions. This within-person relationship was significant even after controlling for daily states of affect. Thus, not only is it the case that people who have many pleasant social interactions and friendships find meaning in their lives, but for the average person, they tend to find their days more meaningful when they engage in pleasant social interactions. This pattern of results was conceptually replicated in a study by Pfund and colleagues (2022), who used a very similar daily measure of purpose in life. Furthermore, in addition to typical pleasant social interactions, people in another study found more meaning in their lives after engaging in sexual intercourse relative to days without engaging in sexual intercourse (Kashdan et al., 2018).

In addition to social events that are naturally viewed as quite pleasant, prosocial events that involve helping other people have also been positively related to daily states of meaning in life. For example, daily states of meaning in life were positively related to both subjective perceptions of prosociality and objective reports of prosociality (Dakin et al., 2022; see also Martela et al., 2018). These relationships were stronger than those involving prosocial behaviors and states of happiness. In a separate study, daily states of meaning in life were positively related to eudaimonic daily activities, which included volunteering, giving money to a person in need, and writing out goals for the future (Steger et al., 2008a). In lagged analyses, daily eudaimonic activities predicted greater states of meaning in life on the following day, but the reverse pathway was not significant. Thus, engaging in prosocial events that may help orient oneself to others could foster a sense of daily meaning in life.

Another way of connecting to something or someone larger than oneself is through religious or spiritual experiences. *Religiosity* has been defined as connecting to the sacred (Pargament et al., 2005), and religious individuals tend to find more meaning and purpose in their lives than nonreligious people do (Newman et al., 2019, 2022; Steger et al., 2006). At a within-person level of analysis, some similar results have been found. On days when people reported higher levels of spirituality, they tended to also find more meaning in their lives relative to days when they felt less spiritual (Kashdan & Nezlek, 2012). In a separate study, daily states of meaning in life were also positively related to daily religious events and they mediated the relationship between religious events and well-being (Steger & Frazier, 2005). Thus, people experience greater well-being when they engage in religious experiences because they find meaning and purpose in those experiences.

Although people tend to report greater well-being and meaning in life on days when they engage in religious experiences, the composite measures of religious experiences may gloss over some important nuances. For example, in a series of daily diary studies about prayer and well-being, prayers of thanksgiving and adoration were positively related to concurrent hedonic measures of well-being (daily life satisfaction and affect), prayers of supplication were negatively related to hedonic well-being, and prayers of confession were inconsistently related to hedonic well-being (Newman et al., 2023). In contrast though, daily meaning in life was positively related to all types of prayer. Thus, although people may not feel particularly happy or satisfied when expressing supplication or confession in prayer, they tend to find their lives meaningful on those days.

Finally, it is worth noting that not all religious experiences are positively associated with daily states of meaning in life at a within-person level of analysis. For instance, when people made various attributions to God for positive and negative events, they were not significantly related to daily meaning in life (Wilt et al., 2024). This nonsignificant within-person relationship was in contrast to the positive between-person relationships between these same constructs.

In addition to religious and spiritual experiences and social events, various feelings and motivational states can help people feel connected to something larger than themselves, which could imbue their lives with meaning. For instance, feeling grateful can help remind people of others in their lives who care for them (Algoe, 2012; Stellar et al., 2017). In line with this, daily states of meaning in life were positively related to daily feelings of gratitude in a diary study that examined within-person relationships (Nezlek et al., 2017). A similar result was found in a diary study that examined within-person relationships between current states of meaning in life and daily states of *experiential appreciation,* which is defined as the extent to which one appreciates and values their experiences (Kim et al., 2022). In addition to gratitude, inspiration often requires an outward focus, as people are often inspired by other people (Thrash, 2021). Daily reports of purpose in life were positively related to daily states of inspiration in a daily diary study that included two reports per day (Thrash et al., 2010). In a similar vein, curiosity often requires attentional focus on others, and daily states of curiosity have been positively associated with daily states of meaning in life (Kashdan & Steger, 2007). In sum, a range of different feelings and states that orient oneself to something outside of oneself may help provide an individual with a sense of meaning and purpose in daily life.

Meaning in Life and Inward Focus

Inward-focused thoughts also have important implications for how people find meaning and purpose in their daily lives, and various EMA methods have shed light on these processes. For instance, how people reflect on their lives during various moments throughout the day can affect their sense of meaning and purpose (Steger et al., 2008b).

Two types of private self-consciousness that have received considerable attention at the trait level include rumination and reflection (Trapnell & Campbell, 1999). *Rumination* refers to a neurotic self-attentiveness, whereas *reflection* refers to an intellectual self-attentiveness. In a daily diary study, daily states of meaning in life were negatively related to daily rumination but were not significantly associated with daily reflection (Newman & Nezlek, 2019). Though these patterns of relationships were in the same direction as prior research conducted at the trait level (Steger et al., 2008b), they represent distinct processes. For example, although people who ruminate often generally find less meaning in their lives than do those who ruminate less frequently, for the average person, when they tend to ruminate they find less meaning in their lives compared to days when they do not ruminate as much.

Another negatively oriented inward thought process that has relevance for meaning in life is *experiential avoidance,* which is considered to be an unwillingness to engage in events and activities or action tendencies to reduce the frequency or occurrence of such events (Hayes et al., 1996). In two separate studies, within-person analyses found that daily states of experiential avoidance were negatively related to states of meaning in life (Machell et al., 2015a; Pavlacic et al., 2021). Experiences can often provide people with meaning in life, so the avoidance of such experiences likely hinders the meaning-making process.

Turning to more positively oriented thoughts and values, daily states of proactive coping were positively related within persons to daily states of meaning in life, and this relationship was mediated by positive affect (Miao et al., 2017). Authenticity, defined as the perception of being true to oneself, has been positively related to daily states of meaning in life and negatively to daily meaning struggles (Wilt et al., 2021). This suggests being true to oneself might be beneficial for one's sense of meaning in life. However, it is important to consider the multifaceted nature of authenticity (Wood et al., 2008). In a daily diary study that examined within-person relationships between different aspects of daily meaning in life and daily facets of authenticity, authentic living was positively related to concurrent meaning in life, whereas self-alienation and accepting external influence were negatively related to daily meaning in life (Lutz et al., 2023a). Lagged analyses suggested that the direction of effects was more consistently linked from authenticity facets to meaning in life rather than the reverse. Thus, certain aspects of authenticity may promote meaning in daily life, whereas other aspects may hinder it.

Finally, various needs and goals may often involve inward thoughts and have relevance to within-person meaning-making processes. According to self-determination theory, autonomy, relatedness, and competence are fundamental human motivations and needs.[1] In one study, daily states of meaning in life were positively related to daily states of autonomy, relatedness, and competence (Martela et al., 2018). Thus, each of these needs seem relevant for the experience of finding meaning in daily life. Similarly, making progress toward goals can be helpful in finding meaning in daily life. In one study, when people made progress toward a goal, they felt as if their life was more meaningful on that particular day, though this effect was most pronounced among those high in social anxiety disorder (Kashdan & McKnight, 2013). Similarly, daily goal progress interference via anxiety was negatively related to daily meaning in life, and this effect was stronger among those high in social anxiety disorder (Goodman & Kashdan, 2021). As noted repeatedly throughout this chapter, it is important to remember that the within-person relationships described here represent advances from between-person findings from prior cross-sectional work that address distinct questions.

CROSS-LEVEL INTERACTIONS

One other advantage of EMA methods is that they allow for cross-level interactions in understanding both trait and daily factors in processes involving meaning in life. In the prior sections, we reviewed within-person relationships between daily states of meaning in life and other constructs. It is possible, though, that trait levels of meaning in life may influence within-person relationships involving other constructs. For example, in one diary study, trait levels of purpose in life moderated the within-person relationship between daily stressors and negative affect and physical symptoms such that the relationships were weaker among those high versus low in trait purpose in life (Hill et al., 2018). In the same dataset, trait purpose in life also moderated the within-person relationship between positive events and positive affect, such that the relationship was weaker among those high in trait purpose in life (Hill et al., 2022b). Taken together, these results show that trait levels of purpose may help people be less reactive to daily events, both good and bad.

CHALLENGES IN MEASURING MEANING IN DAILY LIFE

In the final sections, we discuss some challenges researchers face when measuring meaning in daily life, along with some recommendations and avenues for future research. The first challenge researchers must consider pertains to the interpretations of the questions about meaning and purpose in daily life. Although the topic of understanding how participants interpret questions is important for all methods and for all research topics, there are some unique issues that are specific to the measurement of meaning and purpose in daily life.

The main issues concern the multiple time frames and the focal points participants could consider when answering such questions. For instance, when participants are asked at the end of the day, "How meaningful did you feel your life was today?," some participants may focus quite broadly on their life as a whole (thus ignoring the aspect about today), whereas others might focus solely on their experiences on that day (thus focusing more on the meaningfulness of the events and experiences rather than one's life). Yet others may integrate the two and provide answers that reflect how the day's experiences relate to their larger purpose or sense of meaning in life quite broadly. In the first instance, participants would presumably provide the same response on every single day if they were to only consider their lives as a whole. However, participants may get confused as to why the researchers would ask the same question, as this would violate a conversational norm (Grice, 1975). Participants may provide answers about their life as a whole for the first day or days of the study and then update how they interpret the questions. This could lead to a phenomenon known as the initial elevation bias that has been detected in some daily diary studies (Shrout et al., 2018; though see Cerino et al., 2022, for a critique). In the second instance, participants may focus solely on the meaningfulness of the events that occurred during the day. If someone were in a car accident on a particular day, they might provide a very high score on the daily meaning in life question because the car accident event was highly meaningful in the sense that it had an important impact on their day. Some researchers may not be aware that some of the participants' answers may reflect unintended sources. Although we do not offer any solutions, we urge researchers to consider such issues when designing their questionnaires.

The second challenge facing researchers in this area concerns the conceptualization of meaning in life and the number of facets or aspects of meaning in life one should measure. Many diary and EMA studies commonly adopt the presence and search dimensions captured by Steger and colleagues' (2006) Meaning in Life Questionnaire (MLQ). To assess momentary or daily states of one or both of these dimensions, some researchers have adjusted the instructions of the MLQ to ask participants to rate the items according to the desired level of analysis ("right now"; e.g., Heintzelman & King, 2019). Many diary (e.g., Dakin et al., 2022; Morse et al., 2021; Newman et al., 2018) and some EMA (e.g., Mohideen & Heintzelman, 2023) studies have employed items created by Kashdan and Steger (2007) and Kashdan and Nezlek (2012) to assess presence (sample daily item: "How meaningful did you feel your life was today?") and search (sample daily item: "How much were you searching for meaning in your life today?").

In contrast to these unidimensional measures, some scholars have recently explored tripartite models of meaning in life. In particular, Martela and Steger (2016, p. 534; 2023) suggested that the presence of meaning encompasses a sense of: (1) "comprehensibility and one's life making sense" (coherence); (2) "core goals, aims, and direction in life" (purpose); and (3) "life's inherent value and having a life worth living" (significance). George and Park (2016, 2017; see also Costin & Vignoles, 2020) similarly endorsed a tripartite model, but these researchers replaced significance with "mattering." Research suggests that this distinction may be important, as significance seems to emphasize the value of one's life to the individual, whereas mattering seems to emphasize the value of one's life on a much larger, cosmic scale (Martela & Steger, 2023; but see recent work on different forms of mattering, Gutherie et al., 2024; Prinzing et al., 2023). Diary investigations in particular have either developed items to target a specific tripartite component (e.g., Martela et al., 2018), or adapted items from trait tripartite measures (e.g., George & Park, 2017) for daily use (Gutherie et al., 2024; Kim et al., 2022; Lutz et al., 2023a, 2023b).

Recently, Zambelli and Tagliabue (2024) proposed the Situational Meaning in Life Evaluation (SMILE) that integrates the tripartite components (coherence, purpose, significance) within the dimensions of presence and search, producing six items in total. Each item of the SMILE can be easily adapted to different events and time frames, making it appealing for diary and EMA research. However, caution is warranted given that the scale was developed with a single-assessment method, and more research is needed to validate this measure.

When thinking about different aspects or facets of meaning in life, it is also worth weighing the strengths and weaknesses of each approach. Measuring each specific component of meaning in life increases participant burden, a major concern in EMA studies (Eisele et al., 2022). Given that the facets of meaning in life correlate highly with a composite or general meaning in life scale, it may not be worth increasing the time and effort participants have to spend completing each questionnaire. Moreover, some research has questioned whether the coherence aspect of meaning in life is truly distinct from previously established measures (Hochwälder, 2025). Thus, it might behoove researchers to measure daily or momentary states of meaning in life with one or two items that capture the broader construct of meaning in life unless researchers have specific goals or reasons to capture each individual facet.

FUTURE DIRECTIONS AND RECOMMENDATIONS

Finally, we point to a few fruitful avenues for future research. First, it could be valuable to combine EMA methods with longitudinal designs, sometimes known as burst designs (Hill et al., 2023). In these studies, participants complete an EMA study for a few days or weeks by completing momentary or daily reports about their meaning in life and other experiences. These same participants are then followed and asked to complete the same EMA study at a later time, for example, 6 months or 1 year later. This could be repeated multiple times, which would allow for the examination of how within-person relationships between meaning and daily experiences change over time across the lifespan. People may find meaning from certain types of experiences early in their lives (e.g., moving to a new city, starting a new job or career) and from different kinds of experiences later in their lives (e.g., spending time with family or close friends). A recent study used a similar type of measurement burst design (Pfund et al., 2022), and we believe this can yield promising insights in the future.

Second, the experience of searching for meaning in daily life has been understudied in this field. Most diary and EMA studies focus on the presence of meaning in life, but we know considerably less about daily states of searching for meaning in life. Future research could examine how certain types of daily events and experiences may elicit daily states of searching for meaning as opposed to the presence of meaning. Similar to research at the trait level that has compared the presence of and search for meaning in life (Steger et al., 2008b), it would be interesting to examine how searching for meaning relates to cognitive processes, social interactions, and affective states.

Third, we urge researchers to consider integrating their findings with existing literatures from other fields. For instance, social and personality psychologists have often measured meaning in life from versions of the MLQ (Steger et al., 2006), whereas clinical and health psychologists have often studied purpose in life from Ryff's psychological well-being measures, which have been included in large, publicly available datasets like the Midlife in the United States study. Although some researchers may argue that purpose and meaning may be distinct, the items used to measure them overlap considerably. For example, Machell and colleagues (2015b) examined the within-person relationships between daily events (including social events) and daily meaning in life. One of the items used to measure daily meaning in life was "How much did you feel your life had purpose today?" Pfund and colleagues (2022) examined similar within-person relationships between social events and purpose in life with the item "How much do you think your life had purpose today?" Though the two studies addressed somewhat different questions, they overlapped considerably, and we believe it is good practice to appropriately cite relevant studies from prior research so that readers can understand how recent findings replicate and extend prior research.

Fourth, research examining within-person relationships between daily states of meaning in life and health behaviors and outcomes is rife with possibilities. Most research that has considered the relationships between meaning in life and health has been conducted at a between-person level of analysis, typically with cross-sectional designs. For instance, Kim and colleagues (2014) found that people who reported more purpose in their lives were more likely to go to the doctor for mammograms, colonoscopies, and other health preventive visits compared to those who found less purpose in their lives. Relatedly, during the COVID-19 pandemic, Newman and colleagues (2022) found that meaning and purpose in life predicted greater adherence to health recommendations, such as wearing face masks, washing hands, social distancing, and so forth. However, very little research has examined how daily states of meaning in life may relate to various health outcomes as they naturally occur. We consider this to be a fruitful area for future research.

CONCLUSION

A complete understanding of meaning and purpose in life involves the study of how meaning in life may vary from one time to the next depending on situational contexts. EMA and daily diary methods provide the means to examine these dynamic processes while capturing states of meaning in life and daily experiences as they naturally occur. The conclusions drawn from these methods may challenge conclusions drawn from other methods, and they can also help extend and further research in this important area.

NOTE

1. Admittedly, some of these constructs could also be considered more relational and outward focused in some regards, but we felt it would nevertheless be useful to summarize their findings here.

REFERENCES

Affleck, G., Zautra, A., Tennen, H., & Armeli, S. (1999). Multilevel daily process designs for consulting and clinical psychology: A preface for the perplexed. *Journal of Consulting and Clinical Psychology, 67*(5), Article 5.

Algoe, S. B. (2012). Find, remind, and bind: The functions of gratitude in everyday relationships. *Social and Personality Psychology Compass, 6*(6), Article 6.

Baumeister, R. F., Vohs, K. D., Aaker, J. L., & Garbinsky, E. N. (2013). Some key differences between a happy life and a meaningful life. *Journal of Positive Psychology, 8*(6), 505–516.

Boyle, P. A., Barnes, L. L., Buchman, A. S., & Bennett, D. A. (2009). Purpose in life is associated with mortality among community-dwelling older persons. *Psychosomatic Medicine, 71*(5), 574.

Bradburn, N. M., Rips, L. J., & Shevell, S. K. (1987). Answering autobiographical questions: The impact of memory and inference on surveys. *Science, 236*(4798), Article 4798.

Broderick, J. E., Schwartz, J. E., Vikingstad, G., Pribbernow, M., Grossman, S., & Stone, A. A. (2008). The accuracy of pain and fatigue items across different reporting periods. *PAIN, 139*(1), 146–157.

Brunswik, E. (1956). *Perception and the representative design of psychological experiments.* University of California Press.

Cerino, E. S., Schneider, S., Stone, A. A., Sliwinski, M. J., Mogle, J., & Smyth, J. M. (2022). Little evidence for consistent initial elevation bias in self-reported momentary affect: A coordinated analysis of ecological momentary assessment studies. *Psychological Assessment, 34*(5), 467–482.

Choi, J., Catapano, R., & Choi, I. (2017). Taking stock of happiness and meaning in everyday life: An experience sampling approach. *Social Psychological and Personality Science, 8*(6), 641–651.

Costin, V., & Vignoles, V. L. (2020). Meaning is about mattering: Evaluating coherence, purpose, and existential mattering as precursors of meaning in life judgments. *Journal of Personality and Social Psychology, 118*(4), 864–884.

Curran, P. J., & Bauer, D. J. (2011). The disaggregation of within-person and between-person effects in longitudinal models of change. *Annual Review of Psychology, 62,* 583–619.

Dakin, B. C., Tan, N. P., Conner, T. S., & Bastian, B. (2022). The relationship between prosociality, meaning, and happiness in everyday life. *Journal of Happiness Studies, 23*(6), 2787–2804.

Diener, E., Oishi, S., & Tay, L. (2018). Advances in subjective well-being research. *Nature Human Behaviour, 2*(4), Article 4.

Dwyer, R. J., Dunn, E. W., & Hershfield, H. E. (2017). Cousins or conjoined twins: How different are meaning and happiness in everyday life? *Comprehensive Results in Social Psychology, 2*(2–3), 199–215.

Eisele, G., Vachon, H., Lafit, G., Kuppens, P., Houben, M., Myin-Germeys, I., & Viechtbauer, W. (2022). The effects of sampling frequency and questionnaire length on perceived burden, compliance, and careless responding in experience sampling data in a student population. *Assessment, 29*(2), 136–151.

Fleeson, W. (2001). Toward a structure- and process-integrated view of personality: Traits as density distributions of states. *Journal of Personality and Social Psychology, 80*(6), Article 6.

Fleeson, W., & Jayawickreme, E. (2015). Whole trait theory. *Journal of Research in Personality, 56,* 82–92.

Frankl, V. E. (1963). *Man's search for meaning.* Beacon Press.

Fredrickson, B. L., & Kahneman, D. (1993). Duration neglect in retrospective evaluations of affective episodes. *Journal of Personality and Social Psychology, 65,* 45–55.

George, L. S., & Park, C. L. (2016). Meaning in life as comprehension, purpose, and mattering: Toward integration and new research questions. *Review of General Psychology, 20*(3), 205–220.

George, L. S., & Park, C. L. (2017). The Multidimensional Existential Meaning Scale: A tripartite approach to measuring meaning in life. *Journal of Positive Psychology, 12*(6), 613–627.

Goodman, F. R., & Kashdan, T. B. (2021). The most important life goals of people with and without social anxiety disorder: Focusing on emotional interference and uncovering meaning in life. *Journal of Positive Psychology, 16*(2), 272–281.

Grice, H. P. (1975). Logic and conversation. In P. Cole & J. L. Morgan (Eds.), *Syntax and semantics: Vol. 3. Speech acts* (pp. 41–58). Academic Press.

Guthrie, D., Maffly-Kipp, J., Gause, C., Kim, J., Martela, F., & Hicks, J. A. (2024). Interpersonal mattering and the experience of meaning in life. *Journal of Positive Psychology.*

Hadden, B. W., & Smith, C. V. (2019). I gotta say, today was a good (and meaningful) day: Daily meaning in life as a potential basic psychological need. *Journal of Happiness Studies, 20*(1), 185–202.

Hayes, S. C., Wilson, K. G., Gifford, E. V., Follette, V. M., & Strosahl, K. (1996). Experiential avoidance and behavioral disorders: A functional dimensional approach to diagnosis and treatment. *Journal of Consulting and Clinical Psychology, 64*(6), 1152–1168.

Heintzelman, S. J., & King, L. A. (2014). Life is pretty meaningful. *American Psychologist, 69*(6), 561–574.

Heintzelman, S. J., & King, L. A. (2019). Routines and meaning in life. *Personality and Social Psychology Bulletin, 45*(5), 688–699.

Heintzelman, S. J., & Mohideen, F. (2022). Leveraging the experience sampling method to study meaning in everyday life. In *Proceedings of the Meaning in Life international conference 2022—Cultivating, promoting, and enhancing meaning in life across cultures and life span (MIL 2022)* (pp. 41–56). Atlantis Press.

Hill, P. L., Klaiber, P., Burrow, A. L., DeLongis, A., & Sin, N. L. (2022a). Purposefulness and daily life in a pandemic: Predicting daily affect and physical symptoms during the first weeks of the COVID-19 response. *Psychology and Health, 37*(8), 985–1001.

Hill, P. L., Pfund, G. N., & Allemand, M. (2023). The PATHS to purpose: A new framework toward understanding purpose development. *Current Directions in Psychological Science, 32*(2), 105–110.

Hill, P. L., Sin, N. L., Almeida, D. M., & Burrow, A. L. (2022b). Sense of purpose predicts daily positive events and attenuates their influence on positive affect. *Emotion, 22*(3), 597–602.

Hill, P. L., Sin, N. L., Turiano, N. A., Burrow,

A. L., & Almeida, D. M. (2018). Sense of purpose moderates the associations between daily stressors and daily well-being. *Annals of Behavioral Medicine, 52*(8), 724–729.

Hochwälder, J. (2025). Antonovsky's construct of sense of coherence and the tripartite construct of meaning in life: Comparison and implications. *The Humanistic Psychologist, 53*(1), 163–181.

Jayawickreme, E., Tsukayama, E., Blackie, L. E. R., & Weiss, B. (2021). Examining within-person relationships between state assessments of affect and eudaimonic well-being using multilevel structural equation modeling. *Journal of Positive Psychology, 16*(5), 691–700.

Joshanloo, M. (2016). Revisiting the empirical distinction between hedonic and eudaimonic aspects of well-being using exploratory structural equation modeling. *Journal of Happiness Studies, 17*(5), Article 5.

Kashdan, T. B., Goodman, F. R., Stiksma, M., Milius, C. R., & McKnight, P. E. (2018). Sexuality leads to boosts in mood and meaning in life with no evidence for the reverse direction: A daily diary investigation. *Emotion, 18*(4), 563–576.

Kashdan, T. B., & McKnight, P. E. (2013). Commitment to a purpose in life: An antidote to the suffering by individuals with social anxiety disorder. *Emotion, 13*(6), 1150–1159.

Kashdan, T. B., & Nezlek, J. B. (2012). Whether, when, and how is spirituality related to well-being? Moving beyond single occasion questionnaires to understanding daily process. *Personality and Social Psychology Bulletin, 38*(11), Article 11.

Kashdan, T. B., & Steger, M. F. (2007). Curiosity and pathways to well-being and meaning in life: Traits, states, and everyday behaviors. *Motivation and Emotion, 31*(3), 159–173.

Kim, E. S., Kawachi, I., Chen, Y., & Kubzansky, L. D. (2017). Association between purpose in life and objective measures of physical function in older adults. *JAMA Psychiatry, 74*(10), 1039–1045.

Kim, E. S., Strecher, V. J., & Ryff, C. D. (2014). Purpose in life and use of preventive health care services. *Proceedings of the National Academy of Sciences, 111*(46), 16331–16336.

Kim, E. S., Sun, J. K., Park, N., & Peterson, C. (2013). Purpose in life and reduced incidence of stroke in older adults: "The Health and Retirement Study." *Journal of Psychosomatic Research, 74*(5), 427–432.

Kim, J., Holte, P., Martela, F., Shanahan, C., Li, Z., Zhang, H., . . . Hicks, J. A. (2022). Experiential appreciation as a pathway to meaning in life. *Nature Human Behaviour, 6*(5), 677–690.

King, L. A., & Hicks, J. A. (2021). The science of meaning in life. *Annual Review of Psychology, 72*, 561–584.

King, L. A., Hicks, J. A., Krull, J. L., & Del Gaiso, A. K. (2006). Positive affect and the experience of meaning in life. *Journal of Personality and Social Psychology, 90*(1), 179–196.

Kucinskas, J., Wright, B. R. E., & Riepl, S. (2018). The interplay between meaning and sacred awareness in everyday life: Evidence from a daily smartphone study. *International Journal for the Psychology of Religion, 28*(2), 71–88.

Lutz, P. K., Newman, D. B., Schlegel, R. J., & Wirtz, D. (2023a). Authenticity, meaning in life, and life satisfaction: A multicomponent investigation of relationships at the trait and state levels. *Journal of Personality, 91*(3), 541–555.

Lutz, P. K., Zelenski, J. M., & Newman, D. B. (2023b). Eco-anxiety in daily life: Relationships with well-being and pro-environmental behavior. *Current Research in Ecological and Social Psychology, 4*, 100110.

Machell, K. A., Goodman, F. R., & Kashdan, T. B. (2015a). Experiential avoidance and well-being: A daily diary analysis. *Cognition and Emotion, 29*(2), 351–359.

Machell, K. A., Kashdan, T. B., Short, J. L., & Nezlek, J. B. (2015b). Relationships between meaning in life, social and achievement events, and positive and negative affect in daily life. *Journal of Personality, 83*(3), 287–298.

Martela, F., Ryan, R. M., & Steger, M. F. (2018). Meaningfulness as satisfaction of autonomy, competence, relatedness, and beneficence: Comparing the four satisfactions and positive affect as predictors of meaning in life. *Journal of Happiness Studies, 19*(5), 1261–1282.

Martela, F., & Steger, M. F. (2016). The three meanings of meaning in life: Distinguishing coherence, purpose, and significance. *Journal of Positive Psychology, 11*(5), 531–545.

Martela, F., & Steger, M. F. (2023). The role of significance relative to the other dimensions of meaning in life—An examination utilizing the Three Dimensional Meaning in Life Scale (3DM). *Journal of Positive Psychology, 18*(4), 606–626.

Miao, M., Zheng, L., & Gan, Y. (2017). Meaning in life promotes proactive coping via positive affect: A daily diary study. *Journal of Happiness Studies, 18*(6), 1683–1696.

Mohideen, F., & Heintzelman, S. J. (2023). Routines and meaning in life: Does activity content or context matter? *Personality and Social Psychology Bulletin, 49*(7), 987–999.

Morse, J. L., Prince, M. A., & Steger, M. F.

(2021). The role of intolerance of uncertainty in the relationship between daily search for and presence of meaning in life. *International Journal of Wellbeing, 11*(1), Article 1.

Neubauer, A. B., Scott, S. B., Sliwinski, M. J., & Smyth, J. M. (2020). How was your day?: Convergence of aggregated momentary and retrospective end-of-day affect ratings across the adult life span. *Journal of Personality and Social Psychology, 119*(1), 185–203.

Newman, D. B., & Nezlek, J. B. (2019). Private self-consciousness in daily life: Relationships between rumination and reflection and well-being, and meaning in daily life. *Personality and Individual Differences, 136,* 184–189.

Newman, D. B., Nezlek, J. B., & Thrash, T. M. (2018). The dynamics of searching for meaning and presence of meaning in daily life. *Journal of Personality, 86*(3), Article 3.

Newman, D. B., Nezlek, J. B., & Thrash, T. M. (2023). The dynamics of prayer in daily life and implications for well-being. *Journal of Personality and Social Psychology, 124*(6), 1299–1313.

Newman, D. B., Sachs, M. E., Stone, A. A., & Schwarz, N. (2020). Nostalgia and well-being in daily life: An ecological validity perspective. *Journal of Personality and Social Psychology, 118*(2), Article 2.

Newman, D. B., Schneider, S., & Stone, A. A. (2022). Contrasting effects of finding meaning and searching for meaning, and political orientation and religiosity, on feelings and behaviors during the COVID-19 pandemic. *Personality and Social Psychology Bulletin, 48*(6), Article 6.

Newman, D. B., Schwarz, N., Graham, J., & Stone, A. A. (2019). Conservatives report greater meaning in life than liberals. *Social Psychological and Personality Science, 10*(4), Article 4.

Newman, D. B., Schwarz, N., & Stone, A. A. (2021). Global reports of well-being overestimate aggregated daily states of well-being. *Journal of Positive Psychology, 16*(3), Article 3.

Newman, D. B., & Stone, A. A. (2019). Understanding daily life with ecological momentary assessment. In K. Frank, P. M. Herr, & N. Schwarz (Eds.), *Handbook of research methods in consumer psychology* (pp. 259–275). Routledge.

Nezlek, J. B. (2001). Multilevel random coefficient analyses of event- and interval-contingent data in social and personality psychology research. *Personality and Social Psychology Bulletin, 27*(7), Article 7.

Nezlek, J. B., Forestell, C. A., & Newman, D. B. (2018). Relationships between vegetarian dietary habits and daily well-being. *Ecology of Food and Nutrition, 57*(5), Article 5.

Nezlek, J. B., Newman, D. B., & Thrash, T. M. (2017). A daily diary study of relationships between feelings of gratitude and well-being. *Journal of Positive Psychology, 12*(4), Article 4.

Pargament, K. I., Magyar-Russell, G. M., & Murray-Swank, N. A. (2005). The sacred and the search for significance: Religion as a unique process. *Journal of Social Issues, 61*(4), 665–687.

Park, C. L. (2010). Making sense of the meaning literature: An integrative review of meaning making and its effects on adjustment to stressful life events. *Psychological Bulletin, 136*(2), 257–301.

Pavlacic, J. M., Schulenberg, S. E., & Buchanan, E. M. (2021). Experiential avoidance and meaning in life as predictors of valued living: A daily diary study. *Journal of Prevention and Health Promotion, 2*(1), 135–159.

Pfund, G. N., Hofer, M., Allemand, M., & Hill, P. L. (2022). Being social may be purposeful in older adulthood: A measurement burst design. *American Journal of Geriatric Psychiatry, 30*(7), 777–786.

Prinzing, M. M., Sappenfield, C. A., & Fredrickson, B. L. (2023). What makes me matter?: Investigating how and why people feel significant. *Journal of Positive Psychology, 18*(6), 995–1011.

Schwarz, N. (2012). Why researchers should think "real-time": A cognitive rationale. In M. R. Mehl & T. S. Conner (Eds.), *Handbook of research methods for studying daily life* (pp. 22–42). Guilford Press.

Shiffman, S., Stone, A. A., & Hufford, M. R. (2008). Ecological Momentary Assessment. *Annual Review of Clinical Psychology, 4*(1), Article 1.

Shrout, P. E., Stadler, G., Lane, S. P., McClure, M. J., Jackson, G. L., Clavél, F. D., . . . Bolger, N. (2018). Initial elevation bias in subjective reports. *Proceedings of the National Academy of Sciences, 115*(1), E15–E23.

Steger, M. F., & Frazier, P. (2005). Meaning in life: One link in the chain from religiousness to well-being. *Journal of Counseling Psychology, 52*(4), 574–582.

Steger, M. F., Frazier, P., Oishi, S., & Kaler, M. (2006). The meaning in life questionnaire: Assessing the presence of and search for meaning in life. *Journal of Counseling Psychology, 53*(1), Article 1.

Steger, M. F., & Kashdan, T. B. (2013). The unbearable lightness of meaning: Well-being and unstable meaning in life. *Journal of Positive Psychology, 8*(2), 103–115.

Steger, M. F., Kashdan, T. B., & Oishi, S. (2008a). Being good by doing good: Daily eudaimonic activity and well-being. *Journal of Research in Personality, 42*(1), 22–42.
Steger, M. F., Kashdan, T. B., Sullivan, B. A., & Lorentz, D. (2008b). Understanding the search for meaning in life: Personality, cognitive style, and the dynamic between seeking and experiencing meaning. *Journal of Personality, 76*(2), 199–228.
Stellar, J. E., Gordon, A. M., Piff, P. K., Cordaro, D., Anderson, C. L., Bai, Y., . . . Keltner, D. (2017). Self-transcendent emotions and their social functions: Compassion, gratitude, and awe bind us to others through prosociality. *Emotion Review, 9*(3), 200–207.
Stone, A. A., Broderick, J. E., & Schwartz, J. E. (2010). Validity of average, minimum, and maximum end-of-day recall assessments of pain and fatigue. *Contemporary Clinical Trials, 31*(5), Article 5.
Stone, A. A., & Shiffman, S. (1994). Ecological momentary assessment (EMA) in behavioral medicine. *Annals of Behavioral Medicine, 16*, 199–202.
Thrash, T. M. (2021). The creation and curation of all things worthy: Inspiration as vital force in persons and cultures. In A. J. Elliot (Ed.), *Advances in motivation science* (Vol. 8, pp. 181–244). Elsevier.
Thrash, T. M., Elliot, A. J., Maruskin, L. A., & Cassidy, S. E. (2010). Inspiration and the promotion of well-being: Tests of causality and mediation. *Journal of Personality and Social Psychology, 98*(3), Article 3.
Tov, W., & Lee, H. W. (2016). A closer look at the hedonics of everyday meaning and satisfaction. *Journal of Personality and Social Psychology, 111*(4), Article 4.
Trapnell, P. D., & Campbell, J. D. (1999). Private self-consciousness and the five-factor model of personality: Distinguishing rumination from reflection. *Journal of Personality and Social Psychology, 76*(2), 284–304.
Trope, Y., & Liberman, N. (2010). Construal-level theory of psychological distance. *Psychological Review, 117*(2), Article 2.
Waytz, A., Hershfield, H. E., & Tamir, D. I. (2015). Mental simulation and meaning in life. *Journal of Personality and Social Psychology, 108*(2), 336–355.
Wilt, J. A., Grubbs, J. B., Exline, J. J., & Pargament, K. I. (2021). Authenticity, presence of meaning, and struggle with ultimate meaning: Nuanced between-and within-person associations. *Journal of Research in Personality, 93*, 104104.
Wilt, J. A., Van Tongeren, D. R., & Exline, J. J. (2024). Are daily supernatural attributions to God and the devil/demons linked with meaning in life? *Journal of Positive Psychology, 19*(2), 369–378.
Wirtz, D., Kruger, J., Napa Scollon, C., & Diener, E. (2003). What to do on spring break?: The role of predicted, on-line, and remembered experience in future choice. *Psychological Science, 14*(5), Article 5.
Wong, P. T. P. (2014). Viktor Frankl's meaning-seeking model and positive psychology. In A. Batthyany & P. Russo-Netzer (Eds.), *Meaning in positive and existential psychology* (pp. 149–184). Springer Science + Business Media.
Wood, A. M., Linley, P. A., Maltby, J., Baliousis, M., & Joseph, S. (2008). The authentic personality: A theoretical and empirical conceptualization and the development of the Authenticity Scale. *Journal of Counseling Psychology, 55*(3), 385–399.
Zambelli, M., & Tagliabue, S. (2024). The Situational Meaning in Life Evaluation (SMILE): Development and validation studies. *Journal of Happiness Studies, 25*(1), 2.

CHAPTER 44

The Existential Dynamics of Politics

Understanding the Links between Political Beliefs, Well-Being, and Meaning in Life

Jake Womick, Juliana Ochoa-Peralta, Kevin Flores, Sarahi Lopez Amaro, *and* Andre Martinez

Philosophers, psychologists, and members of the public have long speculated about why people hold particular political views. These questions are rendered salient by historical and modern events. Why did everyday Germans support Adolf Hitler's rise to power? Why did Americans participate in a coup attempt on behalf of President Donald Trump? Psychology has a rich history of studying ideological factors that drive these kinds of behaviors. For instance, the endorsement of right-wing authoritarian attitudes (submission to authorities, conventionalism, and aggression toward dissidents) among everyday people predicts support for authoritarian movements, voting for authoritarian leaders (Womick et al., 2019a), and prejudice toward marginalized groups (Crawford et al., 2015; Sibley et al., 2007; Weise et al., 2012). These findings beg the question, what do people find so appealing about authoritarianism, given such horrific consequences?

As we review in detail, a variety of theoretical perspectives have directly and indirectly provided a similar answer to this question: People find right-wing political views (i.e., conservatism, system justification, just-world beliefs, and right-wing authoritarianism) existentially appealing. Perhaps the earliest of these accounts dates back to World War II. Fromm (1941/1994) was personally impacted by the Holocaust, and his explanation for the popularity of authoritarianism in Nazi Germany was that it serves an existential function, imbuing life with meaning. More contemporary explanations for this link can be derived from frameworks such as terror management theory (Greenberg et al., 1991), uncertainty identity theory (Hogg, 2007), and significance quest theory (Kruglanski et al., 2009), theory of conservatism as motivated social cognition (Jost et al., 2003), and system justification theory (Jost et al., 2004). Integrating across these perspectives, a concrete picture emerges, highlighting the existential nature of the appeal of right-wing political views: Despite their links with social ills, such as racism (e.g., Brandt & Reyna, 2014) and antidemocratic preferences (Osborne et al., 2023), endorsing these beliefs connects a person to a larger group, reduces existential concerns about death (Scott et al., 2021), provides a sense of certainty about identity (Hogg et al., 2010), and makes one feel like a valued member of society (Kruglanski et al., 2018). These experiences in turn promote the feeling that one's life is important and purposeful, makes sense, and ultimately is meaningful (Womick, Ward, et al., 2019).

In this chapter, we first provide an overview of the science of meaning in life and well-being, before outlining three key theories that address the existential appeal of political attitudes and beliefs broadly (terror management theory, uncertainty identity theory, and significance quest theory). We then turn to a sequential review of theoretical perspectives that specifically suggest an existential function of conservatism (the theory of conservatism as motivated social cognition), system justification and just-world beliefs (system justification theory), and right-wing authoritarianism (the existential vacuum hypothesis). We evaluate the existing evidence for the links between each of these, meaning in life, and well-being. Because this is a burgeoning area of existential psychology, we then highlight some pressing questions left unaddressed in this area of research. We conclude by offering a summary of the current state of the science on the existential dynamics of politics.

THE SCIENCE OF MEANING IN LIFE AND WELL-BEING

When people think about the experience of meaning, they often conjure profound questions of human existence: "Who am I, why am I here, what should I do with my time?" However, the science of meaning in life does not attempt to answer these grand questions concerning the meaning *of* life. Instead, the psychology of meaning *in* life studies this experience as a subjective perception (King & Hicks, 2021). Contemporary perspectives commonly define this global experience of overall meaning in life as arising from at least three lower-order facets: Significance (or existential mattering) is of an interpersonal nature and deals with feelings of importance, perceptions that one matters to other people, that one is valued by society, and that one's activities have impact (Martela & Steger, 2023). Purpose is a more explicitly motivational aspect of meaning in life, revolving around goal directedness. People who have a sense of purpose have important goals and feel like their life is organized around the pursuit of these (Crumbaugh & Maholick, 1964). The last facet, coherence (or comprehension), is a comparatively cognitive experience. Life feels coherent when a person feels that their experiences add up to a unified whole, that the reality around them is ordered and predictable, and that they can make sense of their life (Heintzelman & King, 2014a). Although ongoing debates concern the relative importance of these facets as contributors to the global experience of meaning in life (e.g., Costin & Vignoles, 2019), ample empirical evidence supports this tripartite structure (Krause & Heyward, 2014). When people feel their lives are significant, purposeful, and coherent, they experience life as meaningful (George & Park, 2016).

Even though meaning in life is a subjective perception operationalized via self-report, it is an important aspect of human experience that predicts (many objective) positive outcomes in a variety of domains. People who experience their lives as more meaningful have better social connections, more satisfying romantic relationships (Steptoe & Fancourt, 2019), and more social appeal (Stillman et al., 2011). They are also more successful at work (Steptoe & Fancourt, 2019), experience less burnout (Hooker et al., 2020), and make more money (Hill et al., 2016). Perhaps most importantly, people who simply say that their lives are more meaningful live longer lives (Shiba et al., 2022), and have lower risk of health conditions, such as heart disease, stroke, and mortality (Boyle et al., 2009; Kim et al., 2013, 2019). Meaning in life is also a strong protective factor against suicidal ideation (Corona et al., 2019).

Meaning in life is an aspect of psychological well-being. In the research linking existential and political psychology, many researchers have also focused on other aspects of well-being, including life satisfaction, subjective well-being, and self-esteem. Life satisfaction is a cognitive evaluation of one's overall quality of life, and feelings about one's circumstances (Diener et al., 1985). Closely related, subjective well-being refers to a composite of this cognitive evaluation (life satisfaction) with affective judgments of how often one experiences high positive and low negative affect (Diener et al., 1999). Meaning in life is positively correlated with life satisfaction (Disabato et al., 2016) and positive affect (King et al., 2006; although in meaning in life it is less strongly linked with negative affect—people can experience meaning even in the presence of high negative affect [Tov & Lee, 2016]), and subjective well-being (Li et al., 2021). Self-esteem is a relatively existential component of well-being. It reflects positive beliefs about the self that confer a sense of worth and value (Rosenberg, 1965). Meaning in life and self-esteem are also positively correlated (Steger et al., 2006).

Despite being conceptually and empirically separable aspects of well-being, these constructs are all positively associated with each other, and some evidence suggests they can combine to form a higher-order overall well-being factor (Disabato et al., 2016, 2020). Thus, although the primary focus of this chapter is on meaning in life, we also review the associations between politics and these other aspects of well-being, as well as the extent to which those associations are distinct from meaning in life.

WHY WOULD POLITICAL VIEWS SERVE AN EXISTENTIAL FUNCTION?

Meaning in life is promoted by factors such as positive affect (King et al., 2006), social relationships (Hicks & King, 2009), resources that enable a comfortable life (Ward & King, 2016), experiencing order and routine (Heintzelman & King, 2019), and helping others (Martela et al., 2018), which are all positive characteristics of human experience. Compared to these, politics seems out of place, especially those political beliefs and behaviors that restrict the freedoms and safety of other people (e.g., right-wing authoritarianism). Yet views like conservatism, just-world beliefs, and right-wing authoritarianism can connect a person to like-minded others (enhancing significance), outline the kinds of goals that are worthy of pursuing versus avoiding (promoting purpose), and provide tools to make sense of the world (boosting coherence). Beyond these intuitive conceptual links, contemporary theories of existential psychology provide rationale for why political attitudes and beliefs serve an existential meaning function. These include terror management theory, uncertainty identity theory, and significance quest theory.

Terror Management Theory

According to terror management theory (e.g., Greenberg et al., 1991), what makes humans unique from other animals is our self-conscious awareness that our lives will end. Death awareness causes existential anxiety, and human behavior can be understood as motivated to reduce this psychological discomfort (Pyszczynski et al., 2004). People endorse cultural worldviews to ward off death anxiety and gain a sense of symbolic immortality. Specifically, endorsement of cultural worldviews connects a person to a larger group and facilitates the sense that other people value one's life and contributions. These give the person a sense that they can live on through culture after their physical life has ended, thereby reducing existential anxiety about the impermanence of life (Scott et al., 2021). Thus, the endorsement of political attitudes and beliefs can promote meaning in life because they connect the individual to a larger group, give them a sense that members of that group value them (note, this rationale is most relevant to the significance facet of meaning), and provide the person with a sense of symbolic immortality. Indeed, after a reminder of their own mortality, individuals high (vs. low) on right-wing authoritarianism showed more negative evaluations of targets with dissimilar attitudes (Greenberg et al., 1991; see also Weise et al., 2012), suggesting the existential relevance of authoritarian ideals.

Uncertainty management theory (see van den Bos, 2009) is a competing theory that follows similar logic but deemphasizes death anxiety. According to this perspective, instead of defending against death anxiety, political attitudes and beliefs can more generally function to reduce personal uncertainty, which in turn bolsters a person's sense of meaning in life.

Uncertainty Identity Theory

Uncertainty identity theory argues that the central problem driving human behavior is uncertainty about the self and identity (e.g., "Who am I?"). People are averse to identity uncertainty and are motivated to reduce it, often through group membership (Hogg, 2007). The act of endorsing an ideology shared by a group and the sense of identity that results from group belonging reduce uncertainty. For instance, research shows that enhancing the salience of personal uncertainty leads to greater group identification (Hogg et al., 2010). One of the downstream consequences of identity certainty is thought to be enhanced perceptions of life's meaningfulness. Further, groups that are highly entitative (more concretely defined by homogenous members and beliefs) are more effective at reducing uncertainty (an issue we revisit later in this chapter; Hogg et al., 2007). Thus, endorsing a set of political attitudes and beliefs can grant one a sense of membership into an entitative group. Belonging to this group and endorsing shared beliefs can provide an individual with a sense of certainty about who they are. This sense of certainty then promotes the feeling that life is meaningful. Again, the group-based nature of this theoretical rationale implicates the significance facet of meaning most strongly.

Significance Quest Theory

Significance quest theory suggests that feeling undervalued and unappreciated by other members of society is one of the central forces driving (particularly extreme) human behaviors (e.g., Kruglanski et al., 2009). These perceptions of insignificance place individuals at risk for the adoption of extreme beliefs. The theory suggests that commitment to extreme belief systems connects one to a like-minded group, enables one to feel valued by them, and enhances one's sense of significance. Significance quest theory was originally developed to understand the motives of terrorists and is often applied to studying political violence (Kruglanski et al., 2018). However, a version of this process may occur for other less extreme political views. The ideas follow a similar logic to those described above: Endorsing a set of political attitudes and beliefs connects a person to a larger group; these give the person a sense of value and in turn provide them with the feeling that their life is meaningful. Again, this theory impinges most strongly on the significance (vs. purpose or coherence) facet of meaning.

POLITICS, WELL-BEING, AND MEANING IN LIFE

Beyond the broader existential theories reviewed above, scientists and philosophers have spent the past 80 years reasoning about and researching the potential link between politics, well-being, and meaning in life. This work has almost exclusively focused on right-wing ideology—conservatism, system justification, just-world beliefs, and right-wing authoritarianism—an issue we revisit later. We next turn to a sequential review of each of these, as well as the evidence for their relationship with well-being broadly, and meaning in life, specifically.

Conservatism as Motivated Social Cognition

The theory of conservatism as motivated social cognition (Jost et al., 2003) integrated decades of prior sociological, political science, and psychological research to offer two key perspectives: First, conservatism is defined along two continua. One is orientation toward change. Those on the political left tend to be more progressive, holding attitudes and beliefs and engaging in behaviors that are designed to change society (Sheehy-Skeffington & Tomsen, 2019). Conversely, those on the political right support the status quo (Choma et al., 2020). The other continuum is about the distribution of resources, voice, and power in society. Those on the political left tend to support egalitarianism. Their attitudes, beliefs, and behaviors are geared toward fostering a society characterized by greater equality, with a particular concern for advancing equality for people who belong to historically marginalized groups (Kay et al., 2023). By contrast, those on the political right tolerate and actively support inequality (Brandt & Reyna, 2014).

The second major insight offered by the theory of conservatism as motivated social cognition is that there are key motives that drive people to endorse conservatism. People who are especially sensitive to environmental stimuli conveying threat and uncertainty are predisposed to three sets of social-cognitive motives: (1) epistemic motives to dogmatically defend one's beliefs, reject ambiguity, avoid uncertainty, and seek structure and closure (e.g., Choma et al., 2014); (2) ideological motives to defend one's self-interest, protect that status of one's group (and dominate other groups; e.g., Ho et al., 2015), and justify existing sociopolitical systems (e.g., Jost, 2019); and, most importantly for our purposes, (3) existential motives. Jost and colleagues (2003) described these existential motives as concerning the maintenance of self-esteem, minimization of loss, and management of the existential terror that arises from mortality awareness. By extension, these existential motives would also include the experience of meaning in life, significance, purpose, and coherence. The theory suggests that these social-cognitive motives drive people to endorse inequality and resist change, which comprise political conservatism. Taking these ideas one step further, political conservatism would then relate to a set of outcomes that reflect the satisfaction of these motives, including a sense of certainty and dogmatism (e.g., Jessani & Harris, 2018), system justification (e.g., Jost, 2019), support for maintaining a hierarchical group dynamics (e.g., Ho & Ktiely, 2020), as well as existential benefits. For our purposes, these existential benefits should primarily include the enhancement of well-being and the experience of meaning in life.

In what has come to be deemed the "happiness gap," research shows that conservatives experience higher well-being than liberals (Taylor et al., 2006). The majority of this work has focused on life satisfaction (Onraet et al., 2017; Wojcik et al., 2015). The explanation for the happiness gap remains controversial. One perspective focuses on differences in the way liberals and conservatives perceive existing social and political systems. Conservatives justify these more strongly, rationalizing existing social and political problems, such as inequality. These ideological justifications provide conservatives protection against the negative toll the acknowledgment of these social problems could take on one's well-being (Napier & Jost, 2008). The opposing perspective focuses on psychological adjustment. From this view, the happiness gap is explained by left–right political differences in agency, positive outlook, transcendent beliefs, and beliefs in fairness (Schlenker et al., 2012). This perspective suggests conservatives are happier because they are more positively adjusted.

More recently, research has focused on a more decidedly existential component of well-being—meaning in life. Using large cross-sectional, daily diary, and ecological momentary assessment methods, Newman and colleagues (2019) found that conservatism (both the social and the economic components) shares a small but robust positive relationship with meaning in life. These findings were obtained both in the United States and across 15 other Western countries, using data spanning the past four decades (see also Stavrota & Luhmann, 2016). Crucially, multivariate analyses showed that this link was stronger than the relationship between conservatism and life satisfaction. Controlling for meaning in life, conservatism was no longer significantly correlated with life satisfaction (Newman et al., 2019). Thus, the well-being benefits of conservatism are of an existential nature, primarily concerning meaning in life. Those who support the status quo and accept inequality consistently report experiencing their lives as more meaningful.

In response to Jost and colleagues' (2003) theory of motivated social cognition, Greenberg and Jonas (2003) published a reply arguing for what has become the symmetry hypothesis. Instead of factors like dogmatism and cognitive rigidity being uniquely associated with the political right, Greenberg and Jonas argued that these are associated with political extremes on either the left or right. This question has been addressed in many domains, including well-being. Newman and colleagues (2019, Studies 1b and 2) indeed found a quadratic relationship between conservatism and meaning in life. However, it did not look like a U-shaped symmetrical curve. Instead, it showed a more dramatic spike in meaning in life at higher levels of conservatism (and no uptick at the furthest left end of the spectrum). Thus, there is no evidence that the existential benefit of political ideology is symmetrical, or that extreme liberalism promotes meaning in life. Those on the political left consistently report lower meaning.

One important consideration for understanding this relationship is that conservatives are also more religious (e.g., Feldman & Johnston, 2014), and religiosity is a robust predictor of meaning in life (e.g., Dar & Iqbal, 2020). However, the link between conservatism and meaning in life is not explained by religiosity (nor was it explained by demographics such as age, gender, geographical region, income, or education [Newman et al., 2019]; or need satisfaction [Sheldon, 2023]). To date, literature has focused primarily on the link between conservatism and global meaning in life, and the purpose facet of meaning. Less work has specifically focused on the significance and coherence facets. The relative importance of all three facets to the link between conservatism and global meaning in life needs to be empirically addressed. The theories reviewed above suggest that the existential function of conservatism may primarily be about significance.

System Justification Theory and Just-World Beliefs

Closely related to the theory of conservatism as motivated social cognition is system justification theory (Jost & Banaji, 1994). The core tenet of system justification theory is that humans are motivated to defend and bolster the status quo of the systems to which they belong (Jost, et al., 2004; in addition to other key motives of ego and group justification). Many right-wing beliefs, including conservatism, are often coined system-justifying ideologies because they seek to protect the status quo (e.g., Napier & Jost, 2008). Sometimes conservatism is also treated as a moderator of system justification. For instance, perceiving an existing sociopolitical system as under threat produces stronger system justification behaviors, especially among conservatives; and disadvantaged groups show outgroup favoritism (as a means to legitimize existing sociopolitical systems), particularly among conservatives who belong to these groups (Jost, 2019). A rich body of literature, spanning the past three decades, provides support for this theoretical perspective (see Jost, 2019, for a review).

Acknowledging existing systems are unjust is psychologically taxing, so system justification serves a palliative function. It shields people from acknowledging problems in sociopolitical systems (e.g., inequality), and as a result, "justifying the status quo meets basic needs for . . . certainty and meaning" (Osborne et al., 2019, p. 341). The literature supports this view, although it again has primarily focused on life satisfaction. System justification correlates positively with well-being (Henry & Saul, 2006) in the United States (Suppes et al., 2019) and globally (e.g., Bahamondes-Correa, 2016; Vargas-Salfate et al., 2018). System justification also partially mediates the link between conservatism and well-being (Napier & Jost, 2008; Schlenker et al., 2012), providing evidence for the idea that one reason for the happiness gap is that conservatives support the status quo.

This palliative function is thought to be particularly acute for people who belong to historically marginalized groups (Jost & Hunyday, 2003, 2005). Indeed, justifying the status quo also promotes well-being among people who belong to historically marginalized groups (McCoy et al., 2013). Napier and colleagues (2020) reported three studies with over 20,000 participants from 23 different countries showing that gender-based system justification (denying gender discrimination) was positively associated with higher life satisfaction among women, particularly in contexts characterized by high sexism. From this view, system justification can be psychologically palliative because it inoculates people against discrimination toward the groups to which they belong and provides a means to cope with injustice (Osborne et al., 2019; Sengupta et al., 2017).

Although the vast majority of this work has operationalized these palliative outcomes in terms of life satisfaction (e.g., Harding & Sibley, 2013), similar patterns have been obtained for self-esteem (e.g., Godfrey et al., 2018). Notably, the palliative function of system justification has been primarily conceptualized as meaning in life (see Osborne et al., 2019, p. 341), but considerably less research has actually measured it. The existing evidence suggests system justification is positively correlated with meaning in life (Rankin et al., 2009), but there is no evidence this existential benefit is stronger among people who belong to marginalized groups. To date, no research has focused on the links between system justification and the facets of meaning. Future work must also evaluate whether (similar to conservatism) the palliative benefits of justifying the status quo are primarily about meaning in life versus common to other aspects of well-being.

Just-World Beliefs

Belief in a just world is one of the core antecedents of system justification (Jost & Burgess, 2000). Lerner (1980) defined just-world beliefs as a conviction that people get what they deserve for outcomes both positive and negative. Much previous research has shown that just-world beliefs predict negative outcomes, like victim blaming and endorsement of strong punitive punishment (see Hafer & Bègue, 2005, for a review). However, despite its links to negative outcomes, previous research has also linked just-world beliefs to well-being benefits (Dalbert, 1999).

Similar to system justification, previous research has suggested that just-world beliefs function as a positive illusion that facilitate healthy psychological functioning, especially for individuals who are socially disadvantaged (Laurin et al., 2011). Just-world beliefs facilitate life satisfaction (Lipkus et al., 1996) and greater subjective well-being (Dzuka & Dalbert, 2006). Belief in a just world is also associated with adaptive psychological adjustment in the context of adversity, including better adjustment after negative life events (Nasser et al., 2011) and stable life satisfaction following natural disasters (Seker, 2016).

Studies have also linked just-world beliefs to the experience of meaning in life. For example, just-world beliefs are positively correlated with purpose in life (Bègue & Bastounis, 2003). In a sample of cancer survivors, restored belief in a just world was positively associated with ratings of life's meaningfulness (Park et al., 2008). Again, research has yet to examine the links between belief in a just world and the facets of meaning in life or to compare the relative importance of these beliefs to different aspects of well-being. We expect, similar to the other ideological variables considered here, the well-being benefits of just-world beliefs are primarily about meaning in life and centrally concern feelings of significance.

Authoritarianism

Psychological inquiry into authoritarianism dates back to World War II and the rise of the Nazis. Scholars whose lives were directly affected by the war and the Holocaust were interested in understanding how so many everyday people supported Hitler's rise to power and participated in the atrocities that followed. The first scientific attempt to study this issue involved a series of in-depth interviews conducted by Adorno and colleagues (1950). They developed a framework of the authoritarian personality as a psychological disorder characterized by nine components. The paradigm shifted as a result from Altemeyer's (e.g., 1981) seminal studies on authoritarianism. Although Altemeyer operationalized right-wing authoritarianism as a unidimensional construct, he defined it as having three components (and argued that items used to measure it must be double and triple barreled because the three components could not exist independently). In the decades since, researchers have left behind this methodological idiosyncrasy, but have almost uniformly retained the tripartite definition (e.g., Bizumic & Duckitt, 2018): Right-wing authoritarianism involves submission to a strong leader and authorities (e.g., police), conventionalism, or adherence to traditions that are endorsed by those leaders and authorities, and aggression toward those who are seen as deviant to these traditions or dissident to these authorities (e.g., Dunwoody & Funke, 2016; Mavor et al., 2010).

The scientific consensus is that right-wing authoritarian views often result from a predisposition to threat sensitivity (Altemeyer, 2006; Lepage et al., 2022; Onraet et al., 2013). Research shows, for instance, that right-wing authoritarianism is higher in regions with greater threats such as pathogen prevalence (Murray et al., 2013; Zmigrod et al., 2021) or terrorist attacks (Echebarria-Echabe & Fernandez-Guede, 2006). Whether threat causes shifts toward the political right versus political extremism remains a contentious area of debate (e.g., Brandt et al., 2021; Eadeh & Chang, 2020). Yet the idea that a threatening world is one in which people want strong leaders and social traditions, and to root out those who do not conform to these, is supported conceptually (e.g., Altemeyer, 2006) and empirically (e.g., Shaffer & Duckitt, 2013; Stephan, 2014; Stephan et al., 2009).

The role of threat in the endorsement of right-wing authoritarianism is central to the dual-process model of ideology and prejudice (Duckitt, 2001). This theory suggests that punitive socialization creates children who are especially reactive to threat, which in turn predisposes them to support right-wing authoritarianism. Right-wing authoritarianism then leads to prejudice toward groups that are perceived as threatening (Thomsen et al., 2008). The dual-process model also incorporates social dominance orientation (sometimes conceptualized as a second dimension of the authoritarian personality; Altemeyer 1998), which entails a belief that group-based hierarchies are natural and necessary for society to function (Ho et al., 2015). From this view, right-wing authoritarianism and social dominance orientation are two distinct but related constructs that contribute to prejudice through two different paths. In contrast to the process described above for right-wing authoritarianism, tough child rearing predisposes people to be especially sensitive to hierarchy and competition, which in turn enhances both an individual's tendency to endorse social dominance orientation and their prejudice toward those who are perceived to be in competition with that individual's group (Duckitt & Sibley, 2007).

Although a rich body of literature supports these different components of the dual-process model (see Osborne et al., 2023), the perspectives that link authoritarianism to meaning in life tend to be unique to right-wing authoritarianism, rather than social dominance orientation. In fact, no existing research has provided empirical support for an existential function or well-being benefits of social dominance orientation (see Womick et al., 2019b). We expect these differences emerge because right-wing authoritarianism represents a more conceptually rich worldview (e.g., Pyszczynski et al., 2004), and social dominance orientation is more monolithically about group-based hierarchies, the endorsement of which (and related constructs, like racism) are not positively associated with meaning in life (e.g., Florez et al., 2019).

Most theorists who have written about the origins and implications of right-wing authoritarianism have suggested that its psychological appeal lies in its existential function—connecting the individual to a group, giving the person a sense of right and wrong, helping the person make sense of the world—making life feel meaningful. The first psychologist to consider these issues provided the most explicit reasoning for this link. Fromm (1941/1994), who was a German Jewish scholar and fled Nazi Germany to escape the Holocaust, was the first to suggest right-wing authoritarianism might promote meaning in life. His reasoning was steeped in a historical account of the way society had transformed in the decades leading up to Hitler's rise to power. Before the Protestant Reformation, Western life was entirely organized around the church: Everyone had a role that they were born into, and that role provided certainty. One's role determined how one would spend one's days, the career one would pursue, and one's livelihood. Social life, interactions, and relationships were all structured around the church. Following the Protestant Reformation, many people remained religious, but the church played less of a central organizing role in society and everyday life. These basic existential questions of identity, purpose, relationships, structure, and death were less readily answered by an overbearing religion. Thus, Fromm reasoned that people began to experience an existential vacuum—an inner emptiness or void of meaning that was left by the church—and people sought to fill it with something else. For many people, the answer was authoritarianism. This reasoning is consistent with more modern perspectives that characterize political views as a new sort of religion, as rates of religiosity continue to decline (e.g., Finkel et al., 2020). In the absence of religious views, endorsing authoritarian beliefs could provide the same sense of existential security and certainty that had formerly been provided by the church. The capacity for authoritarianism to fill the existential vacuum, Fromm argued, was one of the key factors responsible for the popularity of authoritarian movements in the mid-20th century and may constitute part of their continuing appeal today. One clear implication that follows is that people who endorse right-wing authoritarian attitudes should experience life as more meaningful.

The existential function of political views has been most thoroughly examined with respect to right-wing authoritarianism, compared to the other political constructs reviewed above. Right-wing authoritarianism is positively related to meaning in life in the United States (Steger et al., 2008) and other Western countries (Manzi et al., 2015). As with conservatism and system justification, this relationship is characterized by a small but robust relationship. This link is not explained by a wide range of compelling third variables, including demographics (ranging from age, gender, race, income, to education; nor is it moderated by demographics), other political variables (i.e., protestant work ethic, social dominance orientation, and conservatism), cognitive dispositions (i.e., need for cognition, faith in intuition, cognitive ability), personality traits (neuroticism, extraversion, openness to experience, agreeableness, conscientiousness), or other aspects of well-being (mood, self-esteem, life satisfaction, environmental mastery, self-acceptance, autonomy, personal growth, and social relatedness) (Womick et al., 2019b). Rather, showing a similar pattern to conservatism, meaning in life fully explains the relationship between right-wing authoritarianism and life satisfaction, suggesting the psychological benefits of these beliefs are centrally existential. Importantly, right-wing authoritarianism also buffers meaning in life against existential distress. Among those who more strongly endorse right-wing authoritarianism, aspects of ill-being, such as stress, anxiety, depression, loneliness, and existential isolation, take less of a negative toll on meaning in life (Womick et al., 2019b).

This research has also examined the link between right-wing authoritarianism and the lower-order facets of meaning in life. Recall, each of these links is conceptually plausible, yet existing theories (terror management theory, uncertainty identity theory, and significance quest theory) primarily implicate significance. The evidence shows that right-wing authoritarianism is positively related to all three facets of meaning in life, but this relationship is significantly stronger for significance (vs. purpose and coherence) (Womick et al., 2019b, 2021a). Additionally, significance, but not purpose or coherence, explains the relationship between right-wing authoritarianism and meaning in life (Womick et al., 2019b, 2021a). Thus, right-wing authoritarianism indeed serves an existential function, and this existential function is primarily about making the person feel important, valued, and like they have impact on the world around them.

As with other right-wing views, right-wing authoritarianism is strongly linked to religiosity (Wilkinson, 2004). It is also strongly linked with religious fundamentalism, which Altemeyer and Hunsberger (2004) dubbed a religious type of authoritarianism. Is the existential function of right-wing authoritarianism simply due to its overlap with religion? Similar to conservatism, controlling religiosity (intrinsic or extrinsic) and strength of God belief does not wipe out the relationship between right-wing authoritarianism and meaning in life (Womick et al., 2019b). Structural equation modeling shows that religious fundamentalism accounts for a significant portion of the relationship between right-wing authoritarianism and meaning in life, but even among those who do not endorse religiosity or religious fundamentalism whatsoever, right-wing authoritarianism continues to promote meaning (Womick et al., 2021a). Thus, part of the existential function of right-wing authoritarianism is due to its overlap with religiosity and religious fundamentalism, but right-wing authoritarianism still promotes meaning in life among the nonreligious. (*Note:* Intrinsic religiosity and religious fundamentalism are also more strongly related to significance than the other facets, suggesting the existential function of both religious and political views may primarily be about significance.)

The research reviewed in this chapter has been almost exclusively correlational because it is difficult to manipulate political views, which are dispositional and partly heritable (e.g., Hatemi et al., 2010). However, some experimental evidence speaks to the causal underpinnings of the relationship between right-wing authoritarianism and meaning in life. Using three different experimental paradigms, Womick and colleagues (2021b) showed that exposure to authoritarian values leads to higher meaning in life. First, participants were asked to complete measures of right-wing authoritarianism and meaning in life in counterbalanced order. Those who completed a right-wing authoritarianism scale first reported higher meaning in life than those who completed it after. Second, participants who were exposed to descriptions of authoritarian values reported higher meaning in life than those who read a control passage or a description of egalitarian values. Third, people who were exposed to transcripts of real-world authoritarian speeches (e.g., by Hitler) reported higher meaning in life than did those exposed to a control or to transcripts of speeches from real-world egalitarian leaders (e.g., by Gorbachev). In these studies, there was no evidence that moral outrage, anger, or disagreement explained the effect of condition on meaning in life. A question raised by this work, which is common to all of other variables reviewed in this chapter, is "Why?" Researchers continue to probe the mediational mechanisms that can explain why right-wing authoritarianism (and conservatism, system justification, and just-world beliefs) promotes meaning in life.

Another budding direction for this area of research is to consider the existential function of left-wing authoritarianism. Recently developed scales (Costello et al., 2022) make it possible to test whether right-wing authoritarianism is uniquely associated with meaning in life, or if any kind of authoritarianism serves a similar existential function. Considering the above rationale, many theories would suggest any strongly endorsed ideology (Greenberg & Jonas, 2003) could connect a person to a larger group, reduce their anxiety about death (Greenberg et al., 1991), give them a sense of certainty about their identity (Hogg, 2007), and provide a sense of significance (Kruglanski et al., 2009), thereby enhancing the feeling that life is meaningful. However, all existing evidence consistently shows that those on the political left are slightly lower on meaning in life, and it has failed to show that any left-wing views (e.g., liberalism, progressive values) positively contribute to meaning in life.

OPEN QUESTIONS AND ADDITIONAL CONSIDERATIONS

Although the findings reviewed above are in many ways intuitive and theoretically consistent, there remains a puzzle of understanding meaning in life on the political left. We next turn to additional questions and considerations that can contextualize this problem and chart a course forward.

What about the Political Left?

As noted above, the symmetry perspective argues that correlates of political ideology should not be unique to the political right but be common to the political extremes. From this view, the existential benefits of political attitudes and beliefs should not be specific to right-wing constructs but be common to corresponding left-wing views. Yet across all of the studies reviewed here, no U-shaped curvilinear relationships have been found, and when quadratic relationships exist, they show a bigger existential boost for the most extreme conservatives (e.g., Newman et al., 2019). This pattern is problematic for the core existential theories reviewed above (terror management theory, uncertainty identity theory, and significance quest theory). The existential benefits of politics outlined by each of these is not unique to the political right. Rather, any set of political views should have the capacity to link one to a like-minded group and provide a sense of symbolic immortality, identity certainty, and significance that result in higher perceptions of meaning in life. To be clear, in the research reviewed above, the positive links between right-wing views and meaning in life are small (ranging from $r \sim 0.10$ to 0.30 in samples ranging from $N \sim 200$ to $30{,}000$). Liberals and those who reject system justification and right-wing authoritarianism are not experiencing their lives as meaningless. In fact, one of the most counterintuitive findings from the science of meaning in life is that people broadly experience their lives as pretty meaningful (Heintzleman & King, 2014b; King & Hicks, 2021). Yet we fail to find theoretically consistent evidence that liberalism and left-wing views serve similar existential functions to their right-wing counterparts. One possibility that needs to be empirically addressed is that left-wing views serve entirely different psychological needs or existential functions (e.g., psychological richness; Oishi & Westgate, 2021). However, there remain numerous other possibilities that may contribute to resolving this issue, which we turn to next.

Entitativity

Although uncertainty identity theory (Hogg, 2007) argues that different liberal and conservative groups can be more and less entitative, the political left tends to be more demographically, culturally, and ideologically heterogenous (Pew Research Center, 2024). Thus, conservatism and the groups this ideology can link one to are more entitative than liberalism and left-wing groups. Supporting this idea, dispositional uncertainty about American identity is negatively related to right-wing authoritarianism (Wagoner et al., 2017), suggesting that right-wing beliefs provide more certainty about what it means to be American. Because left-wing ideologies tie individuals to groups that are less entitative, they may be less effective at providing certainty about identity and, ultimately, meaning in life. Research supports this idea. For instance, when exposed to religious pluralism (i.e., there are many valid ways of being religious), participants in one study experienced lower meaning in life than when exposed to a nonpluralistic descriptions of what it means to be religious (i.e., there is only one right way to be religious; Womick & King, 2023). The same may hold true for other aspects of identity, such as what it means to be American. There are many benefits to belonging to diverse groups, including cultural richness, novelty, complexity, and egalitarianism. It may be that those who endorse left-wing beliefs and belong to less entitative groups simply experience these other kinds of benefits at a small cost to perceptions of life's meaningfulness.

Diverse Samples

One strength of political psychology and the different areas of research reviewed above is that the field often assesses cross-cultural generalizability (e.g., Napier er al., 2020). However, many of the studies contributing to this area of knowledge still rely on predominantly White samples. One result of the lower entitativity and higher demographic diversity of the political left is that one's identity may shape the way politics relates to the experience of meaning in life. For instance, the link between political beliefs and meaning in life and the potential moderators of this relationship may differ depending on identity characteristics, such as race, ethnicity, gender, sexual orientation, and the intersections of these. Based on existing work, initial tests suggested that the link between right-wing authoritarianism and meaning in life was not moderated by these demographics in convenience samples (although analyses have not assessed intersectionality); and although most research suggests the palliative function of system justification is stronger for people who belong to marginalized groups, this was not the case for meaning in life. Thus, the field needs to conduct more high-powered tests of these possibilities, focusing on diverse samples and intersectionality.

What Is Political Leftism?

Although no evidence suggests a U-shaped curvilinear relationship between political ideology and meaning in life (or well-being), conservatism is the only political variable for which it makes sense to test such a hypothesis. Everyday people learn and think about political ideology as a spectrum that ranges from liberalism on the left to conservatism on the right. Our operationalizations use corresponding labels. So, low scores on a measure of conservatism convincingly represent liberalism. However, the same is not true for other political constructs, like right-wing authoritarianism, system justification, and just-world beliefs. To illustrate this conceptual ambiguity, consider someone who scores very low on a measure of right-wing authoritarianism. What does that mean about their political views? It could mean that they are not authoritarian at all, or it could mean that they support left-wing authoritarianism, or a host of other potential explanations. Although recent efforts have begun to focus specifically on the political left (Kay et al., 2023) and have resulted in new measures (Costello et al., 2022), there remains a dearth of theory and measurement available to researchers to understand political leftism. Moving forward, the field needs to develop conceptually rich theories (that mirror the rigor of the theory of conservatism as motivated social cognition) that explain the motives and needs relevant to the political left, as well as richer measures of left-wing politics (e.g., socialism, communism, anarchy). Only with a better understanding of what political leftism truly is, can we fully evaluate whether it serves important existential functions.

Beliefs versus Behavior

Endorsing right-wing political views is enough to experience existential benefits. Perhaps the same is not true for left-wing political beliefs. Liberalism is defined by dissatisfaction because the status quo is characterized by inequality (Jost et al., 2003). If this is the core of one's beliefs, then perhaps the mere endorsement of these views may not be enough to make life feel significant, purposeful, and coherent. For left-wing political beliefs to promote meaning, they may need to be paired with behaviors designed to create ideologically consistent social change. Research provides partial support for this idea, showing that expressing anger at injustice can bolster meaning in life for those particularly sensitive to injustice (Rothschild & Keefer, 2021). Future research should integrate existential psychology with collective action to further test these possibilities.

CONCLUSION

Right-wing political beliefs, including conservatism, system justification, just-world beliefs, and right-wing authoritarianism (but not social dominance orientation) are positively related to well-being. This well-being function appears to be primarily of an existential nature, specific to meaning in life. Although more research needs to study the facets of meaning in life, the existential function of right-wing political views seems to be primarily about significance—enhancing feelings that one's life is important, that one is valued by others, and that one's activities have impact—rather than purpose or coherence. Although experimental evidence is generally lacking, longitudinal designs have helped address the temporal order of these associations, and some research suggests right-wing authoritarianism causally leads to higher meaning in life. Yet theoretical inconsistencies and empirical gaps remain. Ultimately, this is a blossoming area of existential psychology, and these remaining open questions strike an important chord in the field.

REFERENCES

Adorno, T., Frenkel-Brunswick, E., Levinson, D., & Sanford, R. (1950). *The authoritarian personality.* Harper.

Altemeyer, B. (1981). *Right-wing authoritarianism.* University of Manitoba Press.

Altemeyer, B. (1998). The other "authoritarian personality." *Advances in Experimental Social Psychology, 30,* 47–92.

Altemeyer, B. (2006). *The authoritarians.* http://members.shaw.ca/jeanaltemeyer/drbob/TheAuthoritarians.pdf.

Altemeyer, B., & Hunsberger, B. (2004). A revised religious fundamentalism scale: The short and sweet of it. *International Journal for the Psychology of Religion, 14,* 47–54.

Bahamondes-Correa, J. (2016). System justification's opposite effects on psychological well-being: Testing a moderated mediation model in a gay men and lesbian sample in Chile. *Journal of Homosexuality, 63,* 1537–1555.

Bègue, L., & Bastounis, M. (2003). Two spheres of belief in justice: Extensive support for the bidimensional model of belief in a just world. *Journal of Personality, 71,* 435–463.

Bizumic, B., & Duckitt, J. (2018). Investigating right wing authoritarianism with a very short authoritarianism scale. *Journal of Social and Political Psychology, 6,* 129–150.

Boyle, P. A., Barnes, L. L., Buchman, A. S., & Bennett, D. A. (2009). Purpose in life is associated with mortality among community-dwelling older persons. *Psychosomatic Medicine, 71,* 574–579.

Brandt, M. H., & Reyna, C. (2014). To love or hate thy neighbor: The role of authoritarianism and traditionalism in explaining the link between fundamentalism and racial prejudice. *Political Psychology, 35,* 207–223.

Brandt, M. H., Turner-Sqinkels, F. M., Karapirinler, B., Van Leeuwen, F., Bender, M., van Osch, Y., & Adams, B. (2021). The association between threat and politics depends on the type of threat, the political domain, and the country. *Personality and Social Psychology Bulletin, 47,* 324–343.

Choma, B., Hodson, G., Hoffarth, M. R., Charlesford, J. J., & Hafer, C. L. (2014). Reasoning ability and ideology: Inaccuracies in hierarchical category relations (but not numerical ability) are associated with right-wing authoritarianism. *Journal of Individual Differences, 3,* 177–183.

Choma, B. L., Hodson, G., Jagayat, A., & Hoffarth, M. R. (2020). Right-wing ideology as a predictor of collective action across four political issue domains. *Political Psychology, 41,* 303–322.

Corona, C. D., Van Orden, K. A., Wisco, B. E., & Pietrzak, R. H. (2019). Meaning in life moderates the association between morally injurious experiences and suicide ideation among US combat veterans: Results from the National Health and Resilience in Veterans Study. *Psychological Trauma, 11,* 614–620.

Costello, T. H., Bowes, S. M., Stevens, S. T., Waldman, I. D., Tasimi, A., & Lilienfeld, S. O. (2022). Clarifying the structure and nature of left-wing authoritarianism. *Journal of Personality and Social Psychology.*

Costin, V., & Vignoles, V. L. (2019). Meaning is about mattering: Evaluating coherence, purpose and existential mattering as precursors of meaning in life judgements. *Journal of Personality and Social Psychology, 118,* 864–884.

Crawford, J. T., Brandt, M. J., Inbar, Y., & Mallinas, S. R. (2015). Right-wing authoritarianism predicts prejudice equally toward "gay men and lesbians" and "homosexuals." *Journal of Personality and Social Psychology.*

Crumbaugh, J., & Maholick, L. T. (1964). An experimental study in existentialism: The psychometric approach to Frankl's concept of noogenic neurosis. *Journal of Clinical Psychology, 20,* 200–207.

Dalbert, C. (1999). The world is more just for me than generally: About the personal belief in a just world scale's validity. *Social Justice Research, 12,* 79–98.

Dar, K. A., & Iqbal, N. (2020). Religious commitment and well-being in college students: Examining conditional indirect effects of meaning in life. *Journal of Religion and Health, 58(6),* 2288–2297.

Diener, E., Emmons, R. A., Larsen, R. J., & Griffin, S. (1985). The Satisfaction with Life Scale. *Journal of Personality Assessment, 49,* 71–75.

Diener, E., Suh, E. M., Lucas, R. E., & Smith, H. L. (1999). Subjective well-being: Three decades of progress. *Psychological Bulletin, 125,* 276–302.

Disabato, D. J., Goodman, F. R., & Kashdan, T. B. (2020). *A hierarchical framework for the measurement of well-being.* https://osf.io/preprints/psyarxiv/5rhqj.

Disabato, D. J., Goodman, F. R., Kashdan, T. B., Short, J. L., & Jarden, A. (2016). Different types of well-being? A cross-cultural examination of hedonic and eudaimonic well-being. *Psychological Assessment, 28,* 471–482.

Duckitt, J. (2001). A dual-process cognitive-motivational theory of ideology and prejudice. *Advances in Experimental Social Psychology, 22,* 41–113.

Duckitt, J., & Sibley, C. G. (2007). Right wing authoritarianism, social dominance orientation and the dimensions of generalized prejudice. *European Journal of Personality, 21,* 113–130.

Dunwoody, P. T., & Funke, F. (2016). The aggression–submission–conventionalism scale: Testing a new three factor measure of authoritarianism. *Journal of Social and Political Psychology, 4,* 571–600.

Dzuka, J., & Dalbert, C. (2006). The belief in a just world and subjective well-being in old age. *Aging and Mental Health, 10,* 439–444.

Eadeh, F. R., & Chang, K. K. (2020). Can threat increase support for liberalism? New insights into the relationship between threat and political attitudes. *Social Psychological and Personality Science, 11*(1), 88–96.

Echebarria-Echabe, A., & Fernandez-Guede, E. (2006). Effects of terrorism on attitudes and ideological orientation. *European Journal of Social Psychology, 36,* 259–265.

Feldman, S., & Johnston, C. (2014). Understanding the determinants of political ideology: Implications of structural complexity. *Political Psychology, 35,* 337–358.

Finkel, E. J., Bail, C. A., Cikara, M., Ditto, P. H., Iyengar, S., Klar, S., . . . Druckman, J. S. (2020). Political sectarianism in America. *Science, 370,* 533–536.

Florez, I. A., Schulenberg, S. E., Lair, E. C., Wilson, K. G., & Johnson, K. A. (2019). Understanding meaning and racial prejudice: Examining self-transcendence and psychological inflexibility in a sample of White college students. *Journal of Contextual Behavioral Science, 12,* 1–6.

Fromm, E. (1994). *Escape from freedom.* Henry Holt. (Original work published 1941)

George, L. S., & Park, C. L. (2016). Meaning

in life as comprehension, purpose, and mattering: Toward integration and new research questions. *Review of General Psychology, 20,* 205–220.

Godfrey, E. B., Santos, C. E., & Burson, E. (2018). For better or worse?: System justifying beliefs in sixth grade predict trajectories of self-esteem and behavior across early adolescence. *Child Development.*

Greenberg, J., & Jonas, E. (2003). Psychological motives and political orientation—The left, the right, and the rigid: Comment on Jost et al. (2003). *Psychological Bulletin, 129,* 376–382.

Greenberg, J., Pyszczynski, T., Solomon, S., Rosenblatt, A., Veeder, M., & Kirkland, S. (1991). Evidence for terror management theory II: The effects of mortality salience on reactions to those who threaten and bolster the cultural worldview. *Journal of Personality and Social Psychology, 58,* 308–318.

Hafer, C. L., & Bègue, L. (2005). Experimental research on just-world theory: Problems, developments, and future challenges. *Psychological Bulletin, 131,* 128–167.

Harding, J. F., & Sibley, C. G. (2013). The palliative function of system justification: Concurrent benefits versus longer-term costs to well-being. *Social Indicators Research, 113,* 401–418.

Hatemi, P. K., Hibbing, J. R., Medland, S. E., Keller, M. C., Alford, J. R., Smith, K. B., . . . Eaves, L. J. (2010). Not by twins alone: Using the extended family design to investigate genetic influence on political beliefs. *American Journal of Political Science, 54,* 798–814.

Heintzelman, S. J., & King, L. A. (2014a). (The feeling of) meaning-as-information. *Personality and Social Psychology Review, 18,* 153–167.

Heintzelman, S. J., & King, L. A. (2014b). Life is pretty meaningful. *American Psychologist, 69,* 561–574.

Heintzelman, S. J., & King, L. A. (2019). Routines and meaning in life. *Personality and Social Psychology Bulletin,* 1–12.

Henry, P. J., & Saul, A. (2006). The development of system justification in the developing world. *Social Justice Research, 19,* 365–378.

Hicks, J. A., & King, L. A. (2009). Positive mood and social relatedness as information about meaning in life. *Journal of Positive Psychology, 4,* 471–482.

Hill, P. L., Turiano, N. A., Mroczek, D. K., & Burrow, A. L. (2016). The value of a purposeful life: Sense of purpose predicts greater income and net worth. *Journal of Research in Personality, 65,* 38–42.

Ho, A. K., & Kteily, N. (2020). The role of group-based egalitarianism in collective action. *Current Opinion in Psychology, 35,* 1–6.

Ho, A. K., Sidanius, J., Kteily, N., Sheehy-Skeffington, J., Pratto, F., Henkel, K. E., . . . Stewart, A. L. (2015). The nature of social dominance orientation: Theorizing and measuring preferences for intergroup inequality using the new SDO_7 scale. *Journal of Personality and Social Psychology, 109,* 1003–1028.

Hogg, M. A. (2007). Uncertainty-identity theory. In M. Zanna (Ed.), *Advances in experimental social psychology* (pp. 69–166). Elsevier.

Hogg, M. A., Meehan, C., & Farquaharson, J. (2010). The solace of radicalism: Self-uncertainty and group identification in the face of threat. *Journal of Experimental Social Psychology, 46,* 1061–1066.

Hogg, M. A., Sherman, D. K., Dierselhius, J., Maitner, A. T., & Moffitt, G. (2007). Uncertainty, entitativity, and group identification. *Journal of Experimental Social Psychology, 43,* 135–142.

Hooker, S., Post, R., & Sherman, M. (2020). Awareness of meaning in life is protective against burnout among family physicians: A CERA study. *Family Medicine, 52,* 11–16.

Jessani, Z., & Harris, P. B. (2018). Personality, politics, and denial: Tolerance of ambiguity, political orientation and disbelief in climate change. *Personality and Individual Differences, 131,* 121–123.

Jost, J. T. (2019). A quarter century of system justification theory: Questions, answers, criticisms, and societal applications. *British Journal of Social Psychology, 58,* 263–314.

Jost, J. T., & Banaji, M. R. (1994). The role of stereotyping in system-justification and the production of false consciousness. *British Journal of Social Psychology, 33,* 1–27.

Jost, J. T., Banaji, M. R., & Nosek, B. A. (2004). A decade of system justification theory: Accumulated evidence of conscious and unconscious bolstering of the status quo. *Political Psychology, 25,* 881–919.

Jost, J. T., & Burgess, D. (2000). Attitudinal ambivalence and the conflict between group and system justification motives in low status groups. *Personality and Social Psychology Bulletin, 26,* 293–305.

Jost, J. T., Glaser, J., Kruglanski, A. W., & Sulloway, F. J. (2003). Conservatism as motivated social cognition. *Psychological Bulletin, 129,* 339–375.

Jost, J. T., & Hunyady, O. (2003). The psychology of system justification and the palliative function of ideology. *European Review of Social Psychology, 13,* 111–153.

Jost, J. T., & Hunyday, O. (2005). Antecedents

and consequences of system-justifying ideologies. *Current Directions in Psychological Science, 14,* 260–265.
Kay, A. C., Ponce de Leon, R., Ho, A. K., & Kteily, N. S. (2023). Motivated egalitarianism. *Current Directions in Psychological Science, 32.*
King, L. A., & Hicks, J. A. (2021). The science of meaning in life. *Annual Review of Psychology, 72,* 561–584.
King, L. A., Hicks, J. A., Krull, J. L., & Del Gaiso, A. K. (2006). Positive affect and the experience of meaning in life. *Journal of Personality and Social Psychology, 90,* 179–196.
Kim, E. S., Delaney, S. W., & Kubzansky, L. D. (2019). Sense of purpose in life and cardiovascular disease: Underlying mechanisms and future directions. *Current Cardiological Reports, 21,* 135.
Kim, E. S., Sun, J. K., Park, N., & Peterson, C. (2013). Purpose in life and reduced incidence of stroke in older adults: "The Health and Retirement Study." *Journal of Psychosomatic Research, 74,* 427–432.
Krause, N., & Hayward, R. D. (2014). Assessing stability and change in a second-order confirmatory factor model of meaning in life. *Journal of Happiness Studies, 15,* 237–253.
Kruglanski, A. W., Chen, X., Dechesne, M., Fishman, S., & Orehek, E. (2009). Fully committed: Suicide bomber's motivation and the quest for personal significance. *Political Psychology, 30,* 331–357.
Kruglanski, A. W., Jasko, K., Webber, D., Chernikova, M., & Molinario, E. (2018). The making of violent extremists. *Review of General Psychology, 22,* 107–120.
Laurin, K., Fitzsimons, G. M., & Kay, A. C. (2011). Social disadvantage and self-regulatory function of justice beliefs. *Journal of Personality and Social Psychology, 100,* 149–171.
Lepage, J., Bègue, L., Zerhouni, O., Dambrun, M., Vezirian, K., Besson, T., . . . Mermillod, M. (2022). Authoritarian attitudes are associated with higher autonomic reactivity to stress and lower recovery. *Emotion, 22,* 536–544.
Lerner, M. J. (1980). *The belief in a just world: A fundamental delusion.* Plenum Press.
Li, J., Dou, K., & Liang, Y. (2021). The relationship between presence of meaning, search for meaning, and subjective well-being: A three-level meta analysis based on the Meaning in Life Questionnaire. *Journal of Happiness Studies, 22,* 467–489.
Lipkus, I. M., Dalbert, C., & Siegler, I. C. (1996). The importance of distinguishing the belief in a just world for self versus other. *Personality and Social Psychology Bulletin, 22,* 666–667.
Manzi, C., Roccato, M., & Russo, S. (2015). Meaning buffers right-wing authoritarian responses to societal threat via the mediation of loss of perceived control. *Personality and Individual Differences, 83,* 117–121.
Martela, F., Ryan, R. M., & Steger, M. F. (2018). Meaningfulness as satisfaction of autonomy, competence, relatedness, and beneficence: Comparing the four satisfactions and positive affect as predictors of meaning in life. *Journal of Happiness Studies, 19,* 1261–1282.
Martela, F., & Steger, M. F. (2023). The role of significance relative to the other dimensions of meaning in life—An examination utilizing the three-dimensional meaning in life scale (3DM). *Journal of Positive Psychology, 18,* 606–626.
Mavor, K. I., Louis, W. R., & Sibley, C. G. (2010). A bias-corrected exploratory and confirmatory factor analysis of rightwing authoritarianism: Support for a 3-factor structure. *Personality and Individual Differences, 48,* 28–33.
McCoy, S. K., Wellman, J. D., Cosley, B., Saslow, L., & Epel, E. (2013). Is the belief in meritocracy palliative for members of low status groups?: Evidence for benefit for self-esteem and physical health via perceived control. *European Journal of Social Psychology, 43,* 307–318.
Murray, D. R., Schaller, M., & Suedfeld, P. (2013). Pathogens and politics: Further evidence that parasite prevalence predicts authoritarianism. *PLOS One, 8,* 1.
Napier, J., & Jost, J. T. (2008). Why are conservatives happier than liberals? *Psychological Science, 19,* 565–572.
Napier, J. L., Suppes, A., & Bettinsoli, M. L. (2020). Denial of gender discrimination is associated with better subjective well-being among women: A system justification account. *European Journal of Social Psychology, 50,* 1191–1209.
Nasser, R., Doumit, J., & Carifio, J. (2011). Well-being and belief in a just world among rest home residents. *Social Behavior and Personality, 39,* 655–670.
Newman, D. B., Schwarz, N., Graham, J., & Stone, A. A. (2019). Conservatives report greater meaning in life than liberals. *Social Psychological and Personality Science, 10,* 494–503.
Oishi, S., & Westgate, E. C. (2021). A psychologically rich life: Beyond happiness and meaning. *Psychological Review.*
Onraet, E., Van Assche, J., Roets, A., Haesevoets, T., & Van Hiel, A. (2017). The happiness gap between conservatives and liberals

depends on country-level threat: A worldwide multilevel study. *Social Psychological and Personality Science, 8,* 11–19.

Onraet, E., Van Heil, A., & Dhont, K. (2013). The relationship between right-wing ideological attitudes and psychological well-being. *Personality and Social Psychology Bulletin.*

Osborne, D., Costello, T. H., Duckitt, J., & Sibley, C. G. (2023). The psychological causes and societal consequences of authoritarianism. *Nature Reviews Psychology, 2,* 220–232.

Osborne, D., Sengupta, N. K., & Sibley, C. G. (2019). System justification theory at 25: Evaluating a paradigm shift in psychology and looking towards the future. *British Journal of Social Psychology, 58,* 340–361.

Park, C. L., Edmondson, D., Fenster, J. R., & Blank, T. O. (2008). Meaning making and psychological adjustment following cancer: The mediating roles of growth, life meaning and restored just-world beliefs. *Journal of Consulting and Clinical Psychology, 76,* 863–875.

Pew Research Center. (2024, April 9). *Changing partisan coalitions in a politically divided nations.* www.pewresearch.org/politics/2024/04/09/changing-partisan-coalitions-in-a-politically-divided-nation/.

Pyszczynski, T., Greenberg, J., Solomon, S., Arndt, J., & Schimel, J. (2004). Why do people need self-esteem?: A theoretical and empirical review. *Psychological Bulletin, 130,* 435–468.

Rankin, L. E., Jost, J. T., & Wakslak, C. J. (2009). System justification and the meaning of life: Are the existential benefits of ideology distributed unequally across racial groups? *Social Justice Research, 22,* 312–333.

Rosenberg, M. (1965). *Society and the adolescent self-image.* Princeton University Press.

Rothschild, Z. K., & Keefer, L. A. (2021). Meaningful outrage: Anger at injustice bolsters meaning for justice sensitive individuals. *European Journal of Social Psychology, 52,* 124–146.

Schlenker, B. R., Chambers, J. R., & Le, B. M. (2012). Conservatives are happier than liberals, but why?: Political ideology, personality, and life satisfaction. *Journal of Research in Personality, 46,* 127–146.

Scott, A., Schimel, J., & Sharp, M. (2021). Long live A(me)rica!: An examination of the interplay between nationalistic-symbolic immortality striving and belief in life after death. *Journal of Personality and Social Psychology, 120,* 861–881.

Seker, B. D. (2016). Evaluation of life satisfaction after the 2011 Van (Turkey) earthquake. *Social Behavior and Personality, 44,* 1409–1418.

Sengupta, N. K., Greaves, L. M., Osborne, D., & Sibley, C. G. (2017). The sigh of the oppressed: The palliative effects of ideology are stronger for people living in highly unequal neighbourhoods. *British Journal of Social Psychology, 56,* 437–454.

Shaffer, B., & Duckitt, J. (2013). The dimensional structure of people's fears, threats, and concerns and their relationship with right-wing authoritarianism and social dominance orientation. *International Journal of Psychology, 48,* 6–17.

Sheehy-Skeffington, J., & Thomsen, L. (2019). Egalitarianism: Psychological and socio-ecological foundations. *Current Opinion in Psychology, 32,* 146–152.

Sheldon, K. M. (2023). Conservatives report less autonomous work motivation and less intrinsic values than liberals, but are happier nonetheless: The explanatory role of psychological need-satisfaction. *Journal of Happiness Studies, 24,* 1533–1547.

Shiba, K., Kubzansky, L. D., Williams, D. R., Vanderweele, T. J., & Kim, E. S. (2022). Purpose in life and 8-year mortality by gender and race/ethnicity among older adults in the U.S. *Preventative Medicine, 164,* 107310.

Sibley, C. G., Wilson, M. S., & Duckitt, J. (2007). Antecedents of men's hostile and benevolent sexism: The dual roles of social dominance orientation and right-wing authoritarianism. *Personality and Social Psychology Bulletin, 33,* 160–172.

Stavrova, O., & Luhmann, M. (2016). Are conservatives happier than liberals? Not always and not everywhere. *Journal of Research in Personality, 63,* 29–35.

Steger, M. F., Frazier, P., Oishi, S., & Kaler, M. (2006). The meaning in life questionnaire: Assessing the presence of and search for meaning in life. *Journal of Counseling Psychology, 53,* 80–93.

Steger, M. F., Kashdan, T. B., Sullivan, B. A., & Lorentz, D. (2008). Understanding the search for meaning in life: Personality, cognitive style, and the dynamic between seeking and experiencing meaning. *Journal of Personality, 76,* 199–228.

Stephan, W. G. (2014). Intergroup anxiety: Theory, research, and practice. Personality and *Social Psychology Review, 18, 239–255.*

Stephan, W. G., Ybarra, O., & Morrison, K. R. (2009). Intergroup threat theory. In T. Nelson (Ed.), *Handbook of prejudice* (pp. 43–59). Erlbaum.

Steptoe, A., & Fancourt, D. (2019). Leading a meaningful life at older ages and its relationship with social engagement, prosperity, health, biology, and time use. *Proceedings of the National Academy of Sciences, 116,* 1207–1212.

Stillman, T. F., Lambert, N. M., Fincham, F. D., & Baumeister, R. F. (2011). Meaning as magnetic force: Evidence that meaning in life promotes interpersonal appeal. *Social Psychological and Personality Science, 2,* 13–20.

Suppes, A., Napier, J. L., & Van der Toorn, J. (2019). The palliative effects of system justification on the health and happiness of lesbian, gay, bisexual, and transgender individuals. *Personality and Social Psychology Bulletin, 45,* 372–388.

Taylor, P., Funk, C., & Craighill, P. (2006). *Are we happy yet?* Pew Research Center. http://pewresearch.org/pubs/301/are-we-happy-yet.

Thomsen, L., Green, E. G. T., & Sidanius, J. (2008). We will hunt them down: How social dominance orientation and right-wing authoritarianism fuel ethnic persecution of immigrants in fundamentally different ways. *Journal of Experimental Social Psychology, 44,* 1455–1464.

Tov, W., & Lee, H. W. (2016). A closer look at the hedonics of everyday meaning and satisfaction. *Journal of Personality and Social Psychology, 111,* 585–609.

van den Bos, K. (2009). Making sense of life: The existential self trying to deal with personal uncertainty. *Psychological Inquiry, 20,* 197–217.

Vargas-Salfate, S., Paez, D., Khan, S. S., Liu, J. H., & de Zuniga, H. G. (2018). System justification enhances well-being: A longitudinal analysis of the palliative function of system justification in 18 countries. *British Journal of Social Psychology, 57,* 567–590.

Wagoner, J. A., Belavadi, S., & Jung, J. (2017). Social identity uncertainty: Conceptualization, measurement, and construct validity. *Self and Identity, 16,* 505–530.

Ward, S. J., & King, L. A. (2016). Poor but happy? Money, mood, and experienced and expected meaning in life. *Social Psychological and Personality Science, 7,* 463–470.

Weise, D. R., Arciszewski, T., Verlhiac, J., Psyzczynski, T., & Greenberg, J. (2012). Terror management and attitudes towards immigrants: Differential effects of mortality salience for low and high right-wing authoritarians. *European Psychologist, 17,* 63–72.

Wilkinson, W. W. (2004). Religiosity, authoritarianism, and homophobia: A multidimensional approach. *International Journal for the Psychology of Religion, 14,* 55–67.

Wojcik, S., Hovasapian, A., Graham, J., Motyl, M., & Ditto, P. (2015). Conservatives report, but liberals display, greater happiness. *Science, 347,* 1243–1246.

Womick, J., Ecklekamp, J., Luzzo, S., Ward, S. J., Salamun, A., Baker, S. G., & King, L. A. (2021). The affective and existential effects of Hitler: Exposure to authoritarian values leads to lower positive affect, higher negative affect, and higher meaning in life. *PLOS One, 16,* 1–30.

Womick, J., & King, L. A. (2023). The existential threat of religious pluralism. *International Journal for the Psychology of Religion.*

Womick, J. J., Rothmund, T., Azevedo, F., King, L. A., & Jost, J. T. (2019). Group-based dominance and authoritarian aggression predict support for Donald Trump in the 2016 U.S. presidential election. *Social Psychological and Personality Science, 10,* 643–652.

Womick, J., Ward, S. J., Heintzelman, S. J., Woody, B., & King, L. A. (2019). The existential function of right-wing authoritarianism. *Journal of Personality, 87,* 1056–1073.

Womick, J., Woody, B., & King, L. A. (2021). Religious fundamentalism, right-wing authoritarianism, and meaning in life. *Journal of Personality, 90*(2), 277–293.

Zmigrod, L., Ebert, T., Gotz, F. M., & Rentfrow, P. J. (2021). The psychological and socio-political consequences of infectious diseases: Authoritarianism, governance, and nonzoonotic (human-to-human) infection transmission. *Journal of Social and Political Psychology, 2.*

CHAPTER 45

Science and Religion

Meaning-Making Tools Competing to Explain the World

Natalia Zarzeczna *and* Roosa Haimila

The relationship between science and religion has been the subject of numerous heated debates, with some arguing that the two are in conflict and others advocating for compatibility. Across history, discussions on the nature and conceptualization of this relationship have permeated academic and public spheres alike (see Rutjens & Preston, 2020, for an overview). In this chapter, we examine the assumption that one crucial reason behind such passionate care about science and religion is that each constitutes an important tool for meaning making.

Reality is difficult to grasp because it is filled with inconsistencies and uncertainties that disrupt one's expectations about life and what the world should look like. People strive for a coherent picture of reality and have existential concerns over how to lead a moral life and deal with the awareness that life inevitably ends. Indeed, a particularly enigmatic aspect of human life that shatters expectations of reality is the awareness of death. The inevitability of death triggers especially strong existential anxieties that may render life meaningless (Proulx & Heine, 2006; Vail & Horner, 2023). However, perceiving meaning is a core route to well-being, and as such, meaning is one of the most fundamental needs that humans strive to fulfill (Heine et al., 2006; King & Hicks, 2021). In this chapter, we examine the assumption that science and religion are powerful meaning-making tools that form belief systems or worldviews and ensure that perceived reality is coherent and existential anxieties are quashed, at least some of the time.

We suggest that science and religion have the power to fulfil the need for meaning by addressing epistemological (e.g., "How do we acquire knowledge?") and ontological questions (e.g., "What is the nature of being?") that aid understanding of human existence (e.g., "What is the meaning of life?"). As science and religion aim to address the same questions, the two may be seen in competition to provide accurate accounts of reality (Preston & Epley, 2009). This competition might be exacerbated by reliance on different epistemologies. But as humans strive for perceptions of coherence and unity, some may be able to resolve the epistemological and explanatory conflict between science and religion and see the two as compatible. Throughout this chapter, we examine how psychological meaning-making mechanisms utilize scientific and religious explanations of reality, ultimately shaping the nature of the relationship between science and religion.

SCIENCE AND RELIGION AS DISTINCT MEANING SOURCES

Science and religion are multifaceted constructs that can be conceptualized in many different ways. At first glance, there seems to be little overlap in the definitions of science and religion, as in principle they cover different areas of knowledge. In sociological terms, religion has been conceptualized as a system of beliefs and practices that establishes moral principles and a sense of community, and emphasizes the importance of sacredness, for example, in terms of connection to a god (Durkheim, 1912). As a belief system, its primary role is therefore to fulfill spiritual needs, guide moral behaviors, and provide existential meaning, but also to address epistemic needs for coherence and order (Geertz, 1973). Religion can also represent institutions that offer places of worship and guidance. In contrast, science is not a belief system by definition, but rather a cultural method of learning to accumulate knowledge and explain the natural world, serving primarily epistemic needs (McCauley, 2013; Rutjens & Preston, 2020). Science can be also conceptualized as an institution, encompassing different organizations engaging in research (Kiikeri & Ylikoski, 2004; Yilmaz & Bahçekapili, 2015). Although science and religion seem quite distinct, there is some overlap between them: Both can function as cultural authorities providing knowledge. Science and religion can therefore address similar needs through different routes. In theory, conceptual definitions of science and religion are largely distinct, like the definitions of other cultural knowledge systems, such as art or philosophy. However, unlike other systems, it seems that it is the relationship between science and religion that evokes disagreements and heated discussions. We suggest that one prominent psychological reason for such disagreements is that people use science and religion as meaning-making tools to understand the world.[1] As meaning-making tools the two become highly valued and personally important. Knowledge produced by science, religion, or both can be incorporated into unique valued worldviews providing meaning, and fulfilling epistemic and existential needs (Davoodi & Lombrozo, 2022; Preston & Epley, 2005, 2009).

Science and religion attempt to describe the world in orderly ways that can enhance perceptions that one's life and the environment make sense. This type of meaning refers to coherence, that is, basic understanding of how different entities in the world, such as events, objects, or people, relate to one another in expected ways (Heine et al., 2006; King & Hicks, 2021). Acquiring coherence can fulfill epistemic needs concerned with causal explanations of the natural environment and having control over it (Rutjens & Preston, 2020). Importantly, the other core facets of meaning are purpose, associated with having valued aims and direction in life, and existential significance, concerned with the belief that one's life matters in the grand scheme of things. Although coherence, purpose, and existential significance are all positively associated, existential significance has been found to be the most important facet in determining people's overall judgments about meaning in life (Costin & Vignoles, 2020). Indeed, as science and religion tap into "big-picture" existential questions concerning the origins and nature of life and the universe ("Where do we come from?"; "What happens when we die?"), the two should be able to fulfill existential needs, as long as they are incorporated into worldviews that provide holistic explanations of reality and a subjective sense of increased meaning (Preston, 2011; Proulx, 2020; Rutjens et al., 2013; Taves et al., 2018). Given this conceptualization, science and religion can be seen as meaning sources that complement each other in providing a complete and comprehensive picture of reality. Although both systems are used to fulfill both types of needs, science tends to serve more epistemic functions than religion does in providing causal explanations for natural phenomena, while religion more so than science provides existential functions concerned with morality and emotional support (Davoodi & Lombrozo, 2022), which we discuss in more detail in the morality section below.

Overall, science and religion are distinct sources of meaning, but each may be able to address epistemic and existential needs.

We argue that the extent to which different types of meaning can be derived from scientific and religious explanations of reality may differ across individuals and their ways of accommodating the salient differences in scientific and religious epistemology and explanation (Zarzeczna & Preston, 2025; Zarzeczna et al., 2024c).

EPISTEMOLOGICAL AND EXPLANATORY CONFLICT

So far, we have reviewed literature suggesting that science and religion have distinct definitions and cover different areas of knowledge, but both can address the need for meaning. However, the two are at times perceived to be in conflict. The point of contention between science and religion often arises because of salient epistemological differences. In principle, scientific epistemology relies on natural mechanisms and reason, logic, and systematic empirical methods to generate knowledge. Any scientific speculation or claims need to be clearly communicated, informed by logic, tested empirically, and independently verified by others to be accepted as true (Hanegraaff, 2013; Rutjens & Preston, 2020). This epistemology by definition thus stands in contradiction to religion, which focuses on supernatural forces, faith, authorities, and sacred scriptures that are believed to provide absolute knowledge communicated by supernatural entities. Religious knowledge can also be derived through personal revelation and intuition of what feels true (Hanegraaff, 2013). These differences in ways of knowing further result in discrepancies between scientific and religious explanations.

Unsurprisingly, the epistemological conflict has often brought contradictory conclusions about the nature of reality that are difficult to reconcile. For example, Charles Darwin's theory of species evolution stands in contradiction to the religious account of a god creating humans and animals in their present form at one point in time (Rutjens et al., 2018a), with recent studies still demonstrating that religious orthodoxy is associated with stronger evolution skepticism (Rutjens et al., 2022; but also see Elsdon-Baker, 2015). Based on such accounts derived from epistemological differences, one could conclude that science and religion are irreconcilable. Nevertheless, scientific and religious explanations do not exist in a psychological vacuum. As one of the most important human needs is to perceive the world as unified and coherent, people are continuously attempting to make meaning in the face of apparent inconsistencies (Proulx et al., 2012). Therefore, perceptions of conflict between science and religion can be either increased or attenuated depending on people's individual needs for meaning and the status of science and religion in society.

A NEED FOR MEANING

The world is inherently incomprehensible and absurd (Camus, 1955). However, there are psychological mechanisms that motivate humans to deal with inconsistencies encountered in the world. Informed by existentialist philosophy, the meaning maintenance model posits that people have a fundamental need for meaning—that is, coherence and perception of unity (Heine et al., 2006). This is reflected in cultural frameworks or worldviews that are constructed to provide coherent accounts of reality, and such frameworks indeed include science and religion. In turn, perceptions of meaning are highly predictive of increased well-being, health, and happiness (King & Hicks, 2021). The model relies on three assumptions. First, meaning is conceptualized as expected relations. In other words, there is a psychological need to form associations between elements in the world, and doing so organizes experiences in an orderly manner. Second, the construction of expected associations represents an innate predisposition to make meaning and see the world as coherent. Because of this innate capacity to impose meaning on the environment, humans are sensitive to meaning violations. Meaning violations happen when people are confronted with contradictions, ranging from basic cognitive inconsistencies, such as perceptual anomalies (playing cards with reverse colors, e.g., black hearts), to existential threats, such as death reminders (Proulx & Heine, 2006). Importantly, the experience of meaning violation is linked to aversive physiological arousal. In turn, this unpleasant state motivates engagement in palliative compensatory activities allowing a restoration of meaning (Proulx et al., 2012; Sleegers et al., 2021).

Third, violations to expected associations in one domain motivate compensatory pursuit of meaning in another intact domain (termed *fluid compensation*). One example of such compensation is increased commitment to or affirmation of one's beliefs following meaning loss in response to experiences not directly related to those beliefs, including existential threats or cognitive inconsistencies (Greenberg et al., 1986; Heine et al., 2006; Sleegers et al., 2015). Both science and religion, independently, provide explanations about the world that can quash such salient inconsistencies. In turn, such explanations can become highly valuable motivating defense strategies (Preston & Epley, 2005; Proulx & Inzlicht, 2012). We therefore suggest that the motivation to pursue and maintain meaning across different domains of life determines the extent to which one is motivated to see science and religion as equally useful or incompatible meaning-making tools.

MEANING SHAPES THE SCIENCE–RELIGION RELATIONSHIP

In the current section, we review literature on how science and religion can each function to satisfy the need for different types of meaning, and how this pursuit of meaning in different psychological domains shapes the relationship between science and religion. First, we discuss literature on how people pursue meaning through the endorsement of worldviews derived from scientific epistemology and religious doctrines. Second, we examine literature on how science and religion can offer existential insights into the nature of death and moral behaviors.

Worldviews: Science and Religion Beliefs

Recently, Zarzeczna and colleagues (2024c) tested whether worldviews built on science and religion, separately, could inform the subjective perception of the relationship between science and religion. Previous work conducted in the United States demonstrated especially strong compatibility perceptions when religious belief was also accompanied by greater belief in science (Johnson et al., 2023). Zarzeczna and colleagues aimed to extend these findings by measuring participants' beliefs in science and religion as distinct and independent meaning systems across three countries, with Christian and Muslim religious traditions: the United Kingdom, Netherlands, and Kazakhstan.

Regarding the researchers' predictions, on the one hand, it was possible to assume that compatibility perceptions were indeed a combination of independent positive attitudes toward science and religion (Johnson et al., 2023). Previously, researchers found that religious individuals in Western countries perceived strong compatibility between science and religion when considering "big-picture" questions (e.g., "What happens when we die?"; explaining the origins of life), with atheists endorsing conflict, and agnostics having moderate views (Leicht et al., 2022). This demonstrates that religious individuals may be able to overcome epistemological or explanatory inconsistencies between science and religion and see them both as useful meaning tools. On the other hand, however, while it was possible for religious believers to also believe in science, it might have been more difficult for strong science believers to endorse religious belief. For example, religious believers have been found to use explanatory coexistence, whereby seemingly contradictory beliefs are integrated or juxtaposed to explain the same phenomena using both supernatural and scientific explanations (Haimila, Metsähinen, et al., 2024; Legare & Shtulman, 2018). In contrast, strong reliance on science as a way of knowing implies strict adherence to physical laws, natural causal mechanisms, and objectivity. This may leave no room to incorporate religious belief focused on supernatural mechanisms and intuition into a knowledge system prioritizing empirical data.

Zarzeczna and colleagues (2024c) therefore hypothesized that religious belief, independently of belief in science, would predict science–religion compatibility perceptions, while belief in science, independently of religious belief, would predict conflict perceptions. They found support for these hypotheses. A subsequent study then replicated these findings using unobtrusive physiological measures that excluded the possibility that belief in compatibility among religious individuals was due to social desirability (Zarzeczna et al., 2024d). Overall, religious believers likely combine science and religion as two explanatory tools to understand reality, while science believers apply science. Exploring this further, they found that intellectual humility, that is, the acknowledgement that one's knowledge has limits, significantly predicted compatibility beliefs when controlling for religiosity. Interestingly, the link between intellectual humility and compatibility beliefs was particularly pronounced for moderately-to-highly religious individuals (Preston et al., 2025).

Zarzeczna and colleagues (2024c) also examined whether compatibility views were a combination of positive attitudes toward science and religion, separately. Yet their analysis revealed that belief in science was negatively related to religious belief, and this association was linear. Indeed, exposure to scientific and religious learning and behaviors in childhood predicts the extent to which one makes sense of the world using either religious or scientific worldviews (Park et al., 2024; also see Ma et al., 2024). The negative association between scientific and religious belief may be because religious individuals see science and religion as accurate ways of knowing, but neither can fully explain the world. In contrast, nonreligious individuals appear to see high value in science only (Jackson et al., 2024; Longest & Uecker, 2021). That is, religious individuals likely use both science and religion as useful meaning-making tools to satisfy epistemic and existential needs, whereas nonreligious individuals seem to only rely on science. However, for nonreligious individuals and those who strongly believe in science, it is unclear whether science alone can actually satisfy their existential needs.

Pursuit of Meaning in Life

Religion Advantage

Folk and colleagues (2024) explored the issue of whether science or religion was associated with stronger existential benefits by measuring the extent to which belief in science (as the best epistemology) and religious belief, among other variables, predicted meaning in life in terms of coherence, purpose, and existential significance. Religious belief strongly predicted all aspects of meaning in life (Folk et al., 2024). Interestingly, belief in science was negatively associated with all dimensions of meaning in life among the general public, while it was not significantly related to any facets of meaning in life among scientists. Although belief in science was not associated with meaning in life, belief in scientific optimism, that is, the idea that science can improve life, predicted greater existential significance and coherence. Indeed, not all aspects of attitudes toward science reduce meaning. It seems that it is scientific materialism--the idea that human life can be broken down into organic components and processes--that leads to lower meaning in life, especially in terms of existential significance (Tracy et al., 2024). In contrast, the same is not true for reminders of scientific progress. Importantly, the effect of scientific materialism on existential significance was only significant for nonreligious individuals. Possibly, religious individuals derive significance from religious belief and hence are buffered from threats to existential meaning posed by scientific materialism and reductionism (Tracy et al., 2024).

Overall, it appears that believers in science might not experience an increased sense of meaning from believing in scientific epistemology or scientific materialism, but an optimistic outlook on science and scientific progress might help gain similar existential advantage to religious believers who gaining meaning from religious epistemology. Importantly, it is also possible that not everyone has a high need to fulfill existential needs through seeing greater meaning in life. In fact, evidence shows that there is a strong association between the need for meaning in life and religious belief (Abeyta & Routledge, 2018), in line with Freud's early suggestions that religious belief encourages and serves the need to find answers to existential questions and the meaning of life (Freud, 1939; Parsons, 2021). In a similar vein, while religiosity is consistently decreasing in Western countries, this decrease has not been accompanied by a similar decline in meaning in life and well-being over time (Zarzeczna et al., 2024a).

Overall, although religious belief is correlated with existential benefits, it might be that religious individuals are inclined to seek existential meaning, with secular individuals and believers in science finding meaning through other routes, including everyday experiences, interpersonal relationships, personal goals, or—importantly—other components of science attitudes, such as scientific optimism. Yet it is clear that scientific materialism reduces existential meaning in nonreligious individuals. Intriguingly, there are also other aspects of attitudes toward science that may contribute to meaning in life, such as viewing science as revealing the beauty of the natural world and highlighting one's tangible connections to it.

Science Advantage

Feelings of connection to the natural world may play a key role in perceptions of greater unity for some individuals. As noted earlier, meaning concerns perceiving elements in the world and oneself to be connected in expected ways. Although science by definition is an epistemology focused on objectivity and empirical observation to causally explain natural phenomena, the experience of uncovering and learning about scientific discoveries is more than that: It can inspire strong emotions of awe, interconnection, and a deep sense of meaning (Preston et al., 2023). These experiences are traditionally attributed to spirituality. In fact, spirituality is typically associated with experiences evoked by religious practices, including prayer, rituals, or religious music. These practices result in highly personal and inner experiences with entities deemed as sacred. In fact, spiritual experiences inspire the impression that one has reached ultimate meaning and connection with entities that transcend the material world (Hanegraaff, 2013; Preston & Shin, 2017).

However, contemporary spirituality has become a meaning system independent from religion and science, as it is primarily focused on individualized, inner, and subjective epistemology, relying on the assumption that truth can be found within oneself (Rutjens et al., 2022; Rutjens & van der Lee, 2020; Zarzeczna et al., 2023a). Although spiritual epistemology rejects scientific and religious ways of knowing, it utilizes religious faith *in practice,* that is, the belief that one can find divine properties within one's soul, and scientific reason *in theory,* as the mind and reason are necessary to take the final step to experiencing ultimate spiritual meaning (Hanegraaff, 2013).

Although spiritual epistemology is linked to supernatural beliefs about reaching meaning that transcends the material world, nonreligious individuals also report experiencing spirituality through secular sources, such as science (Preston & Shin, 2017). Indeed, atheists and agnostics can experience spirituality of science and find existential meaning through science (Preston et al., 2023). Spirituality of science is defined as feelings of awe, interconnection between oneself and the world, and meaning evoked by thoughts about science, scientific theories, or discoveries, illustrating the beauty of the world. Greater spirituality of science is linked to increased meaning in life and emotional well-being, demonstrating that certain components of science attitudes have similar existential benefits to religion. Supporting these findings, another study found that individuals who were science-oriented reported gaining a sense of meaning in life and awe through science (Haimila, 2020).

To summarize, in this section, we reviewed literature on how the need for meaning-making motivates people to use science and religion as tools to explain reality. Evidence demonstrates that the perceived relationship between science and religion depends on how strongly one believes in science and in religion, as separate meaning sources, with belief in science being linked to low religious belief. Although atheists and strong believers in science see science and religion as in conflict, religious believers tend to see high compatibility and hence possibly utilize each as useful meaning sources. Furthermore, religious belief, but not belief in science, predicts stronger meaning in life. At the same time, secular individuals in particular can experience spiritual meaning through science. The way these psychological tendencies interact with religious and scientific meaning-making tools also depends on exposure to science and religion in childhood.

In the next section, we consider the extent to which science and religion interact when utilized as meaning-making tools to alleviate existential concerns surrounding death.

MORTALITY AWARENESS

Few things are as strongly associated with religion in popular and scholarly imaginations as death. In fact, studies on afterlife beliefs and managing fear of death often focus on religious belief and practice (Haimila & Muraja, 2023). This is not surprising, because religious beliefs often offer comforting reassurance and explanation about humans transcending death and continuing life in another dimension (see Vail et al., Chapter 52, this volume, for a thorough discussion on this topic). It could be argued that religion is uniquely helpful in managing death anxiety by giving people meaning and hope for afterlife. This suggests that religion more so than science may be useful in alleviating mortality concerns, with religion tapping into spiritual afterlife directly reducing the fear of death. Yet it is also possible that certain aspects of belief in science may offer existentially comforting responses to the problem of death.

Terror Management Theory

Terror management theory (TMT) posits that the primary motivation underlying human cultural behavior is fear of death—or rather the need to suppress the possibly debilitating awareness of one's own mortality (Greenberg et al., 1986). This is because humans have an innate desire to live, and this desire is threatened by the awareness that death is inevitable. Importantly, TMT argues that to assuage this existential anxiety, humans can lean on a variety of buffers, including socially shared worldviews that offer a type of permanency (Solomon et al., Chapter 6, this volume; Vail et al., Chapter 52, this volume). In typical mortality salience studies, participants are asked to write down their thoughts about feelings evoked by mortality and what happens to them when they physically die. Participants in the control condition are asked to write about a topic that is not related to death, such as dental pain, and after a short delay, a target worldview measure is presented (Arrowood & Cox, 2020).

Religion and Science Alleviate Existential Anxiety

Many have suggested that religious belief is rather unique in offering literal permanency, via existential significance and supernatural afterlife. Accordingly, ample research shows that religious belief can effectively quash anxiety evoked by mortality awareness (e.g., Jong et al., 2012; Vail et al., 2012, 2019). Given that religious belief can alleviate death concerns, we could predict that there should be a strong relationship between levels of religiosity and death anxiety. That is, experiencing death anxiety might motivate religious beliefs, but religious belief in turn reduces death anxiety, altogether resulting in a curvilinear relationship (Ellis & Wahab, 2013). Yet a recent review of the literature suggests mostly a weak or absent association between religious belief and death anxiety (Jong, 2021). In other words, we know that religious belief can reduce death anxiety, but this does not result in a straightforward relationship between death anxiety and religious belief. Indeed, other research indicates that factors such as social learning also contribute to levels of religious belief (Gervais et al., 2021), and people also rely on other culturally shared worldviews for existential relief, as suggested by TMT.

This brings us to belief in science as a potential solution to the existential problem of death. Can people also turn to their science-related beliefs to tackle death anxiety? Some studies have aimed to answer this question, utilizing the mortality salience paradigm and examining whether people turn to science when reminded of mortality. Such studies have investigated whether mortality salience increases trust in science (like it has increased belief in God in religious individuals), or whether affirming scientific concepts decreases reliance on other common defenses following reminders of mortality (Farias et al., 2013; Lifshin et al., 2018; Tracy et al., 2011; Vail et al., 2020). Interestingly, some studies have found that, similar to belief in

God, belief in science increases after people have been reminded of mortality (Farias et al., 2013; Tracy et al., 2011, Study 5).

In a similar vein, affirming science-related concepts can reduce the need to turn to other existential reliefs. For instance, affirming the possibility of medical indefinite life extension (MILE) has reduced the likelihood of increased belief in an afterlife following mortality salience (for nonreligious individuals and atheists, see the latter part of this section; Lifshin et al., 2018; Vail et al., 2020). Similarly, experiencing mortality awareness has increased the endorsement of scientific theories and authority for biology students (Tracy et al., 2011). These results suggest that belief in science (or scientific innovations) can mitigate concern over mortality in similar ways as belief in God or an afterlife.

However, mortality salience has not increased belief in science in all relevant studies (see Rutjens et al., 2016; Tracy et al., 2011). Indeed, it might be that belief in science only alleviates concern over mortality for *some* individuals. More specifically, belief in MILE has (to our knowledge) only buffered existential anxiety in nonreligious individuals (Lifshin et al., 2018), and mortality salience has only bolstered belief in science in samples of individuals who are particularly likely to value scientific research, such as biology students (Tracy et al., 2011) and other academic participants (Farias et al., 2013; Haimila et al., 2024).

Still, why might belief in science alleviate existential concern over death at all, as it is not commonly thought to provide continuity after death (the way religious belief does)? And why might science serve this existential function for some individuals and not others? These questions relate to the possible mechanisms underlying the existential functions of beliefs more generally. One perspective is that belief in science could sometimes "replace" religion. In this "belief replacement hypothesis," belief in science can similarly fulfill the existential function (for nonreligious individuals) that is fulfilled by religion for religious believers (Farias, 2013; Farias et al., 2013; for discussion, see Haimila, 2023b). As we mentioned, some findings indeed suggest that trust in science or scientific innovation only alleviates mortality salience for nonreligious individuals (Lifshin et al. 2018; see also Farias et al., 2013). However, other findings indicate that people can rely on their belief in science regardless of religiosity *if* their worldview and/or social surroundings encourages a science-oriented identity (Tracy et al., 2011)—albeit the research is so scarce there is a need for further evidence (Haimila et al., 2025). In any case, findings on religious individuals at times also turning to science to alleviate death anxiety indicate that social learning and identities might also play a role in the existential function of belief in science (Haimila et al., 2024; Stavrova et al., 2016)—that is, belief in science as an existential relief is not limited to nonreligious individuals "replacing" religion with science or other secular frameworks. Furthermore, it could be said that individuals who were never religious might not need to "replace" religion (which they never had) but rather need *something* that offers a meaningful and permanence-promising worldview (see also Farias et al., 2013). Indeed, aside from science, nonreligious individuals may derive meaning from other secular sources such as humanism or caring for nature (Coleman et al., 2019; van Mulukom et al., 2023).

Interestingly, belief in science as one secular meaning source can also be seen in what nonreligious people think happens upon death. Recent studies suggest that some secular beliefs about continuity after death are intertwined with scientific terminology and theories. These constitute science-oriented beliefs about symbolic (albeit quite physical) immortality, for instance, that humans "live on" in the cycle of nature through the decomposition of the body, or that after death we continue as energy, with a reference to the law of conservation of energy in the universe (Haimila & Muraja, 2023; Manning, 2023; Miller & Beaman, 2024). However, even if people hold beliefs that integrate science into their existential worlds, this does not mean that science answers death-related (or other) existential concerns due to scientific findings being apt for this purpose—humans might simply be motivated to use *any* socially valued content as a meaning-making tool.

In a similar vein, in a recent study, Zarzeczna and Preston (2025) aimed at testing whether components of science attitudes focused on high-level transcendent meaning could alleviate mortality awareness in nonreligious individuals who valued science as a way of knowing. They recruited a large sample of secular individuals from the United States and the United Kingdom and randomly assigned participants to either a mortality salience prime condition (where they wrote about death) or a control condition (where they wrote about dental pain). After a short filler task, the researchers measured spirituality of science. Contrary to their predictions, they found no moderate evidence against differences in spirituality of science between conditions. Hence, the capacity to experience a deep sense of meaning through science may not function to alleviate existential concern over death. After conducting an exploratory post-hoc qualitative analysis of participants' responses in the writing task, they found that only 35% of participants reported being explicitly afraid of death and feeling existentially anxious in response to thoughts about death, and 29% reported being explicitly not afraid, with the rest reporting feelings of sadness, or conflicting feelings (sadness/relief). It is therefore unclear whether the results reflect the inability of deep meaning from science to buffer death anxiety (for the participants) or whether the conventional mortality awareness prime did not suffice to elicit existential anxiety over death (e.g., Treger et al., 2023).

Overall, research indicates that religious beliefs and science-related beliefs may each function as tools to alleviate existential concern over mortality, but only for some individuals under certain circumstances. Religious belief in God can be used to alleviate concern over death in religious individuals, while scientific belief is utilized when science-oriented identities are socially encouraged, and especially in nonreligious individuals when scientific theories are important for one's understanding of reality and provide a sense of life extension. But an emerging study found spirituality of science (awe, interconnectedness, meaning) may not buffer against mortality awareness. These findings suggest a myriad of nuances that certainly warrant additional studies.

MORAL CONCERNS

Morality refers to judgments of what is right or wrong, and moral principles are seen as important guides for human behavior. Religion has commonly been seen as an important source or even the backbone of morality. Many people around the world think that one must believe in God in order to be a moral person (Pew Research Center, 2020, p. 3). This belief about religiosity seems to be in obvious contrast with people's beliefs about science. Science has often been characterized as amoral and an institution not concerned with directing people's values (Rutjens & Heine, 2016). Is there therefore no overlap between religious beliefs and belief in science when it comes to the domain of morality? Although this could be expected, findings in existential psychology indicate that the relationship between religious belief, belief in science, and (other) secular beliefs might be more complex than previously thought when it comes to morality.

Religious Morality

In line with common stereotypes, some research has recently found that scientific explanations might not be associated with a moral function in the same way that religion is associated with morality (Davoodi & Lombrozo, 2022). More specifically, U.S. participants were less likely to associate moral virtue with scientific explanations of suffering, death, and the origin of universe than with religious explanations for the same phenomena. In the study, moral virtue referred to an explanation potentially changing the world for the better in terms of morality ("If everyone believed this, the world would be a kinder place" and "If everyone believed this, the world would be a more moral place"). In other words, based on the findings, it seems likely that U.S. adults perceive agreement about science as less relevant for morality and kindness than agreement about religion. This result does not seem surprising—people might not generally associate science with "kindness" or think that science of our cosmological origins or death would change the world for better if people only believed in them.[2] But is this all there is to belief in science being (or not being) relevant for the domain of morality? And, furthermore, what about people's views about science and its relationship with morality outside the United States?

Scientific Morality

A somewhat differing approach to investigating the relationship between science and morality is presented by studies asking people to indicate what they believe provides them with moral values. Findings indicate that some individuals believe that moral values ("right and wrong") should be informed by science and critical reasoning—we should strive for a "rational morality" (Haimila et al., 2025). One such view leans on the ability of scientific research to inform us about what increases human well-being and decreases suffering. This is seen as key to determining "right" and "wrong" by several nonreligious proponents of science-based morality (Haimila, 2020; Harris, 2010).

How common is it to think that we can use science in this way to decipher what is morally right? In a poll conducted by Pew Research Center (2015), 1 in 10 U.S. adults stated that they mainly rely on science "for guidance on questions of right and wrong" (Galen, 2021). In nonreligious adults, primarily looking to science for guidance on right and wrong was more common, albeit still quite rare (17% of nonaffiliated U.S. Americans). Indeed, it seems to be more likely for nonreligious individuals to lean on other sources of morality instead of science. A recent study (Haimila et al., 2025) investigated what nonreligious individuals who do not believe in God perceive as the source of their morality, with samples recruited from 10 countries. Nontheistic individuals most often thought that "right and wrong" come from others around us or society, for instance from "the social contract." Fewer nontheists mentioned science or related concepts (such as critical reasoning) as the source of their right and wrong (Caldwell-Harris et al., 2011; Haimila et al., 2025).

Morality Tools

Even among nonreligious nontheists, relatively few believe that science provides answers to the questions of right and wrong. Some research indicates that instead of framing science as a source for moral values, it might be more common for people to perceive scientific knowledge as a *tool* for morality (Haimila, 2020). In practice, proponents of such a view have suggested that although people often believe their values do not come from science (but rather, for instance, from humanism or religion), they can use science to determine what actions they should take to *realize* their values—for example, how they should raise their children in order for them to become happy adults or how to best prevent suffering by fighting climate change (Haimila, 2020, 2023). In practice, such views resemble the previously mentioned suggestion that science can help determine what is "right" by informing individuals about actions increasing or decreasing human well-being. The difference seems to be that some of the people endorsing this view regard science as a *tool* for informing or implementing morality, rather than a *source* of "right and wrong." Interestingly, preliminary findings suggest that the view on science as a *tool* for morality could be shared by both nonreligious and religious individuals, at least in cultural contexts where people generally trust science (Haimila, 2020, 2023a). Overall, it might be more common for people to perceive that science plays an important role in moral *actions* rather than deciphering moral *values* (what is good and bad, or right and wrong).

Interestingly, however, looking to scientific knowledge as a source for moral values is not the only narrative where science contributes to the source of morality. One recurring nontheistic view about right and wrong is that morality stems from human evolution (Haimila et al., 2025; Lee, 2015). According to these views, humans have evolved to be a social species, which underlies human empathy and prosocial behavior—our "inherent" ability to distinguish right from wrong. In other words, scientific theories seem to help some individuals understand *why* humans can be moral even when science in itself is not perceived as a source of right and wrong (Haimila et al., 2025; for similar notions in research on phylogeny of morality, see Beit-Hallahmi, 2010; de Waal, 2013).

An additional approach to the possible moral function of belief in science can be found in experimental studies looking into moral sensitivity. More specifically, some work has investigated whether reminders of science bolster people's sensitivity to moral violations, similar to religion (Ma-Kellams & Blascovich, 2013; Yilmaz & Bahçekapili, 2015). As one example, Yilmaz and Bahçekapili (2015) found that in Turkish university students, moral violations were more harshly judged had the participants been reminded of science; for example, students were harsher toward a hypothetical person who, they were told, ran over a cat and then fled the scene. In a replication of their study, Yilmaz and Bahçekapili further found that the effect of science reminders on moral sensitivity was likely driven by perceiving science as a secular authority (as opposed to activating analytical thinking; see Study 3).

If science is generally seen as amoral, why might it function as a secular authority that bolsters moral sensitivity, or a potential source of right and wrong, if only for a small group of individuals? One potential answer might be derived from the findings of Davoodi and Lombrozo (2022), who, as discussed earlier in this chapter, examined belief in science potentially serving epistemic and nonepistemic functions, including one related to moral virtue. Although science was primarily associated with epistemic functions (in practice, epistemic virtue) and religion with nonepistemic functions, Davoodi and Lombrozo noted that some people simply tended to assign nonepistemic functions to explanations they were dedicated to—possibly explaining why scientific explanations were also deemed by some to potentially increase morality in the world. Another option, based on the research presented here, is that some people truly perceive moral virtues in scientific explanations not merely because they believe in science, but because they see the *contents* and methods of science as practically valuable when it comes to determining the underlying causes of morality, moral values, and/or the right course of action. These two options, of course, may not be mutually exclusive (Davoodi & Lombrozo, 2022).

Overall, it looks like science can serve as a tool for making sense of morality and informing moral actions and, at times, act as a morality-related secular authority. The findings on science and morality we have introduced demonstrate that *in some cases* science can fulfill these morality-related existential functions previously associated with religion. Although such cases are interesting, people still are more likely to associate religion than science with morality.

CONSEQUENCES

Evidence suggests that science and religion can each serve as a meaning-making tool to fulfill an important psychological function of quashing the world's incomprehensibility through explanatory frameworks and solving the mysteries surrounding existential concerns over death and morality. Despite these benefits, the nature of the perceived relationship between the two may not always lead to benefits but may sometimes present challenges for societal functioning.

Religion–Science Incompatibility Stereotypes Negatively Impact Believers

Studies investigating intergroup processes demonstrated that perceptions of conflict between science and religion may negatively impact individuals identifying as religious. Importantly, whereas religious individuals view religious scientists as stereotypical, atheists tend to see religious scientists as having a counterstereotypical combination of identities (Sharp et al., 2022). Such perceptions, in turn, can lead to negative consequences. When science was presented as incompatible versus compatible with Christianity, Christian participants underperformed on scientific reasoning tasks due to stereotype threat (Rios, 2021). Further, perceptions of incompatibility between science and Christianity among nonreligious individuals predicted views of Christians as less intelligent and lacking the ability to engage in science. These negative stereotypes were reduced when science–Christianity compatibility was made salient (Mackey et al., 2023). That is, changing the perception that science and religion are always in conflict can reduce the negative impact of stereotypes linking religious individuals with poor scientific ability. Benefits of compatibility views for religious believers extend even further, with a recent large-scale study conducted among believers across 54 countries indicating that beliefs in compatibility between science and religion predict greater well-being (Price & Johnson, 2024).

Religion–Science Incompatibility Belief Can Lead to Science Rejection

Another relevant societal issue associated with perceptions of the science–religion relationship is science skepticism. The systematic and unwarranted rejection of scientific evidence presents a global challenge often leading to catastrophic consequences for many aspects of life (Rutjens et al., 2018a, 2018b; Većkalov et al., 2024).

Historically, scientific theories at times came into explicit conflict with religious doctrines. As a result, religious believers may often be skeptical about science. Many studies have found, however, that religious belief does not systematically predict science skepticism around the globe (Rutjens et al., 2022). While religious individuals have more negative attitudes toward science in the United States, the same is not true in other countries (McPhetres et al., 2020). Interestingly, religious individuals across cultures, similarly to secular individuals, are more likely to trust scientific sources of information as compared to spiritual gurus (Hoogeveen et al., 2022) or governments (Zarzeczna et al., 2024b). In some countries, such as Finland, religious individuals tend to trust science more than the teachings of their own religion (Wellcome, 2018). Yet there seems to be a robust link between religious belief and low belief in science as a way of knowing, as well as between religious orthodoxy and rejection of evolution (Rutjens et al., 2022; Rutjens et al., 2018b; Zarzeczna et al., 2024c). Similarly, traditional spirituality predicts low belief in science, but unlike religiosity, it also involves stronger levels of vaccination rejection uniquely (Rutjens et al., 2022; Zarzeczna et al., 2023a, 2023b).

The underlying mechanisms that drive these negative associations between science skepticism and religious and spiritual beliefs are not well understood. It is possible that these associations are driven by intergroup processes and social-identity concerns, whereby skeptical worldviews become normative among meaningful social groups to religious individuals (Rutjens & Hornsey, 2024). This suggests that religious beliefs may not be inherently opposed to science, but psychological processes involved in a pursuit of meaningful social norms result in religious or spiritual belief overtly predicting science skepticism at times.

To summarize, while religious belief does not systematically predict science rejection, there is evidence demonstrating that religiosity and spirituality entail increased rejection of evolution, vaccination, and belief in science as a way of knowing. Furthermore, although religious individuals themselves perceive a combination of scientific and religious identities as intuitive, they are often negatively stereotyped as having poor scientific abilities. This stereotype, in turn, is associated with perceptions that science and religion are in conflict. Overall, the relationship between science and religion is important not only for individual meaning making but also for societal functioning. These consequences should be explored further in future research.

SUMMARY: IS THE SCIENCE–RELIGION RELATIONSHIP STILL ROCKY?

Previous literature identified four theoretical conceptualizations of the relationship between science and religion (Barbour, 1998; Zein et al., 2024). First, science and religion can be seen as distinct systems that use different epistemologies and are bound to produce conflicting conclusions about the nature of reality. Second, the two can be seen as compatible, with science explaining the processes and religion tapping into distal causes. Third, science and religion can cover different knowledge areas; science, for instance, taps into epistemic needs of understanding the natural world, while religion satisfies the existential need for meaning in life. Fourth, science and religion are neither separate nor in conflict/compatibility but rather should be in dialogue. Importantly, Rutjens and Preston (2020) argued that the relationship between science and religion is rocky because it is shaped by shared psychological functions for understanding, order, and meaning. The way these functions are satisfied through distinct underlying assumptions determines the conceptualization of conflict, compatibility, or separation between the two. These distinct assumptions also result in different levels of success that each system achieves in fulfilling each function.

Our chapter echoes the view that science and religion share important psychological functions. Yet we primarily argue it is the individualized way of meaning making that ultimately shapes the relationship between science and religion. The successful implementation or usefulness of science and religion mainly depends on psychological characteristics involved in pursuing different aspects of meaning, including religiosity, belief in science, intellectual humility, sources of spirituality, and the extent to which one needs meaning in life. In turn, the success of these psychological dispositions in facilitating meaning making through science or religion is shaped by cultural exposure to scientific and religious learning. Further, we argue that neither science nor religion is psychologically superior in alleviating existential concerns over death or informing what is right or wrong. Again, each can be used depending on individualized ways of finding meaning shaped by social and cultural contexts.

In practice, science and religion are tools for meaning making that are unconstrained by their theoretical definitions and predefined roles. As such, some individuals perceive science and religion as compatible and each as useful, while others see the two as in conflict, using just one as a useful tool (Zarzeczna et al., 2024c). One conclusion that emerges from the literature is that when science and religion are conceptualized as belief systems or worldviews, they are negatively associated with each other, resulting in distinct consequences for perceptions of science–religion compatibility. Hence, scientific and religious worldviews are more likely in conflict than they are compatible.

Finally, while science and religion as meaning-making tools can positively satisfy individual needs for meaning, the nature of the perceived relationship between science and religion may, at times, have negative consequences for society, including stereotyping and science rejection. We believe that these consequences should be the focus of future research in the psychology of science and religion.

Overall, we echo Rutjens and Preston's (2020) conclusions and suggest that the science–religion relationship remains rocky, but it is most likely determined by individualized ways of utilizing science and religion as meaning-making tools within one's valued social and cultural context.

CONCLUSION

The question about science–religion compatibility or conflict has been at the center of many heated public and academic debates across history. In theory, science and religion can cover different areas of knowledge, be complementary, be in dialogue, or use conflicting epistemologies depending on how they fulfil psychological needs for meaning, understanding, and explanation (Rutjens & Preston, 2020). In this chapter, we argued that in practice science and religion constitute meaning-making tools that are used to form valued worldviews, alleviate mortality concerns, and inform morality. The question of whether science and religion are compatible or in conflict will remain a philosophical one with no straightforward answer. Nevertheless, psychological evidence indicates that the extent to which science and religion are compatible or in conflict depends on how one utilizes each system as a useful tool to make meaning within their social and cultural environment.

NOTES

1. Beyond psychological motivations, the narrative about science–religion conflict has roots in historical conceptualizations of science in relation to religion in Western countries. In the 19th century, the term *science* was constructed in opposition to *religion*, whereby science was meant to be distinct from natural philosophy and knowledge of the clergy (Harrison, 2010).

2. There is even research indicating people perceive scientists as having an increased risk of moral violation (Rutjens & Heine, 2016).

REFERENCES

Abeyta, A. A., & Routledge, C. (2018). The need for meaning and religiosity: An individual differences approach to assessing existential needs and the relation with religious commitment, beliefs, and experiences. *Personality and Individual Differences, 123*, 6–13.

Arrowood, R. B., & Cox, C. R. (2020). Terror management theory: A practical review of research and application. *Brill Research Perspectives in Religion and Psychology, 2*(1), 1–83.

Barbour, I. G. (1998). *Religion and science: Historical and contemporary issues* (rev., exp. ed.). SCM Press.

Beit-Hallahmi, B. (2010). Morality and immorality among the irreligious. In P. Zuckerman (Ed.), *Atheism and secularity: Global expressions* (Vol. 1, pp. 122–129). Praeger.

Caldwell-Harris, C. L., Wilson, A. L., LoTempio, E., & Beit-Hallahmi, B. (2011). Exploring the atheist personality: Well-being, awe, and magical thinking in atheists, Buddhists, and Christians. *Mental Health, Religion and Culture, 14*(7), 659–672.

Camus, A. (1955). *The myth of Sisyphus*. Penguin Books.

Coleman, T. J., III, Sevinç, K., Hood, R. W., & Jong, J. (2019). An atheist perspective on self-esteem and meaning making while under death awareness. *Secular Studies, 1*(2), 204–228.

Costin, V., & Vignoles, V. L. (2020). Meaning is about mattering: Evaluating coherence, purpose, and existential mattering as precursors of meaning in life judgments. *Journal of Personality and Social Psychology, 118*(4), 864–884.

Davoodi, T., & Lombrozo, T. (2022). Explaining the existential: Scientific and religious explanations play different functional roles. *Journal of Experimental Psychology: General, 151*(5), 1199–1218.

de Waal, F. (2013). *The Bonobo and the atheist: In search of humanism among the primates*. Norton.

Durkheim, E. (1912). *Elementary forms of the religious life, a study in religious sociology*. Lulu Com.

Ellis, L., & Wahab, E. A. (2013). Religiosity and fear of death: A theory-oriented review of the empirical literature. *Review of Religious Research, 55*(1), 149–189.

Elsdon-Baker, F. (2015). Creating creationists: The influence of "issues framing" on our understanding of public perceptions of clash narratives between evolutionary science and belief. *Public Understanding of Science, 24*(4), 422–439.

Farias, M. (2013). The psychology of atheism. In S. Bullivant & M. Ruse (Eds.), *The Oxford handbook of atheism* (p. 17). Oxford University Press.

Farias, M., Newheiser, A.-K., Kahane, G., & de Toledo, Z. (2013). Scientific faith: Belief in science increases in the face of stress and existential anxiety. *Journal of Experimental Social Psychology, 49*(6), 1210–1213.

Folk, D., Rutjens, B. T., Van Elk, M., & Heine, S. J. (2024). Dare to know!: The existential costs of a faith in science. *Journal of Positive Psychology*.

Freud, S. (1939). *Totem and taboo*. Routledge.

Galen, L. (2021). Morality, prosociality, and nonreligion. In J. M. Smith & R. T. Cragun (Section Eds.), *Bloomsbury religion in North America* (pp. 135–141). Bloomsbury.

Geertz, C. (1973). *The interpretation of cultures: Selected essays*. Basic Books.

Gervais, W. M., Najle, M. B., & Caluori, N. (2021). The origins of religious disbelief: A dual inheritance approach. *Social Psychological and Personality Science, 12*(7), 1369–1379.

Greenberg, J., Pyszczynski, T., & Solomon, S. (1986). The causes and consequences of a need for self-esteem: A terror management theory. In R. F. Baumeister (Ed.), *Public self and private self* (pp. 189–212). Springer.

Haimila, R. (2020). Does a science-oriented worldview entail unbelief?: Meaning, morality, and continuity from scientific research in self-reports of Finnish unbelievers and believers. *Secular Studies, 2*(2), 83–116.

Haimila, R. (2023a). *Beyond scientific worldviews: Belief in science and "supernatural" explanations in science-oriented individuals*. Doctoral dissertation, University of Helsinki.

Haimila, R. (2023b). Walking the walk of religion and nonreligion: Notes on Turpin's unholy Catholic Ireland: Religious hypocrisy, secular morality, and Irish irreligion. *Religion, Brain and Behavior*.

Haimila, R., Metsähinen, H., & Sevalnev, M. (2024). Supernatural belief in "scientific" worldviews?: Investigating science-oriented Finns' explanations for origins, death and suffering. *Journal of Cognition and Culture, 24*(1–2), 1–34.

Haimila, R., & Muraja, E. (2023). A sense of continuity in mortality?: Exploring science-oriented Finns' views on afterdeath. *OMEGA: Journal of Death and Dying, 88*(1), 38–65.

Haimila, R., Parkkinen, T. A. M., Kundtová Klocová, E., Maraldi, E., Turpin, H., Farias, M., & van Mulukom, V. (2025). *Understanding the morality of unbelievers: Secular beliefs about right and wrong in ten countries*. Preprint.

Haimila, R., van Mulukom, V., Pauha, T., Taira, T., & Farias, M. (2024). *Death, science and design: Does existential anxiety increase belief in science and design in nature?* Unpublished manuscript.

Hanegraaff, W. J. (2013). *Western esotericism: A guide for the perplexed.* Bloombury.

Harris, S. (2010). *The moral landscape: How science can determine human values.* Free Press.

Harrison, P. (2010). "Science" and "religion": Constructing the boundaries. In T. Dixon, G. Cantor, & S. Pumfrey (Eds.), *Science and religion: New historical perspectives* (pp. 23–49). Cambridge University Press.

Heine, S. J., Proulx, T., & Vohs, K. D. (2006). The meaning maintenance model: On the coherence of social motivations. *Personality and Social Psychology Review, 10*(2), 88–110.

Hoogeveen, S., Haaf, J. M., Bulbulia, J. A., Ross, R. M., McKay, R., Altay, S., . . . van Elk, M. (2022). The Einstein effect provides global evidence for scientific source credibility effects and the influence of religiosity. *Nature Human Behaviour, 6*(4), 523–535.

Jackson, J. C., Jasko, K., Abrams, S., Atkinson, T., Balkcom, E., Kruglanski, A., . . . Halberstadt, J. (2024). Religious people view both science and religion as less epistemically valuable than non-religious people view science. *Religion, Brain, and Behavior.*

Johnson, K. A., Okun, M. A., & Moon, J. W. (2023). The interaction of faith and science mindsets predicts perceptions of the relationship between religion and science. *Current Research in Ecological and Social Psychology.*

Jong, J. (2021). Death anxiety and religion. *Current Opinion in Psychology, 40,* 40–44.

Jong, J., Halberstadt, J., & Bluemke, M. (2012). Foxhole atheism, revisited: The effects of mortality salience on explicit and implicit religious belief. *Journal of Experimental Social Psychology, 48*(5), 983–989.

Kiikeri, M., & Ylikoski, P. (2004). *Tiede tutkimuskohteena: Filosofinen johdatus tieteentutkimukseen [Science as research object: A philosophical introduction to science studies].* Gaudeamus.

King, L. A., & Hicks, J. A. (2021). The science of meaning in life. *Annual Review of Psychology, 72*(1), 561–584.

Lee, L. (2015). *Recognizing the non-religious: Reimagining the secular.* Oxford University Press.

Legare, C. H., & Shtulman, A. (2018). Explanatory pluralism across cultures and development. In M. Fortier & J. Proust (Eds.), *Metacognitive diversity: An interdisciplinary approach* (pp. 415–432). Oxford University Press.

Leicht, C., Sharp, C. A., LaBouff, J. P., Zarzeczna, N., & Elsdon-Baker, F. (2022). Content matters: Perceptions of the science-religion relationship. *International Journal for the Psychology of Religion, 32*(3), 232–255.

Lifshin, U., Greenberg, J., Soenke, M., Darrell, A., & Pyszczynski, T. (2018). Mortality salience, religiosity, and indefinite life extension: Evidence of a reciprocal relationship between afterlife beliefs and support for forestalling death. *Religion, Brain and Behavior, 8*(1), 31–43.

Longest, K. C., & Uecker, J. E. (2021). It all depends on what you want to believe: How young adults navigate religion and science. *Review of Religious Research, 63*(1), 1–21.

Ma, S., Payir, A., McLoughlin, N., & Harris, P. L. (2024). Scientific and religious beliefs are primarily shaped by testimony. *Trends in Cognitive Sciences.*

Mackey, C. D., Rios, K., & Cheng, Z. H. (2023). Christianity-science compatibility beliefs increase nonreligious individuals' perceptions of Christians' intelligence and scientific ability. *Public Understanding of Science, 32*(1), 71–87.

Ma-Kellams, C., & Blascovich, J. (2013). Does "science" make you moral?: The effects of priming science on moral judgments and behavior. *PLOS One, 8*(3).

Manning, C. (2023). Facing death without religion: How non-religious elders imagine death and how that shapes their lives. *Journal of Religion, Spirituality and Aging.*

McCauley, R. N. (2013). *Why religion is natural and science is not.* Oxford University Press.

McPhetres, J., Jong, J., & Zuckerman, M. (2020). Religious Americans have less positive attitudes toward science, but this does not extend to other cultures. *Social Psychological and Personality Science.*

Miller, C., & Beaman, L. G. (2024). Nonreligious afterlife: Emerging understandings of death and dying. *Religions, 15*(1), 104.

Park, C. L., David, A. B., Burke, J. D., & Annunziato, L. (2024). Childhood experiences and personal traits as predictors of reliance on science and on religion to make sense of the world: Results of a national US study. *Religion, Brain and Behavior.*

Parsons, W. B. (2021). *Freud and religion: Advancing the dialogue.* Cambridge University Press.

Pew Research Center. (2015). *U.S. public becoming less religious* (p. 266). https://www.pewforum.org/wp-content/uploads/sites/7/2015/11/201.11.03_RLS_II_full_report.pdf.

Pew Research Center. (2020). *The global god divide.* https://www.pewresearch.org/

global/wp-content/uploads/sites/2/2020/07/PG_2020.07.20_Global-Religion_FINAL.pdf.

Preston, J. L. (2011). Religion is the opiate of the masses (but science is the methadone). *Religion, Brain and Behavior, 1*(3), 231–233.

Preston, J. L., Coleman, T. J., & Shin, F. (2023). Spirituality of science: Implications for meaning, well-being, and learning. *Personality and Social Psychology Bulletin.*

Preston, J. L., & Epley, N. (2005). Explanations versus applications: The explanatory power of valuable beliefs. *Psychological Science, 16*(10), 826–832.

Preston, J. L., & Epley, N. (2009). Science and God: An automatic opposition between ultimate explanations. *Journal of Experimental Social Psychology, 45*(1), 238–241.

Preston, J. L., Hotchin, V., & Zarzeczna, N. (2025). Humility and harmony: The influence of intellectual humility and religiousness on science-religion views. *Personality and Individual Differences, 240,* 113136.

Preston, J. L., & Shin, F. (2017). Spiritual experiences evoke awe through the small self in both religious and non-religious individuals. *Journal of Experimental Social Psychology, 70,* 212–221.

Price, M. E., & Johnson, D. D. P. (2024). Science and religion around the world: Compatibility between belief systems predicts increased well-being. *Religion, Brain and Behavior.*

Proulx, T. (2020). Cosmic Dad or Cthulhu: Why we will always need (religious) absolutes. In K. E. Vail III & C. Routledge (Eds.), *The science of religion, spirituality, and existentialism* (pp. 261–271). Elsevier.

Proulx, T., & Heine, S. J. (2006). Death and black diamonds: Meaning, mortality, and the Meaning Maintenance Model. *Psychological Inquiry, 17*(4), 309–318.

Proulx, T., & Inzlicht, M. (2012). The five "A"s of meaning maintenance: Finding meaning in the theories of sense-making. *Psychological Inquiry, 23*(4), 317–335.

Proulx, T., Inzlicht, M., & Harmon-Jones, E. (2012). Understanding all inconsistency compensation as a palliative response to violated expectations. *Trends in Cognitive Sciences, 16*(5), 285–291.

Rios, K. (2021). Examining Christians' reactions to reminders of religion–science conflict: Stereotype threat versus disengagement. *Personality and Social Psychology Bulletin, 47*(3), 441–454.

Rutjens, B. T., & Heine, S. J. (2016). The immoral landscape?: Scientists are associated with violations of morality. *PLOS One, 11*(4), e0152798.

Rutjens, B. T., Heine, S. J., Sutton, R. M., & van Harreveld, F. (2018a). Attitudes towards science. *Advances in Experimental Social Psychology, 57,* 125–165.

Rutjens, B. T., & Hornsey, M. J. (2024). The psychology of science rejection. *Advances in Experimental Social Psychology.*

Rutjens, B. T., & Preston, J. L. (2020). Science and religion: A rocky relationship shaped by shared psychological functions. In K. E. Vail III & C. Routledge (Eds.), *The science of religion, spirituality, and existentialism* (pp. 373–385). Elsevier.

Rutjens, B. T., Sengupta, N., der Lee, R. van, van Koningsbruggen, G. M., Martens, J. P., Rabelo, A., & Sutton, R. M. (2022). Science skepticism across 24 countries. *Social Psychological and Personality Science, 13*(1), 102–117.

Rutjens, B. T., Sutton, R. M., & van der Lee, R. (2018b). Not all skepticism is equal: Exploring the ideological antecedents of science acceptance and rejection. *Personality and Social Psychology Bulletin, 44*(3), 384–405.

Rutjens, B. T., & van der Lee, R. (2020). Spiritual skepticism?: Heterogeneous science skepticism in the Netherlands. *Public Understanding of Science, 29*(3), 335–352.

Rutjens, B. T., van Harreveld, F., & van der Pligt, J. (2013). Step by step: Finding compensatory order in science. *Current Directions in Psychological Science, 22*(3), 250–255.

Rutjens, B. T., van Harreveld, F., van der Pligt, J., van Elk, M., & Pyszczynski, T. (2016). A march to a better world?: Religiosity and the existential function of belief in social-moral progress. *International Journal for the Psychology of Religion, 26*(1), 1–18.

Rutjens, B. T., Zarzeczna, N., & van der Lee, R. (2022). Science rejection in Greece: Spirituality predicts vaccine scepticism and low faith in science in a Greek sample. *Public Understanding of Science, 31*(4), 428–436.

Sharp, C. A., Leicht, C., Rios, K., Zarzeczna, N., & Elsdon-Baker, F. (2022). Religious diversity in science: Stereotypical and counter-stereotypical social identities. *Group Processes & Intergroup Relations, 25*(7), 1836–1860

Sleegers, W. W. A., Proulx, T., & van Beest, I. (2015). Extremism reduces conflict arousal and increases values affirmation in response to meaning violations. *Biological Psychology, 108,* 126–131.

Sleegers, W. W. A., Proulx, T., & van Beest, I. (2021). Pupillometry and hindsight bias: Physiological arousal predicts compensatory behavior. *Social Psychological and Personality Science, 12*(7), 1146–1154.

Stavrova, O., Ehlebracht, D., & Fetchenhauer, D. (2016). Belief in scientific–technological progress and life satisfaction: The role of personal control. *Personality and Individual Differences, 96*, 227–236.

Taves, A., Asprem, E., & Ihm, E. (2018). Psychology, meaning making, and the study of worldviews: Beyond religion and non-religion. *Psychology of Religion and Spirituality, 10*(3), 207–217.

Tracy, J. L., Hart, J., & Martens, J. P. (2011). Death and science: The existential underpinnings of belief in intelligent design and discomfort with evolution. *PLOS One, 6*(3), e17349.

Tracy, J. L., Hohm, I., & Makridakis, A. (2024). Does science erode meaning? *Current Directions in Psychological Science, 33*(4), 254–260.

Treger, S., Benau, E. M., & Timko, C. A. (2023). Not so terrifying after all?: A set of failed replications of the mortality salience effects of terror management theory. *PLOS One, 18*(5), e0285267.

Vail, K. E., Arndt, J., & Abdollahi, A. (2012). Exploring the existential function of religion and supernatural agent beliefs among Christians, Muslims, atheists, and agnostics. *Personality and Social Psychology Bulletin, 38*(10), 1288–1300.

Vail, K. E., & Horner, D. E. (2023). The captain of my soul: Self-determination and need-satisfaction help manage death-related cognition, anxiety, and well-being. *Journal of Personality and Social Psychology, 125*(6), 1308–1331.

Vail, K. E., Soenke, M., & Waggoner, B. (2019). Terror management theory and religious belief. In C. Routledge & M. Vess (Eds.), *Handbook of terror management theory* (pp. 259–285). Elsevier.

Vail, K. E., Soenke, M., Waggoner, B., & Mavropoulou, I. (2020). Natural, but not supernatural, literal immortality affirmation attenuates mortality salience effects on worldview defense in atheists. *Personality and Social Psychology Bulletin, 46*(2), 312–326.

van Mulukom, V., Turpin, H., Haimila, R., Purzycki, B. G., Bendixen, T., Kundtová Klocová, E., . . . Farias, M. (2023). What do nonreligious nonbelievers believe in? Secular worldviews around the world. *Psychology of Religion and Spirituality, 15*(1), 143–156.

Većkalov, B., Zarzeczna, N., McPhetres, J., Van Harreveld, F., & Rutjens, B. T. (2024). Psychological distance to science as a predictor of science skepticism across domains. *Personality and Social Psychology Bulletin, 50*(1), 18–37.

Wellcome. (2018). *Wellcome Global Monitor: How does the world feel about science and health? Appendix D.* https://wellcome.org/insights/reports/wellcome-global-monitor/2018.

Yilmaz, O., & Bahçekapili, H. G. (2015). When science replaces religion: Science as a secular authority bolsters moral sensitivity. *PLoS ONE, 10*(9), e0137499.

Zarzeczna, N., Bertlich, T., Većkalov, B., & Rutjens, B. T. (2023a). Spirituality is associated with COVID-19 vaccination scepticism. *Vaccine, 41*(1), 226–235.

Zarzeczna, N., Bilgin, A., & Hanel, P. H. P. (2024a). *Trends in religiosity and wellbeing diverge over time.* Unpublished manuscript.

Zarzeczna, N., Hanel, P. H. P., Rutjens, B. T., Bono, S. A., Chen, Y. H., & Haddock, G. (2024b). Scientists, speak up!: Source impacts trust in health advice across five countries. *Journal of Experimental Psychology: Applied, 30*(3), 430–441.

Zarzeczna, N., & Preston, J. L. (2025). Meaning in science as a response to existential threat. *Psychology of Religion and Spirituality.*

Zarzeczna, N., Preston, J. L., Samekin, A., Reinhardt, C. S., Bolatov, A., Mussinova, Z., . . . Rutjens, B. T. (2024c). The feeling is not mutual: Religious belief predicts compatibility between science and religion, but scientific belief predicts conflict. *Psychology of Religion and Spirituality.*

Zarzeczna, N., Većkalov, B., & Rutjens, B. T. (2023b). Spirituality and intentions to engage in COVID-19 protective behaviours. *Social and Personality Psychology Compass, 17*(8), e12765.

Zarzeczna, N., Vogel, E. M., Proulx, T., & Preston, J. L. (2024d). *Compatibility between science and religion is an independent meaning system.* Unpublished manuscript.

Zein, R. A., Altenmüller, M. S., & Gollwitzer, M. (2024). Longtime nemeses or cordial allies?: How individuals mentally relate science and religion. *Psychological Review.*

CHAPTER 46

Making Life Matter

The Role of Sociocultural and Experiential Significance

Lydia M. Needy, Michael A. Day, Xiaobo Xu, *and* Joshua A. Hicks

Humans possess an intrinsic desire to believe their existence matters. This quest for significance is considered a fundamental human motivation (Frankl, 1985; Kruglanski et al., 2022). Empirical studies provide evidence for this claim by demonstrating how perceptions of significance play a crucial role in psychological and physical well-being (Costin & Vignoles, 2020). Conversely, a lack of significance can drive humans to great lengths to restore this feeling (Kruglanski et al., 2015). But what does it truly mean to experience significance? In this chapter, we compare and contrast two interrelated conceptions of significance and explain why each is essential for the attainment of a meaningful existence.

The experience of significance in life is defined as the "sense of life's inherent value and having a life worth living" (Martela & Steger, 2016). On one hand, the perception of significance is closely tied to the desire for people's actions to be valued by others; humans believe that individuals who make a lasting impact on others are significant (Kruglanski et al., 2022). On the other hand, humans also seek to feel, on a phenomenological level, that their experiences are significant to themselves (Li et al., 2021). In particular, they want their lived experiences to feel worthwhile. We refer to these two conceptions as *sociocultural significance* and *experiential significance*, respectively. Sociocultural significance relates to the impact one's actions have on others, reflecting one's desire for social validation, esteem, competence, and recognition. Experiential significance, however, is related to the intrinsic value and meaning one derives from one's actions and experiences oneself, independent of external validation. Both forms of significance serve as pathways to finding meaning in life (Kim et al., 2022).

In this chapter, we first distinguish between these two types of significance and describe how each of these concepts are central to the experience of meaning in life. We then describe common sources of meaning in life and how they are inextricably linked to both forms of significance. Finally, we argue that harmonious levels of sociocultural and experiential significance may contribute to a heightened and stable sense that one's life is meaningful.

SOCIOCULTURAL SIGNIFICANCE: LEAVING AN INDELIBLE MARK ON THE WORLD

Kruglanski and colleagues (2022) defined the quest for significance as "the desire to matter, to feel worthy and appreciated by others whose positive regard one seeks."

This conceptualization of significance is fundamentally social: Humans want to feel that they play an important role in the lives of others and that their contributions are appreciated. This need for sociocultural significance is inherently linked with one's own desire to belong, but also encompasses a sense of contributing to others, which is often guided by the belief that one's actions can have lasting importance, even beyond one's lifetime (George & Park, 2016). Essentially, individuals long to know that they have made a meaningful and potentially lasting impact on the world.

When contemplating a life of significance, we often think of those extraordinary individuals who have left a striking mark on society. People naturally think of those outliers who stand apart and are celebrated in the collective consciousness, such as those listed in *Time* magazine's "Most Influential People in History." Scholars, pioneers, and humanitarians like Aristotle, Sigmund Freud, Joan of Arc, Jonas Salk, Mother Teresa, and Albert Einstein are a few who readily come to mind. These icons have changed the course of history and reshaped how people think and behave. Through groundbreaking discoveries or acts of extraordinary compassion, they have left a lasting mark that still resonates today by inspiring many individuals to make themselves and the world a better place.

Alas, the vast majority of people won't leave a legacy as significant as those of eminent individuals. Instead, they often strive for more attainable forms of significance in their lives. For instance, one might volunteer at a local church or a shelter for unhoused individuals. Although these acts may seem less impressive compared to developing the theory of general relativity, for example, they still provide individuals with reassuring feedback that their lives matter—they are impacting people in lasting ways. Perhaps the most ubiquitous way people achieve sociocultural significance is through their close social relationships. Individuals frequently find fulfillment when they believe they play a meaningful role in the lives of their loved ones.

Believing that one has made an important contribution is one of the main pillars of a meaningful existence. For example, Viktor Frankl (1985) emphasized the importance of possessing "creative values," which involve engaging in significant actions as a primary pathway to finding meaning. Similarly, Irvin Yalom (1980) argued that making an impact and leaving a legacy are essential for people to perceive that their actions are meaningful, which helps mitigate fears of death. Likewise, generativity, the act of nurturing and guiding the next generation, is also believed to provide individuals with the sense that their actions have meaning (de St. Aubin, 2013).

According to terror management theory (TMT; Greenberg et al., 1986), the quest for significance stems from an awareness of mortality and efforts to mitigate this existential concern. According to TMT, human cognitive abilities, which are crucial for survival, have also introduced a host of uniquely human challenges, such as the awareness of one's own vulnerability and mortality. To cope with these concerns, individuals adopt culturally validated worldviews that allow them to believe they can achieve some form of immortality (for more information, see Routledge & Vess, 2019), be it literal (e.g., a belief in the afterlife) or symbolic (e.g., viewing one's children as extensions of oneself). Self-esteem, an evaluation of one's perceived worthiness, hinges on the person believing that they are living up to the standards of their cultural worldview and, in turn, this achievement shelters them from their death anxiety (Pyszczynski et al., 2004). Thus, the pursuit of sociocultural significance may also serve to alleviate death anxiety by affirming one's potential to transcend death through meaningful contributions to one's cultural narrative.

Conversely, experiencing an extreme sense of insignificance can undermine not only one's sense of meaning but also the will to live. Williams and Zadro (2005) describe social insignificance, particularly the feeling of being ostracized, as akin to experiencing death itself. Recent studies on loneliness have introduced the term *anti-mattering* to address this dimension of social insignificance previously overlooked in conceptualizations of loneliness (Flett, 2018; McComb et al., 2020). This is noteworthy given that loneliness is linked to various negative mental and physical health outcomes, prompting the U.S. Surgeon General to release an advisory report in 2023 titled *Our Epidemic of Loneliness and Isolation*, which outlines the devastating effects of loneliness and advocates for changes to foster social connection. Research on ostracism and loneliness underscores the profound psychological and physiological impact of feeling unnoticed and undervalued.

Empirical Evidence

Research supports the role of sociocultural significance in experiencing meaning in life. In fact, many measures of meaning actually include items assessing significance because the concepts are so tied together. For instance, the influential Meaning in Life Questionnaire (Steger et al., 2006) includes an item, "I am always searching for something that makes my life feel significant," designed to assess the search for meaning in life. More recently, Costin and Vignoles (2020) demonstrated that the feeling of existential mattering, such as believing that one's actions will have an impact even after death, is one of the strongest predictors of subjective levels of meaning in life. In their studies, they assessed mattering along with two other constructs related to meaning in life: coherence and purpose. Coherence represents the feeling that life makes sense, and purpose is directly related to having important goals that guide one's behavior. Using diverse methodologies, they showed that existential mattering uniquely predicted subjective judgments of meaning in life, leading them to conclude that meaning is fundamentally about mattering.

Studies also have found that more localized forms of mattering are important to meaning. For example, many studies have shown that generativity is a robust predictor of meaning (e.g., de St. Aubin, 2013). More recently, Guthrie and colleagues (2024) demonstrated that social mattering—the feeling that others think the individual is important—is strongly associated with meaning in life. Similar to Costin and Vignoles's study, they showed that feeling that one plays an important role in another's life predicts subjective judgments of meaning even after controlling for perceptions of coherence, purpose, and existential mattering (i.e., mattering in the grand scheme of things). This suggests that people do not necessarily need to feel a sense of legacy or make an extraordinary contribution to experience meaning in life. Simply being an important part of another's life is enough.

Navigating Cultural and Cognitive Influences on Sociocultural Significance

One caveat is that sociocultural significance is not universally objective; what is deemed significant is shaped by culture and historical context. Moreover, there are times when perceptions of sociocultural significance are influenced by cognitive biases. No matter how influential a person's actions are, a depressed mind may fail to recognize its contribution to others. Edwin Arlington Robinson's infamously timeless poem "Richard Cory" captures this reality well. Richard was objectively successful and respected member of his community. Despite this, he took his own life due to the anguish presumably caused by his inner demons. There are many other examples of esteemed figures throughout history whose lives ended in a similar fate (e.g., Cleopatra, Chris Cornell, Robin Williams). These tragic fates demonstrate how internal perceptions can differ vastly from external realities.

Furthermore, societal or cultural values may not always align with eudaimonic well-being or what is beneficial to the greater good. For example, with the recent rise of social media, cultural norms have shifted, often placing value on contributions that do not always translate into traditional views of significance, such as scientific breakthroughs, medical advances, or helping others. Instead, there is more value placed on individualistic, extrinsic contributions such as wealth, fame, or creating a viral video that offers no meaningful benefit beyond fleeting entertainment. Based on research on intrinsic versus extrinsic aspirations (Kasser & Ryan, 1996), we would predict that seeking significance through more other-focused motives provides a more enduring sense of meaning in life compared to chasing more self-focused forms of significance.

It is likely that the most functional form of sociocultural significance comes from making a positive contribution at the highest level of abstraction. People who ultimately develop a cure for Alzheimer's disease, for example, or provide other types of extraordinary help to humankind exemplify this kind of contribution. This sort of self-transcendent contribution likely leads to a more stable, enduring, and ultimately adaptive sense of significance compared to other forms. Therefore, such contributions not only benefit society but also lead to greater confidence that one's actions truly matter.

EXPERIENTIAL SIGNIFICANCE

While sociocultural significance is highly desirable and often a strong motive for many, it alone does not make life feel worthwhile. In addition to wanting their actions to be of consequence, individuals also have a desire for their experiences to transcend the mundane and feel consequential to them. They want to engage in activities that elicit positive affect, challenge their abilities, provide a sense of peace and contentment, or otherwise add color to their daily lives. We refer to this as the desire for experiential significance. It encompasses moments of solitude, creativity, personal achievements, mindfulness, and any situation that adds value to existence, helping solidify the feeling that life is truly worthwhile (see also Oishi et al., 2020, for a similar perspective on the role of experiences in the good life).

Many experiences are naturally high in experiential value. For instance, Frankena (1973) speculated that a diverse range of variables are intrinsically valuable, such as pleasures, love, friendships, wisdom, self-expression, aesthetic experiences, and novelty, to name just a few (see Zimmerman & Bradley, 2019, for a more detailed examination of intrinsic vs. extrinsic value). The motive to feel that experiences are significant is evident from the money people spend on things such as dining at fancy restaurants, going on vacations, attending sporting events, and enjoying music concerts. Although some people engage in these activities for more extrinsic reasons, most do them with the belief that those experiences will somehow feel consequential.

Experiential Significance and Meaning in Life

Experiential significance, like sociocultural significance, is central to the experience of meaning in life. The scholar Viktor Frankl famously described the importance of experiential significance, which he termed *experiential value*. According to Frankl, three types of values are essential for a meaningful existence. First, creative values provide a sense of meaning through an individual's actions or creations, particularly, as mentioned, when these benefit others. These actions contribute to fulfilling a sense of sociocultural significance. Second, attitudinal values help individuals restore or maintain a sense of meaning in life, especially during difficult times. Finally, experiential values enable individuals to find beauty and significance in life itself.

Empirical Evidence

Research also supports the role of experiential significance in the perception of meaning in life. For instance, many common sources of meaning, such as positive affect, awe and wonder, curiosity, savoring, mindfulness, and mental time travel, are likely to enhance a sense of meaning primarily due to the intrinsic significance of the experiences themselves. More direct evidence comes from two recent studies. First, Li and colleagues (2021) attempted to demonstrate that both external value and internal value contribute to the experience of meaning in life. Their measure of external value was akin to the concept of sociocultural significance, while internal value was similar to the concept of experiential value. They found that both dimensions uniquely predicted self-reports of global meaning in life. Further evidence for the idea of experiential significance comes from Kim and colleagues (2022). Using diverse methodologies, they also found that experiential significance (termed *experiential appreciation* in their studies) uniquely predicted global reports of meaning. For example, cross-sectional and longitudinal studies conducted in China and the United States demonstrated that experiential significance was a robust predictor of meaning in life. More convincingly, experimental findings showed that participants who viewed videos designed to induce experiential significance (awe-inspiring videos) influenced participants' levels of meaning in life through this heightened feeling of significance. Importantly, all of these studies controlled for levels of social mattering as well as other primary contributors to meaning in life, including a sense of coherence and purpose in life.

Detecting and Overlooking Experiential Significance

While we know that some experiences feel more significant than others, there are vast individual differences in how much value we extract from any given experience. For example, one person might not appreciate their walk to their car after a long day of work, while another person might notice all the beauty that surrounds them during the walk, whether it be blooming foliage, the sly nature of squirrels or birds trying to steal discarded food, or receiving an unexpected smile from a complete stranger. Essentially, one does not always need to go to the Grand Canyon to feel a sense of experiential significance; one can cultivate it from almost any experience given the right mindset.

As mentioned, the experiential significance that people extract from their environment can vary tremendously based on many factors. For example, anhedonia, the inability to experience pleasure, is often a characteristic of major depression, Parkinson's disease, schizophrenia, posttraumatic stress disorder, and chronic substance use, among other conditions. For people experiencing anhedonia, it is likely challenging to find any form of significance in their daily lives. During these times, even the most intrinsically rewarding experiences may seem lackluster. Moreover, many aspects of modern society are not conducive to experiencing significance in one's environment. For instance, our overreliance on technology, such as smartphones, keeps us distracted from the present moment (Woodlief, 2017). It is impossible to feel connected to an experience if one is not present in the moment.

In sum, although sociocultural significance seems tied to our perceptions that life is meaningful, it alone does not guarantee the feeling that life is worthwhile. In addition to a yearning to leave a mark on the world, there exists a desire for one's experiences to feel meaningful, leading to a deep appreciation of the beauty and richness of the world. Experiential significance manifests most when one is fully present in the current moment and is actively engaging with and appreciates one's lived experience. This feeling of connection between the self and the outside world contributes significantly to the overall sense that life is meaningful.

Delineating Sociocultural and Experiential Significance in the Literature

The literature on both meaning-making processes and the self aligns well with the dichotomy of these two types of significance. For instance, as previously mentioned, two of Viktor Frankl's values that contribute to our sense of meaning in life—creation and experiential—nicely overlap with the ideas of sociocultural and experiential significance. Others have also distinguished between constructing versus detecting meaning in life (Heintzelman & King, 2014; Hicks & King, 2009). Constructing meaning in life resonates more closely with the concept of sociocultural significance, requiring one to be an active agent in order to exert influence on the world. In contrast, detecting meaning in life is more about recognizing significance in the environment, implying a more passive form of meaning making.

Sociocultural and experiential significance also align well with William James's (1890) conception of the self. The self is often considered the engine that drives meaning-making processes (Baumeister, 1991; Schlegel et al., 2009, 2011). According to James, the self comprises both the "Me" and the "I," representing one's sense of self (e.g., self-esteem) and one's conscious experience, respectively. One's appraisal of one's sociocultural significance is partly a function of a specific aspect of one's sense of self, particularly one's perceived contributions in life, while one's sense of experiential significance is a function of one's connection to one's conscious experience.

To illustrate the importance of both sociocultural and experiential significance in the experience of meaning in life, we briefly discuss how many common sources of meaning likely contribute through their direct influence on both conceptions of significance. This is not an exhaustive list of sources of meaning in life. For a more comprehensive discussion of additional sources, see Hicks and Routledge (2013) or Wong (2013).

Frequent Elicitors of Significance

Positive Affect

It is well documented that *positive affect* (i.e., feelings of happiness, cheerfulness, enjoyment, and fun) is associated with general meaning in life (King et al., 2006). Experimental studies demonstrate that positive mood manipulations—such as listening to uplifting music, writing about a happy memory, imagining an accomplishment, or reading comic strips—can reliably enhance participants' feelings of meaning in life (King & Hicks, 2021). Moreover, some scholars even propose that feelings of joy and pleasure themselves form a core element of meaning in life (Ebersole, 1998). In support of this idea, Lambert and colleagues (2010) found that people ranked happiness as the second most important source of meaning among others (e.g., family, friends, religious faith, achievements, and self-worth).

From a lifelong development perspective, happy individuals are usually more successful across distinctive life domains such as marriage, friendship, income, work performance, and health (Lyubomirsky et al., 2005), making them more likely to contribute to the world with a sense of sociocultural significance. From a more micro perspective, positive affect can help individuals expand their attentional scope and recognize their place on a grand scale (King et al., 2006), motivate them to pursue long-term goals and overcome setbacks proactively (Parker et al., 2010), and direct them to establish close and supportive relationships (Ramsey & Gentzler, 2015); all of these are crucial for achieving sociocultural significance in life.

Positive affect can also enhance individuals' perceptions of experiential significance in daily life. According to the broaden-and-build theory, positive emotions foster curiosity, cognitive flexibility, open-mindedness, and a broader perspective, enabling individuals to explore new interests and discover the unknown that brings meaning and fulfillment (Fredrickson, 2001; King et al., 2006). By appreciating life's immediate joys and constructing a meaningful narrative over time, positive affect can arise from everyday experiences and enhance one's feelings of experiential significance. As evidence, Kim and colleagues (2022) consistently observed medium-level positive associations (with *r*s ranging from .35 to .56) between positive affect and experiential significance across diverse methodologies and samples.

Epistemic Emotions

In addition to general positive affect, specific emotions are linked to meaning. *Epistemic emotions* refer to emotions related to knowledge acquisition, understanding, and reasoning (Nerantzaki et al., 2021). In this section, we focus on three epistemic emotions: curiosity, wonder, and awe, and their links to significance.

Curiosity is a fundamental human emotion that drives the pursuit of knowledge, exploration of the unknown, and engagement with the world (Kashdan & Steger, 2007). With a curious attitude, individuals are more likely to actively seek out new and challenging situations and expand their perspectives and skill sets, which functions as a solid basis for better work performance (Mussel, 2013; Schutte & Malouff, 2020), leading to a higher probability of achieving sociocultural significance. In addition, being curious about something could direct an individual's attention and behavior toward specific activities at the moment and encourage mindfulness (Kashdan et al., 2011), contributing to a greater appreciation of life's nuances and complexities, as it involves a keen understanding of one's environment and experiences, which, in turn, benefits the feeling of experiential significance.

Wonder can be described as a feeling mainly consisting of amazement and admiration that results from witnessing something beautiful, remarkable, or unfamiliar (Wonder, 1928). As an inspiring epistemic emotion, wonder can affect the way people connect to and interact with the surrounding world, transform their perception of life and existence, enhance their feeling of empowerment (i.e., as a participant rather than an onlooker of the world), and motivate them to affect the external circumstances and make a difference in the world (Van de Goor et al., 2020). From this perspective, wonder can potentially increase an individual's sociocultural significance. On the other hand, wonder usually accompanies uplifting emotions (e.g., surprise), prompting individuals to expand their awareness and horizons.[1] This inclination drives people to explore new possibilities in thought and action (Glăveanu, 2019), which can, in turn, enable them to intentionally reassess the ordinary, perceive the extraordinary beauty in daily routines, and appreciate the nuanced meanings of life, leading to augmented feeling of experiential significance (Van de Goor et al., 2020).

Awe typically arises when people encounter something physically or mentally vast and feel a need to change their mental structure to accommodate the experience (Keltner & Haidt, 2003; for a review, see Jiang et al., 2024). Due to its multifaceted nature, awe may contribute to sociocultural significance from opposite directions. On the one hand, awe usually accompanies the inability to fully comprehend vast mysteries, leading to the feeling of a small, humble, and less entitled self, which, in turn, may directly decrease people's feelings of sociocultural significance (Rivera et al., 2020). On the other hand, awe can shift an individual's attention from personal concerns to the needs of others (Keltner & Haidt, 2003), triggering the feeling of interconnectedness and promoting prosocial behaviors (Stamkou et al., 2023), which may increase their interpersonal mattering and sociocultural significance. In contrast, awe has a more straightforward influence on experiential significance. As it can offer a wide-ranging viewpoint that helps individuals integrate their life experiences coherently and connect their identity to broader entities (Jiang et al., 2024), awe can lead people to explore the external world more actively and appreciate the beauty of daily life more extensively, contributing to a feeling of experiential significance.

Creativity

Creativity refers to the ability to generate ideas or solutions that are both novel and appropriate (Runco & Jaeger, 2012). In its many forms, creativity can contribute to people's feelings of significance in life, on both a sociocultural and an experiential level.

In its most impressive manifestations, creativity can emerge as groundbreaking theories, astonishing artworks, or innovative products (Kaufman & Beghetto, 2009). As these landmark creations can provoke thought and inspire others, their creators can undoubtedly gain a wide range of recognition in both the current era and the long-lasting future, contributing to high levels of sociocultural significance. In addition, creativity can occur in more diverse and accessible forms. Whether through writing poetry, composing music, painting landscapes, or crafting furniture, people can produce objects and experiences that foster connections and impact wider communities. For instance, Maya Angelou channeled her childhood and early adulthood experiences into a series of autobiographies, transforming her personal challenges and triumphs into universal insights. Similarly, when Taylor Swift released her self-titled debut album at the age of 16, she explored her teenage perspective through captivating songs that resonated with others. Neither of these now-prominent figures likely anticipated this as the outset of their creative success. Recognition of one's creations by the public can validate personal effort and vision, enhancing the creator's feeling of social significance.

People can also feel elevated experiential significance in life through the process of creating. By definition, creating often involves exploring new ideas, techniques, and concepts and finding novel solutions to problems, which can be profoundly satisfying and intellectually stimulating, contributing to personal competence and value (Han et al., 2023). Creating can help individuals achieve more flow-like states, in which people feel highly concentrated and immensely involved in the task at hand with joyful emotions. This peak experience can help them appreciate existential value (Kaufman, 2018). In addition, creating something—art, music, writing, or any form of craft—allows individuals to express their inner thoughts and emotions (Putney et al., 2024). In summary, whether through professional pursuits or hobbies, creating provides a unique avenue to explore one's potential and construct a life filled with significance; thus, it can be an essential path to meaning in life.

Mindfulness

Mindfulness involves consciously directing attention to present-moment experiences such as thoughts, feelings, and physical sensations, with an attitude characterized by curiosity, openness, and acceptance (Bishop et al., 2004; Brown & Ryan, 2003). Research and theory consistently suggest a positive association between mindfulness and perceiving meaning in life. For example, recent meta-analytic findings from correlational studies and randomized controlled trials indicate that mindfulness-based interventions may enhance one's sense of meaning in life (Chu & Mak, 2020). Moreover, mechanisms like decentering (i.e., viewing one's thoughts as objective events rather than identifying with them), authentic self-awareness, and attention to positive experiences partially explain this relationship. This aligns with the mindfulness-to-meaning theory (Garland et al., 2015), which proposes that mindfulness fosters a sense of meaning by facilitating positive reappraisal of stressful events (e.g., seeing an athletic injury as an opportunity for resilience) and enhancing the savoring of positive emotions (e.g., gratitude for the supportive relationships during recovery).

To our knowledge, no studies have investigated the potential link between mindfulness and sociocultural significance. However, indirect support for such a link can be found in case examples of patients who have derived interpersonal benefits from mindfulness-based interventions. For example, a patient of Eric Garland's, who had recently undergone several mindfulness meditation sessions following cancer-removal surgery, reported paying greater attention to his significant professional accomplishments and increased motivation to spend more time with his family (Garland et al., 2015). Thus, mindfulness may increase one's sense of sociocultural significance by making it easier to bring to mind how one has made a meaningful impact on the world and the lives of others and may promote intentions to continue doing so in the future.

Regardless of how mindfulness influences sociocultural significance, a consistent theme across studies linking mindfulness to perceiving meaning in life is the idea that mindfulness enhances one's appreciation for life, which closely parallels our conception of experiential significance. For example, research testing the mindfulness-to-meaning theory by Garland and colleagues revealed that cancer patients who reported greater mindfulness tended to notice and savor positive experiences and life-affirming events (Garland et al., 2017). Another study found that mindfulness might mitigate suicidal tendencies by increasing one's "zest for life"—characterized by positive and enthusiastic engagement—even under conditions of interpersonal adversity (Collins et al., 2018).

Nostalgia

Nostalgia is defined as "a sentimental longing or wistful affection for the past" (Pearsall, 1998, p. 1266). It is a bittersweet, although more sweet than bitter, emotion that involves reminiscing about personal experiences that are relevant to the self and close others (Sedikides & Wildschut, 2018). It is often evoked by stimuli such as familiar scents, old photographs, or retold stories that remind one of positive or momentous past experiences. Though tinged with a sense of loss or yearning, nostalgia is generally a positive emotion that often generates feelings of comfort, happiness, and belonging. Perceptions of nostalgia have evolved over time. At one point it was labeled as a psychological illness (Hofer, 1688/1934), but more than two decades of empirical findings provide evidence to the contrary—nostalgia is now believed to be a psychological resource that has salutary effects when intentionally invoked (Sedikides & Wildschut, 2018). Furthermore, correlational and experimental evidence suggest that nostalgia may help one perceive one's life as meaningful by enhancing one's sense of social connectedness and self-continuity (Sedikides & Wildschut, 2018).

Nostalgia can evoke a sense of sociocultural significance by recalling significant life accomplishments that have now become treasured memories (e.g., acceptance to a prestigious university). Nostalgia may also enhance one's sense of sociocultural significance by enhancing one's sense of social connectedness and, specifically, promoting a sense of reassurance of worth (i.e., when one's abilities, skills, and value are recognized by others), a social provision identified by Cutrona and Russell (1987). Alternatively, nostalgia can heighten one's sense of experiential significance due to one's enjoyment of the positive and pleasurable experience inherent in nostalgic reminiscence. In a similar vein, nostalgia may enhance positive feelings, in a similar way as mindfulness does, by promoting the savoring of events that one believes will be nostalgic in the future (i.e., anticipatory nostalgia; Sedikides & Wildschut, 2018).

Care

Harry Frankfurt, an influential American philosopher, argued that *care* should be conceptualized as a purely personal matter reflecting one's personal identification with the object of care (1982). The things one cares about are not chosen through rational deliberation, because care is not under one's voluntary control. People can care about many different things—animals, people, policies, institutions—but the common factor in care is that these things are deeply tied to their identity and deemed important to them. Even if what an individual cares about is not in their best interest, they cannot simply stop caring, as it has become interwoven into who they are and is shaped by factors beyond their immediate control. For example, an estranged lover can care about someone they wish they did not care about; and a loving mother cannot readily stop caring for her child despite the child's disrespect. When one cares about someone or something, one is made vulnerable—the object of care is tied to the person extending the care. Hence, when the object of care is harmed or benefited, the extender of the care is affected as well (Colombo, 2014; Frankfurt, 1982). This unconditional and involuntary care is inextricably tied to the self and extends it to the objects of care in a passive way. Rather than creating meaning by mattering to others through sociocultural significance, one who deeply cares feels experiential significance in the sense that caring about something makes their time worthwhile, even if that care is not reciprocated. What value does life hold if one cares about nothing at all? Even the nihilist cares about something or someone.

The present conceptualization of *care* is characterized by its inherent fulfillment as an end in itself; hence, it does not necessitate future-oriented action. Consequently, it does not fall within the purview of *purpose,* which specifies the degree to which valued life goals govern one's future behavior (George & Park, 2016). While *acting* in "caring" ways toward the objects of care is highly probable, as emphasized in past research (Kyle, 1995; Pulcini, 2017; Weiner & Auster, 2007), such action is not obligatory within this current conceptualization. Essentially, the sentiment of care exists irrespective of whether the individual has goals related toward the object of their care. Simply caring about someone or something can impart a sense that life is worthwhile.

Prosocial Behaviors

Prosocial behaviors encompass a wide range of actions that are intended to benefit others (Batson & Powell, 2003). Examples include donating to charities, volunteering, expressing gratitude, helping strangers, and nurturing other sentient beings and the environment. Research by Dakin and colleagues (2022) and Van Tongeren and colleagues (2016) revealed a robust connection between culturally accepted prosocial behaviors and the pursuit of meaning in life, especially when these actions were viewed as "heroic" (e.g., saving a drowning child; Kinsella et al., 2019). At the heart of this connection lies the notion that engaging in prosocial acts transcends the self, offering a pathway to invest one's energy and resources into causes greater than oneself. This can increase both sociocultural and experiential significance. Individuals may perceive their actions as leaving a lasting impact, thereby enhancing their sense of sociocultural significance. Simultaneously, they can also appreciate the personal satisfaction gained from this experience, increasing experiential significance. Engaging in prosocial actions can boost one's perceptions of self-worth and contribute to a greater sense of meaning in life (Klein, 2017). Whether the acts are directed toward individuals, communities, or even broader value systems, these self-transcendent actions serve as a way for a person to feel as though they contributed to the world in a worthwhile manner.

It's crucial to recognize that not all prosocial actions stem from altruism, which entails selfless concern for others' well-being. Prosocial behaviors could be motivated by cultural norms regarding reciprocity, often aimed at promoting cooperation, or from egoistic motives such as seeking approval or honor. Perhaps the key factor distinguishing prosocial behaviors driven by experiential significance from those driven by sociocultural significance may lie in their underlying motivation—whether they are ego-driven or genuinely altruistic. Regardless of the underlying motivation, these actions arguably still serve to augment one's sense of significance through increased perceptions of self-worth and group belonging. Indeed, the subjective sense of belonging is a powerful predictor of meaning (Lambert et al., 2013). Even when engaging in prosocial behaviors driven by nonaltruistic motives, individuals can still foster a sense of belonging and worth.

Authenticity

The word *authenticity* has become ubiquitous in today's society, often invoked to describe various qualities such as trustworthiness, genuineness, realness, and vulnerability. However, even among authenticity researchers, consensus on a unified conceptualization and definition of authenticity remains hard to pin down. Nevertheless, in this chapter, our focus centers on personal authenticity. *Personal authenticity* refers to the authenticity of the self, where the individual is both the subject of evaluation and the source of internal information (Newman & Smith, 2016). As such, it represents a subjective experience wherein an individual feels as though they know who they truly are and aligns their actions accordingly (Jongman-Sereno & Leary, 2019; Kernis & Goldman, 2006; Wood et al., 2008).

Living in a way that feels authentic brings about many positive emotions—contentment, excitement, and compassion—while perceptions of living inauthentically can evoke negative feelings like anxiety, shame, and sadness (Sedikides et al., 2019). Distinctively, though, state authenticity has a feeling component (Sedikides et al., 2019), and this has been positively linked to perceived meaning in life (Schlegel et al., 2011). The state authenticity as fit to the environment (SAFE) model, proposed by Schmader and Sedikides (2018), suggests that state authenticity fluctuates based on external environmental cues. According to SAFE, individuals naturally seek environments where they feel they "fit." Consequently, when a person perceives that their true self aligns with their surroundings, they are likely to experience a heightened sense of authenticity and a more meaningful sense of life as worthwhile, giving rise to experiential significance.

The sociocultural significance of one's endeavors and accomplishments could be enhanced by perceived authenticity. When individuals see their contributions as a reflection of their core essence, they may feel as though "my mark on the world is a reflection of the real me." Research by Lutz and colleagues (2023) supports this idea, as they found a positive link between perceived authenticity and significance. However, this research raises an interesting question: Does an individual with high levels of sociocultural significance attached to a fake persona feel *less* significance than someone who attributes the same level of sociocultural significance to their perceived authentic self? For instance, one could imagine that some well-known public figures may present a cultivated image to the public, receiving accolades and recognition for this persona. Nevertheless, these figures might not perceive this cultivated image as part of who they truly are, potentially leading them to somewhat diminish the sociocultural significance of their accomplishments. It seems there is a qualitative difference between individuals who perceive their significance as based solely on a surface-level or cultivated self compared to those who find significance in their perceived authentic selves.

THE INTERPLAY BETWEEN SOCIOCULTURAL AND EXPERIENTIAL SIGNIFICANCE

Although sociocultural and experiential significance are intertwined, there are occasions when the importance of one surpasses the other. This can happen for various reasons, and we explore a few notable examples below and expand on how a harmonious balance is key.

Developmental Influences

According to socioemotional selectivity theory, an individual's choice of objectives, pursuits, and preferences varies across different age periods (e.g., Charles & Carstensen, 2010; Hicks et al., 2012). For example, teenagers usually place a high emphasis on others' opinions of them. After reaching their 20s, young adults often exhibit a pronounced inclination to establish close personal connections. As individuals transition into mid-adulthood, they often prioritize career progression and self-improvement. Throughout all of these periods, sociocultural significance becomes particularly crucial as people seek recognition and resources through social interaction. Conversely, as people age, the importance of sociocultural significance may lessen as traditional pursuits such as career advancements and seeking status become less salient. Additionally, in cultural settings like the United States, older individuals are sometimes marginalized and viewed merely as diminishing entities rather than contributors capable of growth. Despite these challenges, older individuals can still find value in life through simple daily pleasures, such as engaging with friends, looking after family members, or exploring new hobbies. These activities may help sustain their belief that life is still meaningful and feels worthwhile.

Sociocultural Influences

Humans inherently seek social connections (Martino et al., 2015; Wickramaratne et al., 2022), and these connections exert a greater influence on us than often realized. Relationships with others and group dynamics shape the norms and shared values within the group, which in turn influence individuals' behaviors (Cialdini & Goldstein, 2004; Kallgren et al., 2000). Surrounding oneself with people dedicated to leaving a lasting legacy—whether in innovations, business, the arts, or politics—can inspire a similar pursuit of sociocultural significance. Conversely, being in the company of those who value experiential significance, such as those who embrace a slow-living lifestyle, may lead one to seek similar paths focused on personal feelings of fulfillment and finding life worthwhile. The people one surrounds oneself with matter, as research suggests that those in close relationships tend to perceive and respond to the world similarly, even on a neural basis (Parkinson et al., 2018).

Moreover, in many situations and group settings, there are powerful cues that dictate the norms and expected behaviors for conforming to the group. Conformity may entail a reduced sense of significance. Individuals experiencing heightened conformity or social influence may perceive their behaviors as being less autonomous (Alquist et al., 2013), whereas people who firmly believe in their own autonomy may be more inclined to view their actions as significant. In other words, individuals who hold strong free will beliefs—believing their actions stem from personal thoughts and values rather than external pressures (Baumeister, 2008)—may feel that their contributions carry greater meaning as they lay full claim to them.

Intrapersonal Influences

Characteristic adaptations can also influence which type of significance is emphasized. In the same vein as our previous discussion on mindfulness, possessing a quiet ego might lay the foundation for experiential appreciation. The quiet ego, characterized by balance and a growth orientation, comprises four traits: detached awareness, inclusive identity, perspective taking, and growth mindset (Bauer & Wayment, 2008). Detached awareness involves creating mental space to objectively and nonjudgmentally examine oneself and others, while still recognizing areas for improvement. Inclusive identity is the ability to integrate multiple viewpoints, while perspective taking is the capacity to understand and consider another's perception. Growth mindset views situations or events as opportunities for personal development. By adopting a detached view of oneself and others, while still incorporating other perspectives, individuals can focus on personal growth. The quiet ego is positively linked to various aspects of human flourishing. In particular, it is more strongly associated with humanistic and eudaimonic motives, values, and qualities such as well-being and wisdom (Bauer & Weatherbie, 2023). Individuals with a quieter ego might prioritize experiential significance, often seeking the eudaimonic "good life" and actively pursuing self-growth.

Conversely, the noisy ego bears a striking resemblance to narcissism, marked by an excessive focus on oneself and a need for external validation (Campbell & Buffardi, 2008). Unlike high self-esteem, in which a person sees themselves as inherently worthy, a noisy ego involves perceiving oneself as superior to others while simultaneously harboring feelings of low self-worth (Brummelman et al., 2016). In societies that value agentic traits over others, the egoistic bias of a noisy ego often seeks recognition for agentic traits and behaviors, such as being a confident and powerful CEO, rather than for communal contributions, like starting a nonprofit community garden (Campbell et al., 2002). Hence, individuals with a noisy ego might be more focused on their personal significance in order to achieve validation from others, whereas those who have a quieter ego pursue experiential significance for their own intrinsic reasons.

Balancing Sociocultural and Experiential Significance

We believe that both types of meaning are essential for a fulfilling life, and neither is more important than the other in most situations. Similar to other theoretical perspectives (e.g., Sheldon & Niemiec, 2006), we suggest that maintaining a balanced approach to satisfying each level of significance is optimal. This idea aligns with Baumeister's (1991) assertion that, although focusing on one primary source of meaning can temporarily help individuals feel their lives are fulfilling, they remain vulnerable to meaning threats if there is a deficit in another primary source of meaning. By achieving a healthy balance between both types of significance, individuals are better positioned for an enduring sense of meaning.

There are likely situations that are conducive to achieving a healthy balance between sociocultural and experiential significance (see above). Perhaps the most reliable way to experience both forms of significance is by engaging in activities that benefit other people, animals, or the planet more generally. These types of behaviors foster a sense of connection, which in turn engenders a strong sense of meaning (Baumeister, 1991). One not only feels deeply connected to the experience, enhancing one's sense of experiential significance, but also one experiences a self-transcendent feeling of being part of something larger than oneself that can leave a lasting impact. In these moments, individuals perceive themselves as significant actors in a more holistic web of life.

OTHER PATHWAYS TO MEANING: THE ROLES OF COHERENCE AND PURPOSE

It is noteworthy that our discussion of sociocultural and experiential significance was agnostic to the roles of purpose and coherence in experiencing meaning in life. According to many tripartite models of meaning, significance (or sociocultural mattering specifically), purpose, and coherence represent three distinct dimensions of meaning in life (George & Park, 2016; Martela & Steger, 2016). Purpose reflects having clear and satisfying goals in one's life, while coherence generally refers to the perception that one can make sense of one's life.

It is possible that the two conceptions of significance, along with purpose and coherence, represent four unique dimensions of meaning (see Kim et al., 2022, and Li et al., 2021, for a similar idea). Alternatively, including only sociocultural and experiential significance might represent a more parsimonious model of meaning. For instance, the most satisfying goal pursuits are intrinsic in nature; they feel good and are rewarding in and of themselves. Goals also feel more meaningful when they are abstract and often serve others. These two characteristics correspond to experiential and sociocultural significance, respectively, suggesting that the most optimal forms of purpose in life are those goal pursuits that embody both forms of significance.

Moreover, empirical studies suggest that coherence does not consistently predict general meaning in life after controlling for sociocultural and experiential significance (Kim et al., 2022; Li et al., 2021). This insight indicates that experiencing significance in life might be more central to one's beliefs about meaning compared to coherence (see Costin & Vignoles, 2020, for a similar idea). Of course, situations that undermine one's sense of coherence, such as personal or collective trauma (e.g., Park, 2013), can influence how meaningful one perceives one's life to be. However, it is unclear if this is because the lack of coherence leads to excessive rumination about the trauma, thereby undermining the individual's ability to detect meaning in their everyday life. More research is needed to explore the dynamic relationship between significance, purpose, and coherence, and the overall experience of meaning.

CONCLUSION

In this chapter, we presented a more nuanced perspective on the facet of significance in its relation to meaning in life. Significance has traditionally been conceptualized as "the desire to matter, to feel worthy and appreciated by others whose positive regard one seeks" (Kruglanski et al., 2022), emphasizing a social and appraisal-based approach, which we term *sociocultural significance*. Expanding on this, we highlighted how, at a phenomenological level, people also seek experiences that feel personally significant and contribute to a sense that life is worth living. Although more research needs to be conducted on the dynamics between these two forms of significance, we believe each conception of significance is essential for the experience of meaning in life.

REFERENCES

Alquist, J. L., Ainsworth, S. E., & Baumeister, R. F. (2013). Determined to conform: Disbelief in free will increases conformity. *Journal of Experimental Social Psychology, 49*(1), 80–86.

Batson, C. D., & Powell, A. A. (2003). Altruism and prosocial behavior. In T. Millon & M. J. Lerner (Eds.), *Handbook of psychology: Personality and social psychology* (Vol. 5, pp. 463–484). Wiley.

Bauer, J. J., & Wayment, H. A. (2008). The psychology of the quiet ego. In H. A. Wayment & J. J. Bauer (Eds.), *Transcending self-interest: Psychological explorations of the quiet ego* (pp. 7–19). American Psychological Association.

Bauer, J. J., & Weatherbie, K. J. (2023). The quiet ego and human flourishing. *Journal of Happiness Studies, 24*(8), 2499–2530.

Baumeister, R. F. (1991). *Meanings of life*. Guilford Press.

Baumeister, R. F. (2008). Free will in scientific psychology. *Perspectives on Psychological Science, 3*(1), 14–19.

Bishop, S. R., Lau, M., Shapiro, S., Carlson, L., Anderson, N. D., Carmody, J., . . . Devins, G. (2004). Mindfulness: A proposed operational definition. *Clinical Psychology: Science and Practice, 11*(3), 230–241.

Brown, K. W., & Ryan, R. M. (2003). The benefits of being present: Mindfulness and its role in psychological well-being. *Journal of Personality and Social Psychology, 84*(4), 822–848.

Brummelman, E., Thomaes, S., & Sedikides, C. (2016). Separating narcissism from self-esteem. *Current Directions in Psychological Science, 25*(1), 8–13.

Campbell, W. K., & Buffardi, L. E. (2008). The lure of the noisy ego: Narcissism as a social trap. In H. A. Wayment & J. J. Bauer (Eds.), *Transcending self-interest: Psychological explorations of the quiet ego* (pp. 23–32). American Psychological Association.

Campbell, W. K., Foster, C. A., & Finkel, E. J. (2002). Does self-love lead to love for others?: A story of narcissistic game playing. *Journal of Personality and Social Psychology, 83*(2), 340.

Charles, S. T., & Carstensen, L. L. (2010). Social and emotional aging. *Annual Review of Psychology, 61*(1), 383–409.

Chu, S. T. W., & Mak, W. W. (2020). How mindfulness enhances meaning in life: A meta-analysis of correlational studies and randomized controlled trials. *Mindfulness, 11*, 177–193.

Cialdini, R. B., & Goldstein, N. J. (2004). Social influence: Compliance and conformity. *Annual Review of Psychology, 55*(1), 591–621.

Collins, K. R., Stritzke, W. G., Page, A. C., Brown, J. D., & Wylde, T. J. (2018). Mind full of life: Does mindfulness confer resilience to suicide by increasing zest for life? *Journal of Affective Disorders, 226*, 100–107.

Colombo, M. (2014). Caring, the emotions, and social norm compliance. *Journal of Neuroscience, Psychology, and Economics, 7*(1), 33.

Costin, V., & Vignoles, V. L. (2020). Meaning is about mattering: Evaluating coherence, purpose, and existential mattering as precursors of meaning in life judgments. *Journal of Personality and Social Psychology, 118*(4), 864–884.

Cutrona, C. E., & Russell, D. W. (1987). The provisions of social relationships and adaptation to stress. *Advances in Personal Relationships, 1*(1), 37–67.

Dakin, B. C., Tan, N. P., Conner, T. S., & Bastian, B. (2022). The relationship between prosociality, meaning, and happiness in everyday life. *Journal of Happiness Studies, 23*(6), 2787–2804.

de St. Aubin, E. (2013). Generativity and the meaning of life. In J. A. Hicks & C. Routledge (Eds.), *The experience of meaning in life: Classical perspectives, emerging themes, and controversies* (pp. 241–255). Springer.

Ebersole, P. (1998). Types and depth of written life meanings. In P. T. P. Wong & P. S. Fry (Eds.), *The human quest for meaning: A handbook of psychological research and clinical applications* (pp. 179–191). Erlbaum.

Flett, G. (2018). *The psychology of mattering: Understanding the human need to be significant.* Academic Press.

Frankena, W. K. (1973). The ethics of love conceived as an ethics of virtue. *Journal of Religious Ethics, 1,* 21–36.

Frankfurt, H. (1982). The importance of what we care about. *Synthese,* 257–272.

Frankl, V. E. (1985). *Man's search for meaning.* Simon & Schuster.

Fredrickson, B. L. (2001). The role of positive emotions in positive psychology: The broaden-and-build theory of positive emotions. *American Psychologist, 56,* 218–226.

Garland, E. L., Farb, N. A., Goldin, P., & Fredrickson, B. L. (2015). Mindfulness broadens awareness and builds eudaimonic meaning: A process model of mindful positive emotion regulation. *Psychological Inquiry, 26*(4), 293–314.

Garland, E. L., Thielking, P., Thomas, E. A., Coombs, M., White, S., Lombardi, J., & Beck, A. (2017). Linking dispositional mindfulness and positive psychological processes in cancer survivorship: A multivariate path analytic test of the mindfulness-to-meaning theory. *Psycho-Oncology, 26*(5), 686–692.

George, L. S., & Park, C. L. (2016). Meaning in life as comprehension, purpose, and mattering: Toward integration and new research questions. *Review of General Psychology, 20*(3), 205–220.

Glăveanu, V. P. (2019). Creativity and wonder. *Journal of Creative Behavior, 53,* 171–177.

Greenberg, J., Pyszczynski, T., & Solomon, S. (1986). The causes and consequences of a need for self-esteem: A terror management theory. In R. F. Baumeister (Ed.), *Public self and private self* (pp. 189–212). Springer.

Guthrie, D., Maffly-Kipp, J., Gause, C., Kim, J., Martela, F., & Hicks, J. A. (2024). Interpersonal mattering and the experience of meaning in life. *Journal of Positive Psychology.*

Han, J., Wang, Y., Qian, J., & Shi, M. (2023). Delving into the role of creativity on meaning in life: A multiple mediation model. *Heliyon, 9*(6).

Heintzelman, S. J., & King, L. A. (2014). (The feeling of) meaning-as-information. *Personality and Social Psychology Review, 18*(2), 153–167.

Hicks, J. A., & King, L. A. (2009). Meaning in life as a subjective judgment and a lived experience. *Social and Personality Psychology Compass, 3*(4), 638–653.

Hicks, J. A., & Routledge, C. (2013). *The experience of meaning in life: Classical perspectives, emerging themes, and controversies.* Springer.

Hicks, J. A., Trent, J., Davis, W. E., & King, L. A. (2012). Positive affect, meaning in life, and future time perspective: an application of socioemotional selectivity theory. *Psychology and Aging, 27*(1), 181–189.

Hofer, J. (1934). Medical dissertation on nostalgia (C. K. Anspach, Trans.). *Bulletin of the History of Medicine, 2,* 376–391. (Original work published 1688)

James, W. (1890). *The principles of psychology* (Vol. 1). Holt.

Jiang, T., Hicks, J. A., Yuan, W., Yin, Y., Needy, L., & Vess, M. (2024). The unique nature and psychosocial implications of awe. *Nature Reviews Psychology.*

Jongman-Sereno, K. P., & Leary, M. R. (2019). The enigma of being yourself: A critical examination of the concept of authenticity. *Review of General Psychology, 23*(1), 133–142.

Kallgren, C. A., Reno, R. R., & Cialdini, R. B. (2000). A focus theory of normative conduct: When norms do and do not affect behavior. *Personality and Social Psychology Bulletin, 26*(8), 1002–1012.

Kashdan, T. B., & Steger, M. F. (2007). Curiosity and pathways to well-being and meaning in life: Traits, states, and everyday behaviors. *Motivation and Emotion, 31,* 159–173.

Kashdan, T. B., Weeks, J. W., & Savostyanova, A. A. (2011). Whether, how, and when social anxiety shapes positive experiences and events: A self-regulatory framework and treatment implications. *Clinical Psychology Review, 31*(5), 786–799.

Kasser, T., & Ryan, R. M. (1996). Further examining the American dream: Differential correlates of intrinsic and extrinsic goals. *Personality and Social Psychology Bulletin, 22*(3), 280–287.

Kaufman, J. C. (2018). Finding meaning with creativity in the past, present, and future. *Perspectives on Psychological Science, 13,* 734–749.

Kaufman, J. C., & Beghetto, R. A. (2009). Beyond big and little: The Four C model of creativity. *Review of General Psychology, 13*(1), 1–12.

Keltner, D., & Haidt, J. (2003). Approaching awe, a moral, spiritual, and aesthetic emotion. *Cognition and Emotion, 17,* 297–314.

Kernis, M. H., & Goldman, B. M. (2006). A multicomponent conceptualization of authenticity: Theory and research. In M. P. Zanna (Ed.), *Advances in experimental social psychology* (Vol. 38, pp. 283–357). Elsevier Academic Press.

Kim, J., Holte, P., Martela, F., Shanahan, C., Li, Z., Zhang, H., . . . Hicks, J. A. (2022). Experiential appreciation as a pathway to meaning in life. *Nature Human Behaviour, 6*(5), 677–690.

King, L. A., & Hicks, J. A. (2021). The science of meaning in life. *Annual Review of Psychology, 72*(1), 561–584.

King, L. A., Hicks, J. A., Krull, J. L., & Del Gaiso, A. K. (2006). Positive affect and the experience of meaning in life. *Journal of Personality and Social Psychology, 90,* 179–196.

Kinsella, E. L., Igou, E. R., & Ritchie, T. D. (2019). Heroism and the pursuit of a meaningful life. *Journal of Humanistic Psychology, 59*(4), 474–498.

Klein, N. (2017). Prosocial behavior increases perceptions of meaning in life. *Journal of Positive Psychology, 12*(4), 354-361.

Kruglanski, A. W., Gelfand, M. J., Bélanger, J. J., Hetiarachchi, M., & Gunaratna, R. (2015). Significance quest theory as the driver of radicalization towards terrorism. In J. Jerard & S. M. Nasir (Eds.), *Resilience and resolve: Communities against terrorism* (pp. 17–30). Imperial College Press.

Kruglanski, A. W., Molinario, E., Jasko, K., Webber, D., Leander, N. P., & Pierro, A. (2022). Significance-quest theory. *Perspectives on Psychological Science, 17*(4), 1050–1071.

Kyle, T. V. (1995). The concept of caring: a review of the literature. *Journal of Advanced Nursing, 21*(3), 506–514.

Lambert, N. M., Stillman, T. F., Baumeister, R. F., Fincham, F. D., Hicks, J. A., & Graham, S. M. (2010). Family as a salient source of meaning in young adulthood. *Journal of Positive Psychology, 5,* 367–376.

Lambert, N. M., Stillman, T. F., Hicks, J. A., Kamble, S., Baumeister, R. F., & Fincham, F. D. (2013). To belong is to matter: Sense of belonging enhances meaning in life. *Personality and Social Psychology Bulletin, 39*(11), 1418–1427.

Li, Z., Liu, Y., Peng, K., Hicks, J. A., & Gou, X. (2021). Developing a quadripartite existential meaning scale and exploring the internal structure of meaning in life. *Journal of Happiness Studies, 22,* 887–905.

Lutz, P. K., Newman, D. B., Schlegel, R. J., & Wirtz, D. (2023). Authenticity, meaning in life, and life satisfaction: A multicomponent investigation of relationships at the trait and state levels. *Journal of Personality, 91*(3), 541–555.

Lyubomirsky, S., King, L., & Diener, E. (2005). The benefits of frequent positive affect: Does happiness lead to success? *Psychological Bulletin, 131,* 803–855.

Martela, F., & Steger, M. F. (2016). The three meanings of meaning in life: Distinguishing coherence, purpose, and significance. *Journal of Positive Psychology, 11*(5), 531–545.

Martino, J., Pegg, J., & Frates, E. P. (2017). The connection prescription: Using the power of social interactions and the deep desire for connectedness to empower health and wellness. *American Journal of Lifestyle Medicine, 11*(6), 466–475.

McComb, S. E., Goldberg, J. O., Flett, G. L., & Rose, A. L. (2020). The double jeopardy of feeling lonely and unimportant: State and trait loneliness and feelings and fears of not mattering. *Frontiers in Psychology, 11,* Article 563420.

Mussel, P. (2013). Introducing the construct curiosity for predicting job performance. *Journal of Organizational Behavior, 34,* 453–472.

Nerantzaki, K., Efklides, A., & Metallidou, P. (2021). Epistemic emotions: Cognitive underpinnings and relations with metacognitive feelings. *New Ideas in Psychology, 63,* 100904.

Newman, G. E., & Smith, R. K. (2016). Kinds of authenticity. *Philosophy Compass, 11*(10), 609–618.

Office of the Surgeon General. (2023). *Our epidemic of loneliness and isolation: The U.S. Surgeon General's Advisory on the healing effects of social connection and community.* U.S. Department of Health and Human Services. www.hhs.gov/sites/default/files/surgeon-general-social-connection-advisory.pdf.

Oishi, S., Choi, H., Koo, M., Galinha, I., Ishii, K., Komiya, A., et al. (2020). Happiness, meaning, and psychological richness. *Affective Science, 1*(2), 107–115.

Park, C. L. (2013). Trauma and meaning making: Converging conceptualizations and emerging evidence. In J. A. Hicks & C. Routledge (Eds.), *The experience of meaning in life: Classical perspectives, emerging themes, and controversies* (pp. 61–76). Springer.

Parker, S. K., Bindl, U. K., & Strauss, K. (2010). Making things happen: A model of proactive motivation. *Journal of Management, 36*(4), 827–856.

Parkinson, C., Kleinbaum, A. M., & Wheatley, T. (2018). Similar neural responses predict friendship. *Nature Communications, 9*(1), 332.

Pearsall, J. (Ed.). (1998). *The new Oxford dictionary of English.* Oxford University Press.

Pulcini, E. (2017). What emotions motivate care? *Emotion Review, 9*(1), 64–71.

Putney, H., Silver, S., Silvia, P., Christensen, A. P., & Cotter, K. N. (2024). Why does creativity foster well-being?: Autonomy, competence, and relatedness during everyday creative activities. *Journal of Research in Personality, 113,* 104552.

Pyszczynski, T., Greenberg, J., Solomon, S., Arndt, J., & Schimel, J. (2004). Why do people need self-esteem?: A theoretical and empirical review. *Psychological Bulletin, 130*(3), 435.

Ramsey, M. A., & Gentzler, A. L. (2015). An upward spiral: Bidirectional associations between positive affect and positive aspects of close relationships across the life span. *Developmental Review, 36,* 58–104.

Rivera, G. N., Vess, M., Hicks, J. A., & Routledge, C. (2020). Awe and meaning: Elucidating complex effects of awe experiences on meaning in life. *European Journal of Social Psychology, 50,* 392–405.

Routledge, C., & Vess, M. (Eds.). (2019). *Handbook of terror management theory.* Elsevier Academic Press.

Runco, M. A., & Jaeger, G. J. (2012). The standard definition of creativity. *Creativity Research Journal, 24*(1), 92–96.

Schlegel, R. J., Hicks, J. A., Arndt, J., & King, L. A. (2009). Thine own self: True self-concept accessibility and meaning in life. *Journal of Personality and Social Psychology, 96*(2), 473–490.

Schlegel, R. J., Hicks, J. A., King, L. A., & Arndt, J. (2011). Feeling like you know who you are: Perceived true self-knowledge and meaning in life. *Personality and Social Psychology Bulletin, 37*(6), 745–756.

Schmader, T., & Sedikides, C. (2018). State authenticity as fit to environment: The implications of social identity for fit, authenticity, and self-segregation. *Personality and Social Psychology Review, 22*(3), 228–259.

Schutte, N. S., & Malouff, J. M. (2020). A meta-analysis of the relationship between curiosity and creativity. *Journal of Creative Behavior, 54,* 940–947.

Sedikides, C., & Wildschut, T. (2018). Finding meaning in nostalgia. *Review of General Psychology, 22*(1), 48–61.

Sedikides, C., Lenton, A. P., Slabu, L., & Thomaes, S. (2019). Sketching the contours of state authenticity. *Review of General Psychology, 23*(1), 73–88.

Sheldon, K. M., & Niemiec, C. P. (2006). It's not just the amount that counts: Balanced need satisfaction also affects well-being. *Journal of Personality and Social Psychology, 91*(2), 331–341.

Stamkou, E., Brummelman, E., Dunham, R., Nikolic, M., & Keltner, D. (2023). Awe sparks prosociality in children. *Psychological Science, 34,* 455–467.

Steger, M. F., Frazier, P., Oishi, S., & Kaler, M. (2006). The meaning in life questionnaire: Assessing the presence of and search for meaning in life. *Journal of Counseling Psychology, 53*(1), 80–93.

Van de Goor, J., Sools, A. M., Westerhof, G. J., & Bohlmeijer, E. T. (2020). Wonderful life: Exploring wonder in meaningful moments. *Journal of Humanistic Psychology, 60*(2), 147–167.

Van Tongeren, D. R., Green, J. D., Davis, D. E., Hook, J. N., & Hulsey, T. L. (2016). Prosociality enhances meaning in life. *Journal of Positive Psychology, 11*(3), 225–236.

Weiner, S. J., & Auster, S. (2007). From empathy to caring: Defining the ideal approach to a healing relationship. *Yale Journal of Biology and Medicine, 80*(3), 123.

Wickramaratne, P. J., Yangchen, T., Lepow, L., Patra, B. G., Glicksburg, B., Talati, A., . . . Weissman, M. M. (2022). Social connectedness as a determinant of mental health: A scoping review. *PLOS One, 17*(10), e0275004.

Williams, K. D., & Zadro, L. (2005). Ostracism: The indiscriminate early detection system. In K. D. Williams, J. P. Forgas, & W. von Hippel (Eds.), *The social outcast: Ostracism, social exclusion, rejection, and bullying* (pp. 19–34). Psychology Press.

Wonder. (1928). In *Oxford English dictionary.* Oxford University Press.

Wong, P. T. (Ed.). (2013). *The human quest for meaning: Theories, research, and applications.* Routledge.

Wood, A. M., Linley, P. A., Maltby, J., Baliousis, M., & Joseph, S. (2008). The authentic personality: A theoretical and empirical conceptualization and the development of the Authenticity Scale. *Journal of Counseling Psychology, 55*(3), 385.

Woodlief, D. T. (2017). *Smartphone use and mindfulness: Empirical tests of a hypothesized connection.* Doctoral dissertation. https://scholarcommons.sc.edu/etd/4241.

Yalom, I. D. (1980). *Existential psychotherapy.* Basic Books.

Zimmerman, M. J., & Bradley, B. (2019). Intrinsic vs. extrinsic value. In E. N. Zalta (Ed.), *The Stanford encyclopedia of philosophy.* https://plato.stanford.edu/archives/spr2019/entries/value-intrinsic-extrinsic.

CHAPTER 47

From Conscious Wishes to Nonconscious Actions

Gabriele Oettingen

This chapter examines wishes and daydreams about the future and how they help us fulfill our desires and meet our existential needs. First, I explore where these wishes and fantasies come from and how they can guide us in navigating daily life and addressing deeper questions of meaning and purpose. Next, I introduce a self-regulatory strategy called mental contrasting, which involves imagining a desired future and then reflecting on the reality that stands in the way. This process helps people commit to feasible goals and let go of unfeasible ones, allowing them to conserve energy and focus on more attainable pursuits. Mental contrasting is also helpful when dealing with counterfactual fantasies, the "if only . . ." thoughts about missed opportunities or alternate pasts that never happened. Finally, I compare mental contrasting with other behavior change strategies commonly used in psychology, including those in the areas of work, education, and health. Taken together, these insights show how people can use self-regulation to pursue their most meaningful wishes and manage life in ways that support both everyday functioning and long-term well-being.

WISHES AND FANTASIES ABOUT THE FUTURE

Needs Drive Wishes and Fantasies

While fantasies may appear to originate from external sources—stories we hear, events that happened, or ideas that are pushed upon us—they are primarily rooted in unmet needs (Atkinson & McClelland, 1948; Murray, 1938). The greater the need, the more likely individuals are to generate positive fantasies aimed at satisfying it (H. B. Kappes et al., 2012b). Needs can be physiological and specific, with immediate relevance to survival (e.g., need for water, food, safety; Maslow, 1943), or psychological and vague (e.g., need for esteem, meaning, intimacy). They are thought of as basic to human nature (e.g., need for autonomy, competence, relatedness; Ryan & Deci, 2000, 2017) or acquired through experience (e.g., need for power, achievement, affiliation; McClelland, 1985; Murray, 1938). Regardless of the presumed origin and type, needs shape the content of people's thoughts and daydreams (Atkinson & McClelland, 1948; McClelland et al., 1949; Murray, 1938).

The valence of fantasies and daydreams also plays a role. Across four experiments, H. B. Kappes and colleagues (2012b) showed that inducing specific needs (e.g., lack of water, lack of meaning, lack of interpersonal relations, lack of power) increased the positivity and idealizing attributes of future fantasies to satisfy the needs. For example, participants deprived of water versus satisfied control participants positively fantasized drinking water and enjoying it; those primed with a lack of meaning imagined going for a more meaningful job; those who were deprived of interpersonal relationships positively imagined getting together with their family and friends. Finally, those made to feel powerless yearned for strong leadership and idealized it. These findings suggest that positive fantasies reflect current needs and thus give helpful advice in which direction we want to move. Similarly, indulging in wishful fantasies is linked to greater autonomy motivation than simply stating one's goals, as is commonly asked to do in goal-setting research (Holding & Oettingen, 2025).

The Downside of Positive Fantasies

Despite their appeal, positive fantasies can undermine success. Although they boost mood and encourage exploring future possibilities (Fredrickson, 2004; Oettingen, 2000), they reduce effort and achievement across domains (H. B. Kappes et al., 2012a; Oettingen & Mayer, 2002). Students who fantasized about academic success or romance performed worse or were less likely to initiate relationships. Among job seekers, the more people entertained positive employment fantasies, the less they earned 2 years later and the fewer applications they submitted. Similarly, patients who fantasized about rapid recovery before they underwent hip replacement surgery, healed more slowly after surgery, as reported by their physical therapists. While such positive future fantasies reduced current depressive symptoms in the present moment, they predicted depressive mood over time (Oettingen et al., 2016), a relation that was partially explained by poor performance.

Why do fantasies hinder success? Fantasies mentally simulate achieving the desired future, leading to relaxation and reduced effort. In experiments, participants induced to positively fantasize about winning money were less likely to exert effort in delayed gratification tasks (Sciarappo et al., 2015). Positive fantasies lowered physiological (i.e., systolic blood pressure [SBP]; Wright, 1996) and self-reported energization (H. B. Kappes & Oettingen, 2011) that in turn predicted reduced goal-directed behavior over time.

When fulfilling wishes becomes demanding, the relaxation induced by positive fantasies becomes counterproductive. In two studies, participants read about a charity asking for little versus moderate resources (e.g., $1 vs. $25) to ease a human crisis (e.g., a lack of pain medication in Sierra Leone or the risk of flooding after Hurricane Irene). Inducing positive fantasies about the charity's success (vs. factual or no thoughts) led participants to spend only a little money and made them reluctant to give a moderate amount. Additionally, participants assigned to generate positive fantasies deemed the moderate request overly demanding (H. B. Kappes et al., 2013). These results align with findings on delay of gratification (Mischel, 1974) and ideomotor action theory (James, 1890/1950), suggesting that positive thoughts and images promote acting on easily attainable futures, but that mental effort is needed to meet more challenging future outcomes.

Summary

Unmet needs fuel positive, idealized fantasies about the future. While these fantasies help people identify their unsatisfied needs, they can impair effort and success when reaching the future outcomes is challenging. By simulating having already achieved the desired future, positive fantasies reduce energy and thereby the necessary problem-solving behavior to pursue real-world outcomes.

MENTAL CONTRASTING OF THE FUTURE AND REALITY

If positive fantasies drain energy and reduce effort and success, should we replace them with negative future thoughts? Not quite. Positive fantasies reflect our existential needs and give action direction. They cannot simply be dismissed. Instead, fantasy realization theory (Oettingen, 1999, 2000) proposes that positive fantasies about the future be complemented by a clear view of reality, specifically, the obstacle of reality that stands in the way of fulfilling the wish. By identifying and vividly imagining that obstacle, people recognize that their desired future is not yet attained. This realization mobilizes the energy needed to overcome the obstacle and enables insight into effective action. In other words, mentally contrasting the desired future with current reality provides three key elements for effective goal pursuit: direction, energy, and action. Thus, if the obstacle appears surmountable, people will pursue the direction of the desired outcome with full energy and active striving to attain the outcome. If the obstacle appears too costly or insurmountable, people can adjust by scaling down the wish, postponing it to a more apt point in time, or letting it go entirely, which frees resources for more feasible pursuits. Thus, mental contrasting helps people decide whether to push forward or let go; they engage when the obstacle seems possible to overcome and worth the effort, but disengage when it appears either impossible or not worth surmounting.

The Principle of Mental Contrasting

The principle of mental contrasting is straightforward. By imagining both the desired future *and* the obstacle of reality, two mental representations are simultaneously activated. According to Hebb's law (1949), concurrently activated entities form strong associative links. The link formed between future and reality in mental contrasting is one of obstruction, that is, the respective reality is experienced as standing in the way of the desired future (see also Higgins & Chaires, 1980). The relational construct of "obstacle standing in the way of the desired future" compels people to resolve the inner conflict, by overcoming the obstacle on the way to wish fulfilment. Importantly, if the obstacle is considered before fantasizing about the desired future, the energizing and action-guiding effects do not emerge (Oettingen, 2000, 2012; Oettingen et al., 2001).

Fantasy realization can be framed as problem solving. People face the problem of wanting to reach a future that is not readily attainable. Whether they resolve this problem effectively depends on how accurately their subjective understanding (their "subjective problem space") reflects the actual challenge (see Newell & Simon, 1972). Only when both the desired future and the obstructing reality are represented, and they are understood as conflicting, do people act accordingly. Ignoring either component, future or reality, or failing to see reality as a barrier, leads to ineffective or wasteful behavior, including futile persistence or premature disengagement.

Experimental Findings on Mental Contrasting

In one study (Oettingen et al., 2001, Study 3), for example, participants identified an important interpersonal problem and rated its importance and their expectation of resolution. They then listed four positive outcomes of resolving the problem and four negative aspects of current reality standing in the way. Participants were randomly assigned to four conditions. In the mental contrasting condition, they elaborated two positive future aspects and two negative reality aspects in alternating order, starting with the future. Other participants only indulged in positive outcomes, only dwelled on reality, or engaged in reverse contrasting (reality first, then future). Afterward, all participants reported how energized and motivated they felt to reach the desired future. Two weeks later, they described the actions they had taken to resolve the problem and when they had started acting.

Results showed that only participants in the mental contrasting condition responded according to their expectations (as a proxy for whether their obstacle is surmountable or insurmountable): those with high expectations felt more energized and acted quickly; those with low expectations felt hardly energized and delayed action. In contrast, the other conditions showed no such pattern: Indulging in the desired future failed to provide the energy to reach the desired future, while dwelling on reality failed to point out the future direction in which to act. In reverse contrasting, the desired future served as a relief from reality rather than a reference point—failing to produce goal-directed behavior as well. These findings have been replicated across domains (e.g., achievement, health, interpersonal relations), and across age, SES, and cultural backgrounds (reviews by Oettingen, 2012, 2014; Oettingen & Sevincer, 2018). When obstacles were seen as surmountable and not too costly, people who mentally contrasted engaged fully; when obstacles seemed insurmountable or too costly, they disengaged and redirected efforts toward more realistic endeavors, saving energy and other valuable resources. Recent research shows that even when future thoughts were directed toward negative, feared future outcomes, mental contrasting could translate them into constructive behavior, in this case, to prevent the feared future from occurring (Kim et al., 2024a; Yang et al., 2023).

Cognitive and Motivational Mechanisms of Mental Contrasting

Several series of experiments have investigated the mechanisms by which mental contrasting shapes setting preferences and changing behavior. In short, mental contrasting as a conscious exercise instigates nonconscious processes that drive behavior toward feasible desired futures and away from unfeasible ones.

Future–Reality Associations

In three lexical decision task studies, A. Kappes and Oettingen (2014) showed that mental contrasting creates strong nonconscious links between a desired future and the obstacle standing in the way. The strength of these links depended on whether participants had high expectations of reaching the desired future (i.e., perceived the obstacle as surmountable). Stronger links, in turn, predicted active pursuit of the desired future. Once participants reached the outcome, however, these nonconscious links, and the associated behaviors, dissolved. This finding suggests that such associations serve as a temporary, action-guiding mechanism.

Reinterpreting Reality

In two studies, A. Kappes and colleagues (2013) used task-switching paradigms to demonstrate that mental contrasting prompts people to reinterpret the present reality as an obstacle, particularly when expectations for success are high. For instance, being invited to a party may be construed as an obstacle to performing well on an exam the following day. Building on these findings, Wittleder and colleagues (2019) showed that mental contrasting also leads to more negative implicit evaluations of obstacles—provided they are seen as surmountable. Both the nonconscious reinterpretation of reality as an obstacle and its negative evaluation mediated increases in energization and performance aimed at overcoming the obstacle and achieving the desired future.

Reality–Behavior Associations

In two further studies, mental contrasting has been shown to strengthen nonconscious associative links between the obstacle and instrumental behaviors needed to overcome it (A. Kappes et al., 2012b). These links, formed nonconsciously as well, predicted actual behavior such as taking stairs instead of an elevator to become fitter. The observed effects were again contingent on the surmountability of the obstacle as indicated by participants' respective expectations of success.

Resilience to Negative Feedback

Mental contrasting helps people handle setbacks and negative feedback in a constructive way. Across four studies (A. Kappes et al., 2012a), it promoted careful processing of feedback and the formation of respective plans, while protecting self-views of competence and encouraging constructive interpretations of criticism. These effects depended on expectations of success: When high, mental contrasting turned negative feedback into fuel for pursuing the desired future; when low, it helped people disengage. These findings also suggest that, through mental contrasting, people may have interpreted setbacks as challenges and been sheltered from experiencing them as failures (Dweck & Leggett, 1988).

Energization

Finally, mental contrasting has increased energization when the desired outcome was seen as attainable and reduced it when not. This was shown in two studies (Oettingen et al., 2009; see also Sevincer et al., 2014a) using physiological (e.g., SBP) and self-report measures. Energization mediated the effect of mental contrasting on goal commitment and performance (e.g., rater-assessed performance in giving a talk in front of a camera). When the obstacle was deemed surmountable, mental contrasting provided the level of energy needed to overcome the obstacle and pursue the desired future; when the obstacle was deemed insurmountable, people reduced the energy level so they could save their resources for promising alternative endeavors.

Spontaneous Mental Contrasting

Despite its effectiveness in clarifying what people wish for and how they can go about fulfilling their wishes, spontaneous mental contrasting is surprisingly rare. Most individuals either indulge in positive fantasies or dwell on present reality (Sevincer & Oettingen, 2013). One may surmise that this pattern is particularly common in Western cultures. However, similar patterns have emerged among Chinese university students (Tamim et al., 2022, 2023).

Measuring spontaneous mental contrasting is challenging due to the fluid nature of conscious thought and imagery (James, 1904). However, mental contrasting can be assessed through content analysis of spontaneous thoughts and images associated with a personally meaningful wish (Sevincer & Oettingen, 2013). Across multiple studies, only 10–15% of participants engaged in spontaneous mental contrasting. This rate increased modestly, to around 20%, in contexts that demanded problem solving, such as tight timelines, taking responsibility, or being confronted with actionable opportunities (Sevincer et al., 2018, 2020; Tamim et al., 2024). Mental contrasting has been more common among individuals with high academic achievement, a strong need for achievement, and effective self-regulation skills (Sevincer et al., 2017). It has also been more frequent among successful athletes (Tay et al., 2019) and those with a promotion-focused mindset (Tamim et al., 2023).

Summary

Mental contrasting transforms vague wishes into actionable goals when success seems feasible and helps individuals disengage from unattainable goals. Experiments using different (e.g., lexical decision and task-switching) paradigms suggest it influences behavior via three nonconscious mechanisms: (1) strengthening associative links between the desired future outcome and the obstacle of the current reality; (2) formation of a relational construct where reality is perceived as an obstacle to the future; and (3) strengthening associative links between the obstacles of reality and effective means to overcome them. Additionally, mental contrasting enhances receptiveness to critical feedback while protecting self-esteem and perceived competence. It also increases energization when pursuing feasible future outcomes.

Importantly, mental contrasting is not a default mode of thinking. Instead, people tend to favor less cognitively demanding strategies, such as fantasizing about the future or ruminating about current reality. The cognitive effort required for mental contrasting has been demonstrated in neuropsychological research (Achtziger et al., 2009), as well as in experimental studies showing that its spontaneous use declines under conditions of energy depletion (Sevincer et al., 2015) or cognitive load (Sevincer et al., 2024).

MENTAL CONTRASTING AS A METACOGNITIVE STRATEGY

After discovering that mental contrasting helps people set preferences and fulfill wishes, and after identifying the mechanisms that lead from mental contrasting to behavior change, the question was whether mental contrasting could be taught and applied as a metacognitive self-regulatory strategy to help people satisfy existential needs, master everyday life, and ease long-term decision making. Teaching mental contrasting is particularly important because so few individuals engage in it spontaneously. When applied in everyday life, mental contrasting should enable people to discern central, more existential wishes, differentiate feasible from unfeasible ones, actively pursue the former, and let go of the latter.

Teaching Mental Contrasting

People can be taught to mentally contrast feasible yet challenging wishes, a practice that supports behavior change across a range of domains, including achievement, health, and interpersonal relationships. Because mental contrasting is an imagery-based exercise that involves identifying deep personal wishes, it is crucial to take a calm, uninterrupted moment, that is, a moment where the world can wait for the 5 minutes needed to perform the mental exercise. It involves three main steps: (1) identifying a meaningful, feasible, and challenging wish; (2) finding and imagining the best possible outcome; and (3) switching to reality by identifying the most critical internal obstacle standing in the way of realizing the wish. This obstacle, often an emotion, belief, or habit, is then vividly imagined in its specific time and place.

Even young children benefit from this method. For example, second-grade students taught to mentally contrast (rather than merely indulge in positive future fantasies) were more successful in learning vocabulary in a new language (Gollwitzer et al., 2011). In other studies, students improved their overall school performance (Oettingen et al., 2000), found more constructive negotiation solutions (Kirk et al., 2011), and increased creative output (Oettingen et al., 2012). In the health domain, even brief instructions to use mental contrasting promoted behavior change (Sheeran et al., 2013) and helped people cope with diabetes (Adriaanse et al., 2013), improve diet and exercise (Johannessen et al., 2013), and both seek and offer help (Oettingen et al., 2010b). In the interpersonal domain, couples practicing mental contrasting (vs. indulging) showed more genuine efforts toward reconciliation, with victims perceiving the apologies of their partners who had been taught mental contrasting as more sincere (Schrage et al., 2020). It improved romantic relationship satisfaction by facilitating constructive conflict resolution (Jöhnk et al., 2024). And it fostered support of significant others who were in an existential crises such as being in danger of catching COVID-19 (Kim et al., 2024b).

Mental Contrasting as a Strategy for Setting Preferences

Mental contrasting can also help individuals set preferences and disengage from unrealistic wishes. When applied to wishes of doubtful feasibility, people gain clarity on whether the wish should be pursued or abandoned. These clear insights make mental contrasting a particularly useful tool when people feel uneasy about their short- or long-term future. For instance, during the COVID-19 pandemic, many people wished intensely for the crisis to end, sometimes becoming paralyzed in other areas of life. Mentally contrasting this wish, imagining the relief of a post-pandemic world, and then considering the obstacles of the present reality, quickly revealed that this goal lay largely outside personal control. Consequently, individuals could disengage from this unfeasible wish and redirect their energy toward more actionable wishes, such as protecting themselves and their loved ones.

Early evidence supports this application. In one study, middle managers at a large hospital were taught either mental contrasting or positive future thinking. Two weeks later, those who learned mental contrasting reported greater success in time management, decision making, completing projects, and letting go of unproductive projects (Oettingen et al., 2010a). Letting go of futile projects freed up cognitive and motivational resources to pursue more realistic alternatives.

Mental Contrasting as a Strategy for Letting Go of Counterfactual Pasts

Mental contrasting is also effective for disengaging from idealized pasts, counterfactual scenarios that never came to pass and can no longer be realized. In six studies, participants imagined a longed-for counterfactual past (e.g., "If only I had gotten a PhD") and then mentally contrasted that scenario with present reality, highlighting the impossibility of ever realizing that past (Krott & Oettingen, 2018a). Compared to only fantasizing or only focusing on present reality, mental contrasting led to reduced regret, disappointment, and resentment, indicating lower emotional attachment to the counterfactual past. These effects held across different life domains and time spans, and regardless of whether the loss was attributed to oneself, others, or nonhuman forces. In a different set of experiments, participants who mentally contrasted counterfactual pasts also performed better on unrelated tasks, such as the Raven's Progressive Matrices, suggesting improved cognitive focus and engagement with the present (Krott & Oettingen, 2018b).

Mental contrasting thus seems to support a clear understanding of what can be changed and what lies beyond personal control, enabling people to focus on and successfully solve the tasks in their present moment.

Summary

Mental contrasting can be taught and applied as a metacognitive tool, in daily life and over the long term. It enables people to identify and pursue feasible wishes, set realistic preferences, and let go of unfeasible futures or lost counterfactual pasts. Although it is a conscious, structured imagery exercise, it works through nonconscious mechanisms, allowing people to change behavior without needing to directly challenge attitudes or beliefs. The steps of mental contrasting only provide the structure, while the individuals provide the content: They are the experts of their life. In addition, the three-step structure of mental contrasting stays stable, whereas the content of the wish, outcome, and obstacle is ever changing with the individual's changing needs (wish, outcome) and changing contexts (obstacle). In short, mental contrasting is a highly personal and flexible self-regulatory tool leading to effective and efficient behavior change. The tool can be easily learned and readily applied during everyday life.

MENTAL CONTRASTING WITH IMPLEMENTATION INTENTIONS

Some obstacles, such as strong impulses, intense emotions, or entrenched habits, are difficult to overcome because they involve automatic processes. While mental contrasting builds strong nonconscious associative links between obstacles and instrumental behavior to overcome them (A. Kappes et al., 2012a), these links can be further strengthened by combining mental contrasting with implementation intentions (MCII).

Implementation Intentions

Implementation intentions are "if–then" plans (e.g., "If situation *X* arises, then I will carry out goal-directed behavior *Y*") that link situational cues to goal-directed behaviors (Gollwitzer, 1999, 2014; Gollwitzer & Sheeran, 2025). These plans foster nonconscious associations between the specified cue and behavior, increasing the likelihood of goal-directed responses when the cue is encountered. Meta-analyses confirm their efficacy in goal pursuit ($d = 0.65$; Gollwitzer & Sheeran, 2006, 2025). In the context of mental contrasting, such plans typically take the form: "If [obstacle], then I will [behavior to overcome obstacle]." This plan strengthens the obstacle–behavior associative links even further, which is especially helpful when obstacles are strong impulses or emotionally charged. On the other hand, mental contrasting supports implementation intentions by providing the necessary preconditions for their functioning. It fosters commitment to wish fulfillment, identifies relevant and personalized obstacles (for the "if" part), and facilitates the selection of effective responses (for the "then" part). Additionally, mental contrasting readies people's minds for generating if–then plans (Oettingen et al., 2005). Importantly, in standard implementation intention studies, researchers provide participants with the content of the if–then plans. On the contrary, mental contrasting enables individuals to generate their own personalized, context-specific plans, thereby enhancing both autonomy and real-world applicability.

MCII across Life Domains

MCII is a flexible, content-independent tool applicable to any wish, whether short- or long-term, trivial or existential, and self- or other-serving. The method involves four steps: (1) identifying a feasible yet challenging wish, (2) identifying and imagining the best outcome, (3) identifying and imagining the main inner obstacle, and (4) forming an "if . . . *obstacle*, then I will . . . *act to overcome obstacle*" plan. It is accessible via WOOP (Wish, Outcome, Obstacle, Plan) instructions, available in multiple formats (written, audio, video, etc.) on *woopmylife.org* and via the WOOP app, making it easy to integrate the mental tool into daily life without professional support.

MCII is more effective than mental contrasting or implementation intentions alone in life domains where obstacles are often linked to strong impulses, emotions, or habits. For example, in reducing snacking, MCII outperformed the mere if–then plan (Adriaanse et al., 2010). MCII also enhanced cooperation in negotiation tasks, as mental contrasting encouraged planning of how to cooperate and take the perspective of the partner during the heat of negotiation (Kirk et al., 2013).

In education, MCII improved time management and academic performance in mothers of low socioeconomic status enrolled in vocational training (Oettingen et al., 2015), boosted homework quality for children at risk for attention-deficit/hyperactivity disorder (Gawrilow et al., 2013), and increased test preparation among high school students (Duckworth et al., 2011). It also improved classroom attendance, teacher–student relationships, and grades among middle school students (Duckworth et al., 2013). When integrated into a first-grade curriculum, MCII enhanced academic performance and executive functions over 12 months, and it fostered enrollment in advanced secondary education tracks 3 years later (Schunk et al., 2022).

In the health domain, MCII supported exercise (Stadler et al., 2009), improved diet (Stadler et al., 2010), promoted sports activities and weight loss in stroke patients (Marquardt et al., 2017), and increased physical capacity in chronic back pain patients (Christiansen et al., 2010). It reduced alcohol use, particularly in high-risk drinkers (Wittleder et al., 2019), and it decreased smoking in heavy smokers more effectively than governmental antismoking campaigns (Mutter et al., 2020). In interpersonal relationships, MCII reduced insecurity-driven behaviors (Houssais et al., 2013) and supported spouses of persons suffering from early-stage dementia (Monin et al., 2021; Mroz et al., 2024).

Summary

MCII combines the strengths of mental contrasting and implementation intentions into a single, effective self-regulation tool. Mental contrasting provides the prerequisites for implementation intentions to work, and implementation intentions enhance the associative links previously formed by mental contrasting. Together, they most effectively enable individuals to independently generate personalized behavior change. As brief, imagery-based, content-independent techniques, mental contrasting and MCII can be applied across ages, cultures, and life domains, empowering people to gain clarity and take active steps toward meaningful goals.

MENTAL CONTRASTING AND OTHER BEHAVIOR CHANGE STRATEGIES

Key Differences

Mental contrasting and MCII differ from most behavior change strategies in three key ways: (1) they consciously link future and reality through imagery, (2) they draw on nonconscious mechanisms of action control, and (3) they are content-independent and easily teachable. This section briefly outlines these differences and explores how mental contrasting and MCII may complement other behavior change strategies.

Mental contrasting uses conscious imagery of two independent entities—future and reality—to create nonconscious associative links: between future outcomes and present obstacles, and between those obstacles and the instrumental means to overcome them. Forming implementation intentions additionally strengthens the links between the obstacles and the instrumental behavior to overcome the obstacles via if–then plans. In short, mental contrasting and MCII consciously connect separate elements that are a priori apart. Connecting these elements produces nonconscious associative links that then automatically drive behavior. After engaging in MC or MCII, these nonconscious links allow for fast and effortless action that are resistant to disruption (Bargh, 1994), facilitating the pursuit of desired future outcomes.

Unlike other approaches to the pursuit of future outcomes, such as goal setting, cognitive reappraisal, or growth mindsets, which in-directly influence behavior via changing single entities (e.g., values, beliefs), mental contrasting and MCII address behavior change more directly by creating nonconscious associative mental structures that then predict behavior change without touching values or beliefs. Over time, the behavior changes brought about by mental contrasting or MCII may, in turn, lead to shifts in values and beliefs.

Mental contrasting and MCII can be taught as metacognitive tools that empower individuals to self-regulate and take ownership of their behavior change, shifting agency from external professional sources (e.g., teachers, therapists, counselors) to persons themselves.

Content for mental contrasting and MCII is generated by individuals based on their own needs and wishes and their own past experiences, making it easily teachable and effective across contexts and cultures. Brief written, audio, or video instructions (see *woopmylife.org* and the *WOOP app*) have led to long-term effects in diverse populations, from improved academic performance in first-grade children (Schunk et al., 2022), to increased physical activity in adults (Sheeran et al., 2013), to sustained weight loss in stroke patients (Marquardt et al., 2017).

Performance Accomplishments

Goal Setting

Fantasy realization theory and its construct of mental contrasting are often confused with goal-setting theory (Locke & Latham, 1990, 2002), but the two clearly differ in focus and mechanisms. Mental contrasting concerns how goals and subsequent goal pursuit emerge from wishful thinking via self-regulatory processes, while goal-setting theory emphasizes which attributes of goals (e.g., specificity, moderate difficulty) optimize performance. In addition, mental contrasting fosters commitment through nonconscious mechanisms; goal-setting theory emphasizes conscious effort, strategy, and persistence as mediators of strong performance (Seijts & Latham, 2005). In mental contrasting, commitment is an outcome; in goal setting, it moderates performance. Feedback processing also differs. Mental contrasting leads people to selectively integrate feedback based on whether the critical obstacle can be overcome (expectations of success are high), while goal setting treats feedback as a performance moderator (Locke & Latham, 2019).

In counseling, goal-setting theory is commonly applied using SMART goals—goals that are "specific, measurable, achievable, relevant, and time-bound" (Doran, 1981). Recent reviews in the field of physical activity suggest that the application of SMART goals is not always grounded in theory, is applied inconsistently, often lacks consistent empirical support, and tends to provide insufficient guidance and goal specification. Reviews also caution that using SMART goals may have harmful effects, including greater pressure, stress, or anxiety and reduced enjoyment. They conclude that interventions based on the original goal-setting theory tend to be more effective (Swann et al., 2021, 2023; see also comment by Kwasnicka et al., 2021).

Self-Efficacy

Expectancy–value models (e.g., Ajzen, 1991; Atkinson, 1957; see Oettingen & Gollwitzer, 2010) suggest that goal pursuit depends on two factors: the expected likelihood that a desired outcome will occur if one performs a relevant behavior (outcome expectations), and the value placed on that outcome. In addition, self-efficacy expectations, defined as the belief that one can carry out the behavior needed to achieve a desired outcome, is a strong predictor of goal pursuit across various domains (Bandura, 1977; Schunk & DiBenedetto, 2018). Bandura (1977) identified four main sources of self-efficacy: past performance, vicarious experience, verbal persuasion, and emotional arousal, with past performance being the most influential.

According to Bandura's model of reciprocal determinism, behavior change strengthens efficacy beliefs, which in turn promote further behavior change, creating a positive cycle of "behavior–efficacy–behavior" (Bandura, 1978). However, this cycle may stall when efficacy expectations do not translate into action, such as when individuals indulge in fantasies about the future, dwell on the reality, reverse contrast, or simply drift in their thoughts through daily life (Oettingen, 2000, 2012). Mental contrasting can help activate the positive cycle of behavior–efficacy–behavior by translating high efficacy expectations into actual behavior.

Mental contrasting also addresses outcome expectations. These expectations can be difficult to shift, especially when shaped by experiencing a lack of contingency between behaviors and outcomes, as often happens in uncontrollable or discouraging environments (e.g., Abramson et al., 1978;

Seligman, 1972). By helping individuals distinguish between feasible and unfeasible wishes and goals, mental contrasting prevents wasted effort, directing motivation toward attainable positive future outcomes.

Growth Mindset

Growth mindset refers to beliefs that human attributes are malleable and can be developed through effortful engagement. This mindset fosters learning goals that in turn spur resilience and persistence when setbacks occur (Dweck, 2006; Dweck & Leggett, 1988). In contrast, a fixed mindset assumes that attributes are static, leading to performance goals and avoidance behaviors in response to setbacks, which are seen as personal failures rather than challenges. Mindsets can function both as stable traits and as dynamic states, shaped by social context and performance feedback. Procedural feedback supports growth mindsets, while competence-focused feedback tends to foster fixed mindsets (Park et al., 2016). People with a growth mindset tend to focus on future possibilities, whereas those with a fixed mindset are more attuned to present obstacles (Sevincer et al., 2014b). Mental contrasting may help individuals with a fixed mindset shift their focus toward future opportunities and reinterpret negative feedback as a challenge rather than a failure (A. Kappes et al., 2012a).

Supporting Mental Health

Cognitive-Behavioral Therapy

Cognitive-behavioral therapy (CBT) is a well-established, evidence-based treatment (Beck, 1993, 2019; Butler et al., 2006) used to address depression, anxiety, addiction, interpersonal problems, and personality disorders. CBT improves functioning by identifying and restructuring distorted beliefs about the self, the world, and the future. Sample techniques include fear confrontation, role playing, mental simulation, and relaxation. The primary goal of CBT is cognitive change leading to behavioral change. Mental contrasting shares CBT's emphasis on present realities and personal context but differs in mechanisms. Rather than altering beliefs, mental contrasting links a desired future to current obstacles to mobilize goal-directed behavior. Mental contrasting is brief, structured, and can be self-applied, making it a potential adjunct to CBT, particularly when cognitive change is difficult.

Motivational Interviewing

The client-centered method of motivational interviewing fosters trust and autonomy through empathic dialogue (Miller & Rollnick, 2013). It aims to raise awareness of discrepancies between current behavior and goals in a nondirective way. Both motivational interviewing and mental contrasting avoid imposing content and encourage self-direction. However, motivational interviewing is unstructured and provider-guided, while mental contrasting follows a strict procedural sequence (wish, outcome, obstacle, plan) that can be self-guided. Mechanistically, motivational interviewing promotes reflection, whereas mental contrasting mobilizes action by mentally linking future and reality.

Mindfulness

Mindfulness, increasingly used in clinical contexts, is a form of meditation aimed at reducing stress and enhancing well-being (Kabat-Zinn, 2003, 2023). It involves nonjudgmental awareness of present experiences—what one feels, sees, hears, or senses—without interpreting or evaluating them. Breathing exercises and guided imagery focused on bodily sensations or the immediate environment help calm the mind and body, promoting full immersion in the present.

Mental contrasting also involves guided imagery and a calm setting, but with a different purpose. While mindfulness encourages detachment and passive acceptance, mental contrasting fosters active engagement, guiding individuals to visualize a desired future, confront current obstacles, and identify steps toward goal attainment. In contrast to mindfulness's focus on nonstriving, mental contrasting explicitly promotes behavior change—via either active striving for attaining feasible desired futures or letting go of unrealistic ones to redirect effort toward more promising endeavors.

Coping with Stress

Cognitive Reappraisal

While mindfulness promotes calm acceptance of the present, cognitive reappraisal involves deliberately changing the meaning of a situation to regulate thoughts, impulses, and emotions. It can help create distance, shift focus to alternatives or find meaning and positive aspects in challenging events (Gross, 1998; McRae et al., 2012). In CBT this technique is known as cognitive restructuring—replacing unrealistic, negative thoughts with more accurate, constructive interpretations (Beck et al., 1979). Children have been observed using reappraisal to delay gratification by reframing tempting stimuli (e.g., viewing a pretzel as a wooden log; Mischel, 1974, 2015; see also Gawrilow et al., 2011). By prompting reappraisal of one's personal reality as an obstacle in the way of reaching the desired future, mental contrasting offers insight and clarity, laying a solid foundation for action while conserving resources and avoiding risky decisions.

Cognitive Appraisal

Cognitive reappraisal differs from Lazarus and Folkman's (1984) cognitive appraisal model, which involves assessing the situation (primary appraisal) and assessing one's coping resources (secondary appraisal). When resources are sufficient, problem-focused coping is effective; when resources are not sufficient, emotion-focused coping, often via reappraisal, can reduce stress by finding meaning or alternative perspectives. However, emotion-focused coping has shown mixed effectiveness in dealing with stressors (Ryan, 2013; Schoenmakers et al., 2015). Its limitations may arise from difficulties in recognizing the key obstacles to effective coping with stressful situations, which can hinder the ability to assess whether a problem-focused or emotion-focused approach is more suitable. In this context, mental contrasting may offer a useful tool. By mentally juxtaposing a desired outcome with the primary obstacle, individuals can better evaluate which coping strategy—problem-focused or emotion-focused—is more appropriate for the situation. If the obstacle appears surmountable, problem-focused coping will lead to resolving the issue; if the obstacle does not appear surmountable, emotion-focused coping will lead to accepting the limitation and to redirecting efforts toward more promising futures.

Social Comparison

Social comparison is another form of coping used to manage stressful or threatening situations. People compare themselves with others for reasons of self-evaluation (contrast) or inspiration (assimilation; Unkelbach et al., 2023). Downward contrast comparisons (to those worse off) can boost self-esteem, while assimilation of upward comparisons (to those doing better) can provide models for coping. Taylor (1983) showed that combining downward contrast with upward assimilation in newly diagnosed breast cancer patients helped people feel better, while at the same time learning how to manage their condition. Mental contrasting can help to make use of upward assimilation comparisons by helping individuals personalize the coping behaviors observed in admired role models. For instance, seeing a role model cope by exercising regularly, a person might use mental contrasting to commit to exercising as well, but identify and act on their own preferred form of physical activity.

Self-Affirmation

Beyond social comparison, people can bolster self-worth through self-affirmation, thereby affirming core values to protect self-esteem, particularly in the face of threat (Sherman et al., 2021; Steele, 1988). Affirming personal values, for example, improves academic outcomes and buffers against negative feedback, enhancing resilience and belonging. Self-affirmation works best when it targets a domain that is different from the domain in which the threat occurs. Affirming in the same domain may backfire, reinforcing resistance to change due to strong commitment in the domain of the threatened outcome (Blanton et al., 1997; Sherman & Cohen, 2006). Functionally, self-affirmation resembles emotion-focused coping, offering support and stability rather than resolving the threat itself.

Mental contrasting differs from self-affirmation in targeting problem solving rather than reinforcing self-worth or boosting mood. It prompts individuals either to actively address a threatening situation or to disengage from it when necessary. Given this functional difference, the effectiveness of combining self-affirmation with mental contrasting depends on whether the affirmation and the threat pertain to the same domain. If the affirmation addresses a different domain than the threat, mental contrasting is unlikely to be effective, as the affirmation may reduce the urgency to act. In contrast, when affirmation and threat occur in the same domain, the resulting boost in commitment can ignite a strong desire to actively cope with the threat, thereby enhancing the impact of mental contrasting.

Summary

Mental contrasting should be considered alongside other established behavior change strategies. Drawing on its distinct principles, I outlined how mental contrasting can complement three major types of approaches: enhancing performance, supporting mental health in clinical settings, and managing stress in everyday life. As a conscious technique that activates nonconscious processes to automate behavior, mental contrasting can innovatively enhance existing methods that primarily target beliefs, attitudes, or self-concept.

CONCLUSION

This chapter highlights self-regulatory strategies that enhance everyday functioning and long-term development. Mental contrasting stands out by using conscious imagery to elicit nonconscious processes that drive behavior change, either by promoting action toward feasible wishes or by facilitating disengagement from unrealistic ones. This cognitive procedure helps conserve resources and redirect effort toward desirable and attainable future outcomes. Using conscious thoughts to produce automatic cognition, emotion, and action, mental contrasting enables people to find meaning and direction to act. Additionally, it prepares in advance how to act according to reality with little need for ongoing reflection, thereby easing daily life and reducing mental strain. Integrating mental contrasting, on its own or with if–then plans, into motivational and clinical interventions offers a promising path for advancing research and practice in behavior change.

REFERENCES

Abramson, L. Y., Seligman, M. E., & Teasdale, J. D. (1978). Learned helplessness in humans: Critique and reformulation. *Journal of Abnormal Psychology, 87,* 49–74.

Achtziger, A., Fehr, T., Oettingen, G., Gollwitzer, P. M., & Rockstroh, B. (2009). Strategies of intention formation are reflected in continuous MEG activity. *Social Neuroscience, 4,* 11–27.

Adriaanse, M. A., de Ridder, D. T. D., & Voorneman, I. (2013). Improving diabetes self-management by mental contrasting. *Psychology and Health, 28,* 1–12.

Adriaanse, M. A., Oettingen, G., Gollwitzer, P. M., Hennes, E. P., de Ridder, D. T. D., & de Witt, J. B. F. (2010). When planning is not enough: Fighting unhealthy snacking habits by mental contrasting with implementation intentions (MCII). *European Journal of Social Psychology, 40,* 1277–1293.

Ajzen, I. (1991). The theory of planned behavior. *Organizational Behavior and Human Decision Processes, 50,* 179–211.

Atkinson, J. W. (1957). Motivational determinants of risk-taking behavior. *Psychological Review, 64,* 359–372.

Atkinson, J. W., & McClelland, D. C. (1948). The projective expression of needs: II: The effect of different intensities of the hunger drive on thematic apperception. *Journal of Experimental Psychology, 38,* 643–658.

Bandura, A. (1977). Self-efficacy: Toward a unifying theory of behavioral change. *Psychological Review, 84,* 191–215.

Bandura, A. (1978). The self system in reciprocal determinism. *American Psychologist, 33,* 344–358.

Bargh, J. A. (1994). The four horsemen of automaticity: Awareness, intention, efficiency, and control in social cognition. In R. S. Wyer, Jr., & K. T. Srull (Eds.), *Handbook of social cognition* (pp. 1–40). Erlbaum.

Beck, A. T. (1993). Cognitive therapy: Past, present, and future. *Journal of Consulting and Clinical Psychology, 61,* 194–198.

Beck, A. T. (2019). A 60-year evolution of cognitive theory and therapy. *Perspectives on Psychological Science, 14,* 16–20.

Beck, A. T., Rush, A. J., Shaw, B. F., & Emery,

G. (1979). *Cognitive therapy of depression.* Guilford Press.

Blanton, H., Cooper, J., Slkurnik, I., & Aronson, J. (1997). When bad things happen to good feedback: Exacerbating the need for self-justification with self-affirmations. *Personality and Social Psychology Bulletin, 23,* 684–692.

Butler, A. C., Chapman, J. E., Forman, E. M., & Beck, A. T. (2006). The empirical status of cognitive-behavioral therapy: A review of meta-analyses. *Clinical Psychology Review, 26,* 17–31.

Christiansen, S., Oettingen, G., Dahme, B., & Klinger, R. (2010). A short goal-pursuit intervention to improve physical capacity: A randomized clinical trial in chronic back pain patients. *Pain, 149,* 444–452.

Doran, G. T. (1981). There's a S.M.A.R.T. way to write management's goals and objectives. *Management Review, 70,* 35–36.

Duckworth, A. L., Grant, H., Loew, B., Oettingen, G., & Gollwitzer, P. M. (2011). Self-regulation strategies improve self-discipline in adolescents: Benefits of mental contrasting and implementation intentions. *Educational Psychology, 31,* 17–26.

Duckworth, A. L., Kirby, T. A., Gollwitzer, A., & Oettingen, G. (2013). From fantasy to action: Mental contrasting with implementation intentions (MCII) improves academic performance in children. *Social Psychological and Personality Science, 4,* 745–753.

Dweck, C. S. (2006). *Mindset: The new psychology of success.* Random House.

Dweck, C. S., & Leggett, E. L. (1988). A social-cognitive approach to motivation and personality. *Psychological Review, 95,* 256–273.

Fredrickson, B. L. (2004). The broaden-and-build theory of positive emotions. *Philosophical Transactions of the Royal Society B: Biological Sciences, 359,* 1367–1378.

Gawrilow, C., Gollwitzer, P. M., & Oettingen, G. (2011). If–then plans benefit delay of gratification performance in children with and without ADHD. *Cognitive Therapy and Research, 35,* 442–455.

Gawrilow, C., Morgenroth, K., Schultz, R., Oettingen, G., & Gollwitzer, P. M. (2013). Mental contrasting with implementation intentions enhances self-regulation of goal pursuit in schoolchildren at risk for ADHD. *Motivation and Emotion, 37,* 134–145.

Gollwitzer, A., Oettingen, G., Kirby, T. A., Duckworth, A. L., & Mayer, D. (2011). Mental contrasting facilitates academic performance in school children. *Motivation and Emotion, 35,* 403–412.

Gollwitzer, P. M. (1999). Implementation intentions: Strong effects of simple plans. *American Psychologist, 54,* 493–503.

Gollwitzer, P. M. (2014). Weakness of the will: Is a quick fix possible? *Motivation and Emotion, 38,* 305–322.

Gollwitzer, P. M., & Sheeran, P. (2006). Implementation intentions and goal achievement: A meta-analysis of effects and processes. *Advances in Experimental Social Psychology, 38,* 69–119.

Gollwitzer, P. M., & Sheeran, P. (2025). Psychology of planning. *Annual Review of Psychology, 76*(1), 303–328.

Gross, J. J. (1998). The emerging field of emotion regulation: An integrative review. *Review of General Psychology, 2,* 271–299.

Hebb, D. O. (1949). *The organization of behavior; A neuropsychological theory.* Wiley.

Higgins, E. T., & Chaires, W. M. (1980). Accessibility of interrelational constructs: Implications for stimulus encoding and creativity. *Journal of Experimental Social Psychology, 16,* 348–361.

Holding, A., & Oettingen, G. (2025). *Mental contrasting breeds autonomous motivation for goal pursuit.* Manuscript in preparation.

Houssais, S., Oettingen, G., & Mayer, D. (2013). Using mental contrasting with implementation intentions to self-regulate insecurity-based behaviors in relationships. *Motivation and Emotion, 37,* 224–233.

James, W. (1904). The stream of consciousness. In *Psychology* (pp. 151–175). Holt.

James, W. (1950). *Principles of psychology.* Holt. (Original work published 1890)

Jöhnk, H., Sevincer, A. T., & Oettingen, G. (2024). Mental contrasting and conflict management in satisfied and unsatisfied romantic relationships. *Journal of Social and Personal Relationships, 42*(2), 367–391.

Johannessen, K. B., Oettingen, G., & Mayer, D. (2012). Mental contrasting of a dieting wish improves self-reported health behaviour. *Psychology and Health, 27,* 43–58.

Kabat-Zinn, J. (2003). Mindfulness-based interventions in context: Past, present, and future. *Clinical Psychology: Science and Practice, 10,* 144–156.

Kabat-Zinn, J. (2023). *Wherever you go, there you are: Mindfulness meditation in everyday life.* Hachette UK.

Kappes, A., & Oettingen, G. (2014). The emergence of goal pursuit: Mental contrasting connects future and reality. *Journal of Experimental Social Psychology, 54,* 25–39.

Kappes, A., Oettingen, G., & Pak, H. (2012a). Mental contrasting and the self-regulation of responding to negative feedback. *Personality and Social Psychology Bulletin, 38,* 845–856.

Kappes, A., Singmann, H., & Oettingen, G. (2012b). Mental contrasting instigates goal pursuit by linking obstacles of reality with instrumental behavior. *Journal of Experimental Social Psychology, 48*, 811–818.

Kappes, A., Wendt, M., Reinelt, T., & Oettingen, G. (2013). Mental contrasting changes the meaning of reality. *Journal of Experimental Social Psychology, 49*, 797–810.

Kappes, H. B., & Oettingen, G. (2011). Positive fantasies about idealized futures sap energy. *Journal of Experimental Social Psychology, 47*, 719–729.

Kappes, H. B., Oettingen, G., & Mayer, D. (2012). Positive fantasies predict low academic achievement in disadvantaged students. *European Journal of Social Psychology, 42*, 53–64.

Kappes, H. B., Schwörer, B., & Oettingen, G. (2012). Needs instigate positive fantasies of idealized futures. *European Journal of Social Psychology, 42*, 299–307.

Kappes, H. B., Sharma, E., & Oettingen, G. (2013). Positive fantasies dampen charitable giving when many resources are demanded. *Journal of Consumer Psychology, 23*, 128–135.

Kim, S., Gollwitzer, P. M., & Oettingen, G. (2024a). Mental contrasting of a negative future facilitates COVID-19 preventative behaviors: Two randomized controlled trials. *Psychology and Health, 39*, 1–23.

Kim, S., Gollwitzer, P. M., & Oettingen, G. (2024b). Mental contrasting promotes effective self-regulation for the benefits of groups. *British Journal of Social Psychology.*

Kirk, D., Oettingen, G., & Gollwitzer, P. M. (2011). Mental contrasting promotes integrative bargaining. *International Journal of Conflict Management, 22*, 324–341.

Kirk, D., Oettingen, G., & Gollwitzer, P. M. (2013). Promoting integrative bargaining: Mental contrasting with implementation intentions. *International Journal of Conflict Management, 24*, 148–165.

Krott, N. R., & Oettingen, G. (2018a). Mental contrasting of counterfactual fantasies attenuates disappointment, regret, and resentment. *Motivation and Emotion, 42*, 17–36.

Krott, N. R., & Oettingen, G. (2018b). Mental contrasting of counterfactual fantasies engages people in their present life. *Motivation Science, 4*, 137–157.

Kwasnicka, D., Ntoumanis, N., & Sniehotta, F. F. (2021). Setting performance and learning goals is useful for active and inactive individuals, if goals are personalized and flexible: Commentary on Swann et al. *Health Psychology Review, 15*(1), 51–55.

Lazarus, R. S., & Folkman, S. (1984). *Stress, appraisal, and coping.* Springer.

Locke, E. A., & Latham, G. P. (1990). *A theory of goal setting and task performance.* Prentice Hall.

Locke, E. A., & Latham, G. P. (2002). Building a practically useful theory of goal setting and task motivation: A 35-year odyssey. *American Psychologist, 57*, 705–717.

Locke, E. A., & Latham, G. P. (2019). The development of goal setting theory: A half century retrospective. *Motivation Science, 5*, 93–105.

Marquardt, M. K., Oettingen, G., Gollwitzer, P. M., Sheeran, P., & Liepert, J. (2017). Mental contrasting with implementation intentions (MCII) improves physical activity and weight loss among stroke survivors over one year. *Rehabilitation Psychology, 62*, 580–590.

Maslow, A. H. (1943). A theory of human motivation. *Psychological Review, 50*, 370–396.

McClelland, D. C. (1985). How motives, skills, and values determine what people do. *American Psychologist, 41*, 812–825.

McClelland, D. C., Clark, R. A., Roby, T. B., & Atkinson, J. W. (1949). The projective expression of needs: IV. The effect of the need for achievement on thematic apperception. *Journal of Experimental Psychology, 39*, 242–255.

McRae, K., Ciesielski, B., & Gross, J. J. (2012). Unpacking cognitive reappraisal: Goals, tactics, and outcomes. *Emotion, 12*, 250.

Miller, W. R., & Rollnick, S. (2013). *Motivational interviewing: Helping people change* (3rd ed.). Guilford Press.

Mischel, W. (1974). Processes in delay of gratification. In L. Berkowitz (Ed.), *Advances in experimental social psychology* (Vol. 7, pp. 249–292). Academic Press.

Mischel, W. (2015). *The marshmallow test: Why self-control is the engine of success.* Little, Brown.

Monin, J. K., Oettingen, G., Laws, H., David, D., DeMatteo, L., & Marottoli, R. (2021). A controlled pilot study of the wish outcome obstacle plan strategy for spouses of persons with early-stage dementia. *Journal of Gerontology: Psychological Sciences, 77*(3), 513–324.

Mroz, E. L., Schwartz, A. E., Valeika, S., Oettingen, G., Marottoli, R., David, D., . . . Monin J. K. (2024). "WOOP is my safe haven": A qualitative feasibility and acceptability study of the wish outcome obstacle plan (WOOP) intervention for spouses of people living with early-stage dementia. *International Journal of Geriatric Psychiatry, 39*(5).

Murray, H. (1938). *Explorations in personality.* Oxford University Press.

Mutter, E., Oettingen, G., & Gollwitzer, P. M. (2020). An online randomised controlled trial of mental contrasting with implementation intentions as a smoking behaviour change intervention. *Psychology and Health, 35*, 318–345.

Newell, A., & Simon, H. A. (1972). *Human problem solving.* Prentice-Hall.

Oettingen, G. (1999). Free fantasies about the

future and the emergence of developmental goals. In J. Brandtstädter & R. M. Lerner (Eds.), *Action and self-development: Theory and research through the life span* (pp. 315–342). Sage.

Oettingen, G. (2000). Expectancy effects on behavior depend on self-regulatory thought. *Social Cognition, 18,* 101–129.

Oettingen, G. (2012). Future thought and behaviour change. *European Review of Social Psychology, 23,* 1–63.

Oettingen, G. (2014). *Rethinking positive thinking: inside the new science of motivation.* Penguin/Random House.

Oettingen, G., & Gollwitzer, P. M. (2010). Strategies of setting and implementing goals: Mental contrasting and implementation intentions. In J. E. Maddux & J. P. Tangney (Eds.), *Social psychological foundations of clinical psychology* (pp. 114–135). Guilford Press.

Oettingen, G., Hönig, G., & Gollwitzer, P. M. (2000). Effective self-regulation of goal attainment. *International Journal of Educational Research, 33,* 705–732.

Oettingen, G., Kappes, H. B., Guttenberg, K. B., & Gollwitzer, P. M. (2015). Self-regulation of time management: Mental contrasting with implementation intentions. *European Journal of Social Psychology, 45,* 218–229.

Oettingen, G., Marquardt, M. K., & Gollwitzer, P. M. (2012). Mental contrasting turns positive feedback on creative potential into successful performance. *Journal of Experimental Social Psychology, 48,* 990–996.

Oettingen, G., & Mayer, D. (2002). The motivating function of thinking about the future: Expectations versus fantasies. *Journal of Personality and Social Psychology, 83,* 1198–1212.

Oettingen, G., Mayer, D., & Brinkmann, B. (2010a). Mental contrasting of future and reality: Managing the demands of everyday life in health care professionals. *Journal of Personnel Psychology, 9,* 138–144.

Oettingen, G., Mayer, D., & Portnow, S. (2016). Pleasure now, pain later: Positive fantasies about the future predict symptoms of depression. *Psychological Science, 27,* 345–353.

Oettingen, G., Mayer, D., Sevincer, A. T., Stephens, E. J., Pak, H., & Hagenah, M. (2009). Mental contrasting and goal commitment: The mediating role of energization. *Personality and Social Psychology Bulletin, 35,* 608–622.

Oettingen, G., Mayer, D., Thorpe, J. S., Janetzke, H., & Lorenz, S. (2005). Turning fantasies about positive and negative futures into self-improvement goals. *Motivation and Emotion, 29,* 237–267.

Oettingen, G., Pak, H., & Schnetter, K. (2001). Self-regulation of goal-setting: Turning free fantasies about the future into binding goals. *Journal of Personality and Social Psychology, 80,* 736–753.

Oettingen, G., & Sevincer, A. T. (2018). Fantasy about the future as friend and foe. In G. Oettingen, A. T. Sevincer, & P. Gollwitzer (Eds.), *The psychology of thinking about the future* (pp. 127–149). Guilford Press.

Oettingen, G., Stephens, E. J., Mayer, D., & Brinkmann, B. (2010b). Mental contrasting and the self-regulation of helping relations. *Social Cognition, 28,* 490–508.

Park, D., Gunderson, E. A., Tsukayama, E., Levine, S. C., & Beilock, S. L. (2016). Young children's motivational frameworks and math achievement: Relation to teacher-reported instructional practices, but not teacher theory of intelligence. *Journal of Educational Psychology, 108,* 300–313.

Ryan, K. (2013). *How problem focused and emotion focused coping affects college students' perceived stress and life satisfaction.* https://esource.dbs.ie/handle/10788/1622.

Ryan, R. M., & Deci, E. L. (2000). Self-determination theory and the facilitation of intrinsic motivation, social development, and well-being. *American Psychologist, 55*(1), 68–78.

Ryan, R. M., & Deci, E. L. (2017). *Self-determination theory: Basic psychological needs in motivation development and wellness.* Guilford Press.

Schoenmakers, E. C., Van Tilburg, T. G., & Fokkema, T. (2015). Problem-focused and emotion-focused coping options and loneliness: how are they related? *European Journal of Ageing, 12,* 153–161.

Schrage, J., Schwörer, B., Krott, N. R., & Oettingen, G. (2020). Mental contrasting and conciliatory behavior in romantic relationships. *Motivation and Emotion, 44,* 356–372.

Schunk, D., Berger, E. M., Hermes, H., Winkel, K., & Fehr, E. (2022). Teaching self-regulation. *Nature Human Behavior, 6,* 1680–1690.

Schunk, D. H., & DiBenedetto, M. K. (2018). Expectations in the academic domain. In G. Oettingen, A. T. Sevincer, & P. Gollwitzer (Eds.), *The psychology of thinking about the future* (pp. 153–173). Guilford Press.

Sciarappo, J., Norton, E., Oettingen, G., & Gollwitzer, P. M. (2015). *Positive fantasies of winning money reduce temporal discounting.* Unpublished manuscript, Department of Psychology, New York University.

Seijts, G. H., & Latham, G. P. (2005). Learning versus performance goals: When should each be used? *Academy of Management Perspectives, 19,* 124–131.

Seligman, M. E. (1972). Learned helplessness. *Annual Review of Medicine, 23,* 407–412.

Sevincer, A. T., Busatta, P. D., & Oettingen, G.

(2014a). Mental contrasting and transfer of energization. *Personality and Social Psychology Bulletin, 40,* 139–152.
Sevincer, A. T., Kluge, L., & Oettingen, G. (2014b). Implicit theories and motivational focus: Desired future versus present reality. *Motivation and Emotion, 38,* 36–46.
Sevincer, A. T., Mehl, P. J., & Oettingen, G. (2017). Well self-regulated people use mental contrasting. *Social Psychology, 48,* 348–364.
Sevincer, A. T., Musik, T., Degener, A., Greinert, A., & Oettingen, G. (2020). Taking responsibility for others and use of mental contrasting. *Personality and Social Psychology Bulletin, 46,* 1219–1233.
Sevincer, A. T., & Oettingen, G. (2013). Spontaneous mental contrasting and selective goal pursuit. *Personality and Social Psychology Bulletin, 39,* 1240–1254.
Sevincer, A. T., Schlier, B., & Oettingen, G. (2015). Ego depletion and the use of mental contrasting. *Motivation and Emotion, 39,* 876–891.
Sevincer, A. T., Schroeder, A., Plakides, A., Edler, N., & Oettingen, G. (2024). Low working memory reduces the use of mental contrasting. *Consciousness and Cognition, 118,* 103644.
Sevincer, A. T., Tessmann, P., & Oettingen, G. (2018). Demand to act and use of mental contrasting. *Social Psychology, 49,* 344–359.
Sheeran, P., Harris, P., Vaughan, J., Oettingen, G., & Gollwitzer, P. M. (2013). Gone exercising: Mental contrasting promotes physical activity among overweight, middle-aged, low-SES fishermen. *Health Psychology, 32,* 802–809.
Sherman, D. K., & Cohen, G. L. (2006). The psychology of self-defense: Self-affirmation theory. In M. P. Zanna (Ed.), *Advances in experimental social psychology* (Vol. 38, pp. 183–242). Academic Press.
Sherman, D. K., Lokhande, M., Müller, T., & Cohen, G. L. (2021). Selfaffirmation interventions. In G. M. Walton & A. J. Crum (Eds.), *Handbook of wise interventions: How social psychology can help people change* (pp. 63–99). Guilford Press.
Steele, C. M. (1988). The psychology of self-affirmation: Sustaining the integrity of the self. In L. Berkowitz (Ed.), *Advances in experimental social psychology* (Vol. 21, pp. 261–302). Academic Press.
Swann, C., Jackman, P. C., Lawrence, A., Hawkins, R. M., Goddard, S. G., Williamson, O., . . . Ekkekakis, P. (2023). The (over) use of SMART goals for physical activity promotion: A narrative review and critique. *Health Psychology Review, 17,* 211–226.
Swann, C., Rosenbaum, S., Lawrence, A., Vella, S. A., McEwan, D., & Ekkekakis, P. (2021). Updating goal-setting theory in physical activity promotion: A critical conceptual review. *Health Psychology Review, 15*(1), 34–50.
Stadler, G., Oettingen, G., & Gollwitzer, P. M. (2009). Physical activity in women: Effects of a self-regulation intervention. *American Journal of Preventive Medicine, 36,* 29–34.
Stadler, G., Oettingen, G., & Gollwitzer, P. M. (2010). Intervention effects of information and self-regulation on eating fruits and vegetables over two years. *Health Psychology, 29,* 274–283.
Tamim, M., Gai, X., Wang, G., & Ma, Y. (2022). The relationship between predominant promotion focus and spontaneous mental contrasting. *Social Psychology, 53,* 368–382.
Tamim, M., Wang, G., Gai, X., & Ma, Y. (2023). Big five personality traits and spontaneous mental contrasting among Chinese students. *Current Psychology, 43*(17), 15459–15470.
Tamim, M., Wang, G., Gai, X., & Ma, Y. (2024) Causality orientations and spontaneous mental contrasting. *Journal of General Psychology, 151*(4), 486–511.
Tay, I. Q., Valshtein, T. J., Krott, N. R., & Oettingen, G. (2019). Mental contrasting in DanceSport: The champion's mindset. *Psychology of Sport and Exercise, 45,* 101511.
Taylor, S. E. (1983). Adjustment to threatening events: A theory of cognitive adaptation. *American Psychologist, 38,* 1161–1173.
Unkelbach, C., Alves, H., Baldwin, M., Crusius, J., Diel, K., Galinsky, A. D., . . . Mussweiler, T. (2023). Relativity in social cognition: Basic processes and novel applications of social comparisons. *European Review of Social Psychology, 34,* 387–440.
Wittleder, S., Kappes, A., Oettingen, G., Gollwitzer, P. M., Jay, M., & Morgenstern, J. (2019). Mental contrasting with implementation intentions (MCII) reduces drinking when drinking is hazardous: An online self-regulation intervention. *Health Education and Behavior, 46,* 666–676.
Wright, R. A. (1996). Brehm's theory of motivation as a model of effort and cardiovascular response. In P. M. Gollwitzer & J. A. Bargh (Eds.), *The psychology of action: Linking cognition and motivation to behavior* (pp. 424–453). Guilford Press.
Yang, Z., King, W. C., Oettingen, G., & Sheeran, P. (2023). Evidence that mental contrasting reduces health information avoidance. *Annals of Behavioral Medicine, 57,* 687–692.

CHAPTER 48

Boredom and Meaning

Managing Everyday Existential Dread

Eric R. Igou, Wijnand A. P. van Tilburg, Andrew B. Moynihan, *and* Muireann K. O'Dea

Boredom is an undeniable reality of people's lives. Its deceiving commonality may lull one into treating this experience as harmless, a triviality, or a nuisance. Yet beneath its calm—too calm—surface lurks, in Heidegger's words, an "insidious creature" (quoted in Thiele, 1997, p. 491). Boredom is a manifestation of purposelessness in everyday life. The investigation of boredom spans from historical, philosophical insights into its nature (e.g., Kierkegaard, 1852; Schopenhauer, 1851/1970) to more recent epidemiological, sociological, and psychological assessments of boredom in everyday life (e.g., Britton & Shipley, 2010; Chin et al., 2017), and to the latest psychological process models explaining the causes, characteristics, and consequences of this experience (e.g., Danckert & Elpidorou, 2023; Tam et al., 2021b). Work shows that boredom and its remedies are closely tied to existential processes, including the meaning people ascribe to, gain from, and search for in activities and life in general. Accordingly, boredom threatens a sense of meaning (e.g., Barbalet, 1999; Van Tilburg & Igou, 2017a) and triggers attempts to reinstate meaning or momentarily distract one from this predicament, for better or worse. Studying people's responses to boredom promises the advancement of existential psychological theory and suggests intervention pathways.

BOREDOM

As the cliché in psychology goes, our topic has been defined and characterized in various ways. A popular definition by Eastwood and colleagues (2012) is that boredom is "the aversive experience of wanting, but being unable, to engage in satisfying activity" (p. 482). People consider momentary boredom a mildly unpleasant experience that can be effectively distinguished from other forms of negative affect (e.g., sadness, anger, frustration) based on its comparatively low attentional engagement, low perceived meaning, and low self-reported arousal (Van Tilburg & Igou, 2012, 2017a), but not necessarily low physiological arousal (Merrifield & Danckert, 2014). Boredom is accompanied by task-unrelated mind wandering (Danckert & Merrifield, 2018), preoccupation with thoughts about the lack of purpose of one's (in)activity, and a desire to disengage (Van Tilburg & Igou, 2012).

First authorship is shared by Drs. Igou and Van Tilburg.

Building on Eastwood and colleagues (2012) and recent research, we define boredom as *the aversive experience of insufficient cognitive engagement while perceiving one's (in)activity as subjectively meaningless.*

People experience boredom frequently, with U.S. estimates suggesting that some level of boredom characterizes as much as 2.8% of every 30 minutes of people's waking life on average (Chin et al., 2017), promising each of us will be plagued by boredom for more than 2 years out of an 80-year lifespan. Chin and colleagues also found that young people are more likely to experience boredom, with, in the U.S. context, young unemployed White men being particularly vulnerable to it.

Worryingly, boredom is frequent and affectively unpleasant and often harmful to oneself and society. Specifically, given that attentional failures and feelings of meaninglessness accompany the acute experience of boredom (Eastwood et al., 2012; Van Tilburg & Igou, 2012), it causes impulsiveness, unwarranted risk-taking, and arbitrary decision making (Kılıç et al., 2020; Moynihan et al., 2017; Yakobi & Danckert, 2021). State boredom causes sadistic and bullish behavior, intergroup bias, and political division (Pfattheicher et al., 2021, 2023; Van Tilburg & Igou, 2011, 2016). It fosters unhealthy eating, challenges exercise, causes self-harm, and undermines recovery and treatment in psychiatric settings (Havermans et al., 2015; Moynihan et al., 2015; Seiler et al., 2023; Weich et al., 2022; Yucel & Westgate, 2021). Boredom proneness—the chronic tendency to experience boredom often and intensely and to perceive it as life-encompassing (Tam et al., 2021a)—is notoriously linked to problematic outcomes across the spectrum (see Van Tilburg et al., 2024; Vodanovich & Watt, 2016). Boredom proneness interferes with motivation (e.g., low self-control and academic and occupational disengagement; Grazia et al., 2021; Van Hooff & Van Hooft, 2017; Wolff & Martarelli, 2020) and cognition (e.g., attention problems, unwanted thoughts; Isacescu et al., 2017), accompanies other undesirable affect (e.g., depression, hostility; Dahlen et al., 2004; Weiss et al., 2022), undermines health (e.g., cardiovascular risk; Britton & Shipley, 2010), and comes with a sway of worrisome behaviors (e.g., problem gambling, substance use; Blaszczynski et al., 1990; Cao & An, 2020). This is not to say that boredom is exclusively problematic (Igou & Van Tilburg, 2022); indeed, some work suggests that boredom can be a boon to prosocial intentions (Van Tilburg & Igou, 2017b) and curiosity, balancing the exploration–exploitation tradeoff (Danckert, 2019; Hunter et al., 2016); but, on balance, boredom's undesirable sequelae appear to outweigh its desirable ones. Boredom tends to be dreadful.

Psychological Functions of Boredom

Eastwood and colleagues (2012) captured a fundamental tension within the boredom experience: an assessment of unsatisfactory stagnation on the one hand ("being unable to engage in satisfying activity") alongside a drive for change ("wanting to engage in satisfying activity"). This paradoxical character of boredom, mixing passivity with motivation, has been similarly referred to as being "restless and unchallenged at the same time" (Van Tilburg & Igou, 2012, p. 184) or "under-aroused and restless" (Danckert et al., 2018, p. 24). In keeping with its alleged passivity, the momentary experience of boredom is one characterized by a lack of perceived meaning, attention failures, a perceived lack of challenge and novelty, and the slow passing of time concerning the (in)activity at hand (Danckert & Allman, 2005; Hunter & Eastwood, 2018; Van Tilburg & Igou, 2012). At the same time, those who feel acutely bored seek out sensation and attentional engagement, crave novelty, and, crucially, search for meaningful activities (Bench & Lench, 2019; Dahlen et al., 2004; Tam et al., 2021b). With dull activities unable to satisfy these wants, bored individuals disengage and direct attention and other cognitive efforts elsewhere, for better or worse (Danckert & Elpidorou, 2023; Tam et al., 2021b). Accordingly, boredom can be considered a self-regulatory experience (Barbalet, 1999; Bieleke et al., 2024; Igou et al., 2024); it effectively signals to the person that a change is needed (Bieleke et al., 2024) to redress the momentary lack of novelty, challenge, attentional engagement, and meaning (Danckert, 2019; Tam et al., 2021b). This understanding builds on the general idea that boredom, similar to other experiences, has an informative function (e.g., Clore & Storbeck, 2006; Schwarz, 2001). Specifically, boredom informs about the meaninglessness of activity or life in general, providing a basis for self-regulatory processes that address this existential challenge (Igou et al., 2024).

The restoration of meaning in the face of momentary boredom is pivotal to its psychology, evident from people's self-reports, contemporary boredom theory, and the growing empirical evidence demonstrating close ties between the two (Barbalet, 1999; Fahlman et al., 2009; Moynihan et al., 2021b; Van Tilburg & Igou, 2019; Westgate & Wilson, 2018). The feature of boredom thus feeds into an existential or *meaning*-regulation function, thereby joining the pantheon of existential psychology with boredom as an everyday life existential challenge.

Existential Roots of Boredom

While the psychological science of boredom is booming, its history, especially in systematic empirical study, is relatively young. However, important foundations for studying boredom had already been laid in philosophy (for a review, see Svendsen, 2005), and perhaps especially in existential philosophy. Scholars such as Sartre, Kierkegaard, and Heidegger accused boredom of existential dread, expressing their views with varying degrees of melodrama. Sartre called it a "leprosy of the soul" (quoted in Martin et al., 2006, p. 195). Heidegger viewed it as a pivotal experience in the circular and ultimately unsatisfying pursuit of modernization, demonizing it as an "insidious creature" and "monstrosity in our Dasein [existence]" (quoted in Thiele, 1997, p. 491). Kierkegaard speculated that humans exist because the gods themselves were bored and blamed it for human's subsequent original sin (Kierkegaard, 1852). Thus, Kierkegaard simultaneously portrayed boredom, with divine irony, as the most fundamental existential threat and the very reason for our existence in the first place. Not one to shy away from spectacular exposition either, Schopenhauer pointed to boredom as direct evidence that life is ultimately in error and without meaning (1851/1970, p. 357):

> Human life must be some kind of mistake. The truth of this will be sufficiently obvious if we only remember that man is a compound of needs and necessities hard to satisfy; and that even when they are satisfied, all he obtains is a state of painlessness, where nothing remains to him but abandonment to boredom. This is direct proof that existence has no real value in itself; for what is boredom but the feeling of the emptiness of life?

While Schopenhauer questioned meaningful existence per se, others focused more on boredom as a sociocultural phenomenon, accusing modern societies of breeding boredom by negating core human needs. Fromm (1955, 1968, 1973) held the view that boredom in modern societies is rampant and reflects the alienation of people from themselves and others. Consequently, even without having witnessed recent societal developments, Fromm forewarned in *The Sane Society* (1955, p. 102):

> The danger of the past was that men became slaves. The danger of the future is that men may become robots. True enough, robots do not rebel. But given man's nature, robots cannot live and remain sane, they become "golems." They will destroy their world and themselves because they cannot stand any longer the boredom of a meaningless life.

Philosophical wisdom (and fears) aside, this view of boredom as a lack of purpose incarnate reverberated in contemporary psychological and empirically testable models of boredom, such as the meaning-regulation hypothesis and meaning and attention models.

BOREDOM AS AN EXISTENTIAL EXPERIENCE AND CHALLENGE

Pragmatic Meaning-Regulation Hypothesis

Boredom's existential connotations are central to several influential approaches (e.g., Barbalet, 1999; Fahlman et al., 2009; Westgate & Wilson, 2018; Van Tilburg & Igou, 2011, 2012, 2017a). The pragmatic meaning-regulation hypothesis (Van Tilburg & Igou, 2011, 2012, 2017a) combined existential psychology and self-regulatory principles to investigate boredom and how people manage this existential dread. The hypothesis has served as a useful guide for studying the relationship between boredom and meaning (for reviews, see Igou et al., 2022; Moynihan et al., 2021b; Van Tilburg & Igou, 2019). Yet it was not designed as a comprehensive theory of boredom (or meaning, for that matter), leaving room for other key variables (e.g., attention, challenge; Eastwood et al., 2012; Van Tilburg & Igou, 2012) to explain boredom's psychology.

The pragmatic meaning-regulation hypothesis proposes that boredom is a self-regulatory experience that, at its heart, signals that one's current course of (in)action is subjectively meaningless. This realization is averse, and people subsequently seek to remedy it. This remedial action tends to take one of two forms. On the one hand, people attempt to restore a sense of meaning by searching for and subsequent commitment to more meaningful activities. On the other hand, people may seek to (temporarily) escape their predicament by distracting themselves from the lack of meaning.

The pragmatic meaning-regulation hypothesis builds on the notion that meaning is central to life. This notion follows the sociological treatise of boredom and meaning by Barbalet (1999), who articulated a major role of meaning in understanding boredom's consequences. Specifically, Barbalet proposed that boredom is central to people's meaning-making behavior in life, with this experience providing an essential signal that meaning is lacking and needs to be found. Barbalet thus places boredom at the foundation of how people relate to and seek sense in the world around them. Likewise, the pioneering work of Fahlman and colleagues (2009) showed that low meaning in life predicted subsequent rises in boredom. At a broader level, the pragmatic meaning-regulation hypothesis builds on the notion in terror management theory (Greenberg et al., 1986, 1997) that meaning is closely linked to cultural beliefs and values but, different from that theory, suggests that (also) boredom may trigger attempts at bolstering meaning. In this sense, the pragmatic meaning-regulation hypothesis of boredom rhymes with the meaning maintenance model (Heine et al., 2006), which proposes various existential threats but is silent about boredom.

Meaningful activities tend to be behaviors perceived as instrumental in pursuing subjectively valuable goals. Specifically, committing time and effort toward goals is experienced as meaningful (for the experience of meaning, see also Heintzelman & King, 2014a) as long as doing so effectively progresses one toward a goal (i.e., it is instrumental) and if the goal itself is seen as worthwhile (Van Tilburg & Igou, 2013). For example, charitable giving would be considered meaningful to the extent that giving is appraised as an effective tool for helping others and if helping is appraised as valuable (Van Tilburg & Igou, 2017b). Behavior is perceived as meaningful only if these two conditions (high instrumentality, high goal value) are met. Conversely, noninstrumental activities and/or activities that serve a relatively nondesirable goal lack meaning and may thus invite boredom, following the expectancy × value rationale in decision making and motivation, including self-regulation (e.g., for overviews, see Baron, 2023; Heckhausen & Heckhausen, 2018). Whether the perception of remedial behaviors as meaningful is accurate—that is to say, whether they *actually* make the person feel meaningful—is secondary; boredom will persist if they don't and will vanish if they do, and the motivational consequences of boredom are theorized to remain the same as long as the appraisal of the behaviors' instrumentality and value remains unchanged. The meaning-regulation role ascribed to boredom is beneficial in understanding how people deal with boredom in a cultural context, where rudimentary motives (e.g., optimizing arousal and attentional engagement; Danckert & Elpidorou, 2023; Tam et al., 2021b) may be expressed through actions that are perceived as promising meaning in particular (Van Tilburg & Igou, 2019), with meaningful acts perhaps being more likely to engage our attention (Tam et al., 2025).

In essence, boredom motivates people to engage in activities that are either associated with more meaning or that distract from the boredom experience and its negation of one's needs. Within the regulatory area of conflict between a desired level of meaning and the perceived level of meaning, boredom thus starves actual meaning, enlarging the discrepancy between desired and actual levels of meaning. The need to reduce this discrepancy or its salience is the key to understanding how people manage the meaning threat that boredom represents. Thus, regulating one's sense of meaning is a lens through which responses to and avoidance of boredom can be conceptualized.

Existential Enhancement: Search for Meaning

As Viktor Frankl (1959/2006) put it, "search for meaning is the primary motivation" (p. 99) in life. Barbalet (1999) proposed that boredom sparks this motivation (see also Fahlman et al., 2009), as further captured by the pragmatic meaning-regulation hypothesis (e.g., Van Tilburg & Igou, 2011). The rationale builds on Heine and colleagues' (2006) fluid compensation hypotheses of their meaning maintenance model and Steger and colleagues' (2006) conceptualization of search for meaning. People often attempt to compensate for a threat to one's meaning system with a different source of meaning, thereby enhancing meaning as a response to the threat posed by boredom.

Meaning enhancement can be achieved in various ways, with positive or negative consequences for the self and society. Boredom motivates people to seek sources of meaning in a certain situation or life in general, and people are more likely to engage in self-regulatory behavior that provides meaning (i.e., is desirable) and can succeed (i.e., is feasible; Van Tilburg & Igou, 2013). Consistently, boredom has predicted stronger social identity (e.g., Van Tilburg & Igou, 2011), more nostalgia (e.g., Van Tilburg et al., 2013), a polarization of political attitudes (Van Tilburg & Igou, 2016), and prosocial behavior (Van Tilburg & Igou, 2017b), each putative vessels of meaning. Enhancement-directed effects have been recorded for both state and trait boredom, indicating functional similarity. Indeed, boredom was more likely to have such effects if the engagement in the self-regulatory process would likely enhance meaning (e.g., Van Tilburg et al., 2017b). Further, search for meaning as measured by the Meaning in Life Questionnaire (MLQ; Steger et al., 2006) or a state-focused alternative (e.g., Van Tilburg & Igou, 2016) consistently explained these effects. Further, in line with the meaning-enhancement function we ascribe to boredom, several of these sources of meaning predicted a higher presence of meaning in life (as measured by the MLQ; Steger et al., 2006), for example, through nostalgic reverie (Van Tilburg et al., 2013) and appreciation of heroes (Coughlan et al., 2019).

Existential Escape: Avoidance of Meaninglessness

Defenses against the meaninglessness signaled by boredom are not limited to culturally defined or symbolic sources of meaning (Moynihan et al., 2021b). According to the existential escape hypothesis, Wisman (2006) argued that people may also "lose the self" to deal with threats to meaning in life. Specifically, people may engage in behaviors that render self-awareness low (e.g., Baumeister, 1991) and, in so doing, facilitate an "escape" from experienced meaninglessness. According to objective self-awareness theory (Duval & Wicklund, 1972), self-awareness initiates a self-evaluative process in which one's current state on a salient dimension is compared to ideal standards. Discrepancies between the actual (i.e., meaningless) and ideal self occur when someone experiences a meaning threat (Arndt et al., 1998; Silvia, 2001). These discrepancies arouse negative feelings and may motivate people to avoid self-awareness (Duval & Wicklund, 1972).

Accordingly, subdued self-awareness reduces the salience of such discrepancies, including those related to perceived meaning in life (Skowronski & Sedikides, 2017). Reducing self-awareness thus helps people cope with situations effectively, at least momentarily. Various hedonic and interpersonal behaviors involving low self-awareness function as existential escapes. These responses may be evolutionarily and developmentally more basic (e.g., eating, drinking, sex, anonymity in groups) as they are not specific to culture. Wisman (2006) termed these behaviors *presymbolic* since they can be enacted without the symbolic capacities needed in the more complex cultural world.

A body of research has been conducted on how a lack of meaning in life associated with boredom may prompt existential escape strategies (Moynihan et al., 2021b). These studies centered on eating and sex as existential escapes. Initially, a set of studies focused on how food consumption may be used as an escape (Moynihan et al., 2015). Since eating distracts people from unpleasant self-awareness (Heatherton & Baumeister, 1991; Wheeler et al., 2001), the question was whether boredom promoted consumption as a means of existential escape.

In the first study, a diary procedure measured people's everyday levels of boredom and whether or not increases in state boredom predicted increased food intake. Each day, participants recorded how bored and stressed they felt and how enjoyable they found their day using the 7-Day EPIC-Norfolk diary (Bingham et al., 2001). Consistent with the existential escape hypothesis (Wisman, 2006), state boredom significantly predicted increased calorie, fat, carbohydrate, and protein consumption. These results maintained significance when controlling for stress, enjoyment, and individual differences in boredom proneness, positive and negative affect, and body mass index.

Next, a lab experiment investigated if an adverse state of self-awareness motivates bored people to snack as an escape. Initially, participants completed a trait measure of objective self-awareness (Fenigstein et al., 1975). Afterward, participants were randomly assigned to complete either a simple puzzle to induce high levels of boredom or a more engaging puzzle (as a control condition). Then, participants indicated their desire to snack or eat something healthy. As predicted, participants exposed to the high boredom condition expressed a greater desire to snack, particularly among those who scored higher in self-awareness.

It was also investigated how consuming *exciting* foods may be used to escape boredom. Some foods may be more exciting in terms of appearance or taste (e.g., Craeynest et al., 2008). As boredom encourages sensation seeking (Dahlen et al., 2004), it was predicted that exciting foods, both unhealthy and healthy, would be consumed to a greater extent under high levels of boredom and heightened objective self-awareness. After completing an objective self-awareness measure (Fenigstein et al., 1975), participants were randomly assigned to watch either a boring or a sad film. Beforehand, they were provided with candies (an unhealthy, exciting food), cherry tomatoes (a healthy, exciting food), or crackers (a healthy, unexciting food). Participants were told to eat as many or as few foods as they wished throughout the film. As predicted, participants in the boredom condition ate significantly more candies, particularly at higher levels of self-awareness. No effect was found among those lower in self-awareness or in the control condition. Interestingly, and also as predicted, participants in the high boredom condition consumed significantly more cherry tomatoes at higher levels of self-awareness. Again, this effect did not extend to those lower in self-awareness or who were assigned to the control condition. This research highlights how boredom promotes increased unhealthy and healthy eating, consistent with the existential escape rationale (see also Van Tilburg et al., 2022, on boredom and eating during the COVID-19 pandemic).

Recently, the focus of attention examining existential escape turned to sexual attitudes and behaviors. Sex may be used as a coping mechanism to distract bored people from unpleasant or uncomfortable emotions by providing pleasure and arousal (Gaither & Sellbom, 2003; Reid et al., 2009, 2011). The first set of studies on sex and existential escape from boredom (Moynihan et al., 2021a) recorded that a lack of meaning in life predicted greater boredom susceptibility, and, in turn, boredom was associated with increased interest in sexual sensation-seeking and endorsing an open sociosexual orientation (e.g., favorable attitudes to casual, uncommitted sex). This relationship was significantly explained (i.e., statistically mediated) by using sex as a coping mechanism to deal with unpleasant affective states.

The escape hypothesis also allows for predictions about the consumption of pornography (Moynihan et al., 2022). People may consume pornography to relieve boredom (Böthe et al., 2021). Consistent with existential escape theorizing (Wisman, 2006), pornography may be used hedonically and help disconnect from reality (Reid et al., 2011). In this study, the use of pornography for emotional avoidance was measured and then used as a predictor of pornography as a means for excitement seeking and sexual pleasure. As expected, a lack of meaning in life predicted increased boredom. Subsequently, boredom predicted increased use of pornography for emotional avoidance. Such use significantly predicted increased use of pornography for excitement seeking, sexual pleasure, and more frequent pornography use. In summary, research on existential escape from boredom is a growing and promising area with important real-world applications (e.g., Grubbs & Kraus, 2021).

Existential Buffering: Preventing Boredom via Meaningful Experiences

If boredom encourages meaningful behavior to restore a sense of meaning, then it stands to reason that heightening a sense of meaning prevents boredom. Indeed, the relationship between meaning and boredom is considered bidirectional (Fahlman et al., 2009); therefore, possessing a strong sense of meaning in life should limit the onset of boredom. We refer to this process as *existential buffering*. Consistent with the pragmatic meaning-regulation hypothesis (Van Tilburg & Igou, 2011, 2019) and the meaning maintenance model (Heine et al., 2006), people may protect themselves from a meaning threat by maintaining high levels of meaning through a variety of sources, even when these are not directly related to a boring experience. Since boredom predicts a plethora of undesirable well-being and behavioral outcomes (Goldberg et al., 2011; Moynihan et al., 2017), examining if and how sources of meaning protect against boredom adds to an understanding of boredom and has practical implications.

In recent years, there has been considerable support for the *existential buffering* hypothesis. Van Tilburg and colleagues (2019) found that people who identified as religious or held comparatively stronger religious beliefs experienced less boredom, and this relationship was explained by greater levels of meaning in life. Religiosity is a noteworthy provider of meaning in life (e.g., Steger & Frazier, 2005). However, many individuals do not identify as religious or at least do not practice a religion. Thus, the question arises: Which other sources of meaning could buffer against boredom? Coughlan and colleagues (2019) found that positive evaluations of cultural heroes predicted lower levels of boredom through higher levels of perceived meaning in life. Similarly, O'Dea and colleagues (2024) reported that spontaneous self-affirmation, an inclination to self-affirm in response to psychological threats, was negatively associated with boredom proneness, and this relationship was explained by elevated meaning in life.

Positive affect and social relationships have been recognized as important players in the experience of meaning in life (Hicks & King, 2009; King et al., 2006; Stravrova & Luhmann et al., 2016). Profound sources of meaning are self-transcendent emotions (e.g., Van Cappellen et al., 2013), such as awe, gratitude, and compassion, which typically evoke decreased self-salience and increased feelings of social connectedness (Stellar et al., 2017; Yaden et al., 2017). While meaning can be derived from a multitude of resources (see King & Hicks, 2021), transcending self-oriented concerns appears to play a powerful role in people's perceptions of meaning (Huang & Yang, 2023). Accordingly, a consistent negative association between self-transcendent emotions and boredom may occur.

Following this reasoning, O'Dea and colleagues (2022) examined the relationship between self-compassion, an experience that increases connectedness by reminding us of our common humanity (Neff, 2003), and boredom. In three studies, both dispositional self-compassion and momentary experiences of self-compassion predicted lower levels of boredom by offering higher levels of meaning in life. Consistently, O'Dea and colleagues (2023) demonstrated in a series of studies that gratitude served as a resource for overcoming boredom. Specifically, participants prone to gratitude experienced less state and trait boredom, which was explained by the enhanced perceptions of meaning in life that gratitude begets. Furthermore, in one study adopting an experimental design, participants in the state gratitude condition reported less state boredom compared to the neutral control, and this effect was explained by state perceptions of meaning in life. Awe is another typical self-transcendent experience (Stellar et al., 2017) that helps transcend everyday life's mundane concerns (Jiang & Sedikides, 2022). It is, however, a rather complex experience, evoking feelings of vastness and connectedness but also existential insignificance, which leads to mixed effects on perceptions of meaning in life (Dai et al., 2022; Rivera et al., 2020). Although awe predicts lower levels of boredom through meaning in life and vastness, the overall relationship between awe and boredom may be more complex than for other self-transcendent emotions (O'Dea et al., 2025).

Overall, considerable evidence supports the role of existential buffering in the context of boredom. Experiences that increase meaning in life are likely to prevent boredom experiences, and this relationship holds for both state and trait boredom. One question arising from this research is how this matters for everyday life experiences. Do experiences of meaning reduce the frequency and intensity of boredom in everyday life? Do people learn from such experiences, enabling people to use these relationships (consciously or unconsciously) as a buffer against potential boredom experiences? Daily diary studies, which enable researchers to capture daily emotional experiences in an ecologically valid manner (Nezlek, 2012), could provide some answers to these questions and create a foundation for the development of intervention procedures to reduce chronic boredom in daily life, across a range of applied settings.

DISCUSSION, UNANSWERED QUESTIONS, AND FUTURE DIRECTIONS

Prior and simultaneous work on existential psychological processes (e.g., Greenberg et al., 2004; Heine et al., 2006; Heinzelman & King, 2014b; Sedikides et al., 2008; Wisman, 2006) presented theoretical perspectives and practical tools to examine boredom's characteristics and effects more closely. Equally, the meaning-regulation perspective offers new insights into boredom, existential self-regulatory processes, and considerable implications for well-being.

Boredom, Routines, and Everyday Sources of Meaning

Boredom is a common, often mundane, aspect of daily life (Chin et al., 2017). Nevertheless, it plays an important role in the regulation of perceived meaning. In this sense, our research suggests that the processes through which people find and maintain a sense of meaning are an important aspect of everyday life. Boredom is relevant from an existentialist perspective because it has strong associations with meaning in life, a central human need and experience that is common and accessible, in line with the arguments by Heintzelman and King (2014a, 2014b). Given that mundane experiences, such as daily routines, can make life meaningful (Heintzelman & King, 2019; Mohideen & Heintzelman, 2023), it is interesting to examine how daily routines buffer against boredom or might strengthen boredom if repetitive and overused (Van den Bergh & Vrana, 1998). Behavior may induce boredom if the tasks lack direction or purpose (Van Tilburg & Igou, 2013). If an individual perceives their task as meaningful and goal-directed, it may buffer against boredom, even if the task may be viewed as ostensibly "boring" by others. For instance, in educational settings, researchers have shown that students who reappraised their academic tasks as valuable were less frequently bored (Nett et al., 2010). This highlights the subjective judgment process of both meaning in life and boredom. To bolster meaning as a buffer, it may be useful to employ an approach like the person–activity fit model (Lyubomirsky & Layous, 2013), which considers people's motivations, beliefs, efforts, and personality. Boredom can likely be regulated through an array of meaning sources, above and beyond what current research has documented. Then again, optimism must be limited as the literature reflects that state and trait boredom is associated with severely adverse psychological conditions and states, with strong associations with self-regulatory failures (e.g., Todman, 2003, 2021).

Boredom and Death

Terror management theory (Greenberg et al., 1997) and the research on mortality salience were pioneers in experimental existential psychology. This framework presupposes that people face an existential dilemma: On the one hand, they are biologically and psychologically programmed to live; on the other hand, they are capable of realizing their inevitable death. To manage the threat of one's mortality, people readily use cultural worldviews to instill life with meaning and provide standards against which people can attain purpose and significance (i.e., self-esteem; Harmon-Jones et al., 1997). Accordingly, people may defend against mortality concerns by relying on symbolic representations of the world (i.e., adhering more strongly to cultural worldviews) and the self (i.e., affirming self-esteem from living up to standards of those worldviews; Greenberg et al., 1986). Similarly, affirming cultural sources of meaning is also a psychological tool to cope with boredom and its characteristic sense of meaninglessness (Van Tilburg & Igou, 2017a). Yet the meaning maintenance model (Heine et al., 2006) offers an explanation that directly conceptualizes perceived meaning in life rather than the avoidance of terror associated with mortality salience. Meaning can be compensated through various (interchangeable) core needs (self-esteem, certainty, belongingness, or symbolic immortality). Indeed, Van Tilburg and Igou (2011) showed that bored people identified more strongly with their national ingroups as a defense against a perceived threat to meaning in their lives. Furthermore, other symbolic sources of meaning that bored people have used include engaging in prosocial behavior (Van Tilburg & Igou, 2017b), nostalgic reverie (Van Tilburg et al., 2013), affirming one's political ideologies (Van Tilburg & Igou, 2016), and affirmation of heroes (Coughlan et al., 2019). Where fear of death focuses on a single terminal and terrifying moment, boredom lingers below the surface to rear its monstrous head at any moment if novelty, attention, and excitement are not satisfied sufficiently to lull people into perceived meaning: It is an "insidious creature" (Heidegger, cited in Thiele, 1997, p. 491).

Terror management theory (Greenberg et al., 1997) argues that proximal defenses remove meaning threats from consciousness by distraction or suppression (e.g., Arndt et al., 1997). In contrast, adherence to worldviews operates at the distal (i.e., nonconscious) level of awareness of mortality salience (e.g., Pyszczsynski et al., 1999). Boredom research has highlighted symbolic responses (i.e., worldview defense) to that threat occurring at the proximal (i.e., conscious) level. It has also demonstrated existential escape responses (Wisman, 2006) at the distal level, yet not as a means for self-esteem enhancement or worldview defense. Hence, despite both qualifying as existential threats, boredom seems to operate differently than mortality salience.

Meaning and Attention

Evidence indicates that, in combination, attention and meaning stand out as crucial factors that differentiate boredom from other undesirable states (Van Tilburg & Igou, 2017a). The meaning and attention components (MAC) model of boredom (Westgate & Wilson, 2018) proposes that boredom results from inappropriate attentional engagement and a lack of meaning. In the MAC model of boredom, a lack of meaning involves a mismatch between the task at hand and the goals people hold; activities that do not contribute toward a valued goal lack meaning (see also Van Tilburg & Igou, 2013). Understimulation will occur if external demands exceed one's attention capacity. Low-level attentional engagement will occur if the attentional demands of a task are low and match one's current resources. When attentional demands are matched with high resources, attentional engagement is considered high. Finally, attentional demands exceeding one's capacity result in experienced overstimulation.

Importantly, the MAC model (Westgate & Wilson, 2018) stipulates that meaning and attention are *independent* predictors of boredom; being low in one is sufficient to warrant boredom, and different combinations of the two components can give rise to different forms of boredom. When meaning is lacking, understimulation will be accompanied by boredom and a search for interesting activity, whereas boredom experienced when meaninglessness is combined with low-level attention is characterized by a search for enjoyment. Even when attentional engagement is high, a lack of meaning predicates boredom characterized by the desire to find more interesting activities. Meaninglessness and overstimulation, on the other hand, are expected to feature a bored state accompanied by the search for enjoyment. Thus, a lack of task meaning is expected to trigger boredom, but which motivations accompany this form of boredom depends on the corresponding attentional engagement. When meaning is high, on the other hand, boredom is expected to occur only when understimulation or overstimulation occurs, with resultant boredom then being characterized by the desire to increase task demands and attentional resources, respectively.

Across several studies, Westgate and Wilson (2018) found that a lack of meaning and attentional engagement predicted boredom significantly and simultaneously. The two components did not interact, yet they correlated significantly, though not substantially. These studies suggest that boredom can result from inappropriate attentional engagement, a lack of meaning, or both (cf. Danckert & Elpidorou, 2023; Tam et al., 2021b, 2024).

Boredom and Arousal

The meaning maintenance model (Heine et al., 2006) comprehensively accounts for various existential threats and corresponding psychological processes. Research within this paradigm has suggested that adverse arousal from existential threats drives meaning making (Proulx & Inzlicht, 2012). Does this apply to boredom? Boredom is experienced as both a challenge to meaning (Van Tilburg & Igou, 2012, 2017a) and a self-reported state of *low* arousal (e.g., Mikulas & Vodanovich, 1993; Van Tilburg & Igou, 2017a), albeit context matters (Van Hooft & Van Hooff, 2018) and arousal levels may change over phases of boredom (Goetz et al., 2014). Physiological evidence is more mixed, depending on how it is measured (e.g., Merrifield & Danckert, 2014). Low arousal would challenge the central role ascribed to arousal in the meaning maintenance model. If or when arousal is high, its putative role in meaning-restorative behavior could be tested. Work following the meaning-regulation hypothesis has directly measured meaning motives: search for meaning in life or motivation to engage in meaningful activity (e.g., Van Tilburg & Igou, 2011, 2016; Van Tilburg et al., 2013). As these variables statistically explain the relationship between boredom and existential enhancement, it seems worthwhile to test whether they also explain some consequences of other meaning threats and whether these search processes are associated with arousal.

Boredom and Meaning

As stated above, boredom signals a lack of meaning. Which comes first, boredom or meaninglessness? Perceptions of low meaning in life seem to cause state boredom (Fahlman et al., 2009). Furthermore, some studies indicate that experimental induction of boredom causes a decrease in the momentary sense of meaning (Van Tilburg & Igou, 2011), others show that manipulations of state meaning alter boredom (Tam et al., 2024), and yet others show that boredom elevates search for meaning (Van Tilburg & Igou, 2019). While treating a sense of life's meaninglessness as a precursor to boredom seems reasonable, the same cannot be said for the momentary experience of meaning. The causal positioning of momentary meaning in the context of boredom needs further clarification.

Boring People

Leary and colleagues (1986) reported that boring people are perceived as, for example, self-centered, uninteresting, and overly serious in speech and conversations. Recent research on the beliefs about boring people (Van Tilburg et al., 2023) brought to bear that professions involving money and math (e.g., banking, accountancy), hobbies such as watching birds and TV, and personality traits such as lack of humor and sharing few opinions are characteristics that define this stereotype, at least in the United States and the United Kingdom. Furthermore, boring people are perceived as low in *both* interpersonal warmth and competence, a rare combination that people tend to ascribe to marginalized groups, such as poor people, homeless people, and criminals (Fiske & Cuddy, 2006). Meeting an allegedly boring other causes people to feel superior while at the same time experiencing a lack of meaning, finding it difficult to maintain attention (Gallegos et al., 2023), and trying to avoid the boring person (Van Tilburg et al., 2023). Is the stigmatization of being boring an existential threat? Would people turn to presymbolic and symbolic responses to deal with such a prospect? A greater focus on these matters could lift boredom research further into the spheres of interpersonal and intergroup relations.

CONCLUSION

Boredom plays a vital role in human life, as it is unpleasant and common, and people use strategies to avoid boredom and the associated sense of meaninglessness. As research has established boredom as a distinct experience, the lack of meaning qualifies it as an existential threat. People use various strategies to avoid boredom or its existential connotations or to enhance meaning once boredom strikes. More research is necessary to fully understand how existential processes link with other psychological processes and how boredom operates in the real world, especially interpersonally and in intergroup relations. Hopefully, research on boredom will foster positive solutions to boredom, preventing the human race from turning into destructive golems (Fromm, 1955).

REFERENCES

Arndt, J., Greenberg, J., Simon, L., Pyszczynski, T., & Solomon, S. (1998). Terror management and self-awareness: Evidence that mortality salience provokes avoidance of the self-focused state. *Personality and Social Psychological Bulletin, 24,* 1216–1232.

Arndt, J., Greenberg, J., Solomon, S., Pyszczynski, T., & Simon, L. (1997). Suppression, accessibility of death-related thoughts, and cultural worldview defense: Exploring the psychodynamics of terror management. *Journal of Personality and Social Psychology, 73,* 5–18.

Barbalet, J. M. (1999). Boredom and social meaning. *British Journal of Sociology, 50,* 631–646.

Baron, J. (2023). *Thinking and deciding* (5th ed.). Cambridge University Press.

Baumeister, R. F. (1991). *Escaping the self: Alcoholism, spirituality, masochism, and other flights from the burden of selfhood.* Basic Books.

Bench, S. W., & Lench, H. C. (2019). Boredom as a seeking state: Boredom prompts the pursuit of novel (even negative) experiences. *Emotion, 19,* 242–254.

Bieleke, M., Wolff, W., & Bertrams, A. (2024). On the virtues of fragile self-control: Boredom as a catalyst for adaptive behavior regulation. In M. Bieleke, W. Wolff, & C. Martarelli (Eds.), *Handbook of boredom research* (pp. 133–144). Routledge.

Bingham, S. A., Welch, A. A., McTaggart, A., Mulligan, A. A., Runswick, S. A., Luben, R., . . . Day, N. E. (2001). Nutritional methods in the European prospective investigation of cancer in Norfolk. *Public Health Nutrition, 4,* 847–858.

Blaszczynski, A., McConaghy, N., & Frankova, A. (1990). Boredom proneness in pathological gambling. *Psychological Reports, 67,* 35–42.

Böthe, B., Tóth-Király, I., Bella, N., Potenza, M. N., Demetrovics, Z., & Orosz, G. (2021). Why do people watch pornography?: The motivational basis of pornography use. *Psychology of Addictive Behaviors, 35,* 172–186.

Britton, A., & Shipley, M. J. (2010). Bored to death? *International Journal of Epidemiology, 39,* 370–371.

Cao, Q., & An, J. (2020). Boredom proneness and aggression among people with substance use disorder: The mediating role of trait anger and impulsivity. *Journal of Drug Issues, 50,* 77–88.

Chin, A., Markey, A., Bhargava, S., Kassam, K. S., & Loewenstein, G. (2017). Bored in the USA: Experience sampling and boredom in everyday life. *Emotion, 17,* 359–368.

Clore, G. L., & Storbeck, J. (2006). Affect as information for social judgment, behavior, and memory. In J. P. Forgas (Ed.), *Hearts and minds: Affective influences on social cognition and behavior* (pp. 123–141). Psychology Press.

Coughlan, G., Igou, E. R., Van Tilburg, W. A. P., Kinsella, E. L., & Ritchie, T. D. (2019). On boredom and perceptions of heroes: A meaning-regulation approach to heroism. *Journal of Humanistic Psychology, 59*(4), 455–473.

Craeynest, M., Crombez, G., Koster, H. W. E., Haerens, L., & De Bourdeaudhuij, I. (2008). Cognitive-motivational determinants of fat food consumption in overweight and obese youngsters: The implicit association between fat food and arousal. *Journal of Behavior Therapy and Experimental Psychiatry, 39,* 354–368.

Dahlen, E. R., Martin, R. C., Ragan, K., & Kuhlman, M. M. (2004). Boredom proneness in anger and aggression: Effects of impulsiveness and sensation seeking. *Personality and Individual Differences, 37,* 1615–1627.

Dai, Y., Jiang, T., & Miao, M. (2022). Uncovering the effects of awe on meaning in life. *Journal of Happiness Studies, 23*(7), 3517–3529.

Danckert, J. (2019). Boredom: Managing the delicate balance between exploration and exploitation. In J. Ros Velasco (Ed.), *Boredom is in your mind* (pp. 37–53). Springer International.

Danckert, J. A., & Allman, A. A. (2005). Time flies when you're having fun: Temporal estimation and the experience of boredom. *Brain and Cognition, 59*(3), 236–245.

Danckert, J., & Elpidorou, A. (2023). In search of boredom: Beyond a functional account. *Trends in Cognitive Sciences, 27*(5), 494–507.

Danckert, J., Hammerschmidt, T., Marty-Dugas, J., & Smilek, D. (2018). Boredom: Underaroused and restless. *Consciousness and Cognition, 61,* 24–37.

Danckert, J., & Merrifield, C. (2018). Boredom, sustained attention and the default mode network. *Experimental Brain Research, 236,* 2507–2518.

Duval, T. S., & Wicklund, R. A. (1972). *A theory of objective self-awareness.* Academic Press.

Eastwood, J. D., Frischen, A., Fenske, M. J., & Smilek, D. (2012). The unengaged mind: Defining boredom in terms of attention. *Perspectives on Psychological Science, 7,* 482–495.

Fahlman, S. A., Mercer, K. B., Gaskovski, P., Eastwood, A. E., & Eastwood, J. D. (2009). Does a lack of life meaning cause boredom?: Results from psychometric, longitudinal, and experimental analyses. *Journal of Social and Clinical Psychology, 28*(3), 307–304.

Fenigstein, A., Scheier, M. F., & Buss, A. H. (1975). Public and private self-consciousness: Assessment and theory. *Journal of Consulting and Clinical Psychology, 43,* 522–527.

Fiske, S. T., & Cuddy, A. J. C. (2006). Stereotype content across cultures as a function of group status. In S. Guimond (Ed.), *Social comparison and social psychology: Understanding cognition, intergroup relations, and culture* (pp. 249–263). Cambridge University Press.

Frankl, V. E. (2006). *Man's search for meaning.* Beacon Press. (Original work published 1959)

Fromm, E. (1955). *The sane society.* Rinehart.

Fromm, E. (1968). *The revolution of hope: Toward a humanized technology.* Harper & Row.

Fromm, E. (1973). *The anatomy of human destructiveness.* Holt, Rinehart & Winston.

Gaither, G. A., & Sellbom, M. (2003). The sexual sensation seeking scale: Reliability and validity within a heterosexual college student sample. *Journal of Personality Assessment, 81,* 157–167.

Gallegos, J., Gasper, K., & Schermerhorn, N. E. (2023). Bored and better: Interpersonal boredom results in people feeling not only superior to the boring individual, but also to others. *Self and Identity, 22,* 408–434.

Goetz, T., Frenzel, A. C., Hall, N. C., Nett, U. E., Pekrun, R., & Lipnevich, A. A. (2014). Types of boredom: An experience sampling approach. *Motivation and Emotion, 38,* 401–419.

Goldberg, Y. K., Eastwood, J. D., LaGuardia, J., & Danckert, J. (2011). Boredom: An emotional experience distinct from apathy, anhedonia, or depression. *Journal of Social and Clinical Psychology, 30*(6), 647–666.

Grazia, V., Mameli, C., & Molinari, L. (2021). Being bored at school: Trajectories and academic outcomes. *Learning and Individual Differences, 90,* 102049.

Greenberg, J., Koole, S. L., & Pyszczynski, T. (Eds.). (2004). *Handbook of experimental existential psychology.* Guilford Press.

Greenberg, J., Pyszczynski, T., & Solomon, S. (1986). The causes and consequences of a need for self-esteem: A terror management theory. In R. F. Baumeister (Ed.), *Public self and private self* (pp. 189–212). Springer.

Greenberg, J., Pyszczynski, T., & Solomon, S. (1997). Terror management theory of self-esteem and cultural worldviews: Empirical assessments and conceptual refinements. *Advances in Experimental Social Psychology, 29,* 61–141.

Grubbs, J. B., & Kraus, S. W. (2021). Pornography use and psychological science: A call for consideration. *Current Directions in Psychological Science, 30,* 68–75.

Harmon-Jones, E., Simon, L., Greenberg, J., Pyszczynski, T., Solomon, S., & McGregor, H. (1997). Terror management theory and self-esteem: Evidence that increased self-esteem reduced mortality salience effects. *Journal of Personality and Social Psychology, 72,* 24–36.

Havermans, R. C., Vancleef, L., Kalamatianos, A., & Nederkoorn, C. (2015). Eating and inflicting pain out of boredom. *Appetite, 85,* 52–57.

Heatherton, T. F., & Baumeister, R. F. (1991). Binge eating as escape from self-awareness. *Psychological Bulletin, 110,* 86–108.

Heckhausen, J., & Heckhausen, H. (2018). *Motivation and action.* Springer International.

Heine, S. J., Proulx, T., & Vohs, K. D. (2006). The meaning maintenance model: On the coherence of social motivations. *Personality and Social Psychology Review, 10,* 88–110.

Heintzelman, S. J., & King, L. A. (2014a). (The feeling of) meaning-as-information. *Personality and Social Psychology Review, 18*(2), 153–167.

Heintzelman, S. J., & King, L. A. (2014b). Life is pretty meaningful. *American Psychologist, 69*(6), 561–574.

Heintzelman, S. J., & King, L. A. (2019). Routines and meaning in life. *Personality and Social Psychology Bulletin, 45*(5), 688–699.

Hicks, J. A., & King, L. A. (2009). Positive mood and social relatedness as information about meaning in life. *Journal of Positive Psychology, 4*(6), 471–482.

Huang, M., & Yang, F. (2023). Self-transcendence or self-enhancement: People's perceptions of meaning and happiness in relation to the self. *Journal of Experimental Psychology: General, 152*(2), 590–610.

Hunter, A., & Eastwood, J. D. (2018). Does state boredom cause failures of attention? Examining the relations between trait boredom, state boredom, and sustained attention. *Experimental Brain Research, 236,* 2483–2492.

Hunter, J. A., Abraham, E. H., Hunter, A. G., Goldberg, L. C., & Eastwood, J. D. (2016). Personality and boredom proneness in the prediction of creativity and curiosity. *Thinking Skills and Creativity, 22,* 48–57.

Igou, E. R., O'Dea, M. K., Tam, K. Y. Y., & Van Tilburg, W. A. P. (2024). Boredom and the quest for meaning. In M. Bieleke, W. Wolff, & C. Martarelli (Eds.), *Handbook of boredom research* (pp. 90–105). Routledge.

Igou, E. R., & Van Tilburg, W. A. P. (2022). The existential sting of boredom. In A. Elpidorou (Ed.), *The moral psychology of boredom* (pp. 57–78). Rowman & Littlefield.

Isacescu, J., Struk, A. A., & Danckert, J. (2017). Cognitive and affective predictors of boredom proneness. *Cognition and Emotion, 31,* 1741–1748.

Jiang, T., & Sedikides, C. (2022). Awe motivates authentic-self pursuit via self-transcendence: Implications for prosociality. *Journal of Personality and Social Psychology, 123*(3), 576–596.

Kierkegaard, S. (1852). *A rotation of crops: A venture in the theory of social prudence.* www.sorenkierkegaard.nl.

Kılıç, A., Van Tilburg, W. A. P., & Igou, E. R. (2020). Risk-taking increases under boredom. *Journal of Behavioral Decision Making, 33,* 257–269.

King, L. A., & Hicks, J. A. (2021). The science of meaning in life. *Annual Review of Psychology, 72*(1), 561–584.

King, L. A., Hicks, J. A., Krull, J. L., & Gaiso, A. K. D. (2006). Positive affect and the experience of meaning in life. *Journal of Personality and Social Psychology, 90*(1), 179–196.

Leary, M. R., Rogers, P. A., Canfield, R. W., & Coe, C. (1986). Boredom in interpersonal encounters: Antecedents and social implications. *Journal of Personality and Social Psychology, 51,* 968–975.

Lyubomirsky, S., & Layous, K. (2013). How do simple positive activities increase well-being? *Current Directions in Psychological Science, 22*(1), 57–62.

Martin, M., Sadlo, G., & Stew, G. (2006). The phenomenon of boredom. *Qualitative Research in Psychology, 3,* 193–211.

Merrifield, C., & Danckert, J. (2014). Characterizing the psychophysiological signature of boredom. *Experimental Brain Research, 232,* 481–491.

Mikulas, W. L., & Vodanovich, S. J. (1993). The essence of boredom. *Psychological Record, 43,* 3–12.

Mohideen, F., & Heintzelman, S. J. (2023). Routines and meaning in life: Does activity content or context matter? *Personality and Social Psychology Bulletin, 49*(7), 987–999.

Moynihan, A. B., Igou, E. R., & Van Tilburg, W. A. P. (2017). Boredom increases impulsiveness. *Social Psychology, 48*(5), 293–309.

Moynihan, A. B., Igou, E. R., & Van Tilburg, W. A. P. (2021a). Bored stiff: The relationship between meaninglessness, sexual sensation seeking, and promiscuous attitudes via boredom susceptibility. *Personality and Individual Differences, 168,* 110295.

Moynihan, A. B., Igou, E. R., & Van Tilburg, W. A. P. (2021b). Existential escape of the bored: A review of meaning-regulation processes under boredom. *European Review of Social Psychology, 32,* 161–200.

Moynihan, A. B., Igou, E. R., & Van Tilburg, W. A. P. (2022). Pornography consumption as existential escape from boredom. *Personality and Individual Differences, 198,* 111802.

Moynihan, A. B., Van Tilburg, W. A. P., Igou, E. R., Wisman, A., Donnelly, A. E., & Mulcaire, J. B. (2015). Eaten up by boredom: Consuming food to escape awareness of the bored self. *Frontiers in Psychology, 6.*

Neff, K. (2003). Self-compassion: An alternative conceptualization of a healthy attitude toward oneself. *Self and identity, 2*(2), 85–101.

Nett, U. E., Goetz, T., & Daniels, L. M. (2010). What to do when feeling bored? Students' strategies for coping with boredom. *Learning and Individual Differences, 20*(6), 626–638.

Nezlek, J. B. (2012). *Diary methods.* Sage.

O'Dea, M. K., Igou, E. R., & Van Tilburg, W. A. P., (2023). Preventing boredom with gratitude: The role of meaning in life. *Motivation and Emotion, 48,* 111–125.

O'Dea, M. K., Igou, E. R., & Van Tilburg, W. A. P. (2024). Spontaneous self-affirmation predicts more meaning and less boredom. *Motivation and Emotion, 48*(2), 237–247.

O'Dea, M. K., Igou, E. R., Van Tilburg, W. A. P., & Kinsella, E. L. (2022). Self-compassion predicts less boredom: The role of meaning in life. *Personality and Individual Differences, 186,* 111360.

O'Dea, M. K., Igou, E. R., Van Tilburg, W. A. P., & Kinsella, E. L. (2025). Awe and boredom:

Unravelling dual pathways through meaning in life. *European Journal of Social Psychology, 55*(5), 931–949.

Pfattheicher, S., Lazarević, L. B., Nielsen, Y. A., Westgate, E. C., Krstić, K., & Schindler, S. (2023). I enjoy hurting my classmates: On the relation of boredom and sadism in schools. *Journal of School Psychology, 96,* 41–56.

Pfattheicher, S., Lazarević, L. B., Westgate, E. C., & Schindler, S. (2021). On the relation of boredom and sadistic aggression. *Journal of Personality and Social Psychology, 121,* 573–600.

Proulx, T., & Inzlicht, M. (2012). The five "A" s of meaning maintenance: Finding meaning in the theories of sense-making. *Psychological Inquiry, 23,* 317–335.

Pyszczynski, T., Greenberg, J., & Solomon, S. (1999). A dual-process model of defense against conscious and unconscious death-related thoughts: An extension of terror management theory. *Psychological Review, 106,* 835–845.

Reid, R. C., Harper, J. M., & Anderson, E. H. (2009). Coping strategies used by hypersexual patients to defend against the painful effects of shame. *Clinical Psychology and Psychotherapy, 16,* 125–138.

Reid, R. C., Li, D. S., Gilliland, R., Stein, J. A., & Fong, T. (2011). Reliability, validity, and psychometric development of the pornography consumption inventory in a sample of hypersexual men. *Journal of Sex and Marital Therapy, 37,* 359–385.

Rivera, G. N., Vess, M., Hicks, J. A., & Routledge, C. (2020). Awe and meaning: Elucidating complex effects of awe experiences on meaning in life. *European Journal of Social Psychology, 50*(2), 392–405.

Schopenhauer, A. (1970). *Essays and aphorisms* (R. J. Hollingdale, Trans.). Penguin Books. (Original work published 1851)

Schwarz, N. (2001). Feeling as information: Implications for affective influences on information processing. In L. L. Martin & G. L. Clore (Eds.), *Theories of mood and cognition. A user's guidebook* (pp. 159–176). Erlbaum.

Sedikides, C., Wildschut, T., Arndt, J., & Routledge, C. (2008) Nostalgia: Past, present, and future. *Current Directions in Psychological Science, 17*(5), 304–307.

Seiler, J. P. H., Zerr, K., Rumpel, S., & Tüscher, O. (2023). High state boredom vastly affects psychiatric inpatients and predicts their treatment duration. *Translational Psychiatry, 13,* 350.

Silvia, P. J. (2001). Nothing or the opposite: Intersecting terror management and objective self-awareness. *European Journal of Personality, 15,* 73–82.

Skowronski, J. J., & Sedikides, C. (2017). On the evolution of the human self: A data-driven review and reconsideration. *Self and Identity, 18*(1), 4–21.

Stavrova, O., & Luhmann, M. (2016). Social connectedness as a source and consequence of meaning in life. *Journal of Positive Psychology, 11*(5), 470–479.

Steger, M. F., & Frazier, P. (2005). Meaning in life: One link in the chain from religiousness to well-being. *Journal of Counseling Psychology, 52*(4), 574–582.

Steger, M. F., Frazier, P., Kaler, M., & Oishi, S. (2006). The meaning in life questionnaire: Assessing the presence of and search for meaning in life. *Journal of Counseling Psychology, 53*(1), 80–93.

Stellar, J. E., Gordon, A. M., Piff, P. K., Cordaro, D., Anderson, C. L., Bai, Y., . . . Keltner, D. (2017). Self-transcendent emotions and their social functions: Compassion, gratitude, and awe bind us to others through prosociality. *Emotion Review, 9*(3), 200–207.

Svendsen, L. (2005). *A philosophy of boredom.* Reaktion Books.

Tam, K. Y. Y., Van Tilburg, W. A. P., & Chan, C. S. (2021a). What is boredom proneness?: A comparison of three characterizations. *Journal of Personality, 89,* 831–846.

Tam, K. Y. Y., Van Tilburg, W. A. P., Chan, C. S., Igou, E. R., & Lau, H. (2021b). Attention drifting in and out: The boredom feedback model. *Personality and Social Psychology Review, 25,* 251–272.

Tam, K. Y. Y., Van Tilburg, W. A. P., Chan, C. S., & Inzlicht, M. (2025). Meaning and attention intertwined: Experimental and experience-sampling findings. *Personality and Social Psychology Bulletin.*

Thiele, L. P. (1997). Postmodernity and the routinization of novelty: Heidegger on boredom and technology. *Polity, 29,* 489–517.

Todman, M. (2003). Boredom and psychotic disorders: Cognitive and motivational issues. *Psychiatry: Interpersonal and Biological Processes, 66*(2), 146–167.

Todman, M. (2021). Boredom mismanagement and attributions of social and moral goals. In A. Elpidorou (Ed.), *The moral psychology of boredom* (pp. 133–169). Rowman & Littlefield.

Van Cappellen, P., Saroglou, V., Iweins, C., Piovesana, M., & Fredrickson, B. L. (2013). Self-transcendent positive emotions increase spirituality through basic world assumptions. *Cognition and Emotion, 27*(8), 1378–1394.

Van Den Bergh, O., & Vrana, S. R. (1998). Repetition and boredom in a perceptual fluency/attributional model of affective judgements. *Cognition and Emotion, 12*(4), 533–553.

Van Hooff, M. L., & Van Hooft, E. A. (2017). Boredom at work: Towards a dynamic spillover model of need satisfaction, work motivation, and work-related boredom. *European Journal of Work and Organizational Psychology, 26,* 133–148.

Van Hooft, E. A., & Van Hooff, M. L. (2018). The state of boredom: Frustrating or depressing? *Motivation and Emotion, 42,* 931–946.

Van Tilburg, W. A. P., & Igou, E. R. (2011). On boredom and social identity: A pragmatic meaning-regulation approach. *Personality and Social Psychology Bulletin, 37,* 1679–1691.

Van Tilburg, W. A. P., & Igou, E. R. (2012). On boredom: Lack of challenge and meaning as distinct boredom experiences. *Motivation and Emotion, 36,* 181–194.

Van Tilburg, W. A. P., & Igou, E. R. (2013). On the meaningfulness of behavior: An expectancy × value approach. *Motivation and Emotion, 37,* 373–388.

Van Tilburg, W. A. P., & Igou, E. R. (2016). Going to political extremes in response to boredom. *European Journal of Social Psychology, 46,* 687–699.

Van Tilburg, W. A. P., & Igou, E. R. (2017a). Boredom begs to differ: Differentiation from other negative emotions. *Emotion, 17,* 309–322.

Van Tilburg, W. A. P., & Igou, E. R. (2017b). Can boredom help?: Increased prosocial intentions in response to boredom. *Self and Identity, 16,* 82–96.

Van Tilburg, W. A. P., & Igou, E. R. (2019). The unbearable lightness of boredom: A pragmatic meaning-regulation hypothesis. In J. Ros Velasco (Ed.), *Boredom is in your mind* (pp. 11–35). Springer International.

Van Tilburg, W. A. P., Igou, E. R., Maher, P. J., Moynihan, A. B., & Martin, D. G. (2019). Bored like hell: Religiosity reduces boredom and tempers the quest for meaning. *Emotion, 19*(2), 255–269.

Van Tilburg, W. A. P., Igou, E. R., & Panjwani, M. (2023). Boring people: Stereotype characteristics, interpersonal attributions, and social reactions. *Personality and Social Psychology Bulletin, 49,* 1329–1343.

Van Tilburg, W. A. P., Igou, E. R., & Sedikides, C. (2013). In search of meaningfulness: Using nostalgia as an antidote to boredom. *Emotion, 13,* 450–461.

Van Tilburg, W. A. P., Moynihan, A. B., Chan, C. S., & Igou, E. R. (2024). Boredom proneness. In M. Bieleke, W. Wolff, & C. Martarelli (Eds.), *Handbook of boredom research* (pp. 191–210). Routledge.

Van Tilburg, W. A. P., Pekrun, R., & Igou, E. R. (2022). Consumed by boredom: Food choice motivations and weight changes during the COVID-19 pandemic. *Behavioral Sciences, 12*(10), 366.

Vodanovich, S. J., & Watt, J. D. (2016). Self-report measures of boredom: An updated review of the literature. *Journal of Psychology, 150,* 196–228.

Weich, C., Schüler, J., & Wolff, W. (2022). 24 Hours on the run—Does boredom matter for ultra-endurance athletes' crises? *International Journal of Environmental Research and Public Health, 19,* 6859.

Weiss, E. R., Todman, M., Maple, E., & Bunn, R. R. (2022). Boredom in a time of uncertainty: State and trait boredom's associations with psychological health during COVID-19. *Behavioral Sciences, 12,* 298.

Westgate, E. C., & Wilson, T. D. (2018). Boring thoughts and bored minds: The MAC model of boredom and cognitive engagement. *Psychological Review, 125,* 689–713.

Wheeler, H. A., Adams, G. R., & Keating, L. (2001). Binge eating as a means for evading identity issues: The association between an avoidance identity style and bulimic behaviour. *Identity: An International Journal of Theory and Research, 1,* 161–178.

Wisman, A. (2006). Digging in terror management theory: To "use" or "lose" the symbolic self? *Psychological Inquiry, 17,* 319–327.

Wolff, W., & Martarelli, C. S. (2020). Bored into depletion?: Toward a tentative integration of perceived self-control exertion and boredom as guiding signals for goal-directed behavior. *Perspectives on Psychological Science, 15,* 1272–1283.

Yaden, D. B., Haidt, J., Hood, R. W., Jr., Vago, D. R., & Newberg, A. B. (2017). The varieties of self-transcendent experience. *Review of General Psychology, 21*(2), 143–160.

Yakobi, O., & Danckert, J. (2021). Boredom proneness is associated with noisy decision-making, not risk-taking. *Experimental Brain Research, 239,* 1807–1825.

Yucel, M., & Westgate, E. C. (2021). From electric shocks to the electoral college: How boredom steers moral behavior. In A. Elpidorou (Ed.), *The moral psychology of boredom* (pp. 35–56). Rowman & Littlefield.

CHAPTER 49

Pathways to Meaning and Meaning Maintenance in an Ever-Changing, Complex, and Chaotic World

Pninit Russo-Netzer *and* Stefan E. Schulenberg

Human awareness of the finite nature of existence presents a profound challenge—one that fuels one of humanity's most enduring pursuits: the search for meaning. Existential theories posit the universe is inherently devoid of meaning, leaving humans motivated to search for it, even to create it themselves. Contemporary research supports this premise, with meta-analytic findings demonstrating robust associations between meaning in life (MIL) and various indicators of psychological well-being (e.g., Czekierda et al., 2017; King & Hicks, 2021). Conceptualized as "shared mental representations of possible relationships among things, events, and relationships" (Baumeister, 1991, p. 15), the effects of MIL go beyond mental health to physical well-being and longevity, suggesting that meaning serves as a crucial integrative force in human evolution and continued adaptation (Baumeister & Hippel 2020; King & Hicks, 2021; Russo-Netzer, 2019).

The nature and significance of meaning sources have evolved in response to shifting historical, cultural, and religious contexts. Historically, religious institutions and their associated figures—pastors, priests, rabbis, and imams—served as primary guides in the search for meaning, offering structured systems of belief and moral frameworks that addressed fundamental questions of existence. These institutions provided coherent roadmaps for understanding what was considered true, significant, and purposeful, often grounding individuals in culturally endorsed collective meaning systems that would ensure the individual's legacy. The Enlightenment that began with the Scientific Revolution in the 16th century marked a crucial turning point, introducing a paradigm shift that began to unravel the authority of religious institutions in defining and guiding individual meaning making (Berman, 2009; Vos, 2020). Emphasizing reason, autonomy, and individualism promoted the idea that individuals could pursue meaning independently of institutionalized belief systems. Alternatively, this fundamental change in perspective has caused people to lose interest in the communal setting, and the traditional relation system beyond the self that offered a path toward meaning (Berman, 2009; Vos, 2020). This personalized, introspective shift rewrote the script toward purposeful existence that had endured for millennia. This change in emphasis resulted in a new conceptualization of meaning, and the traditional overarching and more abstract concept of *meaning of life* to be differentiated from the individualized personal conception of *meaning in life*. This shift in thinking also catalyzed a more nuanced discussion about the construction of meaning.

This chapter explores pathways to finding and sustaining MIL through various theoretical lenses, integrating classical and contemporary perspectives with empirical findings. We delve into core theoretical frameworks that illuminate the concept of MIL, with a focus on meaning making and maintenance processes (Heine et al., 2006) and terror management theory's (TMT's; see Solomon et al., Chapter 6, this volume) view that meaning has motivational utility. Then we consider frameworks for the integration of these theories into meaning-centric interventions, such as existential positive psychology's (Wong, 2010, 2020) emphasis on growth through suffering and narrative psychology's (McAdams, 2008) emphasis on personal and cultural stories' relation to coherence and significance.

MIL: CONCEPTUAL FOUNDATIONS AND MEASUREMENT APPROACHES

The concept of MIL introduces both conceptual and empirical challenges in its definition and measurement (George & Park, 2016; Martela & Steger, 2016). One approach differentiates the *presence* of meaning from the *search* for meaning (Frankl, 1959/1985; Schulenberg et al., 2014; Steger et al., 2006), and a meta-analysis has shown that the presence of meaning is clearly linked to subjective well-being while the search for meaning's pattern of associations is much more complicated (Li et al., 2021; Schulenberg et al., 2014; Steger & Marsh, Chapter 51, this volume). The presence of MIL has been widely considered to be comprised of three core concepts. The earliest is Viktor Frankl's (1959/1985; see also Schulenberg et al., 2008) "triangle" of creative, experiential, and attitudinal values pathways. Creative values focus on unique, passionate, and legacy creation; experiential values center around (re)appraisal and finding growth opportunities in our encounters; and attitudinal values stress the resilient and dignified will to attain meaning. More recent empirical testing has led to the development of the tripartite models of MIL (George & Park, 2016; Martela & Steger, 2016), involving *comprehension/coherence* (similar to the experiential values path), *purpose* (similar to the attitudinal values path), and *mattering/significance* (similar to the creative values path). This three-dimensional model of meaning has been conceptualized similarly by Reker and Wong (2013), involving cognitive, motivational, and affective components.

The assessment of meaning has evolved significantly, becoming more nuanced and precise, with new methodological approaches complementing traditional measures. The most prevalent, contemporary self-report measure is the Meaning in Life Questionnaire (MLQ; Steger et al., 2006), which includes two subscales assessing presence of meaning and search for meaning. The brief Purpose in Life Test—Short Form (PIL-SF; Schulenberg & Melton, 2010; Schulenberg et al., 2011) is another measure of perceived meaning that is rooted in 60 years of research, considering the original 20-item form was published by Crumbaugh and Maholick in 1964 (1964, 1969/1981). Recently, a Meaning in Life in Children Questionnaire (MIL-CQ) has been validated (Shoshani & Russo-Netzer, 2017), which assesses three constructs that parallel Frankl's (1959/1985) creative, experiential, and attitudinal values pathways. The Multidimensional Existential Meaning Scale (MEMS; George & Park, 2017) and the Three-Dimensional Meaning in Life Scale (3DM; Martela & Steger, 2023) were developed to measure the three elements of comprehension, purpose, and significance/mattering. Other recent scales include the Prioritizing Meaning Scale (Russo-Netzer, 2019) and the Claremont Purpose Scale (Bronk et al., 2018).

In addition to self-report, neural imaging studies have begun mapping brain networks associated with meaning construction and maintenance, revealing the role of the anterior cingulate cortex (ACC), an area related to conflict and difficult decision making, and relevant in threat and social exclusion (Eisenberger et al., 2003). This brain structure specifically relates to threats that have been connected to concepts relevant to maintaining meaning. Supporting these findings, another study found that people with strong, perceived purpose showed less activity in the dorsal region of the ACC (Kang et al., 2019). MIL has been phenomenologically linked to episodic memory (Sutin et al., 2022), and the medial temporal lobes—involved with high resolution episodic memory (Eichenbaum et al., 2012)—have also been associated with self-reports of MIL (King & Hicks, 2021).

New field research methods, such as experience-sampling methods, measure near-immediate antecedents and consequences in a natural environment, providing new insights into the dynamic nature of meaningful experiences in daily life (Shiffman et al., 2008). Relating to meaning, a study using this method (Choi et al., 2017) showed that in a Korean sample, the degree of happiness and meaning in daily lives was far weaker on a moment-to-moment basis than it was holistically. This finding suggests the connection is more tenuous in our day-to-day lives or that there is a requirement to reflect holistically to connect the two. On this note, another recent experience-sampling study (Chu et al., 2020) showed that low-activation positive affect, in particular, was more strongly related to MIL among older (versus younger) people, indicating that older adults live day to day with greater meaning and happiness. Lastly, naturally occurring routines relate to the momentary feeling of MIL (Heintzelman & King, 2019). These dynamic revelations around the experience of meaning challenge conceptualizations of meaning as a stable trait, demonstrating the importance of situational meaning versus global meaning (Park & Blake, 2020; Reker & Wong, 2013).

CORE THEORETICAL PERSPECTIVES

Descriptive Theories: The Tripartite Models

The two prevailing descriptive theories are the tripartite models of George and Park (2016) and Martela and Steger (2016). The models describe meaning as involving three components: a sense of *coherence* or comprehension; a sense of *purpose;* and a sense of *significance* (Martela & Steger, 2016) or mattering (George & Park, 2016). The sense of coherence or comprehension involves an understanding of how things are related in the world. The sense of purpose involves goals. And the sense of significance/mattering is the "sense of life's inherent value and having a life worth living" (Martela & Steger, 2016, p. 534), and/or "the degree to which individuals feel that their existence is of significance, importance and value in the world" (George & Park, 2016, p. 206). It seems likely that significance and mattering are the same component, and that the different terminology is simply a result of two different author teams describing the same process with different words (Martela & Steger, 2023). These three MIL components bear similarity to what Reker and Wong (2013) described as a cognitive element (coherence), a motivational element (purpose), and an affective element (significance/mattering).

Motivational Theories

The meaning maintenance model (MMM; Heine et al., 2006) argues that people are motivated to maintain the presence of meaning, having developed the ability to adapt when meaning is threatened. According to the MMM, meaning is built on coherent, expected relationships—coherence within oneself and in the external world, as well as between oneself and the external world (Heine et al., 2006). From this perspective, then, meaning comes in many varieties of concrete relationships (e.g., between keys and locks between functional components) and abstract relationships (e.g., self-esteem, group affiliation). Because people are motivated to maintain a sense of MIL, the MMM proposes that if one area of meaning is threatened or undermined, people will increase their reliance on an alternative area of meaning in a process called *fluid compensation.* Therefore, the MMM proposes that fluid compensation ultimately represents a search for a coherent structure of relationships in which one can find solace, mitigating the perceived threat of meaninglessness.

TMT (Arndt et al., 2013; Solomon et al., Chapter 6, this volume) posits that meaning is an important tool that humans use to grapple with their uniquely sophisticated awareness of death. From the TMT perspective, the conscious awareness of mortality motivates direct physical avoidance of death (e.g., applying sunscreen, wearing a seatbelt) whereas nonconscious awareness of mortality motivates people to seek a sense of immortality through symbolic forms (e.g., legacies) or literal forms (e.g., belief in an eternal soul and an afterlife). To successfully achieve those goals, people must be able to understand and navigate the micro- and macrolevel relationships of characteristics within themselves, within the external environment, and between themselves and the environment. Thus, according to TMT, the awareness of death is what motivates people to maintain a meaningful understanding of their place in the world, navigate those meanings to achieve a sense of permanence-promising value, and flexibly adjust as needed (Arndt et al., 2013). Research has shown a robust effect of death awareness on investment in a variety of micro- and macrolevel meaning systems (Arndt et al., 2013; Burke et al., 2010).

Narrative Identity Theories

Research of identity processes and their relationship to meaning has garnered new insights into the meaning literature. Whereas the field originally conceived of meaningful identity development as the integration of social interactions, relationships, norms, and roles into the self (Marcia, 1980), the literature now also views successful identity development as including the project of developing a dynamic, personal story (Bruner, 1991). This personal story is the home of one's identity and develops more solidity over time and experience as it compensates for threats and realigns meaning frameworks. If our identity processes optimally hone the meaning system, then our story compensates for obstacles and reimagines the frameworks that are no longer tenable, updating our prediction of expected relations and the greater narrative web.

Identity integration through cultural identity is often shaped by stories children are told by prior generations about their personal stories and those of their predecessors, shaping the communal and personal narrative of the younger generation (Bruner, 2010). Societal values and stories also dictate the identity one adopts. Some societies may prioritize work identity because of the cultural narrative surrounding work's importance. Other cultures may emphasize familial identity, thus making one's story revolve more around that role. Both examples though, create the overarching identity of the self-narrative and, if inconsistent, incoherent, purposeless, or insignificant, may undermine one's meaning frameworks and values systems (Boucher et al., 2016; Neimeyer & Levitt, 2001).

The life story model of identity (McAdams, 2003) claims that people make a coherent story with plots, characters, and themes, creating a dynamic narrative that they internalize and use to make sense of the world and bring purpose to life (McAdams, 2008). The efficacy of making sense of autobiographical memories has an extensive literature showing how it leads us toward coherence and purpose in our lives (James, 1893; Pasupathi, 2001). This evolving, coalescing life story integrates events and encounters into a larger, coherent arc of meaning and sense making, much as expected relations create meaning frameworks that foster coherence and unity (Heine et al., 2006; King & Hicks, 2021). Narratives enhance our capacity to project ourselves into memories and future possibilities, enabling us to perceive our lives as intentional processes, with these outcomes contributing to the construction of a meaningful life (Baumeister & Hippel, 2020; Rivera et al., 2019; Sutton, 2020).

In addition to the meaning derived through one's personal narrative, shared memories, storytelling, and collective stories have been shown to promote well-being (Einam et al., 2024; Ruini et al., 2022). As an example of such an occurrence, when an elder within the family shares a personal memory, an intergenerational narrative can be created that enriches a family member's identity, improving the coherence of their story and its meaningfulness (Russo-Netzer, 2023). Other examples can also occur within the social identity framework through collective narratives such as religious or nationalistic stories that create purpose and coherence (e.g., the stories surrounding Moses, Jesus, Mohammed, George Washington, Golda Meir). Cultural values and history shape individual narratives (Benet-Martínez, 2021; Benet-Martínez & Oishi, 2008). These cultural *master narratives* inspire individuals to construct their own stories of positivity, world-changing impact, and heroism, fostering coherence and purpose both within themselves and in relation to others (Hammack, 2008; McLean et al., 2018; Neimeyer & Levitt, 2001).

Recently, research has utilized a common master narrative known as the *hero's journey* (Campbell, 2003) to ascertain its therapeutic capabilities. This quest, or monomyth, is a redemptive story arc (Dunlop, 2022; McAdams & McLean, 2013) that is replicated among many cultures and epochs, describing the transformation of the main character into a hero through the facing and the overcoming of adversity. A recent study (Rogers et al., 2023) described the seven stages of the hero's journey, which unfold as follows: (1) the protagonist's initial, stable way of life or normal world; (2) a disruptive shift that upends this familiar existence; (3) the initiation of a quest or path toward a significant goal; (4) the formation of alliances with friends and mentors who assist in the journey; (5) the confrontation of challenges and adversaries; (6) the personal transformation gained through perseverance and overcoming obstacles; and (7) the return to the community or world, bringing back wisdom and a lasting legacy. Utilizing this framework, the study suggested that such cultural narratives are both associated with and causally linked to MIL and well-being, as measured by several indices of meaning (e.g., Costin & Vignoles, 2020; Martela & Steger, 2016; Steger et al., 2008). The results of such research efforts highlight the significant, positive benefit of this powerful narrative, suggesting that for individuals who perceive their own life story as reflecting these stages, they often experience a heightened sense of meaning in their lives. In other words, the hero's journey offers a framework that underscores the significance of seeking coherence, purpose, and a broader sense of MIL. This framework, which highlights the pursuit of these elements, is deeply embedded in cultural narratives that glorify the quest for illumination through hardship—a process that ultimately ensures the creation of one's legacy.

The stages of the hero's journey can also be integrated with the theories we have described to this point. At the onset of a hero's journey, the story describes one's fluid compensation toward a quest in the face of a threat to one's meaning frameworks. This original shift threatens the coherence of the person's meaning and life story, calling them to adventure and the pursuit of purpose through the facing and the conquering of this threat (an example in popular culture of a hero's journey is the evolution of Luke Skywalker in the original 1977 *Star Wars* film). The middle of the story focuses on the importance of connectedness (Ryan & Deci, 2000). Obstacles are encountered, such as enemies and suffering experiences, followed by triumph, transformation, and the realignment of meaning frameworks (Heine et al., 2006). Lastly, the seventh stage refers to symbolic immortality, significance and existential mattering in creating and leaving a legacy, that is, the ability to endure past one's physical demise, to keep alive the unique and creative contribution the individual has brought to life (see Figure 49.1; see also Smith, 2018).

The hero's journey highlights the significant role that a personal story and narrative play in finding MIL, encapsulating the pathways and key experiences that shape an individual's understanding of meaning. This approach aligns closely with TMT, which emphasizes how personal narratives and the quest for meaning help individuals cope with existential anxieties.

Therapeutic Perspectives

The most comprehensive and deeply rooted meaning-oriented therapy is logotherapy (sometimes referred to as logotherapy and existential analysis), pioneered by Austrian neurologist, psychiatrist, and Holocaust survivor Viktor E. Frankl (1905–1997). *Logotherapy* is generally defined as an empirically-based meaning-centered approach to psychotherapy. The framework posits that human beings are primarily motivated by a search for meaning (i.e., the *will to meaning*) rather than by the fulfillment of basic drives or the resolution of past conflicts (Frankl, 1959/1985, 1978/1985). Frankl's theory is based on a three-dimensional view of human existence, comprising the physiological, the psychological, and the noetic (spiritual, or contemplative) dimensions,

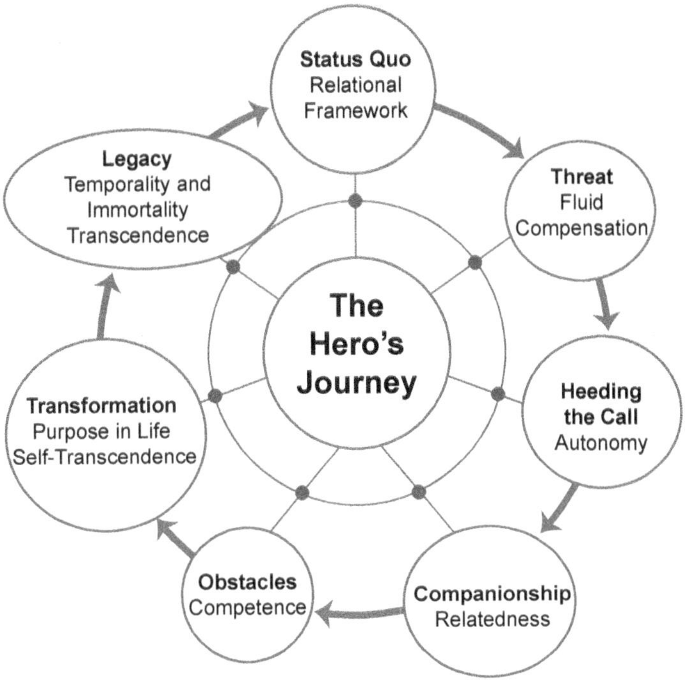
Status Quo
Relational
Framework
Threat
Fluid
Compensation
Heeding
the Call
Autonomy
Companionship
Relatedness
Obstacles
Competence
Transformation
Purpose in Life
Self-Transcendence
Legacy
Temporality and
Immortality
Transcendence
The
Hero's
Journey

FIGURE 49.1. The hero's journey suggested framework.

which interact but remain ontologically separate (Frankl, 1959/1985, 1978/1985; see also Schulenberg et al., 2008). According to logotherapy, symptoms and distress are understood not only in terms of their physical or psychological causes but also through the lens of existential frustration, which arises when individuals fail to find MIL (Frankl, 1959/1985, 1978/1985; Russo-Netzer & Maoz, 2021). The therapeutic process emphasizes the unique capacity of humans to exercise freedom of will, take responsibility, and make intentional choices, which allows them to discover and actualize meaning, even in the face of suffering (Schulenberg, 2020; Schulenberg et al., 2008).

Frankl identified three pathways to meaning: creative values, experiential values, and attitudinal values, which involve what we give to the world, what we take from it, and how we respond to unchangeable situations of adversity and suffering, respectively (Frankl, 1959/1985, 1978/1985; Schulenberg et al., 2008). Central to logotherapy is the concept of tragic optimism, which suggests that individuals can maintain hope, faith, and love despite life's inherent suffering, guilt, and death (Frankl, 1959/1985). This philosophy has been supported by empirical research, highlighting the roles of optimism, hope, and resilience in overcoming adversity and transforming negative experiences into meaningful ones (Schulenberg, 2020; Schulenberg et al., 2008).

Logotherapy and post-Franklian meaning-oriented therapies are commonly categorized under the broader umbrella of "existential therapies," or even more generally as "humanistic therapies." However, many of these post-Franklian approaches have evolved beyond the traditional existential and humanistic schools (see Russo-Netzer & Vos, in press; Schulenberg et al., 2008). For example, existential positive psychology focuses on the integration of positive and negative aspects of life as the foundation of personal flourishing and MIL, describing how meaning transforms the negative into the positive (Wong, 2010, 2020). Existential positive psychology, otherwise known as the second wave of positive psychology (PP 2.0), asserts that effective coping strategies during suffering are creative and proactive—in other words, the approach asserts that reconceiving suffering as a challenge to transform is a better catalyst for fostering meaning making and maintenance. This adaptation of the logotherapy framework as an adaptive coping strategy incorporates prosocial behaviors (Klein, 2017), positive reframing (Park, 2010), and life appreciation (Jans-Beken & Wong, 2021). In an update on the goals of PP 2.0, Wong (2020) pointed out that the ongoing Fourth Industrial Revolution (Schwab, 2018) is driving rapid technological changes and disruptions in global markets, while the forces of nature challenge people's naive conceptions of reality, throwing them into chaos. Such changes can be perceived as radical, volatile, unpredictable, capricious, or otherwise variable, which can result in new kinds of psychological problems, *hikikomori* in Japan being one example (Takano & Wong, 2021). *Hikikomori* is similar to loneliness, a condition experienced by youth characterized by isolating themselves physically from the external world, for a substantial amount of time, only communicating virtually. This trend is paralleled in the Western world as well (Jeste et al., 2020; Twenge et al., 2021). This current state also creates a sense of loneliness that Frankl (1959/1985) pointed to as a cause of meaninglessness.

The shift from traditional structures such as religion, faith communities, and stable homes and neighborhoods to the dominance of media platforms and online communities has contributed to a breakdown in meaningful relationships and the fragmentation of social life. With the rise of digital communication, people can more easily surround themselves with like-minded individuals, often leading to the formation of echo chambers where opposing perspectives are excluded or dismissed. This phenomenon has fueled extremism and political polarization, as individuals become more entrenched in their own beliefs and less open to engaging with differing viewpoints. A naive conception of reality emerges when individuals perceive their online communities or personal networks as representative of the world, failing to recognize the complexity and diversity of perspectives outside their immediate circles. For example, someone might view political issues solely through the lens of their preferred social media group, thus developing a skewed understanding of the broader societal context. This selective exposure to information exacerbates misunderstanding, mistrust, and conflict, as individuals become disconnected from the lived experiences of others. In this environment, meaning becomes essential for anchoring human responsibility, coping with uncertainty, and fostering self-transcendence. Meaning-oriented frameworks offer ways to bridge ideological divides by promoting empathy, critical thinking, and openness to diverse perspectives, helping individuals effectively navigate the complexities of a polarized world.

Wong (2020) asserted that therefore, sustainable well-being is discovered along the course of trials and tribulations, and one must carry with them the Buddhist proverb that "Pain is inevitable, but suffering is a choice." This truth also corresponds with Frankl's attitudinal stance according to which transforming suffering into resilience and meaning is an adoption of voluntary sacrifice for something we love greater than ourselves. This love for something outside of ourselves, beyond the self, gives us courage to persevere, confront, and conquer the suffering experienced, willfully sacrificing the hedonic for the transcendent. In other words, when confronted with profound challenges such as natural or technological disasters, pandemics, terrorism, or extreme values conflicts, our responses can be transformative, enabling us to grow stronger through our experiences. Such events often prompt deep existential questions, particularly the fundamental "why" that compels us to reassess our values, worldviews, and our sense of meaning. When confronted with events that defy understanding or seem inexplicable, our existing frameworks for making sense of the world may become inadequate, prompting a profound restructuring of those frameworks. This process of reworking our worldviews is essential in navigating the chaos and tragedy we encounter. It also sheds light on the search for meaning: When faced with overwhelming experiences, we may find ourselves unable to cope, as our current sense of meaning fails to provide adequate answers. This dissonance drives a deliberate process of rumination, as we seek to reconcile the incomprehensible with our understanding of the world. In this way, the search for meaning becomes not just a passive response, but an active, necessary endeavor to make sense of life in the wake of tragedy and hardship.

CORE CONCEPTS OF MEANING CONSTRUCTION

In this section, we delve into some of the foundational elements of finding, creating, and sustaining meaning, as well as the process of abstracting meaning from our experiences. This endeavor involves selecting key components from existing models and integrating them with ideas that enhance their contribution by linking them together cohesively. We begin with the concept of fluid compensation, a response to the breakdown of structures that sustain the presence of meaning in our lives. From this starting point, we move toward self-determination, reclaiming our sense of agency and locus of control (Lefcourt, 1991). This process involves asserting personal autonomy, fostering connections with others, and discovering our competence in navigating the world. These steps collectively lead to uncovering our sense of purpose. As we inevitably progress through time, we encounter challenges such as feelings of futility, suffering, and the awareness of our mortality. Through these struggles, we experience a transformative process, finding meaning by transcending pain and adopting a broader, more encompassing perspective on life.

Fluid Compensation

The concept of fluid compensation refers to a psychological balancing mechanism that helps individuals maintain a sense of global meaning when a specific meaning framework is threatened (Heine et al., 2006). When one domain—such as social affiliation, which is often central to one's identity and worldview—is challenged, it can disrupt one's overall sense of meaning. In response, individuals may compensate by reaffirming another psychological structure that remains intact, such as self-esteem, thereby preserving a stable sense of meaning. Research supports this dynamic process. For instance, Boucher and colleagues (2016) found that when individuals are highly identified with a particular meaning framework, threats to that framework may lead them to express more polarized views toward members of outgroups. Overall, studies highlight fluid compensation as a key mechanism through which people respond to threats to their meaning systems.

Self-Determination Theory

Self-determination theory discusses the achievement of personal growth and well-being (Deci & Ryan, 1985; Ryan & Deci, 2017), elucidating three core needs: competence, relatedness, and autonomy. *Autonomy* involves the expression of one's internalized thoughts, feelings, and actions, and is related to the concept of authenticity (Baumeister, 2019; Lutz et al., 2023; Sutton, 2020). *Relatedness* involves maintaining positive connections with others (Ryan & Deci, 2017; see also Baumeister & Leary, 1995), which has a positive impact on MIL (Lambert et al., 2013), while loneliness and exclusion have the opposite effect (Eisenberger et al., 2003; Kang et al., 2021). *Competence* relates to mastery over one's actions. The need for competence, relatedness, and autonomy has been demonstrated through experimental and longitudinal studies (Ryan & Deci, 2017) and is related to MIL (Martela et al., 2018).

Purpose in Life

A prevalent construal of MIL inspired by Frankl (1959/1985, 1978/1985) is that meaning arises when people have a clear purpose in life. George and Park defined purpose in life as a "sense of core goals, direction in life, and enthusiasm regarding the future" (George & Park, 2013, p. 371). They distinguished between purpose and MIL in a longitudinal study (George & Park, 2013; Schippers & Ziegler, 2019). Purpose is conceived of as a "goal manager" (Kashdan et al., 2024) that creates a structure of and a motivation toward higher-order goals (Elliot, 2006; McKnight & Kashdan, 2009). Research strongly corroborates this claim, as purpose in life predicts when people feel they are making behavioral progress toward their most important values (Smout et al., 2014).

A growing body of findings shows that purpose has unique psychological benefits in relation to meaning (e.g., Costin & Vignoles, 2020; Li et al., 2021; Martela & Steger, 2023). As a daily diary study of social anxiety disorder found, when people gave extra effort toward a purpose in life, self-esteem and positive emotions increased along with it (Kashdan & McKnight, 2013). In addition, purpose uniquely predicted a high behavioral approach system and a low inhibitory system (Kashdan et al., 2024; Martela & Steger, 2023). Neural imaging research has shown that individuals with a greater sense of purpose showed less activity in conflict-related regions of the brain when facing burdensome health decisions, indicating an ability to handle adversity through heightened purpose (Kang et al., 2019). Overall, these studies illuminate the unique contribution of purpose in constructing meaning and maintaining it, despite adversity, through goals and values that make up our meaning framework between ourselves and the world.

Temporality and Immortality

Human beings are born with the ability to be aware of the concept of time and impermanence. An individual's conception of MIL changes across the lifespan based on what that person has done (past), what they are doing (present), and what awaits them (future). Research has demonstrated the effect mortality salience plays on an individual's implicit processing and meaning creation, specifically through the conception of physical or symbolic immortality (Burke et al., 2010; Koole et al., 2014). Research also demonstrates that anxiety surrounding death is directly associated with MIL among older adults (Zhang et al., 2019), yet the impact of death awareness appears to diminish with age (Maxfield et al., 2016). Similarly, Chu and Mak (2020) found that low-activation positive affect—such as calmness and contentment—enhances the sense of MIL for older individuals. Cross-cultural findings further support this pattern, showing that a sense of coherence tends to increase with age (Russo-Netzer et al., 2023), suggesting that aging may bring with it a more stable and integrated sense of meaning.

In addition, the concept of time itself plays a strong role in meaning and defining what is important from the past and what should be important in the future (Rogers et al., 2023; Shipp et al., 2009). The reframing and reappraisal of the past and future also play an integral role in creating a positive sense of meaning (Rogers et al., 2023). From the past perspective positive meaning relates to flourishing through tragedy (Wong, 2020) and creating coherence out of the chaos of the past. In the present, concepts such as mindfulness and flow (Csikszentmihalyi, 1988; Hölzel et al., 2011) demonstrate how meaning is pursued through observation and transcendence in the moment, stimulating gratitude and creativity (Kaufman, 2018; Lepisto & Pratt, 2017). The future contains goals that fluctuate as people age and range from having offspring to unique creative contributions that connect them to next generations (McAdams & Guo, 2015; Shoshani & Russo-Netzer, 2017). These elements point to the connection between temporal focus (Shipp et al., 2009) and MIL because moving beyond the past to the present and toward the future seems to be related to achieving MIL (Zhou et al., 2022).

Transcendence

Transcendence puts focus outside of the self toward connection with others and the world, giving a sense of existential significance, strength, and MIL. Viktor Frankl (1959/1985) stressed the noetic (i.e., the spiritual or contemplative) aspect as the integral element of life, where people encounter the transcendent and sacred, giving them greater purpose. Meaning therapy (Wong, 2020) stresses transcendental values and overlooking oneself to pursue that which is external and above (Frankl, 1978/1985). A growing body of research specifically in the field of psychedelics (Nichols, 2020) examines how transcendent experiences contribute to meaning construction. William James, in his *Varieties of Religious Experience* (1917), pointed out four principal features of mystical-type experiences—the ineffable, the noetic, the transient, and the passive—creating an experience of access to a more significant plane of existence, above human reality, imbued with significance and meaning. This is emblematic of the transcendent experience and has been implicated in the use of psychedelics (Huxley, 1999). Psychedelics have been shown to enhance meaning and assist in coping with death anxiety and existential suffering (Griffiths et al., 2008; Johnson et al., 2019; Ross et al., 2016). Overall, these concepts underscore essential components of the journey toward meaning, illustrating a path from existential threat to the transcendent self.

CROSS-CULTURAL VARIATIONS

The uniquely human search for meaning is shaped and influenced by forces and frameworks embedded in culture, and, in turn, individuals' search for meaning also simultaneously recreates and affects culture (Chao & Kesebir, 2013). The dynamic interplay between meaning and culture is evident when a shared network of meaning is being constructed, distributed, and reconstructed among a collective of interconnected individuals that constitute a given culture (Chiu & Hong, 2007). Therefore, concepts such as independence and affiliation may vary in content and extent between cultures. Individuals who value individualistic expression versus collectivistic expression may view their affiliation and independence differently and therefore value or express them distinctly (Markus & Kitayama, 1991). For example, Rothbaum and Trommsdorff (2007) made the case that self-coherence in non-Western cultures is tied not to an independent, isolated self but to a self in the context of roles, affiliations, and situations. Therefore, it is essential to broaden an understanding of meaning beyond specific cultural contexts such as the WEIRD (Western, educated, industrialized, rich, and democratic) ones that are usually researched (Henrich et al., 2010; Robustelli & Whisman, 2018). Indeed, each individual hero's journey occurs in its own unique, temporal–sociopolitical–economic–cultural context and is best understood with consideration for a given journey's full range of nuance.

In the context of narratives, culture also plays a crucial role in describing ideal aspirations and identities that make up a meaningful story (Benet-Martínez & Oishi, 2008; Markus & Kitayama, 1991). Illuminating the extent of this role, researchers have found that individuals first appreciate the exceptional efforts of heroes, which, in turn, translates into a personal desire to search for MIL (Coughlan et al., 2019; Kinsella et al., 2017). This indicates that specific cultural heroes and their respective stories are pathways toward cultural conceptions of MIL. This point is corroborated by a study that found collectivistic cultures such as China found patriotism as the most prototypical feature of heroes (Sun et al., 2023). In addition, the authors found that the perception of social heroes (e.g., political figures and religious leaders who lead a nation or inspire a movement for civil rights and freedom) was associated with collectivistic value orientations among Chinese participants (Sun et al., 2023).

Therefore, different values create different pursuits in the search for meaning and within the constructs and concepts that make and maintain meaning. That being the case, MIL has been measured across cultures with 23,641 adults from countries such as the Philippines, Mexico, and the United Arab Emirates, in addition to commonly studied countries such as the United States and Canada (Russo-Netzer et al., 2023). This research indicates the validity of MIL across cultures, though the differences within the concept may indicate important aspects required for finding a coherent, significant, and purposeful life based on culture. In other words, essential meaning-based concepts such as coherence, significance, and purpose, as well as how these concepts are defined and expressed, may vary dramatically across cultures, as well as within cultures. Each individual hero's journey is a unique path. While some journeys may garner some similarities, no two journeys are precisely the same. Heroes have different worldviews, values, strengths, and resources; experience different calls to arms; and confront different antagonists (challenges, obstacles); in addition, contextual circumstances necessitate or otherwise promote different responses from a given individual. There is a huge range of possible responses and experiences in the human enterprise, and there are many different challenges to meaning potentials that one may be called upon to confront and to overcome.

CONCLUSION, WITH AN EYE TO THE FUTURE

By integrating multiple theoretical perspectives—from the tripartite models, to the motivational perspectives of the MMM to TMT, to narrative identity theory and therapeutic perspectives—researchers are developing an increasingly sophisticated understanding of how people construct and sustain meaningful lives. Looking to the future, several key needs and challenges for the field become apparent. First, there is a clear need for the development of meaning-centered interventions, especially as they adapt to digital delivery formats across clinical, educational, organizational, and community contexts. Second, the accelerating pace of social and technological change presents new demands for understanding how meaning systems adapt to rapid transformation. Third, the global scale of contemporary challenges—such as climate change, disasters and pandemics, terrorism, and social and political polarization—necessitates a deeper understanding of collective meaning making and maintenance processes. Fourth, the rise of artificial intelligence and advanced digital technologies raises profound questions about human uniqueness and purpose, which are likely to shape meaning construction in the coming decades.

Despite these needs and challenges, the evidence reviewed in this chapter suggests that human meaning is both resilient and adaptable. It is a coherent story that pursues the call to meaning through autonomy, purpose, and values. This quest requires camaraderie, relatedness, and connection to others, helping us navigate the tumultuous journey of life. The story views the threats posed by modernity as calls to pursue meaning, guiding us toward realizing our goals. In doing so, it brings about a transformation of self and fosters an eternal calm within the finite, facilitating a connection to the self-transcendent and the achievement of a lasting legacy. This process generates significance and existential meaning.

This narrative arc reinvents multiple frameworks, such as affiliation through camaraderie, self-esteem through perseverance in failure, and symbolic immortality through legacy. Integrating such a meaningful narrative into modern dialogue and therapeutic practice can emulate meaning-centered therapy, helping individuals stay afloat amid the turbulent waves of life (Murray, 2003). Research indicates that narrative therapy can enhance one's perception of MIL (Vess, 2019), and it has been suggested that meaning-centered therapists utilize mindfulness to improve personal agency, transcendental thinking, and reappraisal (Hölzel et al., 2011; Vos & Vitali, 2018).

On a broader scale, technological advancements also offer solutions to challenges related to meaning making. For example, as Wong (2020) suggested, artificial intelligence–powered coaches could help individuals discover their skills, interests, and aptitudes, fostering coherence in their lives. Advances in technology also allow us to augment human memory, enabling the pursuit of more coherent and continuous autobiographical stories (McAdams & Jennings, 2024). Even social media can play a positive role in meaning making. Verduyn and colleagues (2017) demonstrated how social networks, when used actively and intentionally, can enhance meaning-making processes by offering new opportunities for connection.

These developments highlight the growing importance of digital literacy programs in education. Such programs teach individuals how to effectively and critically navigate, evaluate, and create information using various digital technologies (e.g., Van Laar et al., 2017). With proper guidance, digital technologies can help people navigate the chaotic world of the internet, foster connectedness, and integrate storytelling that nurtures coherence, purpose, and significance—ultimately helping ascribe meaning to existence (McAdams, 1996; Twenge, 2017; Wong, 2020).

The continued development of both theoretical understanding and practical applications provides invaluable resources for supporting meaning construction across diverse contexts and populations. As research continues to shed light on the intricate processes through which humans create and maintain meaningful lives, the field is well-positioned to contribute crucial insights to addressing contemporary challenges, while also promoting human flourishing in an increasingly complex world.

REFERENCES

Arndt, J., Landau, M. J., Vail, K. E. III, & Vess, M. (2013). An edifice for enduring personal value: A terror management perspective on the human quest for multilevel meaning. In K. D. Markman, T. Proulx, & M. J. Lindberg (Eds.), *The psychology of meaning* (pp. 49–69). American Psychological Association.

Baumeister, R. F. (1991). *Meanings of life.* Guilford Press.

Baumeister, R. F. (2019). Stalking the true self through the jungles of authenticity: Problems, contradictions, inconsistencies, disturbing findings—And a possible way forward. *Review of General Psychology, 23,* 143–154.

Baumeister, R. F., & Hippel, W. V. (2020). Meaning and evolution: Why nature selected human minds to use meaning. *Evolutionary Studies in Imaginative Culture, 4,* 1–18.

Baumeister, R. F., & Leary, M. R. (1995). The need to belong: Desire for interpersonal attachments as a fundamental human motivation. *Psychological Bulletin,* 117(3), 497–529.

Benet-Martínez, V. (2021). Culture and personality processes: Basic tenets and current directions. In J. F. Rauthmann (Ed.), *The handbook of personality dynamics and processes* (pp. 247–271). Academic Press.

Benet-Martínez, V., & Oishi, S. (2008). Culture and personality. In O. P. John, R. W. Robins, & L. A. Pervin (Eds.), *Handbook of personality: Theory and research* (3rd ed., pp. 542–567). Guilford Press.

Berman, M. (2009). *The politics of authenticity: Radical individualism and the emergence of modern society.* Verso Books.

Boucher, H. C., Bloch, T., & Pelletier, A. (2016). Fluid compensation following threats to self-concept clarity. *Self and Identity, 15,* 152–172.

Bronk, K. C., Riches, B. R., & Mangan, S. A. (2018). Claremont Purpose Scale: A measure that assesses the three dimensions of purpose among adolescents. *Research in Human Development, 15*(2), 101–117.

Bruner, J. (1991). The narrative construction of reality. *Critical Inquiry, 18,* 1–21.

Bruner, J. (2010). Narrative, culture, and mind. In D. Schiffrin, A. De Fina, & A. Nylund (Eds.), *Telling stories: Language, narrative, and social life* (pp. 45–55). Georgetown University Press.

Burke, B. L., Martens, A., & Faucher, E. H. (2010). Two decades of terror management theory: A meta-analysis of mortality salience research. *Personality and Social Psychology Review, 14,* 155–195.

Campbell, J. (2003). *The hero's journey: Joseph Campbell on his life and work* (Vol. 7). New World Library.

Chao, M. M., & Kesebir, P. (2013). Culture: The grand web of meaning. In J. Hicks & C. Routledge (Eds.), *The experience of meaning in life: Classical perspectives, emerging themes, and controversies* (pp. 317–331). Springer.

Chiu, C., & Hong, Y.-Y. (2007). Cultural processes: Basic principles. In E. T. Higgins & A. E. Kruglanski (Eds.), *Social psychology: Handbook of basic principles* (pp. 785–806). Guilford Press.

Choi, J., Catapano, R., & Choi, I. (2017). Taking stock of happiness and meaning in everyday life: An experience sampling approach. *Social Psychological and Personality Science, 8,* 641–651.

Chu, S. T. W., Fung, H. H., & Chu, L. (2020). Is positive affect related to meaning in life differently in younger and older adults?: A time sampling study. *Journals of Gerontology: Series B, 75*(10), 2086–2094.

Chu, S. T. W., & Mak, W. W. (2020). How mindfulness enhances meaning in life: A meta-analysis of correlational studies and randomized controlled trials. *Mindfulness, 11,* 177–193.

Costin, V., & Vignoles, V. L. (2020). Meaning is about mattering: Evaluating coherence, purpose, and existential mattering as precursors of meaning in life judgments. *Journal of Personality and Social Psychology, 118,* 864–884.

Coughlan, G., Igou, E. R., Van Tilburg, W. A., Kinsella, E. L., & Ritchie, T. D. (2019). On boredom and perceptions of heroes: A meaning-regulation approach to heroism. *Journal of Humanistic Psychology, 59,* 455–473.

Crumbaugh, J. C., & Maholick, L. T. (1964). An experimental study in existentialism: The psychometric approach to Frankl's concept of noögenic neurosis. *Journal of Clinical Psychology, 20,* 200–207.

Crumbaugh, J. C., & Maholick, L. T. (1981). *Manual of instructions for the Purpose in Life test.* Viktor Frankl Institute of Logotherapy. (Original work published 1969)

Csikszentmihalyi, M. (1988). *The flow experience and its significance for human psychology.* Cambridge University Press.

Czekierda, K., Banik, A., Park, C. L., & Luszczynska, A. (2017). Meaning in life and physical health: Systematic review and meta-analysis. *Health Psychology Review, 11,* 387–418.

Deci, E. L., & Ryan, R. M. (1985). The General Causality Orientations scale: Self-determination in personality. *Journal of Research in Personality, 19,* 109–134.

Dunlop, W. L. (2022). The cycle of life and story: Redemptive autobiographical narratives and prosocial behaviors. *Current Opinion in Psychology, 43,* 213–218.

Eichenbaum, H., Sauvage, M., Fortin, N., Komorowski, R., & Lipton, P. (2012). Towards a functional organization of episodic memory in the medial temporal lobe. *Neuroscience and Biobehavioral Reviews, 36,* 1597–1608.

Einam, H., Mikulincer, M., & Shachar, R. (2024). Shedding a light on the teller: On storytelling, meaning in life, and personal goals. *Journal of Positive Psychology.*

Eisenberger, N. I., Lieberman, M. D., & Williams, K. D. (2003). Does rejection hurt?: An fMRI study of social exclusion. *Science, 302*(5643), 290–292.

Elliot, A. J. (2006). The hierarchical model of approach–avoidance motivation. *Motivation and Emotion, 30,* 111–116.

Frankl, V. E. (1985). *Man's search for meaning.* Washington Square Press. (Original work published 1959)

Frankl, V. E. (1985). *The unheard cry for meaning.* Washington Square Press. (Original work published 1978)

George, L. S., & Park, C. L. (2013). Are meaning and purpose distinct?: An examination of correlates and predictors. *Journal of Positive Psychology, 8,* 365–375.

George, L. S., & Park, C. L. (2016). Meaning in life as comprehension, purpose, and mattering: Toward integration and new research questions. *Review of General Psychology, 20,* 205–220.

George, L. S., & Park, C. L. (2017). The Multidimensional Existential Meaning Scale: A tripartite approach to measuring meaning in life. *Journal of Positive Psychology, 12,* 613–627.

Griffiths, R. R., Richards, W. A., Johnson, M. W., McCann, U. D., & Jesse, R. (2008). Mystical-type experiences occasioned by psilocybin mediate the attribution of personal meaning and spiritual significance 14 months later. *Journal of Psychopharmacology, 22*(6), 621–632.

Hammack, P. L. (2008). Narrative and the cultural psychology of identity. *Personality and Social Psychology Review, 12,* 222–247.

Heine, S. J., Proulx, T., & Vohs, K. D. (2006). The Meaning Maintenance Model: On the coherence of social motivations. *Personality and Social Psychology Review, 10,* 88–110.

Heintzelman, S. J., & King, L. A. (2019). Routines and meaning in life. *Personality and Social Psychology Bulletin, 45,* 688–699.

Henrich, J., Heine, S. J., & Norenzayan, A. (2010). The weirdest people in the world? *Behavioral and Brain Sciences, 33*(2–3), 61–83.

Hölzel, B. K., Lazar, S. W., Gard, T., Schuman-Olivier, Z., Vago, D. R., & Ott, U. (2011). How does mindfulness meditation work?: Proposing mechanisms of action from a conceptual and neural perspective. *Perspectives on Psychological Science, 6,* 537–559.

Huxley, A. (1999). *Moksha: Aldous Huxley's classic writings on psychedelics and the visionary experience.* Simon & Schuster.

James, W. (1893). *The principles of psychology* (abridged ed.). Holt.

James, W. (1917). *The varieties of religious experience: A study in human nature.* Longman.

Jans-Beken, L., & Wong, P. T. P. (2021). Development and preliminary validation of the Existential Gratitude Scale (EGS). *Counselling Psychology Quarterly, 34*(1), 72–86.

Jeste, D. V., Lee, E. E., & Cacioppo, S. (2020). Battling the modern behavioral epidemic of loneliness: Suggestions for research and interventions. *JAMA Psychiatry, 77,* 553–554.

Johnson, M. W., Hendricks, P. S., Barrett, F. S., & Griffiths, R. R. (2019). Classic psychedelics: An integrative review of epidemiology, therapeutics, mystical experience, and brain network function. *Pharmacology and Therapeutics, 197,* 83–102.

Kang, Y., Cosme, D., Pei, R., Pandey, P., Carreras-Tartak, J., & Falk, E. B. (2021). Purpose in life, loneliness, and protective health behaviors during the COVID-19 pandemic. *Gerontologist, 61,* 878–887.

Kang, Y., Strecher, V. J., Kim, E., & Falk, E. B. (2019). Purpose in life and conflict-related neural responses during health decision-making. *Health Psychology, 38,* 545–552.

Kashdan, T. B., Goodman, F. R., McKnight, P. E., Brown, B., & Rum, R. (2024). Purpose in life: A resolution on the definition, conceptual model, and optimal measurement. *American Psychologist, 79,* 838–853.

Kashdan, T. B., & McKnight, P. E. (2013). Commitment to a purpose in life: An antidote to the suffering by individuals with social anxiety disorder. *Emotion, 13*(6), 1150–1159.

Kaufman, J. C. (2018). Finding meaning with creativity in the past, present, and future. *Perspectives on Psychological Science, 13,* 734–749.

King, L. A., & Hicks, J. A. (2021). The science

of meaning in life. *Annual Review of Psychology, 72,* 561–584.

Kinsella, E. L., Ritchie, T. D., & Igou, E. R. (2017). On the bravery and courage of heroes: Considering gender. *Heroism Science, 2*(1), 4.

Klein, N. (2017). Prosocial behavior increases perceptions of meaning in life. *Journal of Positive Psychology, 12,* 354–361.

Koole, S. L., Tjew, A., Sin, M., & Schneider, I. K. (2014). Embodied terror management: Interpersonal touch alleviates existential concerns among individuals with low self-esteem. *Psychological Science, 25,* 30–37.

Lambert, N. M., Stillman, T. F., Hicks, J. A., Kamble, S., Baumeister, R. F., & Fincham, F. D. (2013). To belong is to matter: Sense of belonging enhances meaning in life. *Personality and Social Psychology Bulletin, 39*(11), 1418–1427.

Lefcourt, H. M. (1991). *Locus of control.* Academic Press.

Lepisto, D. A., & Pratt, M. G. (2017). Meaningful work as realization and justification: Toward a dual conceptualization. *Organizational Psychology Review, 7,* 99–121.

Li, J. B., Dou, K., & Liang, Y. (2021). The relationship between presence of meaning, search for meaning, and subjective well-being: A three-level meta-analysis based on the Meaning in Life Questionnaire. *Journal of Happiness Studies, 22,* 467–489.

Lutz, P. K., Newman, D. B., Schlegel, R. J., & Wirtz, D. (2023). Authenticity, meaning in life, and life satisfaction: A multicomponent investigation of relationships at the trait and state levels. *Journal of Personality, 91,* 541–555.

Marcia, J. E. (1980). Identity in adolescence. In R. M. Lerner & L. Steinberg (Eds.), *Handbook of adolescent psychology* (Vol. 9, pp. 159–187). Wiley.

Markus, H. R., & Kitayama, S. (1991). Cultural variation in the self-concept. In J. Strauss & G. R. Goethals (Eds.), *The self: Interdisciplinary* approaches (pp. 18–48). Springer.

Martela, F., Ryan, R. M., & Steger, M. F. (2018). Meaningfulness as satisfaction of autonomy, competence, relatedness, and beneficence: Comparing the four satisfactions and positive affect as predictors of meaning in life. *Journal of Happiness Studies, 19,* 1261–1282.

Martela, F., & Steger, M. F. (2016). The three meanings of meaning in life: Distinguishing coherence, purpose, and significance. *Journal of Positive Psychology, 11,* 531–545.

Martela, F., & Steger, M. F. (2023). The role of significance relative to the other dimensions of meaning in life—An examination utilizing the Three Dimensional Meaning in Life Scale (3DM). *Journal of Positive Psychology, 18,* 606–626.

Maxfield, M., Pyszczynski, T., Greenberg, J., & Bultmann, M. N. (2016). Age differences in the effects of mortality salience on the correspondence bias. *International Journal of Aging and Human Development, 84,* 329–342.

McAdams, D. P. (1996). Narrating the self in adulthood. In J. E. Birren, G. M. Kenyon, J.-E. Ruth, J. J. F. Schroots, & T. Svensson (Eds.), *Aging and biography: Explorations in adult development* (pp. 131–148). Springer.

McAdams, D. P. (2003). Identity and the life story. In R. Fivush & C. A. Haden (Eds.), *Autobiographical memory and the construction of a narrative self* (pp. 203–224). Psychology Press.

McAdams, D. P. (2008). Personal narratives and the life story. In O. P. John, R. W. Robins, & L. A. Pervin (Eds.), *Handbook of personality: Theory and research* (3rd ed., pp. 242–262). Guilford Press.

McAdams, D. P., & Guo, J. (2015). Narrating the generative life. *Psychological Science, 26,* 475–483.

McAdams, D. P., & Jennings, S. C. (2024). Narrative identity in the digital age. *Psychological Inquiry, 35,* 124–130.

McAdams, D. P., & McLean, K. C. (2013). Narrative identity. *Current Directions in Psychological Science, 22,* 233–238.

McKnight, P. E., & Kashdan, T. B. (2009). Purpose in life as a system that creates and sustains health and well-being: An integrative, testable theory. *Review of General Psychology, 13,* 242–251.

McLean, K. C., Lilgendahl, J. P., Fordham, C., Alpert, E., Marsden, E., Szymanowski, K., & McAdams, D. P. (2018). Identity development in cultural context: The role of deviating from master narratives. *Journal of Personality, 86,* 631–651.

Murray, M. (2003). Narrative psychology and narrative analysis. In P. M. Camic, J. E. Rhodes, & L. Yardley (Eds.), *Qualitative research in psychology: Expanding perspectives in methodology and design* (pp. 95–112). American Psychological Association.

Neimeyer, R. A., & Levitt, H. (2001). Coping and coherence: A narrative perspective on resilience. In C. R. Snyder (Ed.), *Coping with stress: Effective people and processes* (pp. 47–67). Oxford University Press.

Nichols, D. E. (2020). Psilocybin: From ancient magic to modern medicine. *Journal of Antibiotics, 73,* 679–686.

Park, C. L. (2010). Making sense of the meaning

literature: An integrative review of meaning making and its effects on adjustment to stressful life events. *Psychological Bulletin, 136,* 257–301.

Park, C. L., & Blake, E. C. (2020). Resilience and recovery following disasters: The meaning making model. In S. E. Schulenberg (Ed.), *Positive psychological approaches to disaster: Meaning, resilience, and posttraumatic growth* (pp. 9–25). Springer International.

Pasupathi, M. (2001). The social construction of the personal past and its implications for adult development. *Psychological Bulletin, 127,* 651–672.

Reker, G. T., & Wong, P. T. P. (2013). Personal meaning in life and psychosocial adaptation in the later years. In P. T. P. Wong (Ed.), *The human quest for meaning* (2nd ed., pp. 433–456). Routledge.

Rivera, G. N., Christy, A. G., Kim, J., Vess, M., Hicks, J. A., & Schlegel, R. J. (2019). Understanding the relationship between perceived authenticity and well-being. *Review of General Psychology, 23,* 113–126.

Robustelli, B. L., & Whisman, M. A. (2018). Gratitude and life satisfaction in the United States and Japan. *Journal of Happiness Studies, 19,* 41–55.

Rogers, B. A., Chicas, H., Kelly, J. M., Kubin, E., Christian, M. S., Kachanoff, F. J., . . . Gray, K. (2023). Seeing your life story as a hero's journey increases meaning in life. *Journal of Personality and Social Psychology, 125,* 752–778.

Ross, S., Bossis, A., Guss, J., Agin-Liebes, G., Malone, T., Cohen, B., . . . Schmidt, B. L. (2016). Rapid and sustained symptom reduction following psilocybin treatment for anxiety and depression in patients with life-threatening cancer: A randomized controlled trial. *Journal of Psychopharmacology, 30,* 1165–1180.

Rothbaum, F., & Trommsdorff, G. (2007). Do roots and wings complement or oppose one another?: The socialization of relatedness and autonomy in cultural context. In J. E. Grusec & P. D. Hastings (Eds.), *Handbook of socialization: Theory and research* (pp. 461–489). Guilford Press.

Ruini, C., Albieri, E., Ottolini, F., & Vescovelli, F. (2022). Once upon a time: A school positive narrative intervention for promoting well-being and creativity in elementary school children. *Psychology of Aesthetics, Creativity, and the Arts, 16,* 259–271.

Russo-Netzer, P. (2019). Prioritizing meaning as a pathway to meaning in life and general well-being. *Journal of Happiness Studies, 20,* 1863–1891.

Russo-Netzer, P. (2023). Building bridges, forging new frontiers: Meaning-making in action. *Social Sciences, 12,* 574.

Russo-Netzer, P., & Maoz, D. (2021). *Meaning in search of a person: Existential analysis and logotherapy in theory and practice.* Shtaim Press. [Hebrew]

Russo-Netzer, P., Niemiec, R. M., & Tarrasch, R. (2023). Developmental, genderial and cross-cultural aspects of meaning. *Journal of Happiness Studies, 24*(8), 2583–2597.

Russo-Netzer, P., & Vos, J. (in press). Meaning interventions: Working with meaning in life in psychological therapies. In L. Hoffman (Ed.), *APA handbook of humanistic and existential psychology.* American Psychological Association.

Ryan, R. M., & Deci, E. L. (2000). Self-determination theory and the facilitation of intrinsic motivation, social development, and well-being. *American Psychologist, 55,* 68–78.

Ryan, R. M., & Deci, E. L. (2017). *Self-determination theory: Basic psychological needs in motivation, development, and wellness.* Guilford Press.

Schippers, M. C., & Ziegler, N. (2019). Life crafting as a way to find purpose and meaning in life. *Frontiers in Psychology, 10,* 2778.

Schulenberg, S. E. (Ed.). (2020). *Positive psychological approaches to disaster: Meaning, resilience, and posttraumatic growth.* Springer International.

Schulenberg, S. E., Baczwaski, B. J., & Buchanan, E. M. (2014). Measuring search for meaning: A factor-analytic evaluation of the Seeking of Noetic Goals test (SONG). *Journal of Happiness Studies, 15,* 693–715.

Schulenberg, S. E., Hutzell, R. R., Nassif, C., & Rogina, J. M. (2008). Logotherapy for clinical practice. *Psychotherapy: Theory, Research, Practice, Training, 45,* 447–463.

Schulenberg, S. E., & Melton, A. M. A. (2010). A confirmatory factor-analytic evaluation of the Purpose in Life test: Preliminary psychometric support for a replicable two-factor model. *Journal of Happiness Studies, 11,* 95–111.

Schulenberg, S. E., Schnetzer, L. W., & Buchanan, E. M. (2011). The Purpose in Life test-Short Form: Development and psychometric support. *Journal of Happiness Studies, 12,* 861–876.

Schwab, K. (2018, October). *The global competitiveness report 2018.* World Economic Forum.

Shiffman, S., Stone, A. A., & Hufford, M. R. (2008). Ecological momentary assessment. *Annual Review of Clinical Psychology, 4,* 1–32.

Shipp, A. J., Edwards, J. R., & Lambert, L. S. (2009). Conceptualization and measurement of temporal focus: The subjective experience of the past, present, and future. *Organizational Behavior and Human Decision Processes, 110,* 1–22.

Shoshani, A., & Russo-Netzer, P. (2017). Exploring and assessing meaning in life in elementary school children: Development and validation of the Meaning in Life in Children Questionnaire (MIL-CQ). *Personality and Individual Differences, 104,* 460–465.

Smith, B. W. (2018). *Positive psychology for your hero's journey: Discovering true and lasting happiness.* Kindle Direct.

Smout, M., Davies, M., Burns, N., & Christie, A. (2014). Development of the Valuing Questionnaire (VQ). *Journal of Contextual Behavioral Science, 3,* 164–172.

Steger, M. F., Frazier, P., Oishi, S., & Kaler, M. (2006). The Meaning in Life Questionnaire: Assessing the presence of and search for meaning in life. *Journal of Counseling Psychology, 53,* 80–93.

Steger, M. F., Kashdan, T. B., Sullivan, B. A., & Lorentz, D. (2008). Understanding the search for meaning in life: Personality, cognitive style, and the dynamic between seeking and experiencing meaning. *Journal of Personality, 76,* 199–228.

Sun, Y., Igou, E. R., & Kinsella, E. L. (2023). From heroism motivation to civic engagement: The role of self-construals. *Journal of Humanistic Psychology.*

Sutin, A. R., Luchetti, M., Stephan, Y., Strickhouser, J. E., & Terracciano, A. (2022). The association between purpose/meaning in life and verbal fluency and episodic memory: A meta-analysis of >140,000 participants from up to 32 countries. *International Psychogeriatrics, 34,* 263–273.

Sutton, A. (2020). Living the good life: A meta-analysis of authenticity, well-being and engagement. *Personality and Individual Differences, 153,* 109645.

Takano, Y., & Wong, P. T. P. (2021). Deterritorialization of shame in Japan during theFourth Industrial Revolution (4IR). In C.-H. Mayer, E. Vanderheiden, & P. T. P. Wong (Eds.), *Shame 4.0: Investigating an emotion in digital worlds and the Fourth Industrial Revolution* (pp. 147–158). Springer Nature.

Twenge, J. M. (2017). *iGen: Why today's super-connected kids are growing up less rebellious, more tolerant, less happy and completely unprepared for adulthood and what that means for the rest of us.* Simon & Schuster.

Twenge, J. M., Haidt, J., Blake, A. B., McAllister, C., Lemon, H., & Le Roy, A. (2021). Worldwide increases in adolescent loneliness. *Journal of Adolescence, 93,* 257–269.

Van Laar, E., Van Deursen, A. J., Van Dijk, J. A., & De Haan, J. (2017). The relation between 21st-century skills and digital skills: A systematic literature review. *Computers in Human Behavior, 72,* 577–588.

Verduyn, P., Ybarra, O., Résibois, M., Jonides, J., & Kross, E. (2017). Do social network sites enhance or undermine subjective well-being?: A critical review. *Social Issues and Policy Review, 11,* 274–302.

Vess, M. (2019). Varieties of conscious experience and the subjective awareness of one's "true" self. *Review of General Psychology, 23,* 89–98.

Vos, J. (2020). *The economics of meaning in life: From capitalist life syndrome to meaning-oriented economy.* University Professors Press.

Vos, J., & Vitali, D. (2018). The effects of psychological meaning-centered therapies on quality of life and psychological stress: A metaanalysis. *Palliative and Supportive Care, 16,* 608–632.

Wong, P. T. P. (2010). What is existential positive psychology? *International Journal of Existential Psychology and Psychotherapy, 3*(1).

Wong, P. T. P. (2020). Existential positive psychology and integrative meaning therapy. *International Review of Psychiatry, 32*(7–8), 565–578.

Zhang, J., Peng, J., Gao, P., Huang, H., Cao, Y., Zheng, L., & Miao, D. (2019). Relationship between meaning in life and death anxiety in the elderly: Self-esteem as a mediator. *BMC Geriatrics, 19,* 1–8.

Zhou, Z., Zheng, L., Qi, W., & Miao, M. (2022). Finding meaning from the present and future: The mediating role of meaning in life between temporal focus and mental health. *Journal of Pacific Rim Psychology, 16.*

CHAPTER 50

Making Meaning of Adversity

A Conceptual and Empirical Overview

Crystal L. Park

The meaning-making model is a conceptual framework rooted in psychological theories of stress and coping and trauma recovery (Park, 2010). This model helps explain people's day-to-day functioning in the world and how they may regain functioning after highly stressful or traumatic events. The model focuses on two levels of meaning: global and situational (Park, 2017). *Global meaning* comprises people's fundamental beliefs and their unique hierarchies of goals and values along with their sense of life as meaningful. *Situational meaning* refers to the influences of global meaning, in conjunction with the context of a particular situation, on one's appraisals of and subsequent responses to a particular situation. This meaning-making model serves as an organizing framework for this chapter, which aims to provide an overview of meaning in the context of adversity. In the chapter, both global and situational meaning are characterized in terms of conceptual models and then recent empirical research on these models is described. Because systematic reviews of such a large body of literature are neither feasible nor appropriate for a book chapter, my aim here is to highlight some recent studies that tested elements of the meaning-making framework.

GLOBAL MEANING SYSTEMS

Conceptual Model of Global Meaning

Global meaning systems consist of individuals' unique constellations of overarching beliefs, global goals, and subjective senses of the meaningfulness of life. Global beliefs comprise the cognitive frameworks through which individuals interpret and assign meaning to life events. These beliefs form the foundation for constructing a coherent and personally significant narrative of one's experiences. The meaning-making model posits that global beliefs are the organizing principles that guide individuals in understanding the world and their place within it. These beliefs encompass broader existential, spiritual, and philosophical perspectives that influence how individuals perceive the purpose and significance of life events, contributing to the formulation and maintenance of a cohesive worldview. Global beliefs also encompass individuals' own identity in that world (Park, 2010).

Global goals represent the overarching cognitive frameworks that individuals construct that serve as the guiding principles shaping their pursuit of fundamental aspirations and overarching life aims. Global goals are organized hierarchically, with one or several ultimate concerns or goals, the major and enduring objectives individuals pursue to give purpose and direction to their lives. For example, ultimate goals can include serving God, serving their country, supporting a family, having a robust social life, being healthy, being happy, and being of service to others (Emmons, 2003). Each overarching goal gives rise to numerous more specific goals and objectives that are served by even more lower-order proximal goals (e.g., pass a course, make it to weekend worship service; Tamir et al., 2020). Individuals' enduring goals contribute to the coherence of their life narrative by providing an ongoing sense of direction and values.

The third component of global meaning, the sense of life as meaningful, is derived from the extent to which one's system of global beliefs and goals works well. Meaning in life has been defined as a subjective sense of meaningfulness that includes three distinct components: (1) a sense of comprehension (coherence and understanding of one's life and experiences provided by one's global beliefs), (2) purpose in life (direction and motivation derived from progressing on one's global life goals and aims; see Hood & Dinsmore, Chapter 57, this volume), and (3) mattering (finding one's life significant and worth living, based on one's global beliefs and goals; George & Park, 2016; see Igou et al., Chapter 48, this volume).

Global meaning, as a comprehensive cognitive framework, plays a pivotal role in shaping individuals' everyday functioning and mental and physical well-being. Further, a well-established and resilient global meaning system can act as a potent protective factor during challenging circumstances. Indeed, a robust meaning framework can buffer the impact of adversity on mental health and contribute to individuals' capacity to navigate and adapt in the face of life's trials. For example, individuals who have strong philosophical or spiritual belief systems that help them view the world as comprehensible and controllable may draw strength from their beliefs, even in the midst of adversity, facilitating psychological adjustment. Further, global meaning can act as a compass, guiding individuals toward constructive actions and coping strategies during crises and thereby contributing to better postcrisis well-being.

Recent Research on Global Meaning

Many researchers have investigated global meaning as a potent determinant of psychological, social, and even physical well-being. Possessing a coherent set of beliefs, values, and aspirations establishes a harmonious internal framework (Wissing et al., 2021). This *coherence* creates a stable psychological foundation by fostering a secure sense of identity and clear direction in life (King & Hicks, 2021). Further, the *content* of specific beliefs and goals relates to well-being. For example, decades of research have established strong relationships between beliefs in control and well-being (Cheng et al., 2013). In terms of global goals, holding transcendent and intrinsic aims are associated with greater interpersonal functioning as well as personal happiness and spiritual growth, while materialistic goals and values focused on wealth, possessions, image, and status are associated with the opposite (see Kasser, 2016, for a review). Finally, myriad studies consistently underscore the positive links between a strong sense of meaning in life and various markers of well-being, including greater life satisfaction, elevated levels of happiness, and enhanced overall mental and physical health (Boreham & Schutte, 2023; King & Hicks, 2021). These studies collectively demonstrate the links between global meaning systems and everyday functioning.

Along with these studies of global meaning and everyday functioning are a growing number of studies focused on global meaning and resilience in the face of adversity. Similar to the literature on global meaning and everyday functioning, however, much of this work is piecemeal, focusing not on the entirety of global meaning systems but rather on a specific aspect. For example, in studies of beliefs, one study of survivors of physical injury (whiplash), bereavement, or childhood sexual abuse showed that high levels of beliefs in self-worth and benevolence of people were related to better adjustment (Ferrajão & Elklit, 2020a). A longitudinal study of survivors of childhood sexual abuse from the beginning of psychotherapeutic treatment to 12 months later found that beliefs in both self-worth and benevolence of the world increased over time and that these increases corresponded with declines in posttraumatic stress symptoms (Ferrajão & Elklit, 2020b). In a study of young adults exposed to interpersonal violence, the impact of the exposure on depressive symptoms was moderated by beliefs in the world as safe, such that the exposure–depressive-symptom link was over three times greater for young adults with low "world-is-safe" beliefs compared to those with high "world-is-safe" beliefs. In that study, other global beliefs did not moderate the impact of exposure to interpersonal violence (Schleider et al., 2021). One set of studies of Chinese adult survivors from the 2008 Sichuan earthquake with high exposure to postearthquake trauma and poverty-stricken adolescents found that beliefs in a just world buffered the impact of these exposures on measures of resilience and life satisfaction (Wu et al., 2011). The authors concluded that even in a relatively collectivistic culture, high endorsement of just-world beliefs protected against the adverse impact of high-magnitude stressors.

Few studies have explicitly focused on the global meaning component of goals as a protective factor in the face of trauma or major life stress. Although many studies have focused on how a sense of purpose may serve as a stress buffer (e.g., Hill et al., 2022), a sense of purpose is derived from commitment to and estimations of progress toward one's goals rather than a measure of one's goals per se (George & Park, 2016). Therefore, a sense of purpose is an appraisal that in part comprises a subjective sense of life as meaningful, as reviewed below. Far rarer are studies that examine how the *specific goals* that individuals pursue affect their ability to withstand high-magnitude stressors. Two exceptions are a study of older adults that found that higher levels of important life goals buffered the impact of lifetime trauma on depression (Krause, 2007) and an older but intriguing study of political activists that found commitment to one's political principles buffered the impact of torture on posttraumatic stress symptoms (Basoglu et al., 1994). Several additional studies have examined commitment specifically to religion, demonstrating that greater religious commitment is related to greater well-being in stressful circumstances such as the COVID-19 pandemic (Hu et al., 2022) and being a refugee (Acquaye et al., 2018).

Relative to beliefs and goals, a veritable trove of research has accumulated examining the potential for subjective sense of meaning in life to protect individuals facing trauma and other negative life circumstances. Hundreds of cross-sectional studies report favorable associations between a subjective sense of meaning in life and a range of mental health and physical health indices such as depression, anxiety, and posttraumatic stress symptoms (Czekierda et al., 2018; He et al., 2023). For example, higher levels of meaning in life were associated with lower concurrent distress in earthquake survivors (Feder et al., 2013), cancer survivors (Sleight et al., 2021), and veterans (see Fischer et al., 2020, for a review). A cross-sectional study of Hurricane Katrina survivors 3–4 months after the event found that meaning buffered the link between trauma intensity and posttraumatic symptoms (Haynes et al., 2017). Emerging cross-sectional research conducted during the COVID-19 pandemic suggests meaning in life showed similar buffering associations between COVID-19 stressors and distress (e.g., Chao et al., 2020; Schnell & Krampe, 2020).

Longitudinal research studies have yielded similar positive associations between meaning in life and psychological adjustment or well-being. For example, in two studies with nearly 20,000 people, individuals who held a higher sense of meaning in life assessed early in the COVID-19 pandemic experienced subsequent increases in well-being, while well-being declined over time among those who possessed lower levels of meaning in life (Ku et al., 2023). Similar findings were reported in a study of German adults assessed early in the pandemic: Higher levels of meaning in life predicted subsequent reductions in distress (Schnell & Krampe, 2022).

However, these studies that assessed meaning in life after trauma and found it to be associated with less distress after trauma are limited in that they cannot rule out the possibility that people who experienced trauma experienced declines in their sense that life is comprehensible or purposeful as a result of the trauma, prior to being assessed. Studies that assessed meaning in life prior to a trauma are more easily interpretable, and evidence is accumulating that meaning in life is prospectively protective of distress when subsequently encountering trauma. For example, in a sample of German college students assessed prior to the COVID-19 pandemic, meaning in life prospectively predicted less depression and anxiety (although *not* posttraumatic stress symptoms) but meaning in life did not buffer the impact of being affected by the pandemic and distress.

Further, the meaning subcomponent of comprehension was most strongly related with distress (tested only cross-sectionally; Seidel et al., 2023). In a sample of U.S. adults assessed prior to the COVID-19 pandemic, meaning in life predicted lower levels of perceived stress during the pandemic when controlling for baseline stress levels (Boylan et al., 2023). A study of U.S. undergraduates found that meaning in life predicted less rumination after a subsequent flood (Ostafin & Proulx, 2020, Study 2).

Similar findings have been reported outside of the COVID-19 pandemic. In a laboratory study, meaning in life predicted experiencing less distress when college students subsequently wrote about their experience of interpersonal trauma (Ostafin & Proulx, 2020, Study 3). In a sample of navy soldiers assessed predeployment to a combat zone, meaning in life predicted postdeployment posttraumatic stress symptoms (Seol et al., 2021). However, a study already in progress prior to Hurricane Katrina, focusing on mostly non-Hispanic Black low-income mothers living in or near New Orleans, found that purpose in life assessed 1 year prior to Hurricane Katrina *did not* predict posttraumatic stress symptoms at 1 or 2 years after the hurricane (Lowe et al., 2013). This growing body of research suggests that meaning in life and its components typically—but not always—act as a resource promoting resilience when people encounter adversity.

Overall, research is accumulating that demonstrates that different aspects of a global meaning system can protect individuals from the worst effects of stressful and traumatic life events. The majority of this research has focused not on the specific characteristics of the meaning system (e.g., the levels or specific types of beliefs, the specific goal commitments) but rather on the subjective sense of life as meaningful. The bountiful literature on this last point indicates that higher levels of subjective meaning (in the form of overall meaning, or by components of comprehensibility, purpose, and mattering) are virtually across the board related to doing better in the face of adversity, regardless of population, type or severity of adversity, timing, or population.

A conclusion that can be drawn from this body of literature suggests that well-functioning meaning systems including high levels of subjective meaning in life promote well-being in stressful or traumatic situations but may not always fully protect individuals from experiencing posttraumatic distress. In fact, situations often arise that present substantial suffering. Thus, while a robust meaning system undoubtedly serves as a protective buffer against psychological distress, at least some traumatic circumstances or events possess an overwhelming capacity to challenge and violate individuals' global meaning frameworks.

The inherent threat and magnitude of trauma may disrupt the coherence and stability of individuals' established meaning systems, rendering them inadequate to accommodate the profoundly distressing nature of the experience. In such instances, individuals face a critical crisis that calls for attempts at meaning making. People recover by restoring harmony between global and situational meaning. Such processes may also influence the strength and flexibility of global meaning in the face of subsequent stressful encounters; thus, meaning making not only influences recovery from an index event but also can influence levels of resilience for responding to future stressful encounters.

SITUATIONAL MEANING: ENCOUNTERS WITH ADVERSITY

Conceptual Model

Situational meaning refers to the set of processes whereby specific situations—usually highly stressful events—challenge individuals' global meaning, initiating a sequence of appraisal, distress, and meaning-making processes that can ultimately lead to changes in global meaning and either enhanced or diminished well-being. Situational meaning encompasses the appraised meanings of these experiences, the potential discrepancies between global and appraised meaning, the processes involved in reconciling those discrepancies (i.e., "meaning making"), and the changes produced through these reconciliation processes (i.e., "meaning made").

When individuals encounter potentially significant stressors, they evaluate and assign meaning to them (e.g., What has happened? What are its implications for me and my life?) in an effort to grasp their personal significance (Lazarus & Folkman, 1984). This *appraised meaning* is shaped by a combination of individuals' overarching beliefs and goals (i.e., their global meaning) and the specific features of the situation at hand. For example, those with a strong sense that stressful situations are amenable to change may try to understand an event in terms of the specific aspects that can be modified, while those who believe in a "just world" might focus more on identifying what prior mistakes they made or offense they committed to deserve the present adversity.

After appraising the meaning of an event, individuals determine the extent to which that appraised meaning is congruent with their global beliefs, goals, and values. According to the meaning-making model, individuals experience distress when they perceive the trauma and its aftermath as conflicting with their deeply ingrained core beliefs and life aims. Traumatic events may violate global beliefs and goals to the point where they feel "shattered" (Janoff-Bulman, 1992). For example, experiencing a traumatic event might violate a person's global beliefs that they are in control of their fate or that God would protect them. Global goals such as being healthy and safe and maintaining relationships with loved ones can be threatened or taken away by traumatic events. Further, individuals who experience interpersonal traumas (e.g., physical or sexual trauma) compared those who experience noninterpersonal traumas (e.g., natural disasters) may be at greater risk for violation of their global beliefs due to feelings of betrayal and disruptions of trust in others along with violations of important goals (Lilly et al., 2011).

Perceiving such violations or discrepancies may initiate individuals' engagement in cognitive and emotional processing efforts—"meaning making"—to rebuild their meaning systems in ways that incorporate their understanding of the trauma (Park, 2010). *Meaning making* involves either reevaluating the traumatic event to bring its appraised meaning in better alignment with their pretrauma beliefs and goals (i.e., altering the situational meaning) or adjusting their core beliefs and goals to incorporate their experiences (i.e., modifying their global meaning). These shifts in meaning, or the meanings made, can reduce the perceived disconnect between their global beliefs and goals and the traumatic event.

According to the meaning-making model, meaning making should be adaptive, especially to the extent that it results in reducing distress and restoring harmony between global meaning and situational meaning (Brown et al., 2019). However, failing to reduce discrepancies between situational and global meaning may lead to rumination, intrusive thoughts, and depression as individuals continue to try to make meaning (Lachnit et al., 2020).

Meaning-making processes may result in a variety of changed meanings (i.e., *meanings made*), including changes in appraisals of the traumatic event (e.g., coming to see it in a more positive light), changes in global meaning (e.g., changing one's global beliefs, identity, values, or life goals), and perceived stress-related or posttraumatic growth (e.g., perceiving one has increased one's appreciation for life, made stronger connections with family and friends, or grew in awareness of one's strengths; Park, 2017). Successfully making meaning reduces perceived discrepancies between appraised and global meanings and restores a sense of a meaningful world and a worthwhile life, ultimately aiding psychological adaptation to the trauma and fostering future resilience.

Recent Research on Situational Meaning

Understanding how individuals navigate the aftermath of highly stressful circumstances and traumatic experiences is crucial for developing effective interventions and support systems. Thus, better understanding the processes involved in recovering from and making meaning of highly stressful or trau-

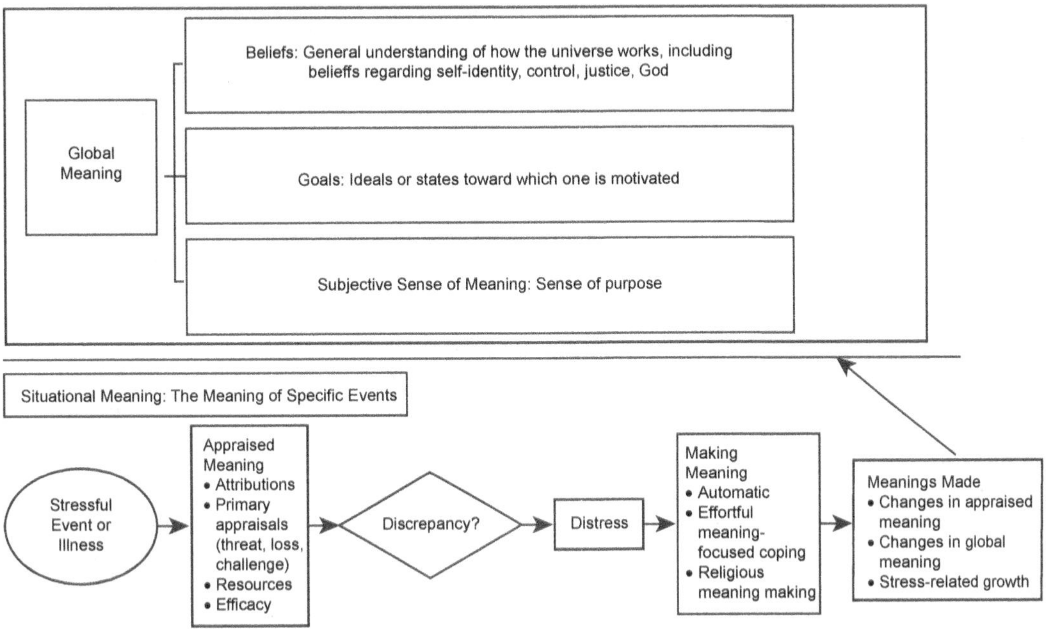

FIGURE 50.1. Schematic of the meaning-making model.

matic events remains a focal point of extensive ongoing research across a range of different types of stressors and sheds light on various aspects of meaning-making processes. The meaning-making model refers to a complex process that unfolds over time. Unfortunately, virtually no research has studied the full model with multiple assessment points of all of its elements, so the research findings in this area are unfortunately piecemeal, with studies tending to examine only one or another part of the linkages shown in Figure 50.1. Results of recent studies that have investigated different aspects of situational meaning are reviewed here, with a focus on four key areas of situational meaning: (1) cognitive appraisals of the situation, (2) violations or discrepancy between global and appraised situational meaning, (3) engagement in meaning making, and (4) meanings made.

Cognitive Appraisals of the Situation

Cognitive appraisals play a pivotal role in shaping individuals' responses to stressors (Lazarus & Folkman, 1984). These appraisals are the cognitive evaluations and interpretations individuals make about the significance of a particular event in relation to their own well-being. These appraisals are not merely objective assessments of external circumstances but involve subjective judgments that reflect an individuals' global meaning systems (e.g., beliefs about their ability to manage the trauma and about their resources for coping). For example, stronger beliefs in internal control or mastery and in the notion that stress can be helpful generally relate to higher appraisals of potentially stressful situations as challenges and lower appraisals of those situations as threats (see Kilby et al., 2018, for a review). One's sense of life as meaningful is also related to more benign appraisals. For example, in a cross-sectional study of survivors of different types of cancer, higher levels of meaning in life related to lower appraisals of threat from their cancer experience and lower levels of belief violation, which were in turn related to lower levels of distress (Curran et al., 2020).

Cognitive appraisals are fairly consistently related to how individuals fare following stressful and traumatic situations. For example, a 3-week longitudinal study of German adults during the COVID-19 lockdown found that increases in appraisal of the pandemic as a threat and decreases in appraisals of the pandemic as a challenge and of one's control and ability to deal with the crisis were associated with increases in mental health symptoms (Brose et al., 2021).

Meaning Violations

The meaning-making model is in essence discrepancy-based; this model posits that distress arises from discrepancies between global meaning and cognitive appraisals of a given situation (George & Park, 2022). Research has only recently begun to explicitly investigate these discrepancies, aided by the development of the Global Meaning Violations Scale (GMVS; Park et al., 2017). Discrepancies are fairly robustly related to distress. For example, a cross-sectional national survey of U.S. adults early in the COVID-19 pandemic found greater belief violation was associated with higher levels of anxiety, depression, and COVID-19 anxiety (Milman et al., 2020), and a replication attempt in a national sample of Italians found virtually the same results (Negri et al., 2023). Similarly, in a cross-sectional study of people in Arkansas early in the COVID-19 pandemic, greater violation of global beliefs by the pandemic was associated with higher levels of stress and helplessness and lower levels of acceptance (Sherman et al., 2022).

Similar findings have been reported in cross-sectional studies of loss. For example, in a sample of bereaved adults during the pandemic whose loved ones had died of COVID-19 and other causes, disrupted beliefs related to greater functional impairment and dysfunctional grief symptoms and partially mediated the relationship between risk factors and impairment/grief (Breen et al., 2022). Cross-sectional studies of survivors of mass shootings at Virginia Tech and the Pulse nightclub also found that belief violations were associated with prolonged grief (Ben-Ezra et al., 2017; Smith et al., 2015).

Fewer studies have included measures of goal violations, even though these are distinct from and potentially as strongly or even more strongly related to distress than are belief violations (Park et al., 2012). For example, in a study of college students who had experienced a recent traumatic event, violations of both beliefs and intrinsic goals—but not extrinsic goals—predicted higher levels of posttraumatic stress symptoms (George et al., 2016), while in a study of young adults dealing with a recent unresolved stressful life event, goal violations—but not belief violations—were positively related to posttraumatic stress symptoms (Appel et al., 2020).

Several studies have identified factors that magnify or attenuate the violations–distress link. For example, the just-mentioned study of recently traumatized college students found that links between violations and posttraumatic stress symptoms were stronger for traumatic events that students rated as more central to their lives (George et al., 2016). Similarly, a study of survivors of the 2016 Louisiana flood found that higher levels of perceiving the flood as violating their global beliefs was related to higher levels of posttraumatic stress symptoms. However, global beliefs about suffering (i.e., in a benevolent, wise, and powerful deity or a deity who suffers along with humans) buffered this link between perceptions of holding certain global beliefs and posttraumatic stress symptoms (McElroy-Heltzel et al., 2018).

Meaning Making

Meaning making refers to the psychological processes wherein individuals actively engage in cognitive and emotional efforts to construct or restore congruence between their global meaning and the appraised meaning of a specific challenging or stressful life event. This type of coping often involves reinterpreting stressors, with a focus on attributing personal meaning to these difficult experiences or casting them in a more positive light. Individuals employing meaning making may engage in cognitive reappraisal, shifting their perspective to find positive or transformative aspects within the adversity. Other meaning-making strategies include searching for meaning and attributing personal growth to challenging experiences. Meaning-making processes can extend beyond adaptation to a given situation to encompass existential exploration as individuals struggle to integrate stressful experiences into a broader and more cohesive life story.

Assessments of meaning making typically include quantitative measures, such as self-report scales, to capture the frequency and intensity of relevant cognitive and emotional processes (Park & George, 2013). Some research also uses qualitative methods, such as narrative analysis, to explore the richness and depth of individuals' meaning-making narratives. Thus, reviewing literature on the full body of meaning making and recovery from stressful experiences is challenging, given the many terms used to describe the various aspects of the process and methods used to capture it.

A core aspect of meaning making is cognitive reappraisal (sometimes called positive reinterpretation or positive reappraisal), the emotion regulation strategy that involves reinterpreting the meaning of situations to modify one's emotional response (Lazarus & Folkman, 1984). A recent systematic review found that using cognitive reappraisal to cope with stressors was generally related to less distress (Riepenhausen et al., 2022). Similarly, a systematic review of positive reappraisal in people diagnosed with HIV found it was often demonstrated to be beneficial for enhancing health promotion and self-management of HIV (Finkelstein-Fox et al., 2020). A recent analysis of midlife adults in the Midlife in the United States (MIDUS) study data spanning 19 years found that, following a trauma, positive reappraisal positively predicted subsequent higher positive affect and lower negative affect; further, all three dimensions of meaning in life (i.e., significance, coherence, and purpose) mediated the effect of positive reappraisal on levels of both positive and negative affect (Fitzke et al., 2021).

Other studies have examined meaning making operationally defined more broadly (e.g., positive reappraisal along with religious coping, acceptance, or searching for meaning). For example, a daily diary study of U.S. undergraduate women with and without sexual violence history found that, across 11 days, sexual violence history was linked to average levels of positive affect through meaning-focused coping, broadly and variously defined (Finkelstein-Fox et al., 2022). A three-wave longitudinal study of Chinese college students assessed 3 months before the COVID-19 pandemic, very early in lockdown, and 3 months after the outbreak in China examined the role of meaning-focused coping as assessed by a measure of explicitly reporting searching for meaning. Results showed that participants reported increased use of meaning-focused coping during the COVID-19 outbreak relative to before the outbreak and that both baseline meaning-focused coping and increased meaning-focused coping predicted less psychological distress during and 3 months after the outbreak. Further, the effects of meaning-focused coping on distress were mediated through increased perceptions of benefits and decreased costs of the COVID-19 pandemic (Yang et al., 2021). In a longitudinal (four-wave) study of U.S. undergraduates who recently experienced a "very stressful event or situation," positive reinterpretation was cross-sectionally associated with better adjustment while higher baseline emotional processing predicted faster declines in goal violations across time (Lachnit et al., 2020). A within-person analysis of these data showed that when participants' appraised-meaning violations increased or decreased, their distress and meaning making also changed in the same direction (George & Park, 2022).

Meaning making as coded from qualitative data has also demonstrated associations with decreased distress. For example, a secondary analysis of data from a trial of a clinical intervention for trauma-exposed adolescents found that constructive processing in the form of accommodation (coded from written narratives) mediated effects of the therapy on posttraumatic stress symptoms (Hayes et al., 2017). In a study using the Pennebaker writing paradigm, meaning making (as coded in the written narratives) predicted lower posttraumatic stress symptoms and depression across three writing sessions (Castiglioni et al., 2023). A study of community adults requiring emergency care following a traumatic event gathered narratives in the Emergency Department and 1 year later; this study showed that narrative structure improved over time and was associated with subsequent decreases in depressive and posttraumatic symptoms. These effects were mediated by greater engagement coping, which predicted increased coherence of the narrative over time (Booker et al., 2020).

Meaning making is considered to be adaptive especially or only to the extent that it results in reducing discrepancies between global beliefs and goals and the appraised meaning of the trauma (Park, 2017). This assertion was demonstrated in the above-cited study of undergraduates who had experienced a recent stressful event: Baseline emotional processing predicted decreased intrusive thoughts for participants who scored high on having made meaning of the event but increased intrusive thoughts for participants who scored low on having made meaning of the event (Lachnit et al., 2020). Similarly, in the earlier-described cross-sectional study of Arkansans early in the COVID-19 pandemic, searching for meaning in the pandemic was related to more distress but feeling one had made meaning of the situation was related to less distress (Sherman et al., 2022).

Meanings Made

Discrepancies can be reduced by making changes in global meaning or in appraisals of the trauma or stressful event. These *meanings made* are outcomes of the meaning-making process and can take many different forms. Changes in global meaning can include shifts in global beliefs, in goals and commitments, and in a sense of meaning in life. In addition, individuals may shift their appraisals of the traumatic event over time, perhaps in a more benevolent direction that helps them more fully integrate the traumatic event into their global meaning system (Park, 2010).

Among the most commonly reported meanings made through the meaning-making process is perceptions of posttraumatic growth or positive changes (e.g., Acquaye et al., 2018; Lowe et al., 2013). These reports of positive changes can include more appreciation for life, improved coping skills, closer relationships with others, increased compassion, greater life meaning, and deeper spirituality along with viewing the world and other people as more benevolent. These perceptions are often taken at face value as indicating genuine positive change (Boals et al., 2023: Park et al., 2023). Yet while these beliefs in positive posttrauma change may be regarded by individuals as genuine favorable outcomes of the trauma, they have been shown to primarily reflect a trait-like positive outlook or efforts to cope rather than accurately reflecting actual positive changes (Frazier et al., 2009; Park et al., 2023). Thus, while reports of growth do not constitute genuine growth, these perceptions may help people feel their trauma was less discrepant with their global meaning and thus help them recover (Boals et al., 2023).

The few prospective studies that have examined changes in global meaning from pretrauma to posttrauma suggest that changes in global meaning are actually fairly uncommon (Frazier et al., 2009). For example, two studies found that major negative life events predicted worldviews becoming, on average, less favorable (e.g., decreased beliefs in benevolence and meaningfulness), but these effects were quite small (Anders et al., 2014; Schuler & Boals, 2016). A sample of U.S. adults provided ratings of their core beliefs about the world before the onset of the COVID-19 pandemic and again several months afterward. On average, no change occurred in 23 of the 26 primal beliefs; small declines were noted in only three beliefs (the world as *Alive*, *Interactive*, and *Acceptable*), although higher personal adversity (e.g., losing family, financial hardship) was associated with greater declines in positive beliefs (Ludwig et al., 2023). In a longitudinal study of a sample of U.S. adults, interim adverse events predicted small average changes in global beliefs; furthermore, different types of adverse events predicted different changes. For example, experiencing violence or adverse relationship events predicted a decline in benevolence beliefs, while experiencing community disasters predicted *increases* in benevolence beliefs (Poulin & Silver, 2019). These studies are consistent with the notion that beliefs may shift as a result of trauma through processes of violation and meaning making, although none of them explicitly examined these processes.

Minimal research has examined changes in global goals or commitments following traumatic events or through the process of meaning making. Some cross-sectional research has shown that adverse life events are related to self-reports of changes in global goals. For example, the abovementioned study of war-zone U.S. veterans from the post-9/11 era who screened positive for spiritual struggle found high levels of retrospectively reported declines in their current religious commitment (Currier et al., 2023). However, prospective research that can determine whether people's goals and commitments actually change following traumatic experiences and meaning-making processes is scant. A study of college students assessed prior to the COVID-19 pandemic found that students' socioeconomic status aspirations assessed in their first year declined when assessed 2 years later and did so at a faster rate than did a group of students assessed in the fall of 2020, after onset of the pandemic (Rogers et al., 2023).

Changes in meaning in life may be another outcome of the meaning-making process. The meaning-making model proposes that one's subjective sense of meaning in life would increase as harmony between global and situational meaning is restored (Park, 2010). Cross-sectional studies support this assertion. For example, a series of studies focusing on the impact of experiences of suffering (self-defined by participants) in U.S. undergraduates found that suffering was related to lower levels of meaning in life, and the more recent the experience that led to suffering, the stronger the negative association. In addition, higher appraisals of one's experience of suffering as meaningful (understandable, significant, and purposeful) related to higher levels of overall meaning in life and life satisfaction (Edwards & Van Tongeren, 2020). Yet again, however, prospective research on changes in meaning in life from prior to following a traumatic encounter is lacking.

In addition to changing one's global meaning, meaning making can result in changes in how one understands or appraises the situation. Very little research has examined changes in appraised meanings of a trauma over time, a surprising omission given the emphasis on reappraisal in the stress and trauma literature (Riepenhausen et al., 2022). Two recent studies of German adults found evidence that shifts in appraised meaning of a recent stressful event were related to subjective well-being. Specifically, over a 3-month period, perceiving events as increasingly externally controlled predicted decreasing life satisfaction and positive affect. Furthermore, increases in perceiving events as threatening one's social status were related to decreasing life satisfaction while appraising events as increasingly threatening predicted decreasing positive affect and increasing negative affect (Studies 1 and 2; Haehner et al., 2023). Thus, this aspect of recovery—changes in appraised meaning of the trauma—appears to be an important area for future research.

LIMITATIONS OF CURRENT RESEARCH ON GLOBAL MEANING, MEANING MAKING, AND WELL-BEING

First, as is true of the trauma literature more broadly, much of the research on meaning making has been conducted at just a single time point. This cross-sectional design leaves researchers attempting to describe longitudinal processes with data that has all been collected at a single time point, which is impossible to temporally model with certainty. At the least, longitudinal studies are needed to better understand relations among meaning and well-being in the context of trauma over time.

A perhaps even greater limitation is that nearly all of the research on the meaning-making model has been carried out after the trauma has occurred. Given the unpredictable nature of trauma, it is understandable that few prospective studies are available to truly test the protectiveness of global meaning to the deleterious impacts of trauma or the changes in global meaning that people experience following it. Yet the extent to which this lack of prospective data precludes truly addressing our research questions cannot be overstated. The very nature of trauma is a violent reordering of global meaning (Park et al., 2017), yet most studies, by necessity, assess "baseline" at some point *after* the trauma has occurred. Furthermore, because the meaning-making model proposes a series of complex processes over time, most studies have focused on a small piece of the model; tests of the complete meaning-making process remain scarce. Further, measurement of different aspects of the meaning-making model in the context of trauma has been overly simplistic. For example, measures of global meaning violation rarely include a consideration of goals, and just a handful of studies have assessed the three distinct components of subjective meaning in life in the context of adversity. All of these limitations make interpreting the extant body of literature challenging; while there is generally support for different parts of the model, more comprehensive and convincing tests of the model await future research efforts.

FUTURE DIRECTIONS FOR RESEARCH ON MAKING MEANING OF TRAUMA

The current state of the literature suggests several avenues for future research. First, prospective longitudinal study designs are ideal for addressing these research questions aiming to understand the potential protective nature of spirituality in the meaning-making process following trauma. However, because researchers cannot predict trauma exposure, it is logistically challenging to obtain baseline measurements prior to individual traumatic events. The rare prospective studies that exist were typically already collecting data for an existing study before a community trauma occurred (e.g., Hurricane Katrina; Lowe et al., 2013). Another possible methodological approach for future research could be to recruit very large, nationally representative samples and follow them over time, knowing that inevitably a significant proportion of the sample will experience a trauma over the course of the study (e.g., Frazier et al., 2009). Another option is to make creative use of large-scale longitudinal studies such as the MIDUS study (e.g., Fitzke et al., 2021).

Second, measurements of the components of the meaning-making model in the context of adversity need to be far more sophisticated and nuanced. Employing measures to empirically assess each aspect of the meaning-making model (Park & George, 2013) could help unpack the roles of each aspect of the model. For example, violations of meaning can be directly assessed with the GMVS (Park et al., 2017), and the three components of meaning in life can be measured separately as well (e.g., George & Park, 2017). Relatedly, although many trauma types were represented throughout this review (e.g., bereavement, combat), many studies focused on a singular trauma type, limiting the comparisons that can be made across different traumatic experiences. Future studies may profitably study samples with a variety of types of trauma in order to make comparisons in meaning-making processes in individuals who experienced different types of trauma (e.g., Poulin & Silver, 2019). In addition, it is common for trauma survivors to experience multiple traumatic events over their lifetime (Kilpatrick et al., 2013), and because effects are often cumulative, taking trauma history into account when assessing meaning-making processes may reveal lasting effects of earlier trauma and meaning-making processes on current meaning making.

Finally, some of the studies reviewed here suggest that making meaning of trauma leads to lasting changes in global meaning, which then suggests that the success of making meaning of trauma may influence individuals' status or preparedness for facing subsequent adversity. For example, if an individual successfully restores beliefs in control and benevolence and reestablishes significant major goals, they would be expected to have a higher sense of meaning in life, all of which would better prepare them for subsequent adverse encounters. Thus, meaning making may be part of an ongoing cycle of adversity and resilience across the lifespan, a possibility that warrants research attention.

By conducting this future work unraveling the complexities of these processes, researchers can contribute to a deeper understanding of the ways that meaning is involved in processes of navigating adversity, fostering a deeper comprehension of the human capacity for resilience and meaning making in the face of significant life challenges. This ongoing scholarly pursuit holds the potential to inform therapeutic practices, public health initiatives, and policies aimed at supporting individuals in their journey toward posttraumatic recovery.

REFERENCES

Acquaye, H. E., Sivo, S. A., & Jones, K. D. (2018). Religious commitment's moderating effect on refugee trauma and growth. *Counseling and Values, 63*(1), 57–75.

Anders, S. L., Frazier, P. A., & Shallcross, S. L. (2014). Changes in functioning following potentially traumatic life events in college students. *Psychological Trauma: Theory, Research, Practice, and Policy, 6*(Suppl. 1), S99–S106.

Appel, J. E., Park, C. L., Wortmann, J. H., & van Schie, H. T. (2020). Meaning violations, religious/spiritual struggles, and meaning in life in the face of stressful life events. *The International Journal for the Psychology of Religion, 30*(1), 1–17.

Basoglu, M., Paker, M., Paker, O., Ozmen, E., Marks, I., Incesu, C., . . . Sarimurat, N. (1994). Psychological effects of torture: A comparison of tortured with nontortured political activists in Turkey. *American Journal of Psychiatry, 151*(1), 76–81.

Ben-Ezra, M., Hamama-Raz, Y., Mahat-Shamir, M., Pitcho-Prelorentzos, S., & Kaniasty, K. (2017). Shattering core beliefs: Psychological reactions to mass shooting in Orlando. *Journal of Psychiatric Research, 85,* 56–58.

Boals, A., Jayawickreme, E., & Park, C. L. (2023). Advantages of distinguishing perceived and veridical posttraumatic growth: Recommendations for future research on both constructs. *Journal of Positive Psychology, 18*(5), 773–783,

Booker, J. A., Fivush, R., Graci, M. E., Heitz, H., Hudak, L. A., Jovanovic, T., . . . Stevens, J. S. (2020). Longitudinal changes in trauma narratives over the first year and associations with coping and mental health. *Journal of Affective Disorders, 272,* 116–124.

Boreham, I. D., & Schutte, N. S. (2023). The relationship between purpose in life and depression and anxiety: A meta-analysis. *Journal of Clinical Psychology, 79*(12), 2736–2767.

Boylan, J. M., Vagnini, K. M., Rush, C. L., Larson, E. K., Adams, M., Wilson, C. L., . . . Masters, K. S. (2023). Meaning salience and meaning in life prospectively predict lower distress during the COVID-19 pandemic. *Annals of Behavioral Medicine, 57*(6), 483–488.

Breen, L. J., Mancini, V. O., Lee, S. A., Pappalardo, E. A., & Neimeyer, R. A. (2022). Risk factors for dysfunctional grief and functional impairment for all causes of death during the COVID-19 pandemic: The mediating role of meaning. *Death Studies, 46*(1), 43–52.

Brose, A., Blanke, E. S., Schmiedek, F., Kramer, A. C., Schmidt, A., & Neubauer, A. B. (2021). Change in mental health symptoms during the COVID-19 pandemic: The role of appraisals and daily life experiences. *Journal of Personality, 89*(3), 468–482.

Brown, L. A., Belli, G. M., Asnaani, A., & Foa, E. B. (2019). A review of the role of negative cognitions about oneself, others, and the world in the treatment of PTSD. *Cognitive Therapy and Research, 43,* 143–173.

Castiglioni, M., Caldiroli, C. L., Negri, A., Manzoni, G. M., & Procaccia, R. (2023). Linguistic predictors of psychological adjustment in healthcare workers during the COVID-19 pandemic. *International Journal of Environmental Research and Public Health, 20*(5), 4482.

Chao, M., Chen, X., Liu, T., Yang, H., & Hall, B. J. (2020). Psychological distress and state boredom during the COVID-19 outbreak in China: The role of meaning in life and media use. *European Journal of Psychotraumatology, 11*(1), 1769379.

Cheng, C., Cheung, S. F., Chio, J. H.-M., & Chan, M.-P. S. (2013). Cultural meaning of perceived control: A meta-analysis of locus of control and psychological symptoms across 18 cultural regions. *Psychological Bulletin, 139*(1), 152–188.

Curran, L., Sharpe, L., MacCann, C., & Butow, P. (2020). Testing a model of fear of cancer recurrence or progression: The central role of intrusions, death anxiety and threat appraisal. *Journal of Behavioral Medicine, 43,* 225–236.

Currier, J. M., Manalo, M., & McDermott, R. C. (2023). Examining the unique role of premilitary religious commitment in posttraumatic symptomatology among post-9/11 veterans. *Traumatology, 29*(1), 1–5.

Czekierda, K., Gancarczyk, A., Park, C. L, & Luszczynska, A. (2018). Meaning in life and physical health: Systematic review and meta-analysis. *Psychology and Health Review, 11,* 387–418.

Edwards, M. E., & Van Tongeren, D. R. (2020). Meaning mediates the association between suffering and well-being. *Journal of Positive Psychology, 15*(6), 722–733.

Emmons, R. A. (2003). *The psychology of ultimate concerns: Motivation and spirituality in personality.* Guilford Press.

Feder, A., Ahmad, S., Lee, E. J., Morgan, J. E.,

Singh, R., Smith, B. W., . . . Charney, D. S. (2013). Coping and PTSD symptoms in Pakistani earthquake survivors: Purpose in life, religious coping and social support. *Journal of Affective Disorders, 147*(1–3), 156–163.

Ferrajão, P. C., & Elklit, A. (2020a). The contributions of different types of trauma and world assumptions to predicting psychological distress. *Traumatology, 26*(1), 137–146.

Ferrajão, P. C., & Elklit, A. (2020b). World assumptions and posttraumatic stress in a treatment-seeking sample of survivors of childhood sexual abuse: A longitudinal study. *Psychology of Violence, 10*(5), 501–508.

Finkelstein-Fox, L., Park, C. L., & Huedo-Medina, T. B. (2022). Appraisal and coping link sexual victimization history to emotional experience: A multilevel daily diary study. *Journal of Interpersonal Violence, 37*(9–10), NP6159–NP6185.

Finkelstein-Fox, L., Park, C. L., & Kalichman, S. C. (2020). Health benefits of positive reappraisal coping among people living with HIV/AIDS: A systematic review. *Health Psychology Review, 14*(3), 394–426.

Fischer, I. C., Shanahan, M. L., Hirsh, A. T., Stewart, J. C., & Rand, K. L. (2020). The relationship between meaning in life and posttraumatic stress symptoms in US military personnel: A meta-analysis. *Journal of Affective Disorders, 277*, 658–670.

Fitzke, R. E., Marsh, D. R., & Prince, M. A. (2021). A longitudinal investigation of the meaning-making model in midlife adults who have experienced trauma. *Journal of Clinical Psychology, 77*(12), 2878–2893.

Frazier, P., Tennen, H., Gavian, M., Park, C. L., Tomich, P., & Tashiro, T. (2009). Does self-reported post-traumatic growth reflect genuine positive change? *Psychological Science, 20*, 912–919.

George, L. S., & Park, C. L. (2016). Meaning in life as comprehension, purpose, and mattering: Towards integration and new research questions. *Review of General Psychology, 20*, 205–220.

George, L. S., & Park, C. L. (2017). The Multidimensional Existential Meaning Scale: A tripartite approach to measuring meaning in life. *Journal of Positive Psychology, 12*, 613–627.

George, L. S., & Park, C. L. (2022). Do violations of global beliefs and goals drive distress and meaning making following life stressors? *Illness, Crisis and Loss, 30*(3), 378–395.

George, L. S., Park, C. L., & Chaudoir, S. R. (2016). Examining the relationship between trauma centrality and posttraumatic stress disorder symptoms: A moderated mediation approach. *Traumatology, 22*(2), 85–93.

Haehner, P., Pfeifer, L. S., Fassbender, I., & Luhmann, M. (2023). Are changes in the perception of major life events associated with changes in subjective well-being? *Journal of Research in Personality, 102*, 104321.

Hayes, A. M., Yasinski, C., Grasso, D., Ready, C. B., Alpert, E., McCauley, T., . . . Deblinger, E. (2017). Constructive and unproductive processing of traumatic experiences in trauma-focused cognitive-behavioral therapy for youth. *Behavior Therapy, 48*(2), 166–181.

Haynes, W. C., Van Tongeren, D. R., Aten, J., Davis, E. B., Davis, D. E., Hook, J. N., . . . Johnson, T. (2017). The meaning as a buffer hypothesis: Spiritual meaning attenuates the effect of disaster-related resource loss on posttraumatic stress. *Psychology of Religion and Spirituality, 9*(4), 446–453.

He, X. X., Wang, X. Q., Steger, M. F., Ji, L. J., Jing, K., Liu, M. F., & Ye, B. J. (2023). Meaning in life and psychological distress: A meta-analysis. *Journal of Research in Personality, 104*, 104381.

Hill, P. L., Sin, N. L., Almeida, D. M., & Burrow, A. L. (2022). Sense of purpose predicts daily positive events and attenuates their influence on positive affect. *Emotion, 22*(3), 597–602.

Hu, X., Cheng, S., & Lai, Y. (2022). Impact of religious involvement and religious commitment on post-pandemic well-being among Chinese university students. *Religious Education, 117*(3), 221–234.

Janoff-Bulman, R. (1992). *Shattered assumptions*. Simon & Schuster.

Kasser, T. (2016). Materialistic values and goals. *Annual Review of Psychology, 67*, 489–514.

Kilby, C. J., Sherman, K. A., & Wuthrich, V. (2018). Towards understanding interindividual differences in stressor appraisals: A systematic review. *Personality and Individual Differences, 135*, 92–100.

Kilpatrick, D. G., Resnick, H. S., Milanak, M. E., Miller, M. W., Keyes, K. M., & Friedman, M. J. (2013). National estimates of exposure to traumatic events and PTSD prevalence using DSM-IV and DSM-5 criteria. *Journal of Traumatic Stress, 26*(5), 537–547.

King, L. A., & Hicks, J. A. (2021). The science of meaning in life. *Annual Review of Psychology, 72*, 561–584.

Krause, N. (2007). Evaluating the stress-buffering function of meaning in life among older people. *Journal of Aging and Health, 19*(5), 792–812.

Ku, X., Lee, S. H., & Choi, I. (2023). Did COVID-19 really change our well-being?: It's up to meaning in life: Evidence from two longitudinal studies. *Social and Personality Psychology Compass*, e12799.

Lachnit, I., Park, C. L., & George, L. S. (2020). Processing and resolving major life stressors: An examination of meaning-making strategies. *Cognitive Therapy and Research, 44*, 1015–1024.

Lazarus, R. S., & Folkman, S. (1984). *Stress, appraisal, and coping*. Springer.

Lilly, M. M., Valdez, C. E., & Graham-Bermann, S. A. (2011). The mediating effect of world assumptions on the relationship between trauma exposure and depression. *Journal of Interpersonal Violence, 26*(12), 2499–2516.

Lowe, S. R., Manove, E. E., & Rhodes, J. E. (2013). Posttraumatic stress and posttraumatic growth among low-income mothers who survived Hurricane Katrina. *Journal of Consulting and Clinical Psychology, 81*(5), 877–889.

Ludwig, V. U., Crone, D. L., Clifton, J. D., Rebele, R. W., Schor, J. A., & Platt, M. L. (2023). Resilience of primal world beliefs to the initial shock of the COVID-19 pandemic. *Journal of Personality, 91*(3), 838–855.

McElroy-Heltzel, S. E., Davis, E. B., Davis, D. E., Aten, J. D., Van Tongeren, D. R., Hook, J. N., & Hwang, J. (2018). Benevolent theodicies protect against PTSD following a natural disaster. *Journal of Psychology and Christianity, 37*, 6–16.

Milman, E., Lee, S. A., Neimeyer, R. A., Mathis, A. A., & Jobe, M. C. (2020). Modeling pandemic depression and anxiety: The mediational role of core beliefs and meaning making. *Journal of Affective Disorders Reports, 2*, 100023.

Negri, A., Conte, F., Caldiroli, C. L., Neimeyer, R. A., & Castiglioni, M. (2023). Psychological factors explaining the COVID-19 pandemic impact on mental health: The role of meaning, beliefs, and perceptions of vulnerability and mortality. *Behavioral Sciences, 13*(2), 162.

Ostafin, B. D., & Proulx, T. (2020). Meaning in life and resilience to stressors. *Anxiety, Stress, and Coping, 33*(6), 603–622.

Park, C. L. (2010). Making sense of the meaning literature: An integrative review of meaning making and its effects on adjustment to stressful life events. *Psychological Bulletin, 136*(2), 257–301.

Park, C. L. (2017). Distinctions to promote an integrated perspective on meaning: Global meaning and meaning-making processes. *Journal of Constructivist Psychology, 30*(1), 14–19.

Park, C. L., Currier, J. M., Harris, J. I., & Slattery, J. M. (2017). *Trauma, meaning, and spirituality: Translating research into clinical practice*. American Psychological Association.

Park, C. L., & George, L. S. (2013). Assessing meaning and meaning making in the context of stressful life events: Measurement tools and approaches. *Journal of Positive Psychology, 8*, 483–504.

Park, C. L., Mills, M. A., & Edmondson, D. (2012). PTSD as meaning violation: Testing a cognitive worldview perspective. *Psychological Trauma: Theory, Research, Practice, and Policy, 4*(1), 66–73.

Park, C. L., Wilt, J., Russell, B. S., & Fendrich, M. (2023). Does perceived post-traumatic growth during the COVID-19 pandemic reflect actual positive changes? *Anxiety, Stress, and Coping, 36*(6), 661–673.

Poulin, M. J., & Silver, R. C. (2019). When are assumptions shaken?: A prospective, longitudinal investigation of negative life events and worldviews in a national sample. *Journal of Research in Personality, 83*, Article 103866.

Riepenhausen, A., Wackerhagen, C., Reppmann, Z. C., Deter, H. C., Kalisch, R., Veer, I. M., & Walter, H. (2022). Positive cognitive reappraisal in stress resilience, mental health, and well-being: A comprehensive systematic review. *Emotion Review, 14*(4), 310–331.

Rogers, J., Shane, J., von Keyserlingk, L., & Heckhausen, J. (2023). Changes in college students' socioeconomic status aspirations during the COVID-19 pandemic. *Social and Personality Psychology Compass, 17*(11), e12859.

Schleider, J. L., Woerner, J., Overstreet, C., Amstadter, A. B., & Sartor, C. E. (2021). Interpersonal trauma exposure and depression in young adults: Considering the role of world assumptions. *Journal of Interpersonal Violence, 36*(13–14), 6596–6620.

Schnell, T., & Krampe, H. (2020). Meaning in life and self-control buffer stress in times of COVID-19: Moderating and mediating effects with regard to mental distress. *Frontiers in Psychiatry, 11*, 983.

Schnell, T., & Krampe, H. (2022). Meaningfulness protects from and crisis of meaning exacerbates general mental distress longitudinally. *BMC Psychiatry, 22*(1), 1–9.

Schuler, E. R., & Boals, A. (2016). Shattering world assumptions: A prospective view of the impact of adverse events on world assumptions. *Psychological Trauma: Theory, Research, Practice, and Policy, 8*(3), 259–266.

Seidel, L. J., Daniels, J. K., & Ostafin, B. D. (2023). The role of meaning in life in psychological distress during the COVID-19 pandemic. *Anxiety, Stress, and Coping, 36*(1), 67–82.

Seol, J. H., Park, Y., Choi, J., & Sohn, Y. W. (2021). The mediating role of meaning in life in the effects of calling on posttraumatic stress symptoms and growth: A longitudinal study of navy soldiers deployed to the Gulf of Aden. *Frontiers in Psychology, 11,* 599109.

Sherman, A. C., Williams, M. L., Amick, B. C., Hudson, T. J., Messias, E. L., & Simonton-Atchley, S. (2022). Adjustment to the COVID-19 pandemic: Associations with global and situational meaning. *Current Psychology,* 1–16.

Sleight, A. G., Boyd, P., Klein, W. M., & Jensen, R. E. (2021). Spiritual peace and life meaning may buffer the effect of anxiety on physical well-being in newly diagnosed cancer survivors. *Psycho-Oncology, 30*(1), 52–58.

Smith, A. J., Abeyta, A. A., Hughes, M., & Jones, R. T. (2015). Persistent grief in the aftermath of mass violence: The predictive roles of posttraumatic stress symptoms, self-efficacy, and disrupted worldview. *Psychological Trauma: Theory, Research, Practice, and Policy, 7*(2), 179–186.

Tamir, M., Vishkin, A., & Gutentag, T. (2020). Emotion regulation is motivated. *Emotion, 20*(1), 115–119.

Wissing, M. P., Schutte, L., Liversage, C., Entwisle, B., Gericke, M., & Keyes, C. (2021). Important goals, meanings, and relationships in flourishing and languishing states: Towards patterns of well-being. *Applied Research in Quality of Life, 16*(2), 573–609.

Wu, M. S., Yan, X., Zhou, C., Chen, Y., Li, J., Zhu, Z., . . . Han, B. (2011). General belief in a just world and resilience: Evidence from a collectivistic culture. *European Journal of Personality, 25*(6), 431–442.

Yang, Z., Ji, L. J., Yang, Y., Wang, Y., Zhu, L., & Cai, H. (2021). Meaning making helps cope with COVID-19: A longitudinal study. *Personality and Individual Differences, 174,* 110670.

CHAPTER 51

The Search for Meaning

A Review of Research and Theory

Michael F. Steger *and* Dylan R. Marsh

"Why are we here?"
"What existed before everything?"
"Where did I come from, and how did I become me?"
"How should I use my lifetime?"

For many, questions like these open the door to the existential corridors of human experience. The balance of fear and exhilaration, of disorientation and exploration, of ease and perturbation that people may feel as they try on such questions intuitively feels important to the way they approach existential meaning. Some may feel enlivened by the bracing, endlessly receding bedrock of certainty at the bottom of these questions. Others may feel lost or diminished by the task of answering questions that have taunted the greatest thinkers for millennia. In the face of trauma or crisis, the search for meaning may occur in people who have never before questioned that their lives are meaningful. Some may latch on to the first answer that comes along while others may toil for years to win their certainty. Still others are bored and befuddled by the exercise, seeing no point in such idle foolishness. It seems likely that these variations should matter.

One characteristic of psychology's approach to existential matters has been to focus more on how settled people appear in their answers to these questions than on what it is like for them to try to answer them, voluntarily or not. At the broadest level, there is a robust set of literature tapping into the dynamics of wrestling with existential questions, such as research on trauma recovery, spirituality, religious quest, even identity formation. The construct of search for meaning is another way of seeking to understand the human confrontation with existential matters. The search for meaning is often contrasted with the finding of meaning, the presumed resolution of that search. Presence of meaning is one way of referring to the degree to which people find meaning in their lives (Steger et al., 2006). Where having meaning seems unassailably good for psychological functioning, is searching for meaning good, bad, or indifferent for individuals? Perhaps the field has overemphasized presence of meaning and neglected the search for it. Within the field of meaning-in-life research, the supposition that presence of meaning has been more researched was borne out by Li and colleagues' (2021) meta-analysis of the most widely used meaning-in-life measure, the Meaning in Life Questionnaire (MLQ; Steger et al., 2006; presence of meaning item: "I have a good sense of what makes my life meaningful"; search for meaning item: "I am always looking to find my life's purpose"). They found 441 effect sizes for presence of meaning and 285 for search for meaning. Still, nearly 300 effect sizes constitute a decent-sized literature, especially considering these effect sizes were generated for scholarship using just one questionnaire. This chapter reviews theoretical perspectives on the search for meaning, presents an overview of research, points out inconsistencies in the research record, and suggests future research that could help resolve some of these inconsistencies.

THE NATURE OF THE SEARCH FOR MEANING

There are a few questions to address regarding the search for meaning. The first, of course, is: What is it? Beyond that are questions around the relationship of searching and experiencing meaning, search for meaning and presence of meaning. The final consideration is whether the search for meaning tells us anything important about people.

The field of meaning in life is beset by a common problem in psychology. Namely, the ideas studied are familiar and common to most people. When people talk about searching for meaning, they can mean any number of things. Frankl (1946/1963) was the first to popularize the idea that searching for meaning was normal, perhaps even definingly human. Frankl discussed the *will to meaning* present in each of us. His writing centered the will to meaning as a primary motivational force, akin to how pleasure or social power might drive humans from the perspective of other psychodynamic theories of the mid-20th century. Maddi (1970) also felt that the search for meaning is a basic motivational impetus.

The will to meaning might be like the search for meaning, or it might be more like a need for meaning. This difference may seem subtle, but it implies different dispositions for the role search for meaning ought to play in well-being. If the will to meaning is a search for meaning, then searching for meaning is a natural human enterprise. Being in touch with and aware of one's fundamental motivational drives would be a good thing for well-being if it is so natural. Essentially, from this perspective, searching for meaning is just how humans are supposed to be. A survey question from this perspective might be read as "Are you in touch with your innate human interest in meaning?" Alternatively, the search for meaning could be natural in the same way that "east" is a natural way to orient. It exists in the natural world, and people can do with that knowledge what they want. In this view, searching for meaning is simply a cardinal direction in the compass of motivation. A survey question from this perspective might be, "Have you been thinking more or less about this thing out there called search for meaning?" However, if the will to meaning reflects a need for meaning, then the more pointedly humans feel that need, the more dire a deprivation of meaning would be. A survey question from this perspective might be, "Are you feeling deprived of meaning and in great need of it?" One could argue that from the start of this field, the search for meaning could be positive, neutral, or negative with regard to adjustment.

Defining the Search for Meaning

An often-used definition of *search for meaning* seemingly tries to bridge this gap. It defines the term as "the strength, intensity, and activity of people's desire and efforts *to establish and/or augment* their understanding of the meaning, significance, and purpose of their lives" (Steger et al., 2008a, p. 200). This definition puts people's search for meaning on a continuum. It suggests people may search for meaning when they have no meaning or when they want to add to the meaning they already have. If this definition is accurate then, again, search for meaning might be a net positive, neutral, or negative for people depending on whether it reflects a growth-oriented process of continually adding to meaning or, alternatively, emerges in the face of a troubling meaning deficit.

HOW ARE THE SEARCH FOR AND PRESENCE OF MEANING RELATED?

With this definition in hand, we have answered the first question—What is search for meaning?—and come to the second question. What is the relation between the two central existential concerns, the search for meaning and the presence of meaning? Steger and colleagues (2008a) called this the search-to-presence model, suggesting that searching may be necessary for finding meaning, at least for some. They also proposed a presence-to-search model wherein a lack of meaning sparks a search for it, indicating that searching is a sign of distress. Both of these models suggest the search for and presence of meaning are related somehow, with the implication that searching creates the finding. However, other research suggests that the presence of meaning may come from ambient features of the environment (Heintzelman et al., 2013) and passively develop. If meaning can develop from the predictability and consistency of key parts of the surrounding world, then it might be the case that the search for meaning is most often activated when these normal, passive modes of building meaning fail. That is, we might anticipate that most of the time, people who experience a lot of meaning will not search for meaning too frequently, and as a corollary, those who are searching for meaning may not feel they have enough of it. If all of this is correct, then from this background information, we might anticipate a moderate negative correlation between search for meaning and presence of meaning. This would allow for people who engage in search for meaning as part of living a meaningful life, as Frankl (1946/1963) and Maddi (1970) argued.

Theoretical Considerations and Models

Another implication of the idea that people might passively accrue meaning by living in a fairly predictable world is that meaning should not be gained only through heroic grappling with intractable ontological matters. Rather, it may be that for most people meaning is automatically perceived and usually abundantly available. Indeed, empirical work suggests that life is generally quite meaningful for most people (Heintzelman & King, 2014). This perspective would suggest that the conscious search for meaning is incited when a circumstance or event catalyzes an experience of meaninglessness, thus supporting Steger and colleagues' (2008a) proposed presence-to-search model. We suggest in a later section of this chapter that there is evidence to sustain the search-to-presence model as well, especially outside of individualistic cultures (and perhaps outside the United States specifically).

Other perspectives also propose people search for meaning when they encounter significant disruptions. For example, Thompson and Janigan (1988) posited that when negative life events impugn one's sense of the world as comprehensible and one's own life as purposeful, the search for meaning ensues. This search serves as a mechanism through which one seeks to reestablish one's sense of one's life scheme or story as meaningful. Steger and colleagues (2006) framed this dynamic in terms of sources of meaning: "We discussed three possible explanations: that people might seek to add to their current sources of meaning, that they might want a deeper understanding of that which already makes their lives feel meaningful, and that they might seek new sources of meaning as existing ones fluctuate in significance" (p. 89). It is the last possibility, perhaps understated as sources of meaning fluctuating, that is understandable in the context of accommodating trauma or other negative life events. Negative life events might take away one's sources of meaning, precious parts one's of life, such as one's career or relationships (Schnell, 2009; Steger et al., 2013, 2014).

Other perspectives might propose that those sources of meaning function because they are constant, helping one maintain a sense of life's meaningfulness in a world that is constantly in flux. The meaning maintenance model (MMM; Heine et al., 2006) argues that while people are automatically detecting, making, and deriving meaning throughout their lives, "humans find it problematic to be correspondingly robbed of meaning, or otherwise confronted with meaninglessness, and therefore seek to reconstruct a sense of meaning" (p. 90). In such cases, MMM suggests that individuals may look to find meaning in areas outside of the framework being threatened by their present circumstance, often entrenching further in standpoints that uphold a framework that provides subjective meaning. Within the MMM, the "search for meaning" is an automatic (not effortful) process, captured in the flexible attachment to alternative meaning sources as other sources become unavailable or are rendered inadequate.

The meaning-making model (Park & Folkman, 1997) provides another example of a framework that assumes meaning is usually unconsciously and constantly detected but search for meaning occurs in the context of distressing events. Though this model was primarily focused on resolving discrepancies between appraised meaning of situations and one's global meaning framework, later iterations of the model accounted for the role of subjective sense of meaning in life (e.g., Park, 2010). Indeed, Park (2013) noted that in the context of the meaninglessness associated with experiencing a traumatic event that catalyzes a search for meaning via the meaning-making process, one possible outcome is the restoration of one's own sense of overall meaning in life. In this way, presence of meaning in life is positioned as an outcome of meaning making, which is supported by empirical evidence (Fitzke et al., 2021; Jim et al., 2006; Park et al., 2008).

Research on the Relation of Search for and Presence of Meaning

There is by now quite a lot of research on the relation between the search for and presence of meaning. As noted above, Li and colleagues (2021) found hundreds of effect sizes for the two scales of the MLQ (Steger et al., 2006). Other ways of assessing search for meaning exist (e.g., Crumbaugh, 1977), or can be approximated (e.g., World Values Survey item "How often if at all do you think about the meaning and purpose of life?" as in Lin, 2019), or there are related ideas, such as crisis of meaning (Schnell, 2009). Nevertheless, the MLQ is used most often. This reliance on the MLQ presents a bit of a conundrum because the scale was developed using confirmatory factor analysis, which optimized distinctiveness of the search for meaning and the presence of meaning subscales. The items that made presence of meaning and search for meaning more different from each other were statistically favored. The advantage of this method is that it yields a psychometrically robust scale and allows for examination of how presence of meaning and search for meaning may interact to reveal different dynamics for meaning seekers at high and low levels of presence of meaning. However, it might be the case that using other methods would reveal stronger or different correlations.

The first pair of measures used to examine the relation of search for meaning and presence of meaning was created by Crumbaugh: the Purpose in Life Test (PIL; Crumbaugh & Maholick, 1964) and the Seeking of Noetic Goals Test (SONG; Crumbaugh, 1977). Crumbaugh (1977) found negative correlations between the PIL and SONG ranging from −0.27 to −0.52 in samples of methadone patients and seminary students among others. These are medium to large effect sizes, roughly equivalent in magnitude to the correlations of the MLQ presence of meaning scale with depression (−0.48), love (0.40), sadness (−0.35), or life satisfaction (0.46; Steger et al., 2006). In contrast, in the original validation of the MLQ (Steger et al., 2006), the reported correlations between search for meaning and presence of meaning ranged from −0.09 to −0.30 across samples. There is some overlap in the correlations reported in Crumbaugh's work and the MLQ's initial results, but later research suggests the negative correlation between the MLQ subscales is small to modest, overall (Abeyta & Routledge, 2018; Dakin et al., 2021; Silva et al., 2024).

There are three major trends that have emerged in research on this association that suggest deeper complexity to the search for meaning and its relation to the presence of meaning. Taken together, they suggest that the experience of searching for meaning differs in its relation to the presence of meaning, depending on who is doing the searching, where, and when. Culture and age appear to moderate the relation between search for meaning and presence of meaning. Further, presence of meaning appears to moderate the relation between search for meaning and other variables. This latter idea was initially proposed by Steger and colleagues (2006), who argued that the MLQ would make it "possible to identify those who feel great meaningfulness yet still seek to further their understanding of life's meaning and compare them with those who feel their life is meaningful and are not engaged in any further search for meaning" (p. 89). Although their focus was entirely on the high presence of meaning end of the spectrum, presumably there might be differences in those who are not searching for meaning who feel their lives are meaningless and those who feel their lives are very meaningful. The former would seem not to care about meaning, and the latter might be happy with the meaning they already have. Steger and colleagues mapped these four combinations onto identity formation, proposing that high presence of meaning coupled with high search for meaning corresponded with identity achievement, positioning that combination to reflect mature psychological functioning.

Interaction of Search for and Presence of Meaning

As noted above, an advantage of the MLQ (and the generally small negative correlation between its subscales) is that it allows for the examination of these interactions between these experiences. That interaction has been tested across a range of variables, such as relatedness, autonomy, rumination, openness to experience, behavioral inhibition and behavioral activation, and life satisfaction (Steger et al., 2008a, 2011). People high in both presence of and search for meaning appear just as well functioning as those high in presence but low in search. Several of these moderation effects have been tested and replicated by independent researchers (Park et al., 2010) and extended to other variables, such as anxiety and depression (Fischer et al., 2021), health anxiety (Yek et al., 2017), and struggle with meaning (Wilt et al., 2018). Generally, research has suggested that at high levels of the presence of meaning, searching is less indicative of poor functioning. In contrast, when searching for meaning occurs in the context of low presence, subjective experience is worse.

For example, research among Belgian pain patients sorted people into five types based on the combination of their search for meaning and presence of meaning scores on the MLQ. The high presence/high search for meaning type showed similar patterns of relations with subjective pain as the high presence/low search for meaning type, with lower pain reported by these types than the others (Dezutter et al., 2015). A second typological study of Belgian prisoners also showed that while the low presence/high search for meaning group had suffered the highest levels of physical abuse during childhood, the high presence/high search and the high presence/low search for meaning types were again very similar, showing lower distress, higher benevolence, and more care for others than the other types (Vanhooren et al., 2016). Taken together, these two studies show that searching for meaning at high levels of experienced meaning may be a companion rather than obstacle to well-being. In contrast, when presence of meaning is low, searching may emerge to resolve that deficit.

Interaction of Search for Meaning and Culture

In keeping with the above review, generally search for meaning has been linked weakly to poorer well-being. In their meta-analysis, Li and colleagues (2021) sought to determine the effect size of the correlations between the search for meaning and the presence of meaning with subjective well-being. At the broadest level, they found search for meaning to have a small negative association with subjective well-being ($ES_z = -0.121$). At a more granular level, search for meaning showed a significant negative association with life satisfaction and a significant positive association with negative affect, while displaying nonsignificant relationships with positive affect and domain-specific satisfaction. Still, Li and colleagues identified nuances in the search for meaning and subjective well-being relationship, such as the moderating influence of the extent to which one's culture is individualistic or collectivistic. Notably, they concluded that search for meaning may be positively associated with subjective well-being for those in highly collectivistic cultures.

This meta-analysis supports work by Steger and colleagues (Steger, Kawabata, et al., 2008) showing that search for meaning was positively related to presence of meaning in Japan but negatively related to it in the United States. Search for meaning and presence of meaning are also positively correlated in Poland (Borawski et al., 2022), China (Chang et al., 2021; Chu & Fung, 2021), Israel (Abu-Raiya et al., 2021), and South

Korea (Lim et al., 2022). Research using the World Values Survey item noted above as a proxy for searching for meaning found that the more collectivistic a culture is, the more positive was the relation of thinking about meaning with well-being indicators such as happiness, life satisfaction, and subjective health (Lin & Chan, 2021). Thus, collectivism is an important dimension to consider alongside search for meaning. It may be that feeling a more expansive connection to others provides support and structure for search for meaning. For example, in a sample of adolescents from Hong Kong, where search for meaning and life satisfaction are positively related, this relationship was stronger among those lower in loneliness (To, 2016). Such results challenge the notion that search for meaning is fundamentally about solving a problem. Rather, it may reflect better functioning, in collectivist contexts. The notion that collectivist cultures may provide a more salubrious context for the search for meaning is suggested in research showing that among Chinese adolescents, search for meaning predicted higher parent–child cohesion and filial piety (Sun et al., 2023).

Interaction with Age

Age is generally negatively related to searching for meaning (Li et al., 2021; Steger et al., 2008a). This negative relation has been found in a variety of samples, including in Spain (Baños et al., 2023), Israel (Bodner et al., 2023), and Turkey (Dakin et al., 2021). Older adults are less likely than younger ones to be engaged in searching for meaning in their lives, which fits with the developmental tasks of these age groups. The trajectory of search for meaning declining over the lifespan tracks the suggestion that meaning in life is related to identity formation (Steger et al., 2006). However, there are some intriguing suggestions that the downward slope of search for meaning across the lifespan might be scalloped, with predictable spikes. Research using an MTurk sample found that people were more likely to search for meaning when entering a new decade, such as at age 29 or 79 (Alter & Hershfield, 2014). This research suggests as well that not only negative or traumatic events spur a search for meaning but also personal landmarks in the lifespan.

Importantly, age also moderates the relation between search for meaning and well-being (Li et al., 2021). Essentially, the negative correlation of search for meaning with well-being and the positive correlation of search for meaning with distress are strengthened in older age groups (Steger et al., 2009). Tying such findings, once again, to the developmental tasks of adulthood suggests that searching for meaning when it is nonnormative for one's age group may reflect a more negative general experience of aging.

THE SEARCH FOR MEANING: A DETRIMENT OR ASSET TO WELL-BEING?

The search for meaning shares a weak correlation with well-being and when Li and colleagues (2021) corrected for publication bias, that weak correlation became even weaker ($ES_z = -0.07$). Thus, the search for meaning may be irrelevant to well-being. The moderator effects reviewed above suggest one reason for this tiny effect—that the search for meaning may unfold differently in different people. Nevertheless, regarding variables relevant to well-being, mental health, and psychopathology, search for meaning has displayed some associations that suggest detrimental aspects to seeking meaning. At the zero-order correlational level in U.S. samples, search for meaning related to higher levels of depression, negative affect, health anxiety, overall anxiety, and rumination (Park et al., 2010; Steger et al., 2006, 2008a, 2008b; Yek et al., 2017). These studies have also found that search for meaning had negative correlations with life satisfaction, positive affect, and subjective happiness. Search for meaning has even been linked to addictive social media use and higher state/trait fear of missing out in a study of 1,152 Germans (Montag et al., 2023).

However, findings showing search for meaning to have deleterious associations may not tell the whole story. To the extent that the search for meaning is propelled by negative circumstances or low feelings of the presence of meaning, these relations may confound a way of coping with such experiences with the distress they cause. Indeed, the search for meaning may have beneficial impacts as well. Identifying these positive impacts may require attention to contexts, life events, and the motivations for seeking meaning. For example, Dursun and colleagues (2016) conducted hierarchical linear regression using data from a sample of 57 survivors of the 2013 Colorado floods to predict posttraumatic growth from several possible antecedents. They found that search for meaning and perceived social support were both *positive* predictors of posttraumatic growth even controlling for posttraumatic stress, gender, and religious status. Such results suggest that the search for meaning in a specific traumatic context can lead to personal growth.

Even in the absence of trauma, searching for meaning can have well-being benefits, when considered in the context of the presence of meaning in life. This point is driven home by within-person analyses conducted on data collected from 254 undergraduate students in the United States (Newman et al., 2018). Daily experiences of search for meaning positively predicted daily well-being through the mediating variable of daily presence of meaning. Such results suggest that when the searching for meaning supports the presence of meaning, it has a (positive) role to play in well-being.

Search for meaning may also be a concomitant of a suite of positive characteristics. For example, Steger and colleagues (2008a) found that search for meaning related to greater trait-level curiosity and openness to experience as well as higher investigative and artistic interests. Their study also showed that search for meaning predicted lower dogmatism and harm-avoidance orientation. In two experiments, Carney and Robertson (2018) found that those higher in search for meaning showed a greater appreciation for literature. These conclusions coincide with Thapa and colleagues' (2023) findings that elucidated search for meaning's connection to reflection inspired by artistic matters, socialization germane to art, and acquisition of skills derived through artistic endeavors. Furthermore, a study of 247 participants from New Zealand found search for meaning to be positively associated with personal growth as a source of meaning (Grouden & Jose, 2015). Taken together, these findings suggest that those high in search for meaning may have a propensity to engage with the world in an inquisitive, open, artistic, and growth-oriented manner.

Searching for meaning may also have social benefits, reflecting a tendency to engage warmly with others. For instance, search for meaning relates negatively to the dark triad trait of psychopathy (Shi et al., 2022). Moreover, research links the search for meaning to costly prosocial behavior. Across five studies, Dakin and colleagues (2021) found that search for meaning predicted greater endorsement of motivation to pursue prosocial action and engagement in prosocial behavior, even if such behavior was detrimental to one's own well-being. Such results cast the negative relation between the search for meaning and well-being in a different light, suggesting that sacrificing personal happiness for others may be a way to satisfy the search for meaning.

Moreover, Dakin and colleagues (2021) compared the search for meaning to the pursuit of happiness and found that pursuing happiness showed no such association with altruistic intention or behavior at the cost of one's own well-being. Based on these results, Dakin and colleagues concluded that meaning seeking, although negatively related to personal well-being, may include "the will to improve the well-being of others" (p. 19). This assertion is supported by research linking the search for meaning to higher levels of civil engagement in the forms of pro-environmental and political engagement (Lin, 2019). Indeed, there may be many positive aspects related to search for meaning—being open, inquisitive, growth-oriented, civically engaged, and altruistic are all desirable characteristics. Nevertheless, these positive features may come at a cost of some degree of subjective well-being, unless other conditions are met (e.g., already having a high presence of meaning, belonging to a collectivistic culture).

PRACTICAL IMPLICATIONS

Numerous scholars have suggested that search for meaning may sometimes be a pleasant and positive experience and, in other cases, an unpleasant and negative experience for individuals. These experiences can be thought of as a relatively healthy search for meaning versus a more dysfunctional one. For example, Steger and colleagues (2008a) posited that "a healthy search is usually depicted as grounded in people's aspirations and insights they derive from engaging life's challenges . . . a dysfunctional search is usually said to be marked by people's inability to engage with and resolve negative or challenging experiences" (p. 203). Similarly, Wong (2019) delineated two kinds of search for meaning. He asserted that the search for meaning could be bifurcated into the two constructs of positively oriented search for meaning and negatively oriented search for meaning. Positively oriented search for meaning is characterized by focusing on a positive future with a primary function of engendering flourishing and making a positive impact. Negatively oriented search for meaning is conceived by Wong to be focused on past or present problems as a reaction to suffering that is rooted in desire to survive or overcome. Such claims are supported by the mixed nature of the findings reviewed above, showing search for meaning's potential to be beneficial or detrimental depending on circumstantial factors. The potential role of traumatic life events in spurring the search for meaning adds yet another layer of complexity to these two ways of searching for meaning. In large part these different orientations to the search for meaning implicate the motivation for that search.

The abovementioned considerations raise questions about the possibility of measuring the positive and negative kinds of search for meaning as separate constructs or dimensions. Indeed, the substantially greater theoretical and empirical attention paid to the construct of presence of meaning relative to that of search for meaning has coincided with a renaissance in operationalization and assessment of presence of meaning. Specifically, most contemporary scholars have come to understand presence of meaning through a tripartite model with dimensions of coherence/comprehension, purpose, and significance/mattering (George & Park, 2016; Martela & Steger, 2016). Correspondingly, more advanced psychometric instruments like the Three-Dimensional Meaning in Life Scale (Martela & Steger, 2023) and Multidimensional Existential Meaning Scale (George & Park, 2017) account for these modern conceptualizations through their factor structure. Nevertheless, the often-acknowledged supposition that search for meaning may be better understood as being composed of two kinds of experience, one healthy and one dysfunctional, has not been reflected through the development of more precise measures for search for meaning.

In addition, scholars have long recognized the distinction between global assessments of the presence meaning (in life) and more situational meanings ascribed to discrete life events (King & Hicks, 2021). The search for meaning may require a similar recognition. To the extent that extraneous circumstances, such as unexpected illness, loss, and so forth, may spur a search for meaning in those events, scholarship on the search for meaning may benefit from considering whether the global search for meaning differs from the pursuit of meaning in circumscribed events that have similar well-being consequences.

It is possible that the often confounding nature of search for meaning's set of relationships with other variables would be better explained through more precise measures of orientations to the search for meaning and context of that search. The development of such psychometric instruments remains an area of need for future research to address.

FUTURE RESEARCH AND CONCLUSION

What, exactly, is packed under the term *search for meaning*? What are we trying to understand, and why are we so far falling short? It is clear from voluminous research that having meaning and seeking meaning are distinct. It is also clear that whereas having meaning is a nearly universally indicator of well-being and flourishing, the search for meaning is sometimes a positive indicator, sometimes a negative indicator, and most often a nonindicator of well-being. The most exciting findings regarding the search for meaning would seem to be the array of variables that interact with search for meaning to moderate its relations with other variables. This suggests an underlying typology that is teased out by these moderators. There are some healthy versions of search for meaning that co-occur with high levels of the presence of meaning. There are positive versions of search for meaning that manifest in collectivistic cultures. There is the trend for search for meaning to be more common and less distressing in youth than in later life. The search for meaning in the context of trauma may promote personal growth through difficult times. The way that search for meaning has been measured thus far seems to require the consideration of additional variables, including the presence of meaning, collectivism, or age, for example. The most common measure, the MLQ, simply asks people if they are searching, not why, how, or how well. Steger and colleagues' (2008a) definition of search for meaning embraces possible differences, but it is up to future research to discover how to coax them into being. Ambitious longitudinal research incorporating a range of dispositions that may predispose people to search for meaning (e.g., rumination but also openness to experience) and track the search and presence of meaning as dynamic experiences in conjunction with life events is required for a comprehensive understanding of this crucial existential quest.

REFERENCES

Abeyta, A. A., & Routledge, C. (2018). The need for meaning and religiosity: An individual differences approach to assessing existential needs and the relation with religious commitment, beliefs, and experiences. *Personality and Individual Differences, 123,* 6–13.

Abu-Raiya, H., Sasson, T., & Russo-Netzer, P. (2021). Presence of meaning, search for meaning, religiousness, satisfaction with life and depressive symptoms among a diverse Israeli sample. *International Journal of Psychology, 56*(2), 276–285.

Alter, A. L., & Hershfield, H. E. (2014). People search for meaning when they approach a new decade in chronological age. *Proceedings of the National Academy of Sciences, 111*(48), 17066–17070.

Baños, R. M., Desdentado, L., Vara, M. D., Escrivá-Martínez, T., Herrero, R., Miragall, M., & Tomás, J. M. (2023). How the COVID-19 pandemic and its consequences affect the presence of and search for meaning of life: A longitudinal study. *Journal of Happiness Studies, 24*(1), 17–33.

Bodner, E., Bergman, Y. S., Shiloh-Levin, S., & Hoffman, Y. S. G. (2023). The interactive effect of aging anxiety and age awareness on meaning in life and psychological distress: A moderated mediation model. *Current Psychology, 42*(10), 8255–8264.

Borawski, D., Nowak, A., & Zakrzewska, A. (2022). Lonely meaning-seekers: The moderating role of search for meaning in the relationship between loneliness and presence of meaning. *Personality and Individual Differences, 190,* 111550.

Carney, J., & Robertson, C. (2018). People searching for meaning in their lives find literature more engaging. *Review of General Psychology, 22*(2), 199–209.

Chang, B., Cheng, J., Fang, J., & Dang, J. (2021). The indirect effect of death anxiety on experienced meaning in life via search for meaning and prosocial behavior. *Frontiers in Psychology, 12.*

Chu, S. T.-W., & Fung, H. H.-L. (2021). Is the search for meaning related to the presence of meaning?: Moderators of the longitudinal relationship. *Journal of Happiness Studies, 22*(1), 127–145.

Crumbaugh, J. C. (1977). The Seeking of Noetic Goals Test (SONG): A complementary scale to the Purpose in Life Test (PIL). *Journal of Clinical Psychology, 33*(3), 900–907.

Crumbaugh, J. C., & Maholick, L. T. (1964). An experimental study in existentialism: The psychometric approach to Frankl's concept of noogenic neurosis. *Journal of Clinical Psychology, 20*(2), 200–207.

Dakin, B. C., Laham, S. M., Tan, N. P.-J., & Brock, B. (2021). Searching for meaning is associated with costly prosociality. *PLOS One, 16*(10), e0258769.

Dezutter, J., Luyckx, K., & Wachholtz, A. (2015). Meaning in life in chronic pain patients over time: Associations with pain experience and psychological well-being. *Journal of Behavioral Medicine, 38*(2), 384–396.

Dursun, P., Steger, M. F., Bentele, C., & Schulenberg, S. E. (2016). Meaning and posttraumatic growth among survivors of the September 2013 Colorado floods. *Journal of Clinical Psychology, 72*(12), 1247–1263.

Fischer, I. C., Secinti, E., Cemalcilar, Z., & Rand, K. L. (2021). Examining cross-cultural relationships between meaning in life and psychological well-being in Turkey and the United States. *Journal of Happiness Studies, 22*(3), 1341–1358.

Fitzke, R. E., Marsh, D. R., & Prince, M. A. (2021). A longitudinal investigation of the meaning-making model in midlife adults who have experienced trauma. *Journal of Clinical Psychology, 77*(12), 2878–2893.

Frankl, V. E. (1963). *Man's search for meaning* (mini book ed.). Beacon Press. (Original work published 1946)

George, L. S., & Park, C. L. (2016). Meaning in life as comprehension, purpose, and mattering: Toward integration and new research questions. *Review of General Psychology, 20*(3), 205–220.

George, L. S., & Park, C. L. (2017). The Multidimensional Existential Meaning Scale: A tripartite approach to measuring meaning in life. *Journal of Positive Psychology, 12*(6), 613–627.

Grouden, M. E., & Jose, P. E. (2015). Do sources of meaning differentially predict search for meaning, presence of meaning, and well-being. *International Journal of Well-being, 5*(1), Article 1.

Heine, S. J., Proulx, T., & Vohs, K. D. (2006). The meaning maintenance model: On the coherence of social motivations. *Personality and Social Psychology Review, 10*(2), 88–110.

Heintzelman, S. J., & King, L. A. (2014). Life is pretty meaningful. *American Psychologist, 69*(6), 561–574.

Heintzelman, S. J., Trent, J., & King, L. A. (2013). Encounters with objective coherence and the experience of meaning in life. *Psychological Science, 24*(6), 991–998.

Jim, H. S., Richardson, S. A., Golden-Kreutz, D. M., & Andersen, B. L. (2006). Strategies used in coping with a cancer diagnosis predict meaning in life for survivors. *Health Psychology, 25*(6), 753–761.

King, L. A., & Hicks, J. A. (2021). The science of meaning in life. *Annual Review of Psychology, 72,* 561–584.

Li, J.-B., Dou, K., & Liang, Y. (2021). The relationship between presence of meaning, search for meaning, and subjective well-being: A three-level meta-analysis based on the Meaning in Life Questionnaire. *Journal of Happiness Studies, 22*(1), 467–489.

Lim, J. I., Yu, J., & Sohn, Y. W. (2022). How does search for meaning lead to presence of meaning for Korean army soldiers?: The mediating roles of leisure crafting and gratitude. *Frontiers in Psychology, 12,* 766798.

Lin, L. (2019). Is searching for meaning in life related to civic engagement?: Individual- and society-level moderators. *Frontiers in Psychology, 10,* 1334.

Lin, L., & Chan, H.-W. (2021). When is search for meaning in life beneficial for well-being?: A cross-national study. *International Journal of Psychology, 56*(1), 75–84.

Maddi, S. R. (1970). The search for meaning. In W. J. Arnold & M. M. Page (Eds.), *The Nebraska Symposium on Motivation* (pp. 134–183). University of Nebraska Press.

Martela, F., & Steger, M. F. (2016). The three meanings of meaning in life: Distinguishing coherence, purpose, and significance. *Journal of Positive Psychology, 11*(5), 531–545.

Martela, F., & Steger, M. F. (2023). The role of significance relative to the other dimensions of meaning in life—An examination utilizing the three dimensional meaning in life scale (3DM). *Journal of Positive Psychology, 18*(4), 606–626.

Montag, C., Müller, M., Pontes, H. M., & Elhai, J. D. (2023). On fear of missing out, social networks use disorder tendencies and meaning in life. *BMC Psychology, 11*(1), 358.

Newman, D. B., Nezlek, J. B., & Thrash, T. M. (2018). The dynamics of searching for meaning and presence of meaning in daily life. *Journal of Personality, 86*(3), 368–379.

Park, C. L. (2010). Making sense of the meaning literature: An integrative review of meaning making and its effects on adjustment to stressful life events. *Psychological Bulletin, 136*(2), 257–301.

Park, C. L. (2013). Trauma and meaning making: Converging conceptualizations and emerging evidence. In J. A. Hicks & C. Routledge (Eds.), *The experience of meaning in life* (pp. 61–76). Springer.

Park, C. L., & Folkman, S. (1997). Meaning in the context of stress and coping. *Review of General Psychology, 1*(2), 115–144.

Park, C. L., Malone, M. R., Suresh, D. P., Bliss, D., & Rosen, R. I. (2008). Coping, meaning in life, and quality of life in congestive heart failure patients. *Quality of Life Research, 17*(1), 21–26.

Park, N., Park, M., & Peterson, C. (2010). When is the search for meaning related to life satisfaction? *Applied Psychology: Health and Well-Being, 2*(1), 1–13.

Schnell, T. (2009). The Sources of Meaning and Meaning in Life Questionnaire (SoMe): Relations to demographics and well-being. *Journal of Positive Psychology, 4*(6), 483–499.

Shi, L., Sun, S., Zhu, X., & Geng, Y. (2022). Meaning in life as a mediator of dark triad with confidence in treatment and subjective evaluation of treatment outcome among male drug abstainers. *Frontiers in Psychiatry, 13,* 928101.

Silva, W. A. D., Alves, G. B. S., & Loureto, G. D. L. (2024). Personality and purpose of life: The moderating role of existential emptiness in the link of ontological perception of time and search for meaning in life. *Current Psychology, 43*(16), 14400–14410.

Steger, M. F., Frazier, P., Oishi, S., & Kaler, M. (2006). The meaning in life questionnaire: Assessing the presence of and search for meaning in life. *Journal of Counseling Psychology, 53*(1), 80–93.

Steger, M. F., Kashdan, T. B., Sullivan, B. A., & Lorentz, D. (2008a). Understanding the search for meaning in life: Personality, cognitive style, and the dynamic between seeking and experiencing meaning. *Journal of Personality, 76*(2), 199–228.

Steger, M. F., Kawabata, Y., Shimai, S., & Otake, K. (2008b). The meaningful life in Japan and the United States: Levels and correlates of meaning in life. *Journal of Research in Personality, 42*(3), 660–678.

Steger, M. F., Oishi, S., & Kashdan, T. B. (2009). Meaning in life across the life span: Levels and correlates of meaning in life from emerging adulthood to older adulthood. *Journal of Positive Psychology, 4*(1), 43–52.

Steger, M. F., Oishi, S., & Kesebir, S. (2011). Is a life without meaning satisfying?: The moderating role of the search for meaning in satisfaction with life judgments. *Journal of Positive Psychology, 6*(3), 173–180.

Steger, M. F., Shim, Y., Barenz, J., & Shin, J. Y. (2014). Through the windows of the soul: A pilot study using photography to enhance meaning in life. *Journal of Contextual Behavioral Science, 3*(1), 27–30.

Steger, M. F., Shim, Y., Rush, B. R., Brueske, L. A., Shin, J. Y., & Merriman, L. A. (2013). The mind's eye: A photographic method for understanding meaning in people's lives. *Journal of Positive Psychology, 8*(6), 530–542.

Sun, P., Yang, Z., Jiang, H., Chen, W., & Xu, M. (2023). Filial piety and meaning in life among late adolescents: A moderated mediation model. *Children and Youth Services Review, 147,* 106837.

Thapa, S., Vaziri, H., Shim, Y., Tay, L., & Pawelski, J. O. (2023). Development and validation of the Mechanisms of Engagement in the Arts and Humanities scales. *Psychology of Aesthetics, Creativity, and the Arts.*

Thompson, S. C., & Janigian, A. S. (1988). Life schemes: A framework for understanding the search for meaning. *Journal of Social and Clinical Psychology, 7*(2–3), 260–280.

To, S. (2016). Loneliness, the search for meaning, and the psychological well-being of economically disadvantaged Chinese adolescents living in Hong Kong: Implications for life skills development programs. *Children and Youth Services Review, 71,* 52–60.

Vanhooren, S., Leijssen, M., & Dezutter, J. (2016). Profiles of meaning and search for meaning among prisoners. *The Journal of Positive Psychology, 11*(6), 622–633.

Wilt, J. A., Stauner, N., Lindberg, M. J., Grubbs, J. B., Exline, J. J., & Pargament, K. I. (2018). Struggle with ultimate meaning: Nuanced associations with search for meaning, presence of meaning, and mental health. *Journal of Positive Psychology, 13*(3), 240–251.

Wong, P. T. P. (2019, November 6). *A two-factor model of search for meaning.* www.drpaulwong.com/a-two-factor-model-of-search-for-meaning.

Yek, M. H., Olendzki, N., Kekecs, Z., Patterson, V., & Elkins, G. (2017). Presence of meaning in life and search for meaning in life and relationship to health anxiety. *Psychological Reports, 120*(3), 383–390.

SECTION VII
RELIGION AND SPIRITUALITY

CHAPTER 52

Death Awareness and Religious Faith

Kenneth E. Vail III, Madhwa S. Galgali, Ashley D. Seeling, *and* Caroline C. Lapish

Not long after the anatomically modern humans emerged, some 300,000 years ago, they began leaving behind evidence of two important mental and social developments. First, evidence of ritualistic burials indicates they had begun thinking about death in more psychologically abstract ways, which some have characterized as "the birth of metaphysical anguish" (Culotta, 2009). For example, nearly 100,000 years ago, the graves at Qafzeh cave in the Jezreel Valley of Galilee, just south of Nazareth, were carved out of the bedrock and the bodies were buried with arms folded across the chest, alongside ochre-painted seashells, deer horns, and other symbolic offerings (Vandermeersch & Bar-Yosef, 2019). Second, modern humans' oldest surviving artistic depictions indicate a corresponding development of spiritual beliefs, focused on the triumph of life over death. Two of humankind's oldest sculptures—40,000-year old mammoth ivory carvings, found in the caves of Germany's Swabian Jura—are the Lowenmensch (Lion-Man) of Hohlenstein-Stadel and the Venus of Hohle-Fels (Conard, 2003, 2009). The Lion-Man is thought to reflect local shamanic spiritual practices regarding predator and prey in the European ice age (Conard, 2003), and the Venus figurine is thought to represent a fertility goddess symbolizing "the hope for survival and longevity" (Dixson & Dixson, 2012, p. 1).

Flash forward several dozen millennia, and humans still retain this inclination toward religion and spirituality. Pew Research Center data from 2015 suggests over 85% of the 7 billion people on Earth are religious in some way, with those proportions projected to remain relatively stable at least through 2060 even as the world's population is projected to climb to nearly 10 billion (Pew Research Center, 2017b). Various theories have attempted to explain why religious beliefs have remained such a fundamental feature of human psychology and culture. Some accounts view religion as justifying existing social hierarchies and dealing with feelings of societal alienation (Jost et al., 2014; Marx, 1843), or explaining seemingly inexplicable natural phenomena and shielding people from their own destructive instincts (Freud, 1927/1961), or providing a sense of interpersonal attachment security with presumed spiritual agents (Cherniak et al., 2021). Others argue religious beliefs are merely a by-product of evolutionarily adaptive cognitive mechanisms (Bering, 2011; Boyer, 2001; Tremlin, 2006), such as when the adaptive ability to attribute activity (e.g., flying spears) to natural world agents (e.g., warriors) also leads people to "see faces in the clouds" and attribute activity (e.g., bolts of lightning) to supernatural agents (e.g., Zeus). Still others argue that religion primarily serves to bind people together into faith communities (Durkheim, 1915; Graham & Haidt, 2010), and that cultural evolutionary pressures led to the flourishing of religious ideas that effectively promoted large-scale cooperation among groups (Norenzayan et al., 2016).

Though such theories offer valuable insights, they do little to explain, for example, why some of the earliest traces of human activity reflect both "the birth of metaphysical anguish" and spiritual ideas focused on the "hope for survival and longevity." The present chapter, however, offers an existential psychological perspective that can explain these—arguing that the awareness of the abstract concept of mortality is what, at least in part, motivates people to believe in eternal spiritual realms inhabited by immortal souls and gods. First, we introduce terror management theory (TMT: Greenberg et al., 1986; Vail et al., 2019) and research on the relationship between death awareness and faith in core religious/spiritual concepts such as afterlife, souls, and gods. Then, we discuss research on the implications for religious worldview defense and explore the variations of religious orientations. In doing so, we explain *why* people are motivated to religious faith, *what* the social consequences are, *who* is impacted by that motivation, and *how* the various orientations shape the motivation to believe.

EXISTENTIAL CONCERN AND FAITH IN RELIGIOUS CONCEPTS

> So far as the unconscious is the result of countless existential experiences, it cannot but resemble the various religious universes. For religion is the paradigmatic solution for every existential crisis. It is the paradigmatic solution not only because it can be indefinitely repeated, but also because it is believed to have a transcendental origin and hence is valorized as a revelation received from an *other*, transhuman world. The religious solution not only resolves the crisis but at the same time makes existence "open" to values that are no longer contingent or particular, thus enabling man to transcend personal situations and, finally, gain access to the world of spirit.
>
> —Mircea Eliade, *The Sacred and the Profane* (1957, p. 210)

A zebra in one moment, fearing for its life, instinctively evades a pouncing lion; and an Adelaide penguin busily searches the shore for a perfectly smooth pebble to woo its mate. Owing to similar evolutionary pressures as these animals, or others, humans similarly adapted to survive and reproduce. However, unlike the zebra or the penguin, human adaptations also led to the particularly sophisticated cognitive capacities for reflective, symbolic, and temporal thought about people's social world (Evans, 2013; Gallup & Anderson, 2020; Skowronski & Sedikides, 2019). Importantly, that adaptation to understand the past, organize in the present, and plan for the future, also introduced a new layer of existential concern: the concept of mortality. Thus, in contrast to the zebra serenely grazing on the grassy plains or the penguin peacefully warming its rocky nest, the human can psychologically defy the relative health and safety of their living room, office job, or date night at the movies, by pondering their impending doom.

Though, because the abstract concept of mortality does not involve any direct physical threat, it cannot be resolved through any direct physical recourse—such as one might do by simply running away from a hunting lion as fast as possible. Instead, humans respond to this abstract mode of existential concern with unique *psychological* adaptations. Building on the works of thinkers such as Otto Rank (Menaker, 1984; Rank, 1936) and Ernest Becker (1971, 1973), TMT argues that humans can manage the awareness of mortality by perceiving themselves as qualifying for some form of permanence. People can do so by developing and participating in *cultural worldviews*: belief systems that imbue one's world with order and articulate the standards and values necessary to successfully navigate one's world. One's *self-esteem* then serves as feedback reflecting the degree to which one judges oneself as successfully or unsuccessfully living up to one's cultural standards and values. Low self-esteem would reflect a judgment that one is struggling or failing to meaningfully live up to one's cultural standards and values, whereas high self-esteem would reflect a judgment that one is successfully meeting or exceeding one's standards and values and is therefore worthy of cultural permanence.

Cultural worldviews offer believers death-denying permanence in the form of nonsupernatural and/or supernatural immortality. With *nonsupernatural immortality*, believers can strive for a sense of symbolic and/or literal permanence. A sense of symbolic immortality involves the impression that one's activities would leave a legacy, such that one achieves a lasting impact on future generations or potentially is even remembered by name. Worldviews placing value on art might lead people to contribute to a valuable innovation in creative medium (e.g., fresco) or style (e.g., renaissance), or to become so inspiringly skilled that they are remembered for many generations (e.g., Michelangelo); worldviews might also place value on making contributions in government, business, education, health care, sports, family, or any of many other available domains. Cultural worldviews might also guide efforts toward nonsupernatural literal immortality, such as modern medical science's efforts to prevent disease, aging, and death—using natural world phenomena to pursue medical indefinite life extension. With *supernatural immortality*, believers can strive for the impression that, despite physical death, their supernatural essence would literally continue to live on in some form of afterlife.

Faith in Supernatural Immortality

Religions are effective at managing the awareness of mortality because religion can offer both symbolic and literal immortality (Vail et al., 2010). Believers can achieve a sense of symbolic immortality by spreading their beliefs to their children and/or proselytizing to others, donating time and money to their religious organization, or generally supporting other members of their faith community, ensuring their beliefs and values are shared by others and are passed along to future generations. But the defining feature of religion is that it offers the idea of spiritual immortality.

Among the world's oldest surviving literature, chiseled on clay tablets in Mesopotamia some 4,000-plus years ago, is the *Epic of Gilgamesh*. Lamenting the death of his friend, Enkidu, Gilgamesh (king of Uruk) embarks on a heroic journey to discover the secret to eternal life. During his journey, he learns how humans must die, how to worship the gods, and how to live a good life so that one might be treated well in the afterlife. Likewise, Hindus believe their actions in the world (*karma*) determine their fate after death: whether they will be sent to heaven (*Svarga*) or hell (*Naraka*), be cursed to another earthly rebirth, or be blessed to achieve the ultimate spiritual release from the cycle of life and death (*moksha*). Similarly, Buddhism provides elaborate descriptions of the afterlife, describing in detail the different levels of eternal spiritual realms floating above the mythical Mount Meru, which one can enter following death. Christians believe their "saved" souls will continue to live an eternal life with God in Heaven, and Muslims believe the faithful will enjoy the pleasures of eternal life in the heavenly gardens (*Jannat al-Na'im*). The common theme, whatever their variations in names and details, is that religions offer the existentially comforting idea that physical death is not the end—one's soul will live on forever.

Several studies have tested the idea that religious concepts about supernatural immortality help manage the awareness of mortality. Here, it's important to introduce a few of the ways researchers typically test ideas related to TMT (see Solomon et al., Chapter 6, this volume, for more detail). First, according to the *mortality salience hypothesis*, if cultural worldview beliefs and self-esteem help provide protection from the awareness of mortality, then heightened awareness of death should motivate increased investment in those beliefs and in positive self-esteem. To test that hypothesis, researchers randomly assign participants to either a non-death-related prime condition or a condition that increases the awareness of death (mortality salience; MS) and then measure the effects of those primes on worldview investment and self-esteem striving. Exploring spiritual immortality beliefs, some initial research (Osarchuk & Tatz, 1973) found religious believers reminded of death (vs. control conditions) increased their belief in afterlife. Other research (Jong et al., 2012) has similarly found that MS led Christians to increase faith in supernatural concepts such as having a soul, a spiritual realm, and heaven.

Second, according to the *buffer hypothesis*, if belief in spiritual immortality helps provide protection from the awareness of mortality, then affirming this belief should provide a buffer against death awareness and thus eliminate MS effects. Indeed, when participants with a strong afterlife belief were confronted with death awareness, they viewed death with stronger positive and weaker negative implications (Schoenrade, 1989). In another series of experiments (Dechesne et al., 2003), half of participants read an article claiming (falsely) that medical researchers had documented over 600 cases of out-of-body experiences after patients had died on the operating table (e.g., floating above one's body, moving toward a light, feeling comfort, seeing old friends and family), which suggested the existence of an afterlife, whereas the other half of participants read an article debunking such experiences as the natural by-products of biological processes (e.g., oxygen deprivation in the brain). In the latter condition, there was no buffer, and MS (vs. control condition) led to increased self-esteem striving. However, that MS effect was eliminated when participants were exposed to information promoting the existence of spiritual life after death.

In the *Yaksha Prashna* passage of the Hindu epic *Mahabharata,* Yudhisthira (king of Indraprastha—modern-day Delhi) is questioned by Yama (god of death and justice), who has taken the form of a crane yaksha (nature spirit). In a surprisingly self-aware exchange, the yaksha asks: "What is most wonderful?" to which Yudhisthira replies: "Day after day, countless creatures go to the abode of Yama, yet those that remain behind believe themselves to be immortal." Indeed, TMT research shows that ideas about supernatural immortality—souls, spiritual realms, and afterlives—offer an effective way to manage the awareness of physical death.

Faith in Supernatural Agents

The idea of spiritual immortality becomes particularly compelling as people's natural cognitive inclinations lead them to also imagine supernatural agents inhabiting the presumed spiritual realms (Bering, 2011; Boyer, 2001; Tremlin, 2006). Indeed, every religion has imagined the universe to be created and governed by spiritual agents—gods, demons, angels, spirits, and souls. Consider the *Enuma Elish*, another of humankind's oldest surviving stories, which tells a Babylonian creation story in which the god *Marduk* struggles against dragon goddess *Tiamat* to create Earth and other supernatural realms. Similarly, the Hindu *Rigveda* offers many creation stories, such as one in which the cosmos was birthed by a god of gods, in the form of a primordial golden womb known as *Hiranyagarbha*. The Maori and the Hebrews each imagined that *Io* and *Yahweh*, respectively, were supreme beings who created the universe out of nothing. Through the ages, people have imagined thousands of similar stories about spiritual agents creating the world (Leeming & Leeming, 1994). As Mircea Eliade (1957) suggested, the presumed existence of these inhabitants of "the world of spirit" makes rather convincing the possibility that peoples' own souls could similarly transcend their corporeal limitations.

From a TMT perspective, the presumed existence of such supernatural agents therefore plays a key role in managing the awareness of death. Some research has tested that idea using the *death-thought accessibility hypothesis*, which suggests that if religious beliefs about gods and other supernatural agents help manage the awareness of mortality, then threatening those ideas should undermine the buffer and allow increased accessibility of death-related thoughts. Increases in death-thought accessibility (DTA) can be measured on a word-stem completion task, when participants complete word-stems such as COFF_ _ in death-related (COFFIN) ways rather than neutral (COFFEE) ways; or in a computerized lexical decision task, when participants more quickly classify death-related words (e.g., grave, killed) compared to other types of words (e.g., desk, phone) as words. In one relevant study (Schimel et al., 2007), researchers recruited participants who either believed or did not believe in the Judeo-Christian account of creation, asked them to read either a pro-evolution/anti-creation article or a neutral article about attitudes, and then administered the word-stem completion DTA measure. Results found heightened DTA among creationists who read the pro-evolution/anti-creation article.

Other research has examined the effect of MS on faith in supernatural agency. In one study (Williams et al., 2012), researchers had creationists and evolutionists read passages presenting scientific information about evolution that threatened creationist ideas and then asked them to complete a reading comprehension test. After MS, creationists were less likely to have engaged with the pro-evolution/anti-creation information, though they still engaged with other nonthreatening information—suggesting that they were motivated to defensively preserve faith in their religious creation myth. Other studies found MS increased general religious faith, belief in god, and divine agency (Norenzayan & Hansen, 2006). Still other research found evidence MS motivates faith in worldview-specific ways (Vail et al., 2012). In one study, MS motivated American Christians to increase their faith in their culturally relevant supernatural agent, Jesus/God, while at the same time increasing their rejection of alternatives such as Allah and Buddha. In another study, MS motivated Iranian Muslims to increase their faith in their culturally relevant supernatural agent, Muhammad/Allah, while increasing rejection of Jesus and Buddha.

Together, these findings show that religious ideas about supernatural agents and agency serve an important existential psychological function by helping manage the awareness of death.

THE SOCIAL SIDE OF EXISTENTIALLY MOTIVATED RELIGIOUS FAITH

At their core, cultural worldviews—including religious ones—are human-made concepts and, therefore, exist outside the realm of falsifiability. With no way to directly observe or substantiate the existence of supernatural agents and phenomena (e.g., gods, souls, heavens), people instead rely on social validation of these concepts to maintain confidence in their worldview and its promises of immortality. When other people agree with one's worldview, the shared consensus increases the worldview's perceived legitimacy, providing reassurance that faith in such beliefs is worthwhile (Berger & Luckmann, 1967). On the other hand, when others reject or hold competing beliefs, it raises concerns that one's own belief system could be an illegitimate pathway to immortality. To maintain the perceived legitimacy of their worldviews, people engage in a variety of psychological defenses as they navigate the social landscape.

Supporting Fellow Believers

From a TMT perspective, supporting fellow believers helps validate one's worldview and secure its death-defying benefits. Indeed, a myriad of studies show that reminders of death (compared to control topics) facilitate greater support of those who share one's worldviews. In the health care field, for example, MS motivated Christian medical students to show greater attentiveness to a Christian patient presenting with cardiac risk compared to a Muslim patient with the same symptoms (Arndt et al., 2009). In more general contexts, MS has been shown to increase American Christians' ratings of a Christian target on traits like intelligence and morality (Greenberg et al., 1990), MS increased participants' positive feelings about a potential long-term dating partner who shared the same (vs. different) religious beliefs (Kosloff et al., 2010), and MS increased Indonesian Muslims' agreement with a fellow Muslim's suggestion that the Indonesian government be run according to Islamic law (Iqbal et al., 2016).

These sorts of preferences affect people's personal and societal preferences outside the lab, as well. Christians prioritize other Christians on a hypothetical waiting list to receive a life-saving kidney treatment (Furnham et al., 1998). U.S. census data suggests that about 7 in 10 married Americans report having a spouse who shares their religious views (Murphy, 2015). And American Christians have overwhelmingly and disproportionately elected fellow Christian candidates to Congress. Compared to the 63% of the general public that identifies as Christian, the current (118th) Congress is nearly 88% Christian (Diamant, 2023). Furthermore, all but two U.S. presidents have openly identified as being Christian, and even those with no formal affiliation still claimed to believe in God (Sandstrom, 2021). National polls suggest this trend is not likely to change anytime soon, as 40% of Americans still assert that they categorically would not vote for a nonreligious presidential candidate even if they were well-qualified for the job (Saad, 2020).

Rejecting the Heathens

In addition to supporting fellow believers, existential concern also leads people to derogate and reject those who threaten the validity of one's own religious worldview. For example, following MS, the American Christians who had favorable impressions of a Christian target, mentioned above, also made harsher judgments of a Jewish person (Greenberg et al., 1990), and the Indonesian Muslim participants who supported the implementation of Sharia law, mentioned above, also increased condemnation of the dissident Ahmadiyya sect as heretics of Islam (Iqbal et al., 2016).

This derogation of religious outgroups is also readily seen outside the lab. While the majority-Christian population in the United States has been slowly warming up to minority religious groups over time, in one study Muslims and atheists still remained lowest on the Americans' "feeling thermometer," particularly among the Protestant respondents (Pew Research Center, 2017a). Additional polls have revealed that substantial portions of Western nations still feel that Muslims pose a threat to their religious beliefs (Gallup, 2011). Exhibiting a similar sentiment, early in his first term, U.S. President Donald Trump signed his first executive order banning refugees and citizens from seven Muslim-majority countries, followed by two additional iterations of the ban in subsequent months (Jarrett & Tatum, 2017), and national polls indicated the majority of Americans supported the Muslim-targeted travel bans (Kirk & Scott, 2017; Shepard, 2017). Likewise, in Canada, groups such as Canadians Against Islamization and Suffragettes Against Silence protested outside of a Toronto mosque, calling for similar bans in Canada (Nasser & McLaughlin, 2017).

Accommodating Compelling Alternatives

Despite bolstering fellow believers and derogating heathens, the continued presence of a compelling alternative worldview can potentially threaten the validity of one's religious beliefs. Under such conditions, people may adjust their religious beliefs to accommodate the alternative belief. Thus, they might preserve the core beliefs of their religious worldview (e.g., the existence of God) and modify some peripheral beliefs to include the compelling alternative idea.

For example, the Bible describes God creating the entire universe, including humankind, from scratch directly into their present forms. However, in 1859 Charles Darwin offered a compelling alternative view in his theory of evolution. Though advances in geological sciences had previously undermined a literal reading of Biblical *genesis*, Darwin's ideas had now directly challenged religious ideas about God being the ex-nihilo creator of humankind. With the theory of evolution supported by a growing body of evidence, American Holy Cross priest and scientist John Augustine Zahm published *Evolution and Dogma* (1896), which tried to reconcile Catholic theology with the theory of evolution. The work was reported to the Church's *Congregation of the Index of Prohibited Books*, and Zahm was required to publicly retract his views and withdraw the book from sale (Kemp, 2021).

Yet, half of a century later, in his encyclical *Humani Generis* (1950), Pope Pius XII urged that scientific research and theological discussions should equally consider both sides of the evolution–creationism debate, so long as they did not overstep the Church's absolute position that human souls are created by God. Following another half century, bowing to growing evidence for evolution, Pope John Paul II (1996) admitted the theory of evolution was more than "a mere hypothesis" and accepted it could very well explain the development of physical human bodies. In the Church's most recent statement on the topic, Pope Francis (2014) completely abandoned the literal reading of Genesis and instead asserted that the theory of evolution, now holding scientific consensus, is not only compatible with Christianity but actually proves the existence of God:

> When we read the account of Creation in Genesis, we risk imagining that God was a magician, complete with an all-powerful magic wand. But that was not so. He created beings and he let them . . . develop and reach their fullness. And thus, Creation has been progressing for centuries and centuries, millennia and millennia, until becoming as we know it today. . . . The Big Bang theory, which is proposed today as the origin of the world, does not contradict the intervention of a divine creator but depends on it. Evolution in nature does not conflict with the notion of Creation, because evolution presupposes the creation of beings who evolve.

The point is that none of these ideas are present in the Bible. Yet, as evidence for evolution became more and more compelling, and threatening to the validity of Biblical creationism, the Catholic Church accommodated evolution in such a way that it could still preserve the core belief in the existence of God.

TMT research has found similar effects among creationists more broadly (Hayes et al., 2015). When exposed to information that supported evolution and refuted creationism, creationists primed with MS reduced their rejection of evolution but not their faith in God. Much like the Catholic Church, participants accommodated the theory of evolution while maintaining their core faith in God.

Assimilating Converts

As Abraham Lincoln reportedly said, the best way to destroy your enemy is to make them your friend. In the context of religion, that strategy means assimilating nonbelievers into one's own religion. The Quran, for example, frequently references *da'wah*, which calls Muslims to "Invite [all] to the way of your Lord with wisdom and kind advice" (Quran 16:125), and the Bible instructs believers to "Go therefore and make disciples of all nations" (Matthew 28:19, NRSV). The Buddha also spoke about the importance of teaching the Dharma, eventually prompting third-century century Indian Emperor Ashoka to send vast numbers of Buddhist missionaries throughout Asia (Najmitdinov, 2021).

Such assimilation efforts can vary widely in their tone, ranging from friendly to violent. In the former, many religious groups proselytize by creating welcoming environments, such as mosque open houses, Hindu ISKCON gatherings, or Christian vacation bible schools. More aggressive assimilation tactics involve, for example, Christians using public demonstrations and "gospel tract" pamphlets to preach that those who do not accept Jesus will be sent to burn for eternity in the flames of Hell. More hostile still are violent efforts to forcibly convert nonbelievers to one's religion, such as those carried out by Christians in the European Inquisitions and the conquest of native American peoples.

Again, TMT research shows the role of existential concern in the efforts to assimilate nonbelievers into one's faith. In one study (Kosloff et al., 2017), researchers exposed Christian participants to MS and provided them opportunities to either derogate or proselytize to an atheist. When the target was portrayed as being steadfast in their atheistic beliefs, MS motivated the Christians to simply derogate the atheist; however, when the atheist was portrayed as being open-minded, MS instead led participants to increase assimilation efforts by advising them to attend church services and read the Bible. These findings show that in the face of threatening worldviews, MS can motivate people to choose assimilation over other defense strategies, provided there is a legitimate possibility of converting the nonbeliever.

Annihilation

Religious believers may also resort to the more extreme strategy of annihilation—eliminating worldview-threatening people and ideas from existence. Even the scriptures themselves may call for it. For example, the infamous sword verse (Quran 9:5) directs Muslims to "kill the unbelievers wherever you find them" and the Bible (Deuteronomy 13:6-9) instructs Christians, "If anyone entices you . . . saying, 'Let us go serve other gods' . . . you shall surely kill them." Throughout history, believers have indeed defended their faith and faith communities through violence, terrorism, military conquest, and even genocide. In fact, policy analysts have found that, compared to secular disputes, religious conflict has historically been more frequent, more devastating, and more likely to reoccur (Toft, 2007).

For example, Martin Luther—father of the Protestant Reformation—initially showed interest in converting Europe's Jews to Christianity through his reforms. But then, after his reforms failed to convert them, he became embittered and penned a 65,000 word treatise *On the Jews and Their Lies* (1543) in which he called for Europe's Christians to burn Jewish synagogues and schools and homes, destroy their prayer books and ban rabbinical preaching, confiscate Jewish property and money, press Jews into forced labor, and ultimately murder all the Jews in Europe. The Protestant population later played a major role in the emergence of German nationalism and support for the Nazi rise to power (Steigmann-Gall, 2003).

The longstanding conflict over the "Holy Land" has also provided abundant examples. After the rise of Islamic Caliphates in the region, a series of medieval Christian Crusades sought to reconquer Jerusalem and the surrounding region from Muslim rule. Later, after Jewish immigration to Mandatory Palestine rose following World War I and World War II, the United Nations partitioned the region in 1947 and numerous conflicts have been fought for control over the region ever since. In the ongoing war in Gaza (2023–present), the Palestinian Islamic militant group Hamas (*Harakat al-Muqawama al-Islamiya*), democratically elected by the residents of Israeli-occupied Gaza, launched a surprise attack against Israel—killing some 1,200 Israeli soldiers and civilians and taking hundreds of hostages (Byman et al., 2023). In response, Israel declared war against Hamas and leveled Gaza, displaced its population of roughly 2 million, and killed over 30,000 of Gaza's civilians in the process (Batrawy, 2024).

TMT research highlights the relationship between death awareness and support for the annihilation of religious outgroups. One study randomly assigned Christians to read an article either about a neutral topic or about how the city of Nazareth (Jesus's hometown) is succumbing to "Islamification" and then measured DTA using the word-stem completion task (Hayes et al., 2008). Compared to the neutral topic, reading the article about the Islamification of Nazareth significantly increased participants' DTA. However, this effect was eliminated if the participants were also exposed to a report showing that a plane full of Muslims had been killed in a crash on their way to Nazareth. In another study (Pyszczynski et al., 2006), MS increased Iranian students' support for Islamic martyrdom missions (suicide terrorism) against the United States, as well as their self-reported willingness to join such causes. Together, these results provide insight into the existential motivations behind the violent religious annihilation efforts seen throughout history.

VARIATION IN ORIENTATION TO RELIGIOUS FAITH

While all the world's religions address death-related existential concerns, there is considerable diversity in whether and how people use religion for this purpose. Some are skeptical or uncertain about religious concepts or reject them altogether. Some turn to religion because they genuinely believe in supernatural religious ideas, while others engage religion for the social opportunities for non-supernatural immortality. And some rigidly adhere to their faith's fundamental teachings, whereas others adopt a more open-minded quest for spiritual enlightenment. Below, we explore how these variations in religious orientations can influence whether and how people use religion as a terror management strategy.

Skepticism

Though religious belief can function as a direct, powerful method of managing death awareness, not all people are religious. Globally, roughly 15% have no religious affiliation (Pew Research Center, 2017b). However, these religious "nones" are not necessarily unbelievers. In the United States, for example, recent data suggests 26.1% were religiously unaffiliated, made up of 4% who reported being atheist, 5.3% as agnostic, and 16.8% who indicated "nothing in particular" (Pew Research Center, 2023). Those groups have important differences in their approach to religious concepts.

Prior work shows that large portions of people claiming "no religion" actually do believe in supernatural spiritual concepts, but they choose to disaffiliate from religious organizations for social reasons that have little or nothing to do with their spiritual beliefs (Baker & Smith, 2009; Vernon, 1968). Thus, although "spiritual but not religious" people may distance themselves from more formally organized religious groups, they may nevertheless still manage death awareness by expressing faith in their culturally familiar supernatural spiritual concepts—god, souls, heaven, and so on. Agnostics and atheists, however, are each more genuinely skeptical and yet they differ in existentially important ways.

Agnosticism (*a- gnostic*, without knowledge) entails uncertainty about religious claims about supernatural concepts, stemming from the fact that the supernatural is, by definition, beyond verification via natural observation (Russell, 1927, 1947; Stephen, 1893). However, as Blaise Pascal (1669) noted in his famous *wager* passage, it is impossible to simultaneously believe and not believe—one must choose. Arguing for Christianity, he noted that if Christianity is wrong, and God does not exist, there are no spiritual gains/losses from betting on faith or disbelief; but if correct, and God does exist, the gain of betting on faith is eternal life and the loss of betting on disbelief is eternal damnation. Therefore, he argued, the agnostic should bet on faith. Indeed, TMT research (Vail et al., 2012) has found that, when faced with existential concerns, agnostics make that bet—though perhaps more robustly than Pascal likely imagined. Whereas agnostics showed skepticism in a baseline condition, after being reminded of death they showed stronger general religiosity, faith in a higher power, and in the spirit of Pascal's *wager* they also "hedged their bets" by increasing faith in Christian, Islamic, and Buddhist supernatural agents.

In contrast, *atheism* (*a- theism*, without belief in god) more plainly entails either the passive absence of faith in supernatural concepts or the assertive rejection of supernatural concepts (Dawkins, 2006). Building on dual-process models of cognition, the death-denying power of religious concepts may indeed be just as appealing to atheists as to anyone else, at least intuitively, but upon reflection atheists may override and reject that existentially intuitive desire for supernatural immortality. A growing body of research is consistent with that idea. Several studies have investigated the intuitive appeal of religious concepts using nonconscious, implicit outcome measures. For example, one study (Jong et al., 2012) found that MS led believers and unbelievers alike to implicitly activate supernatural concepts on a single-target Implicit Association Test (IAT). Other research (Vail et al., 2024a) directly sampled atheists, specifically, and confirmed that MS motivated both Christian and atheist samples to implicitly activate common religious faith concepts as measured on a standard IAT (e.g., soul, god, heaven). However, a different pattern emerged when participants were allowed to consciously reflect on and express their accepted beliefs. Several studies using self-report measures have found that after MS atheists continued to explicitly reject religious concepts (Jong et al., 2012; Vail et al., 2012, 2024a). Together, these findings show that, when managing death awareness, the supernatural immortality offered by religious concepts may indeed be just as intuitively appealing to atheists as to anyone else, but that atheists may ultimately override those intuitions to explicitly reject religious concepts.

One important area for future research would be to better understand how atheists rely on alternative systems of secular terror management. At least in religion-dominated cultural settings, such as the United States, Nigeria, or India, meaningful secular immortality concepts may not be as intuitively available, which may have implications both for maintaining existential well-being and for the search for alternative death-denying concepts. For example, one study found that whereas MS had no impact on meaning in life among Christians, it led to reduced meaning in life among atheists (Vail & Soenke, 2018). Other emerging research (Vail et al., 2024b) suggests MS leads atheists to more strongly reject religious beliefs but also become more open-minded, potentially indicating a cognitive search for viable alternatives. Other work has found that atheists continued to engage in MS-induced secular worldview defense after reading an article claiming evidence for spiritual afterlife (which atheists explicitly reject) but not after reading about the more acceptable, secular path to denial of death through advances in medical indefinite life extension (Vail et al., 2020).

One challenge is that atheism merely indicates the absence of religious faith—not the presence of any secular system of meaning. So, in addition to identifying atheists, future research will need to identify atheists' affirmative secular value systems. Some values commonly associated with secular humanism, which individual atheists may identify and internalize to varying degrees, have already been found to be effective terror management buffers in general population samples, including science-based learning (Farias et al., 2013; Williams et al., 2012), compassion (Gailliot et al., 2008; Vail et al., 2009), love (Mikulincer et al., 2003), work (Yaakobi, 2015), and moral progress (Rutjens et al., 2009), among others. Future research should investigate atheists' process of using cognitive resources to override the intuitively appealing religious supernatural immortality concepts, searching for viable secular death-denying concepts, and relying upon them to maintain existential wellbeing.

Faith Orientations

Among religious believers, the way people approach their religious faith appears to vary in both form and function. In terms of form, believers can and do vary in their focus on both the spiritual and the social rewards of faith. In terms of function, multiple observers have conceptualized the existential psychological approach to religion as lying along a continuum, ranging from closed-minded and rigid faith ("security orientations") at the right to open-minded search for spiritual meaning ("growth orientations") at the left (Vail et al., 2019; Van Tongeren et al., 2016).

Form Orientations

One set of individual differences in the form of religious engagement comprise the dimensions of intrinsic and extrinsic religiosity. The dimension of *intrinsic religiosity* reflects the degree of genuine internalization of a religion's teachings and values, focused on the spiritual rewards of faith, whereas the dimension of *extrinsic religiosity* reflects the degree to which a person participates in religion for the social benefits to be gained through one's religious community.

Illustrative examples can be seen in the difference between composer Johann Sebastian Bach compared to Gustav Mahler and Johannes Brahms. On the intrinsic religiosity side, Bach was a devout Christian who taught Luther's Small Catechism (1529), which influenced much of his composition—*St. Matthew Passion* (1727), *Mass in B Minor* (1749), his many sacred *cantatas,* and numerous others. In the margins of one of his Bibles, next to 2 Chronicles 5:13, he wrote, "In a music of worship, God is always present with his grace." On the extrinsic side, born to Jewish parents and a lifelong agnostic, Mahler pragmatically converted to Catholicism in 1897 to overcome anti-Semitism, gain acceptance in the majority-Christian community, and thus secure the prestigious position as conductor and director of the *Vienna Hofoper* (State Opera House; Carr, 1998). Brahms, too, was an agnostic and humanist, which led his devoutly Catholic counterpart Antonín Dvořák to write about him, "Such a fine man, such a fine soul—and yet, he does not believe!" (Swafford, 1999). Even so, Brahms profitably navigated the majority-Christian cultural landscape with musical compositions such as his famous *German Requiem to the Words of the Holy Scriptures* (1868).

In contrast to extrinsic religiosity, intrinsic believers therefore tend to be "true" believers with internalized faith in the religion's core concepts and in gaining the benefit of existential security and meaning in life (Batson et al., 1993). Some studies have indeed found that among those high in intrinsic religiosity, but not extrinsic religiosity, belief in afterlife is associated with reduced death anxiety (Van Tongeren et al., 2017), and when reminded of death those high in intrinsic religiosity reported an increased sense of self-efficacy and positive emotional experience (Fischer et al., 2006). Other work has found that affirmations of one's intrinsic religious faith can serve that protective function and eliminate the need for further death-denying worldview defenses. In one set of studies, participants were reminded of either death or a control topic, then they either affirmed their religious faith or did not, and then were given an opportunity to engage in secular cultural worldview defense (Jonas & Fischer, 2006). When they didn't affirm their faith, MS led to increased worldview defense. However, that effect was eliminated among those high (but not low) in intrinsic religiosity when they first affirmed their faith. These findings show that an intrinsic form of religious faith can help manage existential concerns about mortality.

Functional Orientations

Individual differences in one's existential psychological approach to religion have been conceptualized as lying along a continuum, ranging from closed-minded and rigid "security orientations" at the right to more open-minded "growth orientations" characterized by a search for spiritual meaning at the left (Vail et al., 2019; Van Tongeren et al., 2016).

Security Orientation. At the right side of the spectrum are *religious fundamentalists*, who believe their religion offers the absolute inerrant truth about natural and spiritual matters, including about how to take meaningful steps on the spiritual path toward eternal life (Altemeyer & Hunsberger, 1992). From that view, any threat to the perceived veracity of one's religion would undermine its existential protection against death awareness. Indeed, compared to reading other materials, when American Christian fundamentalists read an "impeaching paragraph" that highlighted errors and inconsistencies in the gospel's claims of Jesus' resurrection, they subsequently displayed heightened DTA on a word-stem completion task (Friedman & Rholes, 2007).

Because fundamentalists "put all their eggs in one basket" like this, believing their religious texts and teachings are the one and only correct way of life, they rely on their religious ideas about spiritual immortality to the exclusion of other worldviews. For example, when asked to write about what they think happens when they die, participants high (vs. low) on religious fundamentalism spontaneously wrote more about religious afterlife—and whereas low fundamentalists still responded to MS with increased secular worldview defense, high fundamentalists did not (Friedman & Rholes, 2008; Koca-Atabey & Öner-Özkan, 2011). Additionally, they may insist on religious or spiritual "healing" (e.g., prayer) rather than modern science-based medical treatments, such as members of the Pentecostal Followers of Christ do in the U.S. state of Idaho. There, Mariah Walton was born with a congenital hole in her heart, teen Arrian Granden ruptured her esophagus, and many newborns developed typical treatable complications (e.g., simple infections, pneumonia). However, because their fundamentalist parents relied on "faith-based healing" rather than medical treatment, Mariah became permanently disabled, Arrian bled to death, and the child mortality rate of Followers of Christ became 10 times higher than among other Idaho families (Wilson, 2016). TMT research has found existential concerns play a part in motivating these sorts of faith-based medical refusals among fundamentalists (Vess et al., 2009a). Indeed, in that same research, when fundamentalists were reminded of death, they more strongly relied on their religious belief, were more supportive of prayer over medical treatment, and more strongly emphasized relying on faith alone to heal.

Fundamentalists' belief that their religion offers the absolute inerrant truth about the world leads them to believe their scriptures should be strictly followed, and that any deviations represent evil spiritual corruptions that must be forcefully resisted and annihilated. Indeed, fundamentalism is associated with greater prejudice and discrimination against people with different beliefs and greater aggression and militaristic attitudes (Altemeyer & Hunsberger, 1992; Henderson-King et al., 2004). However, most religions instruct believers to follow the humanist "Golden Rule" to treat others with kindness, tolerance, and compassion. The Bible, for example, includes Jesus's instruction to "love your neighbor as yourself" (Mark 12:31) and the Quran includes passages calling believers to "do good unto others as God as done good unto you" (Sura 28:77). In American Christian samples as well as Iranian Shi'a samples, TMT studies have found that a focus on prosocial scriptural teachings might conflict with fundamentalists' otherwise aggressive defense of their religious cultures (Rothschild et al., 2009). When participants read neutral statements or secular expressions of compassionate values, MS led fundamentalists to support extreme military actions against worldview threats abroad, including the use of chemical and nuclear weapons and the killing of thousands of civilians. But when they first read their religious scripture's instructions to be compassionate, MS motivated them to reduce their support for violence.

Growth Orientation. At the other end of the spectrum are the more open-minded religious orientations. Religious *quest orientation*, for example, does not regard any one religious faith as having a monopoly on spiritual truth and thus open-mindedly seeks spiritual insights. For example, Hesse was born to a Swabian family of Lutheran missionaries to India and spent his life exploring the world's religious traditions in search for authenticity, self, and spiritual truth—a search that influenced his many novels and essays, including *Siddhartha* (1922), *Steppenwolf* (1927), and *The Glass Bead Game* (1943). Similarly, syncretic religious denominations, such as Unitarian Universalists and the Baha'i Faith, are based on open-minded pursuit of spiritual truth, connection to god, and moral understanding of the world. Thus, such denominations study scriptures from all the world's faith traditions—whether Jewish, Christian, Muslim, Hindu, Buddhist, Zoroastrian, and so on.

However, because quest orientation involves a skeptical yet open-minded approach rather than confident faith in any one religious worldview, it comes at the cost of greater death-related anxiety, DTA, and vulnerability to MS effects on existential concern (Arrowood et al., 2021). Indeed, those high (but not low) in quest orientation are poorly protected against existential concerns, such that death awareness reduces their well-being (Arrowood et al., 2018). However, people with low need for dogmatic belief structure, which may be a facet of quest orientation, are especially inclined to seek solace in existential exploration through the consideration of novel ideas (Vess et al., 2009b). When people high in quest religiosity were reminded of mortality, they became less likely to believe in or commit to God but became more culturally open-minded—and engaging in a thoughtful exploration of their doubts and uncertainties about religious ideas and spiritual truth, which may be experienced as a step toward spiritual fulfillment, seemed to help alleviate these existential concerns (Arrowood et al., 2021).

On another note, *ecumenical* programs and *interfaith fellowship* are often based on the idea that people around the world share a fundamental spiritual nature and that followers of each religion are therefore spiritual brothers and sisters. Building on that idea, and the common ingroup identity model (Gaertner et al., 1993), some research suggests fostering a sense of common cause among religious groups through ecumenical and interfaith programs might contribute to a more open-minded and peaceful way of managing death-related concerns. In one set of studies (Motyl et al., 2011), American participants read stories about people's favorite childhood memories (e.g., going to the beach, camping) and recalled their own similar experiences. However, in one condition the stories were about other Americans (e.g., Michael from Orlando) whereas in another condition the stories were about people from other nations around the world (e.g., Miguel from Cuernavaca). Among those who recalled experiences similar to others around the world, MS motivated increased tolerance of immigrants, ethnic tolerance, and support for international peacebuilding. Other research similarly found that among those who thought about a common cause (e.g., climate change), compared to a localized problem (e.g., flooding), MS motivated reduced support for militarism and increased support for international peacebuilding; this effect was replicated among samples of Israeli Arabs and Israeli Jews during the 2009 war in Gaza (Pyszczynski et al., 2012). Thus, ecumenical outreach and interfaith fellowship may bend existential motivations toward collective compassion, cooperation, and peace, both domestically and internationally.

CONCLUSION

A growing body of research shows that the fundamental human motivation to manage the awareness of mortality can help explain why religious and spiritual beliefs have been so prevalent throughout human history—and why they still hold such broad appeal today. Such existential concern fuels faith in supernatural immortality (souls, afterlife), fuels faith in myths about supernatural agents and agency (creation, gods, angels, demons, etc.), and drives social behaviors designed to protect the perceived legitimacy of those beliefs—supporting fellow believers, rejecting heathens, accommodating compelling alternatives, assimilating converts, and annihilation. The expression of this existentially motivated religious faith also seems to be profoundly influenced by one's religious orientation. Research among skeptics (e.g., agnostics, atheists) suggests death awareness may implicitly increase the intuitive appeal of religious concepts, but that those intuitions may then be explicitly accepted or rejected by one's more reflective thought and worldview beliefs. Research among believers shows that religious terror management processes can depend on one's religious orientation—it can lead some to dogmatically cling to their faith, some toward more mainstream engagement, and some to a more precarious yet open-minded search for spiritual fulfillment. At their core, each of these religious and spiritual inclinations are motivated by the fundamental human motivation to psychologically manage the awareness of death.

REFERENCES

Altemeyer, B., & Hunsberger, B. E. (1992). Authoritarianism, religious fundamentalism, quest, and prejudice. *International Journal for the Psychology of Religion, 2,* 113–133.

Arndt, J., Vess, M., Cox, C. R., Goldenberg, J. L., & Lagle, S. (2009). The psychosocial effect of thoughts of personal mortality on cardiac risk assessment. *Medical Decision Making, 29*(2), 175–181.

Arrowood, R. B., Coleman, T. J. I., Swanson, S. B., Hood, R. W., Jr., & Cox, C. R. (2018). Death, quest, and self-esteem: Re-examining the role of self-esteem and religion following mortality salience. *Religion, Brain and Behavior, 8*(1), 69–76.

Arrowood, R. B., Vail, K. E., & Cox, C. R. (2021). The existential quest: Doubt, openness, and the exploration of religious uncertainty. *International Journal for the Psychology of Religion.*

Baker, J. O., & Smith, B. (2009). None too simple: Examining issues of religious nonbelief and nonbelonging in the United States. *Journal for the Scientific Study of Religion, 48,* 719–733.

Batrawy, A. (2024, February 29). *Gaza's death toll now exceeds 30,000. Here's why it's an incomplete count.* NPR. www.npr.org/2024/02/29/1234159514/gaza-death-toll-30000-palestinians-israel-hamas-war.

Batson, C. D., Schoenrade, P., & Ventis, W. L. (1993). *Religion and the individual: A social-psychological perspective.* Oxford University Press.

Becker, E. (1971). *The birth and death of meaning: An interdisciplinary perspective on the problem of man* (2nd ed.). Free Press.

Becker, E. (1973). *The denial of death.* Free Press.

Berger, P. L., & Luckmann, T. (1967). *The social construction of reality.* Penguin Books.

Bering, J. (2011). *The god instinct: The psychology of souls, destiny, and the meaning of life.* Nicholas Brealey.

Boyer, P. (2001). *Religion explained: The evolutionary origins of religious thought.* Basic Books.

Byman, D., McCabe, R., Palmer, A., Doxsee, C., Holtz, M., & Duff, D. (2023). *Hamas's October 7 attack: Visualizing the data.* Center for Strategic and International Studies. www.csis.org/analysis/hamass-october-7-attack-visualizing-data.

Carr, J. (1998). *Mahler: A biography.* Overlook Press.

Cherniak, A. D., Mikulincer, M., Shaver, P. R., & Granqvist, P. (2021). Attachment theory and religion. *Current Opinion in Psychology, 40,* 126–130.

Conard, N. J. (2003). Palaeolithic ivory sculptures from southwestern Germany and the origins of figurative art. *Nature, 426,* 830–832.

Conard, N. J. (2009). A female figurine from the basal Aurignacian of Hohle Fels Cave in southwestern Germany. *Nature, 459*(7244), 248–252.

Culotta, E. (2009). On the origin of religion. *Science, 326*(5954), 784–787.

Dawkins, R. (2006). *The god delusion.* Houghton Mifflin.

Dechesne, M., Pyszczynski, T., Arndt, J., Ransom, S., Sheldon, K. M., van Knippenberg, A., & Janssen, J. (2003). Literal and symbolic immortality: The effect of evidence of literal immortality on self-esteem striving in response to mortality salience. *Journal of Personality and Social Psychology, 84*(4), 722–737.

Diamant, J. (2023, January 3). *Faith on the hill.* Pew Research Center. www.pewresearch.org/religion/2023/01/03/faith-on-the-hill-2023/.

Dixson, A. F., & Dixson, B. J. (2012). Venus figurines of the European Paleolithic: Symbols of fertility or attractiveness? *Journal of Anthropology, 2011,* e569120.

Durkheim, E. (1915). *The elementary forms of religious life.* Free Press.

Eliade, M. (1957). *The sacred and the profane: The nature of religion.* Harcourt.

Evans, V. (2013). *Language and time: A cognitive linguistics approach.* Cambridge University Press.

Farias, M., Newheiser, A.-K., Kahane, G., & de Toledo, Z. (2013). Scientific faith: Belief in science increases in the face of stress and existential anxiety. *Journal of Experimental Social Psychology, 49*(6), 1210–1213.

Fischer, P., Greitemeyer, T., Kastenmüller, A., Jonas, E., & Frey, D. (2006). Coping with terrorism: The impact of increased salience of terrorism on mood and self-efficacy of intrinsically religious and nonreligious people. *Personality and Social Psychology Bulletin, 32*(3), 365–377.

Francis. (2014). *Plenary session of the Pontifical Academy of Sciences: Inauguration of the bust in honour of Pope Benedict XVI (27 October 2014).* www.vatican.va/content/francesco/en/speeches/2014/october/documents/papa-francesco_20141027_plenaria-accademia-scienze.html.

Freud, S. (1961). The future of an illusion. In J. Strachey (Ed.), *The standard edition of the complete psychological works of Sigmund Freud.* Norton. (Original work published 1927)

Friedman, M., & Rholes, W. S. (2007). Successfully challenging fundamentalist beliefs results in increased death awareness. *Journal of Experimental Social Psychology, 43*(5), 794–801.

Friedman, M., & Rholes, W. S. (2008). Religious fundamentalism and terror management. *International Journal for the Psychology of Religion, 18*(1), 36–52.

Furnham, A., Meader, N., & McClelland, A. (1998). Factors affecting nonmedical participants' allocation of scarce medical resources. *Journal of Social Behavior and Personality, 13*(4), 735–746.

Gaertner, S. L., Dovidio, J. F., Anastasio, P. A., Bachman, B. A., & Rust, M. C. (1993). The common ingroup identity model: Recategorization and the reduction of intergroup bias. *European Review of Social Psychology, 4*(1), 1–26.

Gailliot, M. T., Stillman, T. F., Schmeichel, B. J., Maner, J. K., & Plant, E. A. (2008). Mortality salience increases adherence to salient norms and values. *Personality and Social Psychology Bulletin, 34*(7), 993–1003.

Gallup. (2011, December 12). *Islamophobia: Understanding anti-Muslim sentiment in the West.* https://news.gallup.com/poll/157082/islamophobia-understanding-anti-muslim-sentiment-west.aspx.

Gallup, G. G., Jr., & Anderson, J. R. (2020). Self-recognition in animals: Where do we stand 50 years later?: Lessons from cleaner wrasse and other species. *Psychology of Consciousness: Theory, Research, and Practice, 7*(1), 46–58.

Graham, J., & Haidt, J. (2010). Beyond beliefs: Religions bind individuals into moral communities. *Personality and Social Psychology Review, 14*(1), 140–150.

Greenberg, J., Pyszczynski, T., & Solomon, S. (1986). The causes and consequences of a need for self-esteem: A terror management theory. In R. F. Baumeister (Ed.), *Public self and private self* (pp. 189–212). Springer.

Greenberg, J., Pyszczynski, T., Solomon, S., Rosenblatt, A., Veeder, M., Kirkland, S., & Lyon, D. (1990). Evidence for terror management theory II: The effects of mortality salience on reactions to those who threaten or bolster the cultural worldview. *Journal of Personality and Social Psychology, 58,* 308–318.

Hayes, J., Schimel, J., & Williams, T. J. (2008). Fighting death with death: The buffering effects of learning that worldview violators have died. *Psychological Science, 19*(5), 501–507.

Hayes, J., Schimel, J., Williams, T. J., Howard, A. L., Webber, D., & Faucher, E. H. (2015). Worldview accommodation: Selectively modifying committed beliefs provides defense against worldview threat. *Self and Identity, 14*(5), 521–548.

Henderson-King, D., Henderson-King, E., Bolea, B., Koches, K., & Kauffman, A. (2004). Seeking understanding or sending bombs: Beliefs as predictors of responses to terrorism. *Peace and Conflict: Journal of Peace Psychology, 10*(1), 67–84.

Iqbal, M., O'Brien, K. S., Bliuc, A.-M., & Vergani, M. (2016). Death reminders increase agreement with extremist views but not violent extremist action in Indonesian Muslims. *Journal of Cross-Cultural Psychology, 47*(6), 891–897.

Jarrett, L., & Tatum, S. (2017, September 24). *Trump administration announces new travel restrictions*. CNN. www.cnn.com/2017/09/24/politics/trump-travel-restrictions/index.html.

Jonas, E., & Fischer, P. (2006). Terror management and religion: Evidence that intrinsic religiousness mitigates worldview defense following mortality salience. *Journal of Personality and Social Psychology, 91*(3), 553–567.

Jong, J., Halberstadt, J., & Bluemke, M. (2012). Foxhole atheism, revisited: The effects of mortality salience on explicit and implicit religious belief. *Journal of Experimental Social Psychology, 48*(5), 983–989.

Jost, J. T., Hawkins, C. B., Nosek, B. A., Hennes, E. P., Stern, C., Gosling, S. D., & Graham, J. (2014). Belief in a just god (and a just society): A system justification perspective on religious ideology. *Journal of Theoretical and Philosophical Psychology, 34*(1), 56–81.

Kemp, K. (2021, May 3). A very short introduction to the history of Catholic evolutionism. *Church Life Journal*. https://churchlifejournal.nd.edu/articles/a-very-short-introduction-to-catholic-evolutionism/.

Kirk, A., & Scott, P. (2017, February 10). Americans still support Donald Trump's immigration ban, poll shows. *The Telegraph*. www.telegraph.co.uk/news/2017/02/10/americans-still-support-donald-trumps-immigration-ban-poll-shows/.

Koca-Atabey, M., & Öner-Özkan, B. (2011). Defensive or existential religious orientations and mortality salience hypothesis: Using conservatism as a dependent measure. *Death Studies, 35*(9), 852–865.

Kosloff, S., Cesario, J., & Martens, A. (2017). *Resistance is futile: Mortality salience increases efforts to assimilate differing others into one's own worldview*. Unpublished manuscript.

Kosloff, S., Greenberg, J., Sullivan, D., & Weise, D. (2010). Of trophies and pillars: Exploring the terror management functions of short-term and long-term relationship partners. *Personality and Social Psychology Bulletin, 36*(8), 1037–1051.

Leeming, M., & Leeming, D. (1994). *Encyclopedia of creation myths*. ABC-CLIO.

Luther, M. (1529). *Martin Luther's small and large catechisms*. Concordia.

Luther, M. (1543). *On the Jews and their lies*. Concordia.

Marx, K. (1843). *Critique of Hegel's "Philosophy of Right"* (J. O'Malley, Ed.; A. Jolin, Trans.). Cambridge University Press.

Menaker, E. (1984). *Otto Rank: A rediscovered legacy*. Columbia University Press.

Mikulincer, M., Florian, V., & Hirschberger, G. (2003). The existential function of close relationships: Introducing death into the science of love. *Personality and Social Psychology Review, 7*(1), 20–40.

Motyl, M., Hart, J., Pyszczynski, T., Weise, D., Maxfield, M., & Siedel, A. (2011). Subtle priming of shared human experiences eliminates threat-induced negativity toward Arabs, immigrants, and peace-making. *Journal of Experimental Social Psychology, 47*(6), 1179–1184.

Murphy, C. (2015). *Interfaith marriage is common in U.S., particularly among the recently wed*. Pew Research Center. www.pewresearch.org/short-reads/2015/06/02/interfaith-marriage/.

Najmitdinov, J. (2021). History and factors of missionary movements in world religions. *JournalNX, 7*(12), 302–309.

Nasser, S., & McLaughlin, A. (2017, February 17). *Protesters outside Masjid Toronto call for ban on Islam as Muslims pray inside*. CBC News. www.cbc.ca/news/canada/toronto/anti-muslim-protest-masjid-toronto-1.3988906.

Norenzayan, A., & Hansen, I. G. (2006). Belief in supernatural agents in the face of death. *Personality and Social Psychology Bulletin, 32*(2), 174–187.

Norenzayan, A., Shariff, A. F., Gervais, W. M., Willard, A. K., McNamara, R. A., Slingerland, E., & Henrich, J. (2016). The cultural evolution of prosocial religions. *Behavioral and Brain Sciences, 39*, e1.

Osarchuk, M., & Tatz, S. J. (1973). Effect of induced fear of death on belief in afterlife. *Journal of Personality and Social Psychology, 27*(2), 256–260.

Pascal, B. (1669). *Pensées*. Penguin Books.

Paul, J., II. (1996). *Messaggio ai partecipanti alla Plenaria della Pontificia Accademia delle Scienze (22 ottobre 1996) | Giovanni Paolo II*. www.vatican.va/content/john-paul-ii/it/messages/pont_messages/1996/documents/hf_jp-ii_mes_19961022_evoluzione.html.

Pew Research Center. (2017a, February 15). Americans express increasingly warm feelings toward religious groups. www.pewresearch.org/religion/2017/02/15/americans-express-increasingly-warm-feelings-toward-religious-groups/.

Pew Research Center. (2017b, April 5). *The changing global religious landscape*. www.pewforum.org/2017/04/05/the-changing-global-religious-landscape/.

Pew Research Center. (2023). National public opinion reference survey (NPORS). www.pewresearch.org/methods/fact-sheet/national-public-opinion-reference-survey-npors/.

Pius XII. (1950). *Humani generis (The origin of humankind)*. www.vatican.va/content/pius-xii/en/encyclicals/documents/hf_p-xii_enc_12081950_humani-generis.html.

Pyszczynski, T., Abdollahi, A., Solomon, S., Greenberg, J., Cohen, F., & Weise, D. (2006). Mortality salience, martyrdom, and military might: The great Satan versus the axis of evil. *Personality and Social Psychology Bulletin, 32*(4), 525–537.

Pyszczynski, T., Motyl, M., Vail, K. E., Hirschberger, G., Arndt, J., & Kesebir, P. (2012). Drawing attention to global climate change decreases support for war. *Peace and Conflict: Journal of Peace Psychology, 18*(4), 354–368.

Rank, O. (1936). *Will therapy and truth and reality*. Knopf.

Rothschild, Z. K., Abdollahi, A., & Pyszczynski, T. (2009). Does peace have a prayer?: The effect of mortality salience, compassionate values, and religious fundamentalism on hostility toward out-groups. *Journal of Experimental Social Psychology, 45*(4), 816–827.

Russell, B. (1927). Why I am not a Christian. In P. Edwards (Ed.), *Why I am not a Christian, and other essays on religion and related subjects*. Simon & Schuster.

Russell, B. (1947). *Am I an atheist or an agnostic*. Haldeman-Julius.

Rutjens, B. T., van der Pligt, J., & van Harreveld, F. (2009). Things will get better: The anxiety-buffering qualities of progressive hope. *Personality and Social Psychology Bulletin, 35*(5), 535–543.

Saad, G. (2020, February 11). *Socialism and atheism still U.S. political liabilities*. Gallup. https://news.gallup.com/poll/285563/socialism-atheism-political-liabilities.aspx.

Sandstrom, A. (2021). *Biden is only the second Catholic president, but nearly all have been Christians*. Pew Research Center. www.pewresearch.org/short-reads/2021/01/20/biden-only-second-catholic-president-but-nearly-all-have-been-christians-2/.

Schimel, J., Hayes, J., Williams, T., & Jahrig, J. (2007). Is death really the worm at the core?: Converging evidence that worldview threat increases death-thought accessibility. *Journal of Personality and Social Psychology, 92*(5), 789–803.

Schoenrade, P. A. (1989). When I die . . . : Belief in afterlife as a response to mortality. *Personality and Social Psychology Bulletin, 15*(1), 91–100.

Shepard, S. (2017, July 5). *Poll: Majority of voters back Trump travel ban*. Politico. www.politico.com/story/2017/07/05/trump-travel-ban-poll-voters-240215.

Skowronski, J. J., & Sedikides, C. (2019). On the evolution of the human self: A data-driven review and reconsideration. *Self and Identity, 18*(1), 4–21.

Steigmann-Gall, R. (2003). *The Holy Reich: Nazi conceptions of Christianity, 1919–1945*. Cambridge University Press.

Stephen, L. (1893). An agnostic's apology. In C. Hitchens (Ed.), *The portable atheist: Essential readings for the nonbeliever*. Da Capo Press.

Swafford, J. (1999). *Johannes Brahms: A biography*. Macmillan.

Toft, M. D. (2007). Getting religion?: The puzzling case of Islam and Civil War. *International Security, 31*(4), 97–131.

Tremlin, T. (2006). *Minds and gods: The cognitive foundations of religion*. Oxford University Press.

Vail, K. E., Arndt, J., & Abdollahi, A. (2012). Exploring the existential function of religion and supernatural agent beliefs among Christians, Muslims, atheists, and agnostics. *Personality and Social Psychology Bulletin, 38*(10), 1288–1300.

Vail, K. E., Arndt, J., Motyl, M., & Pyszczynski, T. (2009). Compassionate values and presidential politics: Mortality salience, compassionate values, and support for Barack Obama and John McCain in the 2008 presidential election. *Analyses of Social Issues and Public Policy, 9*(1), 255–268.

Vail, K. E., Galgali, M., Lapish, C., Seeling, A., Waggoner, B., & Soenke, M. (2024a). *The impact of mortality salience on implicit and explicit activation of religious faith among religious and atheist individuals*. Unpublished manuscript, Cleveland State University.

Vail, K. E., Rothschild, Z. K., Weise, D. R., Solomon, S., Pyszczynski, T., & Greenberg, J. (2010). A terror management analysis of the psychological functions of religion. *Personality and Social Psychology Review, 14*(1), 84–94.

Vail, K. E., Seeling, A., Galgali, M., Lapish, C., & Soenke, M. (2024b). *The impact of mortality salience on closed- and open-mindedness among religious and atheist individuals*. Unpublished manuscript, Cleveland State University.

Vail, K. E., & Soenke, M. (2018). The impact of mortality awareness on meaning in life among Christians and atheists. *Religion, Brain and Behavior, 8*(1), 44–56.

Vail, K. E., Soenke, M., & Waggoner, B. (2019). Terror management theory and religious belief. In C. Routledge & M. Vess (Eds.), *Handbook of terror management theory* (pp. 259–285). Elsevier/Academic Press.

Vail, K. E., Soenke, M., Waggoner, B., & Mavropoulou, I. (2020). Natural, but not supernatural, literal immortality affirmation attenuates mortality salience effects on worldview defense in atheists. *Personality and Social Psychology Bulletin, 46*(2), 312–326.

Van Tongeren, D. R., Davis, D. E., Hook, J. N., & Johnson, K. A. (2016). Security versus growth: Existential tradeoffs of various religious perspectives. *Psychology of Religion and Spirituality, 8*(1), 77–88.

Van Tongeren, D. R., Pennington, A. R., McIntosh, D. N., Newton, T., Green, J. D., Davis, D. E., & Hook, J. N. (2017). Where, O death, is thy sting?: The meaning-providing function of beliefs in literal immortality. *Mental Health, Religion and Culture, 20*(5), 413–427.

Vandermeersch, B., & Bar-Yosef, O. (2019). The Paleolithic burials at Qafzeh Cave, Israel. *PALEO. Revue d'archéologie Préhistorique, 30–1,* Article 30–1.

Vernon, G. M. (1968). The religious "nones": A neglected category. *Journal for the Scientific Study of Religion, 7*(2), 219–229.

Vess, M., Arndt, J., Cox, C. R., Routledge, C., & Goldenberg, J. L. (2009a). Exploring the existential function of religion: The effect of religious fundamentalism and mortality salience on faith-based medical refusals. *Journal of Personality and Social Psychology, 97*(2), 334–350.

Vess, M., Routledge, C., Landau, M. J., & Arndt, J. (2009b). The dynamics of death and meaning: The effects of death-relevant cognitions and personal need for structure on perceptions of meaning in life. *Journal of Personality and Social Psychology, 97*(4), 728–744.

Williams, T. J., Schimel, J., Hayes, J., & Faucher, E. H. (2012). The effects of existential threat on reading comprehension of worldview affirming and disconfirming information. *European Journal of Social Psychology, 42*(5), 602–616.

Wilson, J. (2016, April 13). Letting them die: Parents refuse medical help for children in the name of Christ. *The Guardian.* www.theguardian.com/us-news/2016/apr/13/followers-of-christ-idaho-religious-sect-child-mortality-refusing-medical-help.

Yaakobi, E. (2015). Desire to work as a death anxiety buffer mechanism. *Experimental Psychology, 62*(2), 110–122.

Zahm, J. A. (1896). *Evolution and dogma.* D. H. McBride & Co.

CHAPTER 53

Agency, Free Will Beliefs, and Religion

Implications for Meaning Making, Self-Regulation, Well-Being, and Attributional Thinking

Jeffrey D. Green, Stephanie A. Barrientos, *and* Isabella L. Di Lauro

"Timshel!" is the last uttered word in John Steinbeck's (1952) *East of Eden*, a sprawling, multigenerational epic that recreates the Cain and Abel story. Caleb/Cain has always felt irredeemably evil and responsible for his brother's untimely death and approaches his father on the latter's deathbed. His father merely says "Timshel," Hebrew for "thou mayest." Steinbeck's masterpiece portrays evil as inevitably passing down across several generations, yet the final word suggests hope. Individuals *mayest* override family history and choose to be good. This notion of personal autonomy, of possessing free will, is a universal and deep-rooted notion.

Psychologists and philosophers have proffered various definitions of *free will*, including "free choice," "freedom from suffering," and "unconstrained desire" (Berniūnas et al., 2021), though particular emphasis has been placed on the ability to *choose to do otherwise*, also known as the *principle of alternative possibilities*, or PAP (Baumeister et al., 2010; Baumeister & Monroe, 2014; Feldman, 2017; Nichols, 2004). Some researchers have increased conceptual clarity by proposing that a component distinct from PAP is an uncoerced agent having the ability to deliberate and make a free choice, often labeled *volition* (Baumeister & Monroe, 2014). Of course, empirical approaches bypass the philosophical debates and focus on the phenomenological experience of *belief* in free will and little empirical work has attempted to distinguish volition from PAP. Recently, researchers have delved into more nuanced explorations of free will beliefs and agency, uncovering variations in these conceptualizations across religion or spirituality and culture (Berniūnas et al., 2021; Chopik et al., 2023; Joshanloo, 2022). The personal sense of free will, which we will call *free will beliefs* (FWBs), is an inextricable component of feelings of personal agency, and philosophical arguments aside, appears to be an assumption of human life woven into personal, legal, and moral life across cultures (Genschow et al., 2023). Most importantly, the assumption that individuals are free to choose their own actions is a particular emphasis of most religions (e.g., Igbokwe, 2015).

We propose a framework or hypothesis by which to view the literature on FWBs and religion/spirituality. The self-enhancement and meaning-making (SAMM) hypothesis helps explain disparate findings, from links between FWBs and well-being measures to supernatural attributional patterns that may ostensibly appear to be contradictory or self-debasing. This hypothesis is derived from the SCENT (self-concept-enhancing tactician) model that portrays strivings toward self-enhancement as tactical and contextual (Green et al., 2019; Sedikides et al., 2015), such as utilizing negative emotions for self-enhancement. Individuals focus their self-enhancement seeking on self-aspects that are central and important, which helps explain, for example, "Christian self-enhancement" (Gebauer et al., 2017) and leveraging meditation/yoga practices to augment rather than quiet the self (Gebauer et al., 2018).

The SAMM hypothesis extends its focus to both self-enhancement and meaning-enhancement motivations in religious and spiritual practices. The tripartite approach to meaning has received much recent attention and empirical validation: Meaning may be thought of as providing (1) purpose to life, (2) significance or importance, and (3) coherence or predictability. Much work on religion and spirituality provides myriad pathways to achieve one or more of these dimensions of meaning in life. Beliefs about free will and agency can further support meaning making as well as the enhancement and protection of the self.

FREE WILL BELIEFS

Most people believe that individuals are largely free to decide their fate (e.g., Wisniewski et al., 2022). Underscoring the perceived positivity of such beliefs, people believe that they possess more free will than others (Pronin et al., 2010). Some research suggests that one motivation of FWBs is the desire to hold bad actors morally responsible for their choices, which should lead to a smoother-running society; experiments in which individuals thought about or witnessed immoral behavior (i.e., classroom cheating) led to stronger motivations to punish and, in turn, stronger FWBs (Clark et al., 2014). However, some replication attempts have not been not successful; the opposite causal relation—that FWBs are necessary in order to hold individuals morally responsible for their actions—has been proposed, along with the alternative notion that FWBs are enhanced when norm violations are witnessed (Monroe & Ysidron, 2021). Thus, the relation may be bidirectional.

These lines of research illustrate that individuals vary on the strength of their beliefs. Moreover, these FWBs are malleable and thus can be experimentally manipulated (Alderson & Green, 2025). FWBs are intimately tied to religious and spiritual beliefs, though the relation can be complex. Religious and spiritual individuals endorse FWBs more than less religious individuals do (Wisniewski et al., 2022), though FWBs have not been linked to different religious *orientations* (i.e., intrinsic, extrinsic, quest; Gervais, 2014; Yilmaz et al., 2018) and a more fatalistic determinism occasionally has been positively associated with religiosity (Charzyńska & Wysocka, 2014; Yilmaz et al., 2018). For example, six experiments (Gervais, 2014) found evidence that others attribute less intention and responsibility to more highly religiously motivated individuals relative to less motivated individuals: Both religious and nonreligious observers perceived religiously motivated prosocial behaviors as less moral and autonomously enacted than the same behaviors performed by others for nonreligious reasons. Apparently, religious motivation appears to detract from a person's agency in the eyes of others: Observers see religiously motivated moral behavior as more of an ancillary than a primary goal (Gervais, 2014).

Thus, actor-observer biases likely exist regarding the limits that most religions place on thought and behavior. Though outsiders may attribute less freedom to individuals apparently motivated by their religious and spiritual beliefs, those individuals may see themselves as receiving strength to pursue more noble (and long-term) goals by avoiding temptation. Because religious individuals assert that they possess more free will, we can infer that religious limits on choice and freedom are not viewed as such by adherents. Indeed, these limits may enhance the sense of freedom and autonomy, because the beliefs and community provide support to free adherents from temptations to pursue more cherished, and religiously sanctioned, longer-term goals.

Freedom is one of Yalom's (1980) ultimate life concerns, but FWBs tie to his other cardinal life concerns of meaning versus meaninglessness, isolation versus community, and death. There is a tension between having freedom and thus taking responsibility for one's actions and their consequences, versus the safety and comfort of absolving oneself from responsibility via a religious or spiritual entity. (Indeed, an analogy might be made to the rise of a more fascist populism in many countries around the world that provides comfort in the face of perceived existential threats while removing some freedoms from the movement's own supporters.) We attempt to illustrate empirical findings that demonstrate how individuals strategically deploy FWBs, often via particular attributional strategies (attributing positive and negative events to the self or the divine as well as perceiving overlap between the self or one's conscience and the divine), in the context of their religious and spiritual beliefs, in order to meet foundational existential and self-oriented goals, consistent with our SAMM hypothesis. We also discuss many of the downstream effects of FWBs on psychological outcomes including well-being, decision making, and attributional thinking.

William James (1899/1958), illustrating his pragmatic philosophic orientation, famously proposed that his decision to believe in free will constituted some evidence for free will, because a truly free will should be able to nurture belief in free will itself. James exemplified the notion that humans ardently want to believe that they are free to choose how to act, with minimal constraint. This sense of freedom or autonomy is a centerpiece and often a primary need of many psychological theories, such as self-determination theory (Ryan & Deci, 2000). Yet Fromm (1941) argued that this belief is one of the greatest human illusions. Fromm contended that we have given up our freedom to outside sources yet deluded ourselves into thinking that the decisions are ours, in order to assuage "the fear of isolation and . . . more direct threats to our life, freedom, and comfort" (p. 242). However, other times, we seem to more explicitly and consciously embrace this outsourcing of our freedom, such as by attributing outcomes to supernatural sources (e.g., Exline & Wilt, 2023).

RELIGION, FREE WILL, AND THE AGENTIC SELF

The relationship between free will and religion or spirituality is complex. Many traditional religions seem to take a compatibilist view of free will, in which the ability to act freely coexists in "paradoxical harmony" with God's will or some cosmic principle (Igbokwe, 2015). For example, the Abrahamic religions of Christianity, Judaism, and Islam emphasize the role of God's will on life outcomes while simultaneously asserting that free will is a divine gift bestowed on humans for them to choose virtuous, divine-oriented actions (Joshanloo, 2022). Many African religions also balance both concepts by acknowledging the influence of the spirit world without removing free will (Cordeiro-Rodrigues & Agada, 2022). Hinduism proposes the concept of karma, in which the consequences of past and present actions influence future destiny without obviating free will (e.g., as described in the Bhagavadgītā; Sharma, 1979; Silvestre, 2017). Buddhism offers a fascinating case study of this dual perspective in what has been described as "agentless agency" (Repetti, 2017). The rejection of absolute free will accompanies the absence of a true self, yet it admits some level of free will necessary for adherents to follow the Eightfold Path to enlightenment (Das & Sahu, 2018). Even the issue of knowing whether one is a true adherent of a religion or not (e.g., truly "saved") may fall under this paradox, such as the theology of predestination endorsed by Calvinist Protestants: Some individuals have been chosen by God for salvation or damnation, yet they somehow are not absolved of their moral responsibilities inherent in their choices.

Perceptions of free will appear critical for individuals to feel autonomous, but they also play a critical role in how individuals are perceived by others. Individuals are acutely predisposed to see agency: Individuals attribute agency to computers, hurricanes, and, in a classic study by Heider, even moving simple geometric shapes (Heider & Simmel, 1944). Evolutionary arguments have been made to explain this apparent agency sensitivity, and such arguments have also been extended to try to explain the evolution of religion. One apparatus extensively studied as a possible cognitive precursor of religiosity was labeled a "hyperactive agency detection device" (HADD; Barrett & Lanman, 2008). In the presence of ambiguous data, humans often instinctively fill the gaps by assuming the involvement of an intentional agent. The ability to intuit the motivations, emotions, and desires of "agentic creatures," whether human or not, provides clear adaptive functions, such as a sudden sound being a potential predator. In the social arena, strategic judgments of agency enhance the predictability of one's social world and thus become a valuable tool for group living and survival.

This process is not only hyperactive but exceedingly far-reaching, thus leading to extension to the supernatural realm. Whether constructing and naming constellations from semirandom star clusters, believing in luck, or interpreting everyday events as divine interventions or omens, humans consistently infuse their seemingly arbitrary world with meaning (King et al., 2016; Van Tongeren & Green, 2010), and religious and spiritual interpretations in particular, dealing with divine guidance or eternal life, can fulfill existential needs and confer even higher doses of meaning. HADD is best understood as a dual-process model: detecting the presence of another anthropomorphic entity and then assigning intentionality to its actions. This phenomenon offers insights into another pillar of social cognition, the theory of mind (ToM) or mentalizing, delving into the thoughts, beliefs, and emotions of those around us (Premack & Woodruff, 1978). Since its introduction, researchers have looked at the implications of ToM on religious beliefs, theorizing that mentalizing also can be applied to supernatural actors such as gods or deceased loved ones (McKay & Whitehouse, 2015; Stucky & Gardner, 2022).

In a sample of conservative Christian students in the United States, agency motivation predicted greater religious judgmentalism above and beyond the influence of one's religiosity or conservatism (Beck & Miller, 2000). Given that agency motives align best with endeavors for individuality and control, the researchers argued that individuals with higher agency motives may be more prone to make critical social evaluations of others. In contrast, both communion motives and intrinsic religiosity were associated with less judgmentalism. These findings warrant replication and extension.

Berger (1967) described an existential tradeoff in which economically disadvantaged individuals who rely heavily on religion gain existential security but are alienated from their own agency: Their religiosity may render them more passive and less likely to improve their economic or social situation. Others have suggested the opposite effect of religion, proposing that religion can alleviate feelings of alienation as well as empower those who are socioeconomically disadvantaged. In this view, perceived or actual agency is enhanced via connection to a supportive faith community (Schnabel, 2021). Building on earlier research, Liu and Froese (2020) found that the relationship between religiosity and personal agency is shaped by social status and one's perception of God. In this context, a belief in divine control appears to compensate for the detrimental effects of lower socioeconomic status on an individual's sense of control. Relatedly, perceiving God as judgmental is inversely related to the sense of control across all socioeconomic groups, whereas a secure attachment to God enhances the sense of control, particularly among believers facing challenges. In line with these findings, in a nationally representative sample of Americans facing financial challenges in the aftermath of the COVID-19 pandemic, a religious change toward increased reliance on God was correlated with reduced psychological distress (Upenieks & Ellison, 2022).

An even more crucial set of strategic tradeoffs is evident in the attributions individuals make for life outcomes: Individuals may outsource agency to a divine source yet retain some measure of agency by seeing overlap between themselves or their conscience with the divine.

CAUSALITY ATTRIBUTIONS: THE INTERPLAY BETWEEN SELF AND THE DIVINE

Attribution research has a venerable research history in social psychology to help explain how individuals understand causes of their own and others' actions (e.g., Kelley, 1967), and attributions of causality are intimately tied to beliefs about free will, agency, and even actions of supernatural agents. Moreover, attribution patterns frequently serve to enhance the individual, relational, or collective self (particularly the individual self, even in collectivistic cultures; Gaertner et al., 2012). Attribution theories have been extended to elucidate how individuals meet existential as well as self needs such as perceptions of control and meaning in life via tactical attributions about the self, other individuals, and even supernatural agents or principles (Spilka et al., 1985; Wilt et al., 2024). Even negative life events can be rehabilitated to confer meaning or significance by attributing causes to divine beings or principles (karma), or by attributing them to evil spiritual forces, such as the devil or demons (Routledge, 2018; Wilt et al., 2024).

Several attributional biases about the self as well as others have been well-documented, but religious beliefs may moderate these biases. When individuals evaluate their own actions, they tend to credit successes to themselves, while attributing shortcomings to external circumstances (self-serving bias [SSB]; e.g., Miller & Ross, 1975). Specific religious beliefs appear to moderate the SSB: Self-serving attributions were higher among Taiwanese Mahayana Christians relative to Taiwanese Buddhists (Huang & Wang, 2019). The authors attributed this difference to the Christian emphasis on the soul and the relationship with God, versus the Buddhist focus on interdependence and abolishing the distinction between self and other. In contrast, when observers assess the behaviors of others, they often downplay the situational influences and overattribute actions to stable individual traits or characteristics (i.e., the fundamental attribution error [FAE]; Li et al., 2012). A study found that the FAE was stronger in Protestants than Catholics (Li et al., 2012); this phenomenon was mediated by the stronger belief in a soul among Protestants. Though much more work is needed to further understand these phenomena (such as by using more sophisticated and more direct measures of self-relevant constructs and by studying additional religious and spiritual groups), the role of the self and self-motivations is critical.

What might help balance or explain when individuals willingly cede agency or self-enhancement opportunities to God or fate when good things happen to them? Having a powerful spiritual entity (or even fate) consider their happiness, care enough to intervene, and exert their power to improve their lives is highly flattering and likely confers meaning in life via augmented significance and purpose (Exline & Wilt, 2024). In addition, and consistent with our SAMM hypothesis, close identification or closeness with a deity in particular may be a method of indirect self-enhancement, akin to tactics individuals deploy when they engage in romantic-partner or ingroup enhancement and view their self-concepts as overlapping with such individuals and groups (Aron et al., 2022).

Attributional Tradeoffs between the Self versus the Supernatural

Though certain situational factors, such as the occurrence of rare or unusual events, surely heighten the likelihood of supernatural attributions, motivational factors including the need to confirm existing worldviews, meaning or self-enhancement strivings (such as God intervening personally to render assistance in a crisis), and wanting to see God as both powerful and personal are particularly important (Exline & Pait, 2021). For example, those who see God as more loving or who feel closer to God, also see God as bestowing more gifts to individuals, which enhances their sense of gratitude (Exline & Wilt, 2024). People motivated to see God as active and intervening benevolently in human affairs have indeed reported experiencing such gifts to a greater extent (Exline & Wilt, 2024).

A recent 3-week experience sampling study (Wilt et al., 2024) of supernatural attributions and meaning found that individuals who made more attributions to God for both positive and negative events also reported higher meaning in life, though the findings for positive (versus negative) events were more robust. Attributions to the devil or demons were not associated with meaning in life generally, though those with strong religious views did exhibit this association (Wilt et al., 2024). Though correlational, this pattern of results is consistent with the SAMM: Individuals do not appear to sacrifice their felt meaning in life by liberally attributing the causes of life events to supernatural entities rather than the self. However, future work should attempt to address causality as well as assess more than perceived meaning in life, such as perceptions of agency or life satisfaction.

Complementary research on *God attributions* and *God-serving biases*, in which positive outcomes are attributed to God and negative outcomes are not, is consistent with the aforementioned work by Exline and colleagues and may also provide hints regarding mechanisms and motivations (DeBono et al., 2020; Riggio et al., 2014; Spilka et al., 1985; Wilt et al., 2024). For example, DeBono and colleagues (2020) observed a God-serving attributional bias regarding a game in which U.S. college students were randomly assigned to win or lose via false feedback. God frequently was credited for victories, whereas "other factors" were more often viewed as the causes of losses. Importantly, individuals who perceived God as an integral part of the self (measured via a single face-valid item) tended to exhibit an increased propensity for God-serving biases. The researchers theorized that this attributional strategy might ultimately boost self-esteem by enhancing what they referred to as "God-esteem." Related research that also at least indirectly investigated God–individual overlap examined God's influence on personal *consciences*. Those who endorsed greater divine influence on their conscience also reported following their own conscience more in everyday life (Schutt & Exline, 2025). To be specific, believing that God influences the conscience predicted perceiving one's conscience as more important and reliable, which in turn predicted the prioritization of following one's conscience (Schutt & Exline, 2025). Taken together, beliefs regarding overlap between the self and the divine appear to affect both attributions regarding the cause of major life events and moral choices. Though the theological beliefs may vary considerably regarding the precise nature of intersection with the divine, and much more research is needed, this organizing principle, consistent with the SAMM hypothesis, may help guide future research. While on the surface individuals may be eschewing direct self-enhancement opportunities, such as when they attribute their successes to God, they appear to tactically enhance the self or their meaning in life by endorsing overlap or closeness to God or God acting through them. Thus, the potential loss of agency or loss of esteem opportunities are more than offset by the divine conferring even greater significance to the self.

Supernatural Attributions and Moral Choices and Actions, Both Good and Evil

Beyond their role in personal coping and meaning making, supernatural beliefs are important to moral reasoning as well as moral *action*. For example, research on the classic "trolley problem," involving U.S. Christian and Israeli Jewish individuals found that moral judgments to act or abstain were more influenced by how responsibility was assigned than by participant religiosity (Barak-Corren & Bazerman, 2017). Those who justified avoiding personal responsibility by attributing the outcome to supernatural powers refrained from action, presuming that it was "up to God" to determine which lives would be saved, but those who rejected the idea that the decision was up to God made more utilitarian judgments, intervening to sacrifice one to save several lives (Barak-Corren & Bazerman, 2017). More research is needed linking supernatural attributions and actions, particularly moral actions.

Of course, individuals are remarkably adept at rationalizing and justifying their bad behavior through creative remembering, interpretation, and attention (e.g., Green et al., 2009; Sedikides et al., 2016). They can excuse actions by attributing them not simply to overwhelming situational forces, but to fate or to malevolent spiritual forces. We propose that tactical deployment of supernatural attributions sometimes may be extended to justify immoral behavior at the individual or the group level. For example, beliefs such as perceiving other individuals or groups under demonic influence or thinking that God is clearly on the side of only the ingroup may cultivate not only ingroup favoritism but outgroup demonization. Aggressive acts toward a vilified outgroup may even be sanctified by being cast as protecting the ingroup, which has a chosen and holy role in the world (Reicher et al., 2008). That is, the ingroup may be viewed as chosen by God to redeem the world, which can justify almost any actions (Exline & Wilt, 2023), which we have seen recently in the political realm for countries that are highly politically polarized.

This work might dovetail with research suggesting that a more deterministic outlook may justify the status quo or lead to passivity regarding injustice: Attributing outcomes to fate or a deity may have similar outcomes (Carey & Paulhus, 2013). Certainly, investigating how the overlap between self and God potentially competes with the perceived overlap (or lack thereof) between self and others, and between ingroups and outgroups, could yield valuable insights into a possible dark side to supernatural attributions by sanctifying evil and discriminatory behavior.

Collectively, these studies offer compelling evidence that religious attributions are indeed connected to how individuals perceive themselves, interpret the actions of others, and understand their own experiences relative to the divine. Though some ostensibly self-deprecating attributional patterns may be evident, extant empirical work so far suggests that tactical self-enhancement or meaning making may more than offset this lost opportunity for esteem.

PSYCHOLOGICAL OUTCOMES OF STRONGER FWBs

We have hinted at the psychological benefits of stronger FWBs, but a more systematic review is appropriate that addresses how religious or spiritual beliefs might moderate such outcomes. Correlational research has been mixed and relatively sparse, but the majority of the findings have revealed a positive correlation between high endorsement of FWBs and well-being (Zhao & Huo, 2022). Life satisfaction has been higher in individuals who endorsed FWBs (e.g., Kondratowicz-Nowak & Zawadzka, 2018; Li et al.; 2017; Moynihan et al., 2017). These findings were replicated in collectivistic cultures for life satisfaction as well as positive affect (e.g., Li et al., 2017). Similar research also has found a positive association between FWBs and meaning in life (e.g., Moynihan et al., 2019), and, of course, religiosity has also contributed to higher perceived meaning in life (Prinzing et al., 2023).

Findings from longitudinal studies also have been inconsistent but hinted more strongly at a causal relationship from FWB strength to psychological well-being. One study employing a single item to measure FWBs did not reveal an association (Gooding et al., 2018), but a better designed cross-lagged study did reveal a positive association (Zhao & Huo, 2022).

Largely absent until recently, experimental work has provided the strongest evidence for the psychological benefits of endorsing FWBs (Alderson & Green, 2025; Moynihan et al., 2019). The purpose-imbuing model of FWBs (Alderson & Green, 2025) proposes that endorsing FWBs enhances felt meaning in life, which in turn enhances eudaimonic and hedonic well-being. Of particular note, an experiment manipulated FWBs (three levels: pro-FWBs, anti-FWBs, and control) via a previously used and validated Velten-like procedure (e.g., Alquist et al., 2015; Vohs & Schooler, 2008). Participants read 10 statements in sequence that were neutral, pro-FWB (e.g., "The most current knowledge from physics supports indeterminacy is a core property of reality, making human free will entirely plausible"), or anti-FWB (e.g., "A belief in free will contradicts the known fact that the universe is governed by lawful principles of science"). Participants then spent 30 seconds reflecting on and then writing each statement into their own words. The pro-FWB manipulation enhanced both hedonic and eudaimonic well-being relative to the control, whereas the anti-FWB manipulation diminished both hedonic and eudaimonic well-being relative to the control. In all cases, the effects were mediated by meaning in life (as assessed by the Meaning in Life Questionnaire [MLQ]; Steger et al., 2006).

Believing more strongly in free will has been linked to other salubrious psychological outcomes. Spirituality (but not religiosity) was positively associated with self-efficacy and this link was partially (for females) or fully (for males) mediated by FWB endorsement (Charzyńska & Wysocka, 2014). In fact, for males, religiosity was correlated with fatalistic determinism. It may be that, compared to beliefs in an established monotheistic religion, general spirituality is relatively more potent when it comes to feeling like an effective agent.

Decision making, particularly the subjective ease with which decisions are made as well as the satisfaction or confidence in those decisions, appears to have a bidirectional association with FWBs. Individuals who believed more strongly in free will found decision making to be easier and were more satisfied with their decisions (Feldman et al., 2014). The same authors also found that FWBs were strengthened following making choices or even simply recalling past choices (Feldman et al., 2014). Lay experiences of free will seem to center on more salient perceptions of choice.

In two experiments, participants induced to disbelieve in the existence of free will conformed to a greater extent (Alquist et al., 2013). Stronger FWBs also have been linked to stronger academic performance (Feldman et al., 2016) as well as superior performance at work (Stillman et al., 2010). These effects should be replicated while examining potential correlations with religious constructs; future research also should investigate the overlapping constructs of FWB, agency, and self-efficacy, particularly vis-à-vis religious and spiritual beliefs.

The link between stronger FWBs and religion seems to be well placed: A number of moral behaviors have been positively linked to endorsing such beliefs. Stronger FWBs have been linked to reduced cheating (Vohs & Schooler, 2008), less aggression, and greater helpfulness (Baumeister et al., 2009). Judgments and behaviors directed toward others also reveal some interactions between religious beliefs and FWBs. Those with stronger FWBs, whether at the dispositional level or via experimental manipulation, had more retributive attitudes toward punishment, though consequentialist attitudes were unchanged by a free will manipulation (Shariff et al., 2014). The experimental manipulation focused on reading about the neural bases of behavior (intended to weaken FWBs); such exposure reduced the endorsement of retributive punishment for wrongdoers. Other work has found that religious individuals hold stronger FWBs; thus, one might speculate about the potency of a free will manipulation among the highly religious, who may have more elaborated reasons for wanting to believe in personal responsibility for both theological and sociological reasons.

Related work found a link between beliefs in a powerful and interventionist God and willingness to experience "altruistic punishment," or shouldering a punishment burden for the greater societal good (Laurin et al., 2012). Some evolutionary theories regarding religion have emphasized its role in discouraging and punishing antisocial behaviors, particularly via an omniscient and omnipotent God. Punishment in larger societies is costly (e.g., monitoring behavior, administering punishment, risking retribution) and more transgressors will escape detection in larger societies, which could encourage even more norm violations. Thus, belief in God (or perhaps principles such as karma) might facilitate internalizing avoidance of antisocial behaviors; thus, some roles of monitoring and punishing bad behavior are outsourced to the supernatural. Five studies found that stronger beliefs in God were associated with lower motivation for costly societal punishment, operationalized as the willingness of participants to use their own resources to punish a transgressor. However, FWBs, measured in only one study, did not moderate these findings (Laurin et al., 2012). Future research needs to examine these patterns among adherents of a wider variety of religions across cultures.

Very few negative outcomes of believing in free will have been identified, perhaps because these perceptions about the nature of reality are closely aligned (positively correlated) with beliefs about the self's freedom and autonomy, such as self-efficacy and locus of control, which have established positive psychological benefits. Underscoring how individuals perceive free will to be positive, the aforementioned finding that individuals believe that they possess more free will than others is notable (Pronin et al., 2010).

Religion, Agency, and Self-Control

Religion has been described as a cultural adaptation that emerged to promote self-control for the collective benefit of society. Self-control enables individuals to regulate their behavior in order to avoid more short-term (and often selfish) actions in favor of pursuing longer-term goals, even in the face of tempting alternatives (Baumeister & Exline, 1999; McCullough & Willoughby, 2009). Reviews of religion and self-control (e.g., Marcus & McCullough, 2021; McCullough & Willoughby, 2009) have argued for the impact of religiosity on self-monitoring, self-regulatory strength, and the development of particular self-regulatory skills or rituals. However, just as attributional decisions often involve tradeoffs, restricting one's viable behavioral choices may have varying effects on attention, self-regulation, and goal-setting (Baumeister & Monroe, 2014; Rounding et al., 2012). Ritualistic behaviors and deontological ethics offer religious adherents a more restricted set of options, potentially alleviating the cognitive burden of moral decision making or of choosing among an overwhelming number of options (Barak-Corren & Bazerman, 2017; Baumeister et al., 2010; Friese & Wänke, 2014; Marcus & McCullough, 2021). Therefore, outsourcing personal agency, whether through seeking divine guidance, prayer, or supernatural attributions, may allow individuals to experience compensatory control while also absolving themselves of responsibility (Barak-Corren & Bazerman, 2017; Kay et al., 2009). That is, consistent with the SAMM hypothesis, principles similar to those discussed regarding supernatural attributions may confer psychological as well as tangible benefits, such as divine assistance in reaching valued personal goals: Individuals tactically give up perceptions of agency and control in order to extract higher-value meaning or self-enhancement.

Research on emotion regulation often has been artificially separated from behavior regulation theory and research, but many religious beliefs have clear links to particular emotion regulation strategies and practices (Vishkin, 2021). Religions typically promote the idea that emotions can be controlled; moreover, they advocate the pursuit of positive over negative emotions and other-elevating emotions like awe over self-elevating emotions like pride (Vishkin et al., 2020). Culture as well as specific religious beliefs matter, of course; for example, Christians typically value high-arousal positive affect, whereas Buddhists value low-arousal positive affect (Tsai et al., 2007). Religions also promote emotion regulation strategies such as attentional focus and especially cognitive reappraisal, which changes the interpretation of events in order to alter the emotions and is intimately linked to felt meaning in life (Vishkin et al., 2016). By training individuals to moderate their emotions as well as their cognitions about such emotions, religions alter behaviors that flow from such emotions.

Religiously prescribed or proscribed behavior may have ostensibly paradoxical effects on the sense of free will and autonomy. On the one hand, selfish behaviors are discouraged or even actively punished in the community, limiting personal freedom and perhaps even occasionally sparking reactance. On the other hand, the encouragement of selfless behavior may provide greater motivation as well as social support for individuals to engage in behaviors consistent with their religious identities or long-term goals. Virtually all religious groups, through religious texts and exhortations from leaders and fellow members, place a premium on "ego dampening" (Sasaki & Kim, 2021). In a series of four experiments, when religious cues were made salient, participants exhibited higher self-control, which then led them to make more adaptive decisions, such as exercising patience and delaying gratification (Rounding et al., 2012). Religious involvement also has been associated with decreased impulsive or socially harmful behaviors, such as alcohol use (Meyers et al., 2017) and sexual promiscuity (Schmitt & Fuller, 2015).

In one illustrative study, personal prayer, versus an open-thinking control condition, counteracted depletion for a second task following an initial depleting event (Stroop task following emotion suppression; Friese & Wänke, 2014). Interestingly, religiosity did not moderate the findings, and the overall religiosity of the sample was moderately low. Other work using a highly similar two-task paradigm, however, examined individual differences in religiosity and found that more religious people persevered on a frustrating task longer than less religious people did after depletion, though no differences were found in the absence of depletion (Watterson & Giesler, 2012). These studies were designed in concordance with the ego depletion model that has been seriously questioned in recent years, but other explanations for these patterns of findings might be proffered and tested in future research (Inzlicht et al., 2021). A recent review of experimental and longitudinal work provided evidence that the religiosity to self-control link is not merely correlational but is causal and has pointed primarily to the longer-term influence of religious contexts (church, school) and rituals such as prayer to build self-regulatory habits over time (Marcus & McCullough, 2021).

CONCLUSIONS

Perceptions of free will and agency are crucial to a broad swath of human behavior and emotion, but in many respects research is just beginning, particularly regarding attention to religion and spirituality. FWBs are almost always associated with psychological health as well as religious beliefs, though there are exceptions, particularly for religious beliefs less consistent with traditional monotheistic religions. Self-control also is influenced by FWBs and religious beliefs, almost always positively. Attributions regarding the causes of behavior are a particularly fascinating and important realm affecting perception of self and others, and recent supernatural attribution work suggests tactical tradeoffs regarding perceptions of agency. Moreover, individuals strategically leverage their FWBs in order to directly or indirectly flatter the self, such as when they incorporate aspects of a deity into their self-concepts and attribute positive traits or actions to the deity (Exline & Wilt, 2024).

Though making sweeping generalizations in this complex literature is fraught with danger, our proposed SAMM hypothesis may help organize much of the reviewed work in spite of the fact that direct empirical tests largely are lacking. For example, we proposed that self-regulation choices (choosing religiously prescribed behaviors and avoiding proscribed behaviors) as well as tactical attribution patterns involve tradeoffs: Individuals willingly give up perceptions of agency or control or even tempting behaviors to achieve greater gains in self-enhancement or meaning making. Saying that God is controlling one's destiny may cede some sense of agency or free will, but the benefits of felt closeness to an omnipotent and personally interested God may more than outweigh the loss. We hope that the SAMM and other theoretical frameworks will provide guidance for future research in this rich yet complex area so central to human endeavors.

REFERENCES

Alderson, C. J., & Green, J. D. (2025). Investigating the potential causal relationship between free will belief and well-being. Unpublished manuscript.

Alquist, J. L., Ainsworth, S. E., & Baumeister, R. F. (2013). Determined to conform: Disbelief in free will increases conformity. *Journal of Experimental Social Psychology, 49*(1), 80–86.

Alquist, J. L., Ainsworth, S. E., Baumeister, R. F., Daly, M., & Stillman, T. F. (2015). The making of might-have-beens: Effects of free will belief on counterfactual thinking. *Personality and Social Psychology Bulletin, 41*(2), 268–283.

Aron, A., Lewandowski, G., Branand, B., Mashek, D., & Aron, E. (2022). Self-expansion motivation and inclusion of others in self: An updated review. *Journal of Social and Personal Relationships, 39*(12), 3821–3852.

Barak-Corren, N., & Bazerman, M. H. (2017). Is saving lives your task or God's?: Religiosity, belief in God, and moral judgment. *Judgment and Decision Making, 12*(3), 280–296.

Barrett, J. L., & Lanman, J. A. (2008). The science of religious beliefs: Cognitive science of religion. *Religion (London), 38*(2), 109–124.

Baumeister, R. F., Bauer, I. M., & Lloyd, S. A. (2010). Choice, free will, and religion. *Psychology of Religion and Spirituality, 2*(2), 67–82.

Baumeister, R. F., & Exline, J. J. (1999). Virtue, personality, and social relations: Self-control as the moral muscle. *Journal of Personality, 67*(6), 1165–1194.

Baumeister, R. F., Mele, A. R., & Vohs, K. D. (Eds.). (2010). *Free will and consciousness:*

How might they work? Oxford University Press.
Baumeister, R. F., Masicampo, E. J., & DeWall, C. N. (2009). Prosocial benefits of feeling free: Disbelief in free will increases aggression and reduces helpfulness. *Personality and Social Psychology Bulletin, 35*(2), 260–268.
Baumeister, R. F., & Monroe, A. E. (2014). Recent research on free will: Conceptualizations, beliefs, and processes. *Advances in Experimental Social Psychology, 50,* 1–52.
Beck, R., & Miller, C. D. (2000). Religiosity and agency and communion: Their relationship to religious judgmentalism. *Journal of Psychology, 134*(3), 315–324.
Berger, P. (1967). *The sacred canopy: Elements of a sociological theory of religion.* Doubleday.
Berniūnas, R., Beinorius, A., Dranseika, V., Silius, V., & Rimkevičius, P. (2021). The weirdness of belief in free will. *Consciousness and Cognition, 87,* 103054–103054.
Carey, J. M., & Paulhus, D. L. (2013). Worldview implications of believing in free will and/or determinism: Politics, morality, and punitiveness. *Journal of Personality, 81*(2), 130–141.
Charzyńska, E., & Wysocka, E. (2014). The role of spirituality and belief in free will in the perception of self-efficacy among young adults. *New Educational Review, 36*(2), 194–205.
Chopik, W. J., Confer, J. A., & Motyl, M. (2023). Age differences in free will and control perceptions across the lifespan and around the world. *Current Research in Ecological and Social Psychology, 4.*
Clark, C. J., Luguri, J. B., Ditto, P. H., Knobe, J., Shariff, A. F., & Baumeister, R. F. (2014). Free to punish: A motivated account of free will belief. *Journal of Personality and Social Psychology, 106*(4), 501–513.
Cordeiro-Rodrigues, L., & Agada, A. (2022). African philosophy of religion: Concepts of God, ancestors, and the problem of evil. *Philosophy Compass, 17*(8).
Das, P., & Sahu, V. (2018). Freedom of the will and no-self in Buddhism. *Journal of Indian Council of Philosophical Research, 35*(1), 121–138.
DeBono, A., Poepsel, D., & Corley, N. (2020). Thank God for my successes (not my failures): Feeling God's presence explains a God attribution bias. *Psychological Reports, 123*(5), 1663–1687.
Exline, J. J., & Pait, K. C. (2021). Perceiving messages from the divine and departed: An attributional perspective. In T. G. Plante & G. E. Schwartz (Eds.), *Human interaction with the divine, the sacred, and the deceased* (pp. 245–259). Routledge.
Exline, J. J., & Wilt, J. A. (2023). Supernatural attributions: Seeing God, the devil, demons, spirits, fate, and karma as causes of events. *Annual Review of Clinical Psychology, 19,* 461–487.
Exline, J. J., & Wilt, J. A. (2024). Divine attributions, gift appraisals, and supernatural operating rules as predictors of gratitude to God. *Journal of Positive Psychology, 19*(1), 95–106.
Feldman, G. (2017). Making sense of agency: Belief in free will as a unique and important construct. *Social and Personality Psychology Compass, 11*(1).
Feldman, G., Baumeister, R. F., & Wong, K. F. E. (2014). Free will is about choosing: The link between choice and the belief in free will. *Journal of Experimental Social Psychology, 55,* 239–245.
Feldman, G., Chandrashekar, S. P., & Wong, K. F. E. (2016). The freedom to excel: Belief in free will predicts better academic performance. *Personality and Individual Differences, 90,* 377–383.
Friese, M., & Wänke, M. (2014). Personal prayer buffers self-control depletion. *Journal of Experimental Social Psychology, 51, 56–59.*
Fromm, E. (1941). *Escape from freedom.* Rinehart.
Gaertner, L., Sedikides, C., Luke, M., O'Mara, E. M., Iuzzini, J., Jackson, L. E., . . . Wu, Q. (2012). A motivational hierarchy within: Primacy of the individual self, relational self, or collective self? *Journal of Experimental Social Psychology, 48*(5), 997–1013.
Gebauer, J. E., Nehrlich, A. D., Stahlberg, D., Sedikides, C., Hackenschmidt, A., Schick, D., . . . Mander, J. (2018). Mind-body practices and the self: Yoga and meditation do not quiet the ego but instead boost self-enhancement. *Psychological Science, 29*(8), 1299–1308.
Gebauer, J. E., Sedikides, C., & Schrade, A. (2017). Christian self-enhancement. *Journal of Personality and Social Psychology, 113*(5), 786–809.
Genschow, O., Cracco, E., Schneider, J., Protzko, J., Wisniewski, D., Brass, M., & Schooler, J. W. (2023). Manipulating belief in free will and its downstream consequences: A meta-analysis. *Personality and Social Psychology Review, 27*(1), 52–82.
Gervais, W. M. (2014). Good for God? Religious motivation reduces perceived responsibility for and morality of good deeds. *Journal of Experimental Psychology: General, 143*(4), 1616–1626.
Gooding, P. L. T., Callan, M. J., & Hughes, G. (2018). The association between believing in free will and subjective well-being is confounded by a sense of personal control. *Frontiers in Psychology, 9,* 623–623.

Green, J. D., Sedikides, C., Pinter, B., & Van Tongeren, D. R. (2009). Two sides to self-protection: Self-improvement strivings and feedback from close relationships eliminate mnemic neglect. *Self and Identity, 8*(2–3), 233–250.

Green, J. D., Sedikides, C., Van Tongeren, D. R., Behler, A. M. C., & Barber, J. M. (2019). Self-enhancement, righteous anger, and moral grandiosity. *Self and Identity, 18*(2), 201–216.

Heider, F., & Simmel, M. (1944). An experimental study of apparent behavior. *American Journal of Psychology, 57*(2), 243–259.

Huang, T.-R., & Wang, Y. H. (2019). Perceiving self, others, and events through a religious lens: Mahayana Buddhists vs. Christians. *Frontiers in Psychology, 10,* 217–217.

Igbokwe, A. C. (2015). Freewill and determinism: The African perspective and experience. *Global Journal of Arts Humanities and Social Sciences, 4*(2), 75–82.

Inzlicht, M., Werner, K. M., Briskin, J. L., & Roberts, B. W. (2021). Integrating models of self-regulation. *Annual Review of Psychology, 72,* 319–345.

James, W. (1958). *Talks to teachers.* Norton. (Original work published 1899)

Joshanloo, M. (2022). The relationship between fatalistic beliefs and well-being depends on personal and national religiosity: A study in 34 countries. *Heliyon, 8*(6), e09814–e09814.

Kay, A. C., Whitson, J. A., Gaucher, D., & Galinsky, A. D. (2009). Compensatory control: Achieving order through the mind, our institutions, and the Heavens. *Current Directions in Psychological Science, 18*(5), 264–268.

Kelley, H. H. (1967). Attribution theory in social psychology. In *Nebraska Symposium on Motivation* (Vol. 15, pp. 192–238). University of Nebraska.

King, L. A., Heintzelman, S. J., & Ward, S. J. (2016). Beyond the search for meaning: A contemporary science of the experience of meaning in life. *Current Directions in Psychological Science, 25*(4), 211–216.

Kondratowicz-Nowak, B. B., & Zawadzka, A. M. (2018). Does belief in free will make us feel good and satisfied? *Health Psychology Report, 6*(2), 109–117.

Laurin, K., Shariff, A. F., Henrich, J., & Kay, A. C. (2012). Outsourcing punishment to God: Beliefs in divine control reduce earthly punishment. *Proceedings of the Royal Society: B, Biological Sciences, 279*(1741), 3272–3281.

Li, C., Wang, S., Zhao, Y., Kong, F., & Li, J. (2017). The freedom to pursue happiness: Belief in free will predicts life satisfaction and positive affect among Chinese adolescents. *Frontiers in Psychology, 7,* 2027–2027.

Li, P. F. J., & Wong, Y. J. (2020). Beliefs in free will versus determinism: Search for meaning mediates the life scheme–depressive symptom link. *Journal of Humanistic Psychology.*

Li, Y. J., Johnson, K. A., Cohen, A. B., Knowles, E. D., Williams, M. J., & Zhansheng, C. (2012). Fundamental(ist) attribution error: Protestants are dispositionally focused. *Journal of Personality and Social Psychology, 102*(2), 281–290.

Liu, Y., & Froese, P. (2020). Faith and agency: The relationships between sense of control, socioeconomic status, and beliefs about God. *Journal for the Scientific Study of Religion, 59*(2), 311–326.

Marcus, Z. J., & McCullough, M. E. (2021). Does religion make people more self-controlled?: A review of research from the lab and life. *Current Opinion in Psychology, 40,* 167–170.

McCullough, M. E., & Willoughby, B. L. B. (2009). Religion, self-regulation, and self-control: Associations, explanations, and implications. *Psychological Bulletin, 135*(1), 69–93.

McKay, R., & Whitehouse, H. (2015). Religion and morality. *Psychological Bulletin, 141*(2), 447–473.

Meyers, J. L., Brown, Q., Grant, B. F., & Hasin, D. (2017). Religiosity, race/ethnicity, and alcohol use behaviors in the United States. *Psychological Medicine, 47*(1), 103–114.

Miller, D. T., & Ross, M. (1975). Self-serving biases in the attribution of causality: Fact or fiction? *Psychological Bulletin, 82*(2), 213–225.

Monroe, A. E., & Ysidron, D. W. (2021). Not so motivated after all?: Three replication attempts and a theoretical challenge to a morally motivated belief in free will. *Journal of Experimental Psychology: General, 150*(1), e1–e12.

Moynihan, A. B., Igou, E. R., & van Tilburg, W. A. P. (2017). Boredom increases impulsiveness: A meaning-regulation perspective. *Social Psychology, 48*(5), 293–309.

Moynihan, A. B., Igou, E. R., & van Tilburg, W. A. P. (2019). Lost in the crowd: Conformity as escape following disbelief in free will. *European Journal of Social Psychology, 49*(3), 503–520.

Nichols, S. (2004). The folk psychology of free will: Fits and starts. *Mind and Language, 19*(5), 473–502.

Premack, D., & Woodruff, G. (1978). Does the chimpanzee have a theory of mind? *Behavioral and Brain Sciences, 1*(4), 515–526.

Prinzing, M., Van Cappellen, P., & Fredrickson, B. L. (2023). More than a momentary blip in the universe? Investigating the link between religiousness and perceived meaning in life.

Personality and Social Psychology Bulletin, 49(2), 180–196.

Pronin, E., Kugler, M. B., & Nisbett, R. E. (2010). People believe they have more free will than others. *Proceedings of the National Academy of Sciences, 107*(52), 22469–22474.

Reicher, S., Haslam, S. A., & Rath, R. (2008). Making a virtue of evil: A five-step social identity model of the development of collective hate. *Social and Personality Psychology Compass, 2*(3), 1313–1344.

Repetti, R. (2017). *Buddhist perspectives on free will: Agentless agency?* Routledge.

Riggio, H. R., Uhalt, J., & Matthies, B. K. (2014). Unanswered prayers: Religiosity and the God-serving bias. *Journal of Social Psychology, 154*(6), 491–514.

Rounding, K., Lee, A., Jacobson, J. A., & Ji, L.-J. (2012). Religion replenishes self-control. *Psychological Science, 23*(6), 635–642.

Routledge, C. (2018). *Supernatural: Death, meaning, and the power of the invisible.* Oxford University Press.

Ryan, R. M., & Deci, E. L. (2000). Self-determination theory and the facilitation of intrinsic motivation, social development, and well-being. *American Psychologist, 55*(1), 68–78.

Sasaki, J. Y., &; Kim, H. S. (2021). The ego dampening influence of religion: Evidence from behavioral genetics and psychology. *Current Opinion in Psychology, 40,* 24–28.

Schmitt, D. P., & Fuller, R. C. (2015). On the varieties of sexual experience: Cross-cultural links between religiosity and human mating strategies. *Psychology of Religion and Spirituality, 7*(4), 314–326.

Schnabel, L. (2021). Opiate of the masses?: Inequality, religion, and political ideology in the United States. *Social Forces, 99*(3), 979–1012.

Schutt, W. A., & Exline, J. J. (2025). Do adults believe that god or the devil can influence their conscience?: Links between religion/spirituality, beliefs about the conscience, and attempts to follow one's conscience. *Spirituality in Clinical Practice, 12*(1), 98–113.

Sedikides, C., Gaertner, L., & Cai, H. (2015). On the panculturality of self-enhancement and self-protection motivation: The case for the universality of self-esteem. In A. J. Elliot (Ed.), *Advances in motivation science* (pp. 185–241). Elsevier.

Sedikides, C., Green, J. D., Saunders, J., Skowronski, J. J., & Zengel, B. (2016). Mnemic neglect: Selective amnesia of one's faults. *European Review of Social Psychology, 27*(1), 1–62.

Shariff, A. F., Greene, J. D., Karremans, J. C., Luguri, J. B., Clark, C. J., Schooler, J. W., . . . Vohs, K. D. (2014). Free will and punishment: A mechanistic view of human nature reduces retribution. *Psychological Science, 25*(8), 1563–1570.

Sharma, A. (1979). Fate and free will in the Bhagavadgītā. *Religious Studies, 15*(4), 531–537.

Silvestre, R. S. (2017). Karma theory, determinism, fatalism and freedom of will. *Logica Universalis, 11*(1), 35–60.

Spilka, B., Shaver, P., & Kirkpatrick, L. A. (1985). A general attribution theory for the psychology of religion. *Journal for the Scientific Study of Religion, 24*(1), 1–20.

Steger, M. F., Frazier, P., Oishi, S., & Kaler, M. (2006). The meaning in life questionnaire: Assessing the presence of and search for meaning in life. *Journal of Counseling Psychology, 53*(1), 80–93.

Steinbeck, J. (1952). *East of Eden.* Viking Press.

Stillman, T. F., Baumeister, R. F., Vohs, K. D., Lambert, N. M., Fincham, F. D., & Brewer, L. E. (2010). Personal philosophy and personnel achievement: Belief in free will predicts better job performance. *Social Psychological and Personality Science, 1*(1), 43–50.

Stucky, K., & Gardner, A. (2022). The evolution of religiosity by kin selection. *Religion, Brain, and Behavior, 12*(4), 347–364.

Tsai, J. L., Miao, F. F., & Seppala, E. (2007). Good feelings in Christianity and Buddhism: Religious differences in ideal affect. *Personality and Social Psychology Bulletin, 33*(3), 409–421.

Upenieks, L., & Ellison, C. G. (2022). Changes in religiosity and reliance on God during the COVID-19 pandemic: A protective role under conditions of financial strain? *Review of Religious Research, 64*(4), 853–881.

Van Tongeren, D. R., & Green, J. D. (2010). Combating meaninglessness: On the automatic defense of meaning. *Personality and Social Psychology Bulletin, 36*(10), 1372–1384.

Vishkin, A. (2021). Variation and consistency in the links between religion and emotion regulation. *Current Opinion in Psychology, 40,* 6–9.

Vishkin, A., Bigman, Y. E., Porat, R., Solak, N., Halperin, E., & Tamir, M. (2016). God rest our hearts: Religiosity and cognitive reappraisal. *Emotion, 16*(2), 252–262.

Vishkin, A., Schwartz, S. H., Ben-Nun Bloom, P., Solak, N., & Tamir, M. (2020). Religiosity and desired emotions: Belief maintenance or prosocial facilitation? *Personality and Social Psychology Bulletin, 46*(7), 1090–1106.

Vohs, K. D., & Schooler, J. W. (2008). The value of believing in free will: Encouraging a belief in determinism increases cheating. *Psychological Science, 19,* 49–54.

Watterson, K., & Giesler, R. B. (2012). Religiosity and self-control: When the going gets tough, the religious get self-regulating. *Psychology of Religion and Spirituality, 4*(3), 193–205.

Wilt, J. A., Van Tongeren, D. R., & Exline, J. J. (2024). Are daily supernatural attributions to God and the devil/demons linked with meaning in life? *Journal of Positive Psychology, 19,* 369–378.

Wisniewski, D., Cracco, E., González-García, C., & Brass, M. (2022). Relating free will beliefs and attitudes. *Royal Society Open Science, 9*(2), 202018–202018.

Yalom, I. D. (1980). *Existential psychotherapy.* Basic Books.

Yilmaz, O., Bahçekapili, H. G., & Harma, M. (2018). Different types of religiosity and lay intuitions about free will/determinism in turkey. *International Journal for the Psychology of Religion, 28*(2), 89–102.

Zhao, M., & Huo, Y. (2022). Is free will belief a positive predictor of well-being?: The evidence of the cross-lagged examination. *Personality and Individual Differences, 193,* 111617.

CHAPTER 54

Facing the Existential Chasm

The Nonreligious Quest for Meaning and Existential Security

Daryl R. Van Tongeren

Religion has long been a source of existential meaning and security. However, the number of nonreligious individuals is increasing (Pew–Templeton, 2015). Over the past three decades, the percentage of U.S. adults identifying as Christian decreased from roughly 90% to 63% (Pew Research Center, 2022). Across religions, affiliation is declining (Pew Research Center, 2015a), with younger generations less likely to endorse religious beliefs and practices (Pew Research Center, 2015b). Estimates predict that Christianity will no longer be the majority religion in the United States by 2070, by which time religiously unaffiliated individuals would match or outnumber Christians. Indeed, a 2024 estimate (Pew Research Center, 2024) suggested that the religious unaffiliated became the largest group in the United States at 28%, outpacing Protestant evangelicals (24%) and Catholics (23%). Most of these nonreligious individuals were raised religious before deidentifying (Pew Research Center, 2016)—Pew Research Center indicates that nearly 1 in 3 Christians walk away from their faith by age 30. In contrast, the number of individuals seeking nonreligious spirituality is growing, with recent estimates suggesting that more than 1 in 5 individuals identify as "spiritual but not religious" (Pew Research Center, 2023).

As the population of the United States is becoming increasingly nonreligious, it is important for scholars to attend to the particular nuances of this group. First, who are the nonreligious? And how and in what ways do nonreligious individuals meet their needs for meaning and existential security? How might having been previously religious affect these processes? And are formerly religious individuals more prone to the existential anxiety associated with ultimate concerns? This chapter seeks to better understand the nonreligious quest for meaning and existential security, and the potential threat of the *existential chasm*.

RELIGION AS AN EXISTENTIAL RESOURCE

One of the primary functions of religion is to address existential concerns. Previous research has suggested that humans must come to terms with several givens of human existence (Koole et al., 2006; Yalom, 1980). For example, each person must make challenging decisions in a structureless world where outcomes are not certain and there are many competing alternatives (*freedom/groundlessness*); humans are phenomenologically isolated from one another and fundamentally alone (*isolation*); everyone must navigate a constantly changing sense of self across their lifespan and in relation to others and the world around them (*identity*); the only certainty in life is our eventual death (*death*); and the world lacks a consensually validated objective meaning, rendering many struggling to perceive whether there is any meaning at all (*meaninglessness*). Research suggests that a host of social, cognitive, and emotional motivations are aimed at addressing these concerns (e.g., Pyszczynski et al., 2015), which operate both implicitly and explicitly (e.g., Pyszczynski et al., 1999).

The predominant way that people address their existential concerns is by creating and adhering to cultural worldviews, which are systems of meaning that imbue people's lives with meaning and permanence and provide answers to the origin of the world, the nature of humanity, and what constitutes a life worth living (through the conferral of self-esteem; Pyszczynski et al., 1997, 2004). These systems of meaning are culturally bound and often socially endorsed. Cultural worldviews serve key existential functions by mollifying the anxiety engendered by the confrontation with existential realities. This dual defense system works across levels of consciousness (Pyszczysnki et al., 1999), most often occurring outside of awareness (Van Tongeren & Green, 2010). The effect of these automatic, nonconscious defenses is that people don't have to spend much time consciously contemplating existential uncertainties, rather living blissfully shielded from the potential terror of acknowledging their finitude or the meaninglessness of life.

In many ways, religion is an ideal existential meaning system. Religious worldviews address the origin of the world through creation myths, offer prescriptions and proscriptions for human morality and virtue, and offer a means by which people can attain symbolic or literal immortality (Vail et al., 2010). Indeed, religion reduces death-related anxiety for those for whom it is a central part of their identity (Van Tongeren et al., 2013) through the provision of meaning in life (Van Tongeren et al., 2017). By imbuing death with meaning (Van Tongeren & Green, 2018), religion helps people manage conscious thoughts about death (Van Tongeren, Green, et al., 2022).

More directly, religion can offer people a strong structure for overcoming groundlessness by imbuing the world with order and control (see compensatory control theory; Kay et al., 2010); helps people conquer isolation by promising connection with the transcendent (see God as an attachment figure; Kirkpatrick, 1998); offers religious followers a clear identity (see research on religion as a quest; Klaassen & MacDonald, 2002); promises to vanquish death through the provision of literal immortality (see terror management theory; Dechesne et al., 2003); and religious meaning is often considered to be more meaningful than nonreligious meaning (Newton & McIntosh, 2013). Others have argued that religion is an existential resource that meets myriad human needs (Batson & Stocks, 2004). Thus, religion is a prototypical worldview ideally suited to mitigate existential anxiety and provide comfort in the light of ultimate reminders.

Another helpful framing is to consider religion as a meaning system, designed to offer adherents a sense of *coherence*, *significance*, and *purpose*. Meaning has been defined across these three domains, as people feel as though life is meaningful when the world is predictable and makes sense (coherence), they feel valued and as though they matter (significance), and they are oriented toward a goal or effort (purpose) that is larger than themselves (George & Park, 2016; Martela & Steger, 2016). Here, too, we see that religion offers people a schematic interpretation through which they can make sense of the world (McIntosh, 1995), imbues their life with cosmic mattering and significance (Van Tongeren et al., 2017), and grants them a transcendent connection to something greater toward which they can orient their life (Koenig, 2015). This suggests religion often satisfies an existential need for meaning.

Components of Religion

Religion is a multifaceted construct that has been defined in many ways. One helpful definition is to view religion as a set of *beliefs* about the supernatural that enable emotional and ritualistic *bonding* with the transcendent and outline a code of moral *behaviors*, embedded in a social community that offers *belonging* (Saroglou, 2011). Each of these four components of religion operates via distinct psychological processes and helps address core existential concerns (see Table 54.1).

Beliefs refer to the cognitive part of religion and include the specific and doctrinal assertions that people hold about the supernatural (including, for many, the afterlife). For example, they would include the belief in a god or gods, spirits, supernatural forces, and the existence of heaven, paradise, reincarnation, or hell. Depending on the epistemic exclusivity of such ideologies, many of these supernatural beliefs may give rise to lower-level beliefs, such as viewing one's religious group as special and chosen and nonreligious others as adversarial lost souls in need of conversion for salvation. Most powerfully, these beliefs may help address the persistent fear of death. Indeed, belief in literal immortality has been an effective terror management mechanism that mollifies the dread associated with our own mortality (Dechesne et al., 2003; Van Tongeren et al., 2017, 2022).

Bonding refers to the emotional part of religion and includes the rituals that facilitate a perceived connection with the transcendent. This may include prayer, meditation, singing, reading sacred texts or scriptures, or chanting. This kind of emotional relationship helps individuals overcome isolation by offering an enduring, if not eternal, connection to a powerful and benevolent divine being or through interconnectedness with all sentience or life. What better way to vanquish feelings of aloneness than through engaging in a special and significant relationship with something much greater than themselves? Indeed, this kind of deep religious connection can reduce existential isolation (Arrowood et al., 2021; Pinel et al., 2020).

Behaviors refer to the moral prescriptions and proscriptions outlined by religion. Each religion describes behaviors that its adherents should and should not do, offering a moral framework for making decisions. Some examples include the Eightfold Path, the Ten Commandments, and the Fruits of the Spirit. Indeed, religions often have many rules around the body, particularly around food and sex, aimed at maintaining a sense of purity (Haidt & Graham, 2007). These moral mandates, though restrictive in many cases, offer a firm and reliable lens through which religious people can interpret events and make decisions amid uncertainty or when comparing competing options. In turn, this should reduce groundlessness.

Belonging is the social component of religion and refers to the community of like-minded coreligionists of which one is a part. Most religions are deeply communal and involve gatherings at a temple, mosque, church, or other sacred service. Religion offers its followers a clear identity (Klassen & McDonald, 2002; Ysseldyk et al., 2010). Many religious adherents not only make their religion a central part of their identity, by claiming for example they are Muslim or Christian or Hindu or Jewish, but also because they seek to view themselves as religious adherents. Some view themselves as children of God or place their identity in God. Others seek to orient their life around

TABLE 54.1. Existential Functions of Components of Religion

Component of religion	Psychological domain	Existential concern	Existential palliative function	Deidentification process	Existential chasm
Belief	Cognitive	Death	Afterlife beliefs reduce death anxiety	Disbelief	Fear of death and eternal torment
Bonding	Emotional	Isolation	Connection with transcendent	Disengagement	Cosmic aloneness and despair
Behavioral	Moral	Freedom	Moral framework for decision making	Discontinuance	Groundlessness and loss of values
Belonging	Social	Identity	A group-level sense of who one is	Disaffiliation	Questions of authenticity

TABLE 54.2. The Variety of Nonreligious Identities

In the past	In the present	Descriptor
Religious	Same religion	Currently religious
Religious	Different religion	Religious switcher
Religious	Nonreligious	Religious done
Religious or nonreligious	Nonreligious but spiritual	Spiritual but not religious
Nonreligious	Religious	Religious convert
Nonreligious	Nonreligious	Never religious

enlightenment or a quest for sanctification. Their purpose becomes clear and they know how to spend their time and resources. In this way, belonging helps address pressing concerns of identity.

All four of these interlocking dimensions of religion—beliefs, bonding, behaviors, and belonging—collectively provide ultimate meaning. Religious meaning is special (Newton & McIntosh, 2013): Actions done in the name of religion are often seen as higher or more noble, and they justify lower-level inconveniences or harms. This sets up a hierarchy where people feel justified for their actions as long as they serve the greater good of religion. For example, a pastor may skip a family celebration or reunion to attend to a sick congregant in the name of religious duty, and he may feel justified doing so, and even more meaningful, given the sacrifices incurred to follow his perceived calling. In addition, religion provides a script for the meaning of life: serving God, seeking enlightenment, working toward sanctification, overcoming suffering. People know their purpose and are clear on what makes for a meaningful life. And to be sure, the unity of having met all existential concerns conveys an extra layer of meaning that may be hard to replicate. Yet, as mentioned at the outset, not everyone is religious.

WHO ARE THE NONRELIGIOUS?

There is considerable heterogeneity among nonreligious individuals. Indeed, people who are not religious have various identities. Myriad descriptors might explain one's experience or how one perceives one's spirituality (or lack of spirituality). Below, I offer a framework to clarify the variety of nonreligious individuals (see Table 54.2).

Religious

People who have consistently been religious—who were in the past and are now—are *currently religious*. It's possible that they might change in the future, either to another religion or decide to leave religion altogether, but religion has been and continues to be an important part of their identity. Such individuals still identify as religious (at least for now).

Religious Switcher

Those who previously identified as one religion but now ascribe to a different religion have undergone religious change. We would label such an individual as a *religious switcher*. After having changed religion, they now see the world through a different lens. For some, they make a wholesale change from one tradition (e.g., Christianity) to another (e.g., Buddhism) and work hard to fully integrate this new religion. For others, they blend various aspects of different religious traditions (some of the old, some of the new) into a new worldview. Most people who have switched religion find their religion to be an important part of their identity; after all, they've retained religiousness rather than abandoning it altogether. However, it's possible that it may have changed in intensity. Perhaps they used to be a nominally religious person but now are a fervent follower of a new religion; conversely, they may have abandoned their zealous religious identity and now favor a religious identity that holds a different place in their life.

Religious Done

A *religious done* is someone who once identified as religious but no longer does. For example, this would describe someone who grew up Catholic, Muslim, Jewish, or Evangelical, and later finds that the label no longer fits. It could be that they left because they were hurt, disagreed with the teachings of their religious tradition, felt as though they outgrew their faith, had severe doubts about the truth or veracity of their religious upbringing, disliked the label "religious," or perhaps their religious identity simply lost importance in their life (see Van Tongeren, 2024). In short, religion is no longer central to their identity.

Spiritual but Not Religious

Some people report a spiritual identity but are not religious. These individuals are known as *spiritual but not religious* (or SBNR for short) because they are open to spiritual experiences outside of traditional religious structures. Some were previously religious and others were not. What matters more is that spirituality plays a more important role in their life and identity than religion does. This is a complex and multifaceted group. Some believe in god(s) and others don't. Some believe in the afterlife and others don't. Some integrate aspects of various religions into their beliefs, whereas others staunchly avoid anything resembling religion. For this group, a desire to connect with the divine, transcendent, or something larger than themselves is key—and they do it outside of traditional or formalized religion.

Religious Convert

The opposite of a religious done, a *religious convert* is someone who was previously nonreligious but now identifies as religious. Religion has now become a central part of their identity and worldview, and they view themselves as religious. Researchers tend to think of religious converts as people who came to religion after some time of not being religious in their adult lives (rather than someone who "converted" in early childhood, who they may say was always religious).

Never Religious

Someone whose identity has been consistently nonreligious is *never religious*. This nonreligious group is remarkably heterogenous. It may include atheists (i.e., those who do not believe in gods or supernatural agents), agnostics (i.e., those who are unsure if god exists or do not believe a personal relationship with god is possible), or people for whom religion is simply not at all important. But what they have in common is that they have never identified as religious.

As can be seen, the variety of nonreligious individuals is considerable. Given the recent trends in people leaving religion, I now turn to an increasingly common phenomenon of religious deidentification, with a particular focus on the religious dones. This group is likely to continue to increase in number and face a number of unique existential challenges.

A FRAMEWORK FOR RELIGIOUS DEIDENTIFICATION

Religious deidentification is the process by which individuals no longer identify as religious (Van Tongeren et al., 2021a). As previously mentioned, individuals who were formerly religious—once identified as religious but no longer do—are known as *religious dones,* given that they are "done" with religion (McLaughlin et al., 2022; Van Tongeren et al., 2021a, 2023a). Recently, a theoretical model was proposed that highlights four different features of religious deidentification (Van Tongeren & DeWall, 2023). Working from that theoretical framework, I extend that analysis to consider religion from an existential perspective (see Table 54.1).

Disbelief is the cognitive feature of deidentification and involves no longer believing in supernatural agents or claims of religion. Given that afterlife beliefs often mitigate fears of death, after leaving religion, fears of eternal torment or punishment (e.g., hell and the devil, malevolent spirits) may persist (Van Tongeren et al., 2024) and death-related anxiety may increase.

Disengagement is the emotional feature of deidentification and involves no longer experiencing closeness with the transcendent or engaging in ritualistic behaviors meant to foster relational attachment. Such perceived closeness thwarts isolation, which means that following deidentification, religious dones may feel cosmic loneliness, insignificance, or despair.

Discontinuance is the behavioral feature of deidentification and involves no longer adhering to the moral prescriptions or proscriptions of religion. Such a moral framework offers clear guidance for making decisions, attenuating overwhelming feelings of groundlessness that may accompany freedom. After leaving religion, religious dones may struggle to find a coherent set of values toward which they can orient their lives or help inform their decision making, resulting in increased groundlessness.

Disaffiliation is the social feature of deidentification and involves withdrawing from one's religious community. Given that religion is often a core feature of one's identity, providing one a group-level sense of who one is, leaving religion may undermine feelings of authenticity, leaving religious dones to grapple with finding a new narrative for their life and understanding of themselves as they redefine their self-concept.

Individuals may experience deidentification across any number of these features; for example, a religious done may stop attending church and following the moral mandates of their former religious teaching but may still maintain belief. Or, they may continue to attend mosque and engage in communal rituals while privately disbelieving. It is an open question whether one feature of deidentification is primary. Thus, we see heterogeneity in both the nonreligious (e.g., dones vs. never religious), as well as within smaller subgroups (e.g., types of dones and reasons for deidentifying).

Each component of religious deidentification may undermine the satisfaction of existential needs. To the degree that belief in the supernatural or afterlife ameliorated death-related anxiety (Van Tongeren et al., 2017), disbelief may undermine the buffering effect of these beliefs, rendering people more prone to the terror associated with their own mortality (cf. Van Tongeren et al., 2023b). After having known the comfort of having these concerns attenuated, religious dones who disbelieve may now have an increased fear of death or persistent belief in hell and devil (Van Tongeren et al., 2024). Whereas bonding with the sacred provided emotional connection and a deep, lasting sense of meaning, disengagement may leave individuals prone to feelings of cosmic loneliness and despair. Religious meaning is quite potent (Newton & McIntosh, 2013), and leaving one's religious connection with the transcendent may leave people feeling as though life lacks meaning (Van Tongeren et al., in press). The moral framework of religion that guided behaviors may have mollified concerns of groundlessness by providing a structure through which individuals could make moral decisions; discontinuing adherence to those mandates could leave individuals exposed to the full weight of groundlessness and the concomitant anxiety associated with bearing the responsibility for one's decisions in an uncertain world. And whereas a religious community provided a strong social identity and consensual validation for one's worldview, disaffiliation may surface questions of identity that undermine a quest for authenticity; having left religion, religious dones might question who they are apart from their previous beliefs.

Another contribution of this theoretical model is that it offers a conceptual framework for how religious and spiritual struggles may lead to particular features of deidentification. Drawing from work by Exline (2013; Exline et al., 2014), the six religious and spiritual struggles may map onto these four features. *Doubt-related* struggles may lead to cognitive disbelief. Supernatural struggles, involving *divine* or *demonic* agents, may lead to emotional disengagement. *Moral struggles* may lead to behavioral discontinuance. *Interpersonal struggles* may lead to social disaffiliation. And it is possible that struggles around *ultimate meaning* may pressure all of the four domains. Again, these relationships require empirical validation, as well as conclusive proof if their relationship is predictive and causal, as well as the direction of that relationship (i.e., struggles lead to deidentification *or* deidentification causes struggles), or merely correlative (i.e., something else is leading to both struggles and deidentification).

Religious Residue

It can be difficult to fully, and completely, leave one's religion behind. Research sampling from three countries (United States, Hong Kong, and Netherlands) found that roughly 20% of the sample identified as formerly religious—the religious *dones* (Van Tongeren et al., 2021a). This group of dones differed, in important ways, from those who were never religious. Notably, my colleagues and I found evidence of a *religious residue*: the effects of one's former religion persisted after deidentification. This residue effect was found across a host of religious and religion-adjacent measures, including self-reported explicit attitudes (e.g., attitude toward God, attitude toward religion, religious certainty), implicitly assessed attitudes (e.g., through an Implicit Association Test), self-reported behaviors (e.g., frequency of engaging in religious rituals and practices, frequency of interacting with religious individuals, volunteer behavior), and observed behavior (e.g., donation behavior). An important contribution of this research is that one's religious history matters. Having once been religious affects people in ways that differ from those who have never identified as religious.

To better understand the nature and boundary conditions of this effect, we extended this research on religious residue into several domains. We found evidence for religious residue within the moral foundations (Van Tongeren et al., 2021b). Religious dones more closely resembled currently religious individuals in their endorsement of the moral foundations than never religious participants did, and this was particularly pronounced for the binding foundations (i.e., ingroup/loyalty, hierarchy/authority, and purity/sanctity). Moreover, longitudinal evidence from the National Study of Youth and Religion revealed a *residual decay*: the residual effects of religion were stronger the more recently the person had deidentified, with lingering associations waning over time. We confirmed this with our adult sample, showing that the percentage of time one identified as nonreligious (years nonreligious divided by total age) was positively associated with endorsing the individuating foundations (i.e., harm/care, fairness/justice) and negatively associated with the binding foundations. We also found evidence for religious residue in personal values (Schwadel et al., 2021), consumer behavior (DeWall & Van Tongeren, 2022), and negative religious cognitions (Van Tongeren et al., 2024).

What might explain the religious residue effect? There are (at least) three possible mechanisms. First, we suspect *cognitive factors* play a role. Religion operates as a schema (McIntosh, 1995), and schemas are notoriously resistant to change. Even when presented with counterattitudinal or schema-inconsistent evidence, such beliefs are enduring and persevere. Second, *behavioral factors* likely affect these processes through the development of habits. Habits are internalized knowledge structures (Aarts & Dijksterhuis, 2000) in which people rely on ritualistic behavioral patterns in particular settings. The development of religious habits may persist even once one's outward identity has changed. Finally, we anticipate that *social factors* are important in the lingering effects of religion. As people are embedded in religious communities, they are more likely to think, feel, and act like coreligionists. Indeed, we found that for religious dones, the association between religious identity and endorsement of moral foundations was mediated by frequency of interacting with religious individuals (Van Tongeren et al., 2021b). Being embedded in a religious context intensifies religious residue. Of course, there are likely other pathways to be identified that explain religious residue. Still, religious residue may pose a challenge for religious dones seeking existential security.

THE EXISTENTIAL CHASM

In what ways might religious residue affect the process by which religious dones seek to engage in existential meaning making? I propose that a primary concern for religious dones after leaving religion is what I term the *existential chasm:* the psychological state that arises from forfeiting formerly satisfactory answers for existential questions offered by religion and facing afresh the pressing concerns of human existence (Van Tongeren, 2024). Religious dones are perniciously disposed to this phenomenon in a way that currently religious or never religious individuals are not; religious individuals can draw from their religious and spiritual beliefs to address such concerns and maintain a sense of psychological equanimity in the face of threat. Never religious individuals have not previously embraced the answers offered by religion, and thus do not confront the reality (faced by dones) of the compound emotional state of simultaneously experiencing both *grief* for having lost the existentially soothing comfort offered by these the beliefs and the *fear* of having to address these concerns in new ways without the reliance upon their religious meaning systems or external religious authority or structures. Moreover, it is entirely likely that religious dones may not have developed the necessary skills or capabilities to wrestle with such questions given that, at least in some religious traditions or denominational expressions, relevant answers were offered in comprehensive and coherent packages, requiring only assent and memorization, rather than cooperative development or internalization. Thus, religious dones may be *at particularly high risk of existential anxiety*, navigating ultimate concerns (1) without a completely coherent and existentially satisfying meaning system, (2) without requisite skills to navigate such questions, and (3) with the pangs of remembering what it was like to have satisfactorily quenched those existential longings.

Perhaps more directly, it is possible that facing existential concerns without having developed the skills to do so may underlie a host of negative emotional experiences reported by religious dones. For example, McLaughlin and colleagues (2022) reported that religious dones who were still practicing—engaging in more religious-relevant or -adjacent behaviors—were more likely than those who had completely discontinued to report negative emotional states (e.g., anxiety, depression). However, in another study religious dones, regardless of whether they were still practicing or had completely discontinued, suffered poorer health than currently or never religious individuals, including increased drug and alcohol use (Oosterbaan et al., 2025).

There are clues that religious dones may be at particular risk for such existential anxiety. For example, previous work has identified two groups of religious dones that report higher levels of religious and spiritual struggles: (1) those who have begun pulling away from religion but still report being religious and (2) those who began pulling away from religion but still report being spiritual (Exline et al., 2022). These disengaged dones who still report a lingering connection to their religious or spiritual tradition experience struggles, both at the present and across their lifetime. Given the cross-sectional nature of these data, it is not clear whether such struggles precipitated or caused individuals to pull away from religion, whether disengaging from religion led to the struggles, or if a third factor caused both. Nonetheless, the co-occurrence of religious and spiritual struggles with the process of deidentification is consonant with other work documenting the increased negative affect and adverse mental health indicators associated with deidentification (McLaughlin et al., 2022). Other work has revealed that religious dones reported significantly less meaning in life than currently religious individuals reported (Van Tongeren et al., in press). Indeed, a longitudinal sample of more than 45,000 participants revealed that religious dones and those who were never religious reported significantly lower meaning in life than currently religious individuals reported (though some residue remains for religious dones). The full existential benefits of religion extend only to those who identify as religious and are diminished once one is no longer religious.

A SHEEP IN WOLF'S CLOTHING

A compounding concern for religious dones is the sudden lack of community. Given that religious communities offer significant social support, those religious dones who leave their religious communities may experience loneliness, rejection, or long for other individuals with whom they can share their experience. Formerly religious individuals often share "deconversion narratives" (a mirror obverse to a "testimony" or conversion narrative often shared in church) with other co-non-religionists as a way of validating their own experience and vulnerably connecting with others who share a similar religious journey. This may take the form of "trauma-bonding" (i.e., collective rumination) in which religious dones recount the harms of their previous religious experiences; and whereas this is likely a helpful process for a time, getting stuck in a pattern of collective rumination may exacerbate feelings of trauma and leave people unable to move forward toward new identities or experience personal growth.

To further exacerbate these feelings of loneliness, recent research suggests that religious dones often view themselves differently than they are perceived by other religious groups (Van Tongeren et al., 2023a). Religious dones tend to favor, and view themselves more similarly to, never religious individuals: They are less biased against such individuals, are willing to sacrifice for them, and trust them and include them as part of their ingroup. However, such feelings are not reciprocated. Religious dones are seen by others as a *sheep in wolf's clothing:* inwardly religious while projecting a nonreligious exterior. Currently religious individuals sacrifice for them on the same level as other ingroup members and treat them more favorably than never religious individuals, in part because they think that religious dones will become more religious again in the future (i.e., return to the fold). And the never religious individuals, whom the religious dones envy and aspire to include, do not express mutual admiration; they view religious dones with mistrust. Taken together, religious dones are welcomed by a religious group they have left and do not like, and are unwelcome to a group of never religious individuals they admire. This work highlights some social costs of being a religious done.

BALANCING SECURITY AND GROWTH

Regardless of one's religious identity, when seeking to make meaning and address existential concerns, people typically face two primary motives (Pyszczynski et al., 2003). On the one hand, people desire security; they want to feel safe, having effectively managed the anxiety raised by existential questions. On the other hand, people are self-expansive and desire to grow; they want to learn new skills, forge new relationships, and enlarge the self. Whereas security can stagnate, growth can be unsettling. These competing motives for security and growth present themselves in different religious orientations. Prior work has highlighted the *existential tradeoffs* of security-focused beliefs and growth-focused beliefs in religious motivations (Van Tongeren et al., 2016). *Security-focused beliefs* prioritize certainty, rigidity, and conviction and can offer strong answers to existential questions. These beliefs (such as religious fundamentalism) imbue adherents' lives with meaning, permanence, and significance, and they are able to offer ready answers for the challenging questions raised by existential considerations. Intrapersonally, they are able to effectively reduce existential anxiety and provide comfort and psychological equanimity. However, interpersonally, such beliefs are usually associated with prejudice, intolerance, and defensiveness. On the other hand, *growth-focused beliefs* prioritize questions, evolution of perspectives, and intergroup tolerance and cooperation. These beliefs assume that doubt and uncertainty are natural features of religious belief and emphasize the importance of learning from those who are different. Interpersonally, individuals who hold such beliefs are more tolerant of and cooperative with those from whom they differ. Yet intrapersonally, they experience greater existential anxiety because they are tentative or hold doubts about their existentially relevant beliefs.

So, the tradeoffs appear to be clear: The sure safety and certainty of security-focused beliefs offer psychological benefits but can lead to interpersonal defensiveness and intolerance, whereas the openness of growth-focused beliefs provides greater latitude to engage with and learn from those who are different, but at the cost of existential and psychological well-being. A recent series of studies on intellectual humility amid existential challenges revealed that greater intellectual humility—likely a marker of being more growth-oriented—around one's beliefs in the afterlife was associated with greater death anxiety and predicted poorer religious well-being over time (Van Tongeren et al.,

2023b). That is, holding one's beliefs too loosely undermines existential well-being. This would suggest why particular belief systems that offer strong, compelling narratives may be attractive and might persist over time—they are able to provide their adherents with the requisite psychological and existential security.

TOWARD A SCIENCE OF THE EXISTENTIAL MEANING MAKING OF RELIGIOUS DONES

The desire to address existential concerns and make meaning is a fundamental human motivation. Whereas religious individuals can draw from their religious worldviews, the nonreligious engage these processes differently; and religious dones may feel particular tension, peering into the existential chasm and experiencing enhanced anxiety and distress. To be sure, more research is needed to better understand the motivations for existential meaning making and spiritual growth among the nonreligious. What steps are needed to move research on how nonreligious individuals make meaning in light of existential concerns? What existing areas of work are candidates for deepening our understanding of spiritual longing among those underserved by traditional religion? Below, I highlight several open questions and potential pathways to catalyze work in this area.

Defining and Measuring Spiritual Yearning

A central thrust of existential meaning making may involve *spiritual yearning*: a desire to experience greater spiritual depth or transcendent connection in a way that satisfies existential needs. And for religious dones, this likely now occurs outside of traditional religious structures. This construct requires thorough investigation and definition: What is it? How can it best be assessed? With what is it associated? What behavioral, emotional, and cognitive criteria does it predict? It is possible that spiritual yearning may surface in different arenas: When religious dones face the existential chasm and experience distress, they perceive a lack or deficit—something missing in their lives. Nonreligious individuals may experience a desire to connect to something greater, more meaningful, or deeply transcendent. Even religious individuals may desire spiritual deepening, growth, or maturation. But for the nonreligious (including religious dones), this spiritual yearning occurs outside traditional religious structures. Work can be done to (1) thoroughly define spiritual yearning, (2) develop an assessment strategy for measuring spiritual yearning, (3) identify related and distinct constructs, and (4) establish related cognitive, emotional, and behavioral features associated with spiritual yearning.

Deepening an Understanding of Quest Religiousness

One likely candidate for additional work among religious dones and the nonreligious is the construct known as *quest religiousness* or *religion as a quest*. Pioneered by Daniel Batson and Patricia Schoenrade (1991a, 1991b), this work conceptualized a new religious orientation, beyond intrinsic and extrinsic religiousness, that embraced doubt, uncertainty, and questions as central features of the religious experience. Individuals who endorsed this orientation expected to experience religious change and evolution and were less bothered by an ever-revising set of beliefs. This work was revolutionary in proposing a new way to be religious that extended beyond Allport and Ross's (1967) binary. However, it suffered a few limitations. First, researchers often struggled to determine the degree to which respondents who strongly endorsed quest simply weren't that religious. That is, the scale may have been obscured via conflation with nonreligiousness. Of course, there are simple methodological workarounds to address this concern (e.g., add questions that inquire if respondents believe in a god or identify as religious). Second, there was not sufficient clarity around whether quest is a *state* (i.e., a short-term, transient experience) or a *trait* (i.e., an enduring characteristic or pattern of cognitions, emotions, and behaviors). The differences matter greatly. If quest is a state-level "layover" and not a "destination," it becomes more of a mediating mechanism or dependent variable than a predictor variable. For example, in the absence of meaning, people search for it (depart); but once that search is satisfied, people conclude searching having found a satisfying source of meaning (arrive at their destination). Still, it is possible a small subset of people may continually search; and if some people do remain in a permanent state of religious quest, it may have important ramifications for whether or not they experience religious deidentification, and how they experience that process. Moreover, such findings would need to be brought into account with work on balancing security and growth (Van Tongeren et al., 2016), as well as accounts of seeking and dwelling (Shults & Sandage, 2006). It is possible that investing in a stronger understanding of this construct would prove valuable for efforts to capture the rich variety of spiritual yearning and existential meaning making.

Exploring the Promise of Building Existential Distress Tolerance

Given that nonreligious individuals, and religious dones in particular, may face increased existential anxiety, one potential avenue may involve better understanding how to develop *existential distress tolerance*. Similar to how a skill is developed through practice, or fears are reduced through exposure and habituation, perhaps people differ in their comfort levels with existential anxiety. With practice and over time, it is possible that people may become more accustomed to facing existential concerns, viewing them as "truths and not threats," "facts and not fears" (Van Tongeren & Showalter Van Tongeren, 2020). Research on older adults from a terror management perspective offers clues: Rather than engaging in the typical defensive reactions of younger participants, older participants tended to be more prosocial and generous when reminded of their own mortality (Maxfield et al., 2007, 2014). Likely because older adults have more regularly encountered the existential realities of death as they contemplate their more immediate future while also losing friends and family to death, the ongoing confrontation with mortality becomes more commonplace—and perhaps they are either less distressed or better able to tolerate the concomitant stress accompanied by thinking about death. In the same way, it may be worth examining if there are individual differences in how much existential distress people can withstand before experiencing negative intrapersonal or interpersonal reactions, and whether this is a skill that can be developed through intentional practices or contextual features.

Reconceptualizing Flourishing

Trying to articulate under what conditions some people flourish and some languish in the face of religious change requires clear definitions of each. Flourishing has typically been viewed as a balanced life marked by the presence of eudemonic well-being (Keyes, 2002). However, researchers may need to reconceptualize the role that existential anxiety plays in this process, and how it is viewed. Perhaps existential anxiety is not normatively bad—indeed, William James discussed the *sick soul,* which described a person who honestly accounted for the existential nature of the human condition and walked around with the psychological dis-ease associated with knowing that they might wrong about matters of great spiritual import. Pathologizing anxiety may be counterproductive insofar as it might be a by-product of an intellectually honest and existentially authentic engagement with reality. Toward that end, might flourishing for some be the acknowledgment of persistent distress or nagging doubt and the ability to function in spite, or perhaps because, of such feelings or questions? Overly generalized models of human flourishing likely obscure important diversity in the ways in which individuals experience spiritual realities or engage with religion. Too narrowly defined, prescriptive models that fail to account for necessary nuance will not advance an understanding of those who may experience chronic levels of existential anxiety. It is possible to flourish amid suffering (Van Tongeren & Showalter Van Tongeren, 2020) and outside of religion (Van Tongeren, 2024), and future work should explore how expanding definitions of flourishing to increase inclusivity may better capture the complexities of seeking a good life after leaving one's religion.

Causes and Consequences of Spiritual Yearning and Existential Meaning Making

Most basically, research should be aimed at making incremental progress to better understand the predictors of spiritual yearning and existential meaning making, as well as the trajectories of religious change and development among the nonreligious. Empirical work that emphasizes experimental (where appropriate and feasible) and longitudinal designs can help answer questions related to the antecedents/causes and consequences/outcomes of the process under investigating. Building such a science requires a programmatic approach, with smaller increments deeply investigated and reliably replicated before moving to larger questions.

One fruitful first step may to be examine the role of religious and spiritual struggles (Exline, 2013; Exline et al., 2014), particularly in the process of deidentification and religious change (Exline et al., 2022). Do such struggles predict future change, do they occur alongside such change, or are they outcomes of having undergone religious change? And to what degree might such struggles be more or less beneficial (e.g., struggling with doubt as one reorganizes their worldview), and when might such struggles be associated with poorer intrapersonal and interpersonal outcomes (e.g., greater anxiety or depression, strained social relationships)?

Finally, it would be valuable to better understand the degree to which the experience of existential meaning making among (at least some of) the nonreligious is part of a longer developmental trajectory that may lead to (1) returning to religion, (2) changing religions, (3) deepening one's spiritual maturity and experiencing growth, or (4) remaining nonreligious. Work that can follow individual and societal trends over time could prove insightful.

CODA

Whether the current sociological and psychological trends of religious deidentification indicate a secularization that decentralizes formalized religion or the evolution of a new spiritual ways of engaging the world, an increasing number of people are seeking to make meaning and address existential concerns outside the traditional structures of religion. Those who leave religion may face the *existential chasm*: heightened grief and anxiety from forfeiting religious answers to existential questions and fully facing the terror of ultimate concerns. Many feel a deep sense of spiritual yearning and desire a transcendent connection with something greater than themselves. Some may feel groundless and uncertain, grieving the loss of answers once provided by religion and fearful for the harsh realities of existential threats. Many may feel isolated and may experience poorer mental health. Yet others may experience greater freedom and autonomy, living more squarely in accordance with their values. Better understanding how nonreligious individuals seek to answer some of life's biggest questions can help us provide the resources to meet their needs and ensure a fuller and richer part of our community can flourish—whatever that looks like.

ACKNOWLEDGMENT

This work was supported by Grant No. 62948 from the John Templeton Foundation.

REFERENCES

Aarts, H., & Dijksterhuis, A. (2000). Habits as knowledge structures: Automaticity in goal-directed behavior. *Journal of Personality and Social Psychology, 78*, 53–63.

Allport, G. W., & Ross, J. M. (1967). Personal religious orientation and prejudice. *Journal of Personality and Social Psychology, 5*(4), 432.

Arrowood, R. B., Cox, C. R., & Swets, J. A. (2021). Exploring associations between existential isolation, quest religiosity, and well-being. *Mental Health, Religion and Culture, 24*(10), 1101–1116.

Batson, C. D., & Schoenrade, P. A. (1991a). Measuring religion as quest: 1. Validity concerns. *Journal for the Scientific Study of Religion*, 416–429.

Batson, C. D., & Schoenrade, P. A. (1991b). Measuring religion as quest: 2. Reliability concerns. *Journal for the Scientific Study of Religion*, 430–447.

Batson, C. D., & Stocks, E. L. (2004). Religion: Its core psychological functions. In J. Greenberg, S. Koole, & T. Pyszczynski (Eds.), *Hand-*

book of experimental existential psychology (pp. 141–155). Guilford Press.

Dechesne, M., Pyszczynski, T., Arndt, J., Ransom, S., Sheldon, K. M., Van Knippenberg, A., & Janssen, J. (2003). Literal and symbolic immortality: The effect of evidence of literal immortality on self-esteem striving in response to mortality salience. *Journal of Personality and Social Psychology, 84*(4), 722.

DeWall, C. N., & Van Tongeren, D. R. (2022). No longer religious, but still spending money religiously: Religious rituals and community influence consumer behavior among religious dones. *International Journal for the Psychology of Religion, 32*, 53–70.

Exline, J. J. (2013). Religious and spiritual struggles. In K. I. Pargament, J. J. Exline, & J. W. Jones (Eds.), *APA handbook of psychology, religion, and spirituality: Vol. 1. Context, theory, and research* (pp. 459–475). American Psychological Association.

Exline, J. J., Pargament, K. I., Grubbs, J. B., & Yali, A. M. (2014). The religious and spiritual struggles scale: Development and initial validation. *Psychology of Religion and Spirituality, 6*(3), 208–222.

Exline, J. J., Van Tongeren, D. R., Bradley, D. F., Wilt, J. A., Stauner, N., Pargament, K. I., & DeWall, C. N. (2022). Pulling away from religion: Religious/spiritual struggles and religious disengagement among college students. *Psychology of Religion and Spirituality, 14*, 300–311.

George, L. S., & Park, C. L. (2016). Meaning in life as comprehension, purpose, and mattering: Toward integration and new research questions. *Review of General Psychology, 20*(3), 205–220.

Haidt, J., & Graham, J. (2007). When morality opposes justice: Conservatives have moral intuitions that liberals may not recognize. *Social Justice Research, 20*(1), 98–116.

Kay, A. C., Gaucher, D., McGregor, I., & Nash, K. (2010). Religious belief as compensatory control. *Personality and Social Psychology Review, 14*(1), 37–48.

Keyes, C. L. (2002). The mental health continuum: From languishing to flourishing in life. *Journal of Health and Social Behavior, 43*, 207–222.

Kirkpatrick, L. A. (1998). God as a substitute attachment figure: A longitudinal study of adult attachment style and religious change in college students. *Personality and Social Psychology Bulletin, 24*(9), 961–973.

Klaassen, D. W., & McDonald, M. J. (2002). Quest and identity development: Re-examining pathways for existential search. *International Journal for the Psychology of Religion, 12*(3), 189–200.

Koenig, H. G. (2015). Religion, spirituality, and health: A review and update. *Advances in Mind-Body Medicine, 29*(3), 19–26.

Koole, S. L., Greenberg, J., & Pyszczynski, T. (2006). Introducing science to the psychology of the soul: Experimental existential psychology. *Current Directions in Psychological Science, 15*(5), 212–216.

Martela, F., & Steger, M. F. (2016). The three meanings of meaning in life: Distinguishing coherence, purpose, and significance. *Journal of Positive Psychology, 11*(5), 531–545.

Maxfield, M., Greenberg, J., Pyszczynski, T., Weise, D. R., Kosloff, S., Soenke, M., . . . Blatter, J. (2014). Increases in generative concern among older adults following reminders of mortality. *International Journal of Aging and Human Development, 79*(1), 1–21.

Maxfield, M., Pyszczynski, T., Kluck, B., Cox, C. R., Greenberg, J., Solomon, S., & Weise, D. (2007). Age-related differences in responses to thoughts of one's own death: Mortality salience and judgments of moral transgressions. *Psychology and Aging, 22*(2), 341.

McIntosh, D. N. (1995). Religion as schema, with implications for the relation between religion and coping. *International Journal for the Psychology of Religion, 5*, 1–16.

McLaughlin, A., Van Tongeren, D. R., Teahan, K., Davis, D. E., Rice, K., & DeWall, C. N. (2022). Who are the religious "dones?": A cross-cultural latent profile analysis of formerly religious individuals. *Psychology of Religion and Spirituality, 14*(4), 512–524.

Newton, T., & McIntosh, D. N. (2013). Unique contributions of religion to meaning. In J. A. Hicks & C. Routledge (Eds.), *The experience of meaning in life* (pp. 257–269). Springer Science + Business Media.

Oosterbaan, A., Cheadle, A., & Van Tongeren, D. R. (2025). *Deidentifying from religion enhances risky health behavior.* Manuscript in preparation.

Pew Research Center. (2015a). *The future of world religions: Population growth projections, 2010–2050.* www.pewresearch.org/religion/2015/04/02/religious-projections-2010-2050/.

Pew Research Center. (2015b). *U.S. public becoming less religious.* www.pewresearch.org/religion/2015/11/03/u-s-public-becoming-less-religious/.

Pew Research Center. (2016). *Why America's nones left religion behind.* www.pewresearch.org/short-reads/2016/08/24/why-americas-nones-left-religion-behind/.

Pew Research Center. (2022). *Modeling the future of religion in America.* www.pewresearch.org/religion/2022/09/13/modeling-the-future-of-religion-in-america/.

Pew Research Center. (2023). *Spirituality among Americans.* www.pewresearch.org/religion/2023/12/07/spirituality-among-americans/.

Pew Research Center. (2024). *Religious "nones" in America: Who they are and what they believe.* www.pewresearch.org/religion/2024/01/24/religious-nones-in-america-who-they-are-and-what-they-believe/.

Pew–Templeton. (2015). *Global religious futures project.* www.pewresearch.org/topic/religion/religious-demographics/pew-templeton-global-religious-futures-project/.

Pinel, E. C., Yawger, G. C., & Park, Y. C. (2020). The holy grail of connection: I-sharing, existential isolation, and religion. In K. E. Vail III & C. Routledge (Eds.), *The science of religion, spirituality, and existentialism* (pp. 167–174). Elsevier/Academic Press.

Pyszczynski, T., Greenberg, J., & Goldenberg, J. L. (2003). Freedom versus fear: On the defense, growth, and expansion of the self. In M. R. Leary & J. P. Tangney (Eds.), *Handbook of self and identity* (pp. 314–343). Guilford Press.

Pyszczynski, T., Greenberg, J., & Solomon, S. (1997). Why do we need what we need?: A terror management perspective on the roots of human social motivation. *Psychological Inquiry, 8,* 1–20.

Pyszczynski, T., Greenberg, J., & Solomon, S. (1999). A dual-process model of defense against conscious and unconscious death-related thoughts: An extension of terror management theory. *Psychological Review, 106,* 835–845.

Pyszczynski, T., Greenberg, J., Solomon, S., Arndt, J., & Schimel, J. (2004). Why do people need self-esteem? A theoretical and empirical review. *Psychological Bulletin, 130,* 435–468.

Pyszczynski, T., Solomon, S., & Greenberg, J. (2015). Thirty years of terror management theory: From genesis to revelation. *Advances in Experimental Social Psychology, 52,* 1–70.

Saroglou, V. (2011). Believing, bonding, behaving, and belonging: The big four religious dimensions and cultural variation. *Journal of Cross-Cultural Psychology, 42*(8), 1320–1340.

Schwadel, P., Hardy, S. A., Van Tongeren, D. R., & DeWall, C. N. (2021). The values of religious nones, dones, and sacralized Americans: The links between changes in religious affiliation and Schwartz values. *Journal of Personality, 89,* 867–882.

Shults, F. L., & Sandage, S. J. (2006). *Transforming spirituality: Integrating theology and psychology.* Baker Academic.

Vail, K. E., III, Rothschild, Z. K., Weise, D. R., Solomon, S., Pyszczynski, T., & Greenberg, J. (2010). A terror management analysis of the psychological functions of religion. *Personality and Social Psychology Review, 14,* 84–94.

Van Tongeren, D. R. (2024). *Done: How to flourish after leaving religion.* American Psychological Association.

Van Tongeren, D. R., Brady, I., Casper, C., Fuller, H., & Swanson, C. (2024). To hell with the devil: Lingering negative religious beliefs among religious dones. *Psychology of Religion and Spirituality, 16*(4), 343–351.

Van Tongeren, D. R., Davis, D. E., Hook, J. N., & Johnson, K. A. (2016). Security versus growth: Existential tradeoffs of various religious perspectives. *Psychology of Religion and Spirituality, 8,* 77–88.

Van Tongeren, D. R., Davis, D. E., Sibley, C., & Bulbulia, J. (in press). Life loses some meaning after leaving religion. *Psychology of Religion and Spirituality.*

Van Tongeren, D. R., & DeWall, C. N. (2023). Disbelief, disengagement, discontinuance, and disaffiliation: An integrative framework for the study of religious deidentification. *Psychology of Religion and Spirituality, 15*(4), 515–524.

Van Tongeren, D. R., DeWall, C. N., Chen, Z., Sibley, C. G., & Bulbulia, J. (2021a). Religious residue: Cross-cultural evidence that religious psychology and behavior persist following deidentification. *Journal of Personality and Social Psychology, 120,* 484–503.

Van Tongeren, D. R., DeWall, C. N., Hardy, S. A., & Schwadel, P. (2021b). Religious identity and morality: Evidence for religious residue and decay in moral foundations. *Personality and Social Psychology Bulletin, 47,* 1550–1564.

Van Tongeren, D. R., DeWall, C. N., & Van Cappellen, P. (2023a). A sheep in wolf's clothing?: Toward an understanding of the religious dones. *Journal of Experimental Psychology: General, 152,* 98–119.

Van Tongeren, D. R., & Green, J. D. (2010). Combating meaninglessness: On the automatic defense of meaning. *Personality and Social Psychology Bulletin, 36,* 1372–1384.

Van Tongeren, D. R., & Green, J. D. (2018). Meaning and death-thought accessibility. *British Journal of Social Psychology, 57,* 230–239.

Van Tongeren, D. R., Green, J. D., & Richmond, T. (2022). In the valley of the shadow of death: The existential benefits of imbuing life and death with meaning. *Psychology of Religion and Spirituality, 14*(3), 395–405.

Van Tongeren, D. R., McIntosh, D. N., Raad, J., & Pae, J. (2013). The existential function of intrinsic religiousness: Moderation of effects of priming religion on intercultural tolerance and afterlife anxiety. *Journal for the Scientific Study of Religion, 52,* 508–523.

Van Tongeren, D. R., Pennington, A., McIntosh, D. N., Newton, A. T., Green, J. D., Davis, D. E., & Hook, J. N. (2017). Where, o death, is thy sting?: The meaning- providing function of beliefs in literal immortality. *Mental Health, Religion, and Culture, 20,* 413–427.

Van Tongeren, D. R., Severino, M., Kojima, Y., Miskowski, K., & Blank, S. (2023b). Is there a dark side to humility? Cross-sectional and longitudinal evidence for existential costs of humility. *International Journal for the Psychology of Religion, 33,* 136–150.

Van Tongeren, D. R., & Showalter Van Tongeren, S. A. (2020). *The courage to suffer: A new clinical framework for life's greatest crises.* Templeton Foundation Press.

Yalom, I. (1980). *Existential psychotherapy.* Basic Books.

Ysseldyk, R., Matheson, K., & Anisman, H. (2010). Religiosity as identity: Toward an understanding of religion from a social identity perspective. *Personality and Social Psychology Review, 14*(1), 60–71.

CHAPTER 55

Nonreligious Paths to Existential Fulfillment

Luke W. Galen

The existential concerns confronting humanity—facing the inevitability of death, achieving epistemic certainty, deriving a sense of meaning or purpose, among others, have traditionally been viewed as optimally addressed by religious and spiritual worldviews. But the nonreligious—atheists, agnostics, and those with secular humanist worldviews—must also navigate these problems of living. The following sections will examine how major domains of existential concern are approached from nonreligious perspectives.

ISSUES RELATED TO NONRELIGIOUS PERSPECTIVES

The literature pertaining to existential concerns has often reflected a cultural perspective of religious normativity, which has shaped the framing of research questions, the measurement of constructs, and the interpretation of findings. Therefore, several points must be kept in mind. First, framing the topic as one of "nonreligious approaches" yields a categorization based on what is *not* believed. This results in a high degree of heterogeneity because the organization of concepts (or people) based on the absence of belief in a worldview does not itself represent a unified belief system. Knowing that any two given individuals both lack belief in god(s) may be relatively inconsequential for attempts to discern any shared approach to existential concerns. One nonbeliever may be nihilistic, lacking any coherent worldviews, whereas the other's approach to life may be unified around secular humanist tenets. Therefore, it is important to examine different ways of being secular or nonreligious.

Second, some approaches to existential concerns stem directly from nonreligious metaphysical and philosophical views such as those relating to ontology/cosmology, materialism, logical positivism, and a rejection of supernaturalism (Koltko-Rivera, 2004). However, this does not mean that all existential approaches commonly utilized by the nonreligious originated directly from the rejection of religious concepts. For instance, atheists, on average, tend to adopt liberal sociopolitical attitudes, but liberalism is not an inherent product of nonreligious beliefs. Relatedly, compared to the religious, nonreligious individuals tend to value individualism, self-direction, and universalism as opposed to traditionalism, authoritarianism, and parochialism (Schwartz & Huismans, 1995). Rather than emerging specifically from a nonreligious metaphysical stance, these values may instead arise from other beliefs about human nature, views of determinism/free will, or social and political attitudes (Taves, 2020). Basic underlying cognitive, perceptual, and temperamental traits also lead to the formation of worldviews or ideologies (Zmigrod et al., 2021). Thus, these formative influences likely produce a range of worldviews, including nonreligious ones, as well as other approaches to existential concerns.

It is also important to consider that religious content or the lack thereof may be less relevant to helping people meet existential challenges than the overall strength and coherence of their beliefs. In some domains of existential concern, there are few differences between highly religious and staunchly nonreligious individuals, but both groups differ from those whose worldviews are inchoate or uncertain. The ability to effectively negotiate the tasks of living may be primarily predicated on strongly held convictions that are consensually validated rather than worldviews that are incoherent and held with tepid conviction.

Finally, when studying the connection between worldviews and approaches to existential concerns, it is important to keep in mind that neither domain operates in a static manner. Instead, they vary as a function of interacting dispositional traits and proximal need states. Rather than a simplistic relationship such as "Belief *X* was successfully deployed to address existential concern *Y*," more complicated and fluid patterns are operative, such as "Those who believe *X* are likely to construe an absence or deficit in *Y* as a concern at this time but they may not in other contexts." Those whose beliefs reflect religious perspectives may regard the concept of a literal transcendence of death as essential for ultimate meaning, but this is not the case for the nonreligious. Although a religious fundamentalist is likely to be distressed when contemplating the termination of individual consciousness, an atheist may not view this as being problematic. Likewise, whereas a nonreligious individual's need for security may be satisfied in a stable environment, this may no longer be the case in a chaotic environment. Consequently, the relationship between nonreligious worldviews and the ability to cope with certain existential concerns varies as a function of different states or different contexts.

Death

Perhaps the most fundamental existential task for any comprehensive worldview is the provision of assistance in coping with the inevitability of death. For many, the confrontation with life's termination is inextricably linked with religious concepts. Indeed, some scholars posit that religion itself originated with the desire for death transcendence. Notably, Freud (1927/1961) located the psychological roots of religious belief in its ability to exorcise "the terrors of nature" (p. 17). How can these concerns be addressed by nonreligious worldviews?

According to terror management theory, a necessary feature of any worldview is the ability to assist in maintaining our self-esteem when negotiating existential problems. In the case of death concerns, one method of preserving self-esteem is by framing mortality not as complete annihilation but rather as a process of continuity—of living on in some form (Lifton, 1979). Impersonal forms of continuity include the construal of one's physical body as being recycled, the anticipation of merging with universal consciousness, or a focus on vicarious survival in the form of leaving a legacy. Although these postdeath continuity beliefs can be held by religious and nonreligious individuals alike, theists typically believe in a personal afterlife, whereas for atheists, personal consciousness is viewed as discontinuous (Haimila & Muraja, 2023; Manning, 2023). A similar distinction characterizes the relationship between mind and body. Religious believers tend to be substance dualists for whom the soul (or mind) is irreducible to the physical body, whereas atheists tend to be materialists or monists, for whom the mind is equivalent to the functions of the brain (Riekki et al., 2013). For materialists, brain death is the extinction of personal consciousness.

If the religious concept most essential in assuaging death anxiety is the belief in a literal transcendence, it follows that worldviews lacking this component should be linked with greater personal distress. The absence of any assurance of personal continuity is stereotypically characterized as inherently pessimistic, leaving little room for emotional comfort. And there is some evidence that atheists do not tend to view their deaths as having the same cosmic significance as religious believers do; indeed, the former may even feel their death will inconvenience others (Spitzenstätter & Schnell, 2023). However, it is not evident that belief in the cessation of consciousness necessarily produces a sense of despair. The empirical evidence on religion and death anxiety is notably ambiguous and messy (Jong, 2021). A meta-analysis of approximately 100 studies by Jong and colleagues (2018) yielded a very weak overall association ($r = .06$). The most frequently observed relationship across studies was a null result; relatively few studies demonstrated a negative correlation, and some, a positive correlation.

Aside from direct measurement using self-reports of death anxiety, other methods have examined different forms of reactivity following exposure to increased mortality salience (MS). But results of these compensatory responses are even "messier still" (Jong, 2021). Some studies have not found any impact of MS in nonreligious samples (Norenzayan & Hansen, 2006, Study 4), some have found evidence of defensive worldview bolstering (Norenzayan et al., 2009), and yet others have detected greater religious disbelief following MS induction (Jong et al., 2012; Lifshin et al., 2018). Similar to the latter effect, MS has also been shown to decrease afterlife beliefs for mind–body monists (typically, nonbelievers; Heflick et al., 2015). The amplification of disbelief after MS has been interpreted as representing a worldview defense effect: that is, the compensatory affirmation of nonreligiosity.

The contemplation of mortality by atheists does not rely upon belief in a literal transcendence such as eternal life; rather, symbolic belief systems appear to serve similar needs in striving for immortality (Lifton, 1979; Solomon & Thompson, 2019). These secular methods include devoting time to building a family, finding joy in the present, and connecting with loved ones (Manning, 2023). Abstract forms of legacies include dedication to sociopolitical movements or causes, or to institutions such as government, education, patriotism/nationalism, business, art, science, or sports (Vail et al., 2020). Perhaps not surprisingly, given their affinity for science-based worldviews (see section below), the nonreligious are also more likely to be drawn to the prospect of life extension via medical technology, which may represent one of the only literal forms of immortality-striving available to those with materialist beliefs (Lifshin et al., 2018; Vail et al., 2020). Taken together, these findings suggest that some forms of nonreligious worldviews perform symbolic compensatory functions. In effect, when compared to literal religious methods, one form of a "buffer" takes the place of another.

The existence of disparate (or for some beliefs, mutually exclusive) coping systems raises questions regarding relative efficacy. Does the utilization of symbolic psychological defenses by the nonreligious and literal forms of immortality-striving differ in terms of observable outcomes? One factor complicating such comparisons is that studies have typically framed the issue from a religiously normative perspective, such as examining whether the effects of religion-as-anxiety-buffer increase in efficacy as a function of greater belief conviction in a dose-response relationship. Empirical findings have indicated that this model is incomplete (Jong, 2021). Rather than religious belief being specifically efficacious, the components most relevant to successful existential buffering may represent more fundamental properties—namely, the overall strength and coherence of any worldview—whether religious or secular. This suggests the possibility of a curvilinear relationship between belief in religious concepts and death anxiety. At one end of the religiosity continuum, those with strong religious convictions have effective buffers against existential anxiety due to the robust and comprehensive nature of their worldview. Likewise, at the other end, those with strong secular beliefs, such as humanist atheists, are similarly well-positioned to address existential concerns. By contrast, it is those with weak or incoherent religious beliefs that are least equipped to confront existential anxiety.

Although not a universally obtained finding, there is some empirical evidence supporting a curvilinear theory of religion and death anxiety. Based on Jong and colleagues' (2018) meta-analytic review, of the 11 studies capable of testing a curvilinear relationship, eight found such a pattern. For example, Wink and Scott (2005) found that those who were moderately religious feared death more than individuals who scored high or low on religiousness. Jong and colleagues noted that other studies could have found a similar pattern, but most were not designed or analyzed in a way that could detect a quadratic relationship. Other recent studies have similarly indicated that uncertain beliefs are associated with greater death anxiety relative to firm nonbelief (Haimila & Muraja, 2023; Sawyer et al., 2021). Likewise, agnostics and spiritual-but-not-religious individuals show greater death anxiety and avoidance compared to atheists (Spitzenstätter & Schnell, 2022). Although the limited number of available studies renders this conclusion provisional, supportive evidence continues to accumulate (see Figure 55.1).

How could a curvilinear relationship between degree of religious belief (or self-identity) and death-related constructs be informative regarding nonreligious worldviews? First, it would suggest that previous theories suggesting the inferiority of nonreligious worldviews in addressing existential issues were inaccurate. Such conclusions have been products of methodologically limited study design, notably the conflation of low religion with nonreligion. Relatedly, the evidence of differential responses between atheists and agnostics may have been attributable to forms of residual religious beliefs in the latter. This may explain why, for instance, Vail and colleagues (2012) found that MS increased religious belief among agnostics but not atheists.

Second, a worldview defense perspective posits that the satisfaction of existential needs is a function not only belief content (whether religious, secular, or humanist) but also of a worldview's comprehensiveness and coherence. As mentioned above, the constellation of beliefs held by many nonreligious individuals appear to provide them with a sense of self-esteem, coherence, meaning, and value. Thus, some of the early results pointing to an increase in religious belief following exposure to death (appearing to support the "no atheists in foxhole" trope) may have been attributable to participants with residual levels of religious beliefs rather than to those completely lacking such beliefs, especially those with additional commitments to alternative secular worldviews (e.g., secular humanism).

Third, rather than being solely attributable to religious content, the relative success of worldviews is also a function of individual differences such as holding beliefs with a high degree of self-centrality and relative flexibility (versus rigidity). Solomon and colleagues (2015) illustrated such properties by contrasting "rock" versus "hard place" types of worldviews. Rock worldviews include clear and comprehensive accounts of the universe with explicit prescriptions for actions required to obtain

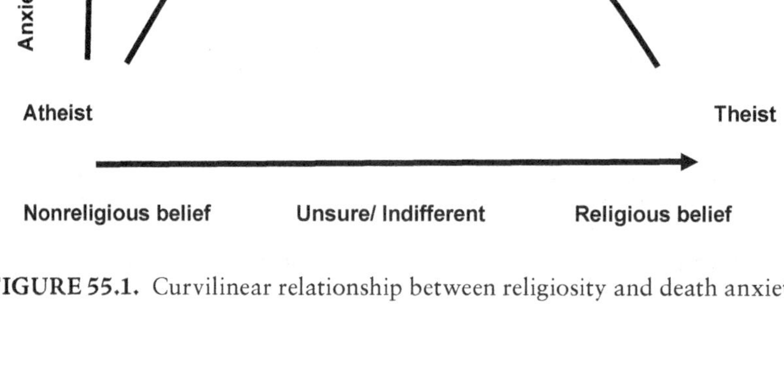

FIGURE 55.1. Curvilinear relationship between religiosity and death anxiety.

literal and/or symbolic immortality (e.g., religious fundamentalism). By contrast, hard place approaches are more malleable conceptions of life allowing ambiguity and uncertainty. Adherents of hard place views are more ecumenical and tolerant of people who are different from themselves, but they may also suffer from anxiety and be drawn to spiritual fads. However, this dichotomy may not fully capture the observed empirical relationship between (non)religious worldviews and death anxiety. On the one hand, as we have seen, those with uncertain or inchoate beliefs (e.g., spiritual-but-not-religious, agnostic) appear to suffer greater anxiety compared to both the strongly religious and atheists. However, religious and secular worldviews can contain mixtures of both belief types (i.e., rigid as well as flexible). Atheists (by definition) have clear convictions regarding metaphysical agents and materialism, but their personalities and sociopolitical views are marked by openness to experience and flexibility, such as moral views that are utilitarian and consequentialist. Likewise, Vail and Soenke (2018) found that MS had the effect of boosting atheists' certainty about their rejection of religion, yet it also increased their ideological open-mindedness (and reduced their dogmatism), which the authors interpreted as a search for viable secular beliefs. The highly religious end of the continuum may also feature paradoxes such as a firm belief in some religious concepts that decrease death anxiety, along with others (e.g., perceived failure in living up to standards, viewing God as punishing) that produce greater anxiety (Bassett & Bussard, 2021). More broadly, if the religious assurance of immortality is predicated on aspects of faith subject to falsification (e.g., literal Biblical historicity), this can generate greater death anxiety when fundamental prior tenets are challenged as compared to more vague, unfalsifiable beliefs. In this sense, firm religious conviction is a "high gain, high risk" combination.

Another body of work providing insight into nonreligious death attitudes is that pertaining to medical end of life (EOL) issues (e.g., advance care planning directives, euthanasia) particularly work featuring the perspectives of the seriously or terminally ill. Many studies have found that religious patients seek and receive more aggressive EOL care, whereas those lowest in religiosity show less desire to prolong their lives if their quality of living is not sufficient (Cicirelli, 1997; Shinall et al., 2014). Relatedly, there are beliefs associated with religion that directly promote a preference for aggressive EOL treatment (Shinall, 2014). Beliefs in potential divine intervention, or that only God should control life's length, or in the use of unrealistically positive religious coping (e.g., "prayer can cure anything") have all been linked to lower rates of advance care planning and more intensive EOL care preferences (Brierley et al., 2013; Colenda & Blazer, 2022; Garrido et al., 2013; Phelps et al., 2009). As mentioned above, atheists may be particularly drawn to the prospect of literal immortality via medical life extension, but nonetheless they are also more likely than the religious to refuse treatment for a terminal illness (van Wijmen et al., 2015).

As with general attitudes regarding death and death anxiety, this work tends to feature a religiously normative perspective, which relegates conclusions regarding the nonreligious to be inferred as the converse of the religious ones. It is reasonable to assume that some differences are attributable to absence of the abovementioned religious beliefs, but other factors such as demographic differences may also play a role (Colenda & Blazer, 2022; Koss, 2018). A seeming paradox is the difference in subjective emotional impact that contemplating mortality has for the nonreligious, compared to the religious. The atheist view of death (i.e., no transcendent literal immortality) is not accompanied by the same negative emotional sequelae compared to when religious people contemplate the same fate. As mentioned above, one reason for a diminished negative impact is that meaningful nonreligious worldviews are enlisted to symbolically fulfill needs. But it also appears that, while many atheists report feeling a sense of insignificance on a cosmic scale, this tends not to be accompanied by despair (Spitzenstätter & Schnell, 2023). A similar effect (mentioned below) is that for atheists, a lack of objective meaning in life does not translate into a perceived crisis of meaning or search for meaning. These findings may also account for the curvilinear patterns of death anxiety in that religious belief systems contain paradoxical or competing influences. On the one hand, strong worldview convictions in an afterlife provide comfort for patients nearing the end of life, but other content can cause distress, such as doubting one's status in the afterlife, or attributing illness as evidence of God's disfavor (Edmondson et al., 2008). In these instances, the belief in an afterlife coupled with a perceived uncertainty of personal salvation may produce a state of distress or what Kirby Farrell referred to as rage for survival or survival greed (Shen, 2003).

In sum, as mentioned previously, there is still much "mess" in the literature on death anxiety and (non)religion, resulting in a weak overall association. There are indications of a curvilinear effect with greater anxiety more characteristic of those with unsure or inchoate beliefs and lower anxiety for both the highly religious and atheists. Another way to conceptualize such a relationship would be as a negative linear relationship between anxiety and the strength of any worldview conviction (i.e., whether religious or atheistic/secular humanist; see Figure 55.2). However, this is based on a limited number of studies and is therefore presently a provisional hypothesis. The religiously normative perspective in the literature has contributed to this lack of clarity. Studies have not included numbers of nonreligious participants sufficient to allow comparisons, and there has been a lack of measurement precision at the low end of religiosity (e.g., overly broad groupings such as "none" or "unaffiliated"). As a result, atheists have been conflated with agnostics even though these self-identity categories significantly differ on many existentially relevant variables. This has contributed to erroneous general conclusions such as "higher death anxiety exists among the nonreligious." Rather than measuring only the presence versus absence of religious belief, studies may benefit from greater detail regarding the presence of nonreligious value systems. As described by Soenke and colleagues (2022), an existentially healthy atheist can compensate for the lack of literal immortality via adopting secular humanist values or participation in larger cultural systems. Many nonreligious individuals may have greater death anxiety not because of a lack of religious belief but because of a lack of corresponding secular humanist worldviews.

Meaning and Purpose

Terror management theory posits that an increased awareness of mortality motivates people to rely on their worldviews to maintain a sense of meaning. From a religious perspective, believers' lives can be imbued with transcendent meaning via aligning their own individual life purposes and goals with those of the deity. Here I focus on how meaning is construed from the secular per-

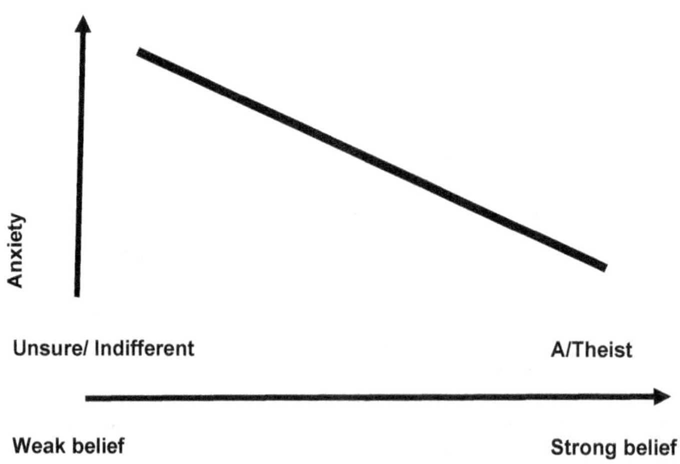

FIGURE 55.2. Negative linear relationship between worldview conviction and death anxiety.

spective, including the sources of meaning most relevant to the nonreligious.

The cultural focus on the importance of religion in providing meaning often implies that the nonreligious must be disadvantaged by their worldviews in obtaining a subjective sense of meaning. Indeed, some differences in experienced meaning as a function of religiosity can be found in the literature. For example, Vail and Soenke (2018) found that atheists, but not Christians, reported lower perceived meaning in life after being reminded of death, suggesting that the nonreligious may feel existentially vulnerable. However, surprisingly, themes of religious meaning do not feature prominently in surveys of the general population, even from those who are religious (apart from measures that specifically prompt religious themes). In a series of Pew Research Center surveys (2018a, 2018b), regardless of respondents' religiosity, the most meaningful aspect of life reported was spending time with family. Other highly ranked sources of meaning (depending on the demographic segment) included relationships with friends, good health, stability, and travel. In surveys of Europeans, religion did not appear in the top 10 sources of meaning. Within the United States, 15% (ranked fifth) of those surveyed mentioned God or religion as a source of meaning. On the other hand, the Pew Research Center surveys indicated that there are differences between religious and nonreligious Americans in both the rank-order importance of meaning sources and the overall rated importance or meaningfulness of the sources. Atheists were particularly likely to list the importance of a range of lifestyle-oriented activities or participation in activism or causes. Atheists were also more likely than Christians to derive fulfillment from finances, leisure activities, hobbies, and traveling. Thus, even among some evidence of differing emphasis of sources of meaning as a function of religiosity, there is nonetheless a substantial level of similarity.

The patterns in sources of meaning resemble those of stated life values. Relative to the religious, nonreligious individuals tend to prioritize self-direction, autonomy, stimulation, and achievement (Saroglou et al., 2004; Schwartz & Huismans, 1995). By contrast, religiosity is associated with greater valuation of obedience, conformity, self-control, tradition, security, and benevolence. Atheists' greater valuation and meaning derived from creative achievement is notable because of the link between creativity and the management of existential concerns. Perach and Wisman (2019) found that at high, but not low, levels of creative goals, creative achievement was associated with low death-thought accessibility under mortality salience. This suggests that for some, creative achievement may be not only a source of meaning but an avenue to symbolic immortality.

For religious and nonreligious individuals alike, some highly meaningful experiences can be imbued with a sense of exceptionality produced by feelings of awe and "small self" (Preston & Shin, 2017). In some cases, the experiences of atheists are described in the literature as "spiritual." However, atheists typically reject supernatural terms and were referring to experiences linked with nature, science, and yoga/meditation (Caldwell-Harris et al., 2011). The endorsement of the term *spiritual* by atheists may also be a methodological artifact produced by framing questions in a way that suggests an equivalence between secular and religious forms of exceptionality or meaning. For example, Preston and Shin asked all participants to recall a time they felt "strong feelings of spirituality and connection to the divine" but added the prompt "If you are not religious, recall a time when you felt a deep connection with the Universe/world around you." Such wording may lead respondents to construe phenomena such as "connecting to something greater" or "purposefulness" as being tantamount to "spiritual" (Preston et al., 2023). Although endorsing themes of meaning, emotional elevation, and connection has led some to conclude "atheists can be spiritual" this doesn't necessarily mean that atheists spontaneously and explicitly select *spiritual* as their preferred descriptor.

Believers and nonbelievers alike may derive meaning from similar foundational qualities within certain existential and epistemic domains, with the differences primarily consisting of the labeling of the content. For example, benefits accrue from worldviews and institutions that provide a sense of control, predictability, and orderliness (Rutjens et al., 2013). One study found that, when exposed to mortality salience, those low in religious belief showed heightened belief in sociomoral progress compared to those high in religious belief, suggesting that the nonreligious may particularly prioritize a sense of teleological progress in their worldviews (Rutjens et al., 2016).

One phenomenon that has attracted much interest and debate pertains to whether religious worldviews provide the most comprehensive sources of meaning, and that therefore, secular sources and experiences of meaning are less "existentially satisfactory" (Park & McNamara, 2006). On the one hand, secular individuals tend to rate a wide range of sources as generally less meaningful, even those unrelated to religious content (Pew Research Center, 2018a). Likewise, Schnell and Keenan (2011) found that atheists reported lower degrees of experienced meaningfulness. By contrast, religion produces a sense of cosmic significance, which in turn fosters a sense of meaning in life (Prinzing et al., 2023). Compensatory models predict that, as with fears of mortality, threats to a sense of meaning result in increased religious beliefs suggesting that atheists may experience chronic deficits of meaning (Routledge et al., 2017).

On the other hand, observed differences may not result from the deficiency of worldviews themselves but in factors such as differences in how individuals construe the concept "meaning," as well as the dispositional need for and desire to search for meaning. Whereas religious individuals primarily derive meaning from sources perceived to be exogenous (i.e., extrinsically produced, transcendent), the nonreligious tend to derive meaning that is endogenous (individually provided; Speed et al., 2018). A related pattern can be observed in the absence of negative psychological sequalae among atheists with low levels of meaning. In other words, despite experiencing a lower presence of meaning, atheists do not experience this as a crisis or source of negative affect (Schnell & Keenan, 2011), whereas strong religious believers experiencing low meaning tend to have lower well-being (Galek et al., 2015). Atheists also display a lower need to search for meaning relative to theists (Abeyta & Routledge, 2018; Nelson et al., 2021). Consequently, the lack of overall meaning for the nonreligious does not appear to manifest in fatalism or nihilism (Speed et al., 2018). Also, as previously mentioned, there are benefits from having firm beliefs in any coherent worldview, whether religious or secular, which are associated with low motivation to search for meaning. Those atheists with higher commitments to secular humanist worldviews may feel little need to search for additional exogenous meaning (Schnell & Keenan, 2011.)

In a pattern similar to that of perceived meaning, the sense of perceived control is attained via different sources as a function of religiosity. Certainly, the belief in a concerned deity can function as a perceived source of external control; however, possessing alternative sources of external control tends to reduce the motivation for religiously based control beliefs. These alternative secular sources of control include stable sociopolitical institutions and effective governance (Kay et al., 2010). I discuss this relationship in greater detail below in the context of existential insecurity theory.

The subjective perceptions of experienced meaning and control also vary as a function of individual differences in dispositional epistemic needs. For instance, although some atheists experience lower meaningfulness, those with high levels of commitment to different sources of meaning experience high levels of meaningfulness as well as well-being (Schnell & Keenan, 2011). The sense of satisfaction with meaning appears to hinge on whether individuals' worldviews are of central rather than of peripheral importance to them. For instance, Steger and Frazier (2005) found that experienced presence of meaning was related to high religious importance (i.e., intrinsic religiosity), not merely with identifying as being religious. This may be yet another instance in which the degree of belief conviction and belief integration is of greater existential relevance than the content of beliefs—whether religious or secular.

Epistemic Needs and the Role of Scientific Worldviews

Humans prefer to live in a coherent, understandable world. This includes the needs for basic epistemic consistency, certainty, and reliability. Religious and scientific worldviews are similar in their claimed status as epistemically "prior"—providing explanation while not being explained (Preston & Epley, 2005). Discussions such as the perennial "science versus religion" debate are often framed in terms of the merits of each general belief system. Clearly, when viewed from the perspective of individuals who define themselves by their rejection of religion, epistemic challenges are more likely to be satisfactorily addressed by a scientific worldview. For secular people, scientific worldviews can function not only in generating explanations and knowledge of specific phenomena, but also by providing a sense of predictability, control, order, and in some cases, meaningful progress.

The nonreligious, particularly atheists, have also been found to have distinct epistemic patterns or modes of thought, such as a greater reliance on analytic cognition (as opposed to intuition), and a greater valuation of rationality (Ståhl & van Prooijen, 2021; Yilmaz, 2021). Conversely, they tend to be less likely to value epistemically questionable belief systems (e.g., conspiracy theories, pseudoscience). The issue of how individuals' religiosity correlates with their typical epistemic processing is a topic of ongoing debate. Whereas the nonreligious have traditionally been regarded as cognitively flexible and open to new ideas, there is some evidence that this may depend upon how these constructs are defined and measured. For example, atheists tend not to be dogmatically certain in general, yet they may exhibit lower appreciation of different perspectives and be less tolerant of ambiguity than others (Uzarevic et al., 2017). Such patterns may also differ as a function of the type or degree of nonreligiosity, with agnostics presenting as more flexible and less certain in their epistemology compared to atheists (Karim & Saroglou, 2023).

The nonreligious consistently report that science plays an important role in their value systems (Van Mulukom et al., 2023), but this valuation can fluctuate, such as when under conditions of existential threat. For instance, Farias and colleagues (2013) found that, in a largely secular sample, mortality salience led to increased belief in science. Likewise, increased valuation of scientific theories can also reflect a motivated need for enhanced order (Rutjens et al., 2018). Rutjens, van der Pligt, and van Harreveld (2010) found that threats to a sense of control increased individuals' endorsement of those scientific theories that specifically promoted order and predictability, such as evolution guided by intelligent agency rather than Darwinian natural selection. These findings imply that framing scientific theories in terms of orderly and predictable processes can reduce belief in supernatural agency, indicating a degree of epistemic substitutability of science for religion. Such effects may be most evident for those who are least religious (Lifshin et al., 2018). For example, increased mortality salience can produce greater acceptance of evolutionary theory among natural science students when naturalism is presented as a source of existential meaning (Tracy et al., 2011). Thus, aspects of science can provide existential meaning specifically when playing a central role in individuals' worldviews.

These findings also suggest that scientific epistemology may be viewed by nonreligious individuals in a qualitatively different way from the religious. Although some nonreligious individuals and indeed some scientists may view scientific and religious worldviews as compatible (Ecklund & Johnson, 2021) or at least occupying different "nonoverlapping magisteria," this varies as a function of the definition of religion as well as the perceiver's degree of (ir)religiosity. The least religious individuals and those with a greater understanding of scientific methods are the most likely to see science and religion as incompatible (Leicht et al., 2022; Pew Research Center, 2015). This is particularly evident for those scientific domains with the greatest existential import, such as human evolution and the creation of the universe. Although some aspects of scientific worldviews are primarily epistemic and control-oriented (e.g., explaining and predicting), others have more relevance to existential meaning (e.g., the purpose of life), with views of the latter diverging the most as a function of religious belief (Haimila, 2020; Rutjens & Preston, 2020). Compatibilists may base their views on framing the issue as one pertaining to compartmentalized aspects such as "a person can be religious and a scientist" or "science covers the how, but religion the why." However, atheists are more likely to focus on the existential implications for scientific findings regarding natural selection, the age of the universe, the implications of neuroscience, or naturalistic models of morality. Thus, although the issue has often been framed as one of the general compatibility of "science" and "religion" as abstract worldviews, this is a separate issue from how compatible (or more accurately, incompatible) scientific and religious methods and the findings they yield are viewed by the nonreligious.

Social and Affiliative Needs

The process of grappling with existential challenges can heighten the desire to affiliate with others, to form close relationships, and to become immersed in groups. These responses help alleviate anxiety. The availability of social support enhances our ability to confront threats, whereas the lack thereof can have deleterious emotional consequences. More generally, as articulated by terror management theory, the validation we derive through meeting culturally prescribed expectations is attributable to the socially constructed basis of self-esteem (Solomon et al., 2015). Traditionally, religious organizations have been an important component in providing normative standards and fostering social and communal ties. In religiously predominant societies, overtly rejecting a religious identity or contradicting prevailing religious values can lead to social exclusion and discrimination. In such contexts, atheists are considered a social "other"—stereotyped as immoral and unworthy of trust (Edgell et al., 2016; Galen et al., 2011). Ironically, although social rejection contributes to a sense of isolation, it may also simultaneously foster a stronger sense of minority identification and a decreased desire to conform. This results in mutual distrust and may lead the nonreligious to view belonging to a community of people with shared values as being relatively unimportant (Pew Research Center, 2018a). Among teens, atheists are the group least likely to believe that it is important to fit in with what other teens think is "cool" (Pearce & Denton, 2011). It is also possible that more individualistic and nonconforming people may gravitate toward, or be more willing to consider, nonnormative worldviews such as atheism. As mentioned above, the nonreligious place a greater valuation on self-direction and individualism and have personalities marked by lower agreeableness (Karim & Saroglou, 2023). Therefore, there may be bidirectional processes operating in religious societies, where atheists are socially ostracized, but also where nonconformists self-select into atheism.

The social components of organized religion are arguably the features most associated with well-being for believers. Mechanisms of positive effects include strong within-group social networks and communal ties (Lim & Putnam, 2010). Not surprisingly those unaffiliated with any religion, particularly in religiously predominant locations, are likely to be socially isolated. However, there has been a steady, if modest, growth of "organized nonreligion" in the form of groups promoting secular humanism (Smith, 2017). These groups are quite heterogeneous, differing in their relative emphasis on informational content (e.g., science and current event lectures) or social activities (e.g., meet-ups, skeptics in the pub). Some, such as the Sunday Assembly, specifically adapt features of religious services, including sharing personal narratives, highlighting prosocial content (e.g., positive messages, opportunities for volunteering), and engaging in shared rituals (communal singing).

Although membership in nonreligious organizations is relatively small, these groups have attracted interest from researchers partly because they allow secular features operating in a social milieu to be distinguished from religious content. This has led to challenges of theories suggesting that religious groups involve sui generis qualities unavailable to secular groups. The previously mentioned heterogeneity makes it difficult to render any blanket conclusion that would pertain to all secular groups; however, some studies have indicated that secular networks and communities can indeed provide a sense of meaning (Smith, 2017). Having a strong nonreligious identification coupled with sharing social connections can increase self-esteem and protect against the harmful effects of marginalization (Brewster et al., 2020; Doane & Elliott, 2015). Secular rituals can play a role similar to religious ones in fostering feelings of social connection (Charles et al., 2021). Outcome studies suggest that socially engaged believers and nonbelievers alike derive equivalent well-being from participation (Shor & Roelfs, 2013). Additionally, patterns of well-being observed as a function of participation in such groups and that include the full range of religion and secularity reflect the previously mentioned curvilinear relationship. Those who are unaffiliated with any religion report low levels of civic involvement and have few meaningful social contacts. However, both the religiously engaged and engaged secularists, atheists, and agnostics have higher levels of such communal involvement (Galen et al., 2015; Pew Research Center, 2024). In sum, individuals, regardless of their religiosity, may benefit from participation in groups featuring content matching their worldviews and that have meaningful engagement, provide consensual validation, and foster a sense of community.

Worldviews can also be evaluated in terms of their association with social and emotional benefits as a function of whether they are normative relative to their broader cultural and regional context. Theories of culture-fit or social-value posit that worldviews, whether religious or secular, matching those of the surrounding milieu are associated with greater well-being relative to nonnormative ones (Stavrova et al., 2013). For example, whereas nonreligious individuals display lower well-being in religiously dominant areas, this is not the case in secular milieus (Gebauer et al., 2017; Stavrova, 2015). When evaluating the existential usefulness of a given worldview, the most relevant properties are those involving the ability to provide a sense of consensual, normative support rather than content-related aspects pertaining to either religion or secularity.

Related findings suggest that many of the functions of religious or secular worldviews are dependent upon, or moderated by, properties of social living conditions. According to existential security theory (Norris & Inglehart, 2011), conditions of living in more secure societies decrease the salience of religion because these buffers against anxiety (e.g., as mentioned above, a sense of control and meaning) are superfluous when other forms (e.g., effective secular institutions) are available. Consequently, secularity is more common in societies with stable living conditions. This relationship exists at the country and state level, as well as across a variety of time periods (Barber, 2011, 2015) and suggests that, under secure conditions, secular worldviews are sufficient to meet various existential needs (Zuckerman et al., 2018). In sum, the association of nonreligious worldviews with successfully meeting affiliative needs varies as a function of normative matching.

SUMMARY

It has often been assumed that nonreligious worldviews are insufficient in their ability to provide resources for optimally negotiating existential tasks, such as preserving a sense of self-esteem and meaning. However, as we have seen across a range of domains, including death, meaning, epistemology, and social affiliation, nonreligious and secular worldviews function similarly to religious ones in many ways, despite having disparate content. Differences between religious and nonreligious content may be less relevant than the relative coherence of worldviews, the conviction with which they are held, and the level of consensual support they receive from the social milieu. Certainly, there are meaningful differences as a function of religious belief, such as in views regarding death or in the construal of concepts of ultimate meaning. However, manifestation of these differences in the form of outcomes such as emotional well-being (e.g., death anxiety, crises of meaning) are quite small. Additionally, it is unclear to what extent these differences derive directly from the (non)religious beliefs themselves or rather from the more fundamental traits related to cognition and personality of the nonreligious, notably their tendency toward individualism and social autonomy. Future work will benefit from a focus on such complexities.

REFERENCES

Abeyta, A. A., & Routledge, C. (2018). The need for meaning and religiosity: An individual differences approach to assessing existential needs and the relation with religious commitment, beliefs, and experiences. *Personality and Individual Differences, 123,* 6–13.

Barber, N. (2011). A cross-national test of the uncertainty hypothesis of religious belief. *Cross-Cultural Research, 45*(3), 318–333.

Barber, N. (2015). Why is Mississippi more religious than New Hampshire?: Material security and ethnicity as factors. *Cross-Cultural Research, 49*(3), 315–325.

Bassett, J. F., & Bussard, M. L. (2021). Examining the complex relation among religion, morality, and death anxiety: Religion can be a source of comfort and concern regarding fears of death. *OMEGA: Journal of Death and Dying, 82*(3), 467–487.

Brewster, M. E., Velez, B. L., Geiger, E. F., & Sawyer, J. S. (2020). It's like herding cats: Atheist minority stress, group involvement, and psychological outcomes. *Journal of Counseling Psychology, 67*(1), 1–13.

Brierley, J., Linthicum, J., & Petros, A. (2013). Should religious beliefs be allowed to stonewall a secular approach to withdrawing and withholding treatment in children? *Journal of Medical Ethics, 39*(9), 573–577.

Caldwell-Harris, C. L., Wilson, A. L., LoTempio, E., & Beit-Hallahmi, B. (2011). Exploring the atheist personality: Well-being, awe, and magical thinking in atheists, Buddhists, and Christians. *Mental Health, Religion and Culture, 14*(7), 659–672.

Charles, S. J., van Mulukom, V., Brown, J. E., Watts, F., Dunbar, R. I., & Farias, M. (2021). United on Sunday: The effects of secular rituals on social bonding and affect. *PLOS One, 16*(1), e0242546.

Cicirelli, V. G. (1997). Elders' end-of-life decisions: Implications for hospice care. *Hospice Journal, 12*(1), 57–72.

Colenda, C. C., & Blazer, D. G. (2022). Review of religious variables in advance care planning for end-of-life care: Consideration of faith as a new construct. *American Journal of Geriatric Psychiatry, 30*(7), 747–758.

Doane, M. J., & Elliott, M. (2015). Perceptions of discrimination among atheists: Consequences for atheist identification, psychological and physical well-being. *Psychology of Religion and Spirituality, 7*(2), 130–141.

Ecklund, E. H., & Johnson, D. R. (2021). *Varieties of atheism in science.* Oxford University Press.

Edgell, P., Hartmann, D., Stewart, E., & Gerteis, J. (2016). Atheists and other cultural outsiders: Moral boundaries and the non-religious in the United States. *Social Forces, 95*(2), 607–638.

Edmondson, D., Park, C. L., Chaudoir, S. R., & Wortmann, J. H. (2008). Death without God: Religious struggle, death concerns, and depression in the terminally ill. *Psychological Science, 19*(8), 754–758.

Farias, M., Newheiser, A. K., Kahane, G., & de Toledo, Z. (2013). Scientific faith: Belief in science increases in the face of stress and existential anxiety. *Journal of Experimental Social Psychology, 49*(6), 1210–1213.

Freud, S. (1961). *The future of an illusion.* Anchor Books. (Original work published 1927)

Galek, K., Flannelly, K. J., Ellison, C. G., Silton, N. R., & Jankowski, K. R. (2015). Religion, meaning and purpose, and mental health. *Psychology of Religion and Spirituality, 7*(1), 1.

Galen, L. W., Sharp, M., & McNulty, A. (2015). Nonreligious group factors versus religious belief in the prediction of prosociality. *Social Indicators Research, 122,* 411–432.

Galen, L. W., Smith, C. M., Knapp, N., & Wyngarden, N. (2011). Perceptions of religious and nonreligious targets: Exploring the effects of perceivers' religious fundamentalism. *Journal of Applied Social Psychology, 41*(9), 2123–2143.

Garrido, M. M., Idler, E. L., Leventhal, H., & Carr, D. (2013). Pathways from religion to advance care planning: Beliefs about control over length of life and end-of-life values. *The Gerontologist, 53*(5), 801–816.

Gebauer, J. E., Sedikides, C., Schönbrodt, F. D., Bleidorn, W., Rentfrow, P. J., Potter, J., & Gosling, S. D. (2017). The religiosity as social value hypothesis: A multi-method replication and extension across 65 countries and three levels of spatial aggregation. *Journal of Personality and Social Psychology, 113,* e18–e39.

Haimila, R. (2020). Does a science-oriented worldview entail unbelief?: Meaning, morality, and continuity from scientific research in self-reports of Finnish unbelievers and believers. *Secular Studies, 2*(2), 83–116.

Haimila, R., & Muraja, E. (2023). A sense of continuity in mortality?: Exploring science-oriented Finns' views on afterdeath. *OMEGA: Journal of Death and Dying, 88*(1), 38–65.

Heflick, N. A., Goldenberg, J. L., Hart, J., & Kamp, S. M. (2015). Death awareness and body–self dualism: A why and how of afterlife belief. *European Journal of Social Psychology, 45*(2), 267–275.

Jong, J. (2021). Death anxiety and religion. *Current Opinion in Psychology, 40,* 40–44.

Jong, J., Halberstadt, J., & Bluemke, M. (2012). Foxhole atheism, revisited: The effects of mortality salience on explicit and implicit religious belief. *Journal of Experimental Social Psychology, 48*(5), 983–989.

Jong, J., Ross, R., Philip, T., Chang, S. H., Simons, N., & Halberstadt, J. (2018). The religious correlates of death anxiety: A systematic review and meta-analysis. *Religion, Brain and Behavior, 8*, 4–20.

Karim, M., & Saroglou, V. (2023). Being agnostic, not atheist: Personality, cognitive, and ideological differences. *Psychology of Religion and Spirituality, 15*(1), 118–127.

Kay, A. C., Gaucher, D., McGregor, I., & Nash, K. (2010). Religious belief as compensatory control. *Personality and Social Psychology Review, 14*, 37–48.

Koltko-Rivera, M. E. (2004). The psychology of worldviews. *Review of General Psychology, 8*, 3–58.

Koss, C. S. (2018). Does religiosity account for lower rates of advance care planning by older African Americans? *Journals of Gerontology: Series B, 73*(4), 687–695.

Leicht, C., Sharp, C. A., LaBouff, J. P., Zarzeczna, N., & Elsdon-Baker, F. (2022). Content matters: Perceptions of the science-religion relationship. *International Journal for the Psychology of Religion, 32*(3), 232–255.

Lifshin, U., Greenberg, J., Soenke, M., Darrell, A., & Pyszczynski, T. (2018). Mortality salience, religiosity, and indefinite life extension: Evidence of a reciprocal relationship between afterlife beliefs and support for forestalling death. *Religion, Brain and Behavior, 8*(1), 31–43.

Lifton, R. J. (1979). *The broken connection*. Simon & Schuster.

Lim, C., & Putnam, R. D. (2010). Religion, social networks, and life satisfaction. *American Sociological Review, 75*(6), 914–933.

Manning, C. (2023). Facing death without religion: How non-religious elders imagine death and how that shapes their lives. *Journal of Religion, Spirituality and Aging*, 1–20.

Nelson, T. A., Abeyta, A. A., & Routledge, C. (2021). What makes life meaningful for theists and atheists? *Psychology of Religion and Spirituality, 13*(1), 111–118.

Norenzayan, A., Dar-Nimrod, I., Hansen, I. G., & Proulx, T. (2009). Mortality salience and religion: Divergent effects on the defense of cultural worldviews for the religious and the non-religious. *European Journal of Social Psychology, 39*(1), 101–113.

Norenzayan, A., & Hansen, I. G. (2006). Belief in supernatural agents in the face of death. *Personality and Social Psychology Bulletin, 32*(2), 174–187.

Norris, P., & Inglehart, R. (2011). *Sacred and secular: Religion and politics worldwide*. Cambridge University Press.

Park, C., & McNamara, P. (2006). Religion, meaning, and the brain. In P. McNamara (Ed.), *Where God and science meet: How brain and evolutionary studies alter our understanding of religion* (pp. 67–89). Praeger.

Pearce, P. L., & Denton, M. L. (2011). *A faith of their own: Stability and change in the religiosity of American adolescents*. Oxford University Press.

Perach, R., & Wisman, A. (2019). Can creativity beat death? A review and evidence on the existential anxiety buffering functions of creative achievement. *Journal of Creative Behavior, 53*(2), 193–210.

Pew Research Center. (2015, October 22). *Religion and science*. www.pewresearch.org/science/2015/10/22/science-and-religion/.

Pew Research Center. (2018a, August 29). *The religious typology*. www.pewresearch.org/religion/2018/08/29/the-religious-typology/.

Pew Research Center. (2018b, November 20). *Where Americans find meaning in life*. www.pewresearch.org/religion/2018/11/20/where-americans-find-meaning-in-life/.

Pew Research Center. (2024, January). *Religious "nones" in America: Who they are and what they believe*. www.pewresearch.org/religion/2024/01/24/religious-nones-in-america-who-they-are-and-what-they-believe/.

Phelps, A. C., Maciejewski, P. K., Nilsson, M., Balboni, T. A., Wright, A. A., Paulk, M. E., . . . Prigerson, H. G. (2009). Religious coping and use of intensive life-prolonging care near death in patients with advanced cancer. *Journal of the American Medical Association, 301*(11), 1140–1147.

Preston, J. L., Coleman T. J., III, & Shin, F. (2023). Spirituality of science: Implications for meaning, well-being, and learning. *Personality and Social Psychology Bulletin*.

Preston, J., & Epley, N. (2005). Explanations versus applications: The explanatory power of valuable beliefs. *Psychological Science, 16*, 826–832.

Preston, J. L., & Shin, F. (2017). Spiritual experiences evoke awe through the small self in both religious and non-religious individuals. *Journal of Experimental Social Psychology, 70*, 212–221.

Prinzing, M., Van Cappellen, P., & Fredrickson, B. L. (2023). More than a momentary blip in the universe?: Investigating the link between religiousness and perceived meaning in life. *Personality and Social Psychology Bulletin, 49*(2), 180–196.

Riekki, T. J. J., Lindeman, M., & Lipsanen, J. (2013). Conceptions about the mind–body problem and their relations to afterlife beliefs, paranormal beliefs, religiosity, and ontological confusions. *Advances in Cognitive Psychology, 9,* 112–120.

Routledge, C., Roylance, C., & Abeyta, A. A. (2017). Further exploring the link between religion and existential health: The effects of religiosity and trait differences in mentalizing on indicators of meaning in life. *Journal of Religion and Health, 56,* 604–613.

Rutjens, B. T., Heine, S. J., Sutton, R. M., & van Harreveld, F. (2018). Attitudes towards science. *Advances in Experimental Social Psychology, 57,* 125–165.

Rutjens, B. T., & Preston, J. L. (2020). Science and religion: A rocky relationship shaped by shared psychological functions. In K. Vail & C. Routledge (Eds.), *The science of religion, spirituality, and existentialism* (pp. 373–385). Elsevier/Academic Press.

Rutjens, B. T., van der Pligt, J., & van Harreveld, F. (2010). Deus or Darwin: Randomness and belief in theories about the origin of life. *Journal of Experimental Social Psychology, 46,* 1078–1080.

Rutjens, B. T., van Harreveld, F., & van der Pligt, J. (2013). Step by step: Finding compensatory order in science. *Current Directions in Psychological Science, 22*(3), 250–255.

Rutjens, B. T., van Harreveld, F., van der Pligt, J., van Elk, M., & Pyszczynski, T. (2016). A march to a better world?: Religiosity and the existential function of belief in social-moral progress. The International *Journal for the Psychology of Religion, 26*(1), 1–18.

Saroglou, V., Delpierre, V., & Dernelle, R. (2004). Values and religiosity: A meta-analysis of studies using Schwartz's model. *Personality and Individual Differences, 37*(4), 721–734.

Sawyer, J. S., Brewster, M. E., & Ertl, M. M. (2021). Death anxiety and death acceptance in atheists and other nonbelievers. *Death Studies, 45*(6), 459–468.

Schnell, T., & Keenan, W. J. (2011). Meaning-making in an atheist world. *Archive for the Psychology of Religion, 33*(1), 55–78.

Schwartz, S. H., & Huismans, S. (1995). Value priorities and religiosity in four Western religions. *Social Psychology Quarterly, 58,* 88–107.

Shen, P. (2003). *Flight from death: The quest for immortality* [Film]. Transcendental Media.

Shinall, M. C., Jr. (2014). Fighting for dear life: Christians and aggressive end-of-life care. *Perspectives in Biology and Medicine, 57*(3), 329–340.

Shinall, M. C., Jr., Ehrenfeld, J. M., & Guillamondegui, O. D. (2014). Religiously affiliated intensive care unit patients receive more aggressive end-of-life care. *Journal of Surgical Research, 190*(2), 623–627.

Shor, E., & Roelfs, D. J. (2013). The longevity effects of religious and nonreligious participation: A meta-analysis and meta-regression. *Journal for the Scientific Study of Religion, 52*(1), 120–145.

Smith, J. M. (2017). Communal secularity: Congregational work at the Sunday Assembly. In R. T. Cragun, C. Manning, & L. Fazzino (Eds.), *Organized secularism* (pp. 151–170). De Gruyter Press.

Soenke, M., Vail, K. E., III, & Greenberg, J. (2022). Investigating the role of normative support in atheists' perceptions of meaning following reminders of death. *Frontiers in Psychology, 13,* 913508.

Solomon, S., Greenberg, J., & Pyszczynski, T. (2015). *The worm at the core: On the role of death in life.* Random House.

Solomon, S., & Thompson, S. (2019). Secular cultural worldviews. In C. Routledge & M. Vess (Eds.), *Handbook of terror management theory* (pp. 287–302). Academic Press.

Speed, D., Coleman, T. J., III, & Langston, J. (2018). What do you mean, "What does it all mean?": Atheism, nonreligion, and life meaning. *Sage Open, 8*(1).

Spitzenstätter, D., & Schnell, T. (2022). The existential dimension of the pandemic: Death attitudes, personal worldview, and coronavirus anxiety. *Death Studies, 46*(5), 1031–1041.

Spitzenstätter, D., & Schnell, T. (2023). The uncertain certainty: A mixed methods exploration of personal meanings of death and preliminary insights into their relationship with worldview. *OMEGA-Journal of Death and Dying.*

Ståhl, T., & van Prooijen, J. W. (2021). Analytic atheism: Valuing epistemic rationality strengthens the association between analytic thinking and religious disbelief. *Personality and Individual Differences, 179,* 110914.

Stavrova, O. (2015). Religion, self-rated health, and mortality: Whether religiosity delays death depends on the cultural context. *Social Psychological and Personality Science, 6,* 911–922.

Stavrova, O., Fetchenhauer, D., & Schlösser, T. (2013). Why are religious people happy?: The effect of the social norm of religiosity across countries. *Social Science Research, 42*(1), 90–105.

Steger, M. F., & Frazier, P. (2005). Meaning in life: One link in the chain from religiousness to well-being. *Journal of Counseling Psychology, 52*(4), 574–582.

Taves, A. (2020). From religious studies to worldview studies. *Religion, 50*(1), 137–147.

Tracy, J. L., Hart, J., & Martens, J. P. (2011). Death and science: The existential underpinnings of belief in intelligent design and discomfort with evolution. *PLOS One, 6*(3), e17349.

Uzarevic, F., Saroglou, V., & Clobert, M. (2017). Are atheists undogmatic? *Personality and Individual Differences, 116,* 164–170.

Vail, K. E., III, Arndt, J., & Abdollahi, A. (2012). Exploring the existential function of religion and supernatural agent beliefs among Christians, Muslims, Atheists, and Agnostics. *Personality and Social Psychology Bulletin, 38*(10), 1288–1300.

Vail, K. E., III, & Soenke, M. (2018). The impact of mortality awareness on meaning in life among Christians and atheists. *Religion, Brain and Behavior, 8*(1), 44–56.

Vail, K. E., III, Soenke, M., Waggoner, B., & Mavropoulou, I. (2020). Natural, but not supernatural, literal immortality affirmation attenuates mortality salience effects on worldview defense in atheists. *Personality and Social Psychology Bulletin, 46*(2), 312–326.

van Mulukom, V., Turpin, H., Haimila, R., Purzycki, B. G., Bendixen, T., Kundtová Klocová, E., . . . Farias, M. (2023). What do nonreligious nonbelievers believe in?: Secular worldviews around the world. *Psychology of Religion and Spirituality, 15*(1), 143–156.

van Wijmen, M. P., Pasman, H. R., Widdershoven, G. A., & Onwuteaka-Philipsen, B. D. (2015). Continuing or forgoing treatment at the end of life?: Preferences of the general public and people with an advance directive. *Journal of Medical Ethics, 41,* 599–606.

Wink, P., & Scott, J. (2005). Does religiousness buffer against the fear of death and dying in late adulthood?: Findings from a longitudinal study. *Journals of Gerontology Series B: Psychological Sciences and Social Sciences, 60*(4), 207–214.

Yilmaz, O. (2021). Cognitive styles and religion. *Current Opinion in Psychology, 40,* 150–154.

Zmigrod, L., Eisenberg, I. W., Bissett, P. G., Robbins, T. W., & Poldrack, R. A. (2021). The cognitive and perceptual correlates of ideological attitudes: A data-driven approach. *Philosophical Transactions of the Royal Society B, 376,* 20200424.

Zuckerman, M., Li, C., & Diener, E. (2018). Religion as an exchange system: The interchangeability of God and government in a provider role. *Personality and Social Psychology Bulletin, 44*(8), 1201–1213.

CHAPTER 56

Religious and Spiritual Struggles

A Brief Overview Highlighting Links with Existential Topics

Julie J. Exline *and* Kenneth I. Pargament

Religion can serve a powerful role in meeting many important human needs, such as needs for meaning (Park, 2013), belonging (Saroglou, 2011), identity (Mavor & Ysseldyk, 2020), attachment (Granqvist, 2020), and comfort (Exline et al., 2000). However, religion can also become a source of strain or struggle. Over the past several decades, scholars have addressed the dark and difficult sides of religion and spirituality through constructs such as spiritual crisis (Piedmont, 2012), meaning crisis (Schnell, 2009), religious/spiritual distress (King et al., 2017; Monod et al., 2010), spiritual pain (Delgado-Guay et al., 2011), spiritual suffering (Bartel, 2004), spiritual dryness (Büssing et al., 2013), spiritual needs (Büssing, 2021), spiritual decline (Cole et al., 2008), and spiritual emergency (Goretzki et al., 2013; Grof & Grof, 1991), to name just a few. In recent years, our research teams have studied *spiritual struggles,* which refer to experiences of tension, strain, or conflict surrounding whatever people view as sacred (Exline, 2013; Pargament, 2007; Pargament & Exline, 2021, 2022). The spiritual struggles concept grew from our earlier work on religious strain (Exline et al., 2000) and negative religious coping (e.g., Pargament, 1997; Pargament et al., 1998). (Note that we use *spiritual struggle* and *negative religious coping* as synonyms rather than separate constructs.)

There is now too much literature on spiritual struggles to review in one chapter. (For more detailed recent reviews and clinical suggestions, see Pargament & Exline, 2021, 2022.) In this chapter, we give a broad overview of key concepts and findings before moving on to emphasize direct connections between spiritual struggles and existential psychology themes.

First, we introduce the topic of spiritual struggles and the six types that we have emphasized in our research. After briefly reviewing several recent measurement approaches, we turn our attention to research that clarifies the importance of spiritual struggles, showing their prevalence and connections to mental and physical health, social relationships, and religious engagement. Next, we touch on the controversial question of whether spiritual struggles lead to growth. After this brief overview of empirical literature, we tie our discussion of spiritual struggles directly to existential themes, such as meaning, freedom, isolation, and death (Yalom, 1980). We highlight points of connection between each struggle and existential issues, and we offer testable ideas about how different existential worldviews might protect against certain struggles while setting the stage for others.

SPIRITUAL STRUGGLE: DEFINITIONS, TYPES, AND MEASUREMENT APPROACHES

We use the term *spiritual* in a broad sense, referring to a search for the sacred (Pargament et al., 2013b). By *search*, we refer to the effort to form, sustain, and perhaps transform a relationship with the sacred. By *sacred*, we refer to something that people see as transcendent, profoundly meaningful, and perhaps (but not necessarily) divine. We use *religion* to refer to attempts to pursue the sacred as part of a specific organization or community—one whose primary goal is to foster these human connections with the sacred (Pargament et al., 2013b). This chapter focuses on *religious/spiritual struggles* (often shortened to *spiritual struggles*), which refer to experiences of tension, strain, or conflict around religion or spirituality (Pargament & Exline, 2021, 2022).

Given the vast number of ways that people could pursue the sacred, along with the many religious belief systems found around the world, we found it impractical (and perhaps not possible) to try to catalog all forms of spiritual struggle within a single measure. Our more modest aim, then, was to focus on a few forms of struggle that we expected to be relatively widespread. As a starting point, we drew from our existing work on negative religious coping (Pargament et al., 1998, 2013) and religious strain (Exline et al., 2000) to develop a measure to assess six types of spiritual struggles that we expected many people to experience: divine, demonic, interpersonal, moral, ultimate meaning, and doubt. We have assessed these struggles through several measures: the original, 26-item Religious and Spiritual Struggles Scale (RSS; Exline et al., 2014b); the shorter RSS-14 (Exline et al., 2023a); and an upcoming six-item screener (Exline et al., 2025c) that taps each type of struggle with one broad item.

We categorize two of these—divine and demonic struggles—as *supernatural* struggles, because they focus on beliefs about specific supernatural entities. *Divine struggles* involve negative thoughts or feelings focused on a deity or one's perceived relationship with a deity, such as anger at God, questioning God's love, feeling isolated or distant from God, or feeling punished by God. (These items could be reworded to focus on multiple gods [Exline et al., 2017a] or a higher power.) *Demonic struggles* refer to concerns about how supernatural evil forces might be involved in one's own life: perceived attacks, temptations, or problems caused by the devil or evil spirits. *Interpersonal religious struggles* involve the social dimension of religion, including conflicts with people around religious issues, feeling hurt, misunderstood, or rejected by religious people, or feeling angry at organized religion. We categorize the last three struggles as *intrapersonal* struggles, as they all focus on issues within the self that do not necessarily involve supernatural beliefs or religious communities. These include *moral struggles* (guilt about perceived moral offenses; wrestling to follow moral guidelines), *ultimate meaning struggles* (questioning the purpose of life in general or one's own life), and *doubt struggles* (feeling confused about one's religious beliefs; concern about correctness of beliefs).

Although the RSS measures seem quite effective for assessing the six domains of struggle that we mentioned above, they are by no means exhaustive. They complement many other tools available in the research and clinical literature, including broadly focused measures of kindred concepts mentioned above, such as spiritual crisis (Piedmont, 2012), religious/spiritual distress (King et al., 2017; Monod et al., 2010), spiritual needs (Büssing, 2021), spiritual pain (Delgado-Guay et al., 2011), and spiritual decline (Cole et al., 2008). Other tools focus on struggles that we did not tap in the RSS, such as fear of hell (Cranney et al., 2018), spiritual dryness (which can involve spiritual lethargy or a lack of energy in one's relationship with God; Büssing et al., 2013), and spiritual emergency (difficulty integrating challenging unusual spiritual experiences; Goretski et al., 2013). Still other measures take a closer look at specific issues that the RSS captures only broadly or indirectly. For example, Koch's measure of spiritual harm and abuse (Koch & Erdstrom, 2022) isolates a specific type of interpersonal religious struggle, whereas moral injury (Jinkerson, 2016) assesses a response to a specific type of moral struggle. The meaning in life construct (Steger, 2021; Steger et al., 2006, 2009) captures a perceived absence of meaning in life, along with ongoing searches for meaning. Altemeyer and Hunsberger's (1997) measure taps various sources of religious doubt. And many measures relate to divine struggle, including tools to assess attachment to God (Beck & McDonald, 2004; Hall, 2015; Rowatt & Kirkpatrick, 2002), God images (Davis et al., 2013), views of God's role in suffering (Hale-Smith et al., 2012), and behaviors toward God in response to spiritual struggle (Exline et al., 2023c), to name just a few.

WHY SHOULD PSYCHOLOGISTS CARE ABOUT SPIRITUAL STRUGGLES?

Prevalence

Many people experience spiritual struggles. Although Christian samples have predominated in research in the United States, spiritual struggles have been documented across many religious traditions (Stauner et al., 2015), including Judaism (Abu-Raiya et al., 2016), Islam (Abu-Raiya et al., 2015a), Buddhism (Phillips et al., 2009), and Hinduism (Exline et al., 2017a; Tarakeshwar et al., 2003). Many atheists and agnostics also report spiritual struggles (e.g., Bradley et al., 2017, 2018; Exline et al., 2014b; Sedlar et al., 2018). In a survey of over 18,000 U.S. adults (Exline et al., 2014a), 70% reported some level of spiritual struggle in the past few weeks. Importantly, these figures may be underestimates: Many people see certain spiritual struggles, such as anger toward God, as morally wrong (Exline et al., 2012), which might lead to underreporting. Others may suppress or repress struggles because they are uncomfortable with them. If people feel ashamed of their spiritual struggles and see such strains as uncommon or pathological, they might also feel more isolated, lonely, and stigmatized when facing these struggles.

Links with Mental Health and Other Indicators of Adjustment

Hundreds of studies have focused on connections between spiritual struggles (including negative religious coping) and mental health—far more than we can review here (see Pargament & Exline, 2022, for a review.) Because items tapping spiritual struggles focus on concerns, conflicts, and worries, it makes sense that one would see consistent links with distress—and this is clearly what the literature shows. Some of the strongest data come from nationally representative surveys, which show consistent positive correlations between spiritual struggles and indicators of depression, anxiety, anger, and stress (Abu-Raiya et al., 2015b; Ellison & Lee, 2010; McConnell et al., 2006), extending in some cases to suicidality (Currier et al., 2018, 2020; Raines et al., 2017).

To date, much of the work on spiritual struggles and mental health has been cross-sectional, which raises questions about timing: Do baseline spiritual struggles predict later increases in distress, or does baseline distress predict later increases in spiritual struggles? To begin to address this question, Pargament and Lomax (2013) presented three models to represent possible relationships between spiritual struggles and distress: In the *primary struggles model*, spiritual struggles predict increased distress. In the *secondary struggles model*, distress predicts increased struggle. And in the *complex struggles model*, spiritual struggle and distress have a reciprocal relationship, building on one another. As we elaborate elsewhere (Pargament & Exline, 2022; Pargament et al., 2024), research suggests strong support for the primary struggles model (e.g., meta-analysis of 32 longitudinal studies by Bockrath et al., 2022), along with some support for the secondary struggles model (e.g., Neimeyer & Burke, 2011; Reynolds et al., 2014) and the complex struggles model (Beeman et al., 2024; Cowden et al., 2022; Lemke et al., 2023). Thus, the answer to the question of whether spiritual struggles cause distress or vice versa may depend on the particular struggle, the type of distress, the challenges the individual is facing, and their social context.

Spiritual struggles also relate to other indicators of mental and physical health. They predict faster progression of HIV symptoms (Ironson et al., 2011), greater hospitalization risk for heart failure patients (Park et al., 2011), and even increased mortality rates (Pargament et al., 2001). Spiritual struggles also show connections with relational strains, such as politically focused anger (Exline et al., 2023b) and poorer adjustment to divorce (Krumrei et al., 2011), and they predict self-regulation difficulties such as alcohol problems (Stauner et al., 2019) and perceived addiction to internet pornography (Grubbs et al., 2017). People reporting more spiritual struggles are also more likely than others to report spiritual decline (Desai & Pargament, 2015; Exline et al., 2023a) and to pull away from religion (Exline et al., 2020).

The Potential for Growth through Struggle

Even though spiritual struggles tend to be distressing, it seems intuitive that they might also lead to growth, given the commonly held idea that struggles make people stronger. Yet data on the connection between spiritual struggles and spiritual growth is mixed: Some studies suggest positive associations, others suggest negative associations, and others suggest no relationship (for reviews, see Pargament et al., 2006; Pargament & Exline, 2021, 2022). Consider, too, what a group of college students said about their spiritual struggles: Nearly half (49%) said that they had grown from their struggles (Desai & Pargament, 2015); yet, in this same sample, 29% of students reported both spiritual growth and decline from their struggles.

There are several methodological challenges in studying the idea that struggle leads to perceived growth. One problem is that many studies to date are cross-sectional, whereas the perception of growth from struggle might take time to develop. There have also been recent debates about what constitutes growth and how best to measure it (Infurna & Jayawickreme, 2019). Value judgments enter here as well: One person might see religious disaffiliation as a path toward growth, while another might frame it as decline.

In short, existing research does not point to a simple conclusion that spiritual struggles lead to growth. In empirical terms, perhaps the best question to ask is not whether struggle, in and of itself, leads to growth, but whether certain responses to struggle might lead to perceptions of growth. Here we have more answers: In the wake of spiritual struggle, people report more growth to the extent that they take a flexible, questing approach to life (Hart et al., 2020), frame their struggle as a spiritual challenge to draw them closer to God (Saritoprak et al., 2018, 2020), see God's intentions as benevolent (Exline et al., 2017b), and view themselves as having a collaborative relationship with God, one in which they partner with God to solve problems (Exline et al., 2017b; Wilt et al., 2019).

HOW DO SPIRITUAL STRUGGLES RELATE TO EXISTENTIAL THEMES?

Next, we move closer to the themes of this handbook by highlighting connections between spiritual struggles and existential issues. Although we cite some studies in this section, our main aim is simply to suggest points of connection and hypotheses that might be fruitful to test in future research. First, we consider each of the six struggle types from our prior work (Exline et al., 2014b; Pargament & Exline, 2022) and suggest ways in which each one could have existential relevance. Then, we speculate about whether different existential worldviews might protect against certain struggles while promoting others.

Existential Relevance of the Six Types of Spiritual Struggles: Seeds for Future Research

The search for the sacred, along with the religious beliefs, meaning structures, and communities that often accompany it, can be fundamental parts of how people make sense of the world and find a sense of deep purpose in their lives (Park, 2013). As such, we propose that each type of struggle has the potential to tap into deep existential concerns. In this section we briefly outline some of these points of connection. We intend to frame many of the ideas here as testable ideas for future research.

Ultimate Meaning Struggles

Of all the spiritual struggles, those involving questions of ultimate meaning show the most obvious, clear connections with existential issues. When people wrestle with core questions about whether their own lives have meaning—or whether life itself has any deep meaning or purpose, they are tapping into fundamental human questions: Why do we exist, and do our lives carry any real significance? How should we spend our limited time and energy, and how much will it all really matter in the long run? Prior work confirms that ultimate meaning struggles relate to a lower perceived presence of meaning but a greater search for meaning (Exline et al., 2014b, 2021; Wilt et al., 2017). We also expect to see connections here with the emerging construct of *spiritual yearning* (Van Tongeren et al., 2025; Wilt et al., 2025), which captures the idea that many nonreligious people seek a deeper sense of existential meaning and security by engaging with something greater than themselves. And what if people conclude that their lives lack meaning? Such conclusions could be very painful or threatening psychologically, as shown in many prior studies (Keesee et al., 2008; Li et al., 2019; Schnell, 2009; Steger et al., 2006, 2009; Wilt et al., 2017; Wong, 2012, 2014, 2016). Our own work also shows that, of the six struggle types, ultimate meaning struggles show the strongest links with distress (Exline et al., 2014b, 2021). In future work, it would be especially helpful to see more applied studies focusing on strategies for helping people cope with these existential struggles.

Divine Struggles

Who created the world, and who is ultimately in charge of it? These are core existential questions related to the existence of God, gods, or some type of higher power. Doubts about God's existence (along with other sources of religious doubt) are associated with elevated distress (Exline et al., 2025a). If people believe that a deity exists (or might exist), do they tend to see this deity as benevolent and forgiving, or harsh and punitive? Is God a reliable source of care, protection, and guidance? (See, e.g., Granqvist, 2020.) Will the afterlife be a place of eternal reward and reconciliation with God, or a place of divine punishment? Such questions, though still understudied from a psychological perspective, may be powerful parts of a person's orienting system (Pargament, 1997) and their fundamental sense of security versus fear in daily life. If people see God as punitive or unloving, or if they feel angry at God, they are more likely to be anxious and depressed and to question whether their lives have deep meaning (Exline et al., 2014b, 2021). If people see God as distant, uncaring, or uninvolved, might they also experience a profound sense of isolation and disconnection? Also, when thinking about the afterlife, might the idea of an angry, cold, or unpredictable God make people fear eternal punishment? Furthermore, might even those who expect to go to heaven have mixed feelings about spending the afterlife with such a God? Such ideas await empirical testing.

Demonic Struggles

Questions about good and evil, like those about the existence of a deity, may be core parts of a person's orienting system. These questions could easily lead to divine struggles, as people try to answer the question of why God allows evil and suffering in the world (Hale-Smith et al., 2012). Belief in supernatural evil—the devil, demons, or evil spirits—may help with meaning making by offering at least a partial answer for why bad things happen. Blaming the devil may also keep people from blaming God (Beck & Taylor, 2008), which in turn could help them feel more relationally and existentially secure. But at the same time, it could be terrifying to see the world embroiled in an epic struggle between good and evil in which human beings are the pawns. Many people believe that the devil has the power to attack them and cause problems in their lives (Exline et al., 2021; Exline et al., 2023d), which could contribute to a fundamental view of the world as unsafe. Despite their psychological importance, demonic struggles have received little research attention to date. This is a wide-open area for future work.

Doubt Struggles

Given that religious beliefs often address core components of human existence, it is easy to see how doubts about religion could threaten core aspects of one's orienting system (cf. Pargament, 1997, 2007) or shake deeply held worldviews (Exline et al., 2023a). As shown in Altemeyer and Hunsberger's (1997) measure, some sources of religious doubt are explicitly existential: Does God exist? Is there an afterlife? Can the authority of one's sacred text be trusted? If people have been raised to believe in these things, and especially if they turn to such belief for security, hope, or comfort, they may find it frightening or disorienting to face questions and doubts about these core beliefs. Many people also doubt religion for interpersonal reasons, such as witnessing hypocrisy, intolerance, or cruelty by religious people (Altemeyer & Hunsberger, 1997; Exline et al., 2025a). As we highlight below, these interpersonal tensions can carry existential relevance. Given that doubts can be frightening, it makes sense that many people gravitate toward fundamentalist beliefs (Hood et al., 2005; Williamson et al., 2010) to shield against doubt and despair. However, religious doubt may also have a bright side: Recent work (Exline et al., 2025a) shows that doubt struggles related positively to an open, inquisitive stance that included intellectual humility, openness to experience, and (especially) a quest orientation to religion (cf. Batson & Schoenrade, 1991; Beck & Jessup, 2004), one in which people embraced doubt and uncertainty as part of their spiritual growth and development. Again, intervention studies would be helpful at this stage: How can people learn to face religious doubts and questions in life-giving ways? (See Pargament & Exline, 2022, for a discussion.)

Moral Struggles

When individuals reflect on the deep values and purposes underlying their lives, moral challenges may take on special significance. For example, as people consider their misdeeds, they may have difficulty forgiving themselves (Woodyatt et al., 2017). They may also question whether God forgives them (Fincham, 2022) or worry about accumulating bad karma (White & Norenzayan, 2019, 2022). Some may see themselves as fundamentally bad, immoral, or sinful, feeding a global sense of shame (Tangney & Dearing, 2002) that could cripple the pursuit of a positive identity and purpose. When trying to discern the most moral choices, existential questions might also arise if people question whether they can trust their own internal compass, the conscience. Some recent work (Schutt & Exline, 2023) has shown that if people see the conscience as divinely inspired, they tend to trust it more; but at the same time, those who see God as an influencer of the conscience also tend to see the devil as having similar abilities—demonic attributions that, in turn, are linked with less trust in the conscience. More attention is needed to these types of questions that link moral struggles with existential concerns.

Interpersonal Religious Struggles

On the surface, interpersonal struggles around religion might seem to be the most earthbound of the struggles, as they focus on relationships with religious communities. But the need to belong is a fundamental human motivation (Baumeister & Leary, 1995). And, as outlined by scholars such as Mahoney (2010, 2013) and Saroglou (2011; see also Saroglou et al., 2020), connections with a religious community can be a powerful way to meet this need to belong. As such, conflicts with and disapproval or rejection from members of a religious community could pose a serious existential threat. Even if people do not see their own status in a religious community as being jeopardized, it could be disorienting or destabilizing to question the veracity of sacred texts or the authority of religious leaders. Those who have been leaning on these sources for guidance might wonder, "Who (or what) is a reliable source of authority for these deep questions in my life?"

How Different Existential Worldviews Might Relate to Spiritual Struggles

Given that so many people experience spiritual struggles and considering the wide array of ways that people see the world and their place in it, we are eager to understand more about the "flavors" of struggle that might characterize different existential worldviews. In this section we offer some testable ideas about how certain religious, spiritual, and secular worldviews might protect against certain struggles while setting the stage for others. Most of the material here is in the realm of idea and hypothesis generation rather than literature review. Also, note that we mention only a few select worldviews here; many other options and nuances are possible.

How Well Do My Beliefs Fit?

Before launching into specific existential beliefs, we first raise some general predictions around how well a person's beliefs and practices fit with those of valued or powerful others. On the one hand, being part of a community brings its own strains. Anyone might find it frustrating, inauthentic, or costly to be part of a group—tendencies that might be strongest for people who highly value individuality, autonomy, or distinctiveness. But at the same time, people open themselves to interpersonal religious struggles when they hold (and express) viewpoints that do not mesh well with those of a dominant group. Such strain should be possible in any type of group, all the way from couple or family units (cf. Mahoney, 2010, 2013) to religious communities to cultures: Those who question or violate norms, especially if they lack power within the group, may open themselves to painful social outcomes ranging from disapproval and judgment to punishment, shaming, and rejection. In extreme authoritarian contexts, dissent might be considered heretical or even criminal. From the imprisonment of early Christians to the brutality of religious wars to the burning of witches at the stake, human beings have repeatedly shown that going against the group can be dangerous.

Atheist, Materialist, and Secular Worldviews

People who do not hold supernatural beliefs could conceivably avoid struggles involving God, the devil, spirits, or afterlife beliefs, and they could avoid the costs of commitment to religious groups that hold such beliefs. Along these lines, some people do report that they stopped believing in God because of divine or interpersonal religious struggles from earlier in their lives (Bradley et al., 2017, 2018). Yet people who have left religion often carry vestiges of prior beliefs, as shown in work on *religious residue* (Van Tongeren et al., 2021). Along these lines, some atheists report divine struggles (Sedlar et al., 2018), based on past religious experiences or hypothetical images of God (Bradley et al., 2015, 2017, 2018). Atheists also report more ultimate meaning struggles than religious believers report (Exline et al., 2014b). If most people in their culture hold religious beliefs, atheists and religious exiters may also find themselves facing stigma (Gervais et al., 2011). And for agnostics, ongoing uncertainty about the nature of ultimate reality might create a different type of stress.

Impersonal Supernatural Forces: Karma, Fate, Destiny, and Luck

Rather than believing in personal or anthropomorphic deities and devils, many people believe in universal laws or forces that order the universe or maintain justice within it. Belief in such entities and their associated laws could provide some sense of meaning and control in a world that might otherwise seem random and chaotic. Psychologically, benefits should be strongest if people believe that they can influence these forces through their behavior—if good deeds can improve karma, for example, or if people can take action to improve their luck or shape their destiny (see Exline & Wilt, 2023, for a review). Yet this is not guaranteed, and some people may see themselves as trapped, helpless, or doomed in the face of these powerful but uncaring forces. Back on the positive side, belief in impersonal supernatural forces could eliminate the fear of wrathful deities; however, because the forces in question are impersonal, believers likely forgo some comforts of relational supernatural beliefs, such as a secure attachment to God/gods or ongoing help from saints, spirit guides, or departed loved ones. In addition, some people might fear dark or evil forces even if they do not believe in a personal devil or demons.

A Personal God, the Devil, Heaven and Hell

Many people find comfort in believing they have a personal, secure relationship with a loving and benevolent God (or god/goddess), as shown in the literature on religious coping (Pargament, 1997; Pargament et al., 2013a) and attachment to God (Beck & McDonald, 2004; Granqvist, 2020; Hall, 2015; Rowatt & Kirkpatrick, 2002). People may also find comfort and meaning if they believe that a deity has given people clear moral guidelines to follow: What constitutes a moral life? How can I go to heaven and avoid hell? If people find a clear moral compass in their religious beliefs and feel confident that they will go to heaven after they die, this should buffer against spiritual struggles. On the other hand, people may open the door for spiritual struggles if they see God as cruel and punitive (Exline et al., 2023a), believe that the devil is active in the world, and worry that they (or others they care about) may end up in hell (Cranney et al., 2018; Shariff & Aknin, 2014). A *cosmic battle mindset*—one including a powerful devil, a warrior God, and many people destined for hell, has also been linked with greater conspiracy thinking (including QAnon beliefs) and stronger tendencies to see political opponents as enemies and as evil (Exline et al., 2025c); such a mindset may open the door to interpersonal religious struggles as well.

An Enchanted World: Ghosts, Angels, Spirits, and Magic

Regardless of whether they believe in deities, people might find a sense of direction, control, or meaning if they believe that they can receive guidance or protection from other supernatural sources: angels, spirit guides, saints, animal or nature spirits, or spirits of deceased loved ones or ancestors, for instance. Some may also turn to occult practices or magic to strive for desired personal ends (Collins, 2015). These supernatural beliefs and practices might help people feel safe, connected, and hopeful without requiring a singular focus on a deity for comfort and assistance—thus reducing the odds of divine struggles. Perceived relationships with those who have died (see Pait et al., 2023, for a review) may also combat ultimate meaning struggles and loneliness by assuring people that life, as well as loving bonds, can continue after the death of the physical body (LaGrand, 2005; McCormick & Tassell-Matamua, 2016). Of course, some perceived spirit encounters could be troubling (Exline & Wilt, 2023; Sabucedo et al., 2023), such as beliefs or experiences involving evil spirits, unfriendly ghosts, or angry or demanding spirits of family members or ancestors. Here we might see overlap with demonic struggles, particularly if people fear harm from spirits.

Everything Is Alive and Has a Spirit: Pantheistic/Animistic/Oneness Beliefs

Another belief that does not invoke personal gods would involve seeing every aspect of nature or creation as sacred and alive, perhaps having a spirit or soul, and fundamentally interconnected as part of a greater whole or "one" (Coomber & Harré, 2022; Deal & Magyar-Russell, 2022; Edinger-Schons, 2020; Garfield et al., 2014; Krause et al., 2018). Such nondualistic, unifying, oneness-oriented beliefs should work against demonic and divine struggles while providing a sense of connection with other people, nature, the Earth, and perhaps beyond; this should be especially true if the ultimate reality that holds everything together is seen as loving or benevolent. A deep sense of interconnectedness or oneness could also provide a deep sense of meaning and purpose, especially if people see themselves as playing a useful role in this broader system. Yet at the same time, belief in profound or ultimate interconnectedness might also trigger ultimate meaning struggles if this belief leaves people feeling powerless, insubstantial (i.e., too small to matter in an infinitely vast universe), or lacking personal identity or autonomy (i.e., mere cogs in a machine). Some might also feel overwhelmed or suffer from compassion fatigue due to their heightened attunement to suffering in the world around them.

CONCLUSION

Our aim was to give a brief overview of the topic of spiritual struggles, emphasizing connections to existential psychology and questions for future research. Not only are spiritual struggles common and strongly linked with mental health; they often involve core parts of people's beliefs, daily lives, and relationships—areas that can carry deep, sacred meaning. We hope that this snapshot of existing literature, along with suggested topics for future research, helps build bridges between people who share interests in these deep issues at the heart of the human condition.

ACKNOWLEDGMENT

We are grateful for funding support from the John Templeton Foundation, Grant Nos. 36094, 59916, and 62948.

REFERENCES

Abu-Raiya, H., Exline, J. J., Pargament, K. I., & Agbaria, Q. (2015a). Prevalence, predictors, and implications of religious/spiritual struggles among Muslims. *Journal for the Scientific Study of Religion, 54*(4), 631–648.

Abu-Raiya, H., Pargament, K. I., Krause, N., & Ironson, G. (2015b). Robust links between religious/spiritual struggles, psychological distress, and well-being in a national sample of American adults. *American Journal of Orthopsychiatry, 85*(6), 565–575.

Abu-Raiya, H., Pargament, K. I., Weissberger, A., & Exline, J. J. (2016). An examination of religious/spiritual struggle among Israeli Jews. *International Journal for the Psychology of Religion, 26*(1), 67–79.

Altemeyer, B., & Hunsberger, B. (1997). *Amazing conversions: Why some turn to faith and others abandon religion.* Prometheus.

Bartel, M. (2004). What is spiritual? What is spiritual suffering? *Journal of Pastoral Care and Counseling, 58*(3), 187–201.

Batson, C. D., & Schoenrade, P. A. (1991). Measuring religion as Quest: I. Validity concerns. *Journal for the Scientific Study of Religion, 30*(4), 416–429.

Baumeister, R. F., & Leary, M. R. (1995). The need to belong: Desire for interpersonal attachments as a fundamental human motivation. *Psychological Bulletin, 117*(3), 497–529.

Beck, R., & Jessup, R. K. (2004). The multidimensional nature of quest motivation. *Journal of Psychology and Theology, 32*(4), 283–294.

Beck, R., & McDonald, A. (2004). Attachment to God: The Attachment to God Inventory, tests of working model correspondence, and an exploration of faith group differences. *Journal of Psychology and Theology, 32*(2), 92–103.

Beck, R., & Taylor, S. (2008). The emotional burden of monotheism: Satan, theodicy, and relationship with God. *Journal of Psychology and Theology, 36*(3), 151–160.

Beeman, C., Davis, E. B., Voytenko, V. L., McConnell, J. M., Lemke, A. W., Douce, T., . . . Pargament, K. I. (2024). The temporal association between religious/spiritual struggles and anxiety symptoms: A longitudinal study of psychiatric outpatients. *Journal of Affective Disorders Reports,* 100709.

Bockrath, M. F., Pargament, K. I., Wong, S., Harriott, V. A., Pomerleau, J. M., Homolka, S., . . . Exline, J. J. (2022). Religious and spiritual struggles and their links to psychological adjustment: A meta-analysis of longitudinal studies. *Psychology of Religion and Spirituality, 14*(3), 283–299.

Bradley, D. F., Exline, J. J., & Uzdavines, A. (2015). The god of nonbelievers: Characteristics of a hypothetical god. *Science, Religion and Culture, 2,* 120–130.

Bradley, D. F., Exline, J. J., & Uzdavines, A. W. (2017). Relational reasons for nonbelief in the existence of gods: An important adjunct to intellectual nonbelief. *Psychology of Religion and Spirituality, 9*(4), 319–327.

Bradley, D. F., Exline, J. J., Uzdavines, A., Coleman, T. J., Grubbs, J. B., & Hood, R. W. (2018). The reasons of atheists and agnostics for nonbelief in God's existence scale: Development and initial validation. *Psychology of Religion and Spirituality, 10*(3), 263–275.

Büssing, A. (2021). The Spiritual Needs Questionnaire in research and clinical application: A summary of findings. *Journal of Religion and Health, 60*(5), 3732–3748.

Büssing, A., Günther, A., Baumann, K., Frick, E., & Jacobs, C. (2013). Spiritual dryness as a measure of a specific spiritual crisis in Catholic priests: Associations with symptoms of burnout and distress. *Evidence-Based Complementary and Alternative Medicine.*

Cole, B. S., Hopkins, C. M., Tisak, J., Steel, J. L., & Carr, B. I. (2008). Assessing spiritual growth and spiritual decline following a diagnosis of cancer: Reliability and validity of the Spiritual Transformation Scale. *Psycho-Oncology, 17*(2), 112–121.

Collins, D. J. (Ed.). (2015). *The Cambridge history of magic and witchcraft in the West: From antiquity to the present.* Cambridge University Press.

Coomber, T., & Harré, N. (2022). Psychological

oneness: A typology. *Review of General Psychology, 26*(1), 49–67.

Cowden, R. G., Pargament, K. I., Chen, Z. J., Davis, E. B., Lemke, A. W., Glowiak, K. J., . . . Worthington, E. L., Jr. (2022). Religious/spiritual struggles and psychological distress: A test of three models in a longitudinal study of adults with chronic health conditions. *Journal of Clinical Psychology, 78*(4), 544–588.

Cranney, S., Leman, J., Fergus, T. A., & Rowatt, W. C. (2018). Hell anxiety as non-pathological fear. *Mental Health, Religion and Culture, 21*(9–10), 867–883.

Currier, J. M., Fadoir, N., Carroll, T. D., Kuhlman, S., Marie, L., Taylor, S. E., . . . Sims, B. M. (2020). A cross-sectional investigation of divine struggles and suicide risk among men in early recovery from substance use disorders. *Psychology of Religion and Spirituality, 12*(3), 324–333.

Currier, J. M., McDermott, R. C., McCormick, W. H., Churchwell, M. C., & Milkeris, L. (2018). Exploring cross-lagged associations between spiritual struggles and risk for suicidal behavior in a community sample of military veterans. *Journal of Affective Disorders, 230*(1), 93–100.

Davis, E. B., Moriarty, G. L., & Mauch, J. C. (2013). God images and god concepts: Definitions, development, and dynamics. *Psychology of Religion and Spirituality, 5*(1), 51–60.

Deal, P. J., & Magyar-Russell, G. M. (2022). A qualitative study of sanctification: How nature becomes sacred for nontheistic environmental activists. *Spirituality in Clinical Practice, 9*(1), 40–54.

Delgado-Guay, M. O., Hui, D., Parsons, H. A., Govan, K., De la Cruz, M., Thorney, S., & Bruera, E. (2011). Spirituality, religiosity, and spiritual pain in advanced cancer patients. *Journal of Pain and Symptom Management, 41*(6), 986–994.

Desai, K. M., & Pargament, K. I. (2015). Predictors of growth and decline following spiritual struggles. *International Journal for the Psychology of Religion, 25*(1), 42–56.

Edinger-Schons, L. M. (2020). Oneness beliefs and their effect on life satisfaction. *Psychology of Religion and Spirituality, 12*(4), 428–439.

Ellison, C. G., & Lee, J. (2010). Spiritual struggles and psychological distress: Is there a dark side of religion? *Social Indicators Research, 98*(3), 501–517.

Exline, J. J. (2013). Religious and spiritual struggles. In K. I. Pargament (Ed.-in-Chief), J. J. Exline, & J. W. Jones (Assoc. Eds.), *APA handbook of psychology, religion, and spirituality: Vol. 1. Context, theory, and research* (pp. 459–475). American Psychological Association.

Exline, J. J., Kamble, S., & Stauner, N. (2017a). Anger toward God(s) among undergraduates in India. *Religions, 8*(9), 194.

Exline, J. J., Kaplan, K. J., & Grubbs, J. B. (2012). Anger, exit, and assertion: Do people see protest toward God as morally acceptable? *Psychology of Religion and Spirituality, 4*(4), 264–277.

Exline, J. J., Keller, Y., Moffitt, A. C., Wilt, J. A., & Pargament, K. I. (2025a). Many reasons for religious doubt: Links with doubt struggles, mental health, and an open, humble, questing orientation. *Psychology of Religion and Spirituality.*

Exline, J. J., Moffitt, A., Wilt, J. A., & Schutt, W. A. (2025b). *The cosmic battle: How belief in a warrior God, a powerful devil, and a serious threat of hell relates to QAnon belief, general conspiracist beliefs, and seeing political opponents as evil.* Manuscript submitted for publication.

Exline, J. J., Pargament, K. I., & Grubbs, J. B. (2014a). [Longitudinal study of religious/spiritual struggles among U.S. adults using Qualtrics panels.] Unpublished raw data.

Exline, J. J., Pargament, K. I., Grubbs, J. B., Wilt, J. A., & Yali, A. M. (2025c). *A brief, broad measure of six spiritual struggles: Initial validation of the RSS-6, comparisons with the new RSS-14-R, and demographic differences using a nationally representative sample from the United States.* Manuscript under review.

Exline, J. J., Pargament, K. I., Grubbs, J. B., & Yali, A. M. (2014b). The Religious and Spiritual Struggles Scale: Development and initial validation. *Psychology of Religion and Spirituality, 6*(3), 208–222.

Exline, J. J., Pargament, K. I., Hall, T. W., & Harriott, V. A. (2017b). Predictors of growth from spiritual struggle among Christian undergraduates: Religious coping and perceptions of helpful action by God are both important. *Journal of Positive Psychology, 5,* 501–508.

Exline, J. J., Pargament, K. I., Wilt, J. A., Grubbs, J. G., & Yali, A. M. (2023a). The RSS-14: Development and preliminary validation of a 14-item form of the Religious and Spiritual Struggles Scale. *Psychology of Religion and Spirituality, 15*(4), 592–604.

Exline, J. J., Pargament, K. I., Wilt, J. A., & Harriott, V. A. (2021). Mental illness, normal psychological processes, or attacks by the devil?: Three lenses to frame demonic struggles in therapy. *Spirituality in Clinical Practice, 8*(3), 215–228.

Exline, J. J., Stauner, N., Wilt, J. A., & Grubbs,

J. B. (2023b). Religious and spiritual struggles around the 2016 and 2020 U.S. presidential elections. *Psychology of Religion and Spirituality, 15*(4), 578–591.

Exline, J. J., Van Tongeren, D. R., Bradley, D. F., Wilt, J. A., Stauner, N., Pargament, K. I., & DeWall, C. N. (2020). Pulling away from religion: Religious/spiritual struggles and religious disengagement among college students. *Psychology of Religion and Spirituality, 14*(3), 300–311.

Exline, J. J., & Wilt, J. A. (2023). Supernatural attributions: Seeing God, the devil, demons, spirits, fate, and karma as causes of events. *Annual Review of Clinical Psychology, 19,* 461–487.

Exline, J. J., Wilt, J. A., Stauner, N., & Pargament, K. I. (2023c). Approach, disengagement, protest, and suppression: Four behaviors toward God in the context of religious/spiritual struggle. *Psychology of Religion and Spirituality. 15*(4), 491–503.

Exline, J. J., Wilt, J. A., Stauner, N., Schutt, W. A., Pargament, K. I., Fincham, F. D., & May, R. W. (2023d). Supernatural operating rules: How people envision and experience God, the devil, ghosts/spirits, fate/destiny, karma, and luck. *Psychology of Religion and Spirituality, 15*(4), 504–514.

Exline, J. J., Yali, A. M., & Sanderson, W. C. (2000). Guilt, discord, and alienation: The role of religious strain in depression and suicidality. *Journal of Clinical Psychology, 56*(12), 1481–1496.

Fincham, F. D. (2022). Towards a psychology of divine forgiveness. *Psychology of Religion and Spirituality, 14*(4), 451–461.

Garfield, A. M., Drwecki, B. B., Moore, C. F., Kortenkamp, K. V., & Gracz, M. D. (2014). The Oneness Beliefs Scale: Connecting spirituality with pro-environmental behavior. *Journal for the Scientific Study of Religion, 53*(2), 356–372.

Gervais, W. M., Shariff, A. F., & Norenzayan, A. (2011). Do you believe in atheists?: Distrust is central to anti-atheist prejudice. *Journal of Personality and Social Psychology, 101*(6), 1189–1206.

Goretzki, M., Thalbourne, M. A., & Storm, L. (2013). Development of a Spiritual Emergency Scale. *Journal of Transpersonal Psychology, 45*(2), 105–117.

Granqvist, P. (2020). *Attachment in religion and spirituality: A wider view.* Guilford Press.

Grof, S., & Grof, C. (1991). *The stormy search for self: Understanding and living with spiritual emergency.* Mandala.

Grubbs, J. B., Exline, J. J., Pargament, K. I., Volk, F., & Lindberg, M. J. (2017). Internet pornography use, perceived addiction, and religious/spiritual struggles. *Archives of Sexual Behavior, 46*(6), 1733–1745.

Hale-Smith, A., Park, C. L., & Edmondson, D. (2012). Measuring beliefs about suffering: Development of the Views of Suffering Scale. *Psychological Assessment, 24*(4), 855–866.

Hall, T W. (2015). *Spiritual Transformation Inventory technical report: Development and validation.* www.spiritualtransformation.org.

Hart, A. C., Pargament, K. I., Grubbs, J. B., Exline, J. J., & Wilt, J. A. (2020). Predictors of self-reported growth following religious and spiritual struggles: Exploring the role of wholeness. *Religions.* www.mdpi.com/2077-1444/11/9/445/htm.

Hood, R. W., Hill, P. C., & Williamson, W. P. (2005). *The psychology of religious fundamentalism.* Guilford Press.

Infurna, F. J., & Jayawickreme, E. (2019). Fixing the growth illusion: New directions for research in resilience and posttraumatic growth. *Current Directions in Psychological Science, 28*(2), 152–158.

Ironson, G., Stuetzle, R., Ironson, D., Balbin, E., Kremer, H., George, A., . . . Fletcher, M. A. (2011). View of God as benevolent and forgiving or punishing and judgmental predicts HIV disease progression. *Journal of Behavioral Medicine, 34*(6), 414–425.

Jinkerson, J. D. (2016). Defining and assessing moral injury: A syndrome perspective. *Traumatology, 22*(2), 122–130.

Keesee, N. J., Currier, J. M., & Neimeyer, R. A. (2008). Predictors of grief following the death of one's child: The contribution of finding meaning. *Journal of Clinical Psychology, 64*(10), 1145–1163.

King, S. D., Fitchett, G., Murphy, P. E., Pargament, K. I., Harrison, D. A., & Loggers, E. T. (2017). Determining best methods to screen for religious/spiritual distress. *Supportive Care in Cancer, 25*(2), 471–479.

Koch, D., & Edstrom, L. (2022). Development of the Spiritual Harm and Abuse Scale. *Journal for the Scientific Study of Religion, 61*(2), 476–506.

Krause, N., Hill, P. C., Pargament, K. I., & Ironson, G. (2018). Do pantheistic, theistic, and deistic views of god moderate the relationship between financial strain and physical health status? *International Journal for the Psychology of Religion, 28*(1), 19–30.

Krumrei, E. J., Mahoney, A., & Pargament, K. I. (2011). Spiritual stress and coping model of divorce: A longitudinal study. *Journal of Family Psychology, 25*(6), 973–985.

LaGrand, L. E. (2005). The nature and therapeutic implications of the extraordinary experiences of the bereaved. *Journal of Near-Death Studies, 24*(1), 3–19.

Lemke, A. W., Davis, E. B., Voytenko, V. L., Cowden, R. G., Chen, Z. J., McConnell, J. M., . . . Wolff, R. P. (2023). Religious/spiritual struggles and suicide ideation among adult psychiatric outpatients: A 12-month longitudinal study. *Journal of Affective Disorders Reports, 14,* 100640.

Li, P. F. J., Wong, Y. J., & Chao, R. C.-L. (2019). Happiness and meaning in life: Unique, differential, and indirect associations with mental health. *Counselling Psychology Quarterly, 32*(3–4), 396–414.

Mahoney, A. (2010). Religion in families, 1999–2009: A relational spirituality framework. *Journal of Marriage and Family, 72*(4), 805–827.

Mahoney, A. (2013). The spirituality of us: Relational spirituality in the context of family relationships. In K. I. Pargament, J. J. Exline, & J. W. Jones (Eds.), *APA handbook of psychology, religion, and spirituality: Vol. 1. Context, theory, and research* (pp. 365–389). American Psychological Association.

Mavor, K. I., & Ysseldyk, R. (2020). A social identity approach to religion: Religiosity at the nexus of personal and collective self. In K. E. Vail III & C. Routledge (Eds.), *The science of religion, spirituality, and existentialism* (pp. 187–205). Elsevier/Academic Press.

McConnell, K. M., Pargament, K. I., Ellison, C. G., & Flannelly, K. J. (2006). Examining the links between spiritual struggles and symptoms of psychopathology in a national sample. *Journal of Clinical Psychology, 62*(12), 1469–1484.

McCormick, B. M. E., & Tassell-Matamua, N. A. (2016). After-death communication: A typology of therapeutic benefits. *Journal of Near Death Studies, 34*(3), 151–172.

Monod, S. M., Rochat, E., Büla, C. J., Jobin, G., Martin, E., & Spencer, B. (2010). The spiritual distress assessment tool: an instrument to assess spiritual distress in hospitalised elderly persons. *BMC Geriatrics, 10,* 88.

Neimeyer, R. A., & Burke, L. A. (2011). Complicated grief in the aftermath of homicide: Spiritual crisis and distress in an African American sample. *Religions, 2*(2), 145–164.

Pait, K. C., Exline, J. J., Pargament, K. I., & Zarrella, P. (2023). After-death communication: Issues of nondisclosure and implications for treatment. *Religions, 4*(8), 985.

Pargament, K. I. (1997). *The psychology of religion and coping: Theory, research, practice.* Guilford Press.

Pargament, K. I. (2007). *Spiritually integrated psychotherapy: Understanding and addressing the sacred.* Guilford Press.

Pargament, K. I., Desai, K. M., & McConnell, K. M. (2006). Spirituality: A pathway to posttraumatic growth or decline? In L. G. Calhoun & R. G. Tedeschi (Eds.), *Handbook of posttraumatic growth: Research and practice* (pp. 121–137). Erlbaum.

Pargament, K. I., & Exline, J. J. (2021). *The psychology of spiritual struggle.* Report prepared for the John Templeton Foundation. www.templeton.org/wp-content/uploads/2021/10/Spiritual-Struggle-Whitepaper_FINAL-10.5.pdf.

Pargament, K. I., & Exline, J. J. (2022). *Working with spiritual struggles in psychotherapy: From research to practice.* Guilford Press.

Pargament, K. I., Exline, J. J., Cowden, R. G., & Wilt, J. A. (2024). *Are spiritual struggles the cause or effect of psychological problems (or both)?* Manuscript submitted for publication.

Pargament, K. I., Falb, M. D., Ano, G. G., & Wachholtz, A. B. (2013a). The religious dimension of coping: Advances in theory, research, and practice. In R. F. Paloutzian & C. L. Park (Eds.), *Handbook of the psychology of religion and spirituality* (2nd ed., pp. 560–579). Guilford Press.

Pargament, K. I., Koenig, H. G., Tarakeshwar, N., & Hahn, J. (2001). Religious struggle as a predictor of mortality among medically ill elderly patients: A 2-year longitudinal study. *Archives of Internal Medicine, 161*(6), 1881–1885.

Pargament, K. I., & Lomax, J. W. (2013). Understanding and addressing religion among people with mental illness. *World Psychiatry, 12*(1), 26–32.

Pargament, K. I., Mahoney, A., Exline, J. J., Jones, J., & Shafranske, E. (2013b). Envisioning an integrative paradigm for the psychology of religion and spirituality. In K. I. Pargament (Ed.-in-Chief), J. Exline, & J. Jones (Assoc. Eds.), *APA handbook of psychology, religion, and spirituality: Vol. 1. Context, theory, and research* (pp. 3–20). American Psychological Association.

Pargament, K. I., Smith, B. W., Koenig, H. G., & Perez, L. (1998). Patterns of positive and negative religious coping with major life stressors. *Journal for the Scientific Study of Religion, 37*(4), 711–725.

Park, C. L. (2013). Religion and meaning. In R. F. Paloutzian & C. L. Park (Eds.), *Handbook of the psychology of religion and spirituality* (2nd ed., pp. 357–379). Guilford Press.

Park, C. L., Wortmann, J. H., & Edmondson, D. (2011). Religious struggle as a predictor of subsequent mental and physical well-being in advanced heart failure patients. *Journal of Behavioral Medicine, 34,* 426–436.

Phillips, R. E., III, Cheng, C. M., Pargament, K. I., Oemig, C., Colvin, S. D., Abarr, A. N., . . . Reed, A. S. (2009). Spiritual coping in American Buddhists: An exploratory study. *International Journal for the Psychology of Religion, 19*(4), 231–243.

Piedmont, R. L. (2012). Overview and development of a trait-based measure of numinous constructs: The Assessment of Spirituality and Religious Sentiments (ASPIRES) Scale. In L. J. Miller (Ed.), *The Oxford handbook of psychology and spirituality* (pp. 104–122). Oxford University Press.

Raines, A. M., Currier, J. M., McManus, E. S., Walton, J. L., Uddo, M., & Franklin, C. L. (2017). Spiritual struggles and suicide in veterans seeking PTSD treatment. *Psychological Trauma: Theory, Research, Practice, and Policy, 9*(6), 746–749.

Reynolds, N., Mrug, S., Hensler, M., Guion, K., & Madan-Swain, A. (2014). Spiritual coping and adjustment in adolescents with chronic illness: A two-year prospective study. *Journal of Pediatric Psychology, 39*(5), 542–551.

Rowatt, W. C., & Kirkpatrick, L. A. (2002). Two dimensions of attachment to God and their relation to affect, religiosity, and personality constructs. *Journal for the Scientific Study of Religion, 41*(4), 637–651.

Sabucedo, P., Evans, C., & Hayes, J. (2023). Perceiving those who are gone: Cultural research on post-bereavement perception or hallucination of the deceased. *Transcultural Psychiatry, 60*(6), 879–890.

Saritoprak, S. N., Exline, J. J., & Abu-Raiya, H. (2020). Spiritual jihad as an emerging psychological concept: Connections with religious/spiritual struggles, virtues, and perceived growth. *Journal of Muslim Mental Health, 14*(2), 109–131.

Saritoprak, S. N., Exline, J. J., & Stauner, N. (2018). Spiritual jihad among U.S. Muslims: Preliminary measurement and associations with well-being and growth. *Religions, 9*(5), 158.

Saroglou, V. (2011). Believing, bonding, behaving, and belonging: The Big Four religious dimensions and cultural variation. *Journal of Cross-Cultural Psychology, 42*(8), 1320–1340.

Saroglou, V., Clobert, M., Cohen, A. B., Johnson, K. A., Ladd, K. L., Van Pachterbeke, M., . . . Tapia Valladares, J. (2020). Believing, bonding, behaving, and belonging: The cognitive, emotional, moral, and social dimensions of religiousness across cultures. *Journal of Cross-Cultural Psychology, 51*(7–8), 551–575.

Schnell, T. (2009). The Sources of Meaning and Meaning in Life Questionnaire (SoMe): Relations to demographics and well-being. *Journal of Positive Psychology, 4*(6),483–499.

Schutt, W. A., & Exline, J. J. (2023). Can God or the devil influence the conscience?: Links between religion/spirituality, beliefs about the conscience, and attempts to follow the conscience. *Spirituality in Clinical Practice.*

Sedlar, A. E., Stauner, N., Pargament, K. I., Exline, J. J., Grubbs, J. B., & Bradley, D. F. (2018). Spiritual struggles among atheists: Implications for psychological distress and well-being. *Religions, 9*(8), 242.

Shariff, A. F., & Aknin, L. B. (2014). The emotional toll of Hell: Cross-national and experimental evidence for the negative well-being effects of Hell beliefs. *PLOS ONE, 9*(1).

Stauner, N., Exline, J. J., Kusina, J. R., & Pargament, K. I. (2019). Religious and spiritual struggles, religiousness, and alcohol problems among undergraduates. *Journal of Prevention and Intervention in the Community, 47*(3), 243–258.

Stauner, N., Exline, J. J., & Pargament, K. I. (2015, October). *The demographics of religious and spiritual struggles in the USA.* Presentation at the annual meeting of the Society for the Scientific Study of Religion, Newport Beach, CA.

Steger, M. F. (2021). Meaning in life: A unified model. In C. R. Snyder, S. J. Lopez, L. M. Edwards, & S. C. Marques (Eds.), *Oxford handbook of positive psychology* (3rd ed., pp. 959–967). Oxford University Press.

Steger, M. F., Frazier, P., Oishi, S., & Kaler, M. (2006). The Meaning in Life Questionnaire: Assessing the presence of and search for meaning in life. *Journal of Counseling Psychology, 53*(1), 80–93.

Steger, M. F., Oishi, S., & Kashdan, T. B. (2009). Meaning in life across the life span: Levels and correlates of meaning in life from emerging adulthood to older adulthood. *Journal of Positive Psychology, 4*(1), 43–52.

Tangney, J. P., & Dearing, R. L. (2002). *Shame and guilt.* Guilford Press.

Tarakeshwar, N., Pargament, K. I., & Mahoney, A. (2003). Initial development of a measure of religious coping among Hindus. *Journal of Community Psychology, 31*(6), 607–628.

Van Tongeren, D. R., DeWall, C. N., Chen, Z., Sibley, C. G., & Bulbulia, J. (2021). Religious residue: Cross-cultural evidence that religious psychology and behavior persist following deidentification. *Journal of Personality and Social Psychology, 120*(2), 484–503.

Van Tongeren, D. R., Wilt, J. A., Exline, J. J.,

Van Cappellen, P., Brady, I., & Van Duinen, C. (2025). *Nonreligious spiritual yearning: The spiritual pursuit of existential fulfillment.* Manuscript submitted for publication.
White, C. J. M., & Norenzayan, A. (2019). Belief in karma: How cultural evolution, cognition, and motivations shape belief in supernatural justice. In J. M. Olson (Ed.), *Advances in experimental social psychology* (Vol. 60, pp. 1–63). Elsevier Academic.
White, C. J. M., & Norenzayan, A. (2022). Karma and God: Convergent and divergent mental representations of supernatural norm enforcement. *Psychology of Religion and Spirituality, 14*(1), 70–85.
Williamson, W. P., Hood, R. W., Jr., Ahmad, A., Sadiq, M., & Hill, P. C. (2010). The Intratextual Fundamentalism Scale: Cross-cultural application, validity evidence, and relationship with religious orientation and the Big 5 factor markers. *Mental Health, Religion and Culture, 13*(7–8), 721–747.
Wilt, J. A., Stauner, N., Harriott, V. A., Exline, J. J., & Pargament, K. I. (2019). Partnering with God: Religious coping and perceptions of divine intervention predict spiritual transformation in response to religious/spiritual struggle. *Psychology of Religion and Spirituality, 11*(3), 278–290.
Wilt, J. A., Stauner, N., Lindberg, M. J., Grubbs, J. B., Exline, J. J., & Pargament, K. I. (2017). Struggle with ultimate meaning: A unique component of the psychological experience of meaning in life. *Journal of Positive Psychology, 13*(3), 240–251.
Wilt, J. A., Van Tongeren, D. R., Van Cappellen, P., & Exline, J. J. (2025). *Spirituality beyond religion: Development of 9-item and 27-item multidimensional measures of spiritual yearning.* Manuscript submitted for publication.
Wong, P. T. P. (Ed.). (2012). *The human quest for meaning: Theories, research, and applications* (2nd ed.). Routledge.
Wong, P. T. P. (2014). Viktor Frankl's meaning seeking model and positive psychology. In A. Batthyany & P. Russo-Netzer (Eds.), *Meaning in positive and existential psychology* (pp. 149–184). Springer.
Wong, P. T. P. (2016). Meaning-seeking, self-transcendence, and well-being. In A. Batthyany (Ed.), *Logotherapy and existential analysis: Proceedings of the Viktor Frankl Institute* (Vol. 1, pp. 311–322). Springer.
Woodyatt, L., Worthington, E. L., Jr., Wenzel, M., & Griffin, B. J. (Eds.). (2017). *Handbook of the psychology of self-forgiveness.* Springer.
Yalom, I. D. (1980). *Existential psychotherapy.* Basic Books.

CHAPTER 57

Guided by the Glimpse

The Psychology of Meaning from Anomalous Experience

Ralph W. Hood, Jr., *and* Jonathan Dinsmore

Throughout the history of psychology, the major focus of the discipline has been on ordinary waking consciousness, and other mental conditions in terms of being disruptive of that preferred state. Yet, the unavoidable fact is that the history of human thought, ways of life, culture, beliefs, and values has been heavily shaped by precisely such divergences from the typical state of mental affairs. From the spirit mediations of "shamanism" in hunter-gatherer societies, to various Abrahamic encounters with God and his angels, the path to enlightenment described by Buddha and other Indic and contemplative traditions, or the impact of the likely psychedelically infused Eleusinian mysteries on the Greek foundations of Western civilization (Juan-Tresserras & Matamala, 2005), we have good reason to think that cultures not heavily shaped by these states are the rare exceptions rather than the general rule, if such indeed exist. Uncomfortable a fact as it may be for some, almost all cultural frameworks are inextricably linked with, if not largely founded upon, what in modern scientific terminology would be called *altered states, anomalous experiences,* or *nonordinary states of consciousness* (Tart, 1975), including the Western cultural context from which psychological science itself arose.[1]

However, a conscious recognition and reconciliation with this fact is also the exception rather than the rule in secular culture and the psychological science embedded in it. While such nonordinary states in a contemporary context have at times inspired fascination, reverence (albeit unwelcomed by many), or excitement for their therapeutic potential, within secular psychology, they have most often been regarded as mere distortions of appropriate mental functioning, and implicitly, any meanings or supposed truths drawn from them the product of faulty thinking. We view this as an extension of a narrative staple of the enlightenment, that of modern humans and their now finally accurate concept of material reality emerging from the dim, deluded predawn millennia of barbarism and superstition.

Therefore, in the overall narrative most widely subscribed to by scientists and academics, and its accompanying ontological model variously referred to as physicalism, naturalism, or materialism, any such meanings gleaned from nonordinary states can be nothing but delusions, a lurking remnant of the hallucinatory phantasmagoria that our hapless ancestors unfortunately took as real and allowed to shape their ways of life. If we, in our now enlightened state, feel we have a firm and fairly exclusive grasp on a tangible universe we are able to sense, measure, and analyze with regularity, then any experience that *seems* to be a glimpse beyond that domain of consistent sensory accessibility must necessarily be nothing more than another pesky mental poltergeist, which, it naturally follows, should be exorcised with the light of rigorous scientific analysis and naturalistic explanation.

Despite this prevailing narrative within science and secular culture, for the majority of the world's people, many historical and contemporary anomalous experiences are still taken as indicative of reality—that is to say, as true *glimpses* of something beyond the scope of our everyday experiential world. This takes the form, for perhaps most people, of belief in the historical glimpses of the founders and subsequent figures of their respective religions, and sometimes, contemporary experiences that are compatible with their tradition. For others, a belief in the veridicality of at least some historical and contemporary reports of such experiences are taken seriously with relatively little filtration according to institutional religious doctrine, including by transpersonal psychologists who regard them as valid experiences that may produce valid ontological claims. The perspective that such nonordinary states and insights gained from them are merely hallucinations magnified by poor critical thinking is therefore undeniably a minority position, in the global scope of human culture and belief.

These phenomena and the *effects of believing in them* are therefore significant facts of psychological life. Consequently, understanding how and why it is that individuals derive meaning from such anomalous experiences, and very often shape the lives of themselves and others according to those meanings, is a critical topic within the purview of psychological science, and particularly existential psychology. How this topic has been addressed in various ways within psychology more broadly, as well as the larger cultural and psychological contexts that have influenced such conceptions, along with potential future directions are addressed succinctly in this chapter.

Finally, before we begin, some clarification is in order: Numerous terms have been introduced and used by various psychologists studying this category of experiences, along with almost equally as various demarcations. In the face of such theoretical cacophony, and in lieu of convenient consensus terminology, an explicit labeling and definition at the outset is warranted. Here, the terms *anomalous* or *religious/spiritual* (R/S) will be used interchangeably depending on context,[2] although both have shortcomings.[3] In terms of demarcation, it is important to be clear what *we regard* as the best working definition and demarcation, from the outset: (1) anomalous or nonordinary experiences, which are (2) interpreted by the experiencer to have significant metaphysical or ontological (and therefore existential) implications. In other words, phenomenologically highly unusual experiences interpreted as actual glimpses of significant, typically (but not necessarily) metaphysical aspects or dimensions of reality not normally available to everyday modes of experience, frequently because the qualities and content of the experience directly indicate such.[4] Those who have such experiences will simply be referred to as *experiencers*.

A (VERY) BRIEF HISTORY OF THE PSYCHOLOGY OF ANOMALOUS EXPERIENCES

A comprehensive review of the history of psychology's treatment of this category of experiences is more appropriate for several large volumes than a portion of one chapter. Luckily, such volumes exist, as there is a massive literature that Hood has contributed to for decades and that we can but reference and build upon (Hood et al., 2018; Streib & Hood, 2016; Streib & Hood, in press). Our brief, partial account of this history here, then, focuses only on what we regard as the most important or prominent lenses through which this category of experiences has been studied, especially per their relevance to the larger theoretical and methodological issues we then address.

Some of the earliest psychologists were fascinated by nonordinary states and their potential philosophical implications. We regard the quintessential example to be William James, whose early treatise on the subject, *The Varieties of Religious Experi-*

ence (James, 1902/1985) is *widely* regarded as among the great classics of psychology, and the Western intellectual tradition more broadly. While James's initiation of the psychological study of these experiences (here dubbed religious) was simultaneously broad and cautious, it was notably uncommitted to a reductive naturalistic framework and made heavy use of detailed qualitative interpretation. James, like many of his contemporaries, also took a great interest in parapsychology, and the related perspective that these experiences at least sometimes provided empirical evidence for actual "supernatural"[5] phenomena with ontological status. In an early memorial in praise of James's contribution to psychology, Troeltsch (1912) emphasized that after the *Principles of Psychology*, "James repeatedly and positively . . . professes to supernaturalism and dualism, and by no means rejects miracles" (p. 402).

It is worth pausing for a moment on James, as we feel that he represented not only an attempt to strike the balance between psychology, philosophy, and faith, but also an orientation to the phenomenon that we hope psychology may return to. James's *The Varieties of Religious Experience* was largely a response to issues alluded to in his previous monumentally influential *Principles of Psychology* (1890/1981), whose 1,700-plus pages were reduced by two-thirds at the behest of his editors, primarily to remove his discussion of conceptual and philosophical concerns about the empirical data presented. This resulted in the significantly shorter, philosophically muzzled text referred to by his students as *Jimmy*.

James was not convinced that trying to treat psychology as a natural science would prove to be productive. He reminded readers of the Jimmy, speaking of the actual existential content of what psychologists explore, in this worthwhile extended quote:

> This is no science, it is only the hope of a science . . . at present psychology is in the condition of physics before Galileo and the laws of motion, of chemistry before Lavoisier and the notion that mass is preserved in all reactions. The Galileo and the Lavoisier of psychology will be famous men [or women!] indeed, as come they surely will, or past successes are no index of the future. When they do come, however, necessities of the case will make them "metaphysical." Meanwhile the best way in which we can facilitate their advent is to understand how great is the darkness in which we grope, and *never to forget that the natural-science assumptions with which we started are provisional and reversable things.* (1892, p. 478, emphasis added)

While many might assert that this nascent description of psychology was only accurate at the time that James wrote it, we suggest that it is still relevant. In James, we see data derived from scientific positivism (existential roots) in dialogue with philosophy (spiritual fruits). In the story of *Principles of Psychology* and its editors' procrustean demands, we also see an early example of a common approach of the majority of psychologists, committed to making their discipline an extension of the positivist endeavor, in dealing with those who wish to expand beyond it. Then, as now, scientific positivism restricts dialogue and stops conversation.

Contemporary to James was E. D. Starbuck (1911), whose work represented possibly the earliest attempt at studying these experiences statistically. John Dewey (1934) contributed to theoretical discussion of the topic and attempted to separate religious experience from religion and its supernatural interpretive frameworks, even while acknowledging its importance for psychological life. Many who came after James were inclined to view this category of experiences exclusively in a pathological or otherwise hallucinatory light. Leuba (1925), as an example, provided extensive discussion of mystical experience both as reducible to psychophysiological mechanisms and as central to human nature and culture. Although Leuba recognized the value and even positive outcomes of religious experience, he nevertheless rejected religious interpretation bound to supernaturalism. Freud gave an interpretation of mystical experience,[6] here referred to as "oceanic feeling," which he theorized to be a reversion to a "primitive ego feeling" from infancy, where the child felt itself to be unified with the mother. Despite this attempt at interpretation in terms of his own theories, he also remarked that there seemed to be little place in psychology for such experiences (Freud, 1927/1961, Parts V and VI; Parsons, 1998).

In the era during which behaviorism dominated the discipline (1915–1955), little focus was given to the topic of religious experience within mainstream empirical psychology, due to the fact that subjective experience in general was specifically excluded from the methodological paradigm (Wagenaar, 1973). During this period, most academic work on the topic took place not in psychology, but in comparative religion and philosophy, where figures like Stace, Zaehner, and Otto studied and attempted to categorize the experiences in qualitative and theoretical ways (Kim & Ferrari, 2022). Thus, this can be considered a time during which the study of religious experience was pushed outside the domain of psychology, a trend that was not to end entirely with the fall of the reign of behaviorism. This extensive lull in the psychological study of religious experience was disrupted in the mid-20th century by scholarship such as Allport's (1950) discussion of the experiences' potential relationship to religious maturity, Maslow's (1964) incorporation of peak experiences into his theories of self-realization, Fromm's (1950) attempt to separate them from supernaturalism and to differentiate between self-oriented or other-oriented forms, and Jung's (1958) interpreting them to be numinous encounters with the unconscious. Despite their differences, these all represent a resurgence of interest in this class of experiences in psychology, around this time.

More significantly for their scientific study, early attempts at assessing the prevalence of these experiences were undertaken by Hardy (1979), Back and Bourque (1970), Greeley (1975), and Hay and Morisy (1978), all of whom included brief items in surveys of the general population that, although vague, could be considered to approximate R/S experience, and found 20–50% having reported such experiences. Later, the topic was brought out of the realm of theory and single survey items, and into more rigorous measurement, primarily by Hood, who created the first psychometrically validated and widely used measure of mystical experience, the Hood Mysticism Scale (Hood, 1975; Hood et al., 2001). The development of this scale represented not only a major methodological landmark of measurement, notably accomplished via phenomenologically descriptive items, but also a move toward separating the concept of experiences from their interpretive context, typically religion. This is an example of the evolving understanding of the relationship between meaningful interpretation, cultural frameworks by which interpretation happens, and the experiences themselves, in psychological thought. However, the separability of culture and experience spearheaded by Stace/Hood would not go unchallenged for long. Hood's precedent was followed by others such as Greyson's (1983) Near-Death Experience Scale, as well as the altered states of consciousness scale developed by Dittrich (1998), and later, many others.

The later portion of the mid-20th-century period around the 1970s represented both a proliferation and fragmentation of the study of anomalous experiences. A set of alternative theoretical perspectives were gaining popularity in the milieu of the humanities, which here we overgeneralize as *constructivisms* (Hood, 2019). These centered on the contention that such experiences are wholly or partially determined by language and culture, and began to challenge perennialist accounts of religious experience, as exemplified by Katz's (1978) critique of Stace/Hood's common core model. The debate over the extent to which these experiences are interpreted or even caused by cultural beliefs, in our view, much resembles the nature–nurture debate in general psychology: a false dilemma that will inevitably be recognized as such by all reasonable scholars. While apparently quite different from positivism, a less obvious similarity is that both constructivism and positivism support the physicalist orthodoxy, and its necessarily hallucinatory interpretation of anomalous experience.[7]

During the same era and shortly after, more in the mainstream of psychology, the further development of cognitive approaches and advances in neuroscience and neuroimaging were also emerging, and began to be applied to R/S experiences, in what would eventually come to be known as the cognitive science of religion, which would become a major force in the psychology of religion. Before advancements in neuroimaging, theoretical explanations from this perspective on the topic of R/S experiences were proposed sparsely in the early days (Horowitz, 1975; Hunt, 1984), but would eventually come to be applied more prominently, such as by the application of event cognition concepts to the recall of such experiences (Taves & Asprem, 2017), and of course, neuroimaging studies of the brain during psychedelic and contemplative experiences (Barrett et al., 2020; Gattuso et al., 2023; Tagliazucchi, 2021) and subsequent theories derived from them (Carhart-Harris et al., 2024; d'Aquili & Newberg, 1993; Woollacott & Shumway-Cook, 2020). This neurocognitively oriented vein is discussed more below.

Another perspective that emerged in the mid-20th century and hit its stride in the late 20th century was existential psychology. Despite some more recent work, there is relatively little to say of how this branch of psychology has approached the topic of R/S experiences. Although clearly within its purview, relatively little has been done to study the topic in this niche field, beyond some isolated qualitative studies (Irwin, 2015; Kelly, 1995; Wilde & Murray, 2010) or, more recently, quantitative studies. This may be due to the methodological association of existential psychology with phenomenology[8] and the tendency of the phenomenological tradition of research to focus on everyday experience, rather than exceptional or anomalous experiences. However, like other areas of psychology, psychologists in the newer experimental existential vein have more recently begun to take existentially inspired theories previously applied elsewhere (Koole et al., 2006), such as terror management theory, and apply them in experimental research of anomalous experiences and their life impacts (Moreton et al., 2020; Piotrowski et al., 2020; Sielaff, 2021; Sielaff et al., 2022, 2023).

While other branches of psychology have often attempted to fit R/S experience into the naturalistic secular picture, like fitting a round peg into a square hole,[9] at least one has wholeheartedly embraced the more expansive metaphysical ontologies seemingly implied by many anomalous experiences: transpersonal psychology. Beginning with the work of Stanislav Groff (1973, 1992) and others on altered states of consciousness and therefore having been concerned with such from its inception, naturalism here is abandoned in favor of a more metaphysically rich if not always empirically oriented exploration. The subfield currently has a handful of independent colleges and psychology departments that operate according to its principles. A steadily growing (Hartelius, 2021) stream of empirical research of anomalous experiences and their meaningful implications has taken place in this area, which continues up to today (Lukoff et al., 1998, 1990; Nardini-Bubols et al., 2019). It is interesting to note that the eclectic form of spirituality characteristic of transpersonal psychologists, though different in flavor, has some resonance with existential thought, in the sense of its eclecticism.

As previously mentioned, more contemporary mainstream research has been very neurocognitively focused. This has included the proliferation of contemplative (Gamma & Metzinger, 2021), psychedelic (Vollenweider & Preller, 2020), and even what is being called neurotheology (Newberg, 2016) research threads, among others. The therapeutic potential of psychedelics has particularly brought this topic back into the domain of clinical psychology, where it largely started, when researchers in the 1950s studying them as psychotomimetics eventually began to discover their positive mental health impacts (Masters & Houston, 2000). In some instances, an attempt at studying the interpretation of the experiences has been made in various ways, such as by measuring spiritual transcendence in psilocybin studies (Griffiths et al., 2006, 2008), discussing how to integrate the experiences in a clinical context (Rabeyron, 2022), assessing changes to beliefs as a result of psychedelic experiences (Nayak et al., 2023), consideration of the potential role of applied philosophy in psychedelic therapy (Sjöstedt-Hughes, 2023), and using qualitative methods to assess why, in participants' own words, psychedelic therapy is so much more efficacious than standard modalities (Breeksema et al., 2020).

The last branch of psychology mentioned here is one that I (Hood) have had extensive involvement with throughout my career, which has been recounted in greater detail elsewhere (Hood, 2022), and also, one that serves as perhaps the closest analog to the neutral ground we recommend existential psychology should strive to be: the psychology of religion (and spirituality). Here, more than anywhere else in psychology, the tension and dialogue between secular science and the faithful[10] has been apparent, yet the very fact that such tension was even able to occur, because of the presence of both perspectives being allowed to coexist, we regard as progress. Partially in response to such debates, Hood (2022) has also proposed a theistic psychology,[11] which acknowledges the possible existence of the transcendent and thereby engages ontological questions, as one way of solving this problem. It is also in this domain that we find much fruitful treatment of the phenomena at hand, and these studies have at times taken place with a degree of impartiality that is rare in most of those subfields we have reviewed here, and notably, often without ignoring the philosophical and religious implications of the experiences.

This review is by no means comprehensive but is a high-level survey of various prominent or relevant approaches to anomalous experiences within psychology. Not only have a variety of theoretical and methodological lenses been applied, but for the most part, no consensus or theoretical clarity has been achieved. Also, various methodological problems have arisen. In the remainder of the chapter, our focus is thus heavily conceptual and methodological, in the spirit of Wittgenstein's (1953) claim that often in psychology, empirical methods and conceptual confusions are heavily entangled.

ISSUES WITH EXISTING APPROACHES

In the review of theoretical lenses thus far discussed, a pattern may be noted: With some exceptions, each approach that remains within the mainstream of psychology attempts in some way to reduce or explain the experiences within the scope of ontological assumptions most prevalent within the social sciences and the academy at large, that is, naturalism or physicalism; conversely, the few that do not are generally relegated to the periphery of the discipline.[12] Types of reduction are ostensibly different: The cognitive neuroscience approach attempts to reduce them to hallucinatory patterns of neural activity, the constructivist approach attempts to reduce them to manifestations of language and culture, and some psychodynamic approaches attempt to reduce them to compensatory mechanisms. However, upon deeper inspection, we view these as essentially iterations of the ultimately singular attempt to account for this class of experiences in terms of the orthodox philosophical framework in the academy, and the intellectual subculture that flows out from it.

This explanatory strategy is significant not because it is unique or uncharacteristic of the social sciences, but because in this case, it is being applied to the one category of experiences that is most indicative of that framework's insufficiency. Further, it is the category that has been the primary source of faith for virtually all other belief systems—the religions and spiritualities to which the majority of the world's population subscribe. In this sense, it might best be viewed cautiously, in a light similar (though not identical) to how we might regard apologetic theologians attempting to explain experiences that contradict their chosen doctrines. That is, we might expect to see certain familiar cognitive biases or fallacies come into play, such as a certain cherry-picking emphasis on those elements that are amenable to preferred explanatory frameworks, and underemphasis or even complete disregard of those details that are not and therefore contradict them. In fact, such lapses in unpartisan analysis are easily identified by any uncommitted review of the literature.

The clearest example is the case of near-death experiences, which are probably the most difficult subcategory here to explain naturalistically (Greyson, 2010). In the positivistic treatment of this class of experiences, explanatory leaps are frequently made to models based on alleged resemblance to pathological or hallucinatory phenomena, such as anoxic tunnel vision (Blackmore, 1998), dimethyltryptamine entity encounters (Timmerman et al., 2018), or ocular reperfusion (Bókkon et al., 2013). Upon closer examination, these can only be considered phenomenological matches when abstracted virtually into caricatures of each, which we call the *abstraction-matching fallacy.*[13] Other aspects for which there is no adequate naturalistic explanation available, or sometimes even none that is conceivable,[14] are simply ignored or disregarded.

In the case of hard constructivisms, the fact that experiencers frequently describe a problematic lack of cultural context for their "ineffable" mystical or otherwise anomalous experiences, making them difficult to interpret and socially hazardous to share, is likewise contradictive of prevailing theory, and selectively underemphasized. A less selective examination reveals that the occurrence of troubling aftereffects, which have been dubbed spiritual emergency by Groff (1989), are often specifically a consequence of the fact that the experience shatters previous culturally embedded, existentially meaningful frameworks, resulting in some existential disorientation as well as isolation. Such culturally unsupported experiences are also by no means limited to contemporary contexts, but are frequently the historical origin point for the branching off of a new religious group, such as the emergence of Buddhism originating from Gautama Buddha's experiential insights that contradicted elements of the Vedic context from which he emerged, or more recently, the creation of the Mormon church due to the experiences of Joseph Smith.

We view the primary source of science's value as its specifically uncommitted approach to theory or existing beliefs.[15] What prevented the priests from gazing through Galileo's proverbial telescope was just such commitment, and what most fundamentally differentiates scientific reasoning from other types and makes it so incredibly useful is specifically that it submits conceptual models to the acid test of rigorous observation, experimentation, and reasoning. Therefore, if scientific reasoning has anything that might be considered equivalent to a "mortal sin," or a most critical way in which scientists might "miss the mark" or operate in opposition to the essential spirit of science, we suggest it is the distortion of observation and reasoning in the name of preserving a preferred theory or theoretical framework, a "sin" that they are particularly tempted to commit with phenomena that most threaten their worldview, as with many anomalous experiences.

Additionally, we assert that corresponding epistemological and methodological commitments, despite being ostensibly a separate matter, are very much directly related to the ontological commitment to physicalism. This is because physicalism and scientism typically go hand in hand; they are ontological and epistemological sides of the same coin; physicalism is what the world looks like when viewed through the lens of scientism. Therefore, to adhere to naturalism's epistemological prescriptions is essentially to wear physicalism's ontological blinders. These restrict psychologists' ability to consider alternative ontological perspectives or phenomena that extend beyond the image of the world painted by scientistic physicalism, by classifying any methods of research that might indicate such as invalid or inadequate.

This also notably alienates researchers from their participants and the wider public, in that it transforms what would otherwise be an open inquiry into an enigmatic phenomenon widely regarded as existentially significant outside of the academy, into a half-cloaked debunking exercise in which reductive explanations, whose inadequacy is obvious to *anyone* who has carefully studied the first-hand reports, are offered up with grossly overestimated explanatory power. On the other hand, by acknowledging the limitations of physicalism and its methodological prescriptions, and embracing a more inclusive stance, a holistic approach that leaves room for diverse ontological perspectives in a philosophical "neutral ground" can be fostered. This approach would undoubtedly be regarded as more compatible with the sensibilities of experiencers and the wider public, making researchers open and empathetic inquirers, rather than suspicious and dogmatic inquisitors.

Finally, a critical question for existential psychologists considering the above issues is whether this newer subdiscipline might fall prey to some of the same mistakes outlined in others. Although existential thought places a great deal of emphasis on individual meaning making over assertions of objective truth, it is nevertheless also the case that, at least in the minds of some, many concepts inherited from existential philosophers have come to take on *nearly* objective truth status, most notably, a human condition that is essentially characterized by constructs such as meaninglessness, existential anxiety, and radical freedom. Because of this, there is a real risk that such theoretical concepts, like naturalist or transpersonal ones, might be too strongly adhered to, or have their explanatory value overestimated.[16] Additionally, an argument can be made that existentialist thought often presumes physicalism, even when it purports not to, since its concept of the human condition only emerged in response to scientific materialism usurping religion (among intellectuals), historically. A spiritual transformation following an R/S experience may be viewed by an existential psychologist as a coping mechanism with the harsh realities of a brief and meaningless existence, but this presumes physicalism. What receives less attention is that physicalism itself may be equally viewed as just such a coping mechanism, as outlined by Kastrup (2016). Conversely, it may also be that the experiencer is simply and reasonably believing their own experience, and further, that they may be correct. So, while existential psychologists ostensibly focus on personal meaning making and refrain from claiming objective truth, to whatever extent an ontology is implicitly assumed while *apparently* bracketed, the assumed ontology is indirectly supported (Hood & Dinsmore, in press).

That being said, we might simply suggest that existential psychology is not immune to the risk of being too attached to certain theoretical concepts rooted in existential philosophy. Like constructivisms, it also risks assuming and thereby indirectly supporting the naturalist orthodoxy in how it approaches anomalous experiences. Such support or compatibility, while no doubt politically expedient in the ivory tower, is nevertheless problematic for a truly open existential research approach to the topic, in our view.

ADVANCING THE STUDY OF ANOMALOUS EXPERIENCES: SUGGESTIONS FOR FUTURE RESEARCH

In moving forward as a field, we inevitably come up against science's own existential dilemma: the demarcation problem. Most discussions of psychology assume methodological naturalism as the central "dogma" of psychological *science*[17] (Leahey, 1991, p. 379). Wiggens (2009), on the other hand, has argued that if quantification is essential for science, psychology produces truths that are necessarily nonscientific, and we regard the qualitative/quantitative debate as proxy for the fact that epistemological and ontological issues are always interrelated (Proctor, 2002). In particular, the exclusion of qualitative methods from the scope of science has often resulted in problematic details for naturalistic explanations conveniently seeming to disappear (Dinsmore, 2025). We suggest that rather than adjusting itself to become more aligned with science as it is currently conceptualized, existential psychology could contribute to an effort at expanding the scope of what is considered to be scientific.

Methodological agnosticism has been proposed as a solution to some of the problems so far discussed here (Hood, 2012; Porpora, 2006). In contrast to methodological naturalism or atheism, which takes naturalistic assumptions as a given, methodological agnosticism recognizes that such commitments are unnecessary at best, and a source of bias or distortion at worst, in that they incline scientists to engage in the types of distortions of observation and reasoning outlined in the previous section, again particularly where studying phenomena that most threaten their theoretical (and ideological) commitments. Additionally, we regard a phenomenological focus, in terms of an overall orientation toward the study of subjective experience, as critical in the study of anomalous experiences. Combining an agnostic theoretical approach with phenomenological orientation and pragmatic mixed methodologies has also been proposed by Pekala and Cardeña (2000), and similarly by others (Moreira-Almeida & Lotufo-Neto, 2017), and we find we are fundamentally aligned with this broad proposal. In the interest of having a working title for this broad, somewhat neo-Jamesian approach, we suggest methodologically agnostic phenomenological pragmatism (MAPP).

Another critical MAPP solution to the problems and biases currently facing the field would be an expansion of what are regarded as valid and valuable scientific methods of observation, most notably to include phenomenology[18] and other qualitative methodologies as valid routes of inductive data collection that have an important role to play in existential psychological science. We suggest that there is no need to leave the rich information of firsthand accounts on the cutting-room floor when studying these phenomena, such as when converting rich experiences into measurable theoretical abstractions. It is possible to maintain some of the nuanced detail that is otherwise lost in the process of measurement using mixed methods, which can be critical for understanding quantitative findings. While there are signs that the methods wars are increasingly recognized as the mostly unnecessary polarization that we have long thought them to be (Johnson & Onwuegbuzie, 2004; Morgan, 2013), the importance of mixed-methods approaches has not been widely enough recognized in the field, which is heavily dominated by purely quantitative, mostly neurocognitive approaches.

While the time-consuming nature of qualitative methods may seem a hindrance in the short term, we are confident that their ability to provide critical supplementary details to quantitative observations will nevertheless ultimately result in a swifter overall approach to accurate theoretical models, in that they can remove much of the uncertainty in the speculative gap between one study's results and another study's formulation, and thereby reduce "wrong turns" or sometimes costly testing of unlikely, misfit hypotheses, which can easily be recognized as such by a careful study of reported phenomenological details (Dinsmore, 2024). Various practical challenges with qualitative methods also increasingly have solutions; time-consuming analytic procedures will no doubt soon be greatly alleviated by large language models and other rapidly advancing machine-learning solutions assisting human researchers, for instance. Beyond this more pragmatic procedural advantage, taking qualitative observations seriously in psychological science can also be considered a solution to some of the bias problems already mentioned, such as addressing the abstraction-matching fallacy by taking phenomenological details as consequential data that cannot be ignored.

Specific solutions to key problems such as these are merely manifestations of a deeper shift in the ethos of scientific study represented by a MAPP approach, just as the problems solved are manifestations of that which is shifted away from. This deeper shift we identify as a scientific adoption of the principle of *fidelity to the phenomenon*, in the sense of making the subjective description of such experiences the primary focus and observational foundation[19] *against which* all theoretical interpretations or hypotheses must be hung in somewhat suspended judgment and assessed. It is to place not only rigorous but *robust* data and observation first, to make these the anchor that prevents the boat of theory from being unmoored by the abstraction of operational definition and measurement, and risk being carried away by the undercurrent of ideological commitments. Incidentally, we regard this state of theoretical flux or superposition as also not too dissimilar from the fundamental ethos of existential philosophy. However, science's pursuit of the objective and existentialism's pursuit of the personal can also be regarded as being in a state of tension. We believe these can function alongside one another or even be integrated.

A MAPP MODEL FOR EXISTENTIAL PSYCHOLOGY

So, a working model of the key principles of MAPP that we propose for existential psychology might be summarized as the following:

1. *Theoretical agnosticism:* commitment to minimizing the intrusion of preferred theoretical frameworks in the whole scientific process, particularly when ideologically problematic data emerges.
2. *Phenomenological orientation:* focusing on subjective experience, both in terms of the reported experiences themselves and their meaningful life impacts, rather than moving prematurely to neurocognitive explanations.
3. *Theoretical superposition:* allowing not just individual hypotheses but entire frameworks to coexist in suspended judgment and be continuously assessed based on their support by the evidence. Philosophically, this is an application of classical pragmatist principles, as well as intellectual humility.

4. *Methodological pluralism:* pragmatic integration of whatever methods of inquiry and observation are appropriate to the phenomenon, including various types of qualitative methods; to strive to know the phenomenon in whatever ways it is most amenable to being known.
5. *Epistemic caution:* a conservatism in interpretation that is necessitated by item 4 (above), striving for clarity and prudence about the inferences that may be justifiably drawn from various types of data and analyses.[20]
6. *Ontological pragmatism:* bracketing of the ontological question wherever it is unnecessary for the research at hand, without abandoning engagement with it where it is more appropriate, such as in theoretical and philosophical discussions of findings.
7. *Interdisciplinary cooperation:* integration and dialogue in how the research bridges to other disciplines, such as philosophy, anthropology, or religious studies, as well as how their conceptual products may be worthwhile for psychological study.[21]

The primary obstacles we see in the adoption of the MAPP approach in existential psychology are simply existential versions of the same issues faced elsewhere, such as potential overcommitment to certain concepts derived from existential philosophy. There is little reason in our opinion, for instance, to call solely upon terror management explanations as to why someone who had a vivid out-of-body experience came to believe that their consciousness has an existence independent of their body, in spite of the obvious potential hallucinatory explanation;[22] a more parsimonious interpretation is likely (in our view) that this is rather an interpretation of their experience in a manner comparable to interpretations of other veridical perceptions (that is, as a true glimpse), particularly when amplified by the powerful noetic sense of being "realer than real" (Yaden et al., 2017). When one interviews experiencers, as both authors have, one typically does not get the sense that they are wanting and trying to believe, but rather, that they are struggling with something that is difficult to believe or even understand,[23] but that was so potent an experience that they cannot deny its significance, and so must try to. So, while terror management theory may play a role, a richer phenomenological familiarity with the phenomenon gives ample reason to think that this role may be at risk of overestimation.[24] In this and many other cases, existential psychologists may need to decide whether their subfield should be a scientific extension of existential philosophy or a more philosophically open psychological investigation of existential matters. Obviously, we recommend the latter, as it is more aligned with the fundamental telos of the scientific endeavor.

CONCLUDING THOUGHTS

Experimental existential psychology, though small, is perhaps the most well-positioned branch of psychology to truly assume the MAPP orientation in the study of anomalous experiences. Being at a meeting point between qualitative and quantitative, sacred and secular, there is a real possibility here of the so needed and yet tragically so scarce philosophically neutral ground for this peculiar niche area of study. While it faces potential pitfalls, if these issues can be dealt with, we regard the possibility of an existential psychology operating according to MAPP principles as possibly the most promising way forward in the study of anomalous experiences.

NOTES

1. Judeo-Christian, and to some extent Greco-Roman culture.

2. In the former case, to emphasize their anomalistic character, in the latter, to emphasize their R/S (or metaphysical) interpretation.

3. Many experiences are anomalous, that is, beyond the scope of ordinary human experience, but do not have features that intrinsically indicate ontological discoveries pertinent to ontological worldview, such as a feeling of oneness or perception of nonphysical entities; many experiences may also be deemed religious or spiritual but are not sufficiently anomalous as to fit the category to which we are referring. Rather than dwell on the persistent labeling/demarcation issue here, we prefer to simply make ours explicit and get on with the heart of the matter.

4. For example, having an out-of-body experience directly indicates that consciousness is separate from the body, in a manner comparable to how seeing a view of the Earth from space directly indicates that we float in a sea of stars.

5. This and other commonly used terms are sometimes in quotations to indicate that they are problematic in our opinions but used for the familiarity of their signification.

6. As it is known today, an experience of cosmic unity with additional qualities such as a noetic sense of true insights and profound positive affect.

7. That is, in order for culture to determine the content of an anomalous experience, said experience must necessarily be an internal, presumably hallucinatory phenomenon whose content, being entirely mental, is capable of being shaped by culture and language to an extent that veridical perceptions would not be.

8. More or less exclusively before the emergence of experimental existential psychology.

9. A particularly apt metaphor, given that the features of anomalous experiences that cannot be explained naturalistically must be removed or ignored in order for the phenomenon to fit the procrustean bed of their explanatory model.

10. As well as, at times, what we identify here as constructivist approaches and other perspectives.

11. This being used as a placeholder term.

12. Despite this differential in intellectual political status, it is noteworthy that although we primarily focus on the most widespread theoretical commitments of naturalism considered problematic here, these arguments apply equally to transpersonal, existential, and other theoretical commitments, as well.

13. For instance, the resemblance of the tunnel described by near-death experiencers (when details are given) can only be said to resemble anoxic tunnel vision in the sense that a pile of raked leaves may be said to resemble a mountain: not to any extent worthy of comment by serious scientists or scholars.

14. Such as out-of-body perceptions verified by third parties, and in some cases, under conditions in which they could not possibly have occurred via sensory channels in the dying body, such as at distant locations or in the operating theater when sensory organs were blocked, the latter being famously exemplified by the case of Pam Reynolds.

15. Other than those requisite for its most fundamental principles, of course.

16. We suggest that an example of the latter may be seen in the sweeping explanatory narratives woven by some terror management theorists, inspired by existential thinkers, who posit that human activities as diverse and complex as religion, career, family, art, and science are all fundamentally motivated by death anxiety.

17. An addended compensation that no other scientific discipline finds necessary. We regard this as a somewhat humorous manifestation of psychology's longstanding insecurity about being truly "scientific," a "complex" that Dinsmore enjoys referring to as *test tube envy*.

18. In the sense of making detailed description of subjective experience the focus of investigation, as well as phenomenological qualitative methodologies; integrating the philosophical concepts of the continental tradition of phenomenological philosophy is not considered here essential, and maybe not desirable, for conducting psychological science phenomenologically.

19. Even when measured via Likert responses on phenomenologically descriptive items.

20. It is, of course, not without reason that the methods wars occurred, and integrating qualitative methods into psychological science must be accompanied by a healthy degree of caution about how much confidence we should feel about the implications and generalizability of any given study, apropos to the method(s) that it used.

21. Since existentialism is already at the intersection of philosophy and psychology, it is already engaged in such dialogue and interdisciplinary research; this is one more reason that MAPP is appropriate.

22. Critically, experiencers are rarely, if ever, unaware of this hallucinatory explanation, and frequently have it asserted to them by both priest and psychiatrist, with varying degrees of dogma, and sometimes at threat of damnation or institutionalization.

23. Because it often contradicts their existing conceptual frameworks, as well as all prior experience.

24. We concede that terror management theory could certainly motivate a reduced skepticism about the experience's implications.

REFERENCES

Allport, G. W. (1950). *The individual and his religion*. Macmillan.

Back, K. W., & Bourque, L. (1970). Can feelings be enumerated? *Behavioral Science, 15*, 487–496.

Barrett, F. S., Krimmel, S. R., Griffiths, R. R., Seminowicz, D. A., & Mathur, B. N. (2020). Psilocybin acutely alters the functional con-

nectivity of the claustrum with brain networks that support perception, memory, and attention. *Neuroimage, 218,* 116980.
Blackmore, S. (1998). Experiences of anoxia: Do reflex anoxic seizures resemble near-death experiences? *Journal of Near-Death Studies, 17*(2), 111–120.
Bókkon, I., Mallick, B. N., & Tuszynski, J. A. (2013). Near death experiences: A multidisciplinary hypothesis. *Frontiers in Human Neuroscience, 7,* 56377.
Breeksema, J. J., Niemeijer, A. R., Krediet, E., Vermetten, E., & Schoevers, R. A. (2020). Psychedelic treatments for psychiatric disorders: A systematic review and thematic synthesis of patient experiences in qualitative studies. *CNS Drugs, 34,* 925–946.
Carhart-Harris, R. L., Leech, R., Hellyer, P. J., Shanahan, M., Feilding, A., Tagliazucchi, E., . . . Nutt, D. (2014). The entropic brain: A theory of conscious states informed by neuroimaging research with psychedelic drugs. *Frontiers in Human Neuroscience, 8,* 20.
d'Aquili, E. G., & Newberg, A. B. (1993). Religious and mystical states: A neuropsychological model. *Zygon: Journal of Religion and Science, 28*(2), 177–200.
Dewey, J. (1934). *A common faith.* Yale University Press.
Dinsmore, J. R. (2024). *Mystical luminosity experience: An initiation of a construct grounded in phenomenology.* Brill.
Dinsmore, J. (2025). The abstraction matching fallacy: A procrustean problem in the science of anomalous experiences. *Journal of Anomalous Experience and Cognition, 5*(2), 234–249.
Dittrich, A. (1998). The standardized psychometric assessment of altered states of consciousness (ASCs) in humans. *Pharmacopsychiatry, 31*(Suppl. 2), 80–84.
Freud, S. (1961). *The future of an illusion* (J. Strachey, Trans.). Norton. (Original work published 1927)
Fromm, E. (1950). *Psychoanalysis and religion* (Vol. 12). Yale University Press.
Gamma, A., & Metzinger, T. (2021). The Minimal Phenomenal Experience questionnaire (MPE-92M): Towards a phenomenological profile of "pure awareness" experiences in meditators. *PLOS One, 16*(7), e0253694.
Gattuso, J. J., Perkins, D., Ruffell, S., Lawrence, A. J., Hoyer, D., Jacobson, L. H., . . . Sarris, J. (2023). Default mode network modulation by psychedelics: A systematic review. *International Journal of Neuropsychopharmacology, 26*(3), 155–188.
Greeley, A. M. (1975). *The sociology of the paranormal: A reconnaissance* (Vol. 3). Sage.
Greyson, B. (1983). The near-death experience scale: Construction, reliability, and validity. *Journal of Nervous and Mental Disease, 171*(6), 369–375.
Greyson, B. (2010). Implications of near-death experiences for a postmaterialist psychology. *Psychology of Religion and Spirituality, 2*(1), 37.
Griffiths, R. R., Richards, W. A., Johnson, M. W., McCann, U. D., & Jesse, R. (2008). Mystical-type experiences occasioned by psilocybin mediate the attribution of personal meaning and spiritual significance 14 months later. *Journal of Psychopharmacology, 22*(6), 621–632.
Griffiths, R. R., Richards, W. A., McCann, U., & Jesse, R. (2006). Psilocybin can occasion mystical-type experiences having substantial and sustained personal meaning and spiritual significance. *Psychopharmacology, 187,* 268–283.
Grof, S. (1973). Theoretical and empirical basis of transpersonal psychology and psychotherapy: Observations from LSD research. *Journal of Transpersonal Psychology, 5*(1), 15–53.
Grof, S. (1989). *Spiritual emergency: When personal transformation becomes a crisis.* Penguin.
Grof, S. (1992, June 20–25). *Theoretical and empirical foundations of transpersonal psychology.* Revised paper presented at the 12th International Transpersonal Conference "Science, Spirituality, and the Global Crisis: Toward a World with a Future," Prague, Czechoslovakia.
Hardy, A. (1979). *The spiritual nature of man: A study of contemporary religious experience.* Clarendon Press.
Hartelius, G. (2021). Transpersonal psychology: Trends in empirical research and diversity during the first five decades of the field. *International Journal of Transpersonal Studies, 40*(1), 6.
Hay, D., & Morisy, A. (1978). Reports of ecstatic, paranormal, or religious experience in Great Britain and the United States: A comparison of trends. *Journal for the Scientific Study of Religion, 17,* 255–268.
Hood, R. W., Jr. (1975). The construction and preliminary validation of a measure of reported mystical experience. *Journal for the Scientific Study of Religion, 14*(1), 29–41.
Hood, R. W., Jr. (2012). Methodological agnosticism for the socials sciences?: Lesson from Sorokin's and James's allusions to psychoanalysis, mysticism, and Godly love. In M. T. Lee & A. Young (Eds.), *The science and theology of Godly love* (pp. 121–140). Northern Illinois University Press.

Hood, R. W., Jr. (2019). Constructivism and mystical experience. *Constructivist Foundations, 15*(1), 1–9. *http://constructivist.info/15/1/001.gash.*

Hood, R. W., Jr. (2022). William James and the (non) replication crisis in psychology: Conjectures and controversy in the psychology of religion. *Research in the Social Scientific Study of Religion, 32,* 373–398.

Hood, R. W., Jr., & Dinsmore, J. (in press). Commentary on the varieties of spiritual experience: Jimmy or James? Act III cannot have two directors. *Religion, Brain and Behavior.*

Hood, R. W., Jr., Ghorbani, N., Watson, P. J., Ghramaleki, A. F., Bing, M. N., Davison, H. K., . . . Williamson, W. P. (2001). Dimensions of the mysticism scale: Confirming the three-factor structure in the United States and Iran. *Journal for the Scientific Study of Religion, 40*(4), 691–705.

Hood, R. W., Jr., Hill, P. C., & Spilka, B. (2018). *The psychology of religion: An empirical approach* (5th ed.). Guilford Press.

Horowitz M. (1975). Hallucinations: An information-processing approach. In R. Siegel & S. West (Eds.), *Hallucinations: Behavior, experience, theory* (pp. 163–195). Wiley.

Hunt, H. (1984). A cognitive psychology of mystical and altered-state experience. *Perceptual and Motor Skills, 58*(2), 467–513.

Irwin, L. (2015). Mystical knowledge and near-death experience. In T. Cattoi & C. Moreman (Eds.), *Death, dying, and mysticism: The ecstasy of the end* (pp. 153–175). Palgrave Macmillan.

James, W. (1892). *Psychology: The briefer course.* Holt.

James, W. (1981). *The principles of psychology.* Harvard University Press. (Original work published 1890)

James, W. (1985). *The varieties of religious experience: A study in human nature.* Harvard University Press. (Original work published 1902)

Johnson, R. B., & Onwuegbuzie, A. J. (2004). Mixed methods research: A research paradigm whose time has come. *Educational Researcher, 33*(7), 14–26.

Juan-Tresserras, J. J., & Matamala, J. (2005). Estudio de residuos microscópicos y compuestos orgánicos en utillaje de molido y de contenido de las vasijas. *El dolmen de Toledo,* 235–241.

Jung, C. G. (1958). *Psychology and religion: West and east* (R. F. C. Hull, Trans). Pantheon Books.

Kastrup, B. (2016). The physicalist worldview as neurotic ego-defense mechanism. *SAGE Open, 6*(4).

Katz, S. T. (1978). Language, epistemology, and mysticism. In *Mysticism and philosophical analysis* (pp. 22–74). Oxford University Press.

Kelly, C. R. (1995). *Transformative experience: A phenomenological/psychological study.* California Institute of Integral Studies.

Kim, J. J., & Ferrari, M. (2022). On the third day . . . : The death and resurrection of the study of religious experience. *The Humanistic Psychologist, 50*(2), 199.

Koole, S. L., Greenberg, J., & Pyszczynski, T. (2006). Introducing science to the psychology of the soul: Experimental existential psychology. *Current Directions in Psychological Science, 15*(5), 212–216.

Leahey, T. A. (1991). *A history of psychology: From antiquity to modernity.* Prentice Hall.

Leuba, J. H. (1925). *The psychology of religious mysticism.* Harcourt, Brace.

Lukoff, D., Lu, F., & Turner, R. (1998). From spiritual emergency to spiritual problem: The transpersonal roots of the new DSM-IV category. *Journal of Humanistic Psychology, 38*(2), 21–50.

Lukoff, D., Zanger, R., & Lu, F. (1990). Transpersonal psychology research review: Psychoactive substances and transpersonal states. *Journal of Transpersonal Psychology, 22*(2), 107–148.

Maslow, A. H. (1964). *Religions, values, and peak experiences.* Ohio State University Press.

Masters, R., & Houston, J. (2000). *The varieties of psychedelic experience: The classic guide to the effects of LSD on the human psyche.* Simon & Schuster.

Moreira-Almeida, A., & Lotufo-Neto, F. (2017). Methodological guidelines to investigate altered states of consciousness and anomalous experiences. *International Review of Psychiatry,* 29(3), 283–292.

Moreton, S. G., Szalla, L., Menzies, R. E., & Arena, A. F. (2020). Embedding existential psychology within psychedelic science: Reduced death anxiety as a mediator of the therapeutic effects of psychedelics. *Psychopharmacology, 237*(1), 21–32.

Morgan, D. L. (2013). *Integrating qualitative and quantitative methods: A pragmatic approach.* Sage.

Nardini-Bubols, M., da Silva, D. S., dos Santos-Silva, A., Stagnaro, O. K., Irigaray, T. Q., & Alminhana, L. O. (2019). The altered states of consciousness in transpersonal approach psychotherapy: Systematic review and guidelines for research and clinical practice. *Journal of Religion and Health, 58,* 2175–2194.

Nayak, S. M., Singh, M., Yaden, D. B., & Griffiths, R. R. (2023). Belief changes associated with psychedelic use. *Journal of Psychopharmacology, 37*(1), 80–92.

Newberg, A. B. (2016). *Principles of neurotheology*. Routledge.

Parsons, W. B. (1998). The oceanic feeling revisited. *Journal of Religion, 78*(4), 501–523.

Pekala, R. J., & Cardeña, E. (2000). Methodological issues in the study of altered states of consciousness and anomalous experiences. In E. Cardeña, S. J. Lynn, & S. Krippner (Eds.), *Varieties of anomalous experience: Examining the scientific evidence* (pp. 47–82). American Psychological Association.

Piotrowski, J. P., Żemojtel-Piotrowska, M., & Clinton, A. (2020). Spiritual transcendence as a buffer against death anxiety. *Current Psychology: A Journal for Diverse Perspectives on Diverse Psychological Issues, 39*(3), 994–1000.

Porpora, D. V. (2006). Methodological atheism, methodological agnosticism and religious experience. *Journal for the Theory of Social Behavior, 36, 59–75.*

Proctor, G. (2002). *The dynamics of power in counselling and psychotherapy: Ethics, politics and practice*. PCCS Books.

Rabeyron, T. (2022). When the truth is out there: Counseling people who report anomalous experiences. *Frontiers in Psychology, 12,* 693707.

Sielaff, A. (2021). *Investigating the potential for mystical-type experiences and related phenomena to shift existential perspectives*. Doctoral dissertation, University of Arizona.

Sielaff, A., Horner, D. E., & Greenberg, J. (2022). The moderating role of mystical-type experiences on the relationship between existential isolation and meaning in life. *Personality and Individual Differences, 186,* 111347.

Sielaff, A., Horner, D. E., & Greenberg, J. (2023). Differences in existential perspectives as a function of having a mystical-type experience. *Journal of Humanistic Psychology*.

Sjöstedt-Hughes, P. (2023). On the need for metaphysics in psychedelic therapy and research. *Frontiers in Psychology, 14,* 1128589.

Starbuck, E. D. (1911). *The psychology of religion: An empirical study of the growth of religious consciousness* (3rd ed.). Scribner's.

Streib, H., & Hood, R. W., Jr. (Eds.). (2016). *Semantics and psychology of spirituality: A cross-cultural analysis comparing Germany and America*. Springer.

Streib, H., & Hood, R. W., Jr. (in press). *Faith in development: Mixed-method studies the development of worldview and religious styles*. Springer International.

Tagliazucchi, E. (2021). Human neuroimaging studies of serotonergic psychedelics. In C. S. Grob & J. Grigsby (Eds.), *Handbook of medical hallucinogens* (pp. 121–133). Guilford Press.

Tart, C. (1975). Science, state of consciousness, and spiritual experiences: The need for state-specific sciences. In C. Tart (Ed.), *Transpersonal psychologies* (pp. 9–58). Harper & Row.

Taves, A., & Asprem, E. (2017) Experience as event: Event cognition and the study of (religious) experiences. *Religion, Brain and Behavior, 7*(1), 43–62.

Timmermann, C., Roseman, L., Williams, L., Erritzoe, D., Martial, C., Cassol, H., . . . Carhart-Harris, R. (2018). DMT models the near-death experience. *Frontiers in Psychology, 9,* 395026.

Troeltsch, E. (1912). Empiricism and Platonism in the philosophy of religion: To the memory of William James. *Harvard Theological Review, 5,* 401–422.

Vollenweider, F. X., & Preller, K. H. (2020). Psychedelic drugs: Neurobiology and potential for treatment of psychiatric disorders. *Nature Reviews Neuroscience, 21*(11), 611–624.

Wagenaar, J. (1973). *Behaviorism and religious experience: An investigation of B. F. Skinner through William James*. Doctoral dissertation, University of Chicago.

Wiggins, B. J. (2009). William James and methodological pluralism: Bridging the qualitative and quantitative divide. *Journal of Mind and Behavior, 30,* 164–184.

Wilde, D., & Murray, C. D. (2010). Interpreting the anomalous: Finding meaning in out-of-body and near-death experiences. *Qualitative Research in Psychology, 7*(1), 57–72.

Wittgenstein, L. (1953). Philosophical investigations (G. E. M. Anscombe, Trans.). Routledge & Kegan Paul. (Original work published 1945–1949)

Woollacott, M., & Shumway-Cook, A. (2020). The mystical experience and its neural correlates. *Journal of Near-Death Studies, 38*(1).

Yaden, D. B., Le Nguyen, K. D., Kern, M. L., Wintering, N. A., Eichstaedt, J. C., Schwartz, H. A., . . . Newberg, A. B. (2017). The noetic quality: A multimethod exploratory study. *Psychology of Consciousness, 4*(1), 54–62.

SECTION VIII

AWE, GROWTH, AND THE GOOD LIFE

CHAPTER 58

Awe

Megan E. Edwards *and* Patty Van Cappellen

Imagine standing on the edge of the Grand Canyon. The vast expanse stretches out before you like a painted canvas with more colors of red, orange, and brown than you could have ever imagined. The sheer size and depth of your surroundings are beyond comprehension, and for a moment, time seems to stand still. You're filled with emotions beyond admiration, and a deep sense of reverence and wonder fills your entire being. The world suddenly feels vast and interconnected through the majestic beauty it provides, a reflection of the sublime and the mysterious. You look at your friend, to share in this moment, but there are no words to describe what you are feeling. Yet you can see in their eyes that this moment has also touched them at their core, leaving an indelible mark of wonder that will stay with them forever. That is the feeling of awe.

From being moved by music and art to witnessing the worldly wonders or human acts of bravery, awe can be found all around us. The emotion of awe is triggered by an encounter with something vast and extraordinary that transcends everyday understanding. It is an existential emotion that can lead to a reevaluation of an individual's place in the universe, prompting existential questions and reflections about that individual's self, life, and the interconnectedness of all things. In this chapter, we highlight awe's existential effects, ranging from a reevaluation of the place of the self in the grand scheme of things to a sense of interconnectedness, transcendence, and meaning.

AWE

Keltner and Haidt (2003) formulated a definition of *awe* drawing from fields such as psychology, religious studies, philosophy, and sociology, that has very much shaped the empirical research on awe in the past two decades. Their definition highlights two key characteristics of awe-inspiring stimuli: perceived vastness and the need for accommodation. The perception of vastness refers to something that is perceived as dramatically surpassing the individual's usual frame of reference, which could refer to an entity's immense physical dimensions, such as the Grand Canyon. However, vastness can also be perceived in other forms: It could be in the form of a highly influential theory in physics, the significant societal impact of a person or historical event, the intricate details in a musical or visual masterpiece, or the expansive and innovative ideas in art or literature. Such experiences demand cognitive accommodation. Awe-inspiring stimuli are so vast, complex, or novel that they do not immediately fit into one's existing mental frameworks. To make sense of the experience, one's worldview needs to expand.

One may question previously held beliefs, reassess values, or see the interconnectedness of life in a new light. Awe prompts a shift away from relying on established mental models and shortcuts when processing new information. This process reflects a potentially adaptive function of awe, promoting the absorption and integration of new information, essential for survival. In addition, this process of accommodation can lead to a profound personal transformation. Overall, awe involves cognitive processing enfolded in a rich emotional experience that has a number of mental and physical benefits (see Monroy & Keltner, 2023). These benefits include promoting other positive emotions (Shiota et al., 2017; Sturm et al., 2022), humility (Stellar et al., 2017), curiosity (Anderson et al., 2020), prosocial behaviors (Piff et al., 2015), and life satisfaction (Bai et al., 2021).

The subjective experience of the emotion of awe is complex. American participants in one study, asked to recall an event that elicited awe, mostly focused on positive experiences that fit with the definition of Keltner and Haidt (2003; Shiota et al., 2007). Indeed, awe is often considered a positive emotion, creating a pleasurable experience. Yet, other experiences of awe can take on a different emotional tone. Researchers have studied "negative awe" or "threat-based awe" to account for experiences of awe that involve being confronted with some threatening element, producing both amazement and fear. When asked to recall an experience in which participants felt intense awe, about 21% of the experiences involved threatening stimuli such as an extreme weather event (Gordon et al., 2017). In sum, awe experiences can vary on a continuum from positive to negative affect, including many that can be considered as mixed and involving both pleasure and terror. Interestingly, people also vary in their predisposition to feel the positive or negative side of awe (Nakayama et al., 2020). The subjective experience of awe can also vary in its intensity, ranging from mundane everyday experiences to high-intensity and exceptional experiences.

Awe is expressed in both face and body. In a study examining facial and upper body expressions associated with awe, participants first recalled a personal experience of awe (and other positive emotions) and then were asked to show how they would express this feeling to other people. The expressions they typically demonstrated included inner eyebrows lifted (while outer eyebrows remained neutral), eyelids raised, a slightly open mouth with lips apart, and a gentle leaning forward in their posture. Interestingly, the awe expression typically does not include any form of smile—typically an affiliative cue—which may signal the more cognitive rather than affiliative aspect of awe (Campos et al., 2013). Another study shed light on how the rest of the body expresses awe. Participants freely posed a small mannequin to show how they would express in their full body the emotion of awe (and other affective dimensions and emotions). Postures of awe were objectively as expansive as those of dominance (while less expansive than postures of joy) but displayed a signature arm position with the hand(s) touching the head, perhaps reflecting the appraisal of extraordinariness and distinct cognitive activity associated with awe (Van Cappellen et al., 2023).

AWE AND SELF-TRANSCENDENCE

The emotion of awe involves psychological changes that are relevant to existential concerns. In particular, we highlight its transcendent nature and its effect on the self-concept. Awe belongs to the family of self-transcendent positive emotions, which are defined by their ability to expand an individual's usual sense of self and foster a connection to something larger (Haidt, 2003; Stellar et al., 2017). This family of emotions, including gratitude, love, compassion, and admiration, is elicited by the witnessing of greater good or beauty outside the self. These emotions are characterized by a shift from self-centeredness to outward focus. The self and the pursuit of its goals take a backseat in favor of the appreciation of an external stimulus. In doing so, such emotions draw one's attention to something greater than ourselves and invite one to transcend day-to-day experiences. As such, self-transcendent emotions are often present in self-transcendent experiences, which transcend the self and one's ordinary perceptions, leading to a sense of interconnectedness (Yaden et al., 2017). The second characteristic of self-transcendent positive emotions relates to the activation of care for others and prosocial behaviors. Evidence supports the idea that awe, like other self-transcendent positive emotions, encourages people to engage in actions that benefit others and society at large (Piff et al., 2015; Prade & Saroglou, 2016; Rudd et al., 2012).

Awe's transcendent nature, or expansion beyond the self, in a sense dissolves the self. This is most commonly described as two intertwined experiences. First, awe leads to a sense of vastness: a sense of something larger than one's self. Second, awe leads to a sense of smallness: where there is lower attention on the self and even feelings of smallness (Stellar, 2021). Many studies have documented the effects of awe on a diminished sense of the self, often called the *small self,* and suggested its role in eliciting downstream consequences of awe such as oneness, prosociality, or creativity (Chirico et al., 2018; Piff et al., 2015; Zhang et al., 2021). The small self has been measured in a variety of ways, from survey items such as "I feel small or insignificant" (Shiota et al., 2007), to pictorial measures such as drawings of various-sized people or freely drawn representations of the self. Across these studies, feelings of awe, but not other positive emotions such as joy or amusement, predicted a smaller perceived self-size. These effects applied to members of both individualistic and collectivistic cultures (Bai et al., 2017). However, the phenomenology of such small self and the nature of the self itself are still debated. Some have argued that awe promotes more precisely a "quiet ego," a self characterized by an appreciation of self–other interdependence, motivation to behave prosocially, and an orientation toward personal growth (Perlin & Li, 2020). Along these lines, Jiang and Sedikides (2022) found that awe promotes authentic-self pursuit, defined as the perception that one is in alignment with one's true or genuine self. Although the concept of the small self in the context of awe experiences is a topic of ongoing debate, it is proposed that by reducing the reliance on the self, awe may facilitate a reorientation toward others and the grand scheme of things. This shift may be a gateway to the existential qualities of awe, to which we now turn.

INTERCONNECTEDNESS

Awe's transcendent nature suggests that as people become less interested and focused on themselves, they similarly begin to perceive themselves as part of a community or greater network of beings. In other words, they become more interdependent beings and even self-sacrificing beings. Humans have a need for social relationships and a desire to connect with others to reduce a sense of loneliness or isolation that they may face (Hawkley & Cacioppo, 2010). Therefore, awe's potential to connect humans with others is a key existential resource. As we unpack below, awe has the capacity to boost a sense of interconnectedness (Chen & Mongrain, 2021) and need for relatedness (Wu et al., 2023) that can, by extension, even influence feelings of existential connectedness or isolation (Edwards et al., 2024).

In one such study participants were randomly either assigned to an awe experience or placed in a neutral control group. All participants then completed a self-concept task, where they were asked to give 20 statements in response to the question "Who am I?" In response to this question, participants in the awe condition, compared to the control group, were more likely to use descriptor words that reflected they were a part of a universal group. For example, they described themselves as being "a person" or "an inhabitant of the Earth" rather than "one-of-a-kind" (Shiota et al., 2007).

Much research has continued to find support for awe's collective nature, documenting effects of awe on closeness to others (Bai et al., 2017; Edwards et al., 2024; Van Cappellen & Saroglou, 2012) and even on a sense of interconnectedness with the larger world as a whole (Shiota et al., 2007; Stepanova et al., 2019).

Beyond a closeness to others, awe also leads the individual to feel they are a part of their larger community. Dispositional awe is related to greater social connectedness to others and society (Zhao & Zhang, 2023). Furthermore, in two studies, awe, compared to amusement or shame, led to greater collective engagement (Bai et al., 2017). In one study, collective engagement was measured as the number of social ties, which increased among a U.S. sample, and greater closeness to others, which increased among a Chinese sample. In a second study, collective engagement was assessed as feeling more included in one's community. This was enhanced by more negative elicitors of awe. For example, awe induced by natural disasters led to a greater sense of global community (Wang et al., 2023).

To a large extent, awe has the capacity to make one feel a greater connection not just with others in one's community, but to all of humanity or nature—a general sense of interconnectedness between all things. Indeed, awe leads people to feel more connected to nature (Stepanova et al., 2019; Yang et al., 2018). However, this is most evident in extreme experiences of awe. Astronaut Edgar Mitchell (2008, p. 58) experienced an extraordinary level of interconnectedness when viewing Earth from space.

> Then, looking beyond the Earth itself to the magnificence of the larger scene . . . My understanding of the separate distinctness and the relative independence of movement of those cosmic bodies was shattered. There was an upwelling of fresh insight coupled with a feeling of ubiquitous harmony—a sense of interconnectedness with the celestial bodies surrounding our spacecraft.

This feeling of interconnectedness with the universe is a consequence of many experiences of what is considered the overview effect—viewing the world from space. In one study, after experiencing the overview effect using virtual reality, participants reported more holistic views of the world and noticed greater "connection between things that are otherwise separate" (Stepanova et al., 2019).

Disconnectedness: Existential Isolation

Although the majority of research on awe and interconnectedness has highlighted the positive effects of awe, other research has shed light on its mixed effects on the experience of existential isolation. Existential isolation corresponds to the subjective experience that one's perception is not shared by others (Pinel et al., 2017), thus creating a feeling of separateness from others. Yalom (1980) described existential isolation as the awareness of the unbridgeable gap between the self and others, as one cannot truly understand the experiences of another. Similarly, awe can be an ineffable experience that creates further separation from others with whom one can't even share in words what one has experienced (Edwards et al., 2024). Across three studies, inducing awe through virtual reality or a recall experience (compared to a neutral or amusement experience) simultaneously led to greater and reduced feelings of existential isolation via opposing pathways. On the one hand, as awe led to greater feelings of smallness, perceived connectedness was reduced, and thus greater feelings of existential isolation ensued. On the other hand, as awe led to greater feelings of vastness (a sense of something larger than one's self), perceived connectedness was increased and thus lower feelings of existential isolation ensued (Edwards et al., 2024).

The small self plays a mixed role in eliciting feelings of existential isolation (Edwards et al., 2024) or interconnectedness. Indeed, in other studies, awe led to greater (not lower) collective engagement and sense of global community via feelings of a smaller self (Bai et al., 2017; Wang et al., 2023). Moreover, feelings of self-diminishment (not vastness) from awe predicted greater prosocial behaviors (Piff et al., 2015; Wang et al., 2023). These seemingly conflicting findings on the effects of feeling small point back to the issue of what the experience of the small self actually entails. Indeed, it remains confusing as to why feeling small, which is associated with lower self-esteem (Tyson et al., 2022), would make people feel more connected or more willing to help others. It is possible that the two aspects of "smallness"—feeling small and lower attention on the self—are important to distinguish. On the one hand, that feeling of being smaller in comparison to the vastness one is being confronted with likely predicts more negative consequences, including lower connectedness (e.g., Edwards et al., 2024). On the other hand, the reduced attention on the self or quieting of the ego allows for a shift not only away from the self, but toward the collective; a shift from "me" to "we" thinking (Perlin & Li, 2020), that enables those feelings of interconnectedness (e.g., Bai et al., 2017; Piff et al., 2015; Wang et al., 2023). It reflects how one's self-concept broadens to larger circles of inclusion. This is also partially picked up in feelings of vastness, which have also led to greater feelings of connectedness (Edwards et al., 2024), self-sacrificing behaviors (Naclerio & Van Cappellen, 2022), and even moral expansiveness (Song et al., 2023). We believe this is an important and ripe area for future research.

Overall, awe connects people to their close others, their community, and even all of humanity. The implications of such connections have been documented to lead people to behave more prosocially (Piff et al., 2015), conform with their ingroup (Prade & Saroglou, 2023), and even sacrifice their self (Naclerio & Van Cappellen, 2022).

TRANSCENDENCE, RELIGION, AND SPIRITUALITY

A feeling of awe, evoked by the mysteries and vastness of the universe, can inspire a belief in a deeper, often spiritual dimension of existence beyond the visible and tangible world. Scholars of religion have written profusely about awe as an emotional source for the transcendent and the sacred (Fuller, 2007). The very subjective experience of awe is akin to self-transcendent experiences: feeling that the self is small or insignificant, sensing the presence of something greater than the self, being unaware of normal day-to-day concerns, feeling connected with the surrounding world, and wanting to prolong the experience as long as possible (Yaden et al., 2017).

It is therefore not surprising that awe is central to religious experiences, both arising from and promoting them. Indeed, this emotion is not only valued but also experienced more frequently by those who hold religious and spiritual beliefs or actively engage in religious and spiritual practices (Kearns & Tyler, 2022; Vishkin et al., 2019). The design of many worship spaces, with their monumental architecture, serves to facilitate spiritual experiences and evoke awe (Joye & Verpooten, 2013). Religious and mystical experiences are often accompanied by intense emotions, including awe (Hardy, 1979; Hood & Chen, 2013). Moreover, research has shown that among both religious and nonreligious participants, recalling spiritual experiences leads to more awe as explained by the small self (Cohen et al., 2010; Preston & Shin, 2017).

Awe experienced in a religious context (e.g., religious experiences or ceremonies) is consequential for religious people's sense of connectedness and commitment to their group. In one study, participants were given either an awe of childbirth, awe of nature, or humor induction. Among those high in religiosity/spirituality, awe of childbirth led to greater oneness with their friends, while awe of nature led to greater oneness with others in general (Van Cappellen & Saroglou, 2012). Awe also builds a sense of connectedness with one's religious group. Indeed, in one study, greater awe of God promoted greater sense of congregational cohesiveness (having a shared sense of values and beliefs), which further predicted greater belongingness with the congregation (Krause & Hayward, 2015). In addition, awe's effect on religious-group cohesiveness has been found to lead to forms of group signaling, such as sacrificing the self for the group. Specifically, dispositional awe was associated with greater sacrificing of the self in a trolley dilemma, in order to save five people who shared their religious identity (Naclerio & Van Cappellen, 2022).

Experiencing awe and other closely related self-transcendent positive emotions further promotes transcendent experiences and spirituality. Van Cappellen and Saroglou (2012) observed that individuals with higher levels of spirituality and religiousness exhibited increased spirituality-related feelings and behaviors when induced with awe (e.g., intention to visit a spiritual place). These findings were echoed in a series of experimental studies that set out to test the effects of such emotions on spirituality and belief in Gods (Saroglou et al., 2008; Valdesolo & Graham, 2014; Van Cappellen et al., 2013). In one study, participants randomly assigned to experience awe reported greater spirituality (e.g., "There is a higher plane of consciousness or spirituality that binds all people") than did participants assigned to experience either amusement or no particular emotion (control condition; Saroglou et al., 2008). In another series of studies, Valdesolo and Graham (2014) further found that awe increased agency detection and belief in God, as explained by awe's effect on tolerance for uncertainty. Following a compensation model, Valdesolo and Graham found that awe decreased tolerance for uncertainty, explaining the greater reliance on a belief in God and supernatural control. In contrast, two other experiments documented a positive—not compensatory—process through which inducing self-transcendent positive emotions (elicited by witnessing other people exemplifying moral beauty or extraordinary talents and skills) led to increased spirituality, relative to amusement and control conditions (Van Cappellen et al., 2013). In addition, perceived meaning in life and positive worldviews (e.g., a basic belief in the benevolence of others) explained the relationship between self-transcendent positive emotions and spirituality. Interestingly, the effect on spirituality was more pronounced among participants who were initially less religious (Van Cappellen et al., 2013). Together, these findings align with the notion that awe challenges individual-centric worldviews, prompting a reevaluation of one's place in the universe and fostering a sense of spirituality (Shiota et al., 2017; Van Cappellen, 2017).

The cognitive process of accommodation along with the perceived vastness may likely be partly responsible for awe's promotions of transcendent beliefs. This adjustment of mental schemas to accommodate awe-inspiring stimuli is essential for belief revision but does not automatically lead everyone toward spiritual responses. Indeed, research has shown that a disposition toward experiencing awe also correlates positively with scientific thinking, including a more accurate understanding of scientific processes, rejection of creationism, and avoidance of unwarranted teleological explanations (Gottlieb et al., 2018). Thus, awe not only enriches religious and spiritual life but also supports a scientific worldview by facilitating openness to new ideas and curiosity.

MEANING IN LIFE

Awe is often described as a meaning-making emotion (Dai et al., 2022; Danvers et al., 2016; Ihm et al., 2019). Indeed, as found in general cross-sectional studies, people who experienced awe more often also perceived life as more meaningful (Zhao et al., 2019). Such perceptions that life has meaning are considered a subjective experience (Steger et al., 2006), composed of feelings that one's life has significance, coherence, and purpose (Costin & Vignoles, 2020; Heintzelman & King, 2014; Martela & Steger, 2016). *Significance* involves the feeling that one's life matters and has value in the grand scheme of things, *coherence* involves feeling that one's experiences make sense and fit into one's framework of the world, and *purpose* involves having a sense of direction and goals to strive for. As awe experiences can challenge one's view of the self (significance), one's mental schemas (coherence), and one's values or day-to-day priorities (purpose), awe may have the ability to influence not only a global sense of meaning but also its three distinct facets.

Studies investigating awe's causal influence on perceptions of global meaning, and these facets of meaning, depict a nuanced portrait of the existential benefits of awe. Once again, we see the importance of the small self as a psychological consequence of awe when considering global meaning in life. Awe (compared to a neutral or positive control) has indirectly reduced global meaning in life via feelings of smallness (Rivera et al., 2020). Thus, in so far as awe diminishes the self, awe indirectly lowers one's sense of meaning in life. Yet awe does more than just diminish one's sense of the self. At the most basic level, awe is a positive emotion. Positive emotions are an important precursor to meaning in life (King et al., 2006), and awe invokes greater feelings of other positive emotions as well (Sturm et al., 2022). When awe was induced (vs. a control), awe indirectly enhanced meaning via greater feelings of happiness (Rivera et al., 2020). However, the effect via happiness was only found when awe was compared to a neutral control, but not when it was compared to another positive emotion (amusement), suggesting no added value to awe than its positive valence. Furthermore, when awe was elicited using threatening stimuli, thereby amplifying its negative component, awe no longer predicted meaning in life via happiness (compared to a control condition). Rivera and colleagues' (2020) studies showed that these two effects, increasing and decreasing global meaning via differing pathways, can occur simultaneously. Awe implies both positive affect that supports meaning in life and feelings of smallness that reduce meaning in life.

Awe's influence on the self also has implications for significance. Smallness is often defined and measured as a sense of insignificance (e.g., Piff et al., 2015; Tyson et al., 2022). Moreover, induced awe was found to directly reduce feelings of significance (Dai et al., 2022). Both Rivera and colleagues (2020) and Dai and colleagues (2022) showed that these feelings of insignificance (whether measured within a sense of smallness or a direct measure of significance) reduced more global reports of meaning in life.

Yet both the measurement and definition of significance and smallness need more methodological preciseness. Significance has been measured as mattering "even in the grand scheme of the universe" (Costin & Vignoles, 2020) or as "my life is full of value" (Martela & Steger, 2023). These two forms of significance feel like they carry different weight and thus are affected differently by experiences of awe (and smallness). Feelings of smallness seem to reduce a sense of value *in the grand scheme of the entire universe* (Dai et al., 2022), as one becomes aware of the largeness of the universe and the small role one has to play in it. Yet perceived significance may not be totally lost in awe experiences. Indeed, by increasing a sense of connectedness to one's community (Bai et al., 2017), awe may enhance perceived mattering to other people in one's life and hence perceived value.

Another characteristic of awe—perceived vastness and the need for accommodation—plays a role in meaning-making processes. Awe involves an experience so new and incomprehensible that it requires accommodative shifts in one's previous mental structures. As a result, one's sense of coherence of the world may be affected. One possibility is that as one's mental structures need reevaluating and restructuring, one's sense of coherence would be momentarily lowered. Dai and colleagues (2022) referred to this experience as coherence seeking: Awe elicits the need to seek a sense of coherence again and while this process unfolds, one's sense of meaning in life is lowered. There is much support for awe's influence on accommodative processing, including feeling like the awe experience was more challenging to comprehend (Yaden et al., 2019), and seeking coherence through a tendency to seek order and patterns (Valdesolo & Graham, 2014). However, only one study to date has aimed to directly examine the effects of awe on coherence, and it did not find evidence that awe led to coherence seeking (Dai et al., 2022). Perhaps because humans are motivated to create meaning (Becker, 1973; Frankl, 1946/1992), the threat awe poses to one's coherence is quickly accommodated or compensated for. Capturing this process of coherence lost, sought, rebuilt, and expanded may prove methodologically challenging but worth pursuing in future research.

Finally, awe can affect the sense that life has a purpose and can motivate people to pursue their goals according to their values. While experiencing awe, day-to-day concerns fade into the background (Shiota et al., 2007), presumably allowing an individual to better identify what really matters to them and pursue more authentic goals. Research found that awe led to a greater sense of purpose—awe motivated people to pursue their goals, which, in turn, further boosted greater global meaning in life (Dai et al., 2022). Moreover, awe was also found to motivate authentic self-pursuits (i.e., acting in alignment with one's true self; Jiang & Sedikides, 2022), which in turn further predicted finding greater meaning in life (Yuan et al., 2024). Together, such research shows distinct effects of awe on the self—finding clarity on one's values and goals, which promote purpose and general meaning.

In sum, awe involves a complex subjective experience that both promotes and hinders the perception that life is meaningful. To disentangle the divergent effects of awe on meaning, it seems particularly important to zoom in on the specific characteristics of awe (perceived smallness, vastness, need for accommodation) and the valence of awe (is the experience positive or threatening; involving what type of experience for the self?). Similarly, meaning should be studied in all its facets (significance, etc.), which seem to be uniquely influenced by awe. Finally, the timing of the measurement of meaning might be important. One currently understudied possibility is that awe momentarily lowers meaning (significance and coherence are challenged) but then involves processes that restore and enhance meaning (boosting authentic, purposeful pursuits; enhancing connectedness that can further increase significance; reestablishing coherence with accommodative processes).

FUTURE RESEARCH ON AWE'S EXISTENTIAL IMPACTS

Personal accounts of awe describe events from the mundane to powerfully intense experiences. We wonder if there exists a threshold for the subjective experience of awe to reap its existential benefits. We also wonder if the quality of the subjective experience of awe is key in distinguishing between positive and negative existential consequences. One interesting possibility is that for the experience of awe to remain positive, a subjective sense of existential security may be key (Konecni, 2005). Individual differences in security may moderate the impact of awe events. Moreover, using more intense awe manipulations may better capture the range of awe's existential qualities more clearly. Novel research approaches including virtual reality (Chirico et al., 2018), naturalistic settings (Anderson et al., 2018), and psychedelics (Yaden et al., 2017) might be particularly promising for the study of existential awe.

Moreover, while awe has many positive benefits, it is unclear how lasting these benefits are. In addition, more research on understanding what is happening when the self becomes small is required: Do feelings of insignificance and lower salience of the self have different psychological consequences? This question becomes particularly important when investigating outcomes such as interconnectedness and meaning in life. Much of the conflicting evidence appears to be the result of the many ways through which awe affects the self and has opposing effects on these main outcomes. Additional research would also benefit an understanding of awe's influence on self-growth. Unpacking the small self, its differing consequences, and how the elements are all intertwined and coexist would benefit the science of awe and understanding awe's existential nature.

CONCLUSION

This chapter explores the emotion of awe from an existential perspective, examining both its theoretical foundations and empirical research. Awe is defined as the emotional response to something perceived as vast and that requires a process of cognitive accommodation to fit the experience into existing mental schemas. If existential psychology is the science of being and becoming, then awe acts as a catalyst for the accommodation and reevaluation of the self and its place in the universe. Indeed, being confronted with vaster stimuli reminds an individual of their smallness. We highlighted how a quieted and transcended self allows for key psychological consequences to occur following awe. Awe promotes a sense of connectedness to things greater than oneself, triggering prosocial orientations and interdependence with one's group. Awe also deepens the perception of a larger, often spiritual, or universal, reality. Finally, awe affects the core existential question of whether life has purpose and is meaningful. Recognizing the complex subjective experience of awe, ranging from truly positive and grounding to threatening and self-diminishing, we discussed how awe can both support meaning and authentic self-pursuits and sometimes be a source of existential angst. Disentangling the many aspects of the subjective experience of awe, and particularly as they may lead to opposing effects on existential outcomes, is a ripe area for future research.

REFERENCES

Anderson, C. L., Dixson, D. D., Monroy, M., & Keltner, D. (2020). Are awe-prone people more curious?: The relationship between dispositional awe, curiosity, and academic outcomes. *Journal of Personality, 88*(4), 762–779.

Anderson, C. L., Monroy, M., & Keltner, D. (2018). Awe in nature heals: Evidence from military veterans, at-risk youth, and college students. *Emotion, 18*(8), 1195.

Bai, Y., Maruskin, L. A., Chen, S., Gordon, A. M., Stellar, J. E., McNeil, G. D., . . . Keltner, D. (2017). Awe, the diminished self, and collective engagement: Universals and cultural variations in the small self. *Journal of Personality and Social Psychology, 113*(2), 185.

Bai, Y., Ocampo, J., Jin, G., Chen, S., Benet-Martinez, V., Monroy, M., . . . Keltner, D. (2021). Awe, daily stress, and elevated life satisfaction. *Journal of Personality and Social Psychology, 120*(4), 837–860.

Becker, E. (1973). *The denial of death*. Free Press.

Campos, B., Shiota, M. N., Keltner, D., Gonzaga, G. C., & Goetz, J. L. (2013). What is shared, what is different?: Core relational themes and expressive displays of eight positive emotions. *Cognition and Emotion, 27*(1), 37–52.

Chen, S. K., & Mongrain, M. (2021). Awe and the interconnected self. *Journal of Positive Psychology, 16*, 770–778.

Chirico, A., Glaveanu, V. P., Cipresso, P., Riva, G., & Gaggioli, A. (2018). Awe enhances creative thinking: An experimental study. *Creativity Research Journal, 30*(2), 123–131.

Cohen, A. B., Gruber, J., & Keltner, D. (2010). Comparing spiritual transformations and experiences of profound beauty. *Psychology of Religion and Spirituality, 2*(3), 127–135.

Costin, V., & Vignoles, V. L. (2020). Meaning is about mattering: Evaluating coherence, purpose, and existential mattering as precursors of meaning in life judgments. *Journal of Personality and Social Psychology, 118*(4), 864–884.

Dai, Y., Jiang, T., & Miao, M. (2022). Uncovering the effects of awe on meaning in life. *Journal of Happiness Studies, 23*(7), 3517–3529.

Danvers, A. F., O'Neil, M. J., & Shiota, M. N. (2016). The mind of the "happy warrior": Eudaimonia, awe, and the search for meaning in life. In J. Vitterrsø (Ed.), *Handbook of eudaimonic well-being* (pp. 323–335). Springer.

Edwards, M. E., Helm, P. J., Pratscher, S., Bettencourt, B. A., & Arndt, J. (2024). The Impact of awe on existential isolation: Evidence for contrasting pathways. *Personality and Social Psychology Bulletin, 50*(5), 715–732.

Frankl, V. E. (1992). *Man's search for meaning: An introduction to logotherapy* (4th ed.). Beacon Press. (Original work published 1946)

Fuller, R. C. (2007). Spirituality in the flesh: The role of discrete emotions in religious life. *Journal of the American Academy of Religion, 75*(1), 25–51.

Gordon, A. M., Stellar, J. E., Anderson, C. L., McNeil, G. D., Loew, D., & Keltner, D. (2017). The dark side of the sublime: Distinguishing a threat-based variant of awe. *Journal of Personality and Social Psychology, 113*(2), 310.

Gottlieb, S., Keltner, D., & Lombrozo, T. (2018). Awe as a scientific emotion. *Cognitive Science, 42*(6), 2081–2094.

Haidt, J. (2003). The moral emotions. In R. J. Davidson, K. R. Scherer, & H. H. Goldsmith (Eds.), *Handbook of affective sciences* (pp. 852–870). Oxford University Press.

Hardy, A. (1979). *The spiritual nature of man: A study of contemporary religious experience*. Clarendon Press.

Hawkley, L. C., & Cacioppo, J. T. (2010). Loneliness matters: A theoretical and empirical review of consequences and mechanisms. *Annals of Behavioral Medicine, 40*(2), 218–227.

Heintzelman, S. J., & King, L. A. (2014). (The feeling of) meaning-as-information. *Personality and Social Psychology Review, 18*(2), 153–167.

Hood, R. W., Jr., & Chen, Z. (2013). Mystical, spiritual, and religious experiences. In R. F. Paloutzian & C. L. Park (Eds.), *Handbook of the psychology of religion and spirituality* (2nd ed., pp. 422–440). Guilford Press.

Ihm, E. D., Paloutzian, R. F., van Elk, M., & Schooler, J. W. (2019). Awe as a meaning-making emotion: On the evolution of awe and the origin of religions. In J. R. Feierman & L. Oviedo (Eds.), *The evolution of religion, religiosity and theology: A multi-level and multi-disciplinary approach*. Routledge.

Jiang, T., & Sedikides, C. (2022). Awe motivates authentic-self pursuit via self-transcendence: Implications for prosociality. *Journal of Personality and Social Psychology, 123*(3), 576.

Joye, Y., & Verpooten, J. (2013). An exploration of the functions of religious monumental architecture from a Darwinian perspective. *Review of General Psychology, 17*(1), 53–68.

Kearns, P. O., & Tyler, J. M. (2022). Examining the relationship between awe, spirituality, and religiosity. *Psychology of Religion and Spirituality, 14*(4), 436.

Keltner, D., & Haidt, J. (2003). Approaching awe, a moral, spiritual, and aesthetic emotion. *Cognition and Emotion, 17*(2), 297–314.

King, L. A., Hicks, J. A., Krull, J. L., & Del Gaiso, A. K. (2006). Positive affect and the experience of meaning in life. *Journal of Personality and Social Psychology, 90*(1), 179.

Konecni, V. J. (2005). The aesthetic trinity: Awe, being moved, thrills. *Bulletin of Psychology and the Arts, 5*(2), 27–44.

Krause, N., & Hayward, R. D. (2015). Assessing whether practical wisdom and awe of God are associated with life satisfaction. *Psychology of Religion and Spirituality, 7*(1), 51.

Martela, F., & Steger, M. F. (2016). The three meanings of meaning in life: Distinguishing coherence, purpose, and significance. *Journal of Positive Psychology, 11*(5), 531–545.

Martela, F., & Steger, M. F. (2023). The role of significance relative to the other dimensions of meaning in life–an examination utilizing the three dimensional meaning in life scale

(3DM). *Journal of Positive Psychology, 18*(4), 606–626.

Mitchell, E. D. (2008). *The way of the explorer: An Apollo astronaut's journey through the material and mystical world.* New Page Books.

Monroy, M., & Keltner, D. (2023). Awe as a pathway to mental and physical health. *Perspectives on Psychological Science, 18*(2), 309–320.

Naclerio, M., & Van Cappellen, P. (2022). Awe, group cohesion, and religious self-sacrifice. *International Journal for the Psychology of Religion, 32*(3), 256–271.

Nakayama, M., Nozaki, Y., Taylor, P. M., Keltner, D., & Uchida, Y. (2020). Individual and cultural differences in predispositions to feel positive and negative aspects of awe. *Journal of Cross-Cultural Psychology, 51*(10), 771–793.

Perlin, J. D., & Li, L. (2020). Why does awe have prosocial effects?: New perspectives on awe and the small self. *Perspectives on Psychological Science, 15*(2), 291–308.

Piff, P. K., Dietze, P., Feinberg, M., Stancato, D. M., & Keltner, D. (2015). Awe, the small self, and prosocial behavior. *Journal of Personality and Social Psychology, 108*(6), 883–899.

Pinel, E. C., Long, A. E., Murdoch, E. Q., & Helm, P. (2017). A prisoner of one's own mind: Identifying and understanding existential isolation. *Personality and Individual Differences, 105,* 54–63.

Prade, C., & Saroglou, V. (2016). Awe's effects on generosity and helping. *Journal of Positive Psychology, 11*(5), 522–530.

Prade, C., & Saroglou, V. (2023). Awe and social conformity: Awe promotes the endorsement of social norms and conformity to the majority opinion. *Emotion, 23*(7), 2100–2104.

Preston, J. L., & Shin, F. (2017). Spiritual experiences evoke awe through the small self in both religious and non-religious individuals. *Journal of Experimental Social Psychology, 70,* 212–221.

Rivera, G. N., Vess, M., Hicks, J. A., & Routledge, C. (2020). Awe and meaning: Elucidating complex effects of awe experiences on meaning in life. *European Journal of Social Psychology, 50*(2), 392–405.

Rudd, M., Vohs, K. D., & Aaker, J. (2012). Awe expands people's perception of time, alters decision making, and enhances well-being. *Psychological Science, 23*(10), 1130–1136.

Saroglou, V., Buxant, C., & Tilquin, J. (2008). Positive emotions as leading to religion and spirituality. *Journal of Positive Psychology, 3*(3), 165–173.

Shiota, M. N., Keltner, D., & Mossman, A. (2007). The nature of awe: Elicitors, appraisals, and effects on self-concept. *Cognition and Emotion, 21*(5), 944–963.

Shiota, M. N., Thrash, T. M., Danvers, A., & Dombrowski, J. T. (2017). Transcending the self: Awe, elevation, and inspiration. In M. M. Tugade, M. N. Shiota, & L. D. Kirby (Eds.), *Handbook of positive emotions* (pp. 362–377). Guilford Press.

Song, J. Y., Klebl, C., & Bastian, B. (2023). Awe promotes moral expansiveness via the small-self. *Frontiers in Psychology, 14,* 1097627.

Steger, M. F., Frazier, P., Oishi, S., & Kaler, M. (2006). The meaning in life questionnaire: assessing the presence of and search for meaning in life. *Journal of Counseling Psychology, 53*(1), 80.

Stellar, J. E. (2021), Awe helps us remember why it is important to forget the self. *Annals of the New York Academy of Sciences, 1501*(1), 81–84.

Stellar, J. E., Gordon, A. M., Piff, P. K., Cordaro, D., Anderson, C. L., Bai, Y., . . . Keltner, D. (2017). Self-transcendent emotions and their social functions: compassion, gratitude, and awe bind us to others through prosociality. *Emotion Review, 9*(3), 200–207.

Stepanova, E. R., Quesnel, D., & Riecke, B. E. (2019). Understanding AWE: Can a virtual journey, inspired by the overview effect, lead to an increased sense of interconnectedness? *Frontiers in Digital Humanities, 6.*

Sturm, V. E., Datta, S., Roy, A. R., Sible, I. J., Kosik, E. L., Veziris, C. R., . . . Keltner, D. (2022). Big smile, small self: Awe walks promote prosocial positive emotions in older adults. *Emotion, 22*(5), 1044.

Tyson, C., Hornsey, M. J., & Barlow, F. K. (2022). What does it mean to feel small?: Three dimensions of the small self. *Self and Identity, 21*(4), 387–405.

Valdesolo, P., & Graham, J. (2014). Awe, uncertainty, and agency detection. *Psychological Science, 25*(1), 170–178.

Van Cappellen, P. (2017). Rethinking self-transcendent positive emotions and religion: Insights from psychological and biblical research. *Psychology of Religion and Spirituality, 9*(3), 254.

Van Cappellen, P., Edwards, M. E., & Shiota, M. N. (2023). Shades of expansiveness: Postural expression of dominance, high-arousal positive affect, and warmth. *Emotion, 23*(4), 973–985.

Van Cappellen, P., & Saroglou, V. (2012). Awe activates religious and spiritual feelings and behavioral intentions. *Psychology of Religion and Spirituality, 4*(3), 223.

Van Cappellen, P., Saroglou, V., Iweins, C.,

Piovesana, M., & Fredrickson, B. L. (2013). Self-transcendent positive emotions increase spirituality through basic world assumptions. *Cognition & emotion, 27*(8), 1378–1394.

Vishkin, A., Schwartz, S. H., Ben-Nun Bloom, P., Solak, N., & Tamir, M. (2019). Religiosity and desired emotions: Belief maintenance or prosocial facilitation? *Personality and Social Psychology Bulletin, 46*(7), 1090–1106.

Wang, M., Qu, X., Guo, C., & Wang, J. (2023). Awe elicited by natural disasters and willingness to help people in afflicted areas: A meditational model. *Current Psychology, 42*(24), 20883–20889.

Wu, Q., Cui, L., Han, X., Ding, W., & He, W. (2023). Awe and wise reasoning in adolescents: The mediating role of small-self and need for relatedness. *Heliyon, 9*(4).

Yaden, D. B., Haidt, J., Hood, R. W., Jr., Vago, D. R., & Newberg, A. B. (2017). The varieties of self-transcendent experience. *Review of General Psychology, 21*(2), 143–160.

Yaden, D. B., Kaufman, S. B., Hyde, E., Chirico, A., Gaggioli, A., Zhang, J. W., & Keltner, D. (2019). The development of the Awe Experience Scale (AWE-S): A multifactorial measure for a complex emotion. *Journal of Positive Psychology, 14*(4), 474–488.

Yalom, I. D. (1980). *Existential psychotherapy.* Basic Books.

Yang, Y., Hu, J., Jing, F., & Nguyen, B. (2018). From awe to ecological behavior: The mediating role of connectedness to nature. *Sustainability, 10*(7), 2477.

Yuan, W., Du, Y., & Jiang, T. (2024). How and when awe improves meaning in life: The role of authentic-self pursuit and trait authenticity. *Emotion, 24*(2), 412–430.

Zhang, J. W., Howell, R. T., Razavi, P., Shaban-Azad, H., Chai, W. J., Ramis, T., . . . Keltner, D. (2021). Awe is associated with creative personality, convergent creativity, and everyday creativity. *Psychology of Aesthetics, Creativity, and the Arts,* online publication.

Zhao, H., & Zhang, H. (2023). Why dispositional awe promotes psychosocial flourishing?: An investigation of intrapersonal and interpersonal pathways among Chinese emerging adults. *Current Psychology, 42*(15), 12682–12694.

Zhao, H., Zhang, H., Xu, Y., He, W., & Lu, J. (2019). Why are people high in dispositional awe happier?: The roles of meaning in life and materialism. *Frontiers in Psychology, 10,* 1208.

CHAPTER 59

The Transformative Self

How the Narrative Architecture of Identity Frames Humane Flourishing and Authenticity

Jack J. Bauer

The transformative self is a growth-oriented, largely narrative identity that helps a person cultivate human flourishing for the self and others (Bauer, 2021). Before diving into details, I wish to say that the power of a transformative self is *not* the striving for "improvement" or "continual growth." The transformative self does carry an abiding orientation toward growth, but not always explicitly—and in any case it's a humanistic and humane growth, not an onerous push toward improvement for improvement's sake. The power of a transformative self lies in its thematic motives toward *engaged experiencing* (which fosters well-being) and *curiosity-driven reflection* (which fosters wisdom).

This chapter takes the position that the specific goods and meanings in people's lives come in countless forms and from countless sources, all of which vary from person to person and from culture to culture—and furthermore change over time developmentally and historically. Despite this diversity of meaning, *all* these forms and sources of meaning depend in no small part on how one interprets one's life. And perhaps the primary place people interpret meaning in their lives is in the *stories* that they tell each other (and tell themselves) about their lives. Through life stories people create a *narrative identity* by using abstract ideas of cultural goods in life to thread together the events, people, and experiences of their actual lives into a meaningful understanding of themselves. Or at least that's what they're *trying* to do with their narrative identities. One's evolving narrative identity is one's attempt to create a *good life,* as understood and shaped in *story* form.

In this chapter I explore how the architectural elements of narrative identity convey both desires for and actualizations of cultural goods in life, such as well-being, purpose, wisdom, and authenticity. The transformative self is a prototype of self-identity in largely narrative form that features themes of humanistic (versus materialistic or egoistic) growth. As a prototype, the transformative self is illustrated in the *bildungsroman* genre of literature, which provides simultaneously a cultural master narrative of a good life (with master narratives' potential for oppression) and an alternative, countercultural narrative (with potential for humane liberation). As both an individual and cultural prototype of narrative identity, the transformative self aims to cultivate flourishing not merely for oneself but for others as well. This type of flourishing is a *humane* flourishing, one that deepens in interiority and expands inclusively in relationality as one's ego quiets and one's self-authorship becomes more existentially authentic over time.

That's a lot. But it's all tied together: the self, others, and culture; epistemology and ethics; pleasure and meaning; experiencing and identifying; wanting and having; having and hegemony; development toward maturity and authenticity. A transformative self is not just about happiness—and neither is a good life (Bauer, 2021). Wisdom, caring, and becoming wiser and more caring—regardless of "how much" wisdom or love (or happiness) one has—also matter, among other things. The transformative self identifies with the deepening and broadening of capacities to experience and to think about human existence.

THEORIES OF NARRATIVE IDENTITY AND THEORIES OF "THE" GOOD LIFE

Goods may make sense theoretically in the abstract, but a good life makes sense primarily in the context of *lives.* Two features of a life that goods in the abstract typically fail to capture are *time* and *lived experience,* which require *narrative* to understand. As for time, the psychologist George Kelly (1955/1963) lays the foundation for his theory of personal constructs and constructive alternativism by noting that "life has to be seen in the perspective of time if it is to make any sense at all." Goods do not function as pure, abstract forms; they exist in time, in terms of actions that are experienced and narrated over personal, not just chronological, time (Ricoeur, 1990). As for lived experience, the philosopher Alasdair MacIntyre (1981) famously claimed that the good life is the life spent pursuing the good in life. Like Aristotle, he argues that the good life is an *activity.* Unlike Aristotle, MacIntyre argues that one's subjective interpretation of the experience of activity matters greatly—and that the interpreted pursuit of a good life is "a *narrative* quest" (p. 219). The philosopher Charles Taylor (1989) explains how this narrative construction of identity is a culturally and morally yoked quest of meaning making.

Most theories of a good life provide an abstract view from 30,000 feet. However, the problems of and threats to meaning and a good life that we face directly—the problems that drive us existentially bananas—happen on the ground, where we live and breathe, and where we create and live out our stories. In this way, theories of a good life in psychology tend to have a *meaning-making* problem; they generally lack an account of how people actually create meaning in their lives as they develop their capacities to do so. However, theories of narrative identity in psychology tend to have an *ethical* problem; they generally lack an account of how abstract principles of the good inform the meanings that people make.

The term *narrative identity* refers to one's evolving, autobiographical sense of what's meaningful in one's life (McAdams & McLean, 2013). By late adolescence, personal identity becomes not only a primary concern in life (Erikson, 1968), and not only an abstract belief or theory about oneself, but also a *story* that reflects the kind of *autobiographical reasoning* that yields a *narrative* identity (Habermas & Bluck, 2000). Late adolescence also seems to be the time that, across cultures, autobiographical reasoning begins to correspond to well-being (Reese et al., 2017). From then on, for the rest of our lives, we *reconstruct* our narrative identities as our lives unfold over time (McLean et al., 2007). Simultaneously we *co-construct* our narrative identity with others. For example, we modify our interpretations of events in response to others' input on the everyday stories we tell about our lives (Fivush et al., 2006; McLean & Mansfield, 2012; Pasupathi et al., 2007). For another example, we construct our narrative identity by drawing the *master narratives* that surround us, such as in our family stories (McLean & Syed, 2016) and in our culture's literature, movies, and dialogue in religion and politics (Hammack, 2008; McLean & Syed, 2016). In all this reconstruction and co-construction of narrative identity, we use our life stories in an attempt to cultivate not only well-being but also other qualities of good life, such as wisdom, moral virtue, generativity, self-actualizing, and authenticity (Bauer et al., 2008). Whether these goods become actualized in our lives is another question, but the varying ways and degrees that they do are conveyed in our narrative identities.

In an entirely different body of theory, *the good life* refers to a life well lived, which can be defined in countless ways across cultures and individuals but which generally involves some set of ideals for human flourishing. Two competing models in Western philosophy and psychology are *hedonia* and *eudaimonia* (e.g., Huta & Waterman, 2014; Ryan & Deci, 2001; Waterman, 2013). Hedonists argue that *pleasure* is the ultimate good in life, where *pleasure* refers to both subjective experiences of pleasure and subjective evaluations of satisfaction (Haybron, 2008), both of which constitute *hedonic well-being* (see Diener et al., 2006). In contrast, eudaimonists argue that *meaning* is the ultimate good in life, where the term *meaning* here serves as an imperfect term that refers to a sprawling array of goods that includes not only a subjectivist and internalist sense of meaningfulness (which itself encompasses a wide range of phenomena known as *eudaimonic well-being;* e.g., Steger, 2016) but also more objectivist and externalist conditions like moral virtue, wisdom, and self-actualizing growth (e.g., Bauer, 2016, 2021; Tiberius, 2013; Vittersø, 2016). Hedonists and eudaimonists tend to argue for the unique importance of either pleasure or (very broadly defined) meaning—typically by claiming that one set of goods reduces to the other as primary or ultimate. I have developed a model of the good life that shows how the goods of hedonia and eudaimonia are compatible as simultaneously ultimate and irreducible to each other, as they function on different levels of context (Bauer, 2016, 2021). Space prohibits elaboration here, but this model plays behind the scenes of this chapter.

Research and theory on the interface of narrative identity and the good life has been growing, as a recent special issue in the *Journal of Personality* attests (Bauer & Thomsen, 2022). The articles in that special issue explored not only the ways that features of narrative identity correspond to features of a good life but also—and especially—how narrative inquiry challenges the notions of what is good, and for whom (think: marginality, culture, disability), and how and when goods arise in the first place, both ontogenetically and culturally, and how research designs skew what we know about it all.

How Narrative Identity Conveys Goods in Life

Narrative identity and the good life both deal with concerns of *value*—what people identify with and what makes life worth living. Narrative identity and the good life complement each other. Indeed they are two sides of the same coin—the coin of valuing a life. Theories of narrative identity are relatively stronger on explaining processes of meaning making but weaker on modeling goods in life, which are often assumed to be humanistic and humane in value orientation. In contrast, theories of the good life are relatively stronger on modeling goods in life but weaker on explaining processes of meaning making, particularly how they develop over time within social ecologies.

In my two decades of studying the interface of narrative identity and the good life, I have attempted to clarify elemental qualities within each body of theory by exploring how the elements of narrative identity convey the goods of hedonia and eudaimonia. McAdams (1985) had laid a foundation for the scientific study of narrative elements—notably tone, theme, and structure. Yet these terms have often been used interchangeably, reflecting their interlaced use in natural language. Empirical measures also commonly confound these terms (especially tone and theme), even as efforts have been made theoretically and empirically to distinguish them (Adler et al., 2016; Blagov et al., 2022; Graci et al., 2018; McLean et al., 2020). However, my research team and I have recently demonstrated theoretically and empirically how three nonoverlapping elements of narrative identity specifically reflect three broad categories of goods in life (Bauer, Graham, et al., 2019; Bauer et al., 2022). The result is a model of a *good life story* that bridges theories of narrative identity with theories of a good life (and then within developmental, cultural, and transdisciplinary contexts; Bauer, 2021). Value lies at the foundation of that bridge.

Value Orientation and Actualization

More precisely, a framework of value, which I call value orientation and actualization (VOA; Bauer, 2016, 2021), bridges narrative identity and the good life. VOA starts with a relatively simple claim: It's one thing to want goods in life, and it's another to have them. VOA distinguishes these two conditions as value orientation and value actualization. First we consider the dimensions of VOA and then how they lie at the heart of both three superordinate goods in life and three basic elements of narrative identity.

A value *orientation* itself *is* an idea of a good in life, which is to say, a good as the person sees it—something one wants and uses as a criterion of evaluation, whether consciously or unconsciously, regardless of whether the good pans out or not. *Value orientations* come in many forms, such as values, motives, needs, purposes, drives, pleasures, meanings, beliefs, reasons, sakes, or bases for justification—each of which comes in myriad forms (see Baumeister, 1991; Rohan, 2000; Schwartz & Bilsky, 1990). A value orientation may lean toward a hedonic or eudaimonic value actualization, whether as the actualization of pleasure (notably including satisfaction) or as the actualization of any of the myriad forms of meaning (notably including meaningfulness, wisdom, and moral virtue).

A value *actualization* is the manifestation or demonstration of a value orientation in one's life, which may be assessed subjectively or objectively. Value actualization comes in two broad but orthogonal forms: value fulfillment and value perspectivity.

Value fulfillment deals with the *subjective* sense that one's value orientations are *satisfied* in one's life. Value fulfillment is the distinguishing feature of well-being in psychology (DeYoung & Tiberius, 2023). Value fulfillment comes in forms of hedonic (e.g., positive experience and life satisfaction; Diener et al., 2006) or eudaimonic well-being (which involve various forms of meaningfulness; Ryff & Singer, 2008).

Value perspectivity deals with the *objective* degree to which one thinks *coherently* and (especially) *complexly* about matters of value in one's life. Value perspectivity is the structural dimension of value, to complement the orientation and fulfillment dimensions (cf. coherence [but not complexity] as a dimension of meaning in Martela & Steger, 2016, where their purpose and significance dimensions also correspond closely to the present value orientation and value fulfillment). Value perspectivity is the distinguishing feature of wisdom as expert reasoning (Baltes & Staudinger, 2000) and of wisdom as *phronesis*, at least when combined with humanistic value orientations (Kristjánsson & Fowers, 2024).

VOA yields an integrative model of goods in life that integrates hedonia and eudaimonia, where both function in concert, neither collapses into the other, and eudaimonia includes internalist, externalist, subjectivist, and objectivist criteria (Bauer, 2016, 2021; Bauer et al., 2022; Bauer & Weatherbie, 2023). As an abstract model of goods, value orientation, value fulfillment, and value perspectivity lie at the heart of three broad goods in life, respectively: purpose (the orienting or motivating quality of either pleasure or meaning), well-being (whether hedonic or eudaimonic), and wisdom (which is primarily eudaimonic).

However, goods are not lived in the abstract. Goods come alive in our life stories. VOA helps explain how this happens, notably by helping deconstruct narrative identity into nonoverlapping elements. These deconstructed elements of narrative identity convey specific facets of VOA and thus key elements of superordinate categories of goods in life, in a nutshell:

- Narrative *tone* conveys hedonic value fulfillment and thus degrees of hedonic satisfaction and well-being.
- Narrative *theme* conveys hedonic and/or eudaimonic value orientations and thus types of purpose.
- The combination of tone and a eudaimonic theme convey degrees of *eudaimonic* meaningfulness and well-being.
- Narrative *structure* conveys value perspectivity and thus degrees of wisdom, particularly when combined with a humanistic theme (see Table 59.1).

How Narrative Tone Conveys the Good of (Hedonic) Well-Being

When we listen to a person talk about their lives, and we conclude whether they're relatively satisfied and happy or not, we're primarily paying attention to their narrative tone. Narrative tone refers to the posi-

TABLE 59.1. How VOA Differentiates Narrative Elements and Goods in Life

Value facets	Narrative elements	Salient qualities of those elements	Goods in life conveyed by those qualities
Value orientation	Theme	Motive for pleasure/satisfaction	Hedonic motive
		Motive for a type of meaning	Eudaimonic motive
Value fulfillment	Tone[a]	Positive affect[a]	Hedonic well-being (satisfaction)[a]
	Tone × Theme	Positive affect × Humanistic motive[b]	Eudaimonic well-being (meaningfulness)[c]
Value perspectivity	Structure.	Coherence	
		Complexity	Eudaimonic wisdom as expert reasoning
	Theme × Structure	Humanistic motive × Complexity[d]	Eudaimonic wisdom as *phronesis*

Note. Adapted from Bauer et al. (2022).

[a]Measures of narrative tones (i.e., degrees of positive and negative affect) and scale measures of hedonic well-being both signal hedonic value fulfillment, that is, the degree to which events are satisfying (but not why they are meaningful).

[b]Humanistic/experiential motives versus egoistic/status-oriented motives.

[c]Measures of tone–theme combinations (i.e., degrees to which particular kinds of themes are satisfactorily enacted) and scale measures of eudaimonic well-being both signal eudaimonic value fulfillment (i.e., the degree to which events are specifically meaningful and not merely satisfying).

[d]Measures of theme-structure combinations (here as degrees to which humanistic themes are conveyed/interpreted with relatively high levels of structural complexity) and measures of wisdom (notably those employing open-ended responses and researcher-assessed depth of processing) both signal wisdom as *phronesis*.

tive and negative affect of a story. In other words, narrative tone in a personal narrative conveys the person's degree of value fulfillment—but not value orientation. In a personal narrative, tone signals the narrator's levels of satisfaction (i.e., hedonic value fulfillment) with the events of the story (Bauer, 2016). A personal narrative uses positive and negative affect to evaluate events, people, and experiences as relatively good or bad.

Researchers can assess narrative tone as global affect (the general positivity and negativity of a story) or as an "affective sequence" that captures changes in affect over time within the story (Adler et al., 2016). Among the most widely studied affective sequences are various forms of positive outcomes, such as *redemption sequences*—a personal story starts out bad but ends good (McAdams et al., 2001), happy endings, and positive resolution (Adler & Poulin, 2009; King et al., 2000). Affective sequences also include contamination sequences, in which events turn from good to bad (McAdams et al., 2001). Redemption sequences correlate with well-being, but it depends on the narrative event: Redemption seems to be a healthy way to narrate life's difficulties, but narrating a good event by starting with negative emotionality before turning out well seems to have little to do with well-being (Bauer, Graham, et al., 2019; Bauer et al., 2022; Dunlop, 2021; McLean & Lilgendahl, 2008).

Narrative tone is typically fused with at least one theme (such as power or love) in personal narratives, but tone and theme can be disentangled, intuitively and empirically. For example, all redemption sequences are about changes from negative to positive affect, regardless of whether they deal with themes of, for example, wealth (rags to riches), health (illness to wellness), pleasure (unhappiness to happiness), meaning (aimlessness to purposefulness), morality (sin to salvation, selfishness to caring), or wisdom (ignorance to enlightenment).

Most measures of narrative tone capture positive and negative affect without reference to specific contexts of meaning in the story (which are conveyed in themes). Thus, narrative tone is how we express and know (and feel) our own degree of hedonic well-being. Tone is the narrative counterpart to self-report-scale measures of hedonic or subjective well-being (e.g., Diener et al., 2006). Importantly, narrative tone conveys a person's level of hedonic well-being implicitly rather than by asking the person explicitly to rate how satisfied they are with their life. Narrative tone is how we hedonically evaluate our life events when reliving them in our stories (e.g., Adler et al., 2016; Bauer et al., 2022).

How Narrative Theme Conveys the Good of Purpose

When we listens to a person talk about their lives, and we can say what they value and identify with (what motivates them, what they view as the purpose of an action), we're paying attention to their narrative *themes*. Narrative themes convey the purpose of a story—what the narrator values about the story's events. However, themes do not—when distinguished from narrative tone—convey how satisfied we area with them (only tone conveys that). In other words, whereas narrative tone conveys *whether* the narrator is satisfied or dissatisfied (to varying degrees) with this or that event, narrative theme conveys the specific *purpose* for or reason why this satisfaction is important. Like with any value or motive, people narrate their lives with themes sometimes consciously or explicitly but often unconsciously or implicitly. Narrative themes convey the specific meanings (i.e., value orientations) of our life—notably as we see them when reliving our life events in stories.

Two overarching themes in both life stories and literature are *agency* and *communion* (McAdams, 1985; McLean et al., 2020). Agency refers to value orientations of power, mastery, victory, status, and having an impact, whereas communion refers to value orientations of love, intimacy, friendship, dialogue, communication, and other forms of social bonding (McAdams et al., 1996). A third great theme is found in the overarching value orientation of *growth*. As I explain later, the particular value orientation of growth that promotes humane flourishing is *humanistic growth motivation*, which serves as the featured theme of a transformative self (Bauer, 2021).

As value orientations, these superordinate categories of themes refer to the types of purpose in the narrator's life, but not to the (degrees of) fulfillment of those purposes—at least in my model of narrative tone and theme. Most measures of narrative theme operationally confound motive with affective evaluations of those motives in context, as we see next. So as not to misconstrue the research: My hard distinction between tone as affect but not value/motive and theme as value/motive but not affect is largely unique to my deconstructed model of the elements of narrative identity (e.g., Bauer, Graham, et al., 2019; Bauer et al., 2022).

How Narrative Tone and Theme Together Convey the Good of Eudaimonic Well-Being

When we listens to a person talk about their lives, and we concludes that they find their lives not merely satisfied but meaningful in specific ways, we're primarily paying attention to the combination of narrative tone and theme. Whereas narrative tone alone conveys a sense of satisfaction in life, neither narrative tone nor narrative theme alone conveys a sense of meaningfulness in life (Steger, 2016; Wolf, 2010). In other words, neither tone nor theme alone conveys eudaimonic value fulfillment. To convey (and to construct) the sense of eudaimonic meaningfulness in life, a narrative fuses tone and theme in a way that shows both what a person values but also the degree to which the person feels that that value orientation is fulfilled.[1] For example, a person in an interview spoke about the birth of a child (from Bauer et al., 2022):

> We're in the room and the pediatrician comes in. . . . And it was like a freight train hit me right at that point because [now] I had a child with Down syndrome. . . . I had all these visions of terrible, terrible things. . . . But in the end, it's turned out to be one of the best blessings we've ever had in our life. So, I mean, I'm not sure many people have a 22-year-old who comes in from work and comes in, and gives you a big ol' hug and says, "You're the best." . . . boy, he's very loving, very wonderful. But you know. . . . All the kids are out, they're empty nesters. We're not. We still have a child that will be a child for a long time. But he is just a wonderful soul and is a blessing in many ways.

The theme of this narrative is communal, and the tone specifically involves a redemption sequence, combining to create a sense of meaningfulness in the narrator's life. This narrative also shows how narrative methods allow researchers to measure how people's assessments of a single event involve a mix of both satisfactions and dissatisfactions.

I wish to note that most measures of narrative theme confound thematic motives and tonal affect. Most measures of narrative themes involve positively valenced appraisals. For example, the following narrative would generally not be coded for communion, despite the fact that a thematic value orientation of communion is clearly present (from Bauer et al., 2022):

> I was [in school]. Things at home were really awful. . . . Mom had just had [a life-changing event], and . . . that was [unexpected and] that sort of changed the whole family. . . . I was now an adolescent and . . . things just got really difficult at home. . . . It [was] a form of depression that [my mom] was going through, and . . . we didn't . . . understand a whole lot about [it] . . . and Dad . . . wasn't around. And so mom . . . was just [at] a point of exhaustion [and it] was a really hard time for the whole family.

This narrative features the lack of a sense of communion in the person's life ("Dad wasn't around"), that is, a lack of communal value fulfillment. But the value orientation is clearly communal, specifically about the family relationships. The reason that this narrative typically would not be coded as having a theme of communion is that the theme is associated with a negatively valenced tone, specifically a *negative-outcome affect*. Most measures of communion are operationally defined as a narrative's not merely conveying the value orientation of communion but also conveying the value fulfillment of communion, typically via a positive-outcome affective tone. Again, most measures of theme confound theme and tone.

The most comprehensive study of narrative elements to date found that tones and themes load onto the same factor (McLean et al., 2020), which seemingly contradicts my claim that tone and theme are distinct narrative expressions of value fulfillment and value orientation. However, that study uses widely used measures of themes that themselves confound tone and theme. When using deconstructed, nonoverlapping measures of narrative elements, themes of experiential growth tend to predict well-being when controlling for positive tones, but the combination of positive-outcome tones and experiential growth themes are especially predictive of eudaimonic well-being (Bauer, Graham, et al., 2019; Bauer et al., 2022).

How Narrative Structure Conveys the Good of Wisdom

When we listen to a person talk about their lives, and we conclude that they're wise, we're primarily paying attention to their narrative *structure*. Narrative content and structure are interfused, but narrative structure can be deconstructed from narrative content. Narrative content involves the facts, tones, and themes of a narrative—the who, what, where, when, why, and whether it's all good or bad. In contrast, narrative structure involves how the various elements of content are organized (McAdams, 1985). Here we focus on the structural elements of *coherence* and *complexity*. Narrative structural coherence refers to degrees of integration (i.e., how much a story "makes sense"), whereas structural complexity refers to degrees of differentiation (i.e., how many points of view a story presents). As such, structure is how a narrative conveys value perspectivity. Narrative coherence tends to correlate with well-being (for a review, see Adler et al., 2016), whereas narrative complexity tends to correlate with wisdom, psychological maturity, and adjustment to life's difficulties but not to general well-being (e.g., Bauer et al., 2022; Booker et al., 2020; Lilgendahl & McAdams, 2011; Mansfield et al., 2010; Weststrate & Glück, 2017).

However, narrative structure (or value perspectivity) alone does not convey wisdom as *phronesis*—the kind of practical wisdom involved in, say, making effectively and morally good decisions (e.g., Kristjánsson & Fowers, 2024). Instead, value perspectivity conveys only an especially broad form of wisdom akin to "expert knowledge" (e.g., Baltes & Staudinger, 2000). To convey the more personal and practical forms of wisdom, narratives employ a combination of structural complexity with themes of humanistic or humane (versus materialistic or egoistic) value orientations (Bauer, King, & Steger, 2019; e.g., Booker & Dunsmore, 2016; Grossmann et al., 2016; Mansfield et al., 2015), which we examine later.

How might value perspectivity and narrative structure (especially complexity) differentiate wise from unwise thinking? Consider how two people might narrate how the value orientation of freedom takes on different meanings, depending on structural complexity. For the first person, freedom means "I can do whatever I want." For the second person, freedom means "I can do what I want, but only after I consider how my actions affect others' ability to act freely." The first interpretation reveals a structurally simplistic, uniperspectival, and egocentric definition of freedom, whereas the second interpretation reveals a structurally complex, multiperspectival, and expressly principled definition of freedom. In this way, the narrative structure (i.e., value perspectivity) of a theme (i.e., a value orientation) shapes the very meaning of a single theme (i.e., value orientation).[2]

THE TRANSFORMATIVE SELF: HOW NARRATIVES CULTIVATE HUMANE FLOURISHING

Most characteristics of "the good life" in the sense of human flourishing, let alone humane flourishing, require cultivation and development. The transformative self is the largely narrative identity of someone who is motivated to cultivate a good life through a process of humanistic growth.

Three ideas here are important to note. First, the transformative self is not a person; it is a self-identity—a subjective, mental model of oneself as a person. A person *has* a transformative self in the way that a person has any kind of self-identity. Second, as a narrative identity, the transformative self features narrative themes of humanistic growth, which are the narrative expressions of the value orientation of *growth motivation* (Bauer, Graham, et al., 2019; Bauer et al., 2015). Third, as with other forms of motivation (and value orientations more generally), a person might not be aware of having a growth motivation; the motive (and narrative theme) may be unconscious or implicit. Thus, a person who has a transformative self might not be trying to foster growth as an explicit goal. Instead, the person who has a transformative self interprets the past and plans the future in ways that are likely to cultivate humane flourishing, even if the person is not thinking of "improvement" explicitly. In this way, themes of humanistic growth are the heart of the transformative self, beating even when the person isn't thinking about it.

Narrative Themes of the Transformative Self

The person who has a transformative self does not value just any kind of growth. Rather, this person values *humanistic growth*. The word *growth* in the term *humanistic growth* is somewhat superfluous because a humanistic value orientation is inherently growth-promoting—that is, inherently likely to cultivate humane flourishing—both theoretically and empirically (e.g., Bauer & McAdams, 2010; Kasser & Ryan, 1996; Ryan & Deci, 2004; Sheldon, 2004). Humanistic (or humane) value orientations are contrasted with materialistic (or egoistic) value orientations. Humanistic value orientations emphasize *humane experiences* (such as the nonegoistic experience of an activity or a relationship), whereas materialistic/egoistic value orientations emphasize *evaluations* of a person (such as how well one has performed or how high one's social status is). Humanistic themes come in myriad forms and may be agentic or communal. A transformative self is no monolithic prototype. Furthermore, a transformative self is not devoid of materialistic and egoistic themes; they're just balanced by humanistic and humane themes.

As a narrative identity, the transformative self features themes of humanistic growth (or just "growth themes"), which I have also called themes of *eudaimonic growth,* which itself is defined notably by a humanistic value orientation (e.g., Bauer, 2021; Bauer et al., 2005; see also Reischer et al., 2021).[3] Themes of humanistic growth come in two broad forms: experiential and reflective (Bauer, Graham, et al., 2019; Bauer et al., 2005, 2022). Themes of *experiential* growth involve humanistic (versus materialistic/egoistic) motives as just mentioned. They are rooted in growth versus safety orientations (Maslow, 1968) and the motives of self-determination theory (Bradshaw, Conigrave, et al., 2023; Deci & Ryan, 2012). Experiential themes feature motives for experientially meaningful activities, experientially meaningful relationships, and caring for others. Themes of *reflective* growth are also humanistic in value orientation but more specifically emphasize the motive to learn or to explore intellectually new conceptual points of view in psychosocial life—to seek new perspectives and insights on the self and others, to engage in critical reflection on the self, others, and the world. Reflective growth themes are rooted in the mechanisms of cognitive development (e.g., assimilation and accommodation in Piaget, 1970) and structural, social-cognitive development (e.g., Loevinger, 1976). Importantly, themes of eudaimonic growth are not abstract statements of value orientations. Rather, narrative themes of eudaimonic growth tie humanistic value orientations to concrete actions in one's life, in a manner of integrative, self-event connections (Bauer & Bonanno, 2001; Pasupathi & Mansour, 2006).

Experiential growth themes aim toward value fulfillment and well-being, whereas reflective growth themes aim toward value perspectivity and wisdom. Empirically, experiential growth themes (and closely related constructs) predict well-being and moral concerns, whereas reflective growth themes (and closely related constructs) predict wisdom and maturity, even prospectively across years and when controlling for narrative tones and Big Five traits (e.g., Bauer et al., 2005, 2022; Bauer & McAdams, 2004a, 2004b, 2010; Booker et al., 2020; King & Noelle, 2005; King et al., 2000; Lilgendahl & McAdams, 2011; Mansfield et al., 2010; Philippe et al., 2011).

Importantly, growth motivation is *not* the same thing as self-improvement motivation. Self-improvement motivation refers to a general class of value orientations for personal progress (O'Brien & Kardas, 2016; Sedikides & Hepper, 2009) but not to the specifically humanistic value orientation of growth motivation (Bauer et al., 2015). As such, self-improvement in narratives has been shown to predict well-being, but themes of eudaimonic, humanistic growth mediate that relation (Bauer, Graham, et al., 2019).

Narrative Tones of the Transformative Self

The prototypical transformative self has a narrative tone that conveys hedonic well-being via an optimal balance of positivity and negativity in global affect—and not exclusive positivity (Bauer, 2021; Bauer & Bonanno, 2001). This optimal balance seems to reflect that the person is taking into account life's difficulties (rather than either glossing over or drowning in them), while keeping in mind a rosier big picture. As for affective sequences, the transformative self features narrative tones of redemption (McAdams et al., 2001), self-improvement (Bauer, Graham, et al., 2019), and (more generally) positive-outcome affect. As noted earlier, positive-outcome narrative tones predict well-being but do so better when coupled with themes of experiential growth (all while controlling for globally positive tones, themes of agency and communion, and structural coherence and complexity; Bauer, Graham, et al., 2019; Bauer et al., 2022). Again, positive-outcome narrative tones alone convey only affective gains or improvements. Thus I have called positive tones "growthy"—hinting at a vague sense of growthiness but not actually delivering the goods of humanistic growth.

Narrative Structure of the Transformative Self

The prototypical transformative self has a narrative structure that conveys wisdom through structural complexity coupled with themes of humanistic growth. In the study just mentioned, narrative complexity alone predicts an aggregate measure of wisdom, controlling for narrative tones and themes (although growth themes also predicted wisdom independently). However, structural complexity combined with themes of reflective growth is especially predictive of wisdom.

The Prototypical Transformative Self

Life stories with the aforementioned qualities of narrative identity convey the prototypical transformative self (see also Park & Moon, 2022). However, a transformative self need not have them all. (And a transformative self is not necessary for a good life.) A person can have a good life and be happy but not especially wise, wise but not especially happy, and so on.

Narrative themes of humanistic growth are at the heart of a transformative self, which alone predicts eudaimonic meaningfulness and wisdom. To the degree those themes are tied to narrative tones with positive outcomes, we find higher levels of hedonic satisfaction. To the degree those themes are framed by a relatively complex and coherent narrative structure, those themes tie to wisdom more strongly.

But again: A good life is not just about happiness and need not have a happy ending (e.g., Bluck et al., 2022). Wisdom, love, moral aspirations, and humanistic growth itself are other candidate goods in life; a transformative self involves a model of personhood that deeply accounts for this fact (Bauer, 2021).

CULTURAL NARRATIVES OF A TRANSFORMATIVE SELF

Humane flourishing does not emerge suddenly out of the blue. It develops in social contexts, and so does narrative identity. The transformative self, like any narrative identity, draws from cultural stories—called *cultural master narratives*—about how to live a good life (Hammack, 2008; McLean & Syed, 2016; Schwab, 2020). We grow up in a narrative ecology of stories in literature, movies, politics, religion, and beyond. These stories convey value orientations like wealth, happiness, or love that are often tied to the institutions that purvey them, such as education, religion, politics, commerce, and mass media. In creating our own life story, we draw on the tones, themes, structures, scripts, character prototypes, and other features of these cultural narratives. On the one hand, this process is partly how a culture perpetuates itself from generation to generation, even as the stories and their values change somewhat over time. On the other hand, cultural master narratives can be oppressive, enforcing a rigidity and hegemony of the power structure's notions of "good" (Syed & McLean, 2022). To the degree that people do not share in the power structure and resources of a society, owing to various intersections of their demographic identities, they have fewer freedoms in fact to actualize the ideals of their cultural master narratives (e.g., Westberg, 2022). In these cases, individuals may seek out or develop alternative or countercultural narratives from which to draw models for their own, marginalized life stories.

The cultural master narrative of personal growth (and a transformative self) can be found in the bildungsroman genre of fiction (Bauer, 2021). As a cultural master narrative, the bildungsroman carries certain oppressive forces of cultural ideals for a good life that represent the privileged concerns of its historically mostly White, male protagonists (e.g., Stephen Dedalus in Joyce's *Portrait of the Artist as a Young Man*, Larry Darrell in Maugham's *The Razor's Edge*). These protagonists have historically come from middle-class or upper-class circumstances.

However, the bildungsroman has functioned *also* as an *alternative* or *countercultural* narrative since its origin in Goethe's *Wilhelm Meister's Apprenticeship* (see Jeffers, 2005). The genre's humanistic and deeply humane value orientations focus on humanity's inner experience and rail against societal and authoritarian tendencies to neglect inner experience. The bildungsroman protagonist, although born privileged, quickly rejects their bourgeois life of materialism and keeping up with the Joneses. The typical bildungsroman protagonist comes to realize the oppressive nature of those values and charts a life path of artistic, intellectual, or spiritual exploration (think characters like Jane Eyre or Harry Potter). Often the protagonist moves away from home, seeks adventures and wise (often quirky) mentors, encounters challenges to their skills and beliefs, and ends on or often far along a path toward self-actualizing. The bildungsroman offers a model of examined freedom and humane individuation, set against the materialistic conventions and power structures of society.

To sift through the simultaneously hegemonic and humane tendencies of the bildungsroman protagonist, I have distinguished hard and soft marginality. The *hard margins* are defined largely by social power and demographics—margins such as those drawn by socioeconomic status, race, ethnicity, gender, and sexual orientation. Those who live with hard marginality face, on average, greater oppression and unfreedoms (Sen, 1999). Those who live in the hard margins are, on average, less likely to have the social and material resources to live out their culture's ideals for a good life (Bradshaw, DeHaan, et al., 2023; Nussbaum, 2011; Tay & Diener, 2011)—including those of the bildungsroman, even with its humane aspirations. Despite its historically unmarginalized protagonists, the bildungsroman genre has long and increasingly featured protagonists who live with hard marginality, such as Ellison's *Invisible Man* and Munro's *Lives of Girls and Women*, which examine the inner and outer struggles of personal growth for Black and female Americans, respectively (for examples of how these novels illustrate the cultural master narrative of personal growth and a good life, see Bauer, 2021). These protagonists are no Pollyannas; their paths reflect the physical, social, and psychological dangers and violence of hard marginality.

In contrast, the *soft margins* are defined by personal intentions and actions. Whereas the person in the hard margins seeks to escape or minimize their marginality by gaining resources, the person in the soft margins actually seeks marginality by shedding resources.[4] In the bildungsroman genre, the protagonist rejects the bourgeois and hegemonic comforts of their upbringing and seeks the margins of society to pursue a life of humanistic, self-actualizing growth. The difference in the margins is clear: Hard marginality is more entrenched; soft marginality is chosen. The bildungsroman protagonist who starts from fewer of the hard margins can often return to their original social milieu. Still, the social and material risks are not trivial; they commonly include cutting ties to social connections and money. The reward for the protagonist is a life of one's own, shaped by rigorous self-exploration, a strong work ethic (although not in socially valued ways, e.g., artistic or intellectual), and critical examination of societal values (Jeffers, 2005)—an existentially authentic life.

AUTHENTIC SELF-AUTHORSHIP

The bildungsroman protagonist strives to live an authentic life. Like the person who has a transformative self, this protagonist strives mightily to reconstruct their narrative identity in their own voice. This process in real life may take years of trial and error, years of exploration and taking risks, and years of narrative identity reconstruction and development, through which one both discovers and creates an authentic voice of one's own—an increasingly more *authentic self-authorship*.

Essentialist versus Existentialist Authenticity

Authenticity is generally understood to mean being "true" to oneself. But what are the criteria for truth? It is generally agreed that these criteria lie "within" the person. The debate in psychology in recent decades (e.g., Hicks et al., 2019; McGregor et al., 2006; Sheldon et al., 1997) has asked: Is authenticity a matter of being what we were *born* to be or of being what we *want* to be? Is authenticity a matter of being true to our deeply sown *traits* or of being true to our self-determined *values?* In other words, is authenticity a matter of discovery or creation? Or is it both, and if so, how? To answer these questions, I have proposed the distinction between essentialist versus existentialist authenticity (Bauer, 2021; Bauer & Shanahan, 2019).

Essentialist authenticity emphasizes being *true to your traits*, especially the most deeply embedded traits within us (as we perceive them)—what we were born or brought up to be. The idea is that, if we act in accord with characteristics that are deeply engrained, then we're being authentic. It doesn't matter how our actions or words affect others, so long as our actions and words match "who we are" in some *primitive* sense—that kernel of a self that was given, as if from nature, nurture, soul, or daimon. Essentialist authenticity is about being true to one's "categories" of personality rather than to one's "values" (see Newman, 2019). To be authentic from the essentialist perspective, we needs not be concerned about others. Morality and ethics have little to do with whether we act with essentialist authenticity. One need only exert our "essence" in the world. From the essentialist perspective, if Donald is a belligerent and power-hungry soul, then he *should* disparage and coerce others in his outgroup, and he is justified in doing so because he is simply being authentic: "It's just Donald being Donald." Essentialist authenticity is perhaps the more basic or boilerplate view of authenticity, where to be authentic we need only express deeply felt emotions and impulses, without the "varnish" (as it is viewed from the essentialist perspective) of moral concern for others.

Existentialist authenticity emphasizes being true to your examined values. Here authenticity is not merely a matter of acting on our impulses. Loosely, existentialist authenticity is about being true to one's "values" rather than to one's "categories" or traits of personality (Newman, 2019). More specifically, existentialist authenticity requires that we examine our values in relation to others and their potential authenticity. The philosopher Charles Guignon (2004, p. 155) writes, "Authenticity requires something more than making a decision to identify with something, where *what* we identify with is irrelevant. . . . Instead, we need to see that our identity-conferring identifications are drawn from, and are answerable to, the shared historical commitments and ideals that make up our communal life-world." Here we must examine ourselves—our value orientations, our beliefs, our narrative identities. Existentialist authenticity involves a relatively higher level of value perspectivity as well as a more humane value orientation—much in the manner of practical wisdom or *phronesis,* as mentioned earlier. In existentialist philosophy, the construction of self-identity inherently includes ethical concern and responsibility for the welfare of others and not just oneself (Sartre, 1943/1993). From this perspective, essentialist authenticity is too simplistic and too egoistic a conception of authenticity. Existentialist authenticity echoes the philosopher Charles Taylor (1991, p. 41), who writes, "Authenticity is not the enemy of demands that emanate from beyond the self; it *supposes* such demands."

However, existentialist authenticity can also be conceptualized in too simplistic and—not egoistic but—idealistic a manner. Existentialist authenticity requires development and psychological maturity. Youthful existentialist authenticity believes that authenticity as "being what one values" means that one can be whatever one wants to be. But experience suggests otherwise. Here something of essentialism obtains: We do have deeply embedded characteristics and a given range of capabilities and environmental affordances. We cannot be anything we want to be. Thus, mature existentialist authenticity believes not only that we must examine our lives and responsibilities with others' welfare in mind but also that we must "live wisely within our limits" (Tiberius, 2008). Fortunately, we can cultivate and exercise various moral virtues like the cultivation of other skills (Annas, 2011). As we do so, we become more existentially authentic. Thus, existentialist authenticity does not dismiss the importance of deeply embedded traits but rather incorporates and transcends the principles of essentialist authenticity in a developmentally layered manner. Existentialist authenticity is part self-discovery and part self-creation (May, 1969/2007).

The Poiesis Principle

Both essentialist authenticity and existentialist authenticity adhere to what I call the "matching principle" of authenticity. Both forms of authenticity involve a *matching* of one's "actual" self with some criterion of a "true" self (e.g., Schlegel et al., 2011; Wood et al., 2008). However, authenticity involves something else that *generates* the comparisons of one's actual self to one's concept of a true self. This generating function involves an authentic manner of identifying more than of the concepts of identity or self themselves (e.g., Vess, 2019)—a manner of meaning making more than a matching of meanings made. Authenticity in this sense deals more with self-making or *poiesis.* In contrast to the matching principle, I call this approach to defining authenticity the *poiesis principle* (Bauer, 2021).

The poiesis principle addresses how we *frame* the matching of our perceived actual self to our desired true self. The poiesis principle claims that authenticity emerges from a mindset that authors the self and others wisely—that is, with structural complexity and humane themes. The poiesis principle defines authenticity more as a verb than a noun: We can think relatively authentically or inauthentically, according to the degree to which we consider the situation at hand from greater or fewer points of view, where those perspectives are focused on humanistic concerns of the lived experience of both the self and others. The capacity for poiesis develops in degrees of authenticity that parallel ego development (Loevinger, 1976), yielding growth in one's working self-concept (Chen, 2019) from a more youthful authenticity (e.g., defining freedom in terms of independence from contexts) to a more mature authenticity (e.g., defining freedom within contexts of interdependence). As a form of thinking about the self and others, mature existentialist authenticity emerges from a *quiet ego* (Bauer, 2021).

The Quiet Ego

The quiet ego characterizes the mind when thinking about the self and others with a combination of humility and equanimity, compassionate interdependence, curiosity and perspective taking, and humanistic growth-mindedness (Bauer & Wayment, 2008; Wayment et al., 2015). In contrast, the noisy ego clamors for attention, pines for praise, and sets out to establish its dominance over others. The quiet ego balances concerns for the self and others and fosters their growth toward humane flourishing (Bauer & Weatherbie, 2023). A relatively quiet ego is the ego that authors a transformative self—noting that a quiet versus noisy ego is very much a matter of degree.

With the quiet ego we reach the end of this chapter, even though a relatively quiet ego is what generates a transformative self in the first place. Neither the quiet ego nor the transformative self is a static phenomenon. Each develops over time, such that a child's quiet ego is quite noisy by adult standards, and adult egos can be noisy by more psychologically mature standards. Indeed, the ego quiets as it grows, in stages (Bauer, 2008). So does a transformative self (Bauer, 2021). When thinking about our life from the perspective of a quiet ego—notably while reconstructing our narrative identity as we go about our daily lives in a world of others—we approach our lives and its story with greater existential authenticity, which in turn helps us to foster growth toward happiness, love, and wisdom in the self and others.

Easier said than done. The transformative self is no walk in the park. Growth is not for the faint-hearted (Rogers, 1961). However, the quiet ego cuts through the thicket and fog of life's paths, seeing beyond concerns for one's own egoistic ideals and strivings, seeking with curiosity and compassion to see beyond one's assumptions and egotism. In this way, the quiet ego both constructs a transformative self and has the courage and compassion to put it to action and to reconstruct its story along the way, thereby cultivating existentially authentic self-authorship and humane flourishing for self and others.

NOTES

1. When a narrative theme is hedonic in nature (e.g., the value orientation emphasizes pleasurable experience as a good), the idea of pleasure itself serves as an orienting purpose, and thus as a meaning. When a hedonic theme is paired with a positive-outcome tone, the narrative conveys the satisfaction of the value of the pleasure as a meaning, that is, meaningfulness. See Waterman and colleagues (2008) as an example of how intrinsically pleasurable experiences serve as sources of eudaimonic meaningfulness.

2. Note here why value perspectivity is a value *actualization*; perspectivity represents a *demonstrated* capacity to think complexly, not just the desire to do so. Also, narrative structure conveys value perspectivity, not fulfillment, because this is not an assessment of whether the person thinks subjectively that they're thinking complexly; it is an assessment of whether they *are* thinking relatively complexly, objectively.

3. Eudaimonic and humanistic value orientations are not the same, but they are often assumed to be connected empirically and theoretically (e.g., Bauer et al., 2015; Deci & Ryan, 2012).

4. Hard and soft margins are not as clearly cut as this brief presentation might suggest. A person's overall marginality is a matter of degree and intersectionality. The capacities and risks of pursuing humanistic growth vary by the person.

REFERENCES

Adler, J. M., Lodi-Smith, J., Philippe, F. L., & Houle, I. (2016). The incremental validity of narrative identity in predicting well-being: A review of the field and recommendations for the future. *Personality and Social Psychology Review, 20,* 142–175.

Adler, J. M., & Poulin, M. J. (2009). The political is personal: Narrating 9/11 and psychological well-being. *Journal of Personality, 77,* 903–932.

Annas, J. (2011). *Intelligent virtue.* Oxford University Press.

Baltes, P. B., & Staudinger, U. M. (2000). Wisdom: A metaheuristic (pragmatic) to orchestrate mind and virtue toward excellence. *American Psychologist, 55,* 122–136.

Bauer, J. J. (2008). How the ego quiets as it grows: Ego development, growth stories, and eudaimonic personality development. In H. A. Wayment & J. J. Bauer (Eds.), *Transcending self-interest: Psychological explorations of the quiet ego* (pp. 199–210). American Psychological Association.

Bauer, J. J. (2016). Eudaimonic growth: The development of the goods in personhood (or: cultivating a good life story). In J. Vittersø (Ed.), *Handbook of eudaimonic well-being* (pp. 147–174). Springer.

Bauer, J. J. (2021). *The transformative self: Personal growth, narrative identity, and the good life.* Oxford University Press.

Bauer, J. J., & Bonanno, G. A. (2001). Doing and being well (for the most part): Adaptive patterns of narrative self-evaluation during bereavement. *Journal of Personality, 69,* 451–482.

Bauer, J. J., Graham, L. E., Lauber, E. A., & Lynch, B. P. (2019). What growth sounds like: Redemption, self-improvement, and eudaimonic growth across different life events in relation to well-being. *Journal of Personality, 87,* 546–565.

Bauer, J. J., Graham, L. E., Mooney, S. E., Geisz, A. M., & Mueller, M. (2022). A good life story: Deconstructing (and integrating) elements of narrative identity and a good life, with an emphasis on humanistic growth. *Journal of Research in Personality, 101,* 1–14.

Bauer, J. J., King, L. A., & Steger, M. F. (2019). Meaning-making, self-determination theory, and the question of wisdom in personality. *Journal of Personality, 87,* 82–101.

Bauer, J. J., & McAdams, D. P. (2004a). Growth goals, maturity, and well-being. *Developmental Psychology, 40,* 114–127.

Bauer, J. J., & McAdams, D. P. (2004b). Personal growth in adults' stories of life transitions. *Journal of Personality, 72,* 573–602.

Bauer, J. J., & McAdams, D. P. (2010). Eudaimonic growth: Narrative growth goals predict increases in ego development and subjective well-being three years later. *Developmental Psychology, 46,* 761–772.

Bauer, J. J., McAdams, D. P., & Pals, J. L. (2008). Narrative identity and eudaimonic well-being. *Journal of Happiness Studies, 9,* 81–104.

Bauer, J. J., McAdams, D. P., & Sakaeda, A. R. (2005). Interpreting the good life: Growth memories in the lives of mature, happy people. *Journal of Personality and Social Psychology, 88,* 203–217.

Bauer, J. J., Park, S. W., Montoya, R. M., & Wayment, H. A. (2015). Growth motivation toward two paths of eudaimonic self-development. *Journal of Happiness Studies, 16,* 185–210.

Bauer, J. J., & Shanahan, C. (2019). Gratitude, authenticity, and self-authorship. In R. C. Roberts & D. Telech (Eds.), *The moral psychology of gratitude* (pp. 217–242). Rowman & Littlefield.

Bauer, J. J., & Thomsen, D. K. (2022). Introduction to the special issue on "Storying the good life: Pathways and pitfalls to adaptive narrative identity." *Journal of Research in Personality.*

Bauer, J. J., & Wayment, H. A. (2008). The psychology of the quiet ego. In H. A. Wayment & J. J. Bauer (Eds.), *Transcending self-interest: Psychological explorations of the quiet ego* (pp. 3–19). American Psychological Association Books.

Bauer, J. J., & Weatherbie, K. J. (2023). The quiet ego and human flourishing. *Journal of Happiness Studies, 24,* 2499–2530.

Baumeister, R. F. (1991). *Meanings of life.* Guilford Press.

Blagov, P. S., Singer, J. A., Oost, K. M., & Goodman, J. A. (2022). Self-defining memories—Narrative features in relation to adaptive and maladaptive personality traits (replication and extension of Blagov & Singer, 2004). *Journal of Personality, 90,* 457–475.

Bluck, S., Mroz, E. L., Cogdill-Richardson, K., McDarby, M., & Carpenter, B. (2022). Even the good life has an ending: Virtue in the face of finitude. *Journal of Research in Personality, 99.*

Booker, J. A., & Dunsmore, J. C. (2016). Profiles of wisdom among emerging adults: Associations with empathy, gratitude, and forgiveness. *Journal of Positive Psychology, 11,* 315–325.

Booker, J. A., Fivush, R., Graci, M. E., Heitz, H., Hudak, L. A., Jovanovic, T., . . . Stevens, J. S. (2020). Longitudinal changes in trauma narratives over the first year and associations with coping and mental health. *Journal of Affective Disorders, 272,* 116–124.

Bradshaw, E. L., Conigrave, J. H., Steward, B. A., Ferber, K. A., Parker, P. D., & Ryan, R. M. (2023). A meta-analysis of the dark side of the American Dream: Evidence for the universal wellness costs of prioritizing extrinsic over intrinsic goals. *Journal of Personality and Social Psychology, 124,* 873–899.

Bradshaw, E. L., DeHaan, C. R., Parker, P. D., Curren, R., Duineveld, J. J., Di Domenico, S. I., & Ryan, R. M. (2023). The perceived conditions for living well: Positive perceptions of primary goods linked with basic psychological needs and wellness. *Journal of Positive Psychology, 18,* 44–60.

Chen, S. (2019). Authenticity in context: Being true to working selves. *Review of General Psychology, 23,* 60–72.

Deci, E. L., & Ryan, R. M. (2012). Motivation, personality, and development within embedded social contexts: An overview of self-determination theory. In R. M. Ryan (Ed.), *The Oxford handbook of human motivation* (pp. 85–108). Oxford University Press.

DeYoung, C. G., & Tiberius, V. (2023). Value fulfillment from a cybernetic perspective: A new psychological theory of well-being. *Personality and Social Psychology Bulletin, 27,* 3–27.

Diener, E., Lucas, R. E., & Scollon, C. N. (2006). Beyond the hedonic treadmill: Revising the adaptation theory of well-being. *American Psychologist, 61,* 305–314.

Dunlop, W. L. (2021). Everything you wanted to know about redemptive stories* (*but were afraid to ask). *Journal of Research in Personality, 92,* 1–14.

Erikson, E. H. (1968). *Identity: Youth and crisis.* Norton.

Fivush, R., Haden, C. A., & Reese, E. (2006). Elaborating on elaborations: Role of maternal reminiscing style in cognitive and socioemotional development. *Child Development, 77,* 1568–1588.

Graci, M. E., Watts, A. L., & Fivush, R. (2018). Examining the factor structure of narrative meaning-making for stressful events and relations with psychological distress. *Memory, 9,* 1220–1232.

Grossmann, I., Gerlach, T. M., & Denissen, J. J. A. (2016). Wise reasoning in the face of everyday life challenges. *Social Psychological and Personality Science, 7,* 611–622.

Guignon, C. (2004). *On being authentic.* Routledge.

Habermas, T., & Bluck, S. (2000). Getting a life: The emergence of the life story in adolescence. *Psychological Bulletin, 126,* 748–769.

Hammack, P. L. (2008). Narrative and the cultural psychology of identity. *Personality and Social Psychology Review, 12,* 222–247.

Haybron, D. M. (2008). *The pursuit of unhappiness: The elusive psychology of well-being.* Oxford University Press.

Hicks, J. A., Schlegel, R. J., & Newman, G. E. (2019). Introduction to the special issue: Authenticity: Novel insights into a valued, yet elusive, concept. *Review of General Psychology, 23,* 3–7.

Huta, V., & Waterman, A. S. (2014). Eudaimonia and its distinction from hedonia: Developing a classification and terminology for understanding conceptual and operational definitions. *Journal of Happiness Studies, 15,* 1425–1456.

Jeffers, T. L. (2005). *Apprenticeships: The bildungsroman from Goethe to Santayana.* Palgrave Macmillan.

Kasser, T., & Ryan, R. M. (1996). Further examining the American dream: Well-being correlates of intrinsic and extrinsic goals. *Personality and Social Psychology Bulletin, 22,* 281–288.

Kelly, G. A. (1963). *A theory of personality: The psychology of personal constructs.* Norton. (Original work published 1955)

King, L. A., & Noelle, S. S. (2005). Happy, mature, and gay: Intimacy, power, and difficult times in coming out stories. *Journal of Research in Personality, 39,* 278–298.

King, L. A., Scollon, C. K., Ramsey, C., & Williams, T. (2000). Stories of life transition: Subjective well-being and ego development in parents of children with Down syndrome. *Journal of Research in Personality, 34,* 509–536.

Kristjánsson, K., & Fowers, B. J. (2024). *Phronesis: Retrieving practical wisdom in psychology, philosophy, and education.* Oxford University Press.

Lilgendahl, J. P., & McAdams, D. P. (2011). Constructing stories of self-growth: How individual differences in patterns of autobiographical reasoning relate to well-being in midlife. *Journal of Personality, 79,* 391–428.

Loevinger, J. (1976). *Ego development.* Jossey-Bass.

MacIntyre, A. (1981). *After virtue.* University of Notre Dame.

Mansfield, C. D., McLean, K. C., & Lilgendahl, J. P. (2010). Narrating traumas and transgressions: Links between narrative processing, wisdom, and well-being. *Narrative Inquiry, 20,* 246–273.

Mansfield, C. D., Pasupathi, M., & McLean,

K. C. (2015). Is narrating growth in stories of personal transgressions associated with increased, well-being, self-compassion, and forgiveness of others? *Journal of Research in Personality, 58,* 69–83.

Martela, F., & Steger, M. F. (2016). The three meanings of meaning in life: Distinguishing coherence, purpose and significance. *Journal of Positive Psychology, 11,* 531–545.

Maslow, A. H. (1968). *Toward a psychology of being.* Van Nostrand.

May, R. (2007). *Love and will.* Norton. (Original work published 1969)

McAdams, D. P. (1985). *Power, intimacy, and the life story: Personological inquiries into identity.* Guilford Press.

McAdams, D. P., Hoffman, B. J., Mansfield, E. D., & Day, R. (1996). Themes of agency and communion in significant autobiographical scenes. *Journal of Personality, 64,* 339–377.

McAdams, D. P., & McLean, K. C. (2013). Narrative identity. *Current Directions in Psychological Science, 22,* 233–238.

McAdams, D. P., Reynolds, J., Lewis, M., Patten, A. H., & Bowman, P. J. (2001). When bad things turn good and good things turn bad: Sequences of redemption and contamination in life narrative and their relation to psychosocial adaption in midlife adults and in students. *Personality and Social Psychology Bulletin, 27,* 474–485.

McGregor, I., McAdams, D. P., & Little, B. R. (2006). Personal projects, life stories, and happiness: On being true to traits. *Journal of Research in Personality, 40,* 551–572.

McLean, K. C., & Lilgendahl, J. P. (2008). Why recall our highs and lows: Relations between memory functions, age, and well-being. *Memory, 16,* 751–762.

McLean, K. C., & Mansfield, C. D. (2012). The co-construction of adolescent narrative identity: Narrative processing as a function of adolescent age, gender, and maternal scaffolding. *Developmental Psychology, 48,* 436–447.

McLean, K. C., Pasupathi, M., & Pals, J. L. (2007). Selves creating stories creating selves: A process model of self-development. *Personality and Social Psychology Review, 11,* 262–278.

McLean, K. C., & Syed, M. (2016). Personal, master, and alternative narratives: An integrative framework for understanding identity development in context. *Human Development, 58,* 318–349.

McLean, K. C., Syed, M., Pasupathi, M., Adler, J. M., Dunlop, W. L., Drustrup, D., . . . McCoy, T. P. (2020). The empirical structure of narrative identity: The initial Big Three. *Journal of Personality and Social Psychology, 119,* 920–944.

Newman, G. E. (2019). The psychology of authenticity. *Review of General Psychology, 23,* 8–18.

Nussbaum, M. C. (2011). *Creating capabilities: The human development approach.* Belknap.

O'Brien, E., & Kardas, M. (2016). The implicit meaning of (my) change. *Journal of Personality and Social Psychology, 111,* 882–894.

Park, S. W., & Moon, H. (2022). Assessing identity formation in narratives. *Current Psychology, 41,* 4066–4078.

Pasupathi, M., Alderman, K., & Shaw, D. (2007). Talking the talk: Collaborative remembering and self-perceived expertise. *Discourse Processes, 43,* 55–77.

Pasupathi, M., & Mansour, E. (2006). Adult age differences in autobiographical reasoning in narratives. *Developmental Psychology, 42,* 798–808.

Philippe, F. L., Koestner, R., Beaulieu-Pelletier, G., & Lecours, S. (2011). The role of need satisfaction as a distinct and basic psychological component of autobiographical memories: A look at well-being. *Journal of Personality, 79,* 905–938.

Piaget, J. (1970). Piaget's theory. In P. Mussen (Ed.), *Carmichael's manual of child psychology* (pp. 703–732). Wiley.

Reese, E., Myftari, E., McAnally, H. M., Chen, Y., Wang, Q., Jack, F., & Robertsom, S.-J. (2017). Telling the tale and living well: Adolescent narrative identity, personality traits, and well-being across cultures. *Child Development, 88,* 612–628.

Reischer, H. N., Roth, L. J., Villarreal, J. A., & McAdams, D. P. (2021). Self-transcendence and life stories of humanistic growth among late-midlife adults. *Journal of Personality, 89,* 305–324.

Ricoeur, P. (1990). *Time and narrative* (Vol. 3) (K. Blamey & D. Pellauer, Trans.). University of Chicago Press.

Rogers, C. R. (1961). *On becoming a person.* Houghton Mifflin.

Rohan, M. J. (2000). A rose by any name?: The values construct. *Personality and Social Psychology Review, 4,* 255–277.

Ryan, R. M., & Deci, E. L. (2001). On happiness and human potentials: A review of research on hedonic and eudaimonic well-being. *Annual Review of Psychology, 52,* 141–166.

Ryan, R. M., & Deci, E. L. (2004). Overview of self-determination theory: An organismic dialectical perspective. In E. L. Deci & R. M. Ryan (Eds.), *Handbook of self-determination research* (pp. 3–36). University of Rochester.

Ryff, C. D., & Singer, B. H. (2008). Know thyself and become what you are: A eudaimonic approach to psychological well-being. *Journal of Happiness Studies, 9,* 13–39.

Sartre, J.-P. (1993). *Being and nothingness.* Washington Square Press. (Original work published 1943)

Schlegel, R. J., Hicks, J. A., King, L. A., & Arndt, J .(2011). Feeling like you know who you are: Perceived true self-knowledge and meaning in life. *Personality and Social Psychology Bulletin, 37,* 745–756.

Schwab, J. R. (2020). What is the good life?: A master narrative approach to the study of morals and values in American emerging adults. *Journal of Adult Development, 27,* 108–117.

Schwartz, S. H., & Bilsky, W. (1990). Toward a theory of the universal content and structure of values: Extensions and cross-cultural replications. *Journal of Personality and Social Psychology, 58,* 678–891.

Sedikides, C., & Hepper, E. G. D. (2009). Self-improvement. *Social and Personality Psychology Compass, 3*(6), 899–917.

Sen, A. (1999). *Development as freedom.* Anchor.

Sheldon, K. M. (2004). *Optimal human being: An integrated multi-level perspective.* Erlbaum.

Sheldon, K. M., Ryan, R. M., Rawsthorne, L. J., & Ilardi, B. (1997). Trait self and true self: Cross-role variation in the Big-Five personality traits and its relations with psychological authority and subjective well- being. *Journal of Personality and Social Psychology, 73,* 1380–1393.

Steger, M. F. (2016). Hedonia, eudaimonia, and meaning: Me versus us; fleeting versus enduring. In J. Vittersø (Ed.), *Handbook of eudaimonic well-being* (pp. 175–182). Springer.

Syed, M., & McLean, K. C. (2022). Who gets to live the good life?: Master narratives, identity, and well-being within a marginalizing society. *Journal of Research in Personality, 100,* 1–7.

Tay, L., & Diener, E. (2011). Needs and subjective well-being around the world. *Journal of Personality and Social Psychology, 101,* 354–365.

Taylor, C. (1989). *Sources of the self: The making of the modern identity.* Harvard University Press.

Taylor, C. (1991). *The ethics of authenticity.* Harvard University Press.

Tiberius, V. (2008). *The reflective life: Living wisely within our limits.* Oxford University Press.

Tiberius, V. (2013). Recipes for a good life: Eudaimonism and the contribution of philosophy. In A. S. Waterman (Ed.), *The best within us: Positive psychology perspectives on eudaimonia* (pp. 19–38). American Psychological Association.

Vess, M. (2019). Varieties of conscious experience and the subjective awareness of one's "true" self. *Review of General Psychology, 23,* 89–98.

Vittersø, J. (2016). The most important idea in the world: An introduction. In J. Vittersø (Ed.), *Handbook of eudaimonic well-being* (pp. 1–24). Springer.

Waterman, A. S. (2013). Introduction: Considering the nature of a life well lived—intersections of positive psychology and eudaimonist philosophy. In A. S. Waterman (Ed.), *The best within us: Positive psychology perspectives on eudaimonia* (pp. 3–17). American Psychological Association.

Waterman, A. S., Schwartz, S. J., & Conti, R. (2008). The implications of two conceptions of happiness (hedonic enjoyment and eudaimonia) for the understanding of intrinsic motivation. *Journal of Happiness Studies, 9,* 41–79.

Wayment, H. A., Bauer, J. J., & Sylaska, K. (2015). The quiet ego scale: Measuring the compassionate self-identity. *Journal of Happiness Studies, 16,* 999–1033.

Westberg, D. W. (2022). Stories off the beaten path: Exploring the content and correlates of cultural deviation narratives. *Journal of Research in Personality.*

Weststrate, N. M., & Glück, J. (2017). Hard-earned wisdom: Exploratory processing of difficult life experience is positively associated with wisdom. *Developmental Psychology, 53,* 800–814.

Wolf, S. (2010). *Meaning in life and why it matters.* Princeton University Press.

Wood, A. M., Linley, P. A., Maltby, J., & Baliousis, M., & Joseph, S. (2008). The authentic personality: A theoretical and empirical conceptualization and the development of the Authenticity Scale. *Journal of Counseling Psychology, 55,* 385–399.

CHAPTER 60

Familiarity Seeking

Growing and Learning from Repeat Experiences

Yuji K. Winet *and* Ed O'Brien

Modern life offers evermore opportunity for novel experiences. The appeal of finding new and exciting experiences is powerful, with a large psychological literature attesting to people's attraction to novelty's gleam (Garcia-Rada et al., 2024; Lyubomirsky et al., 2005; McAlister & Pessemier, 1982; Ratner et al., 1999; Read & Loewenstein, 1995; Sheldon et al., 2012). And yet, people instead often choose to relive experiences they have already had. People watch the same movies and TV shows, listen to the same songs, eat at the same restaurants, visit the same travel destinations, and so on. Why might people prefer repetition even when novelty seems to promise more? In this chapter, we unpack the psychology of familiarity seeking: when and why people are drawn away from novelty and toward reliving familiar experiences (i.e., *repeat consumption*).

The critical difference between novel and repeat experiences is simply that one has experienced the latter before, holding constant the objective features of the stimulus (O'Brien, 2022a). Having consumed the experience before (i.e., *reconsuming* the experience) transforms its experiential value and psychological significance compared to one's initial consumption experience. The psychological distinctions between reliving an experience and having it for the first time have important implications for the types of value an experience can offer.

Novelty and repetition offer different types of experiential value at different points in the consumption process. Prior to consumption, the value of an experience includes the appeal of novelty; after consumption, it includes the value of having already invested one's time and energy into the experience. During initial consumption, novelty makes experiences more exciting and stimulating, which makes them more enjoyable (Berlyne, 1970). During *reconsumption*, people have already consumed at least some of its novelty, built familiarity, gathered information, created memories, and incorporated it into their personal narrative (at least to some degree). Holding constant the experience itself, as well as ancillary factors like time, cost, and accessibility, the mere fact of having consumed an experience before matters.

People constantly decide between new and old experiences (Mehlhorn et al., 2015). When doing so, different experiential benefits and drawbacks become relevant. Novelty's benefits reside mainly in the hedonic pleasure domain—because novelty is inherently more uncertain than repetition (Mehlhorn et al., 2015; Speekenbrink & Konstantinidis, 2015), it tends to be more exciting (Raju, 1980), which can boost hedonic pleasure (Berlyne, 1970). However, because people also lack past experience with novel experiences by definition, such experiences tend to be less personally meaningful (Winet & O'Brien, 2022). By contrast, the benefits of repeat experiences reside in both the hedonic pleasure and personal meaning domains. Because repeats are more certain than novel experiences (Mehlhorn et al., 2015; Speekenbrink & Konstantinidis, 2015), repeats are a more dependable source of hedonic pleasure (Reber et al., 1998, 2004), and because they involve past personal experience by definition, they also tend to be more personally meaningful (Heintzelman & King, 2019; Routledge et al., 2011; Winet & O'Brien, 2022). Past experience gives reconsumption an experiential advantage because it both allows one to tap into the meaningful relationships one has already built while also providing valuable hedonic information, making repeat experiences a potent source of both types of value.

In what follows in this chapter, we unpack and expand upon these ideas in detail. We review three key questions:

1. What is valuable about repeat consumption?
2. When, why, and for whom is repeat consumption valuable?
3. What research remains on repeat consumption?

WHAT IS VALUABLE ABOUT REPEAT CONSUMPTION?

The appeal of novelty is self-evident. In contrast to already familiar experiences, novel experiences are more stimulating (Raju, 1980). They capture attention, making them more absorbing, immersive (O'Brien & Smith, 2019; Quoidbach et al., 2015; Sansone et al., 1992), and inherently more exciting experiences. Novelty makes experiences more intense—and more likely to reach peak enjoyment—because there is no prior exposure from which to hedonically adapt. Hedonic adaptation (and related constructs, e.g., satiation and habituation) reflect the idea that repeated exposure to stimuli weakens their intensity (Brickman et al., 1978; Campbell et al., 2014; Frederick & Loewenstein, 1999). Insofar as people seek to maximize pleasure and enjoyment (Hornsey et al., 2018), have experiences that leave a rosy trace in memory (Ratner et al., 1999), and expand their "experiential CV" (Keinan & Kivetz, 2011), novel experiences offer clear hedonic benefits over repeat experiences.

In contrast, repetition offers different and potentially more complex experiential benefits that make it less repetitive than one might think. While prior exposure may make repeat experiences less likely to reach peak hedonic value compared to novel ones, it also allows them to yield other, less obvious forms of value. Specifically, repeating experiences enables people to derive meaning from deeper personal connections, to derive enjoyment from a better understanding of their hedonic value, and to better extract their embedded novelty. O'Brien (2021) highlighted two primary pathways that well capture each of these ideas: one is "stimulus-level novelty" (i.e., finding missed or new nuances in an experience upon repeat consumption) and the other is "self-level novelty" (i.e., finding missed or new nuances *about oneself* by virtue of repeatedly consuming an experience; e.g., "I must *really* like this; this is *me*"). Below, we summarize and expand upon each of these kinds of benefits.

Meaningful Personal Connection

Relived experiences provide benefits beyond hedonic pleasure. Indeed, not every experience's value comes from hedonic pleasure alone—people spend time caring for their elderly grandparents instead of having fun times with friends, they wake up early to train for marathons instead of sleeping in their cozy beds, and they go to therapy to work through difficult personal issues instead of scrolling endlessly on social media. People regularly seek experiences that are *meaningful,* even at the expense of hedonic pleasure (Vohs et al., 2019), because meaning is a separate but substantial source of experiential value (Wolfram, 2023). Meaning often comes from psychologically connecting one's present to one's past (Klein & O'Brien, 2017; Kristal et al., 2019; O'Brien et al., 2012; O'Brien & Kardas, 2016) and/or to one's future (O'Brien, 2015a, 2015b, 2022b, 2022c).

In turn, personal meaning is an especially powerful source of value (Ariely et al., 2008; Baumeister, 1991; Baumeister et al., 2013; King & Napa, 1998; Proulx & Inzlicht, 2012). Meaning has long been a difficult concept to define precisely (Leontiev, 2013), but scholars generally agree that it revolves around a sentimental link to "who you are," and the sense that one's understanding of the world and one's place in it make sense (Chater & Loewenstein, 2016; van den Bos, 2009). Key tenets involve a sense of purpose, mattering, and coherence (Heintzelman & King, 2013; Martela & Steger, 2016), giving foundation to the belief that one's life holds some significance beyond merely existing (Steger, 2012). Meaning is a value that connects to one's identity (Schlegel et al., 2011), relationships (Lambert et al., 2013), and the broader narrative of one's life (Baumeister & Newman, 2016; Rogers et al., 2023). Meaningful experiences are those that provide a sense of personal significance as answers to the questions of "Who am I?" and "How do the things in my life make sense?"

Repeat experiences lend themselves to personal meaning in ways that novel experiences do not (Carstensen, 2006; Carstensen et al., 1999; Ersner-Hershfield et al., 2008; Routledge et al., 2011). Whereas novel experiences often lend themselves to hedonic pleasure, which is immediately gratifying at face value, repeat experiences often lend themselves to personal meaning, which typically requires past investment of time and energy to harvest meaning in the present. That is, repetition makes experiences meaningful by tapping into existing relationships with those experiences. Rewatching a cherished movie from one's childhood may be very meaningful, for example, as one reflects on one's relationship with that movie and how it may have changed or stayed the same since one's previous time watching it (Libby et al., 2005).

Nurturing one's relationships creates emotional attachment (Aron et al., 1997). Much in the same way that people build meaningful and intimate relationships with social partners (Altman & Taylor, 1973; Kardas et al., 2022; O'Brien & Kassirer, 2019), they can also grow emotionally attached to material possessions (Lastovicka & Sirianni, 2011; Wheeler & Bechler, 2021) and experiences (Arnould & Price, 1993; Carmon et al., 2003). Experiences often predict greater happiness than material goods do precisely because they hold more meaning (Carter & Gilovich, 2012; Weingarten et al., 2023). Repeated interactions open the door in this way because they allow one to become more emotionally invested (Routledge et al., 2011). Emotional investment may not necessarily provide hedonic value but it does provide a basis for creating meaningful relationships. Tellingly, having a sentimental connection to a possession considerably slows the decline in how happy it makes a person as they interact with it repeatedly over time (Yang & Galak, 2015).

Having consumed an experience in the past can mean one's past investments of time and energy have had time to grow and mature into a meaningful relationship that one can tap into through repeated interaction. A repeat experience may not necessarily yield more hedonic pleasure than a novel experience, but it will generally carry more personal meaning as it becomes increasingly integrated into one's life and personal narrative (Vohs et al., 2019).

Reliving experiences thus often involves an existential process of meaning making, as it ties the past to the present and the present to the past (Russell & Levy, 2012). Implicitly or explicitly, reconsumption must be understood through the psychological linking of past consumption with present reconsumption of the same experience—without this link, repeats are functionally novel. Importantly, meaning is created by comparing past and present experiences, whether they are similar or different. The significance of a relived experience is defined in part by its meaning to the experiencer in the past. For example, hearing a lullaby from one's childhood may be meaningful not only because the song is powerful, but because it prompts one to reflect on its prior meaning and how much has changed (or not) since then.

Repetition creates opportunities to create and consume meaning, even when experiences seem to be mundane, *because* they are so often repeated. Meaning is not limited to special occasions and unusually powerful moments—people experience meaning throughout everyday life (Choi et al., 2017; Heintzelman & King, 2014), as meaning can grow from mere familiarity (Noble, 1953). Even daily routines and merely familiar experiences tend to hold meaning (Heintzelman & King, 2019; Winet & O'Brien, 2022). This is not to say every repeat experience is meaningful or every novel one is meaningless. Repeat experiences can be meaningless simply because they go unnoticed (e.g., blinking), and novel experiences can be meaningful because they are deeply connected to one's life story (e.g., meeting the love of one's life). However, in general, repeat experiences are more likely to be meaningful because familiarity makes it easier to connect them with one's personal identity and life narrative.

Embedded Novelty

Relived experiences are also opportunities to consume embedded novelty that remains within an experience. Experiences contain some amount of novel experiential value that can be consumed, but it may not always be possible to consume all of their available novelty on a first pass. Rather, experiences can contain embedded novel elements that go unexperienced and can only be consumed by repeating the experience one or more times. By reliving an experience one has already had, one can attend to different psychologically valuable elements with each repetition (Forest et al., 2022; Russell & Levy, 2012).

When experiences are richer and more complex, there may be too many novel elements to fully consume in one sitting (e.g., museums: O'Brien, 2019), or their novel elements may not be easily accessible on a first pass. For example, movies with twist endings often contain clues throughout the movie that are only decipherable upon a rewatch and not during a first viewing.

Indeed, repeat experiences can contain elements that offer valuable novelty that one has not yet consumed. As when exploring museum exhibits, amusement parks, and video game worlds, one can gain access to an overwhelming breadth of opportunities to experience stimulating enjoyment, which can simply be too much to consume in one initial consumption experience. But without returning to museums, amusement parks, and video game worlds numerous times, exhibits go unseen, rollercoaster rides go unridden, and side quests go unanswered. Only through repeat consumption can one fully experience the many valuable novel elements that can be embedded within experiences (whether they are hedonically enjoyable or personally meaningful). Webs of interconnected elements can also create layers of meaning that allow one to interpret experiences at multiple levels. Doing so is a crucial element of the meaning-making process, as people seek to form a coherent understanding of the world (Chater & Loewenstein, 2016; Heintzelman & King, 2014; Martela & Steger, 2016). Reconsuming experiences allows for a better understanding of both the experience and oneself (Russell & Levy, 2012), enabling one to tap into deeper, more nuanced forms of meaning through repetition. For example, on a first pass of F. Scott Fitzgerald's classic novel *The Great Gatsby*, one may follow the events of the plot and note how each moment connects to the next—but only by rereading the book might one more easily look past the straightforward plot points and begin to appreciate how each moment connects to deeper underlying themes (such as the decline of the American Dream; Cain, 2020).

An Implication beyond Existential Ones: Hedonic Certainty

As people scroll through the TV looking for something to watch, they might want to find something highly enjoyable that they have not watched before. Indeed, people can spend hours looking for a potentially good fit. People do this because they intuitively understand that novel experiences offer a hedonic boost of stimulation and excitement (Raju, 1980) from having not been hedonically adapted to yet. They also likely intuit that the stimulation of novelty can serve as a hedonic buffer—if the experience turns out to be unenjoyable, they know that at least it will have the hedonic boost of being novel. Despite this advantage, novel experiences also have the disadvantage of being inherently more uncertain. As uncertainty tends to be aversive (Ellsberg, 1961), repeat experiences can be more attractive for their hedonic certainty.

Having already consumed an experience before makes it feel more hedonically certain. Merely being exposed to something repeatedly makes it less taxing on a person's cognition, which reduces perceived uncertainty (O'Brien, 2013; Song & Schwarz, 2009; Zajonc, 1968), which in turn makes people feel more positively toward it (i.e., the mere exposure effect and processing fluency; Alter & Oppenheimer, 2009; Reber et al., 1998, 2004). Moreover, past experience yields valuable hedonic information that reduces uncertainty about what the experience has to offer. For example, watching a TV show allows one to learn how enjoyable the show is. More specifically, past experience increases certainty about the experience's general hedonic value, its variability in dispensing that value, and the malleability of that value.

Expected Hedonic Value

Reliving an experience has the hedonic advantage of giving people a more well-defined sense of how enjoyable reconsumption will be beforehand. When deciding whether to reconsume an experience, a person already has prior knowledge of what to expect in terms of hedonic pleasure because they have had that exact experience before. This past experience makes relived experiences more hedonically predictable than novel experiences by helping preview its *expected hedonic value.* For example, a person considering whether to watch a movie will have a clearer expectation of how enjoyable it will be if they have (vs. have not) seen it before.

In practice, people have expectations about the hedonic value of many novel experiences, but these are formed using nonexperiential information. For example, one might expect to enjoy a movie for which one has read positive reviews or seen attractive promotional materials. Such descriptive information is insufficient to fully communicate the qualia of an experience (i.e., the internal, subjective, perceptual aspects of an experience; see Jackson's [1986] "Mary, the Color Scientist" thought experiment). Ultimately, the gap between *learning* about an experience and *having* it is a psychologically substantial one that can influence the kinds of decisions people make (Kardas & O'Brien, 2018; Klein & O'Brien, 2018; Li et al., 2023; O'Brien & Ellsworth, 2012a; O'Brien et al., 2018; O'Brien & Roney, 2017; Wald & O'Brien, 2022).

Having even a single instance of past experience changes one's certainty about it. Whereas novel experiences may meet, exceed, or fall short of expectations, repeat experiences are relatively more certain, as prior experience serves as a rich and reliable source of hedonic information.

Expected Hedonic Variance

Reliving experiences also gives people a more well-defined sense of how variable enjoyment might be from one consumption event to the next. Just as past experience makes repeat consumption more hedonically predictable by setting clearer expectations about its hedonic value, it does the same by helping define the *expected hedonic variance.* For example, if a person has socialized with someone before, they will have a clearer expectation of how enjoyable interacting with them will be on average *and* of the possible range of enjoyment from the experience.

Having multiple instances of past experience changes the degree of certainty regarding the various possible hedonic values one could experience. For experiences that one recognizes will be perfectly replicable from one consumption event to the next, expected hedonic variance is not relevant (e.g., a movie will be exactly the same in each repeat viewing). For experiences that will differ in some way from one consumption event to the next, however, multiple past experiences can allow for stronger predictions about how good or bad the experience might possibly be (e.g., going to a restaurant will be a similar but not perfectly identical experience on each visit and repeated experiences clarify the possible range of enjoyment). The hedonic variance information provided by past experiences adds a layer of hedonic certainty with which a person could set more accurate hedonic expectations. This benefit is something repeat experiences can provide that novel experiences generally cannot.

Hedonic Curation

Reliving experiences also makes it possible to selectively experience their more rewarding elements (Russell & Levy, 2012). When deciding whether to relive an experience, people can use their existing knowledge of its hedonic landscape to *curate* their reconsumption experience (i.e., to focus on the enjoyable parts and avoid the unenjoyable parts).

The process of curation could involve strategically shifting one's attention—but the "strategic" part can come only from repetition. Because attention is selective, one can pick and choose which aspects of an experience to attend to. For example, when rewatching a movie in theaters that one has seen before, one can pay close attention to one's favorite scenes and deliberately not pay attention during unpleasant ones. Repeat experiences have the advantage of making it possible to use prior knowledge of the hedonic highs and lows to shape the reconsumption experience to one's liking, which is a benefit that novel experiences generally cannot provide.

WHEN, WHY, AND FOR WHOM IS REPEAT CONSUMPTION VALUABLE?

As reviewed in the first section of this chapter, repeat experiences differ from novel ones because they offer unique hedonic and meaning-related benefits. This begs the question of what factors increase or decrease the "repeat value" of an experience. Next, we review how some candidate factors—stimulus complexity, cognitive effort and risk preferences, control over reconsumption, experiential timing, experiential architecture, memory and attention, and social forces—bear on when, why, and for whom repeat consumption is valuable.

Complexity

Many experiences have some degree of consumable novelty contained within them, and complex experiences have a high degree of such novelty (Berlyne, 1970; Cox & Cox, 2002; O'Brien, 2019). Complex experiences can be so rich with novel elements and interwoven relationships that they cannot all be consumed on a first pass. Thus, complexity is a crucial feature of experiences that impacts their reconsumability (O'Brien, 2019). Simpler experiences, like watching paint dry, being stuck in traffic, and waiting on hold, will yield less meaning or hedonic pleasure upon reconsumption, whereas more complex experiences, like rewatching movies with plot twists, traveling to a major city, or getting to know a new person, will yield relatively more meaning, hedonic pleasure, or both.

Reconsumption provides more experiential value for complex experiences because it makes it possible to consume more novelty of different types. Reliving complex experiences can provide access to novelty of greater breadth (e.g., trying all of the wines at a restaurant), or greater depth (e.g., learning to appreciate the specific notes of a given wine). Complex experiences can also contain embedded novelty that is hedonic (e.g., delicious foods on the menu that one has not yet eaten), or meaningful (e.g., learning the history behind each dish). Whether a complex experience's novelty lies in its breadth or depth, or in its hedonic or meaningful elements, such experiences benefit from reconsumption because additional experiential value is contained within their abundance of novelty.

Cognitive Effort and Risk Preferences

Cognitive Fluency

Reconsumption is attractive in part because it is easier on the mind. People are cognitive misers who tend to find repeat experiences more pleasurable than novel ones because they require less cognitive effort to process (Alter & Oppenheimer, 2009; Zajonc, 1968), adding to a sense of comfortable familiarity. As such, repeat consumption should be more attractive when one is unwilling or unable to dedicate cognitive resources to the experience (e.g., cooking a reliable go-to meal may be more appealing than trying a new recipe when one is preoccupied with stressful life events). Among people who feel cognitively overloaded or distracted, reliving experiences should thus be especially attractive.

Status Quo and Flights to Familiarity

Difficult decisions put people in the unenviable position of not knowing what to choose (Chernev et al., 2015). In such cases, people often flock to the familiar by preferring to preserve the status quo, thus choosing to repeat past experiences (Samuelson & Zeckhauser, 1988). Similarly, decision pressure, such as stress and time pressure, causes people to prefer familiar experiences over novel ones (Vanbeselaere, 1980), even when the novel ones would be more enjoyable (Litt et al., 2011). Choice difficulty can push people to return to the familiar because it is perceived as a more emotionally comfortable option.

Risk Preferences

Individual differences and contextual factors also impact people's willingness to take risks, which should influence the appeal of reconsumption. Factors like personality and domain can predict preferences for riskier versus safer options, such as by taking a chance on novel experiences over familiar ones. When people face the prospect of loss (Tversky & Kahneman, 1992), focus less on the future (Boyd & Zimbardo, 2005), or are more extraverted or disagreeable (Joseph & Zhang, 2021), they are more likely to exhibit risk-taking behavior. Thus, when disposition or context leads to a low tolerance for uncertainty or increased risk aversion, people may become more interested in repeat consumption.

Control over Reconsumption

The degree of control one has over reconsumption can shape the experience. Thus far, most of this chapter has focused on volitional reconsumption—meaning experiences that one chooses to repeat. However, it is also possible to repeat experiences without control, either because it is forced upon a person or because one does not realize repetition is happening. Even when reconsumption is volitional, the degree of control one has over the experience can vary. The sense of control a person has over the initial choice to reconsume, or the way the experience is reconsumed, or both may affect the appeal of repeating experiences relative to consuming novelty.

Volitionality

Many reconsumption experiences are volitional, but this is not necessarily the case, and the degree of volitionality can also vary. Some reconsumption is involuntary because it is stumbled upon unexpectedly, or happens below conscious awareness, as with habitual behavior (Neal et al., 2006; Wood et al., 2002). Other reconsumption is involuntary because one's brain chemistry makes it hard to resist (e.g., as with obsessive–compulsive disorder; Rosa-Alcazar et al., 2008). And perhaps most commonly, many repeat experiences are nonvolitional because they are imposed by external factors, such as when doing repetitive labor at work or in school in order to earn money and higher grades. In principle, repeat consumption should offer greater experiential value when it is volitional.

Malleability

Another way that people can exert control over reconsumption is through hedonic curation, as discussed in the first section of this chapter. During reconsumption, people can use their prior knowledge of the experience to modify their experience to emphasize preferred elements and deemphasize less preferred ones (Russell & Levy, 2012). Reconsumption experiences whose composition can be more easily or more effectively modified to suit the experiencer's tastes will be more appealing (e.g., rewatching a movie at home may be more desirable than rewatching in a movie theater because one can fast-forward and rewind to one's heart's content). One can also selectively grant attention to certain elements and not others (e.g., by closing one's eyes when anticipating a jump scare in a scary movie or by paying closer attention during one's favorite scenes). The ability to shape one's experience is unique to repeat experiences because with novel experiences, one lacks the prior knowledge necessary to curate effectively. Thus, the extent to which a given experience is malleable (i.e., *can be* curated) should change its repeat value.

Building Expertise

Repeating experiences allows people to master them. People play games, learn to play instruments, and practice free-throws, which all require repetition. Building competencies like these can foster a sense of meaning in life (Martela et al., 2018), and they require repetitive practice. Experiences that become enriched by mastery through reconsumption should have especially high repeat value.

Experiential Timing

Gaps and Spacing

As the gap between an initial consumption event and a later reconsumption event grows, reconsumption may feel more novel due to disrupted hedonic adaptation. Similar to how inserting interruptions within an experience can keep experiences fresh by slowing hedonic adaptation (Nelson & Meyvis, 2008; Quoidbach & Dunn, 2013), spacing out consumption and reconsumption may do the same. Presumably, longer gaps would allow hedonic adaptation to slow even more, and may even reset it completely.

Another reason that longer gaps might keep experiences fresh is that people's memories of initial consumption events fade with time. Once information about an experience has been consumed, it can be hard to return to a preexperience state (e.g., curse of knowledge, hindsight bias; Birch & Bloom, 2007; Roese & Vohs, 2012). However, the passage of time may enable one to forget the familiar elements of an experience to reenjoy them later as if they were new again (Russell & Levy, 2012). In fact, even merely perceiving temporal distance can make repeat experiences feel more novel (Galak et al., 2014).

Digesting Ideas

Allowing time to pass can also be important for mentally or emotionally processing an experience. Sometimes the meaning of an experience takes time to digest, so to speak. The "spiral curriculum" details this concept, which posits that students learn better when topics are revisited intermittently (as opposed to all at once) and with increasing depth because this structure allows students to better integrate the material into their existing schemas (Harden, 1999). Relatedly, complex matters can be better understood by allowing time for unconscious processing (Dijksterhuis & Nordgren, 2006). To repeat some experiences immediately would be to do them a disservice because time allows their meaning to coalesce in order to make sense. For complex experiences that require longer periods of digestion, reconsumption might feel premature without enough time in the interim.

Sequence and Architecture

Streaks

Reconsumption can be more appealing when it is part of a streak. When occurrences happen repeatedly as part of an unbroken chain of events, this can motivate people to stay on track with their goals and behave consistently (Klein & O'Brien, 2016, 2023; O'Brien, 2020, 2022b; O'Brien & Klein, 2017). Because continuing an intact chain of repeat experiences can be meaningful in and of itself (Silverman & Barasch, 2023), repeating experiences may be more appealing when doing so prolongs a streak.

Variety and Sequential versus Simultaneous Choice

All else equal, people generally prefer more stimulation over less, and the degree to which reconsumption is stimulating can differ as a function of how it is ordered. Variety can provide appealing stimulation (Kahn, 1995; McAlister & Pessemier, 1982; Ratner et al., 1999), even among already familiar experiences, with many positive psychologists proposing that incorporating variety into people's daily lives will help combat hedonic adaptation and maximize happiness (Sheldon et al., 2012).

Reconsumption can be made more appealing by adding variety to its ordering. For example, among two familiar restaurants, one may find it more appealing to alternate between them because it adds variety and provides a break (Quoidbach & Dunn, 2013). How choices are constructed can also influence repeat value. For example, people prefer more of the same candy bar when choosing sequentially (i.e., one at a time in the moment) compared to when choosing simultaneously (i.e., all at once for the future; Simonson, 1990).

Endings

Another important structural factor is the point at which reconsumption occurs within the span of the entire consumption and reconsumption process—particularly whether it occurs during an ending. People prefer endings that end "well"—enjoyably (Diener et al., 2001; O'Brien & Ellsworth, 2012b; Ross & Simonson, 1991) and/or meaningfully (e.g., "full-circle endings"; Schwörer et al., 2020; Winet & O'Brien, 2022). As endings approach, surer sources of value, and meaning in particular, become more attractive. People nearing the end of life, for example, increasingly prefer to spend time with close family and friends over interesting new strangers (Carstensen, 2006; Carstensen et al., 1999; Fredrickson & Carstensen, 1990). In the face of endings big and small, reliving experiences becomes more attractive because doing so is more certain to provide enjoyable and meaningful endings.

Knowing the Architecture

Beyond changing one's in situ experience, prior knowledge of an experience's structure can also increase the appeal of reconsumption. Much like having an event program at a wedding, knowing where one is within an experience changes how the experience feels and what to expect. Having a road map allows people to organize their understanding of an upcoming experience into a broader framework, which can increase its experiential value. For example, counterintuitively, story spoilers often do not spoil stories (despite ruining the surprise) because having an overarching framework helps make sense of the experience and is rewarding in its own right (Leavitt & Christenfeld, 2011).

Attention and Memory

Attention

For a reconsumption event to be recognized as a repeat experience, one must notice and attend to the initial consumption event. Without having paid attention in the first place, reconsumption becomes no different from first-time consumption. For example, someone passing through a national park without looking up from their phone is not consuming the national park experience; for them to revisit the park later would be functionally equivalent to visiting for the first time. Experiences that were simply missed (e.g., by attending to something else), or that failed to reach some minimum threshold of conscious awareness (e.g., inconspicuous experiences like blinking), are technically repeat experiences but are not perceived as such. When an experience captures less attention initially, its repeat value should be higher. Even so, purely habitual or otherwise boring repeat experiences should offer little repeat value due to a lack of sufficient attention being paid at any stage (Neal et al., 2006; Smith, 1981; van Tilburg & Igou, 2012).

Savoring offers an antidote to various attention-related issues with reconsumption—by attending closely to the positive aspects of an experience, one can increase their experiential value (Bryant & Veroff, 2017). Through savoring, one can extract embedded layers of novelty and appreciate the meaning and connections one has to those experiences (as found in, for example, research on mindfulness: Siegel, 2007). If one savors an initial consumption experience, this may allow one to develop a stronger personal connection that could provide more meaning upon reconsumption. For example, by savoring a walk through a familiar park, one might be more attuned to how the flowers have grown and the seasons have changed, thus strengthening one's sense of meaning and emotional connection.

Memory

Memory is crucial for reconsumption because repeat value necessarily depends on remembering (or not remembering) past consumption events. Without such memory, one cannot reap the benefits of one's existing hedonic knowledge or existing relationship with the experience. Poorly remembered experiences may thus be more stimulating when reexperienced, but may also lack the deeper benefits of familiarity. For example, a person who visited a national park as a child but does not remember it may find revisiting the park hedonically exciting, but not so personally meaningful. Well-preserved memories should further deepen the meaningful value of repeat consumption. It could also be argued that reconsumption can occur using *only* one's memories. For example, one cannot actually spend time with loved ones who have passed away, but one may still be able to relive those experiences in one's mind (e.g., the "replay value" of cherished memories). The experiential benefits of this memory-based reliving of experiences will be different than actually reliving those experiences because they are limited by the details available via memory. No new information will be available, meaning that hedonic certainty will be amplified and the control one has over one's own memory may allow for particularly effective hedonic curation. Revisiting memories in this way may also strengthen one's personal connection to these experiences, leading people to become especially protective of them (Zauberman et al., 2009).

Social Forces

Relationship Building

Having meaningful social relationships is crucial for well-being, and repetition plays a vital role in fostering such relationships. People bond by sharing both a breadth and a depth of experiences with each other, through which they become increasingly vulnerable and interpersonally connected (Altman & Taylor, 1973; Taylor & Altman, 1987; Vanlear, 1987). This process necessarily involves repeatedly sharing experiences, like joint activities and conversation. Certainly, a healthy social life involves balancing the exploration of new social connections with reinvesting in one's existing relationships. This tendency changes over time, such that people tend to focus on their existing relationships as they get older by spending time with close friends and family instead of with new and interesting strangers (Carstensen, 2006; Carstensen et al., 1999; Fredrickson & Carstensen, 1990). It is perhaps telling that people who face major life endings (e.g., death) rely most on the relationships they have built most firmly through decades of repeated interactions.

Vicarious Experience

Another more indirect form of reconsumption involves incorporating other people's perspectives into one's own. The ability to empathize with others and incorporate their perspective into a collective "we"-perspective can make novel experiences feel like reconsumption experiences and vice versa. Novel experiences can feel like repeats when they have already been experienced by someone else because it feels redundant at the broader group level (Winet et al., 2022). Repeat experiences can also feel novel again when reexperiencing them alongside someone who is experiencing them for the first time because one tends to adopt the other person's inexperienced perspective (Jung et al., 2020). When consuming experiences with social partners, others' perspectives can influence the appeal of reconsumption because they can make familiar experiences feel novel and novel experiences feel familiar.

WHAT RESEARCH REMAINS ON REPEAT CONSUMPTION?

Despite this quickly growing literature, there is much left to be understood about the psychology of familiarity and repeat reconsumption. We end this chapter by highlighting some of the most interesting and pressing directions from our view.

Practical Directions

Encouraging Repeat Consumption

In the preceding section of this chapter, we discussed various factors that make repeat experiences more or less appealing, but much is left to learn about which strategies work best and when. Future research should pit various strategies against each other to determine their benefits and drawbacks.

One promising direction seems to be emphasizing the novelty that remains embedded within experiences. By making salient how much novelty is left untapped within experiences, people may become more likely to repeat those experiences, rather than seek out new ones. Akin to how video games communicate the percentage of their worlds the player has explored, businesses and organizations might consider a similar strategy. For linear games, this percentage score is merely a progress marker, but for open-world games (which better reflect real life), this is a measure of unexplored optional novelty. Simply making people aware of the amount of untapped novelty contained within an experience may increase the likelihood with which people choose to repeatedly explore things like websites, menus, and tourist attractions. For example, local tourism boards could encourage people to spend more time in the area by making it easier for people to keep track of which local attractions they have and have *not yet* experienced. These boards could distribute local attraction checklists and email people a percentage marker highlighting how many of the local attractions they have experienced and how many they still have left to experience.

Climate Change Action

There is growing global awareness of the importance of minimizing the harms of climate change, which promises to have grave implications for human society and well-being (Masud et al., 2015). As Earth's resources become increasingly strained, the need to reconsume and eschew novelty has become more important than ever. Understanding the psychological drivers of climate-friendly forms of repeat consumption, like repair and reuse, may prove invaluable.

Waste is created in the process of buying and disposing of products. Indeed many companies create products that are meant to be disposed of, as with fast fashion and products created using single-use plastics. Cheap materials degrade quickly, making them difficult to reuse. However, emerging research seeks to explore the psychology driving consumers' desire to prolong the lives of their products, rather than replace them with new ones. Recent work has explored how to encourage repair behaviors, investigating which factors lead people to reinvest in their existing possessions by bringing them back into usable condition (Godfrey et al., 2022). Other work explores the psychology underlying perceptions of degradation, revealing the qualities that lead consumers to believe items retain value, as opposed to categorizing them as trash, such as whether they are physically distorted (Trudel et al., 2016). This work speaks to a broader understanding of how people may be convinced of the enduring value of reconsumption opportunities, thereby encouraging more sustainable behavior. One actionable strategy was documented by O'Brien and Smith (2019), who found that reexperiencing the same consumption object using novel *methods* of consumption (e.g., eating the same old popcorn, but with chopsticks) can help revive people's enjoyment. Strategies like these could be scaled up to encourage familiarity seeking and reuse behaviors more broadly.

Conceptual Directions

Experiences provide different kinds of experiential value at different points in the reconsumption process. Future research could explore how repeat value may be impacted by the architecture of embedded experiential value, the ways in which that value can be accessed, and the time course over which that value may be extracted.

Enjoyment–Meaning Tradeoffs

In the first section of this chapter, we discussed how reconsumption allows one to tap into both meaningful and hedonic benefits, but it remains unclear how these values potentially interact over time. Hedonic adaptation predicts enjoyment will diminish with repeated experience, but how might a growing sense of meaning counterbalance this decline? Future research could chart the progression of both types of value for different types of experiences to determine where they intersect, and considering both hedonic pleasure and meaning combined, which points are the most and least valuable overall. For example, perhaps going to a baseball game for one's hometown team is most enjoyable during one's very first game because that is when the experience is most new and exciting, but with each subsequent game, it becomes gradually less enjoyable due to hedonic adaptation. Simultaneously, that first game may also be when it is least meaningful because one has not yet become emotionally invested in the team—but by attending more games, this personal connection grows and each subsequent game becomes increasingly meaningful. To understand when fandom might be at its peak, one could calculate when people's combined sense of enjoyment and meaning tends to be highest over time. Potential fans could use this understanding to recognize ex ante how much time they should expect to invest before becoming a true fan, and marketers (for example) could use this same information to anticipate lucrative marketing opportunities.

Bottom-Up versus Top-Down Processing

An alternative framework for thinking about repeat consumption is through the lens of bottom-up versus top-down processing. As people relive the same experience over and over, they may turn their attention away from the concrete, sensory elements of an experience and begin to incorporate an *interpretation* of the experience that gets continually reshaped through repeated exposure. Perhaps this framework could help explain why certain experiences are "acquired tastes," which start out being hedonically *unpleasant*, but eventually become enjoyable through repeated experience. Common examples include sophisticated media (e.g., jazz and classical music) and beverages with stimulating properties (e.g., coffee and alcohol). Embedded novelty may play a key role, but a shift from bottom-up to top-down processing may provide another explanation. When people first try coffee, for example, they may only notice its bitterness from a bottom-up perspective. But after having many cups over time, they may begin to associate the taste, however bitter, with the pleasant feeling of being caffeinated. Eventually they may grow to "enjoy the taste," but not because of its literal taste—rather, they enjoy the expectation and background knowledge their minds overlay onto the taste. This tendency to shift to a top-down mode of processing suggests a potential psychological mechanism of repeat consumption that may help explain other related patterns as well. For example, as people repeat experiences, they may increasingly value more abstract elements, such as by choosing to read an analysis of a movie before rewatching it in order to better understand and appreciate its themes on a second viewing (see also Redden, 2008).

Within-Experience Reconsumption

The current research on novelty- and familiarity seeking focuses on what people prefer at a between-experience level (i.e., from one discrete consumption experience to the next)—but future research could also explore how preferences for consumption and reconsumption operate at a *within-experience* level. A single experience may deliver both novelty and familiarity dynamically as it unfolds over time. For example, a movie may contain both scenes with fast-paced novelty (e.g., by introducing new characters and plot points) and ones that return to familiarity (e.g., by having existing characters address familiar plot points). In ongoing research, we are exploring how narrative techniques like "callbacks" (i.e., referencing older material anew) use reconsumption at the within-experience level to imbue media experiences with new meanings, thus increasing their experiential value (Winet & O'Brien, 2025). Future work should continue to explore how other forms of repetition at the within-experience level can change and potentially improve experiences.

Meta-Novelty and Meta-Familiarity

Finally, can the experience of novelty itself feel repetitive, and can the experience of repetition itself feel novel? Uncertainty and novelty are intrinsically linked. The appeal of novelty comes from its relative unpredictability, and yet when one expects the unexpected, this may create a sense of *meta-familiarity* that is distinct from how novel the content itself is. Likewise, an unexpected familiar experience may create a sense of *meta-novelty* that is distinct from how familiar the content itself is. For example, social media offers endless novel content to scroll through—and yet, it may begin to feel repetitive to consume such a continuous stream of novel content. Meanwhile, to stumble upon something familiar in one's feed could be more unexpected than encountering yet more novelty and thus may feel more "novel" at a meta-level. Might repeat experiences receive a hedonic boost from feeling "novel" at a meta-level? Could novel experiences receive any of reconsumption's unique benefits by feeling "familiar" at a meta-level? These are questions that arise from the idea that the novelty and familiarity of *novelty and familiarity* might be consumable, which may be worth exploring in future research.

CONCLUDING THOUGHTS

All told, the current chapter highlights the exciting state of research on familiarity and repeat consumption. The literature on meaning and personal growth has pointed to the obvious value of gaining exposure to new stimuli and new experiences, but what is perhaps less obvious is that meaning and personal growth can also be gained from repeating and reliving familiar experiences. In the years to come, we look forward to seeing continued new discoveries about the power of the old and the familiar.

REFERENCES

Alter, A. L., & Oppenheimer, D. M. (2009). Uniting the tribes of fluency to form a metacognitive nation. *Personality and Social Psychology Review, 13,* 219–235.

Altman, I., & Taylor, D. A. (1973). *Social penetration: The development of interpersonal relationships.* Holt, Rinehart & Winston.

Ariely, D., Kamenica, E., & Prelec, D. (2008). Man's search for meaning: The case of Legos. *Journal of Economic Behavior and Organization, 67,* 671–677.

Arnould, E. J., & Price, L. L. (1993). River magic: Extraordinary experience and the extended service encounter. *Journal of Consumer Research, 20,* 24–45.

Aron, A., Melinat, E., Aron, E. N., Vallone, R. D., & Bator, R. J. (1997). The experimental generation of interpersonal closeness: A procedure and some preliminary findings. *Personality and Social Psychology Bulletin, 23,* 363–377.

Baumeister, R. F. (1991). *Meanings of life.* Guilford Press.

Baumeister, R. F., & Newman, L. S. (2016). How stories make sense of personal experiences: Motives that shape autobiographical narratives. *Personality and Social Psychology Bulletin, 20,* 676–690.

Baumeister, R. F., Vohs, K. D., Aaker, J. L., & Garbinsky, E. N. (2013). Some key differences between a happy life and a meaningful life. *Journal of Positive Psychology, 8,* 505–516.

Berlyne, D. E. (1970). Novelty, complexity, and hedonic value. *Perception and Psychophysics, 8,* 279–286.

Birch, S. A. J., & Bloom, P. (2007). The curse of knowledge in reasoning about false beliefs. *Psychological Science, 18,* 382–386.

Boyd, J. N., & Zimbardo, P. G. (2005). Time perspective, health, and risk taking. In A. Strathman & J. Joireman (Eds.), *Understanding behavior in the context of time: Theory, research, and application* (pp. 85–107). Erlbaum.

Brickman, P., Coates, D., & Janoff-Bulman, R. (1978). Lottery winners and accident victims: Is happiness relative? *Journal of Personality and Social Psychology, 36,* 917–927.

Bryant, F. B., & Veroff, J. (2017). *Savoring: A new model of positive experience.* Psychology Press.

Cain, W. E. (2020). American dreaming: Really reading *The Great Gatsby. Society, 57,* 453–470.

Campbell, T., O'Brien, E., Boven, L. V., Schwarz, N., & Ubel, P. (2014). Too much experience: A desensitization bias in emotional perspective taking. *Journal of Personality and Social Psychology, 106,* 272–285.

Carmon, Z., Wertenbroch, K., & Zeelenberg, M. (2003). Option attachment: When deliberating makes choosing feel like losing. *Journal of Consumer Research, 30,* 15–29.

Carstensen, L. L. (2006). The Influence of a sense of time on human development. *Science, 312,* 1913–1915.

Carstensen, L. L., Isaacowitz, D. M., & Charles, S. T. (1999). Taking time seriously: A theory of socioemotional selectivity. *American Psychologist, 54,* 165–181.

Carter, T. J., & Gilovich, T. (2012). I am what I do, not what I have: The differential centrality of experiential and material purchases to the self. *Journal of Personality and Social Psychology, 102,* 1304–1317.

Chater, N., & Loewenstein, G. (2016). The under-appreciated drive for sense-making. *Journal of Economic Behavior and Organization, 126,* 137–154.

Chernev, A., Böckenholt, U., & Goodman, J. (2015). Choice overload: A conceptual review and meta-analysis. *Journal of Consumer Psychology, 25,* 333–358.

Choi, J., Catapano, R., & Choi, I. (2017). Taking stock of happiness and meaning in everyday life: An experience sampling approach. *Social Psychological and Personality Science, 8,* 641–651.

Cox, D., & Cox, A. D. (2002). Beyond first impressions: The effects of repeated exposure on consumer liking of visually complex and simple product designs. *Journal of the Academy of Marketing Science, 30,* 119–130.

Diener, E., Wirtz, D., & Oishi, S. (2001). End effects of rated life quality: The James Dean effect. *Psychological Science, 12,* 124–128.

Dijksterhuis, A., & Nordgren, L. F. (2006). A theory of unconscious thought. *Perspectives on Psychological Science, 1,* 95–109.

Ellsberg, D. (1961). Risk, ambiguity, and the savage axioms. *Quarterly Journal of Economics, 75,* 643–669.

Ersner-Hershfield, H., Mikels, J. A., Sullivan, S. J., & Carstensen, L. L. (2008). Poignancy: Mixed emotional experience in the face of meaningful endings. *Journal of Personality and Social Psychology, 94,* 158–167.

Forest, T. A., Siegelman, N., & Finn, A. S. (2022). Attention shifts to more complex structures with experience. *Psychological Science, 33,* 2059–2072.

Frederick, S., & Loewenstein, G. (1999). Hedonic adaptation. In D. Kahneman, E. Diener, & N. Schwarz (Eds.), *Wellbeing: The foundations of hedonic psychology* (pp. 302–329). Russell Sage Foundation.

Fredrickson, B. L., & Carstensen, L. L. (1990). Choosing social partners: How old age and anticipated endings make people more selective. *Psychology and Aging, 5,* 335–347.

Galak, J., Redden, J. P., Yang, Y., & Kyung, E. J. (2014). How perceptions of temporal distance influence satiation. *Journal of Experimental Social Psychology, 52,* 118–123.

Garcia-Rada, X., John, L. K., O'Brien, E., & Norton, M. I. (2024). *The revised-is-quality heuristic: Why consumers prefer products labeled as revised.* Manuscript under review.

Godfrey, D. M., Price, L. L., & Lusch, R. F. (2022). Repair, consumption, and sustainability: Fixing fragile objects and maintaining consumer practices. *Journal of Consumer Research, 49,* 229–251.

Harden, R. M. (1999). What is a spiral curriculum? *Medical Teacher, 21,* 141–143.

Heintzelman, S. J., & King, L. A. (2013). On knowing more than we can tell: Intuitive processes and the experience of meaning. *Journal of Positive Psychology, 8,* 471–482.

Heintzelman, S. J., & King, L. A. (2014). (The feeling of) meaning-as-information. *Personality and Social Psychology Review, 18,* 153–167.

Heintzelman, S. J., & King, L. A. (2019). Routines and meaning in life. *Personality and Social Psychology Bulletin, 45,* 688–699.

Hornsey, M. J., Bain, P. G., Harris, E. A., Lebedeva, N., Kashima, E. S., Guan, Y., . . . Blumen, S. (2018). How much is enough in a perfect world?: Cultural variation in ideal levels of happiness, pleasure, freedom, health, self-esteem, longevity, and intelligence. *Psychological Science, 29,* 1393–1404.

Jackson, F. (1986). What Mary didn't know. *Journal of Philosophy, 83,* 291–295.

Joseph, E. D., & Zhang, D. C. (2021). Personality profile of risk-takers: An examination of the Big Five facets. *Journal of Individual Differences, 42,* 194–203.

Jung, M. H., Gonzalez, F. J., & Critcher, C. R. (2020). The vicarious construal effect: Seeing and experiencing the world through different eyes. *Journal of Personality and Social Psychology, 118,* 617–638.

Kahn, B. E. (1995). Consumer variety-seeking among goods and services. *Journal of Retailing and Consumer Services, 2,* 139–148.

Kardas, M., & O'Brien, E. (2018). Easier seen than done: Merely watching others perform can foster an illusion of skill acquisition. *Psychological Science, 29,* 521–536.

Kardas, M., Schroeder, J., & O'Brien, E. (2022). Keep talking: (Mis)understanding the hedonic trajectory of conversation. *Journal of Personality and Social Psychology, 123,* 717–740.

Keinan, A., & Kivetz, R. (2011). Productivity orientation and the consumption of collectable experiences. *Journal of Consumer Research, 37,* 935–950.

King, L. A., & Napa, C. K. (1998). What makes a life good? *Journal of Personality and Social Psychology, 75,* 156–165.

Klein, N., & O'Brien, E. (2016). The tipping point of moral change: When do good and bad acts make good and bad actors? *Social Cognition, 34,* 149–166.

Klein, N., & O'Brien, E. (2017). The power and limits of personal change: When a bad past does (and does not) inspire in the present. *Journal of Personality and Social Psychology, 113,* 210–229.

Klein, N., & O'Brien, E. (2018). People use less information than they think to make up their minds. *Proceedings of the National Academy of Sciences, 115,* 1322–13227.

Klein, N., & O'Brien, E. (2023). Threshold violations in social judgment. *Journal of Personality and Social Psychology, 125,* 284–315.

Kristal, A. C., O'Brien, E., & Caruso, E. M. (2019). Yesterday's news: A temporal discontinuity in the sting of inferiority. *Psychological Science, 30,* 643–656.

Lambert, N. M., Stillman, T. F., Hicks, J. A., Kamble, S., Baumeister, R. F., & Fincham, F. D. (2013). To belong is to matter: Sense of belonging enhances meaning in life. *Personality and Social Psychology Bulletin, 39,* 1418–1427.

Lastovicka, J. L., & Sirianni, N. J. (2011). Truly, madly, deeply: Consumers in the throes of material possession love. *Journal of Consumer Research, 38,* 323–342.

Leavitt, J. D., & Christenfeld, N. J. S. (2011). Story spoilers don't spoil stories. *Psychological Science, 22,* 1152–1154.

Leontiev, D. A. (2013). Personal meaning: A challenge for psychology. *Journal of Positive Psychology, 8,* 459–470.

Li, X., Hsee, C. K., & O'Brien, E. (2023). "It could be better" can make it worse: When and why people mistakenly communicate upward counterfactual information. *Journal of Marketing Research, 60,* 219–236.

Libby, L. K., Eibach, R. P., & Gilovich, T. (2005). Here's looking at me: The effect of memory perspective on assessments of personal change. *Journal of Personality and Social Psychology, 88,* 50–62.

Litt, A., Reich, T., Maymin, S., & Shiv, B. (2011). Pressure and perverse flights to familiarity. *Psychological Science, 22,* 523–531.

Lyubomirsky, S., Sheldon, K. M., & Schkade, D. (2005). Pursuing happiness: The architecture of sustainable change. *Review of General Psychology, 9,* 111–131.

Martela, F., Ryan, R. M., & Steger, M. F. (2018). Meaningfulness as satisfaction of autonomy, competence, relatedness, and beneficence: Comparing the four satisfactions and positive affect as predictors of meaning in life. *Journal of Happiness Studies, 19,* 1261–1282.

Martela, F., & Steger, M. F. (2016). The three meanings of meaning in life: Distinguishing coherence, purpose, and significance. *Journal of Positive Psychology, 11,* 531–545.

Masud, M. M., Akhtar, R., Afroz, R., & Al-Amin, A. Q., & Kari, F. B. (2015). Pro-environmental behavior and public understanding of climate change. *Mitigation and Adaptation Strategies for Global Change, 20,* 591–600.

McAlister, L., & Pessemier, E. (1982). Variety seeking behavior: An interdisciplinary review. *Journal of Consumer Research, 9,* 311–322.

Mehlhorn, K., Newell, B. R., Todd, P. M., Lee, M. D., Morgan, K., Braithwaite, V. A., . . . Gonzalez, C. (2015). Unpacking the exploration–exploitation tradeoff: A synthesis of human and animal literatures. *Decision, 2,* 191–215.

Neal, D. T., Wood, W., & Quinn, J. M. (2006). Habits—A repeat performance. *Current Directions in Psychological Science, 15,* 198–202.

Nelson, L. D., & Meyvis, T. (2008). Interrupted consumption: Disrupting adaptation to hedonic experiences. *Journal of Marketing Research, 45,* 654–664.

Noble, C. E. (1953). The meaning-familiarity relationship. *Psychological Review, 60,* 89–98.

O'Brien, E. (2013). Easy to retrieve but hard to believe: Metacognitive discounting of the unpleasantly possible. *Psychological Science, 24,* 844–851.

O'Brien, E. (2015a). Feeling connected to younger versus older selves: The asymmetric impact of life stage orientation. *Cognition and Emotion, 29,* 678–686.

O'Brien, E. (2015b). Mapping out past versus future minds: The perceived trajectory of rationality versus emotionality over time. *Journal of Experimental Psychology: General, 144,* 624–628.

O'Brien, E. (2019). Enjoy it again: Repeat experiences are less repetitive than people think. *Journal of Personality and Social Psychology, 116,* 519–540.

O'Brien, E. (2020). When small signs of change add up: The psychology of tipping points. *Current Directions in Psychological Science, 29,* 55–62.

O'Brien, E. (2021). A mind stretched: The psychology of repeat consumption. *Consumer Psychology Review, 4,* 42–58.

O'Brien, E. (2022a). Look back, not ahead?: Time use and the value of revisiting past experiences. In C. Hoerl, T. McCormack, & A. Fernandes (Eds.), *Temporal asymmetries in philosophy and psychology.* Oxford University Press.

O'Brien, E. (2022b). Losing sight of piecemeal progress: People lump and dismiss improvement efforts that fall short of categorical change—despite improving. *Psychological Science, 33,* 1278–1299.

O'Brien, E. (2022c). The "next" effect: When a better future worsens the present. *Social Psychological and Personality Science, 13,* 456–465.

O'Brien, E., & Ellsworth, P. C. (2012a). More than skin deep: Visceral states are not projected onto dissimilar others. *Psychological Science, 23,* 391–396.

O'Brien, E., & Ellsworth, P. C. (2012b). Saving the last for best: A positivity bias for end experiences. *Psychological Science, 23,* 163–165.

O'Brien, E., Ellsworth, P. C., & Schwarz, N. (2012). Today's misery and yesterday's happiness: Differential effects of current life-events on perceptions of past well-being. *Journal of Experimental Social Psychology, 48,* 968–972.

O'Brien, E., & Kardas, M. (2016). The implicit meaning of (my) change. *Journal of Personality and Social Psychology, 111,* 882–894.

O'Brien, E., & Kassirer, S. (2019). People are slow to adapt to the warm glow of giving. *Psychological Science, 30,* 193–204.

O'Brien, E., & Klein, N. (2017). The tipping point of perceived change: Asymmetric thresholds in diagnosing improvement versus decline. *Journal of Personality and Social Psychology, 112,* 161–185.

O'Brien, E., Kristal, A. C., Ellsworth, P. C., & Schwarz, N. (2018). (Mis)imagining the good life and the bad life: Envy and pity as a function of the focusing illusion. *Journal of Experimental Social Psychology, 75,* 41–53.

O'Brien, E., & Roney, E. (2017). Worth the wait?: Leisure can be just as enjoyable with work left undone. *Psychological Science, 28,* 1000–1015.

O'Brien, E., & Smith, R. W. (2019). Unconventional consumption methods and enjoying things consumed: Recapturing the "first-time" experience. *Personality and Social Psychology Bulletin, 45,* 67–80.

Proulx, T., & Inzlicht, M. (2012). The five "A"s of meaning maintenance: Finding meaning in the theories of sense-making. *Psychological Inquiry, 23,* 317–335.

Quoidbach, J., & Dunn, E. W. (2013). Give it up: A strategy for combating hedonic adaptation. *Social Psychological and Personality Science, 4,* 563–568.

Quoidbach, J., Mikolajczak, M., & Gross, J. J. (2015). Positive interventions: An emotion regulation perspective. *Psychological Bulletin, 141,* 655–693.

Raju, P. S. (1980). Optimum stimulation level: Its relationship to personality, demographics, and exploratory behavior. *Journal of Consumer Research, 7,* 272–282.

Ratner, R. K., Kahn, B. E., & Kahneman, D. (1999). Choosing less-preferred experiences for the sake of variety. *Journal of Consumer Research, 26,* 1–15.

Read, D., & Loewenstein, G. (1995). Diversification bias: Explaining the discrepancy in variety seeking between combined and separated choices. *Journal of Experimental Psychology: Applied, 1,* 34–49.

Reber, R., Schwarz, N., & Winkielman, P. (2004). Processing fluency and aesthetic pleasure: Is beauty in the perceiver's processing experience? *Personality and Social Psychology Review, 8,* 364–382.

Reber, R., Winkielman, P., & Schwarz, N. (1998). Effects of perceptual fluency on affective judgments. *Psychological Science, 9,* 45–48.

Redden, J. P. (2008). Reducing satiation: The role of categorization level. *Journal of Consumer Research, 34,* 624–634.

Roese, N. J., & Vohs, K. D. (2012). Hindsight bias. *Perspectives on Psychological Science, 7,* 411–426.

Rogers, B., Chicas, H., Kelly, J., Kubin, E., Christian, M., Kachanoff, F., . . . Gray, K. (2023). Seeing your life story as a hero's journey increases meaning in life. *Journal of Personality and Social Psychology, 125,* 752–778.

Rosa-Alcazar, A., Sanchez-Meca, J., Gomez-Conesa, A., & Marin-Martinez, F. (2008). Psychological treatment of obsessive–compulsive disorder: A meta-analysis. *Clinical Psychology Review, 28,* 1310–1325.

Ross, W. T., & Simonson, I. (1991). Evaluations of pairs of experiences: A preference for happy endings. *Journal of Behavioral Decision Making, 4,* 273–282.

Routledge, C., Arndt, J., Wildschut, T., Sedikides, C., Hart, C. M., Juhl, J., . . . Schlotz, W. (2011). The past makes the present meaningful: Nostalgia as an existential resource. *Journal of Personality and Social Psychology, 101,* 638–652.

Russell, C. A., & Levy, S. J. (2012). The temporal and focal dynamics of volitional reconsumption: A phenomenological investigation of repeated hedonic experiences. *Journal of Consumer Research, 39,* 341–359.

Samuelson, W., & Zeckhauser, R. J. (1988). Status quo bias in decision-making. *Journal of Risk and Uncertainty, 1,* 7–59.

Sansone, C., Weir, C., Harpster, L., & Morgan, C. (1992). Once a boring task, always a boring task?: Interest as a self-regulatory mechanism. *Journal of Personality and Social Psychology, 63,* 379–390.

Schlegel, R., Hicks, J., King, L., & Arndt, J. (2011). Feeling like you know who you are: Perceived true self-knowledge and meaning in life. *Personality and Social Psychology Bulletin, 37,* 745–756.

Schwörer, B., Krott, N. R., & Oettingen, G. (2020). Saying goodbye and saying it well: Consequences of a (not) well-rounded ending. *Motivation Science, 6,* 21–33.

Sheldon, K. M., Boehm, J. K., & Lyubomirsky, S. (2012). Variety is the spice of happiness: The hedonic adaptation prevention (HAP) model. In I. Boniwell & S. David (Eds.), *Oxford handbook of happiness* (pp. 901–914). Oxford University Press.

Siegel, D. (2007). *The mindful brain.* Norton.

Silverman, J., & Barasch, A. (2023). On or off track: How (broken) streaks affect consumer decisions. *Journal of Consumer Research, 49,* 1095–1117.

Simonson, I. (1990). The effect of purchase quantity and timing on variety-seeking behavior. *Journal of Marketing Research, 27,* 150–162.

Smith, R. P. (1981). Boredom: A review. *Human Factors, 23,* 329–340.

Song, H., & Schwarz, N. (2009). If it's difficult to pronounce, it must be risky: Fluency, familiarity, and risk perception. *Psychological Science, 20,* 135–138.

Speekenbrink, M., & Konstantinidis, E. (2015). Uncertainty and exploration in a restless bandit problem. *Topics in Cognitive Science, 7,* 351–367.

Steger, M. F. (2012). Making meaning in life. *Psychological Inquiry, 23,* 381–385.

Taylor, D., & Altman, I. (1987). Communication in interpersonal relationships: Social penetration processes. In M. E. Roloff & G. R. Miller (Eds.), *Interpersonal processes: New directions in communication research* (pp. 257–277). Sage.

Trudel, R., Argo, J. J., & Meng, M. D. (2016). Trash or recycle?: How product distortion leads to categorization error during disposal. *Environment and Behavior, 48,* 966–985.

Tversky, A., & Kahneman, D. (1992). Advances in prospect theory: Cumulative representation of uncertainty. *Journal of Risk and Uncertainty, 5,* 297–323.

Vanbeselaere, N. (1980). Mere repeated exposure and experimental stress as determiners of stimulus evaluations. *Motivation and Emotion, 4,* 61–69.

van den Bos, K. (2009). Making sense of life: The existential self trying to deal with personal uncertainty. *Psychological Inquiry, 20,* 197–217.

van Tilburg, W. A. P., & Igou, E. R. (2012). On boredom: Lack of challenge and meaning as distinct boredom experiences. *Motivation and Emotion, 36,* 181–194.

Vanlear, C. A., Jr. (1987). The formation of social relationships: A longitudinal study of social penetration. *Human Communication Research, 13,* 299–322.

Vohs, K. D., Aaker, J. L., & Catapano, R. (2019). It's not going to be that fun: Negative experiences can add meaning to life. *Current Opinion in Psychology, 26,* 11–14.

Wald, K., & O'Brien, E. (2022). Repeated exposure to success harshens reactions to failure. *Journal of Experimental Social Psychology, 103,* 1–18.

Weingarten, E., Duke, K., Liu, W., Hamilton, R. W., Amir, O., Appel, G., . . . Sun, M. (2023). What makes people happy?: Decoupling the experiential-material continuum. *Journal of Consumer Psychology, 33,* 97–106.

Wheeler, S. C., & Bechler, C. J. (2021). Objects and self-identity. *Current Opinion in Psychology, 39,* 6–11.

Winet, Y. K., & O'Brien, E. (2022). Ending on a familiar note: Perceived endings motivate repeat consumption. *Journal of Personality and Social Psychology, 124,* 707–734.

Winet, Y. K., & O'Brien, E. (2025). *Reinterpret the familiar: Consumers prefer experiences that use callbacks.* Manuscript in preparation.

Winet, Y. K., Tu, Y., Choshen-Hillel, S., & Fishbach, A. (2022). Social exploration: When people deviate from options explored by others. *Journal of Personality and Social Psychology, 122,* 427–442.

Wolfram, H. J. (2023). Meaning in life, life role importance, life strain, and life satisfaction. *Current Psychology, 42,* 29905–29917.

Wood, W., Quinn, J. M., & Kashy, D. A. (2002). Habits in everyday life: Thought, emotion, and action. *Journal of Personality and Social Psychology, 83,* 1281–1297.

Yang, Y., & Galak, J. (2015). Sentimental value and its influence on hedonic adaptation. *Journal of Personality and Social Psychology, 109,* 767–790.

Zajonc, R. B. (1968). Attitudinal effects of mere exposure. *Journal of Personality and Social Psychology, 9,* 1–27.

Zauberman, G., Ratner, R. K., & Kim, B. K. (2009). Memories as assets: Strategic memory protection in choice over time. *Journal of Consumer Research, 35,* 715–728.

CHAPTER 61

The Pursuit of Happiness

Toxic Positivity or an Existentially Worthy Goal in Life?

Frank Martela

It is likely that no previous historical era has placed so much emphasis on personally experienced happiness as modern, individualistic, and consumeristic Western culture. Happiness is represented as something desirable and worth pursuing, with research and national policy initiatives on happiness blooming and newspapers offering advice on "the five tricks to make you happy." Companies like Amazon, Google, and SAP now employ chief happiness officers, and the United Arab Emirates even has a minister of happiness. McKinsey (2021) estimated the global wellness industry at $1.5 trillion, while the global mental wellness industry is estimated at $130 billion (Global Wellness Institute, 2024). At the same time, advertisements bombard people with attempts to make an implicit association between their products and happiness, featuring campaigns about "Happy Meals" and "Open Happiness." Happiness has become an industry and a buzzword used to sell self-help books, courses, and employee well-being programs.

Accordingly, it is about time to set the record straight: Is happiness a good goal in life? Should we strive for happiness as individuals and as a culture? Sometimes aiming to be happy is offered as a self-evident life goal, something we all pursue and ought to pursue. "The very purpose of our life is to seek happiness. That is clear," the 14th Dalai Lama (2010, p. 3) declared. This sounds plausible; who would not want to be happy? On the other hand, sometimes striving to be happy is depicted as an empty hedonic pursuit that stands in the way of more noble purposes. Thus, we find Nietzsche (1997, p. 6) exclaiming that "humanity does *not* strive for happiness; only the English do." Among certain intellectual circles, and many existentialist thinkers belong to this group, seeking happiness is easily seen as a trivial pursuit, a mere distraction standing in the way of truly worthwhile ways of living. As Rosten (1962) put it, "The purpose of life is not to be happy—but to matter, to be productive, to be useful, to have it make some difference that you lived at all." While some existentially oriented writers have complaints even against the state of *being* happy, the bulk of this critique targets the *seeking of* happiness.

In the present chapter, I investigate the role of happiness in good life, and the benefits and drawbacks of the pursuit of happiness. Building on empirical research, I investigate what are the positive and negative outcomes of being happy, what ways of approaching one's (lack of) happiness are beneficial, and what practices of pursuing happiness tend to backfire, being detrimental for one's well-being. However, because attitudes toward happiness are not only an individual matter but to a large degree determined through societal ideals and expectations, I also engage in a more historical and philosophical analysis of how Western culture has defined and approached happiness in the past, and how the Enlightenment generated a new way of thinking about happiness. This historical analysis reveals that happiness is not as self-evident a life goal as the modern, Western self-help industry would want you to believe. This Western view on happiness is then contrasted with the way happiness is approached in some other cultures, and empirical research about the impact of such cultural factors on well-being is reviewed. I show that some cultural ideals and expectations about happiness can be beneficial for happiness, while others can be detrimental. I conclude by trying to make sense of these various lines of inquiry, aiming to offer some advice about how to approach happiness as individuals and as societies.

THE DEFINITION, BENEFITS, AND DRAWBACKS OF BEING HAPPY

How happiness is defined and understood differs across historical periods and cultures, as we see later in this chapter. Yet to start discussing it, we need a working definition. Following the modern understanding of happiness as a positive subjective state, I see happiness as being about the presence of positive emotional states, the relative lack of negative emotional states, and that the person in question evaluates their own life positively. This is in line with dictionary definitions of happiness across the world, where the state of pleasantness, satisfaction, joyfulness, and/or positive mood is part of every definition across 30 countries (Oishi et al., 2013). It also aligns with psychological research that sees subjective well-being as consisting of positive affect, lack of negative affect, and positive life evaluation (Diener, 1984; Diener et al., 1999). Happiness can thus be seen as a psychological state of well-being characterized by mainly positive feelings in and evaluations about one's life.

Empirical research has demonstrated that happiness, operationalized as positive affect, life satisfaction, positive affective balance, or similar, is associated with many benefits for mental and physical health as well as various life outcomes (Howell et al., 2007; Lyubomirsky et al., 2005). Positive affect has favorable associations with blood pressure, heart rate, and inflammatory markers (Steptoe et al., 2009), while predicting recovery of ill patients (Lamers et al., 2012) and longevity (Petrie et al., 2018). Happiness also predicts various life outcomes, such as better work performance (Bellet et al., 2023), career success (Walsh et al., 2018), higher income later in life (Neve & Oswald, 2012), probability of getting married and having children (Luhmann et al., 2013), and higher relationship quality (Moore et al., 2018). These and other benefits of happiness have been extensively reviewed (De Neve et al., 2013; Diener et al., 2018; Howell et al., 2007; Lyubomirsky et al., 2005).

Notwithstanding the long line of evidence of the positive effects of happiness, it is worth noting that extreme levels of happiness can also have drawbacks (Oishi et al., 2007). Negative emotions signal us that there is something wrong in our situation, leading to attempts to alter the situation (Baumeister et al., 2001). Thus, unhappiness can work as a crucial trigger to leave an abusive relationship or an oppressive work, while unbridled cheerfulness can make one ignore various risks. For example, one study showed that extremely cheerful people may engage in riskier behavior and be more careless about health and safety (Martin et al., 2002), and another found that those believing that positive self-talk and "manifestation" will attract success in life were more likely to engage in risky investments and have experienced bankruptcy (Dixon et al., 2025). A person's happiness should thus stay responsive to environmental conditions. Feeling happy in situations where one should not feel happy can be maladaptive and hinder the person from making the necessary changes or from taking the necessary precautions.

Finally, besides all the potential benefits, it is worth remembering that it also feels good—by definition—to experience positive emotions, making happiness into a pleasant state to be in. It is simply nicer to be happy than to be suffering. Thus, while extreme and unresponsive levels of happiness can become maladaptive, being relatively happy and content with life seems to be a situation worth having in life.

THE COMPLEX RELATIONSHIP BETWEEN PURSUING HAPPINESS AND BEING HAPPY

While being happy is by and large a good thing, pursuing happiness has received more criticism. First, people may not always be very skillful in their pursuit of happiness, seeking it in the wrong places utilizing the wrong strategies. Research on affective forecasting—the attempt to estimate the emotional consequences of various life events—has shown that people often mispredict how much and how durable pleasure or displeasure certain future events will bring about (Wilson & Gilbert, 2005). For example, the happiness benefits of material purchases tend to be small and short-lived (Van Boven & Gilovich, 2003), yet people often imagine that they would be happier if they just owned a certain product. At worst, this pursuit of happiness through material dreams can turn into a hedonic treadmill, where happiness is always behind the next purchase, which when acquired disappoints in its ability to bring about happiness, leading to an increased attempt to pursue the next material goal. Focus on personal happiness might also make people ignore other people and their needs, which easily can turn detrimental for one's personal happiness, as high-quality relationships and the ability to do good to others are one of the most robust sources of happiness. Conscious pursuit of happiness may thus fail because people may do it in the wrong way.

In addition to identifying poor strategies to attain happiness, the attempt to pursue happiness has been more directly challenged by a stream of research. In 2011, an experimental study on the paradoxical effects of valuing happiness made the headlines (Mauss et al., 2011). Half of the participants were made to read a passage about the benefits of being happy to induce them to value happiness before watching a video clip about a female skater winning a gold medal and celebrating afterward. Despite trying harder to feel positive, those in the valuing happiness condition reported less positive affect after watching the film compared to a neutral control condition. Their willingness to be happy seemed to stand in the way of them actually feeling happy. Other research showed that a similar manipulation made participants feel lonelier after watching a film clip activating intimacy and affiliation themes (Mauss et al., 2012), while cross-sectional research has shown that extremely valuing happiness is associated with less subjective well-being (Mauss et al., 2011), more self-reported and clinician-rated depressive symptoms (Ford et al., 2014), and more depressive symptoms also in youth samples (Gentzler et al., 2019). One study found that this relationship was moderated by participants' expectations about whether they could alleviate their negative moods such that valuing happiness was associated with depressive symptoms only when individuals believed they could not alter their negative mood (Fergus & Bardeen, 2016). These studies have led to the suggestion that the pursuit of happiness can backfire, paradoxically making the person less happy (Gruber et al., 2011; Zerwas & Ford, 2021). However, it is worth noting that a factor analysis of the scale used in these studies revealed that the negative associations with well-being seem to be mostly driven by items focusing on the worry about the possibility of being unhappy (Luhmann et al., 2016). So it could be that avoiding unhappiness is more detrimental to well-being than mere desire for happiness. In line with this, Humphrey and colleagues (2022) noticed that the tendency to avoid depressive or anxious feelings was associated with more symptoms of depression.

Other research has shown that the mere monitoring of one's own happiness can be detrimental for the happiness itself. When students were asked to report their current happiness three or six times daily, this had a detrimental effect on the happiness of those participants higher in depressive symptoms or neuroticism (Conner & Reid, 2012), supposedly because frequent reporting reminded them of their not-so-good mood, which further sank their mood. Introspecting about one's reasons for a consumer choice can also, in some conditions, reduce post-choice satisfaction (Wilson et al., 1993). Also, entertaining positive fantasies about one's future, while soothing in the moment, can impede the hard work necessary to make that future happen, and thus contribute to more depression over time (Oettingen et al., 2016). We also know that people experiencing major depressive disorder tend to have a discrepancy between how they are feeling and how they think they should be feeling (Thompson et al., 2016).

Too much focus on one's own happiness and too urgent striving to be happy and avoid unhappiness can thus make one less happy. However, such negative effects depend on how one is pursuing happiness. Catalino and colleagues (2014) argued that trying to change one's emotions in the moment—by striving to maximize the happiness one is experiencing, for example—tends to not work. Research has shown that expressive suppression of emotions is associated with depressive symptoms (Fergus & Bardeen, 2016). Catalino and colleagues suggested that a more effective strategy for pursuing happiness would have people "putting themselves in situations in which they are likely to experience happiness" (p. 1556). They provided cross-sectional (Catalino et al., 2014) and daily diary study (Catalino & Tov, 2022) evidence that this strategy of *prioritizing positivity* is positively correlated with well-being, while extreme valuing of happiness is indeed negatively correlated with well-being (replicated in Hansenne, 2021).

Overall, there is a need for more research before firm conclusions can be made. However, current research seems to show that attempting to suppress negative emotions and force one's feelings to be positive is a maladaptive emotion regulation strategy that easily has the opposite outcome than intended. Negative emotions serve an important function in human self-regulation by alerting us that something may be wrong (Carver & Scheier, 1990; Roth et al., 2019). Thus, instead of attempting to change one's emotions directly, it seems better to treat emotions as signals that could trigger one to make changes to one's behavior, attitudes, or environment that are causing the negative emotions. Integrative emotion regulation, involving a nonjudgmental, receptive attention to one's emotional experience where one explores one's emotions as potentially relevant signals about how well the current situation aligns with one's goals and needs, has been shown to be a beneficial way of approaching one's emotions (Roth et al., 2019). For example, a compassionate and accepting attitude toward oneself and one's own emotions—especially the negative ones—has been shown to be good for one's well-being (Neff, 2011, 2023). Instead of either ignoring or actively suppressing negative emotions, individuals are better off when they attend to them in an accepting and curious way, trying to learn from them.

A BRIEF HISTORY OF THE (WESTERN) PURSUIT OF HAPPINESS

Has humankind always pursued happiness? In a certain sense, definitely. Something feeling pleasant and another thing feeling unpleasant originally served the evolutionary purpose of making some experiences attractive and other experiences avoidable. Avoiding pain and seeking pleasure is part of our biological makeup, an instinct we humans share with most other animals. On the other hand, happiness as a conscious goal, something one should value and aim for in life, is a relatively recent invention (McMahon, 2004; Oishi et al., 2013). Even the whole concept of happiness, as referring to a positive internal psychological state, is something that took some time to be invented.

Croesus, the wealthy king of Lydia, asked Solon, supposedly the wisest man of his time, whether he was the happiest man on Earth. "Man is entirely what befalls him. . . . I cannot say of you yet, until I hear that you have brought your life to an end well," Solon replied (Herodotus, 1987, 1.32). In *The History* by Herodotus, written around 430 B.C.E., one finds a very different conception of happiness than in the modern era. In fact, translating *eudaimonia,* the term that Herodotus used, as "happiness" will mislead the reader, and thus a better translation would be "flourishing." Eudaimonia was not a psychological concept focusing on some inner state of the person in question but rather focused on a "broad idea of a life's going well" (Annas, 1995, p. 44). In Herodotus's case, eudaimonia was mainly about good fortune in life in the sense of being able to fulfill one's role and avoiding any great misfortunes that may befall a human being (McMahon, 2006).

This intimate connection between happiness and having a good lot in life is visible in the etymology of happiness. *Happiness* has its root in the Middle English *happ*, which meant chance, fortune, and what *happ*ens in the world, while Italian, Spanish, and Portuguese *felicità*, *felicidad*, and *felicidade* all originate from the Latin *felix*, meaning luck and fate. The French *bonheur* combines *bon* (good) and *heur* (fortune or luck), the German *Glück* has still the double meaning of referring to both happiness and luck, and the same is true of the Finnish *onni*. As Darrin McMahon concluded, "happiness at the dawn of Western history was largely a matter of chance" (McMahon, 2006, p. 7), something befalling a human being based on external factors largely beyond one's control.

Aristotle, living a century after Herodotus, challenged the external focus of eudaimonia, by bringing human conduct to the fore (Aristotle, 2012). Human *telos*, meaning the specific human good or goal, stems from humans having a unique ability to live in accordance with reason, with the most complete way to live according to reason being living virtuously (Ryan & Martela, 2016). Thus Aristotle, while giving some role to the external factors as well, came to emphasize living virtuously as the core of eudaimonia, famously arguing that eudaimonia is about a "certain activity of soul in accord with complete virtue" (Aristotle, 2012, p. 23). For external events one can't control, one can decide how one conducts one's self. This focus on one's way of living is also visible in, for example, the Stoics. Although the ancient Greek and Roman philosophers talked to some degree about emotions, mainly about how to temper them, the main focus was on virtuous conduct and fulfilling one's role, rather than on the pursuit of positive feelings as its own goal.

The modern Western conception of happiness started to take shape during the Enlightenment. Especially central was John Locke's contribution, who argued that humans are born *tabula rasa*, without innate ideas, guided simply by the sensations of pleasure and pain (Locke, 2014, p. 220): Pleasure in humans "is that we call good, and what is apt to produce pain in us, we call evil." Thus, as part of an overall turn toward individualism and focus on self and one's emotions (Baumeister, 1987), Locke elevated happiness to something we humans strive for and should strive for. While having been mainly a distraction from or at best a side effect of virtuous living, happiness itself became something valuable by itself (McMahon, 2004). Here Locke can be seen as a symptom of and articulator of an overall individualization of Western culture. One's personal opinions and how one feels acquired much more weight in people's life choices and ideas about how one should live. In previous more collectivistic societies, one's role in the community and the duties emerging from it took precedence over individual feelings and preferences. One should contain one's feelings in order to fulfill one's role. In contrast, in the Enlightenment view what one personally wants and what one personally feels are given much more moral weight (Baumeister, 1987). It became acceptable and even recommended to pursue happiness. This was true as a societal goal, as famously inscribed in the U.S. Declaration of Independence, where each human is declared to have unalienable rights for "life, liberty, and the pursuit of happiness." But happiness also became increasingly seen as a relevant individual goal, something we all have the right to pursue—and often also something that we should pursue. All of this contributed to the development where "this option would make me happy" has become a much more weighty argument in situations of choice (Oishi et al., 2013).

It is important to realize that this modern conception of the role of happiness involves a few separate theses. It is important to explicate them, as they easily are taken for granted in modern Western culture.

1. *Everyone has the right to pursue happiness.* This is a liberating ideal that emphasizes that all human beings should have the freedom to pursue happiness in their own life. Instead of having to accept one's role and its duties—which especially for women tended to be very narrowly defined—one's own happiness is relevant and worthy of being defended. Taking each individual's happiness seriously and giving it weight in (political) decision making was a rather radical idea in the 17th century and was closely tied with the rise of modern democratic societies. Through this development, a person's own feelings, values, and dreams have acquired more weight and value. Instead of

just emphasizing what one ought to do given one's social position, modern individualistic societies give voice to individuals, allowing them to have much more say in their personal life choices. This has likely had a significant positive influence on people's happiness. For example, political scientists Inglehart and colleagues (2008) and Welzel (2013) have found empirical support for their theses that increased freedom in societies contributes to increased happiness among their citizens.

2. *Happiness and morality are two separate factors in a good life.* In many worldviews, such as in many philosophical systems of ancient Greeks and Romans, happiness was an inevitable side-product of virtuous living, and Christianity promised that virtuous behavior is rewarded by happiness and bliss in the afterlife (McMahon, 2006). When happiness started to be seen as valuable by itself, its separation from other values, especially moral obligations, became more evident. This thesis, especially clearly articulated by Immanuel Kant, argues that we humans sometimes face choices where the morally right option is not the one making us happy. While doing the morally right thing is often rewarding in itself and often rewarded by others, sometimes making the virtuous choice entails pain and suffering.

3. *Everyone ought to pursue happiness.* The right to pursue happiness easily transforms into a duty to pursue happiness. If happiness indeed is something everyone should value, is it not also something everyone ought to pursue? Robert Ringer's (1977) bestseller *Looking Out for Number 1* sold 2 million copies in the United States, preaching the gospel of self-interest and pursuit of the greatest amount of happiness for yourself. In their classic study, sociologist Robert Bellah and his colleagues (1985) noticed that some persons in the United States whom they researched tended to behave prosocially but—when asked about it—they tended to invent explanations for their behavior that dismissed altruistic motives and instead framed the behavior as serving themselves. These people thus seemed reluctant to admit that their behavior followed other than self-serving motives, arguably because they had learned in their culture that one should "always look after number one." This kind of cultural ideal thus aims to reduce the plurality of human motives and values into one, the pursuit of personal happiness.

While highly contested even in the most individualistic countries—most see the naked pursuit of self-interest as a vice rather than a virtue—such concerns carry more moral weight in individualistic countries, leading some to take this to the extreme. Furthermore, the assumptions behind modern economic theories upon which our market society is built tend to emphasize self-interest as a key explanation for human behavior. It is emblematic that students of economics behave more selfishly in various monetary experiments compared to other students—mainly because they expect everyone else to behave more selfishly (Gerlach, 2017). Self-interest has thus become more accepted in individualistic consumer societies, with some even seeing it as a virtue.

4. *Everyone ought to be happy.* The normative weight we place on happiness can easily translate into an individual duty to always be happy. If it is "good to feel good," does it not follow that it is "bad to feel bad," or even that sadness is a sin (McMahon, 2004, p. 15)? Traces of this attitude are plentiful in modern culture. For example, at workplaces low employee well-being is often treated as an individual problem, solved through giving individual employees training in, for example, mindfulness, instead of a structural problem solved through changing the conditions of work (Spicer, 2024). If we start to blame individuals for failing to be happy, we put a double burden on them: Not only are they sad but they have also failed to live up to the standards of our culture. When sadness amounts to a personal failure, this is a harmful cultural ideal that is prone to make miserable moments in life more intolerable.

How dominant these four ideals are in modern Western societies remains to be debated. They all carry some weight, but at the same time, humans are moved by other ideals derived from religion and tradition that recognize other virtues and put less emphasis on personal happiness (MacIntyre, 2007). Yet it can be argued that each of the four theses is more strongly present in modern Western societies than in almost any other era. By making them explicit, one can become more aware of the normative assumptions one easily makes about happiness.

The Role of Existentialism in the History of Happiness

Having offered a very brief historical account of how people's relation to happiness has changed in modern individualistic societies, it is worth noting that existentialism as a philosophical tradition has played an important role in this development. While the definition and history of existentialism is examined in more detail in other chapters, one way of understanding this tradition is to see it as a reaction to the possibility that life might lack any lasting value or meaning (Martela, 2023). The human being is "cast into this world . . . condemned to be free" without any "luminous realm of values" providing "justification or excuse" as Sartre (2007, p. 27) famously summarized the existentialist human condition. Key themes in this philosophical and literary tradition include the lack of predetermined values and meaning, a direct confrontation with the absurdity of human existence, the inescapability of human freedom, and the importance of living authentically (Solomon, 2005; Warnock, 1970). While the kernel of the movement took place in post-World War II France and included thinkers like Sartre, de Beauvoir, and Camus, existentialist themes were already discussed in the 19th century by authors like Kierkegaard, Nietzsche, Tolstoy, and Dostoyevsky, among others. They were inspired by and contributed to a shift in worldview taking place during that era, where humans were slowly liberated from predetermined roles and God-given duties, and instead were encouraged to take their own feelings, dreams, and values into account when deciding how to live their lives. The rise of the scientific worldview challenged religious doctrines and the God-given purpose of life, leading to a relatively widespread spiritual crisis in educated circles (Gilmour, 1993; Martela, 2023). Existentialist thinkers felt this crisis and aimed to offer completely new ways of addressing questions about purpose and meaning, by suggesting that meaning could be found "from within," through soul-searching and listening to one's own values.

Existentialists thus significantly contributed to the development of individualism by emphasizing personal freedom and reliance on one's own values and ideals, rather than blind conformity to externally given norms. However, the way of living they offered was not narrowly focused on personal happiness. Finding meaning in life, rather than happiness, tended to be the main concern of existentialist writers. Instead of focusing just on oneself, one was to find something valuable to do with one's life, which often meant various prosocial pursuits in the service of humankind. The difference to other thought traditions was that these valuable pursuits were not given from outside but found from within. One was free, yet in search of something valuable to do with this thing called life—and pursuits we tend to find valuable tend to involve other people (Martela, 2020).

As a very rough characterization, I could separate two questions of individualism: Who decides what you should do in your life—you or others? And who should your life serve—you or others? The key message of existentialism was to awaken people to take their lives into their own hands, thus emphasizing personal freedom as regards the first question. However, this should not be interpreted as entailing a self-focused answer to the second question—one can be free yet voluntarily choose to serve others (Wuthnow, 1991). As the protoexistentialist Thomas Carlyle (1991, pp. 148–149) put it in 1834, "Do the Duty which lies nearest thee . . . the Ideal is in thyself."

HOW DIFFERENT CULTURES APPROACH HAPPINESS—AND HOW THAT AFFECTS PEOPLE'S HAPPINESS IN THOSE CULTURES

The foregoing analysis of the historical conceptions of happiness in Western societies highlights that societies can have different ideals about what kind of emotions one should seek out and experience. This is something recent cross-cultural research has confirmed. For example, a comparison of 27 nations demonstrated differences in participants' ideal levels of happiness and pleasure, with participants from more holistic Asian cultures that emphasize moderation and acceptance of contradictions having lower estimates of their ideal levels (Hornsey et al., 2018). A comparison of U.S., Australian, Chinese, and Taiwanese samples showed that people in the two former nations were more likely to view all positive emotions as desirable and appropriate than were people from the latter two (Eid & Diener, 2001). Furthermore, in individualistic cultures life satisfaction and positive emotions tend to correlate more than in collectivistic cultures, signaling that in individualistic cultures people put more emphasis on their own feelings when evaluating their lives (Suh et al., 1998). In contrast, in collectivistic cultures, cultural norms about the desirability of life satisfaction were a more important predictor of life satisfaction than they were in individualistic cultures. There are also differences as regards ideal affects, with American cultures valuing more high-arousal positive affective states such as excitement and enthusiasm, and East Asian cultures valuing more low-arousal positive affective states like calmness and sense of harmony (Tsai, 2007; Tsai et al., 2006). Interestingly, a comparison of bestselling storybooks for small children in the United States and in Taiwan revealed that the former contained wider smiles and more excited than calm faces, thus contributing to the socialization of ideal affect already from a young age (Tsai et al., 2007). Comparing European American and Asian American U.S. students, Wirtz and colleagues (2009) found that the former emphasized positive affect more, when evaluating vacations, friendships, and life in general. A similar comparison of Canadian students of European and East Asian backgrounds found that the latter put less weight on expected enjoyment in making decisions about various options (Falk et al., 2010). In interpreting these results, however, it is important to note that besides differences between nations, the studies tended to find significant intranational variance (e.g., Eid & Diener, 2001), indicating that within any single nation, there might be people with a variety of cultural ideals and norms.

Recently, empirical research has started to investigate what effects such societal ideals and expectancies about well-being have on individual well-being. One study examined societal pressures to be happy and societal pressures to not be sad in 40 countries, finding that especially the latter led to lower average well-being, with this relationship being particularly strong in happier countries (Dejonckheere et al., 2022). Bastian and colleagues (2012) found both correlational and experimental evidence for their thesis that participants perceiving social expectancies to not feel negative emotions have more negative self-evaluations, and consequently experience less well-being. In a daily diary study, they found that such social expectancies led to a stronger link between depressive symptoms and feelings of loneliness (Bastian et al., 2015). Similarly, Dejonckheere and colleagues (2017) found in a diary study among individuals with elevated depression scores that perceived social pressure not to feel depressed predicted increases in the severity of symptoms of depression. Such social pressures not to feel negative emotions were also associated with a more negative self-concept (Dejonckheere & Bastian, 2021). McGuirk and colleagues (2018), in turn, conducted an experiment to show that when participants were placed in a context emphasizing the value of positive feelings, they tended to ruminate more and experience more negative emotions after failing at a task compared to a control group.

On the other hand, Bastian and colleagues (2014) found, in a sample of college students from 47 countries, that higher average life satisfaction was associated with higher perceptions of positive emotions being valued in one's society, thus suggesting that placing cultural value on positive emotions might not have a negative effect on individual well-being. Societal valuing of negative emotions, in contrast, was not associated (either positively or negatively) with well-being. Joshanloo and colleagues (2014) found in a study of 14 nations that fear of happiness—beliefs that being happy might have negative consequences—was associated with attempts to dampen one's emotions and with lower levels of life satisfaction on an individual level, while cultural levels of fear of happiness also predicted lower subjective well-being. Fear of happiness has also been associated with depressive symptoms (Jordan et al., 2021). Ford and colleagues (2015), in turn, found that while the strong valuing of happiness was negatively associated with well-being in the United States, it had a positive association with well-being in Russia and combined Japan-Taiwan sample. The researchers reasoned that this was likely due to more socially engaged ways of pursuing happiness in the latter, more collectivistic contexts.

WHERE TO FIND HAPPINESS? AND WHERE NOT?

Different cultures and historical eras both define and value happiness differently. However, if one still concludes that it is a worthwhile pursuit, where can one most reliably find happiness, according to research?

Most importantly, a person needs to make sure they are born in the right country. International comparisons using representative samples from various countries have made it clear that society plays a major role in people's well-being and happiness. The Cantril Ladder asks people to evaluate their lives on a scale from 0 to 10, where 0 is the worst possible life and 10 is the best possible life. The average responses by country vary dramatically, with people in Finland, Denmark, and Iceland having average scores of 7.8, 7.6, and 7.5, respectively (Helliwell et al., 2023). Only 3% of Finnish respondents had life satisfaction below the midpoint of the scale (0–4) (Organization for Economic Co-operation and Development, 2021). Compare this with Afghanistan, where the *average* life satisfaction was 1.9, meaning that most everyone rated their life as close to the worst possible life. In Lebanon, life satisfaction was 2.4, in Sierra Leone 3.1, and in Zimbabwe and Congo 3.2. Given that these are country averages, these data tell that there is a dramatic difference in happiness depending on where one lives one's life—in some countries most citizens are relatively happy with their lives, in others most are miserable. No amount of gratitude diaries, mindfulness exercises, small acts of kindness, or other popular "happiness habits" are able to outdo the impact of living in a war-torn country without access to basic health care and with one's children starving. On average, relatively wealthy countries with free speech, free press, and free elections, low corruption, strong rule of law, relatively extensive welfare benefits, and relatively good gender equality are the ones where one has the best chance of being happy (Audette et al., 2019; Helliwell et al., 2018; Martela et al., 2020).

Another relatively stable factor in well-being is one's personality. Twin studies and other evidence have highlighted that there is a genetic component to happiness, with the heritability of subjective well-being estimated to be in the .30 to .40 range (Bartels, 2015; Nes & Røysamb, 2017), correlating negatively with neuroticism, and positively with extraversion and openness to experience (Weiss et al., 2008) but in general being somewhat more fluctuating than such personality traits (Anusic & Schimmack, 2016).

However, despite such relatively stable factors in well-being, the once popular "happiness set-point," "hedonic adaptation," and "hedonic treadmill" approaches to happiness have been shown to have exaggerated their case (Diener et al., 2006; Luhmann & Intelisano, 2018). Such models suggested that while various life events could temporarily make people more or less happy, people's happiness tends to return to a stable set point (e.g., Brickman et al., 1978). Later research has shown that people indeed have had a tendency to adapt to various life events such as a divorce, making their effect wear off after a few years. In contrast, incidents such as becoming unemployed, suffering a spinal cord injury, or becoming widowed have tended to lead to a relatively permanent decrease of well-being (see Diener et al., 2006; Luhmann & Intelisano, 2018). Various positive and negative events and factors in life thus influence people's levels of happiness.

In identifying what kind of life conditions tend to bring about happiness, research on human basic needs is especially useful. It is fairly obvious that one's physical needs being unmet or threatened tends to bring about unhappiness (Maslow, 1943): Hunger, lack of shelter, and lack of protection against various threats such as predators or robbery cause suffering. Accordingly, data from 123 countries showed that deficits in basic physical needs are strongly correlated with lower life satisfaction and more negative emotions across the world (Tay & Diener, 2011; see also Diener et al., 2010).

More positively, the presence of certain psychological needs tends to bring about happiness. There is especially robust evidence about the importance of autonomy, competence, and relatedness for human well-being (Martela & Ryan, 2023; Ryan & Deci, 2000, 2017). *Autonomy* is about a sense of volition and self-endorsement of one's actions; *competence* is about a sense of mastery, effectance, and accomplishment; and *relatedness* is about a sense of caring close relationships. Research from contexts ranging from workplaces (Van den Broeck et al., 2016) and education (Jang et al., 2016) to sports coaching (Curran et al., 2016), including cross-cultural work (Chen et al., 2015; Chirkov et al., 2003; Martela et al., 2023), has shown that the satisfaction of these three psychological needs is a key determinant of people's well-being and happiness. Accordingly, individuals interested in their own well-being are wise to migrate to need-satisfying contexts to the extent that they have a choice as regards these contexts.

Besides the circumstantial factors and genetic personality factors, there is also room for individual habits, attitudes, and activities to make a difference to a person's happiness levels (Sheldon & Lyubomirsky, 2021). Especially robust and cross-culturally validated experimental evidence suggests that engaging in prosocial acts like helping other people increases one's own happiness (Aknin et al., 2013; Hui et al., 2020). Accordingly, often the best intentional strategy to improve one's own happiness is to make someone else happy. Furthermore, having some personal goals in life and being able to successfully pursue them tends to increase happiness, with a meta-analysis finding an attenuation-corrected population correlation of .43 between goal progress and well-being (Klug & Maier, 2015).

Besides engaging in certain activities, cultivating certain attitudes toward life has also been found to be beneficial for well-being. Engaging in mindfulness—defined as a state of being attentive to and aware of what is taking place in the present without judgment or appraisal (Brown & Ryan, 2003; Shapiro et al., 2006)—has been found to improve well-being in many interventions across the world (Galante et al., 2021; Reangsing et al., 2021). Also, many other types of interventions have been tested and found to improve people's well-being, such as expressing gratitude, practicing self-compassion, or using one's strengths in a new way (for meta-analyses, see Bolier et al., 2013; White et al., 2019). Thus, there are individual strategies one can engage in to increase one's happiness, including engaging in prosocial behavior, identifying personally valued goals to pursue, or building more mindfulness.

Before closing, it is worth noting that science has a hard time capturing the dramatic changes in life outlook that philosophical contemplation and spiritual practice can sometimes cause. Stories have been passed on for generations about spiritually enlightened individuals, and life-philosophical schools like Stoicism, Epicureanism, Theravāda-Buddhism, or Sufism have devised contemplative exercises and lifelong paths toward a new orientation to life that Buddhists call *nirvana* and Stoics call *ataraxia*. The experience of saints and sages is hard to capture with large-*N* empirical studies. So, we should not dismiss the anecdotal evidence of exceptional individuals being able to find happiness even under the direst conditions. Indeed, while positive psychology interventions tend to be temporary and small-scale, there is a mostly untouched frontier to study what the long-term practice of a life-philosophical school does to a person's happiness. Here would also be room to study the influence of existentialism on happiness. Reading Nietzsche, Sartre, de Beauvoir, Camus, or Dostoyevsky has been, anecdotally, a transformative experience for many people across generations. Capturing what changes to a person's attitudes, worldview, and well-being such transformative experiences cause would open up a new way to understand the impact that existentialism can have on people.

CONCLUSION: HAPPINESS AS A SIDE EFFECT OF A LIFE WELL LIVED

What should we conclude about the role of happiness in a life well lived? Is happiness an empty hedonic pipe dream or a central building block of a good life? Having reviewed the evidence and historical developments, it is time to attempt an answer. In Aristotelian spirit, I would suggest that a balanced view where one is not obsessed with happiness but not indifferent to it either is recommendable. It is advisable to take one's own happiness into account in life choices but it—especially short-term happiness—should not be the only factor that counts. A balanced human life tends to require goals beyond oneself and one's own happiness, and as social animals, we tend to care about the happiness of others as well. Humans can have values and ideals that they find more worthy than the mere focus on their personal happiness—and paradoxically, by putting more emphasis on these, they can actually become happier. John Stuart Mill (1874, p. 142) realized this already more than a century ago when he noted that "Those only are happy (I thought) who have their minds fixed on some object other than their own happiness," such as "the happiness of others" or "the improvement of mankind."

Accordingly, I find the individualization development of the last few centuries both important and liberating. Instead of pawns in a social group that takes precedence over them, individual human beings have value, and their own interests, dreams, and feelings are recognized and valued. The democratization of societies builds on the ideal that each citizen matters and should have the right and freedom for self-determination and pursuit of their own ideal of happiness. These ideals are worth defending and have contributed to the liberation of many previously oppressed groups.

However, the recognition of the importance of each individual's happiness can turn detrimental, when it leads to societal obligation to be happy. Everyone should be free to pursue their own happiness, but people should not be obliged to pursue happiness—and they should not feel pressured to be happy. When happiness becomes a norm, that becomes a burden on individuals, as nobody is going to be happy all the time. Such a norm easily leads to dysfunctional emotion regulation strategies, such as attempts to suppress one's negative emotions. Thus, on a societal level, freedom to pursue happiness should not be combined with a normative pressure to constantly be happy.

Furthermore, on the societal level, it is important to recognize that structural factors to a large degree determine individual happiness. While it is good to identify strategies that individuals can use to increase their own well-being, this should not come at the cost of ignoring the social and structural context within which individuals aim to pursue happiness. "The risk is that this science ends up blaming—and medicating—individuals for their own misery, and ignores the context that has contributed to it," as Davies (2015, p. 6) put it. The pursuit of happiness, on a societal level, should be first and foremost an attempt to build institutions, regulations, and social conditions that are most conducive to happiness.

On an individual level, a healthy way of approaching one's own happiness involves accepting negative emotions as an inevitable part of life, and recognizing that sadness, grief, and even anger are inevitable parts of life and the appropriate emotional reactions in certain life situations. Much of what happens in one's life—starting with one's genetic makeup, the country one was born in, and who one's parents were—is beyond one's personal control. Accordingly, a significant chunk of one's personal happiness is determined by factors that one doesn't have much influence over. Whatever starting point they give for one's personal pursuit of happiness, it is advisable to learn to accept one's situation. It is also important to understand that sadness, disappointment, and other negative emotions are an inevitable part of any life, and thus the best one can do is accept them as part of one's own life, too, when the occasion arises.

At the same time, one should not ignore one's own feelings in decision making, as they give us valuable information about how well one's life is going. Positive and negative feelings, more tied with one's biological makeup, give one signals about how well one's basic physical and psychological needs are fulfilled—but also how one is doing against implicitly internalized societal norms (Roth et al., 2019). More evaluative measures such as meaning in life and life satisfaction provide information about how well one's life is going as regards one's more consciously upheld goals, values, and standards of living. This all is valuable information and also valuable as such—it feels good to feel good. In my lectures, I often advise students to approach their happiness as a tool, a kind of thermometer, that it is wise to observe and follow, as in most cases it conveys important information about how well one's life is going. However, it is good to realize that sometimes an individual's feelings can trick them, giving them wrong kinds of signals. For example, one might become upset by something one's spouse said—but mainly because it triggered some bad memory from a past relationship. Trusting the negative emotion in that situation would lead to behavior harmful in the present relationship. Thus, while attending to one's feelings, one should also retain a critical distance to them, not blindly following them.

From an existential point, I would argue that humans aim to live a good life. And happiness in most cases is a by-product of life going well—one's basic needs being satisfied and one's goals and values being realized. Thus, happiness mostly accompanies a good life. However, the modern problem is that "rather than being the by-product of a life well lived, feeling happy has become a goal in itself" (McGuirk et al., 2018, p. 755). Here I would suggest to focus more directly on the factors that tend to make life good and let happiness accompany them when it so happens.

As regards the factors that make life good, let me not downplay the importance of other people. Like John Stuart Mill cited above, I believe that often the best way to make oneself happy is to pursue goals that feel more valuable than one's personal happiness. This involves identifying causes worth fighting for and thinking how one could make a prosocial impact through one's own life. Gioconda Belli (2003, p. 91) recounted her participation in the revolutionary movement against the Somoza dictatorship in Nicaragua in the 1970s as a life-threatening and exhausting struggle. And yet, "What I found most bewildering and extraordinary was the real happiness and fulfillment that came along with commitment. . . . In the struggle for everyone's happiness, the first happiness one found was one's own."

REFERENCES

Aknin, L. B., Barrington-Leigh, C. P., Dunn, E. W., Helliwell, J. F., Burns, J., Biswas-Diener, R., . . . Norton, M. I. (2013). Prosocial spending and well-being: Cross-cultural evidence for a psychological universal. *Journal of Personality and Social Psychology, 104*(4), 635–652.

Annas, J. (1995). *The morality of happiness.* Oxford University Press.

Anusic, I., & Schimmack, U. (2016). Stability and change of personality traits, self-esteem, and well-being: Introducing the meta-analytic stability and change model of retest correlations. *Journal of Personality and Social Psychology, 110*(5), 766–781.

Aristotle. (2012). *Nicomachean ethics* (R. C. Bartlett & S. D. Collins, Trans.). University of Chicago Press.

Audette, A. P., Lam, S., O'Connor, H., & Radcliff, B. (2019). (E)quality of life: A cross-national analysis of the effect of gender equality on life satisfaction. *Journal of Happiness Studies, 20*(7), 2173–2188.

Bartels, M. (2015). Genetics of wellbeing and its components satisfaction with life, happiness, and quality of life: A review and meta-analysis of heritability studies. *Behavior Genetics, 45*(2), 137–156.

Bastian, B., Koval, P., Erbas, Y., Houben, M., Pe, M., & Kuppens, P. (2015). Sad and alone: Social expectancies for experiencing negative emotions are linked to feelings of loneliness. *Social Psychological and Personality Science, 6*(5), 496–503.

Bastian, B., Kuppens, P., De Roover, K., & Diener, E. (2014). Is valuing positive emotion associated with life satisfaction? *Emotion, 14*(4), 639–645.

Bastian, B., Kuppens, P., Hornsey, M. J., Park, J., Koval, P., & Uchida, Y. (2012). Feeling bad about being sad: The role of social expectancies in amplifying negative mood. *Emotion, 12*(1), 69–80.

Baumeister, R. F. (1987). How the self became a problem: A psychological review of historical research. *Journal of Personality and Social Psychology, 52*(1), 163–176.

Baumeister, R. F., Bratslavsky, E., Finkenauer, C., & Vohs, K. D. (2001). Bad is stronger than good. *Review of General Psychology, 5*(4), 323–370.

Bellah, R. N., Sullivan, W. M., Tipton, S. M., Swidler, A., & Madsen, R. P. (1985). *Habits of the heart.* University of California Press.

Bellet, C. S., De Neve, J.-E., & Ward, G. (2023). Does employee happiness have an impact on productivity? *Management Science, 70*(3), 1656–1679.

Belli, G. (2003). *The country under my skin*. Anchor Books.

Bolier, L., Haverman, M., Westerhof, G. J., Riper, H., Smit, F., & Bohlmeijer, E. (2013). Positive psychology interventions: A meta-analysis of randomized controlled studies. *BMC Public Health, 13*(119), 1–20.

Brickman, P., Coates, D., & Janoff-Bulman, R. (1978). Lottery winners and accident victims: Is happiness relative. *Journal of Personality and Social Psychology, 36*(8), 917–927.

Brown, K. W., & Ryan, R. M. (2003). The benefits of being present: Mindfulness and its role in psychological well-being. *Journal of Personality and Social Psychology, 84*(4), 822–848.

Carlyle, T. (1991). *Sartor resartus*. Oxford University Press.

Carver, C. S., & Scheier, M. F. (1990). Origins and functions of positive and negative affect: A control-process view. *Psychological Review, 97*(1), 19–35.

Catalino, L. I., Algoe, S. B., & Fredrickson, B. L. (2014). Prioritizing positivity: An effective approach to pursuing happiness? *Emotion, 14*(6), 1155–1161.

Catalino, L. I., & Tov, W. (2022). Daily variation in prioritizing positivity and well-being. *Emotion, 22*(5), 874–879.

Chen, B., Vansteenkiste, M., Beyers, W., Boone, L., Deci, E. L., Van der Kaap-Deeder, J., . . . Verstuyf, J. (2015). Basic psychological need satisfaction, need frustration, and need strength across four cultures. *Motivation and Emotion, 39*(2), 216–236.

Chirkov, V. I., Ryan, R. M., Kim, Y., & Kaplan, U. (2003). Differentiating autonomy from individualism and independence: A self-determination theory perspective on internalization of cultural orientations and well-being. *Journal of Personality and Social Psychology, 84*(1), 97–110.

Conner, T. S., & Reid, K. A. (2012). Effects of intensive mobile happiness reporting in daily life. *Social Psychological and Personality Science, 3*(3), 315–323.

Curran, T., Hill, A. P., Ntoumanis, N., Hall, H. K., & Jowett, G. E. (2016). A three-wave longitudinal test of self-determination theory's mediation model of engagement and disaffection in youth sport. *Journal of Sport and Exercise Psychology, 38*(1), 15–29.

Dalai Lama. (2010). *The art of happiness: A handbook for living* (H. C. Cutler, Ed.). Riverhead Books.

Davies, W. (2015). *The happiness industry*. Verso Books.

De Neve, J.-E., Diener, E., Tay, L., & Xuereb, C. (2013). The objective benefits of subjective well-being. In J. F. Helliwell, R. Layard, & J. D. Sachs (Eds.), *World happiness report 2013* (pp. 54–79). Sustainable Development Solutions Network.

Dejonckheere, E., & Bastian, B. (2021). Perceiving social pressure not to feel negative is linked to a more negative self-concept. *Journal of Happiness Studies, 22*(2), 667–679.

Dejonckheere, E., Bastian, B., Fried, E. I., Murphy, S. C., & Kuppens, P. (2017). Perceiving social pressure not to feel negative predicts depressive symptoms in daily life. *Depression and Anxiety, 34*(9), 836–844.

Dejonckheere, E., Rhee, J. J., Baguma, P. K., Barry, O., Becker, M., Bilewicz, M., . . . Bastian, B. (2022). Perceiving societal pressure to be happy is linked to poor well-being, especially in happy nations. *Scientific Reports, 12*(1514).

Diener, E. (1984). Subjective well-being. *Psychological Bulletin, 95*(3), 542–575.

Diener, E., Lucas, R. E., & Oishi, S. (2018). Advances and open questions in the science of subjective well-being. *Collabra: Psychology, 4*(1), 1–49.

Diener, E., Lucas, R. E., & Scollon, C. N. (2006). Beyond the hedonic treadmill: Revising the adaptation theory of well-being. *American Psychologist, 61*(4), 305–314.

Diener, E., Ng, W., Harter, J. K., & Arora, R. (2010). Wealth and happiness across the world: Material prosperity predicts life evaluation, whereas psychosocial prosperity predicts positive feeling. *Journal of Personality and Social Psychology, 99*(1), 52–61.

Diener, E., Suh, E., Lucas, R., & Smith, H. (1999). Subjective well-being: Three decades of progress. *Psychological Bulletin, 125*(2), 276–302.

Dixon, L. J., Hornsey, M. J., & Hartley, N. (2025). "The secret" to success?: The psychology of belief in manifestation. *Personality and Social Psychology Bulletin, 51*(1), 49–65.

Eid, M., & Diener, E. (2001). Norms for experiencing emotions in different cultures: Inter-and intranational differences. *Journal of Personality and Social Psychology, 81*(5), 869–885.

Falk, C. F., Dunn, E. W., & Norenzayan, A. (2010). Cultural variation in the importance of expected enjoyment for decision making. *Social Cognition, 28*(5), 609–629.

Fergus, T. A., & Bardeen, J. R. (2016). Negative mood regulation expectancies moderate the association between happiness emotion goals and depressive symptoms. *Personality and Individual Differences, 100*, 23–27.

Ford, B. Q., Dmitrieva, J. O., Heller, D., Chentsova-Dutton, Y., Grossmann, I., Tamir, M., . . . Uhrig, M. (2015). Culture shapes whether the pursuit of happiness predicts higher or lower well-being. *Journal of Experimental Psychology: General, 144*(6), 1053–1062.

Ford, B. Q., Shallcross, A. J., Mauss, I. B., Floerke, V. A., & Gruber, J. (2014). Desperately seeking happiness: Valuing happiness is associated with symptoms and diagnosis of depression. *Journal of Social and Clinical Psychology, 33*(10), 890–905.

Galante, J., Friedrich, C., Dawson, A. F., Modrego-Alarcón, M., Gebbing, P., Delgado-Suárez, I., . . . Jones, P. B. (2021). Mindfulness-based programmes for mental health promotion in adults in nonclinical settings: A systematic review and meta-analysis of randomised controlled trials. *PLOS Medicine, 18*(1), e1003481.

Gentzler, A. L., Palmer, C. A., Ford, B. Q., Moran, K. M., & Mauss, I. B. (2019). Valuing happiness in youth: Associations with depressive symptoms and well-being. *Journal of Applied Developmental Psychology, 62,* 220–230.

Gerlach, P. (2017). The games economists play: Why economics students behave more selfishly than other students. *PLOS One, 12*(9), e0183814.

Gilmour, R. (1993). *The Victorian period: The intellectual and cultural context of English literature 1830–1890.* Longman Group.

Global Wellness Institute. (2024). *Wellness economy statistics and facts. https://globalwellnessinstitute.org/press-room/statistics-and-facts/.*

Gruber, J., Mauss, I. B., & Tamir, M. (2011). A dark side of happiness?: How, when, and why happiness is not always good. *Perspectives on Psychological Science, 6*(3), 222–233.

Hansenne, M. (2021). Valuing happiness is not a good way of pursuing happiness, but prioritizing positivity is: A replication study. *Psychologica Belgica, 61*(1), 306–314.

Helliwell, J. F., Huang, H., Grover, S., & Wang, S. (2018). Empirical linkages between good governance and national well-being. *Journal of Comparative Economics, 46*(4), 1332–1346.

Helliwell, J. F., Layard, R., Sachs, J. D., De Neve, J.-E., Aknin, L. B., & Wang, S. (Eds.). (2023). *World Happiness Report 2023.* Sustainable Development Solutions Network.

Herodotus. (1987). *The history* (D. Grene, Trans.). University of Chicago Press.

Hornsey, M. J., Bain, P. G., Harris, E. A., Lebedeva, N., Kashima, E. S., Guan, Y., . . . Blumen, S. (2018). How much is enough in a perfect world?: Cultural variation in ideal levels of happiness, pleasure, freedom, health, self-esteem, longevity, and intelligence. *Psychological Science, 29*(9), 1393–1404.

Howell, R. T., Kern, M. L., & Lyubomirsky, S. (2007). Health benefits: Meta-analytically determining the impact of well-being on objective health outcomes. *Health Psychology Review, 1*(1), 83–136.

Hui, B. P. H., Ng, J. C. K., Berzaghi, E., Cunningham-Amos, L. A., & Kogan, A. (2020). Rewards of kindness?: A meta-analysis of the link between prosociality and well-being. *Psychological Bulletin, 146*(12), 1084–1116.

Humphrey, A., Szoka, R., & Bastian, B. (2022). When the pursuit of happiness backfires: The role of negative emotion valuation. *Journal of Positive Psychology, 17*(5), 611–619.

Inglehart, R., Foa, R., Peterson, C., & Welzel, C. (2008). Development, freedom, and rising happiness: A global perspective (1981–2007). *Perspectives on Psychological Science, 3*(4), 264–285.

Jang, H., Kim, E. J., & Reeve, J. (2016). Why students become more engaged or more disengaged during the semester: A self-determination theory dual-process model. *Learning and Instruction, 43,* 27–38.

Jordan, D. G., Collins, A. C., Dunaway, M. G., Kilgore, J., & Winer, E. S. (2021). Negative affect interference and fear of happiness are independently associated with depressive symptoms. *Journal of Clinical Psychology, 77*(3), 646–660.

Joshanloo, M., Lepshokova, Z. K., Panyusheva, T., Natalia, A., Poon, W.-C., Yeung, V. W.-I. . . . Jiang, D.-Y. (2014). Cross-cultural validation of Fear of Happiness Scale across 14 national groups. *Journal of Cross-Cultural Psychology, 45*(2), 246–264.

Klug, H. J. P., & Maier, G. W. (2015). Linking goal progress and subjective well-being: A meta-analysis. *Journal of Happiness Studies, 16*(1), 37–65.

Lamers, S. M. A., Bolier, L., Westerhof, G. J., Smit, F., & Bohlmeijer, E. T. (2012). The impact of emotional well-being on long-term recovery and survival in physical illness: A meta-analysis. *Journal of Behavioral Medicine, 35*(5), 538–547.

Locke, J. (2014). *An essay concerning human understanding.* Wordsworth.

Luhmann, M., & Intelisano, S. (2018). Hedonic adaptation and the set point for subjective well-being. In E. Diener, S. Oishi, & L. Tay (Eds.), *Handbook of well-being* (pp. 1–25). DEF Publishers.

Luhmann, M., Lucas, R. E., Eid, M., & Diener, E. (2013). The prospective effect of life satisfaction on life events. *Social Psychological and Personality Science, 4*(1), 39–45.

Luhmann, M., Necka, E. A., Schönbrodt, F. D., & Hawkley, L. C. (2016). Is valuing happiness associated with lower well-being?: A factor-level analysis using the Valuing Happiness Scale. *Journal of Research in Personality, 60,* 46–50.

Lyubomirsky, S., King, L., & Diener, E. (2005). The benefits of frequent positive affect: Does happiness lead to success? *Psychological Bulletin, 131*(6), 803–855.

MacIntyre, A. (2007). *After virtue* (3rd ed.). University of Notre Dame Press.

Martela, F. (2020). *A Wonderful life: Insights on finding a meaningful existence.* Harper Design.

Martela, F. (2023). Crisis of meaning in Sartor Resartus—Thomas Carlyle's pioneering work in articulating and addressing the existential confrontation. *The Pluralist, 18*(2), 80–106.

Martela, F., Greve, B., Rothstein, B., & Saari, J. (2020). The Nordic exceptionalism: What explains why the Nordic countries are constantly among the happiest in the world. In J. F. Helliwell, R. Layard, J. Sachs, & J.-E. De Neve (Eds.), *World Happiness Report 2020* (pp. 129–146). Sustainable Development Solutions Network.

Martela, F., Lehmus-Sun, A., Parker, P. D., Pessi, A. B., & Ryan, R. M. (2023). Needs and well-being across Europe: Basic psychological needs are closely connected with well-being, meaning, and symptoms of depression in 27 European countries. *Social Psychological and Personality Science, 14*(5), 501–514.

Martela, F., & Ryan, R. M. (2023). Clarifying eudaimonia and psychological functioning to complement evaluative and experiential well-being—Why basic psychological needs should be measured in national accounts of well-being. *Perspectives on Psychological Science, 18*(5), 1121–1135.

Martin, L. R., Friedman, H. S., Tucker, J. S., Tomlinson-Keasey, C., Criqui, M. H., & Schwartz, J. E. (2002). A life course perspective on childhood cheerfulness and its relation to mortality risk. *Personality and Social Psychology Bulletin, 28*(9), 1155–1165.

Maslow, A. H. (1943). A theory of human motivation. *Psychological Review, 50*(4), 370–396.

Mauss, I. B., Savino, N. S., Anderson, C. L., Weisbuch, M., Tamir, M., & Laudenslager, M. L. (2012). The pursuit of happiness can be lonely. *Emotion, 12*(5), 908–912.

Mauss, I. B., Tamir, M., Anderson, C. L., & Savino, N. S. (2011). Can seeking happiness make people unhappy? Paradoxical effects of valuing happiness. *Emotion, 11*(4), 807–815.

McGuirk, L., Kuppens, P., Kingston, R., & Bastian, B. (2018). Does a culture of happiness increase rumination over failure? *Emotion, 18*(5), 755–764.

McKinsey. (2021, August 4). *The future of the $1.5 trillion wellness market.* www.mckinsey.com/industries/consumer-packaged-goods/our-insights/feeling-good-the-future-of-the-1-5-trillion-wellness-market.

McMahon, D. M. (2004). From the happiness of virtue to the virtue of happiness: 400 B.C.–A.D.2 1780. *Daedalus, 133*(2), 5–17.

McMahon, D. M. (2006). *The pursuit of happiness: A history from the Greeks to the present.* Allen Lane.

Mill, J. S. (1874). *Autobiography.* Longmans, Green, Reader, and Dyer.

Moore, S., Diener, E., & Tan, K. (2018). Using multiple methods to more fully understand causal relations: Positive affect enhances social relationships. In E. Diener, S. Oishi, & L. Tay (Eds.), *Handbook of well-being* (pp. 1–17). Noba Scholar.

Neff, K. D. (2011). Self-compassion, self-esteem, and well-being. *Social and Personality Psychology Compass, 5*(1), 1–12.

Neff, K. D. (2023). Self-compassion: Theory, method, research, and intervention. *Annual Review of Psychology, 74,* 193–218.

Nes, R. B., & Røysamb, E. (2017). Happiness in behaviour genetics: An update on heritability and changeability. *Journal of Happiness Studies, 18*(5), 1533–1552.

Neve, J.-E. D., & Oswald, A. J. (2012). Estimating the influence of life satisfaction and positive affect on later income using sibling fixed effects. *Proceedings of the National Academy of Sciences, 109*(49), 19953–19958.

Nietzsche, F. (1997). *Twilight of the idols* (R. Polt, Trans.). Hackett.

Oettingen, G., Mayer, D., & Portnow, S. (2016). Pleasure now, pain later: Positive fantasies about the future predict symptoms of depression. *Psychological Science, 27*(3), 345–353.

Oishi, S., Diener, E., & Lucas, R. E. (2007). The optimum level of well-being: Can people be too happy? *Perspectives on Psychological Science, 2*(4), 346–360.

Oishi, S., Graham, J., Kesebir, S., & Galinha, I. C. (2013). Concepts of happiness across time and cultures. *Personality and Social Psychology Bulletin, 39*(5), 559–577.

Organization for Economic Co-operation and Development. (2021). *COVID-19 and well-being: Life in the pandemic: Finland.* www.oecd.org/wise/covid-and-well-being-country-note-Finland.pdf.

Petrie, K. J., Pressman, S. D., Pennebaker, J. W., Øverland, S., Tell, G. S., & Sivertsen, B.

(2018). Which aspects of positive affect are related to mortality?: Results from a general population longitudinal study. *Annals of Behavioral Medicine, 52*(7), 571–581.
Reangsing, C., Rittiwong, T., & Schneider, J. K. (2021). Effects of mindfulness meditation interventions on depression in older adults: A meta-analysis. *Aging and Mental Health, 25*(7), 1181–1190.
Ringer, R. (1977). *Looking out for #1.* Fawcett Crest.
Rosten, L. (1962, April 8). On finding truth: Abandon the strait jacket of conformity (text of an address by Leo Rosten at the National Book Awards in New York). *The Sunday Star,* p. E-2.
Roth, G., Vansteenkiste, M., & Ryan, R. M. (2019). Integrative emotion regulation: Process and development from a self-determination theory perspective. *Development and Psychopathology, 31*(3), 945–956.
Ryan, R. M., & Deci, E. L. (2000). Self-determination theory and the facilitation of intrinsic motivation, social development, and well-being. *American Psychologist, 55*(1), 68–78.
Ryan, R. M., & Deci, E. L. (2017). *Self-determination theory: Basic psychological needs in motivation, development, and wellness.* Guilford Press.
Ryan, R. M., & Martela, F. (2016). Eudaimonia as a way of living: Connecting Aristotle with self-determination theory. In J. Vittersø (Ed.), *Handbook of eudaimonic well-being* (pp. 109–122). Springer.
Sartre, J.-P. (2007). Existentialism is a humanism. In C. Macomber (Ed. & Trans.), *Existentialism is a humanism* (pp. 17–72). Yale University Press.
Shapiro, S. L., Carlson, L. E., Astin, J. A., & Freedman, B. (2006). Mechanisms of mindfulness. *Journal of Clinical Psychology, 62*(3), 373–386.
Sheldon, K. M., & Lyubomirsky, S. (2021). Revisiting the sustainable happiness model and pie chart: Can happiness be successfully pursued? *Journal of Positive Psychology, 16*(2), 145–154.
Solomon, R. C. (2005). Introduction. In R. C. Solomon (Ed.), *Existentialism* (2nd ed., pp. xi–xx). Oxford University Press.
Spicer, A. (2024, January 17). Work "wellness" programmes don't make employees happier—But I know what does. *The Guardian.* www.theguardian.com/commentisfree/2024/jan/17/work-wellness-programmes-dont-make-employees-happier-but-i-know-what-does.
Steptoe, A., Dockray, S., & Wardle, J. (2009). Positive affect and psychobiological processes relevant to health. *Journal of Personality, 77*(6), 1747–1776.
Suh, E., Diener, E., Oishi, S., & Triandis, H. C. (1998). The shifting basis of life satisfaction judgments across cultures: Emotions versus norms. *Journal of Personality and Social Psychology, 74,* 482–493.
Tay, L., & Diener, E. (2011). Needs and subjective well-being around the world. *Journal of Personality and Social Psychology, 101*(2), 354–365.
Thompson, R. J., Kircanski, K., & Gotlib, I. H. (2016). The grass is not as green as you think: Affect evaluation in people with internalizing disorders. *Journal of Affective Disorders, 203,* 233–240.
Tsai, J. L. (2007). Ideal affect: Cultural causes and behavioral consequences. *Perspectives on Psychological Science, 2*(3), 242–259.
Tsai, J. L., Knutson, B., & Fung, H. H. (2006). Cultural variation in affect valuation. *Journal of Personality and Social Psychology, 90*(2), 288–307.
Tsai, J. L., Louie, J. Y., Chen, E. E., & Uchida, Y. (2007). Learning what feelings to desire: Socialization of ideal affect through children's storybooks. *Personality and Social Psychology Bulletin, 33*(1), 17–30.
Van Boven, L., & Gilovich, T. (2003). To do or to have?: That is the question. *Journal of Personality and Social Psychology, 85*(6), 1193–1202.
Van den Broeck, A., Ferris, D. L., Chang, C.-H., & Rosen, C. C. (2016). A review of self-determination theory's basic psychological needs at work. *Journal of Management, 42*(5), 1195–1229.
Walsh, L. C., Boehm, J. K., & Lyubomirsky, S. (2018). Does happiness promote career success?: Revisiting the evidence. *Journal of Career Assessment, 26*(2), 199–219.
Warnock, M. (1970). *Existentialism.* Oxford University Press.
Weiss, A., Bates, T. C., & Luciano, M. (2008). Happiness is a personal (ity) thing: The genetics of personality and well-being in a representative sample. *Psychological Science, 19*(3), 205–210.
Welzel, C. (2013). *Freedom rising—Human empowerment and the quest for emancipation.* Cambridge University Press.
White, C. A., Uttl, B., & Holder, M. D. (2019). Meta-analyses of positive psychology interventions: The effects are much smaller than previously reported. *PLOS One, 14*(5), e0216588.
Wilson, T. D., & Gilbert, D. T. (2005). Affective forecasting. *Current Directions in Psychological Science, 14*(3), 131–134.

Wilson, T. D., Lisle, D. J., Schooler, J. W., Hodges, S. D., Klaaren, K. J., & LaFleur, S. J. (1993). Introspecting about reasons can reduce post-choice satisfaction. *Personality and Social Psychology Bulletin, 19*(3), 331–339.

Wirtz, D., Chiu, C., Diener, E., & Oishi, S. (2009). What constitutes a good life?: Cultural differences in the role of positive and negative affect in subjective well-being. *Journal of Personality, 77*(4), 1167–1196.

Wuthnow, R. (1991). *Acts of compassion: Caring for others and helping ourselves.* Princeton University Press.

Zerwas, F. K., & Ford, B. Q. (2021). The paradox of pursuing happiness. *Current Opinion in Behavioral Sciences, 39,* 106–112.

CHAPTER 62

Exploring Psychological Richness and Its Implications for a Good Life

Elizabeth A. Janey *and* Shigehiro Oishi

Determining whether a life is a life well lived poses a difficult question, yet, as any good scientist would, we search for an answer. In this pursuit, we delve into the records of various belief systems and conceptualizations of a good life. For instance, the ancient Egyptians believed in harmony, which denoted equilibrium with the will of the gods and the surrounding community through a stable and productive life. A life well lived was one that fostered the community's joy and successes (Mark, n.d.). Judgement of whether an individual had lived a good life by these standards was decided in the afterlife by weighing their heart on a scale against a feather (Carelli, 2011). The ancient Egyptian ethos offered a distinct framework for how a life may be deemed to be a good life. While a universal, modern definition of this idea may be elusive, by expanding the parameters of a good life in psychology one can embrace the diversity of human experiences.

This chapter seeks to dive into the history of studying a good life within psychology by defining *eudaimonic* and *hedonic well-being* and aims to present evidence for a third category of a good life, a *psychologically rich life*, defined as a life characterized by complex and interesting experiences, ultimately resulting in a perspective change (Oishi et al., 2019; Oishi & Westgate, 2022). We argue that psychological richness may connect to but is ultimately distinct from eudaimonic and hedonic well-being. Consequently, psychological richness broadens the scope of the study of well-being to include individuals who may have lived a good life but are not captured in the prevailing definitions in psychology.

DEFINING A GOOD LIFE, A HAPPY LIFE, A MEANINGFUL LIFE, AND A PSYCHOLOGICALLY RICH LIFE

In pursuit of defining a good life, we turn to the reflections of philosophers on existence. In what stands as one of the most significant works of Aristotle's life, *Nicomachean Ethics,* Aristotle opened by discussing *eudaimonia*, often translated as happiness (Aristotle, 2004). Aristotle argued that the good of a human being is done by acting in accordance with virtues, which leads to living a good life. Aristotle outlined various contenders for living a virtuous life, including a life of pleasure, a life of honor, a life of wealth and eminence, and a life of health. By delineating these diverse paths, Aristotle laid out types of lives that could be considered a good life, helping lay the foundations for theories on psychological well-being and happiness (Fowers, 2016).

In psychology, well-being research has been focused predominately on two of Aristotle's concepts: hedonic well-being, or a happy life (Diener et al., 2018; Kahneman et al., 1999), and eudaimonic well-being, or the development and exercise of one's virtues and excellence (Rogers, 1995; Ryan & Deci, 2001; Ryff, 1989; Waterman, 1993). In this chapter, we discuss a happy life and a meaningful life as an indicator of hedonic and eudaimonic well-being, respectively. Research has demonstrated that a happy life is a life in which a person is satisfied with their life and feels positive emotions often and negative emotions infrequently (Diener, 1984). In practice, a happy life is often measured in terms of life satisfaction (Diener et al., 1985), the frequency of positive and negative emotions (Diener et al., 2010), and subjective happiness (Lyubomirsky & Lepper, 1999). Furthermore, happiness in life is related to many circumstantial factors, such as higher socioeconomic status (Anderson et al., 2012), greater job security (Helbling & Kanji, 2018), higher perceived financial security (Ruberton et al., 2016), living in a country without major conflicts (Diener & Diener, 1995), high satisfaction in a marriage (Margelisch et al., 2017), regular interactions with friends and neighbors (Helliwell & Putnam, 2004), and regular exercise (Mochon et al., 2008). In terms of personality traits, happiness is positively correlated with extraversion, agreeableness, and conscientiousness, and happiness is inversely related to neuroticism (Steel et al., 2008). Considering these factors and traits together, a happy life is a secure life, where an individual is satisfied with their circumstances, relatively financially blessed, participates in fun activities, has stable interpersonal relationships, and is a conscientious, emotionally stable, extraverted, and agreeable person.

Different than a happy life, we define a *meaningful life* as the subjective appraisal that one's life and experiences have significance, coherence, and purpose. As seen in Vittersø's (2016) review, eudaimonic well-being is measured by diverse concepts, including self-expressiveness (Waterman et al., 2008); authenticity (Schlegel et al., 2009); the satisfaction of basic human needs such as autonomy, competence, and relatedness (Ryan & Deci, 2001); psychological well-being such as autonomy, environmental mastery, and personal growth (Ryff, 1989); and meaning in life (Steger et al., 2006). Although concepts and measurements associated with eudaimonic well-being are diverse, meaning in life is highly correlated with many of these eudaimonic well-being measures (Martela et al., 2018). That is, people tend to feel that their lives are meaningful when their fundamental needs are fulfilled and their potentials are realized.

In psychological literature, a meaningful life has frequently been defined with three common elements: The first is *significance*, or the subjective sense that one's life matters (George & Park, 2016). The second is *coherence*, the extent to which one's life roles and experiences fit together into a coherent whole (Baumeister, 1991). The third is *purpose*, the perception that one's life has direction and contributes to something greater than the self (Reker et al., 1987). Meaning in life has also been positively related to extraversion, conscientiousness, and agreeableness and inversely related to neuroticism (Steger et al., 2006). Research has shown that living a meaningful life includes making sense of life, feeling that one's life is significant (Heintzelman & King, 2014), practicing self-acceptance, pursuing positive relationships and personal growth (Steger et al., 2006), and engaging in activities that foster authenticity across one's lifespan (Steger et al., 2009).

Beyond hedonic and eudaimonic well-being, insights from additional philosophical texts point to other dimensions of a good life, such as psychological richness. Just as we turn to philosophy for evidence of hedonic and eudaimonic well-being, we can also look there for evidence of psychological richness. In Nietzsche's *Thus Spoke Zarathustra* (2012), the titular character, Zarathustra, advocated for the life of a wanderer, casting happiness and meaning as banal and lamenting how the doctrine of happiness and virtue had made people smaller. Tangentially, in *Either/Or*, Kierkegaard (2004) critiqued the monotony and boredom inherent in an ethical life, a life that adhered to moral principles, portraying a secure life as lacking liveliness.

Zarathustra's and Kierkegaard's rejection of conventional notions of happiness and ethical living illustrates their unique perspectives on a good life, diverging from the mainstream psychological paradigms. Thus, psychological paradigms of well-being are missing concepts that could capture the lives of Zarathustra and Kierkegaard, such as adventure, artistic endeavors, and novel intellectual experiences. There is philosophical evidence of these concepts being considered components of a good life if we look again at *Nicomachean Ethics*. Aristotle would have considered a life guided by intelligence, adventure, and artistic endeavors as components of eudaimonia (Aristotle, 2004; Fowers, 2016); however, these concepts have rarely been included in the existing measures of eudaimonic well-being. Arguably, eudaimonia, frequently measured as meaning in life (Steger et al., 2009), may not be the best indicator of these concepts, as meaning in life can be related to right-wing authoritarianism (Womick et al., 2021) and political conservatism (Newman et al., 2019), concepts seemingly in conflict with those we wish to capture. Therefore, to expand upon well-being paradigms, a third dimension to a good life must be incorporated: *psychological richness*.

Current research on psychological richness has addressed phenomena related to novelty, complexity, perspective change, and the desirability of a psychologically rich life. Specifically, research has shown that a psychologically rich life is desirable to a portion of individuals across different countries, even at the expense of a happy or meaningful life (Oishi et al., 2020) and that psychological richness is associated with system-defying tendencies (Oishi & Westgate, 2022) and increased pro-environmental behaviors (Xinni et al., 2023), as measured with the Psychologically Rich Life Questionnaire (Table 65.1; Oishi et al., 2019). Furthermore, a daily diary study showed that psychological richness was significantly higher on days when individuals took a short trip (Oishi et al., 2021). Among personality traits, psychological richness has been best predicted by openness to experience and extraversion (Oishi & Westgate, 2022). In short, those who live a psychologically rich life seek out new experiences, are relatively open, and may be willing to sacrifice happiness for complexity.

TABLE 62.1. Sample Items from the Full 17-Item Psychologically Rich Life Questionnaire (PRLQ)

1. My life has been psychologically rich.
4. I have a lot of interesting experiences.
7. My life consists of rich, intense moments.
11. On my deathbed, I am likely to say "I had an interesting life."
15. I often feel bored with my life. (reverse scored)

Note. The 12-item and 17-item scales were both tested within Oishi et al. (2019) and found to be a reliable measure of psychological richness.

The concept of psychological richness can be linked to existing psychological constructs such as interest, curiosity, and cognitive restructuring. It has been theorized that factors such as novelty, complexity, conflict, and uncertainty, which align closely with the definition of psychological richness (Oishi et al., 2019; Oishi & Westgate, 2022), are fundamental determinants of both interest and curiosity (Berlyne, 1949). Further research on interest claims that interest arises when individuals feel they have the capacity to make sense of complex stimuli (Silvia, 2005, 2008). Extending this theory to psychological richness, we propose that a psychologically rich life is characterized by interesting experiences featuring novelty and complexity, coupled with a change in perspective.

Research has drawn a parallel between a change in perspective and the established psychological concept of cognitive restructuring (Clark, 2013). Cognitive restructuring involves revising mental representations, closely resembling the process of experiencing a change in perspective. Moreover, cognitive restructuring aligns with research on emotional theory, which argues that the greater the distance between one's current and revised mental representation, the more intense an emotional experience one will have (Clore, 2011). Similarly, we hypothesize that the more novel an experience is, the more psychological richness and perspective changes one may experience. Overall, psychology has captured some aspects of psychological richness previously, such as interest, curiosity, and perspective change, but has yet to connect them to well-being.

Looking outside of well-being literature, a change in perspective can also be understood in the physical world through the concept of intuitive physics: humans' intuition about a situation based on dynamic relationships (Kubricht et al., 2017). For example, when an intuition about whether or not a stack of precariously stacked dishes will fall is incorrect, an individual must adapt and update their understanding of the physical world (Battaglia et al., 2013). Updating this complex system of intuitions about physics using real-world perceptions is very comparable to a change in perspective. Thus, various psychological concepts allow one to understand a change in perspective and its relationship to experience.

In sum, a happy life, dependent upon stability and security, a psychologically rich life, dependent upon novelty and complexity, and a meaningful life, dependent upon authenticity and significance, can all be forms of a good life according to the individual. Thus, we define a *good life* as a life well lived from the perspective of the person who is living it. Accordingly, a good life may be happy, meaningful, rich, a combination of these concepts, or something completely different, depending on the person. From this perspective, it is necessary to ask the individual what type of life they would like to lead to determine whether they are living a good life.

HUMAN VALUES: WHAT IS MISSING FROM A HAPPY LIFE AND A MEANINGFUL LIFE?

Research has considered the types of lives people would want to live in terms of human values, which are often defined as superordinate goals that are guiding principles of life (Schwartz, 1992). For instance, Vernon and Allport (1931) proposed six values: theoretical, economic, aesthetic, political, social, and religious (Figure 62.1B). From these values one could derive six types of a good life: an intellectual life, a materially wealthy life, an artistic/creative life, an influential life, a loving/caring life, and a religious life. Likewise, Schwartz (1992) argued for the existence of 10 universal values: power, achievement, hedonism, stimulation, self-direction, universalism, benevolence, conformity, tradition, and security (Figure 62.1A). From these, one could derive 10 forms of a good life: a powerful/influential life, a successful life, an enjoyable life, a stimulating life, an autonomous life, a peaceful life, a caring life, a conforming life, a traditional/religious life, and a secure life. Thus, Schwartz and Vernon and Allport identified human values that serve as the guardrails for an individual's life.

While this approach might suggest an infinitude of possible lives, we note that many of these lives are systematically related to a happy life and a meaningful life. For instance, from Vernon and Allport's (1931) six values, two of these values, economic and social, map neatly onto a happy life, as economic security and stable social relationships are central to a happy life. Likewise, Vernon and Allport's religious and political values fit nicely with a meaningful life, as religious values give people a sense of purpose and coherence while political values give them social influence or a sense of significance as well as societal contribution. In contrast, Vernon and Allport's theoretical and aesthetic values do not neatly fit into a happy or meaningful life.

Turning to Schwartz's (1992) universal human value theory, hedonism, conformity, security, and benevolence capture empirical findings from happiness research, as hedonism encourages enjoyment in life, benevolence encourages positive social relationships, and conformity and security provide a sense of stability (see Napier & Jost, 2008, for the correlation between conservatism and happiness). Similarly, traditional values are associated with religious values, which in turn are associated with a meaningful life. People also gain a sense of meaning in life by making a difference in the world (power and achievement). Three remaining values that do not clearly fit a happy life and a meaningful life are stimulation, self-direction, and universalism.

In sum, Vernon and Allport's (1931) theoretical and aesthetic values and Schwartz's (1992) stimulation, self-direction, and universalism values are not well-captured by the dominant views of well-being. In terms

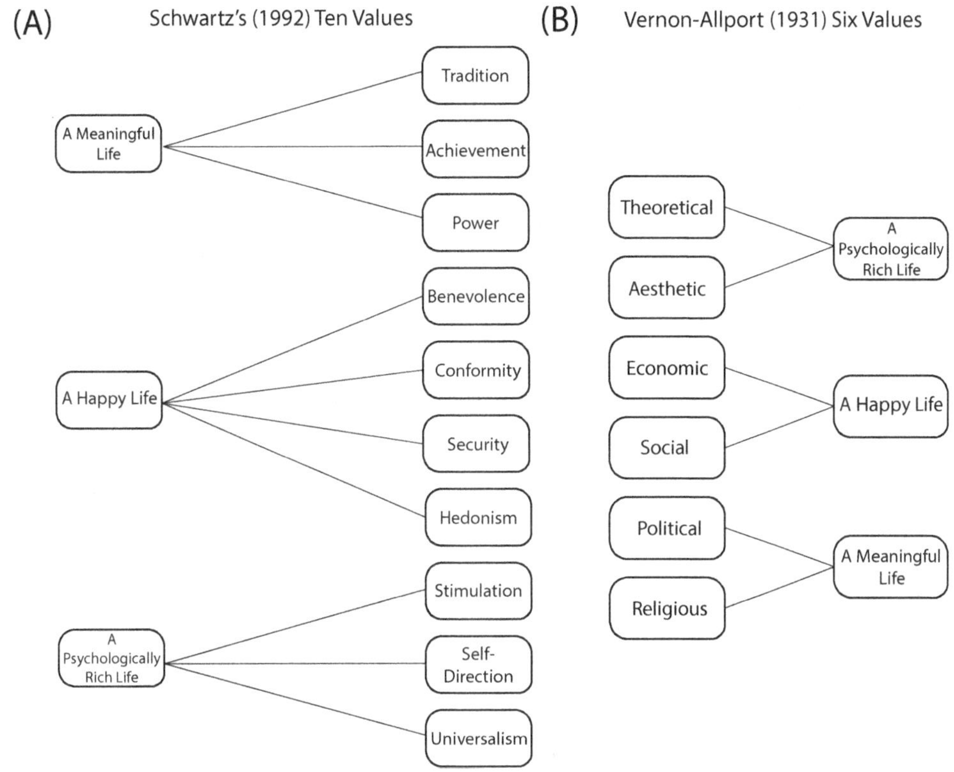

FIGURE 62.1. (A) Schwartz's 10 values, from which one can derive the three forms of a good life. (B) Vernon-Allport's (1931) six proposed values, which one can relate to the three types of a good life.

of the Big Five personality traits, these values are most strongly associated with openness to experiences (Roccas et al., 2002). Interestingly, a recent meta-analysis found that openness to experience was least strongly associated with happiness and meaning among the Big Five personality traits (Anglim et al., 2020). A happy life and a meaningful life capture much of the diversity of human values and the major dimensions of personality traits, but we can build upon them with psychological richness.

MEASURING PSYCHOLOGICAL RICHNESS AND ITS DESIRABILITY

Psychological richness describes how a life of complexity, adventure, artistry, and interestingness can be defined as a good life (Oishi et al., 2019; Oishi & Westgate, 2022). To capture psychological richness at the level of the individual, the PRLQ (see Table 62.1; Oishi et al., 2019) was developed, validated, and compared to responses from questionnaires on a happy life and meaningful life across four studies. In one of these studies, the PRLQ was administered to a sample of college students over a 2-week period (Oishi et al., 2019, Study 1). The fit of the PRLQ to a one-factor model, its test–retest stability, and its self–other agreement were all tested during this study. A one-factor model of fit was confirmed; the scale had high test–retest stability; a multitrait–multimethod matrix confirmed that happiness, richness, and meaning were related but distinct constructs, and self-reports of psychological richness were associated with informant reports of psychological richness.

Additional studies served to replicate this main finding across different samples. Specifically, these results were replicated in a nonstudent U.S. population (Oishi et al.,

2019, Study 2), in a large national probability sample in the United States (Oishi et al., 2019, Study 3), and in a non-Western sample from India (Oishi et al., 2019, Study 4). Among different populations, the PRLQ was shown to be a reliable method for capturing psychological richness and demonstrated that meaning in life, richness, and happiness, were three unique concepts. However, the PRLQ does not capture whether people seek a psychologically rich life.

To determine whether a psychologically rich life is desirable, individuals across nine different countries were asked what type of life they would like to lead (Oishi et al., 2020). Specifically, they were asked to describe the ideal life they would like to lead and to select items from a list that related to the life they described. The list contained adjectives related to a happy life, a psychologically rich life, and a meaningful life. The self-described lives of individuals were characterized by a happy life, a meaningful life, and to a lesser extent, a psychologically rich life. When given a forced-choice scenario where individuals had to choose whether they would want to live a happy life, a meaningful life, or a psychologically rich life, the majority preferred a happy life (49.7–69.9%), a moderate number preferred a meaningful life (14.2%–38.5%), and a minority preferred a psychologically rich life (6.7–16.8%), even at the expense of a happy or meaningful one (Figure 62.2). Among the countries surveyed, European countries, India, Japan, and Korea were those where living a psychologically rich life was the most popular, demonstrating that a psychologically rich life is desirable and valued, even across geographic borders. However, the accuracy of an individual's self-report on the type of life they desire is unclear.

To grapple with the question of whether the type of life people want to live can be inferred indirectly, participants across the United States and Korea were asked what their biggest regret in life was and what their life would look like if they could undo this regret (Oishi et al., 2020, Study 2). They were given the opportunity to choose between a happier life, a more meaningful life, or a more psychologically rich life. Answers in the United States were equally split: 35.7% (n = 575) said their life would have been happier, 36.7% (n = 592) said it would have been more meaningful, and the remaining 27.6% (n = 444) said it would have been more psychologically rich. Answers in Korea were similar to those in the United States: 27.6% (n = 188) said their life would have been happier, 37.4% (n = 254) said it would have been more meaningful, and the remain-

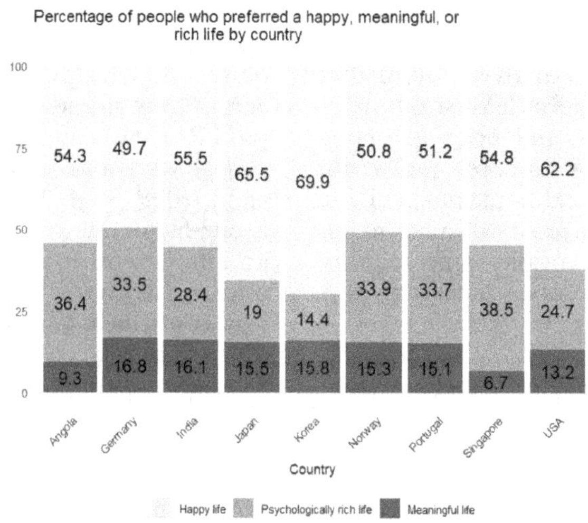

FIGURE 62.2. Percentage of individuals who prefer a happy life, a psychologically rich life, or a meaningful life in a force-choice task, by country. From Oishi et al. (2020).

ing 35% (n = 238) said it would have made their lives more psychologically rich. From these findings, we conclude that the type of life people want to live can be inferred indirectly, with a third of people preferring a psychologically rich life over a happy or a meaningful life.

PSYCHOLOGICAL RICHNESS ACROSS MULTIPLE DAYS

Psychological richness may be defined across various levels of time, a single event, a day, a year, or across a lifespan. To compose a larger picture of what psychological richness looks like and how one may experience psychological richness, research has been done to establish richness across multiple days using the daily diary method. When University of Virginia students were asked to answer various questions about their day, the activities they engaged in, and their well-being for 14 days, daily psychological richness was higher on a more atypical day, a day when they met someone new, ate something new, or did something new (Oishi et al., 2021). Days high in psychological richness were also those with routine activities and less free time. These results suggest that a psychologically rich day is a day that has routine activities as well as a few atypical activities and a full schedule.

Looking more closely at psychological richness at the daily level, research has looked more specifically at the activities that culminate into a rich day. Richness was higher on days when individuals participate in activities such as artistic activities, club activities, exercise, going on a trip, attending a sporting event, shopping, and partying (Oishi et al., 2021). The best predictor of psychological richness at the daily level was going on a short trip. Travel was consistently identified as being related to increased psychological richness (Oishi & Westgate, 2022). Even recalling a travel event can act as a manipulation of psychological richness and lead to more experienced perspective change (Xinni et al., 2023). This work suggests that one way of making a day more psychologically rich may be to go on a short trip, or as was written in the *New York Times*, a "micro-adventure" (Pennington, 2021).

Looking beyond the time frame of a day, another study evaluated richness across a couple of months. Studying abroad is one type of experience that involves travel and spans a couple months or more, and it is therefore an ideal scenario to learn more about psychological richness. Over a period of 12 weeks, psychological richness was recorded in a U.S. population of students who traveled abroad and a group of students who remained on campus (Oishi et al., 2021). These two groups of students were not different in happiness, meaning, or psychological richness at the beginning of the semester. At the end of the semester, however, the ratings of psychological richness for students who studied abroad were significantly higher than they were for those who stayed on campus (in contrast, they were not different in happiness or meaning). Furthermore, changes in richness for the study abroad students occurred at a higher rate than they did for those who stayed on campus, partially due to the study abroad students' engagement in artistic activities. These results further confirm that traveling, practicing art, and doing novel activities are accompanied by increases in psychological richness.

Apart from the unusual experience of travel, illness has also affected psychological richness. Self-reports from individuals in Sweden who contracted COVID-19 and recovered showed higher levels of psychological richness than did self-reports from those who did not contract the disease (Dahlen & Thorbjørnsen, 2022). This offers a silver lining to getting sick, suggesting that increases in an aspect of well-being can occur even with decreases in immediate physical health. Furthermore, another study during the COVID-19 pandemic established the negative effect of boredom on well-being (Lin et al., 2023). As social interactions decreased during the pandemic, boredom increased, leading to worse well-being across measures of happiness, meaning, and richness. Looking at these studies together, they provide evidence for how an event's positive or negative valence and the interpretation of the event can impact perceived richness.

DEFINING PSYCHOLOGICAL RICHNESS ACROSS THE LIFESPAN

We have captured what it means to live a psychologically rich day and couple of months but have yet to discuss what it means to live a psychologically rich life. The construction of a psychologically rich life can start early in life. Factors one may not expect, like the books one reads as a young adult, can contribute to psychological richness later in life. A link has been established between reading literature over time early in life and present-day increases in psychological richness (Buttrick et al., 2023). However, whether or not reading led to increased psychological richness later in life was dependent on the genre of books read. Reading by itself did not increase psychological richness, but reading literary fiction predicted the highest increases in richness later in life while reading essays and chick-lit predicted the least. Thus, previous actions can impact present-day levels of psychological richness.

Looking beyond early life to the entire lifespan, obituaries contain the summation of one's life, capturing information deemed worthy to represent the individual. Coding for richness, happiness, and meaning within obituaries then tells the type of life the individual lived. Consistent across obituary sources within the United States and Singapore, the more psychologically rich an individual's life was, the more meaningful it was (meta-analytic $r = 0.28$), while happiness was negatively related to richness (meta-analytic $r = -0.17$ in Oishi & Westgate, 2022). In obituary ratings, meaning in life was also associated with happiness (meta-analytic $r = 0.21$). Overall, then, obituary studies showed that a psychologically rich life is clearly distinct from a happy life but may contain aspects of a meaningful life throughout the lifespan.

WHO LIVES A PSYCHOLOGICALLY RICH LIFE?

We have covered the events that make up a psychologically rich life, how psychological richness compares to happiness and meaning in life, and whether a psychologically rich life is a life people desire. We have yet to consider deeply who exactly lives a psychologically rich life. To start, we relate richness to the Big Five personality traits. A psychologically rich life is positively associated with extraversion, openness to experience, sensation seeking, agreeableness, and conscientiousness, and negatively associated with neuroticism (Oishi et al., 2019). A meta-analysis of seven studies relating psychological richness, meaning in life, and happiness to personality traits showed that living a psychologically rich life was best predicted by openness to experience and extraversion (Oishi & Westgate, 2022). In contrast, happiness was best predicted by extraversion, then conscientiousness, and finally low neuroticism, while meaning in life was associated evenly with all Big Five traits. Extraversion and openness appear to be the most important traits for predicting tendencies to live a psychologically rich life. We suggest that perhaps through novelty-seeking (Gocłowska et al., 2019), extraverted and open individuals experience more complex and perspective-changing experiences, leading to richer lives.

THE OUTCOME OF A PSYCHOLOGICALLY RICH LIFE

We argue that the overarching potential outcome of living a rich life, characterized by interesting, complex, and perspective-changing experiences, may be wisdom. *Wisdom* is a complicated concept, defined often as factual and procedural knowledge about the pragmatics of life, involving insight into matters of life, judgments, and good advice on difficult problems (Bangen et al., 2013). Beyond this definition, colloquially, wisdom involves having deep but malleable knowledge learned from experiences that comes with an unbiased perspective. Considering these definitions, psychological richness should then be accompanied by holistic thinking styles, attributional complexity, and low levels of discrete essentialism, which recent work has found (Oishi et al., 2024). Thus, individuals with high psychological richness may consider multiple points of view in their attributions, have complex reasoning styles, and be less likely to believe a couple of traits explain differences between people.

FUTURE DIRECTIONS

Novelty, complexity, and changes in perspective lead to a psychologically rich experience and an overall psychologically rich life. We have presented pieces of psychological richness here, but there is ample opportunity for expansion. For example, the definition of a *good life* is culturally construed. A good life in one culture may be a poor life in another. Documenting what a good life looks like cross-culturally is the next step in applying a life well lived to diverse geographic communities.

Tragedy and Adversity

Tragedy, adversity, and difficult challenges may contribute to a good life by fostering resilience, despite these events leading to lower levels of subjective well-being (Nussbaum, 2001; Seery et al., 2010). Coping with tragedy and reflecting on adverse events may be important for fostering psychological richness in tough situations through opportunities for perspective change. Thus, to receive the benefits of perspective change it is necessary to recall the adverse event to reflect on it. The ability to form a coherent story surrounding trauma has been shown to lead to improved health (Pennebaker, 1997). We theorize that experiencing richness may be intrinsically tied to the same coping mechanisms as used for traumatic events.

Identifying Rich Locations

We have been able to identify traveling as an event that consistently leads to increases in psychological richness; however, it is important to test how the location of travel affects the level of psychological richness experienced. For example, the cultural distance (Demes & Geeraert, 2014) between an individual's home and the place they are traveling to may lead to more or less novel experiences, determining the amount of perspective change available. Additionally, certain environmental features have been identified as being either beneficial or harmful to subjective well-being (Jimenez et al., 2021). Determining if experienced psychological richness is affected similarly by environmental features and cultural distance is an important consideration.

Exploration and Exploitation

Exploration is the act of searching through the unknown; it can be goal-directed or random and is demonstrated through explorative actions, such as examining the alternatives of a decision before making a commitment (Cohen et al., 2007) or randomly interacting with individuals to make friends (Tsang et al., 2023). Furthermore, explorative actions can serve as the basis of learning. Children explore the world and collect information from it in rational and spontaneous ways (Gopnik, 2020). However, exploration may be resource-intensive, requiring time to assess options and their profitability. In contrast to exploration, exploitation, in the context of decision making, is the act of turning to the familiar (Cohen et al., 2007), lending itself to stability. By turning to the familiar, exploitation can lead to suboptimal but low-risk outcomes with reduced uncertainty. For example, an act of exploitation would be turning to friends with whom one has an established relationship instead of seeking out new relationships. Thus, across different contexts and situations, exploration and exploitation may be used at different rates, leading to different outcomes at the level of the individual and ultimately different types of lives.

We can relate the context surrounding when exploitation, exploration, or a combination of the two is used, and the type of life an individual lives. For example, a meaningful, psychologically rich, and/or happy life may be tied to enjoyable experiences across the lifespan and explorative knowledge seeking, while only a meaningful and/or happy life may be heavily tied to exploitation through taking advantage of social ties and familiar environments, resulting in stable and comfortable relationships. Identifying the situations that benefit from exploration and exploitation would allow us to answer important questions about their relationship with different types of a good life.

CONCLUSION

We have given definitions of a *good life* in the context of psychology, how this definition may be lacking, and work that demonstrates the need for psychological richness. When considering a good life, it is important to consider what the individual values, the identities they hold, the culture they live in, and the way a good life is measured to capture the breadth of a life well lived. Expanding the scope of the well-being literature to include psychological richness will contribute to a more inclusive framework of psychology and further empirical investigation of the importance of novel and perspective-changing experiences.

REFERENCES

Anderson, C., Kraus, M. W., Galinsky, A. D., & Keltner, D. (2012). The local-ladder effect: Social status and subjective well-being. *Psychological Science, 23*(7), 764–771.

Anglim, J., Horwood, S., Smillie, L. D., Marrero, R. J., & Wood, J. K. (2020). Predicting psychological and subjective well-being from personality: A meta-analysis. *Psychological Bulletin, 146*(4), 279–323.

Aristotle. (2004). *The Nicomachean ethics* (Further revised ed.; J. A. K. Thomson, Trans.). Penguin Books.

Bangen, K. J., Meeks, T. W., & Jeste, D. V. (2013). Defining and assessing wisdom: A review of the literature. *American Journal of Geriatric Psychiatry, 21*(12), 1254–1266.

Battaglia, P. W., Hamrick, J. B., & Tenenbaum, J. B. (2013). Simulation as an engine of physical scene understanding. *Proceedings of the National Academy of Sciences, 110*(45), 18327–18332.

Baumeister, R. F. (1991). *Meanings of life*. Guilford Press.

Berlyne, D. E. (1949). Interest as a psychological concept. *British Journal of Psychology. General Section, 39*(4), 184–195.

Buttrick, N., Westgate, E. C., & Oishi, S. (2023). Reading literary fiction is associated with a more complex worldview. *Personality and Social Psychology Bulletin, 49*(9), 1408–1420.

Carelli, F. (2011). The book of death: Weighing your heart. *London Journal of Primary Care, 4*(1), 86–87.

Clark, D. A. (2013). Cognitive restructuring. In S. G. Hofmann (Ed.), *The Wiley handbook of cognitive behavioral therapy* (pp. 23–44). Wiley.

Clore, G. L. (2011). Psychology and the rationality of emotion. *Modern Theology, 27*(2), 325–338.

Cohen, J. D., McClure, S. M., & Yu, A. J. (2007). Should I stay or should I go?: How the human brain manages the trade-off between exploitation and exploration. *Philosophical Transactions of the Royal Society B: Biological Sciences, 362*(1481), 933–942.

Dahlen, M., & Thorbjørnsen, H. (2022). An infectious silver lining: Is there a positive relationship between recovering from a COVID infection and psychological richness of life? *Frontiers in Psychology, 13*. www.frontiersin.org/articles/10.3389/fpsyg.2022.785224.

Demes, K. A., & Geeraert, N. (2014). Measures matter: Scales for adaptation, cultural distance, and acculturation orientation revisited. *Journal of Cross-Cultural Psychology, 45*(1), 91–109.

Diener, E. (1984). Subjective well-being. *Psychological Bulletin, 95*(3), 542–575.

Diener, E., & Diener, M. (1995). Cross-cultural correlates of life satisfaction and self-esteem. *Journal of Personality and Social Psychology, 68*, 653–663.

Diener, E., Emmons, R. A., Larsen, R. J., & Griffin, S. (1985). The Satisfaction with Life Scale. *Journal of Personality Assessment, 49*(1), 71–75.

Diener, E., Lucas, R. E., & Oishi, S. (2018). Advances and open questions in the science of subjective well-being. *Collabra Psychology, 4*(1), 15.

Diener, E., Wirtz, D., Tov, W., Kim-Prieto, C., Choi, D., Oishi, S., & Biswas-Diener, R. (2010). New well-being measures: Short scales to assess flourishing and positive and negative feelings. *Social Indicators Research, 97*(2), 143–156.

Fowers, B. J. (2016). Aristotle on eudaimonia: On the virtue of returning to the source. In J. Vittersø (Ed.), *Handbook of eudaimonic well-being* (pp. 67–83). Springer International.

George, L. S., & Park, C. L. (2016). Meaning in life as comprehension, purpose, and mattering: Toward integration and new research questions. *Review of General Psychology, 20*(3), 205–220.

Gocłowska, M. A., Ritter, S. M., Elliot, A. J., & Baas, M. (2019). Novelty seeking is linked to openness and extraversion, and can lead to greater creative performance. *Journal of Personality, 87*(2), 252–266.

Gopnik, A. (2020). Childhood as a solution to explore–exploit tensions. *Philosophical Transactions of the Royal Society B: Biological Sciences, 375*, 20190502.

Heintzelman, S. J., & King, L. A. (2014). Life is pretty meaningful. *American Psychologist, 69*(6), 561–574.

Helbling, L., & Kanji, S. (2018). Job insecurity: Differential effects of subjective and objective measures on life satisfaction trajectories of workers aged 27–30 in Germany. *Social Indicators Research, 137*(3), 1145–1162.

Helliwell, J. F., & Putnam, R. D. (2004). The social context of well-being. *Philosophical Transactions of the Royal Society of London. Series B, Biological Sciences, 359*, 1435–1446.

Jimenez, M. P., DeVille, N. V., Elliott, E. G., Schiff, J. E., Wilt, G. E., Hart, J. E., & James, P. (2021). Associations between nature exposure and health: A review of the evidence. *International Journal of Environmental Research and Public Health, 18*(9), Article 9.

Kahneman, D., Diener, E., & Schwarz, N. (Eds.). (1999). *Well-being: Foundations of hedonic psychology*. Russell Sage Foundation.

Kierkegaard, S. (2004). *Either/or: A fragment of life* (A. Hannay, Trans.). Penguin.

Kubricht, J. R., Holyoak, K. J., & Lu, H. (2017). Intuitive physics: Current research and controversies. *Trends in Cognitive Sciences, 21*(10), 749–759.

Lin, Y., LePine, S. E., Krause, A. N., & Westgate, E. C. (2023). A little help from my friends: Lack of social interaction predicts greater boredom during the COVID-19 pandemic. *Social and Personality Psychology Compass, 17*(11), e12871.

Lyubomirsky, S., & Lepper, H. S. (1999). A measure of subjective happiness: Preliminary reliability and construct validation. *Social Indicators Research, 46*(2), 137–155.

Margelisch, K., Schneewind, K. A., Violette, J., & Perrig-Chiello, P. (2017). Marital stability, satisfaction and well-being in old age: Variability and continuity in long-term continuously married older persons. *Aging and Mental Health, 21*(4), 389–398.

Mark, J. J. (n.d.). Social structure in ancient Egypt. *World History Encyclopedia*. www.worldhistory.org/article/1123/social-structure-in-ancient-egypt/.

Martela, F., Ryan, R. M., & Steger, M. F. (2018). Meaningfulness as satisfaction of autonomy, competence, relatedness, and beneficence: Comparing the four satisfactions and positive affect as predictors of meaning in life. *Journal of Happiness Studies, 19*(5), 1261–1282.

Mochon, D., Norton, M. I., & Ariely, D. (2008). Getting off the hedonic treadmill, one step at a time: The impact of regular religious practice and exercise on well-being. *Journal of Economic Psychology, 29*(5), 632–642.

Napier, J. L., & Jost, J. T. (2008). Why are conservatives happier than liberals? *Psychological Science, 19*(6), 565–572.

Newman, D. B., Schwarz, N., Graham, J., & Stone, A. A. (2019). Conservatives report greater meaning in life than liberals. *Social Psychological and Personality Science, 10*(4), 494–503.

Nietzsche, F. (2012). *Thus spoke Zarathustra: A book for all and none* (A. Del Caro, Trans.). Cambridge University Press.

Nussbaum, M. C. (2001). *The fragility of goodness: Luck and ethics in Greek tragedy and philosophy*. Cambridge University Press.

Oishi, S., Choi, H., Buttrick, N., Heintzelman, S. J., Kushlev, K., Westgate, E. C., . . . Besser, L. L. (2019). The psychologically rich life questionnaire. *Journal of Research in Personality, 81*, 257–270.

Oishi, S., Choi, H., Koo, M., Galinha, I., Ishii, K., Komiya, A., . . . Besser, L. L. (2020). Happiness, meaning, and psychological richness. *Affective Science, 1*(2), 107–115.

Oishi, S., Choi, H., Liu, A., & Kurtz, J. (2021). Experiences associated with psychological richness. *European Journal of Personality, 35*(5), 754–770.

Oishi, S., & Westgate, E. C. (2022). A psychologically rich life: Beyond happiness and meaning. *Psychological Review, 129*(4), 790–811.

Oishi, S., Westgate, E. C., & Cha, Y. (2024). The cognitive complexity of a happy life, a meaningful life, and a psychologically rich life. *Journal of Research in Personality, 110*, 104475.

Pennebaker, J. W. (1997). Writing about emotional experiences as a therapeutic process. *Psychological Science, 8*(3), 162–166.

Pennington, E. (2021, July 5). Who needs the Grand Canyon?: Try a microadventure. *New York Times*. www.nytimes.com/2021/07/05/well/live/awe-microadventure-exploration.html.

Reker, G. T., Peacock, E. J., & Wong, P. T. P. (1987). Meaning and purpose in life and well-being: A life-span perspective. *Journal of Gerontology, 42*(1), 44–49.

Roccas, S., Sagiv, L., Schwartz, S. H., & Knafo, A. (2002). The Big Five personality factors and personal values. *Personality and Social Psychology Bulletin, 28*(6), 789–801.

Rogers, C. R. (1995). *On becoming a person: A therapist's view of psychotherapy*. Houghton Mifflin Harcourt.

Ruberton, P. M., Gladstone, J., & Lyubomirsky, S. (2016). How your bank balance buys happiness: The importance of "cash on hand" to life satisfaction. *Emotion, 16*(5), 575–580.

Ryan, R. M., & Deci, E. L. (2001). On happiness and human potentials: A review of research on hedonic and eudaimonic well-being. *Annual Review of Psychology, 52*(1), 141–166.

Ryff, C. D. (1989). Happiness is everything, or is it?: Explorations on the meaning of psychological well-being. *Journal of Personality and Social Psychology, 57*(6), 1069–1081.

Schlegel, R. J., Hicks, J. A., Arndt, J., & King, L. A. (2009). Thine own self: True self-concept accessibility and meaning in life. *Journal of Personality and Social Psychology, 96*(2), 473–490.

Schwartz, S. H. (1992). Universals in the content and structure of values: Theoretical advances and empirical tests in 20 countries. In M. P. Zanna (Ed.), *Advances in experimental social psychology* (Vol. 25, pp. 1–65). Academic Press.

Seery, M. D., Holman, E. A., & Silver, R. C. (2010). Whatever does not kill us: Cumulative lifetime adversity, vulnerability, and resilience. *Journal of Personality and Social Psychology, 99*(6), 1025–1041.

Silvia, P. J. (2005). What is interesting?: Exploring the appraisal structure of interest. *Emotion, 5*(1), 89–102.

Silvia, P. J. (2008). Interest: The curious emotion. *Current Directions in Psychological Science, 17*(1), 57–60.

Steel, P., Schmidt, J., & Shultz, J. (2008). Refining the relationship between personality and subjective well-being. *Psychological Bulletin, 134*(1), 138–161.

Steger, M. F., Frazier, P., Oishi, S., & Kaler, M. (2006). The meaning in life questionnaire: Assessing the presence of and search for meaning in life. *Journal of Counseling Psychology, 53*(1), 80–93.

Steger, M. F., Oishi, S., & Kashdan, T. B. (2009). Meaning in life across the life span: Levels and correlates of meaning in life from emerging adulthood to older adulthood. *Journal of Positive Psychology, 4*(1), 43–52.

Tsang, S., Barrentine, K. J., Chadha, S., Oishi, S., & Wood, A. (2023). *Social exploration: How and why people seek new connections.* PsyArXiv Preprints. https://osf.io/preprints/psyarxiv/2wx9t_v1.

Vernon, P. E., & Allport, G. W. (1931). A test for personal values. *Journal of Abnormal and Social Psychology, 26*(3), 231–248.

Vittersø, J. (Ed.). (2016). *Handbook of eudaimonic well-being.* Springer International.

Waterman, A. S. (1993). Two conceptions of happiness: Contrasts of personal expressiveness (eudaimonia) and hedonic enjoyment. *Journal of Personality and Social Psychology, 64*(4), 678–691.

Waterman, A. S., Schwartz, S. J., & Conti, R. (2008). The implications of two conceptions of happiness (hedonic enjoyment and eudaimonia) for the understanding of intrinsic motivation. *Journal of Happiness Studies, 9*(1), 41–79.

Womick, J., Eckelkamp, J., Luzzo, S., Ward, S. J., Baker, S. G., Salamun, A., & King, L. A. (2021). Exposure to authoritarian values leads to lower positive affect, higher negative affect, and higher meaning in life. *PLOS One, 16*(9), e0256759.

Xinni, W. E. I., Feng, Y. U., Kaiping, P., & Nian, Z. (2023). Psychological richness increases behavioral intention to protect the environment. *Acta Psychologica Sinica, 55*(8), 1330.

CHAPTER 63

Tangled Integration

Weaving Together Philosophy, Science, and Practice to Advance Existential Ideas

Kevin Aho, Natalie Fraser, *and* Carol D. Ryff

In this chapter we bring together three distinct perspectives—existential philosophy (past and present), current scientific research on well-being and health inspired by existential thinking, and ongoing practice to bring existentialism to the public square and increase its accessibility outside of academia. A guiding premise is that existentialism calls for a broad multidisciplinary approach, and that the juxtaposition of these differing perspectives reveals useful insights as well as needed future directions. The larger objective is to usher in a new era of existential thinking that draws on the past and engages with contemporary societal challenges to sharpen the value of existential ideas to improve the human condition.

What follows is organized into four parts. The first section, written by an existential philosopher, examines core meanings of existentialism, drawing on the writings of seminal thinkers from the 19th and 20th centuries. Foremost among these is the idea that *existence precedes essence*, along with other themes: *transcendence*, *freedom*, *authenticity*, and *ethics*. These ideas are explicated with a commitment to clarify how they were a response to the historical and cultural conditions in which they emerged. This return to original sources is important, given that many trained in subfields of psychology may not have had in-depth exposure to foundational writings of existentialism.

The second section, written by a research psychologist, examines how existential ideas were brought to the scientific arena via a eudaimonic model of psychological well-being, which drew on clinical, developmental, existential, and humanistic views about positive psychological functioning. Key components in this model are described, followed by a selective look at research findings, such as how meaning making matters for diverse aspects of health and how long people live. Also addressed are current societal stressors that are undermining purposeful life engagement and self-realization for many, particularly those who are socioeconomically disadvantaged.

The third section, written by a clinical practitioner, addresses initiatives to take existential ideas beyond the sequestered halls of academia into the public square. The focus is on a series of global existential summits offered over recent years via online prerecorded interviews with wide-ranging scholars and practitioners who actively use existential ideas in their work. Rich are the lived experiences of those interviewed, some of whom offer insightful critiques of existentialism as the purview of privileged players from the West. The need to decolonize European existential perspectives is elaborated from multiple vantage points.

A fourth section examines the insights revealed from this tangled integration of philosophy, science, and practice. These include the need to (1) recognize Western and privileged biases in much existential philosophy and science; (2) acknowledge tensions, sometimes constructive, between philosophy and science as well as the need to broaden the focus beyond the individual; and (3) spotlight contemporary societal problems, especially widening inequality fueled by greed in some sectors. These realities call for a return to themes of virtue, ethics, and morality, longstanding priorities in classical existential philosophy.

Below we briefly set the stage for what follows by underscoring a core existential principle—that all human experience is historically and contextually bound. This recognition calls for an understanding of the contextual factors that led to the emergence of existential thinking in the mid-19th century and its sociocultural expansion in the mid-20th century. These past contexts are later juxtaposed with our current context to sharpen appreciation of timeliness of existential ideas amid changing realities.

THE HISTORICAL CONTEXT OF EXISTENTIALISM

Existential philosophy began to take shape in Europe in the mid-19th century with the pioneering work of the Danish philosopher Kierkegaard and the German philosopher Nietzsche. These ideas gained purchase in German universities and scholarly circles in the first two decades of the 20th century under the influence of prominent figures such as Husserl, Heidegger, and Jaspers. By the 1950s and 1960s, the ideas erupted beyond the cloistered walls of the academy under the newly coined moniker "existentialism" and were popularized by influential French figures such as Sartre and Beauvoir. Existentialism spilled into the streets of Paris in the form of student and worker protests, in counterculture revolutions, in the civil and women's rights movements, in the radical politics of the New Left in Britain and the United States, and in anticolonial activism protesting, among other things, the French occupation of Algeria and Vietnam. By the mid-20th-century existentialism had become one of the most significant cultural and political movements in the intellectual history of the West.

What was notable about that historical context? Turning to Nietzsche's (1882/2001) groundbreaking work *The Gay Science*, we find the Madman announcing that God is dead. Jumping into the midst of a bustling crowd gathered in the marketplace, he shouted, "I seek God! I seek God . . . Where has God gone? I'll tell you where! We've killed him—you and I! We are all his murderers!" (p. A 125). This proclamation struck his European audience like a lightning bolt, especially the claim that they were somehow responsible for his murder. The context for the Madman's announcement was an entire generation living through a period of radical sociocultural transformation, where earlier ways of life rooted in a close-knit sense of community, belongingness, and social integration were being destroyed and replaced by an increasingly alienating and impersonal social order ruled by principles of science, mechanization, and technology. For Nietzsche, a pernicious faith in God was replaced with an equally pernicious faith in science. Other utopian advocates, including Marx, J. S. Mill, and N. Chernyshevsky embraced this scientific vision to rationally redesign and automate society in accordance with naturalistic and mathematical laws, thereby releasing human beings from unnecessary labor and maximizing human happiness.

Built into this emergent secularism was the materialist assumption that humans are physical beings and thus subject to the laws of nature, causally responding to environmental stimuli. According to this view, the primary motivation for all human action, despite its apparent complexity, was the desire to avoid pain and pursue pleasure. Nonetheless, amid the optimism to modify human behavior based on scientific principles to create a happier, well-ordered society, the seeds of revolt were being sown. Along with Nietzsche, a renegade group of philosophers, theorists, and literary figures began to push back against the ascendant scientism, pointing out how nihilistic and corrosive an uncritical faith in the power of scientific progress and technique were, especially when it came to the deepest, most unsettling problems of the human condition. Put simply, positivism could not address the ultimate questions of existence: "Who am I?"; "How should I live?"; and "What is the purpose and meaning my life?" For these thinkers, a different kind of science was needed, a human or existential science whose concerns could not be mathematized and assigned a truth-value based on empirical verification. It was this historical backdrop that gave birth to existentialism and, subsequently, to existential psychology.

WHAT IS EXISTENTIALISM?

Unlike Marxism, existentialism does not have an orthodoxy and does not refer to a fixed ideology or system. This may help explain why none of the major figures self-identified with the word *existentialism*. As Beauvoir wrote, "My inspiration came from my own experience, not from a system" (1963/1992, p. 38). Existentialism, in this view, is best understood *not* as a philosophical school or system but as an affective and embodied orientation (or way of seeing) that pays close attention to lived experience and confronts (and works to accept and integrate) the painful givens of the human condition. Rather than proceeding from a set of ready-made principles, the methodological starting point proceeds from the "I am"—from the first-person experience of existence itself.

From the perspective of empirical science this can be viewed as heresy in at least two important ways. First, existentialism begins not from a perspective of scientific detachment and objectivity but from within the concrete struggle of life *as it is lived*, where the researcher pays attention, listens, and documents, however imperfectly, the experiences of human beings in their own worldly contexts. It adopts an "insider's perspective" (Aho, 2020) to illuminate the flesh and blood particulars of individual and collective experience and exposes the ways in which social, political, and economic conditions limit and constrain the possibility of realizing one's own potential, what classical existentialists refer to as *authenticity* (*authenticité*, *Eigentlichkeit*) and what we will be calling *eudaimonic well-being* (Ryff, 1989, 2018). Because it begins from within the situated activity of existence itself, the science of existential psychology is inherently flawed and incomplete because the subject matter is irreducibly complex. The best it can do is describe experience by attending to the stories and narratives of human beings as they confront who they are and struggle with their situation. The goal, as the French philosopher Merleau-Ponty wrote, is "not one of explaining or analyzing" existence; it is, rather, "a matter of describing" existence in its full concreteness by attending to the phenomena in all its richness, mystery, and diversity (1945/1962, p. viii).

This awareness leads to the second existential heresy, namely, that it explodes the boundaries of the academy and the rigid disciplinary silos that separate the arts, sciences, and humanities. Indeed, many of the most powerful expressions of the human condition are found not in the dry and turgid prose of academic philosophy or psychology, but in literary figures. For example, those created by the Russian novelist Fyodor Dostoevsky, the German poet Rainer Maria Rilke, and the Irish dramatist Samuel Beckett. Indeed, many of existentialism's most influential philosophers were best known not for their jargon-filled tomes, but for their accessible fiction, novels, plays, and short stories. Sartre and Camus both won Nobel Prizes in Literature and Beauvoir won the prestigious literary award, *le Prix Goncourt*. But the reach of existentialism stretched far beyond the written word. We see core ideas played out on the big screen by Swedish filmmaker Ingmar Bergman, Italian director Michelangelo Antonioni, and American moviemaker Terrence Malik. We witness the horror and flux of the human condition displayed on the canvases of the Norwegian painter Edvard Munch, the French modernist Marcel Duchamp, and the American "drip-style" work of Jackson Pollack. Documentaries and long-form journalism also give voice to the lived experience of the migrant worker, Indigenous peoples, those who are mentally ill, those who are aged and disabled, impoverished classes in the racialized South and urban ghettos, and those left alienated in the hollowed-out cities of the postindustrial rust belt, where opioid addiction and "deaths of despair" are destroying countless lives.

This broad interdisciplinary approach allows existential psychology to expand beyond its Eurocentric origins. As we document, one of the significant developments of contemporary existentialism is the way it is being decolonized, challenging the socioeconomically privileged, White, and (mostly) male representation by engaging the experience of those who have traditionally been underrepresented and marginalized, especially those in the Global South (Aho et al., 2024). Existentialism's critique of methodological detachment and its focus on the concrete particulars of everyday life provides access to the situated and oppressive nuances of colonialism in Latinx (Ortega, 2016), Black (Gordon, 2020), and aboriginal (Coulthard, 2014) experience. This integration opens fresh paths to expand understanding of alterity within Euro-American culture, including experiences of marginalization and oppression in queer (Ahmed, 2006), aging (Aho, 2022) chronically ill (Toombs, 1995), and disabled (Reynolds, 2022) identities.

The Core Ideas

Despite the disjointed wellspring of sources that engage and reflect existential concerns, there is nonetheless a set of unifying ideas that existential psychology draws on to articulate what is unique about the human condition, beginning with the recognition that human existence is a temporal activity, a finite process of becoming who we are. Understanding human existence as a temporal, historically situated, activity or *way of being* means there is no pregiven nature or essence that determines who and what we are. This sets up what is arguably existentialism's most significant contribution to our understanding of what it means to be human.

Existence Precedes Essence

Existentialism reverses the traditional idea that a pregiven essence necessarily grounds existence, and this leads to the central principle: *existence precedes essence.* Individuals are thrown into an existence that they did not choose, and it is only then that they begin to create who they are through moment-to-moment choices and actions. Sartre (1946/2001) called this the "first principle of existentialism," namely that "man first exists, turns up, appears on the scene, and, only afterwards, defines himself" (pp. 292–293). As self-defining beings, humans are unique among other animals because humans alone exist *for ourselves.* Humans are self-conscious and free to create themselves through their own meaning-giving projects and commitments. This means humans are always *other* than who they are because they are ceaselessly negating former identities and self-interpretations through their choices. Existence, on this view, is an ongoing process of self-making, but this process is not unrestricted or absolute. It is always mediated or conditioned by the facts of the situation they've been thrown into. Humans exist, then, in a state of relational tension with the freedom of self-creation on the one hand and factical determinations that limit them on the other.

Transcendence

Existence is always conditioned by social, economic, political, and biophysical circumstances, but one is not wholly at the mercy of these circumstances. As a self-conscious being, one can surpass or "transcend" them by confronting them, giving them meaning, and taking action to transform them. This tension between "facticity" and "transcendence" means that one freely makes oneself, but it is also true that one is already made. Recognizing existence as a tension is especially instructive for existential psychology, as it allows for a more granular, nuanced, and qualitative understanding of the ways in which the process of self-creation is restricted and confined by social conditions related to intersectional issues such as race, class, gender, religious orientation, physical and mental (dis)ability, gender identity, and sexual orientation.

Freedom

The human capacity to transcend or rise above facticity points to a uniquely human form of suffering or anguish that arises from human's inescapable freedom. If there is no pregiven essence that defines who humans are, this also means there are no moral absolutes that can provide security, guidance, and direction in their lives. This is what Nietzsche (1882/2001) meant when he referred to "God's death." In the secular age, one is left abandoned and adrift, facing what he called "a terrifying infinity" (p. A 124). This uncanny feeling of anguish was described by the existentialists in different ways—as dread (Kierkegaard), anxiety (Heidegger), nausea (Sartre), absurdity (Camus)—but they all referred to the same unsettling realization, that existence is fundamentally insecure, unstable, and groundless, and that from the moment of birth one's being is threatened by the possibility of nonbeing, by death. This focus on the revelatory power of moods reveals another break with the tradition of mainstream science. Knowledge of the human condition is disclosed to humans not by adopting a perspective of theoretical detachment (or "view from nowhere"); rather individuals understand who they are by means of how they feel, and these feelings have the power to shatter their worlds, shaking them out of comfortable routines and ready-made identities. When the world collapses in this way, humans are awakened to the groundlessness and absurdity of the human condition and forced to confront the ultimate questions: "Who am I?" and "What is the meaning of my life?" It is here, amid the collapse, that the journey of self-becoming truly begins.

Authenticity

The transformative power of existential feelings reveals that humans spend most of their lives living in shallow self-deception, blindly conforming to the norms, values, and expectations of the public world. They live, in Nietzsche's (1889/1998, p. 106) words, as "herd animals," believing that they are living well because they are doing what everyone else is doing. This way of life may be predictable and comforting, but it is mired in inauthenticity (or "bad faith") because it compels humans to turn away from who they are and become a "they-self." For the existentialist, a valuable or praiseworthy life has little to do with social convention, happiness, or even being a good person. The aim is to be authentic, to *be true* to oneself, to realize one's own unique potential as a form of eudaimonic well-being. As Kierkegaard illustrated by drawing on the biblical figure of Abraham, there may be (and usually are) times in life when one must, in a state of "fear and trembling," decide between being a good person (being moral) and being true to oneself (being authentic). The existentialist demands that one choose the latter, confront who one is and, in doing so, temporarily suspend one's obligations to socially prescribed moral principles for the sake of something higher, namely one's own personal truth. This explains why themes of revolt, rebellion, and deliverance from the crowd are common in existential philosophy and literature. Being authentic does not, however, mean that one stops caring for others or stops working to transform oppressive social conditions. It is quite the opposite, although there is a risk to other-directed behavior. It can manifest as a form of self-evasion disguised as moral action, where one distracts oneself, fleeing from one's own groundlessness by immersing oneself in the service of knowing and helping others. For the existentialist, the point in privileging authenticity over conventional morality is one of ontological priorities.

Ethics

Prioritizing authenticity over morality suggests there are no moral absolutes, no enduring ethical prescriptions or values that one ought to adhere to. But this does not mean human existence is an amoral event. The point for the existentialist is that it is not God, but existence *qua* freedom that is the source of all value. Being a professor or husband, for example, has worth and value one chooses for it. But choices do not take place in isolation because existence is fundamentally relational; they are bound up in the lives and choices of others. This relational ontology suggests that one is not a solitary, voluntaristic subject but a "being-in-the-world" and a "being-with-others" that invariably places moral demands on oneself. It entails responsibility and obligations to care for others so they can realize and accept their freedom. Here we see that being authentic and being moral are two sides of the same coin. The goal then is to help others confront and accept the painful givens of freedom and finitude but also work to expose socioeconomic and political conditions that prevent this authentic confrontation and the possibility for eudaimonic well-being. We suggest that the capacity to be true to oneself, to flourish as an individual is a privilege when most human beings are thrown into conditions of oppression, subjugation, and material scarcity where the possibility for self-realization is severely restricted. In these conditions, individuals are unable to follow Nietzsche's (1882/2001) imperative, one that commands, "You shall become who you are!" (p. A 270).

To address conditions that restrict an individual or group's capacity for eudaimonic well-being, we contend that the science of existential psychology casts a wide interdisciplinary net. It is an inherently messy and disheveled science that draws on and integrates the insights not just of philosophers, social scientists, public policy experts, and allied health professionals but of writers, poets, artists, filmmakers, documentarians, and journalists. This tangled integration is essential to illuminate complexities of the human condition and constraints and forms of oppression unique to each situation. Most importantly, it opens a discursive space that allows for what Sartre (1968, p. 94) called "social possibles" to be lived, creating a crack in the wall where underrepresented and underprivileged classes can finally emerge from the shadows to be recognized and heard, making it possible to glimpse at a future of deep meaning and self-realization that is no longer blocked off.

In the next section we explore psychological research on eudaimonic well-being from a broad multidisciplinary perspective that draws on existential, humanistic, and developmental perspectives to articulate ideas of meaning and purpose, growth and self-realization, autonomy and mastery. These, as empirical findings show, are contoured by sociodemographic factors and life experiences, and they are also consequential for diverse aspects of health.

EXISTENTIAL IDEAS IN SCIENCE: STUDIES OF PSYCHOLOGICAL WELL-BEING AND HEALTH

More than two decades ago, Ryan and Deci (2001) partitioned the science of well-being into two broad traditions: one dealing with happiness (hedonic well-being) and the other dealing with human potential (eudaimonic well-being). Both are part of wide-ranging research on "subjective well-being" that has been studied empirically since the middle of the last century—for over 70 years (Ryff, 2024a). Much early work examined Americans' reports of their happiness and life satisfaction (Andrews & Withey, 1976; Campbell et al., 1976) and linked such perceptions to various economic indicators. Similar questions were later the focus of psychological research on subjective well-being (Diener et al., 1999), framed as hedonic psychology (Kahneman et al., 1999). Little of this work engaged with existential ideas, theory, or philosophy.

Eudaimonic well-being, in contrast, attends to theories and philosophies about the human condition, including existentialism. Here we focus on a model of well-being (Ryff, 1985, 1989) that grew out of clinical, developmental, existential, and humanistic frameworks as well as seminal insights from Aristotle's *Nicomachean Ethics* (1925). Addressed below are key components of well-being in this model, how they have been studied, and what kinds of findings have grown up around them. The latter offer evidence for how well-being matters, both in individual lives and in terms of broader societal functioning. Parenthetically, we note another eudaimonic approach, namely, self-determination theory (SDT; Ryan & Deci, 2000), which is concerned with human motivation. Three basic psychological needs are posited: autonomy, competence, and relatedness. A key idea in SDT research is that satisfaction of these needs fosters both hedonic and eudaimonic well-being. SDT is thus not a theory about well-being; rather, it is a theory about basic human needs thought to matter for subjective well-being, broadly defined.

What Is Eudaimonic Well-Being?

Center stage in the model put forth by Ryff (1989; Ryff & Singer, 2008) were ideas about human growth, development, and self-realization. Multiple sources were drawn on to explicate what human becoming is, such as Erikson's (1959) formulation of ego development, Buhler's writings about the basic life tendencies (Bühler, 1935; Bühler & Massarik, 1968), and Neugarten's (1968, 1973) descriptions of personality development in middle and later adulthood. Also relevant were Maslow's (1968) views of self-actualization, Rogers's (1961) formulation of the fully functioning person, Allport's (1961) conception of maturity, and Jung's (1933; von Franz, 1964) description of individuation. Existential thinking was strongly evident in Frankl's (1959/1985) emphasis on meaning making in the face of adversity. Jahoda (1958) drew on some of these perspectives to distill the nature of positive mental health.

In the background were enduring ideas from Aristotle's (1925) *Ethics*, where he asserted that happiness was the highest of all human goods achievable by human action. However, he emphasized differences in what "the general run of men and people of superior refinement" say that happiness is. For the former, it is some "plain and obvious thing, like pleasure, wealth, or honor," but Aristotle likened this to a life suitable for beasts. Instead, he defined the highest human good as "activity of the soul in accord with virtue" (see Ryff & Singer, 2008, pp. 15–16). He then asked what was the highest of all virtues and proposed that eudaimonia was the answer. Defined as achieving the "best thing in us," eudaimonia is thus a kind of personal excellence unique to each person's talents and capacities. As we saw earlier, much of what existentialists refer to as "authenticity" is manifestation of a virtuous and praiseworthy life grounded in one's capacity to "realize" and "be true" to oneself. Johnston (1997) captured this telos of self-realization when he wrote, "The excellence of the human being is thus going to be associated with growth towards some final realization of his or her true and best nature" (p. 6).

The central contribution of Ryff (1989; Ryff & Singer, 2008) was to identify points of convergence in these many formulations. Rather than build a eudaimonic model of well-being around a single conceptualization, the aim was to show that many of them pointed toward similar aspects of positive psychological functioning. These were distilled as six key dimensions of well-being: autonomy, environmental mastery, personal growth, positive relations with others, purpose in life, and self-acceptance. Definitions for each of these dimensions came from the underlying conceptual frameworks—that is what makes the model theory-driven. Many of these aspects of well-being address key existential challenges of living: having goals to live for, finding meaning and purpose in life, living authentically according to one's inner convictions, knowing and being true to oneself, and above all, making the most of one's talents and capacities. Despite their appeal in articulating the upside of the human condition, these ideas had been absent in scientific studies of well-being because tools to assess them did not exist.

Thus, a second key contribution of Ryff (1989) was to construct self-report scales designed to measure these various aspects of well-being. Self-descriptive items were written to capture the meaning of high and low scorers for each dimension. The items were then subjected to extensive psychometric evaluation (Keyes et al., 2002; Ryff, 1989; Ryff & Keyes, 1995), including numerous assessments of item-to-scale correlations, multiple types of validity (face, content, convergent and discriminant, factorial) and reliability (internal consistency, test–retest). Measurement of inner experience is inherently imperfect, although extensive evidence supports the psychometric qualities of these instruments, when scales of sufficient length are used.

What Scientific Findings about Eudaimonic Well-Being Have Revealed

Translated in 40 languages, more than 1,950 publications have been generated with the above model of well-being. Much work has been conducted within the MIDUS (Midlife in the United States) national longitudinal study as well as its sister study MIDJA (Midlife in Japan) (see *https://midus.wisc.edu*). These endeavors are deeply multidisciplinary in scope: Included are many subfields of psychology (cognition, emotion, personality, stress and coping) as well as population-based disciplines (demography, epidemiology, sociology) and biological/physiological domains, genomics, and neuroscience. Importantly, MIDUS and MIDJA data are publicly available—researchers from all over the world can access the data (no permissions required). The response from the scientific community has been dramatic: Over 2,200 publications covering 34 different topic areas have been generated by the 30,000-plus users of the data.

Before highlighting select findings, it is useful to reflect on why this model of well-being has attracted so much attention (see Ryff, 2018). One answer may be that the model integrates intellectually vital ideas and ideals about what constitutes the best within humans (as emphasized by Aristotle). Another reason may be these diverse aspects of well-being have wide-ranging relevance and versatility—the scales have been used to study adult development, work and family life, health and biology, and neuroscience. A third reason, not articulated by Ryff (2018) but emphasized here, is that the model engages with core existential challenges of life: finding meaning and purpose, striving to realize personal capacities, knowing one's strengths and weaknesses, and living authentically according to personal convictions. These qualities resonate with researchers and practitioners around the globe.

Multiple prior reviews have summarized wide-ranging findings from the above model (Miyamoto & Ryff, 2022; Ryff, 2014, 2024b; Ryff et al., 2021). We select examples of findings below, including factors that may compromise the well-being and health of many. The latter reveals the need to bring social equity and justice to studies of well-being.

Factors That Influence Experiences of Well-Being

How well-being changes as individuals journey across the decades of adult life has garnered extensive attention. Findings show downward trajectories for personal growth and purpose from midlife into old age, thus pointing to conditions of agism and unique challenges faced by contemporary elders to remain meaningfully engaged in life. Alternatively, upward age trajectories have been observed for environmental mastery and positive relations. Educational status also matters: Better-educated adults have higher levels of all aspects of eudaimonic well-being. Such disparities also endure over time, with recent evidence showing persistent disadvantage in well-being over 20 years among the less educated (Boylan et al., 2025). Minority status (Blacks compared to Whites) has surprisingly emerged as a positive predictor of well-being, suggesting that the challenges of racism may hone qualities of purpose and growth.

Family experience also matters, as helping others in family roles is linked with enhanced reports of purpose and self-acceptance. Married adults show higher well-being, compared to divorced, widowed, or never married individuals, although single women showed higher profiles on autonomy and personal growth compared to married women. Parenting is linked with enhanced well-being, whereas the loss of a child predicts impaired well-being decades later. Loss of a parent in childhood predicts lower adult well-being. Childhood adversity predicts lower purpose in life in adulthood; purpose also moderates the link between early emotional abuse/neglect and depressive symptoms in adulthood.

Studies Linking Psychological Well-Being to Health

Eudaimonic well-being has been linked with a wide array of biological measures, including better glycemic regulation, reduced inflammatory profiles, better lipid profiles, lower risk of metabolic syndrome, and lower allostatic load (a summary index of physiological risk). These biological assessments, in turn, are linked with reduced risk for various disease outcomes such as type 2 diabetes, cardiovascular disease, stroke, and osteoporosis. Eudaimonia has also been linked with brain assessments: Those with higher eudaimonic well-being showed less amygdala activation in response to negative stimuli and more activation of brain regions that help regulate emotions. Those with higher eudaimonia also showed sustained activation of reward circuitry in response to positive stimuli, which was further linked with lower stress hormones (cortisol output) over the course of the day. Other work has linked eudaimonic well-being with greater insular cortex volume that is involved in an array of higher-order cognitive functions. Taken together, these wide-ranging linkages between inner experiences of well-being with diverse biological and brain-based measures underscore the fundamental importance of human subjectivity in making sense of variation in physiological systems as well as the structure and function of parts of the brain. Effectively, the work demonstrates how one's inner self and biological workings are tied together in ways that matter fundamentally for health.

Arguably the most dramatic findings of relevance for existentialists pertain to what has been learned about links between purpose in life and longevity. Extensive science in population-based disciplines (demography, epidemiology, sociology) is built around the study of death—that is, mortality and its causes. This is ground zero for existentialists. A stunning finding is that those with higher purpose in life live longer. This protective benefit of perceiving one's life as having meaning and direction has been documented in multiple large datasets that control for numerous confounds, such as prior health status. The first such result emerged from a community-based study of memory and aging, but later work from numerous national and international studies, including a meta-analysis involving data from 10 prospective studies, has shown that higher purpose in life is a protective factor against death.

Illuminating how this benefit for longevity might work, other studies have shown that those with higher levels of purpose in life have reduced risk of multiple disease outcomes (Alzheimer's disease, heart disease, stroke), and relatedly, that those with higher eudaimonic well-being are more likely to use preventive health care services and to practice better health behaviors (diet, exercise). What then is the larger import of findings showing protective health benefits from perceiving one's life as meaningful and purposeful? Essentially it is this: Although decades of past health research have focused on pathways to illness and disease, eudaimonic well-being, with its strong ties to existential and humanistic thinking, brings knowledge of the upside to the fore—namely, what keeps people healthy and well so they can enjoy long lives. Such benefits require, however, well-functioning societies that protect citizens from undue stress. Growing evidence shows that life is increasingly difficult for those who are disadvantaged.

CONTEMPORARY EXISTENTIAL CHALLENGES: WIDENING INEQUALITY AND THE PANDEMIC

Sadly, socioeconomic inequality has grown ever more dramatic of late, particularly in the United States. Recent historical stressors, such as the Great Recession and the COVID-19 pandemic, have further exacerbated problems of inequality (Ryff, 2023). Extensive research has examined what discrepant life opportunities mean for well-being and health. In MIDUS, focus has been on two national samples, one recruited in 1995 and another in 2012. Over this period of time, educational attainment in the United States improved. Yet despite such gains, the later sample had less household income, lower financial stability, worse general health, more chronic conditions, more functional limitations, and lower levels of well-being (autonomy, personal growth, self-acceptance, positive affect, and life satisfaction) than the baseline sample (Kirsch et al., 2019). Additional findings showed that poorer mental health in the later sample occurred among those of lower socioeconomic status (Goldman et al., 2018).

These findings bring into high relief troublesome realities of the larger societal context—that is, the opioid epidemic, growing alcoholism, and increased deaths due to suicide, collectively referred to as "deaths of despair" (Case & Deaton, 2015, 2020). Others have brought attention to growing homelessness (evictions) (Desmond, 2016) and the extent to which many (employers, landlords, banks, payday lenders) profit from the poor (Desmond, 2023). Other current science shows an increased sense of entitlement, narcissism, and tendency to behave unethically among upper-class compared to lower-class individuals (Piff, 2014). A large panel study of over 65,000 U.S. students (Mendelberg et al., 2017) revealed that those from affluent backgrounds were more likely to disagree with the statement "wealthy people should pay a larger share of taxes than they do now."

Philanthropy, traditionally thought to exemplify commitment among elites to do good in the world, is also under scrutiny (Giridharadas, 2018). The Sackler family, contributors to major art museums around the world, owned Purdue Pharma that created oxycontin, the highly addictive, overprescribed opioid painkiller. Purdue Pharma also marketed new drugs to treat the opioid addiction they helped create. From 1999 to 2021, over half a million people in the United States died from overdoses involving opioids (Centers for Disease Control and Prevention, 2021). Nan Goldin's 2022 documentary, *All the Beauty and the Bloodshed* (*www.imdb.com/title/tt21374850/*), enacts advice from the ancient Greeks to publicly censure greed, as has the removal of the Sackler family name from art museums around the world.

The worldwide COVID-19 pandemic exacerbated problems of ever widening inequalities (Ryff, 2023). The main message is that current existential challenges are not evenly distributed across the social order but disproportionately accrue to those who are disadvantaged. Effectively, eudaimonic well-being is increasingly sequestered among privileged, well-educated, economically comfortable segments of society (Ryff, 2024b), while feelings of anger and shame (Mishra, 2017), along with heightened stress exposures, are concentrated among the disadvantaged. These realities demand attention—in philosophical circles, in scientific inquiry, and in wider public awareness. The next section brings these challenges and others out of the shadows into the public sphere via the global existential summits.

THE PRACTICE AND GLOBAL DISSEMINATION OF EXISTENTIAL IDEAS

Existential philosophies have the potential to offer wisdom, inspiration, and hope for humanity, yet academia's technical and ostracizing jargon regulates their dissemination. Projects such as the global existential summits (GESs; 2025) and Existential Offerings (n.d.) prioritize representation and accessibility, recognizing that while different existential philosophies have *similar themes*, each philosopher contributes unique perspectives providing different "existential offerings" with which one may or may not resonate.

Real life is not in textbooks or journals; it is lived. These projects actively seek to illuminate the human behind the theory, emphasizing the importance of theory being disclosed alongside personal experience, moving the viewer in a human-to-human resonance, which dry academic prose cannot. The GES speakers' personal journeys reveal a common relationship that many develop toward existential philosophies: They give words to something within one that one feels but cannot express—a sense of home. However, the stories of many illuminated a darker side of existential traditions. Many were led by personal and intergenerational histories of existential agony, and stark lived realities of marginalization and oppression.

Obvious were the differing explanations of the origins of existential ideas. GES speakers trained in Eurocentric Western canons near-exclusively referenced the "Eurocentric Elite": Kierkegaard, Nietzsche, Husserl, Heidegger, Camus, Sartre, Beauvoir, Merleau-Ponty, and Frankl. Speakers hailing from outside the Eurocentric Western canons told a different story. Theoretically, they shared influences throughout history from across the globe and notably emphasized transdisciplinary contributions such as artists, musicians, activists, and spiritual leaders. Personally, they shared lived experience and awareness of colonization within today's world, many directly impacted by elitism and racism inherent in academia and engrained within collective consciousness. The following considers what these existential summits have brought into focus.

Existential Perspectives on Elitism: Privilege and Knowledge Hoarding

Existential curiosity is historically and universally a human attribute unbound by demographics such as race, class, or gender, yet the privileges of existing within elitist professions like academia are disproportionately unavailable to most of humanity, resulting in sociocultural disparities in the production and hoarding of knowledge (Fraser, 2024). The dominant culture situates the geography of reason in the West (Gordon, 2023), producing and disseminating knowledge to and from specific sociocultural systems that benefit from disproportionate research and funding. This system directly impedes developing countries that fall victim to the ramifications of academic capitalism (Ellers et al.,

2017). Knowledge hoarding is a small but significant area of investigation, referring to the accumulation of power to dominate over other professions. Knowledge is colonized by neglecting and subordinating a plethora of global contributions, rarely reflected upon in part because it is often invisible to White Western researchers (Marchais et al., 2020). Yang (GES 3) stressed the value of knowledge sharing as a two-way bridge: "There's a lot of, to an extreme, kind of a worship of what's from the West. And I'm troubled by that, and saddened by that. . . . The bridging work I'm trying to do is to bring people from the West who with humility are *gifting*, rather than *instructing* their expert knowledge."

The value of existential psychology can only be felt by those who have access to it, resonate with it, and feel represented by it. "I could intuit some of their moves but the spirit of it just wasn't me, even though I could commiserate intellectually," reflected Haile III (GES 1) about key mainstream philosophers. Among other speakers at the summits, McKenzie (GES 3) and Haile III (GES 1) highlighted the resistance they experienced from senior lecturers in the field when citing sources outside the mainstream literature, raising the question of why there is an unspoken expectation for existential scholarship to be validated via the traditional Eurocentric Elite, despite the vast quantity of global contributions and the potential irrelevance of traditional existentialists of privileged White Western males.

Many of the words, references, and names of people articulated by existential psychology do not exist in the worlds of those it studies. A movement toward the humanization of knowledge is thus required, emancipating ideas from the prison of epistemology, removing methodological and linguistic barriers that ostracize and colonize human minds, and instead facilitate access to new insights through creative and representative transdisciplinary pursuits. Humanizing knowledge includes making existential philosophies accessible and personal so that they can genuinely support and guide the people whom it sets out to guide and support. This is a question of professional humanity and ethics. Worth (2017) warned of the human tendency to act on autopilot rather than as a mark of one's own values. The dedicated efforts of several speakers at the summits provided tangible evidence of stepping beyond the norms to make accessibility possible, including through the arts, publishing popular public blogs, and forming communities of dialogue.

Decolonizing Existential Education

While "existentialism" is considered a fundamentally European historical phenomenon, the GESs reminded us that it is fundamental to discern between "existentialism" and "existential philosophies." Existential philosophies or "philosophies of existence" refer to philosophical questioning premised upon existential concerns (Gordon, 2013). Notably identifiable are the culturally specific responses to existential themes that philosophers offer: isolation, meaning, freedom, and death (American; Yalom, 1980); freedom, anguish, responsibility, embodied agency, sociality, and liberation (Afro-Caribbean; Gordon, 2013); ethical vacuity, forlornness, the crisis of insufficiency, the conundrum of choice, and the enigma of authentic being (Latin American; Murillo, 2023); *wu wei*, authenticity, focusing, surrender, trusting the process/the Tao, getting back to the basics, steadiness amid chaos, listening for the unheard, being fully present, humility and awe, bearing witness, following the flow, letting go, stillness and going nowhere (Asian; Yang, 2020); time, identity, essence, stability and change, creation, knowledge and seeing, and the nature of being and world (Mesoamerican; McLeod, 2023).

Contributions have been offered by every culture during every era of humanity (Robles, 2015) yet remain largely marginalized within the dominant Euro-American canon. By not teaching the full story, the full truth remains suppressed, thus oppressing human realities. Vété-Congolo (GES 3) highlighted the dehumanizing reality of this experience, noting that "de-existentialisation is not taught . . . that's left outside of the curriculum." Inadvertently showcased by the summits was the invisible harm resulting from privileged elitism and oppression occurring within the field. McKenzie (2023) has highlighted that it's not just about *what* is being taught, but *who* is doing the teaching.

Confronting ignorance within privileged cultures, McKenzie unveiled that even seemingly innocent training exercises, such as introducing oneself, have a darker, silenced meaning for those who carry their slave name.

The summits have emphasized the lived reality of education being disproportionately harder for Black students. One example by Haile III (GES 1) emphasized the recurring experience of Black students' theses being systematically rejected, and the challenges of fighting for credibility and acceptance within academia by publishing rejected theses as books (Haile III, 2012), an experience shared by Charles Johnson, who independently published *Being and Race: Black Writing since 1970* (2013), and Frantz Fanon, whose rejected doctoral thesis was later published as *Peau Noire, Masques Blancs* ("Black Skin, White Masks"; 1952). The GESs have revealed that little has changed over the decades, and while academia claims to be more "inclusive," educational spaces are experienced radically differently by people of different races and backgrounds. "One group seeks justification while the other is self-justified," reflected Gordon (GES 1), whose story reflects many whose experiences in academia were interwoven with an inherent awareness that their contributions may be rejected due to their race and nonconformist focus.

The key existential theme of freedom is fundamentally different when discussed from a place of one's existence being self-justified in contrast to one's existence fighting for validation and liberation. While there is a dominant culture choosing whom and whom not to include, there is no global freedom.

Existential Perspectives on Knowledge Trafficking: History, Language, and Translation

Existentialism is often recognized as emerging postwar, yet it also developed following the Atlantic slave trade and imperial movements. Colonists not only steal, traffic, and trade people . . . they steal, traffic, and trade people's skills and wisdoms. Existential history blatantly traces the timeline of influence among the Existential Elite, building on and opposing each other's contributions, yet this history exiles wider global influences. As experts in the GESs explicated, it is no coincidence that scholars are discovering compatibility between Eastern and European philosophies (Kalmanson, 2020). Heidegger (as one example) directly collaborated with Asian scholars and texts, reappropriating many concepts yet rarely citing sources and impeded by his limited multilingualism (Nelson, 2023).

English marketed as the *lingua franca* is often taken for granted by native speakers yet notably was not originally the *lingua franca* of existentialism—all classic thinkers being non-native English speakers. Rarely acknowledged is that the vast majority of existential psychology is taught and conducted by academics who have only studied translated texts. Multilingual speakers at the GESs iterated the limitations and vast potential for mistranslation of meaning, unveiling that (for example) a key concept of Sartre's "freedom" contributions are based on a misreading of Dostoyevsky *Notes from the Underground*, critiqued within Russian academia (e.g., Lesevitskii, 2016) yet a matter of obliviousness to most existential scholars.

Ubuntu: Toward an Ethical Transdisciplinary Existential Movement

An existentially grounded social psychology is uniquely equipped to investigate, illuminate, and disseminate the profound contemporary existential challenges raised in this chapter. For this, we argue for transdisciplinary collaboration. The humanistic African philosophy *Ubuntu*, meaning "humanity," "I am because you are," offers a powerful guide toward this, emphasizing the interconnectedness of all individuals within their societal and physical surroundings; supporting collectivism over individualism; promoting peace, unity, and solidary; and recognizing community as one of the building blocks of society. Humanity is intrinsically bound together and individuals' choices in each moment have great impact, whether they collaborate or isolate, share or hoard, listen or silence. "Who you are as a person, what you live and bring, will affect everything that you do," wrote Worth (2017, p. 3), reminding us that the first intervention is the self.

Getting out of our own disciplinary silos is fundamental, for without a transdisciplinary epistemological awakening, the field risks overreliance and fetishization of its methods leading toward a path of solitude and disciplinary decadence (Gordon, 2023). We call on academics who have access to existential philosophies to connect with creative professionals such as artists, musicians, poets, and directors to share existential insights widely. Connection, music, film, literature, and the beauty of art and nature: These are the truly existential remedies. Thus, tangible creative examples of how scientific and philosophical ideas can become part of common knowledge and subsequently be used to negotiate one's way through difficult life challenges are presented.

Art Transcends Words

Art activities have been evidenced to develop personal, social, cultural, aesthetic, and moral values (Ibrahim, 1999), providing a universal language that transcends words and annihilates language barriers, as evidenced by all speakers at the GESs. Ceylan (GES 3) proved the timelessness of poetry, sharing how verses passed down between generations within the illiterate Turkish (outcast) community he was raised in preserved their culture's wisdom. Evangelista (GES 4) described how ancient Filipino traditional tattooing practices preserve Indigenous culture. Speakers used theater, movement, and documentaries to impart messages of liberation and pay homage to victims and survivors of genocide. Many described the grounding value of nature and creative arts, articulating how cinematics and music have the capacity to express what words cannot. Others promoted comedy and meditation as resources for self-inquiry and unlearning colonized messages. Finally, Soren (GES 3) united philosophies of eudaimonia and yoga practice as a journey toward eudaimonic well-being.

WHAT COMES OF A TANGLED INTEGRATION OF PHILOSOPHY, SCIENCE, AND PRACTICE?

In this section we highlight insights that follow from bringing the above three topics together. A first observation is to recognize Western and privileged biases evident in existential philosophy and science. A second observation underscores tensions, sometimes constructive, between philosophy and science, as well as the need to move beyond a primary focus on the individual. A third observation spotlights contemporary societal problems, particularly widening inequalities and related concerns about greed. These realities call for a return to virtue, ethics, and morality—longstanding themes in existential philosophy.

Addressing Biases in Existential Philosophy and Science: A Need to Decolonize

Humans naturally develop biases to navigate and survive the extraordinary complexities of their uncertain worlds. Yet in existentially inspired endeavors, practitioners and researchers must actively develop reflexive awareness of their biases as a means of discerning between subjectivity and emergent meanings and truths (Fraser, 2023). That same reflexivity is necessary for existential psychology, whose work is sometimes shrouded in colonizing, racist, individualistic, patriarchal, and privileged biases.

Nietzsche reckoned that "God is dead," yet he did not predict that existential philosophers would themselves replace the deity for many devoted followers. The Existential Elite became compounded as the core source of existential wisdom, with their taglines and key concepts sensationalized for their ability to speak to the masses. Yet these "masses" were not universally representative but, rather, constituted the collective consciousness of a comparatively privileged few. Interwoven within these ideas and concepts are contextually and subjectively situated biases, ethics, and values that have seeped through generations of existential psychology. Only by addressing and challenging the sexism, racism, and oppressive biases inherent in the canon can the field evolve into the humane, representative, and ethical source of wisdom that is so desperately needed in today's world.

Constructive Tensions and Moving beyond the Individual

Existential thinking emerged at a time of emergent secularism that embraced positivism and science as the way forward. Such perspectives regarded humans as little more than machines responding to external stimuli in predictable ways, hence the vision of social engineers seeking to rationally design and automate society in accordance with scientific and mathematical laws. This view was strongly challenged by the renegade philosophers, theorists, and literary figures who created the existential movement. They pushed back on scientism, pointing out its incapacity to engage with the deepest and most unsettling problems of the human condition.

Few, if any, contemporary scientists have embraced positivism—indeed, that distant perspective is largely dead, a relic of the past. Similarly, few embrace Skinner's (1971) behaviorist conception of psychology, which framed human experience exclusively in terms of observable behaviors and external inputs—there was no inner being in his stimulus–response reductionism. In contrast, current efforts to bring existential ideas to psychological science show rich varieties of inner experience.

Nonetheless, existential psychology inherited from classical existentialism a narrow focus on the freedom and self-realization *of the individual.* Sartre (1945/2001) went so far as to conflate existentialism with subjectivism, where "subjectivity must be the starting point" (p. 292). This individualistic view failed to acknowledge the fact that existence is not an isolated, solitary affair; it is fundamentally intersubjective and relational. The reality that individuals exist in relation to others invariably places moral demands on them. By focusing on themes of individual freedom, finitude, and self-realization, what often goes missing in existential psychology is an account of moral responsibility to others as central to a virtuous and praiseworthy life. To this end, the call to be authentic, to heroically confront one's own freedom and death, seems privileged and selfish when one sees that the majority of humanity struggles for the basic material goods to avoid *actual death.* Existential psychology needs to be mindful of this lacuna and come to grips with the fact that human existence is bound up with social, political, and ethical implications.

Widening Inequalities and Greed: Return to Virtue and Ethics

We noted that scientific research has described disturbing realities—increased deaths of despair (due to addictions, alcoholism, suicide), growing homelessness and poverty—all exacerbated by the worldwide COVID-19 pandemic. In the background of these problems is the destructive force of greed, which has longstanding presence in human history. The ancient Greeks saw greed and injustice as violating virtues of fairness, generosity, and equality and thereby contributing to civic strife (Balot, 2001). They called for public criticism and censuring of greed and anticipated later admonishments by Jesus Christ, who told his followers, "Watch out! Be on your guard against all kinds of greed; life does not consist in an abundance of possessions" (Luke 12:15). In the 14th century, Dante's *Divine Comedy* (1308/2006) famously placed sins of greed and gluttony, along with fraud and dishonesty, in his nine circles of hell. In the 18th century, Adam Smith's *Wealth of Nations* (1776/1981) made the case for self-interest and capitalism, but at the same time, recognized the problem of greed, framed as limitless appetites of the vain and insatiable. And in the 19th century, Dostoevsky warned readers of *The Brothers Karamazov* (1880/1990) of the "terrible individualism" that was emerging in the modern age, creating a state of self-destructive egoism and greed, where "man only trembles for fear that he should lose his money and the privileges he has won for himself" (p. 276).

Viewing greed as an enduring vice in human history, we underscore that eudaimonic well-being focuses not only on traditional ends of freedom, autonomy, and self-realization, but also prioritizes a life of virtue. Excellence, as originally conceived by Aristotle, regarded the virtuous life as synonymous with human flourishing, but it is not the usual virtues of courage, temperance, or even truthfulness that matter today, but generosity—freely and willingly giving to and caring for others. Nietzsche, in his typical prescience, pointed this out in his later writings, recognizing that the character trait of generosity was becoming increasingly rare as European culture was in the throes of degeneration and sickness, careening toward hedonism, crass materialism, and the mechanized exploitation of the human being.

Although Nietzsche was a starkly antidemocratic thinker who praised exceptional individuals or "higher types" who were preternaturally equipped with traits of courage, creativity, and power, he was acutely aware that the higher types have a moral obligation to treat the less fortunate with tenderness, generosity, and mercy. In *Thus Spoke Zarathustra* (1883/1966), Nietzsche referred to generosity and compassionate gift-giving as "the highest virtue" (p. 74). Later, in *The Anti-Christ* (1888/1990), he described the duty for the privileged, writing, "When the exceptional human being treats the mediocre more tenderly than himself and his peers, this is not mere politeness of the heart—it is simply his duty" (p. 57). Referring to the masses as "mediocre" is unfortunate and typical of Nietzsche elitism, but the message is clear. Nietzsche recognized that it is those in power who have the highest obligation to be generous.

We argue this kind of virtue is crucial to eudaimonic well-being because it reminds us that we are not isolated individuals but communal beings who share the same home. As Zarathustra said to his disciples, "Let your gift-giving love . . . serve the meaning of the earth . . . that it may give the earth a meaning, *a human meaning* (1883/1966, p. 76, emphasis added). Embodying generosity in this way not only creates a more equitable and just society, it addresses the myriad toxicities of late-stage capitalism. To be generous is to be receptive to the expression of existential ideas beyond the rarified halls of the academy and White, Eurocentric dominance. It is to recognize the Zulu principle of *Ubuntu*, that across cultures and histories, we humans are all bound together in the shared project of "humanity."

REFERENCES

Ahmed, S. (2006) *Queer phenomenology: Objects, orientations, others.* Duke University Press.

Aho, K. (2020). *Existentialism: An introduction.* Polity Press.

Aho, K. (2022). *One beat more: Existentialism and the gift of mortality.* Polity Press.

Aho, K., Altman, M., & Pedersen, H. (Eds.). (2024). *The Routledge handbook of contemporary existentialism.* Routledge.

Allport, G. W. (1961). *Pattern and growth in personality.* Holt, Rinehart & Winston.

Andrews, F. M., & Withey, S. B. (1976). *Social indicators of well-being: America's perception of life quality.* Plenum Press.

Aristotle. (1925). *The Nicomachean Ethics* (W. D. Ross, Trans.). Oxford University Press.

Balot, R. K. (2001). *Greed and injustice in classical Athens.* Princeton University Press.

Beauvoir, S. (1992). *After the war: The force of circumstance: Vol. 1. 1944–1952* (R. Howard, Trans.). Paragon House. (Original work published in 1963)

Boylan, J. M., Choi, J. H., Kirsch, J. A., & Ryff, C. D. (2025). Educational disparities in 20-year trajectories of psychological well-being in a national sample. *Scientific Reports, 15,* Article 11437.

Bühler, C. (1935). The curve of life as studied in biographies. *Journal of Applied Psychology, 43,* 653–673.

Bühler, C., & Massarik, F. (Eds.). (1968). *The course of human life.* Springer.

Campbell, A., Converse, P. E., & Rodgers, W. L. (1976). *The quality of American life: Perceptions, evaluations, and satisfactions.* Russell Sage Foundation.

Case, A., & Deaton, A. (2015). Rising morbidity and mortality in midlife among white non-Hispanic Americans in the 21st century. *Proceedings of the National Academy of Sciences, 112*(49), 15078–15083.

Case, A., & Deaton, A. (2020). *Deaths of despair and the future of capitalism.* Princeton University Press.

Centers for Disease Control and Prevention (2021). *Understanding the opioid overdose epidemic.* https://www.cdc.gov/overdose-prevention/about/understanding-the-opioid-overdose-epidemic.html.

Coulthard, G. S. (2014). *Red skin, white masks: Rejecting the colonial politics of recognition.* University of Minnesota Press.

Dante Alighieri. (2006). *The divine comedy* (H. W. Longfellow, Trans.). Chartwell Books. (Original work published 1308)

Desmond, M. (2016). *Evicted: Poverty and profit in the American city.* Crown.

Desmond, M. (2023). *Poverty, by America.* Crown.

Diener, E., Suh, E. M., Lucas, R. E., & Smith, H. L. (1999). Subjective well-being: Three decades of progress. *Psychological Bulletin, 125*(2), 276–302.

Dostoevsky, F. (1990). *The brothers Karamazov.* Penguin. (Original work published 1880)

Ellers, J., Crowther, T. W., & Harvey, J. A. (2017). Gold open access publishing in mega-journals: Developing countries pay the price of Western premium academic output. *Journal of Scholarly Publishing, 49*(1), 89–102.

Erikson, E. H. (1959). Identity and the life cycle: Selected papers. *Psychological Issues, 1,* 1–171.

Existential Offerings. (n.d.). *About us | Our history.* www.existentialofferings.com/about.

Fanon, F. (1952). *Black skin, white masks.* Grove Press.

Frankl, V. E. (1985). *Man's search for meaning.* Simon & Schuster. (Original work published 1959)

Fraser, N. (2023). Structural existential analysis (SEA)—A step-by-step guide for application to research. *Counselling Psychology Review, 38*(2), 4–19.

Fraser, N. (2024). Decolonizing existential philosophy: Considering disciplinary decadence within Western existential thought. *Existential Analysis, 35*(1).

Giridharadas, A. (2018). *Winners take all: The elite charade of changing the world.* Knopf.

Global Existential Summits. (2025). (GES 1 [2022]–GES 4 [2025]). https://existentialsummit.com.

Goldman, N., Glei, D. A., & Weinstein, M. (2018). Declining mental health among disadvantaged Americans. *Proceedings of the National Academy of Sciences, 115*(28), 7290–7295.

Gordon, L. (2020). *Freedom, justice, and decolonization.* Routledge.

Gordon, L. R. (2013). *Existentia Africana: understanding Africana existential thought.* Routledge.

Gordon, L. R. (2023). *Black existentialism and decolonizing knowledge: Writings of Lewis R. Gordon.* Bloomsbury.

Haile, J. B. III. (2012). *Philosophical meditations on Richard Wright.* Rowman & Littlefield.

Ibrahim, M. N. (1999). *The development of value awareness through art education.* Master's thesis, McGill University.

Jahoda, M. (1958). *Current concepts of positive mental health.* Basic Books.

Johnson, C. (2013). *Being and race: Black writing since 1970.* Simon & Schuster.

Johnston, I. (1997). *Lecture on Aristotle's Nicomachaean ethics.* https://johnstoniatexts.x10host.com/lectures/ethicslecture.htm.

Jung, C. G. (1933). *Modern man in search of a soul* (W. S. Dell & C. F. Baynes, Trans.). Harcourt, Brace & World.

Kahneman, D., Diener, E., & Schwarz, N. (Eds.). (1999). *Well-being: The foundations of hedonic psychology.* Russell Sage Foundation.

Kalmanson, L. (2020). *Cross-cultural existentialism: On the meaning of life in Asian and Western thought.* Bloomsbury.

Keyes, C. L. M., Shmotkin, D., & Ryff, C. D. (2002). Optimizing well-being: The empirical encounter of two traditions. *Journal of Personality and Social Psychology, 82*(6), 1007–1022.

Kirsch, J. A., Love, G. D., Radler, B. T., & Ryff, C. D. (2019). Scientific imperatives vis-à-vis growing inequality in America. *American Psychologist, 74*(7), 764–777.

Lesevitskii, A. V. (2016). К вопросу феноменологии понимания свободы у Ф.М. Достоевского И Ж.-П. http://samlib.ru/a/aw_lesewickij/raprma12.shtml.http://samlib.ru/a/aw_lesewickij/raprma12.shtml.

Marchais, G., Bazuzi, P., & Amani Lameke, A. (2020). "The data is gold, and we are the gold-diggers": Whiteness, race and contemporary academic research in eastern DRC. *Critical African Studies, 12*(3), 372–394.

Maslow, A. H. (1968). *Toward a psychology of being* (2nd ed.). Van Nostrand.

McKenzie, D. (2023). *From behind the veil.* YouTube. www.youtube.com/watch?v=5TVQBjlYrKA.

McLeod, A. (2023). *An introduction to Mesoamerican philosophy.* Cambridge University Press.

Mendelberg, T., McCabe, K. T., & Thal, A. (2017). College socialization and the economic views of affluent Americans. *American Journal of Political Science, 61*(3), 606–623.

Merleau-Ponty, M. (1962). *Phenomenology of perception* (C. Smith Trans.). Routledge. (Original work published 1945)

Mishra, P. (2017). *Age of anger: A history of the present.* Farrar, Straus & Giroux.

Miyamoto, Y., & Ryff, C. D. (2022). Culture and health: Recent developments and future directions. *Japanese Psychological Research, 64*(2), 90–108.

Murillo, E. (2023). *Latin America and existentialism: A pan-American literary history (1864–1938).* University of Wales Press.

Nelson, E. S. (2023). *Heidegger and Dao: Things, nothingness, freedom.* Bloomsbury.

Neugarten, B. L. (1968). *Middle age and aging.* University of Chicago Press.

Neugarten, B. L. (1973). Personality change in late life: A developmental perspective. In C. Eisodorfer & M. P. Lawton (Eds.), *The psychology of adult development and aging* (pp. 311–335). American Psychological Association.

Nietzsche, F. (1966). *Thus spoke Zarathustra* (W. Kauffman, Trans.). Penguin. (Original work published 1883)

Nietzsche, F. (1990). *The anti-Christ* (R. J. Hollingdale Trans.). Penguin. (Original work published 1888)

Nietzsche, F. (1998). *Twilight of the idols, or how to philosophize with a hammer* (D. Large, Trans.). Oxford University Press. (Original work published 1889)

Nietzsche, F. (2001). The gay science (R. Polt, Trans.). In C. Guignon & D. Pereboom (Eds.), *Existentialism: Basic writings* (2nd ed., pp. 123–171) Hackett. (Original work published 1882)

Ortega, M. (2016). *In-between: Latina feminist phenomenology, multiplicity, and the self.* SUNY Press.

Piff, P. K. (2014). Wealth and the inflated self: Class, entitlement, and narcissism. *Personality and Social Psychology Bulletin, 40*(1), 34–43.

Reynolds, J. M. (2022). *The life worth living: Disability, pain, and morality.* University of Minnesota Press.

Robles, Y. A. M. (2015). *Existential therapy: Relational theory and practice for a post-Cartesian world* (B. Cornejo, Trans.). Circulo de Estudios en Psicoterapia Existencial.

Rogers, C. R. (1961). *On becoming a person.* Houghton Mifflin.

Ryan, R. M., & Deci, E. L. (2000). Self-determination theory and the facilitation of intrinsic motivation, social development, and well-being. *American Psychologist, 55,* 68–78.

Ryan, R. M., & Deci, E. L. (2001). On happiness and human potentials: A review of research on hedonic and eudaimonic well-being. *Annual Review of Psychology, 52,* 141–166.

Ryff, C. D. (1985). Adult personality development and the motivation for personal growth. In D. Kleiber & M. Maehr (Eds.), *Advances in motivation and achievement: Vol. 4. Motivation and adulthood* (pp. 55–92). JAI Press.

Ryff, C. D. (1989). Happiness is everything, or is it?: Explorations on the meaning of psychological well-being. *Journal of Personality and Social Psychology, 57*(6), 1069–1081.

Ryff, C. D. (2014). Psychological well-being revisited: Advances in the science and practice of eudaimonia. *Psychotherapy and Psychosomatics, 83*(1), 10–28.

Ryff, C. D. (2018). Well-being with soul: Science in pursuit of human potential. *Perspectives on Psychological Science, 13*(2), 242–248.

Ryff, C. D. (2023). Meaning-making in the face of intersecting catastrophes: COVID-19 and the plague of inequality. *Journal of Constructivist Psychology, 36*(2), 185–203.

Ryff, C. D. (2024a). Decades of scientific research on human happiness: Questions, findings, and urgent future directions. In K. Barclay, D. M. McMahon, & P. N. Stearns (Eds), *The Routledge history of happiness* (pp. 408–428). Taylor & Francis.

Ryff, C. D. (2024b). The privilege of well-being in an increasingly unequal society. *Current Directions in Psychological Science, 33(5),* 300–307.

Ryff, C. D., Boylan, J. M., & Kirsch, J. A. (2021). Eudaimonic and hedonic well-being: An integrative perspective with linkages to sociodemographic factors and health. In M. T. Lee, L. D. Kubzansky, & T. J. VanderWeele (Eds.), *Measuring well-being: Interdisciplinary perspectives from the social sciences and humanities* (pp. 92–135). Oxford University Press.

Ryff, C. D., & Keyes, C. L. M. (1995). The structure of psychological well-being revisited. *Journal of Personality and Social Psychology, 69*(4), 719–727.

Ryff, C. D., & Singer, B. H. (2008). Know thyself and become what you are: A eudaimonic approach to psychological well-being. *Journal of Happiness Studies, 9*(1), 13–39.

Sartre. J-P. (1968). *The search for a method* (H. Barnes, Trans.). Vintage Books. (Original work published 1957)

Sartre, J-P. (2001). Existentialism is a humanism (B. Frechtman, Trans.). In C. Guignon & D. Pereboom (Eds.), *Existentialism: Basic writings* (2nd ed., pp. 290–308). Hackett. (Original work published 1946)

Skinner, B. F. (1971). *Beyond freedom and dignity.* Knopf.

Smith, A. (1981). *An inquiry into the nature and causes of the wealth of nations.* Liberty Classics. (Original work published 1776)

Toombs, K. (1995). The lived experience of disability. *Human Studies, 18*(1), 9–23.

Von Franz, M. L. (1964). The process of individuation. In C. G. Jung (Ed.), *Man and his symbols* (pp. 158–229). Doubleday.

Worth, P. (2017). Positive psychology interventions: The first intervention is our self. In C. Procter (Ed.), *Positive psychology interventions in practice* (pp. 1–12). Springer.

Yalom, I. D. (1980). *Existential psychotherapy.* Basic Books.

Yang, M. (2020). *Lighting the candle: Taoist principles in supervision conducted from an existential–humanistic perspective.* University Professors Press.

CHAPTER 64

Existential–Humanistic Psychotherapy

An Integrative, Multicultural Perspective

Kirk J. Schneider, Theopia R. Jackson, *and* Louis Hoffman

The recent motion picture *Barbie* (Gerwig, 2023), with over $1 billion in box office sales (Reuters, 2023), is a striking, if ironic, testament to existentialism's sudden resurgence. The moment that Barbie (the "perfect" and serene doll played by Margot Robbie) blurts out to her fellow Barbies, "Do you guys ever think about dying?" one of the core questions of life thunders into the collective consciousness—and not just in Barbieland but in real audiences worldwide: How are we to live, and not just live but thrive, in the face of our fleeting time on this planet?

What prompted this abrupt—and massive—fascination with "existential *Barbie*"?

Perhaps the film reminds us, after decades of distraction, of our ill-fated tendencies to look away from ourselves and from the perils that abound; or perhaps it shakes us out of our consumerist-technicist mindsets that give us cheerful illusions but fail in the end to address underlying realities. Whatever the metaphor, the overarching message of *Barbie* is stark: We need to wake up, break out of our collective slumber, and revitalize our lives!

But *Barbie* is not the only sign of an existential revival in our world. The field of psychotherapy is rife with enthusiasm about the potential for existential practices to expand and advance the discipline. Witness the voice of leading psychotherapy researcher, Bruce Wampold (2008). "It could be," he wrote in his review of the book *Existential–Integrative Psychotherapy: Guideposts to the Core of Practice*, that "an understanding of the principles of existential therapy is needed by all therapists, as it adds a perspective that might . . . form the basis of all effective therapies" (p. 6). Or consider Shahar and Schiller's (2016) statement in a special issue on existential–humanistic integrations of practice in the *Journal of Psychotherapy Integration*:

> In the last few decades, the existential–humanistic tradition in psychology—also known as the third force—has taken over the field of clinical psychology. . . . Like a Ninja, dressed by the shades of the natural environment, the humanistic–existential movement has infiltrated not only the fortress of clinical psychology, but also mainstream academic psychology in general and has assumed a quiet, albeit steadfast, *control*. (p. 1)

Think what one may about the veracity of the above assertions, they do nevertheless reflect a growing consensus within the field of mainstream psychotherapy. This consensus is robust and stresses that well beyond isolated techniques, it is the *personal* and *interpersonal* qualities of the relationship—the contextual–relational factors—that account for the lion's share of successful therapeutic outcome (Elkins, 2015; Norcross & Lambert, 2019; Wampold & Imel, 2015; Yalom, 1980). For existential therapists, and in particular existential–humanistic (EH) and existential–integrative (EI) therapists (e.g., Bugental, 1987; Geller & Greenberg, 2012; Schneider, 2015), these contextual–relational factors are closely connected to the core dimension of *presence*. Presence can be understood as the holding and illuminating of that which is palpably significant within the client and between client and therapist and for EH and EI therapists it is at the hub of the contextual–relational factors cited in the above outcome literature. We explore therapeutic presence later in this chapter, but suffice it to say that it is foundational, both at the developmental level of people's emergence into life and in the consulting room. This is because it is the balm or salve that enables many clients to feel the emotional security necessitated to make meaningful changes in their lives, those that deeply matter to their lives. It should also be apparent how presence is integral to the specific conditions that contextual–relational researchers, such as Wampold and Norcross, cite as the most salient (Geller & Greenberg, 2012; Schneider, 2015). Consider, for example, how the building of the therapeutic alliance, the cultivation of therapeutic empathy, the provision of genuineness and warmth, the fostering of attunement and collaboration, and the provision of a sense of hope could occur *without* therapeutic presence.

But presence contributes another element that is not often made explicit in mainstream therapy outcome literature—the foundational skill to cope with and make the best of the trials and uncertainties of life. We now elaborate on these dimensions.

EXISTENTIAL PSYCHODYNAMICS BEGIN AT BIRTH

Existential psychology begins with life, literally individuals' "thrownness" into life (Heidegger, 1962, p. 321). But it also begins with the awareness of death (Yalom, 1980), and all its associated dimensions—danger, the radically unknown, and the radically different. Put another way, existential psychology is like a plunge into a vast unknown sea. This sea is filled with strange and wondrous creatures—notably humans—dark and deep crevices, and menacing objects. Humans are awhirl in this maelstrom, groundless and helpless, and lacking in all but the most rudimentary equipment to survive, and not all that well at that. But fast on the heels of this turbulence, individuals begin to experience elements of curiosity, intrigue, and even wonder at the vast mystery into which they have immersed. Like eyes adjusting to a poorly lit room, they gradually begin to see possibilities in people and things that just moments earlier appeared monstrous and poised to thrash them.

Psychoanalyst Otto Rank (1924) called this existential awakening the "trauma of birth," or "urground" (source) for virtually all future anxiety (see also Janus, 2001). But he also recognized—albeit less explicitly—an element of wonder that appeared to follow the trauma. To make this element of wonder more explicit, Schneider (2023) proposed replacing the concept of "trauma of birth" with "drama of birth." That way, Schneider elaborated, elements of both terror and wonder can be recognized for their foundational role in human development. They are critical not only for the development of human capacity for presence but also for human capacity to live a rich and meaningful life (for comparable perspectives, see DeRobertis & Bland, 2020; Kramer, 2019, 2023; May, 1981).

Moreover, in the drama of birth, which humans all arguably share, we shift from a state of relative nonbeing and unity (i.e., with the mother/cosmos) to sudden abrupt being and pandemonium! We shift from a state of passive reception to active scrambling, and from the safe and familiar to the fretful and unknown. We can barely assimilate these states let alone accommodate them. This massive break from the familiar, furthermore, is what Rank (1924) referred to as the "psychology of difference;" and that psychology, he proposed, sets the tone for virtually all subsequent encounters with "otherness" both within oneself and toward the world (see also Kramer, 1996).

The psychology of difference and the radically unknown appears to have a major impact on virtually all major aspects of personality formation. It is evident in one's capacity to express oneself, to venture out and explore the world, to deal with novelty (e.g., in people, places, and things), to give and receive love, and to experience a spiritual dimension that Schneider (2009, 2023) called "awe"—or the humility and wonder, sense of adventure toward living. Furthermore, the psychology of difference appears to play a pivotal role in how individuals conduct not only their individual lives but their collective lives as well (Fanon, 1963; Hoffman et al., 2020; Kramer, 1996). This is precisely why existentially oriented clinicians the world over recognize mystery—birth, death, the indefiniteness of the cosmos—as the basis for a fuller and more comprehensive psychology; a psychology that informs but also underlies all the bona fide orientations (e.g., Becker, 1973; May, 1983; Rank 1924; Schneider, 2023; van Deurzen et al., 2019; Yalom, 1980).

In sum, Rank's position on the trauma of birth has arguably led to the most fundamental principle of existential psychodynamics. This principle is that the *groundlessness* and *helplessness* people experience at birth (or at any point of rupture from the envelopment of cosmic-fetal life) are at the core of virtually all future prejudices, fears (e.g., of specific people or objects), and anxiety, including death anxiety. Correspondingly, this principle elucidates that the *wonder* that is experienced at birth is at the crux of virtually all future capacities to manage those latter anxieties, including presence, openness to experience, and awe (see also Becker, 1973; Kramer, 1996; Schneider, 2023).

It is one thing, however, to identify basic conditions that underlie human behavior and experience, and quite another to address how they are dealt with and shaped throughout the life cycle. The whole question of how one is *met* following one's plunge into life, therefore, is a central one for an existential theory of practice, and in the balance of this chapter we probe it. Focusing mainly on the contemporary U.S. modalities of EH and EI psychotherapies, we detail the theory, research, and applications that attend.

The question of how an individual is met, then, both by their caretakers and the culture that surrounds them is a critical one; it can mean the difference between the influences of an environment that is fear-based and debilitated or love-based and invigorated.

EH THERAPY: ITS ROOTS AND CONTEMPORARY APPLICATIONS

EH therapy, coined by James F. T. Bugental (1978) but inspired and elaborated by Otto Rank (Kramer, 2023), Rollo May and colleagues (1958), and Irvin Yalom (1980), is a mixture of European existential philosophy originated by Søren Kierkegaard, Friedrich Nietzsche, and Martin Heidegger (van Deurzen et al., 2019), and American humanistic psychology led by Abraham Maslow (1971), Carl Rogers (1961), and again Rollo May (1983). Although both humanistic and existential modalities addressed big picture questions about the human experience—namely the human relationship to existence as a whole—they pursued different emphases. Whereas European existential philosophy stressed the *structural* aspects of human beings' relationship to existence—such as one's thrownness toward death, one's quest for meaning in an absurd (or radically puzzling) world, one's biological dimension (*umwelt*), one's social dimension (*mitwelt*), and one's individual or subjective dimension (*eigenwelt*)—American humanistic psychology stressed the *experiential* aspects of one's relationship to existence. That is, American humanistic psychology tended to aver abstract or philosophical formulations *about* the human relation to existence and to prioritize lived and embodied engagement *with* existence. As such, humanistic psychology, and in particular EH psychology, pursued a lineage that had strong ties to the phenomenological heritage of European philosophy. Luminaries of that heritage, such as Edmund Husserl and Maurice Merleau-Ponty, certainly were concerned with anatomizing the structure of human experience, but they also, at base, prized the "lived (or experiential) world" as much or more than conceptions about that world (Merleau-Ponty, 1962). To be sure, both the existential philosophical lineage and the American humanistic lineage embraced many aspects of phenomenology; but here we are highlighting their differences in emphasis.

Finally, whereas the European existential tradition tended to stress life's tragic dimensions—for example, death, the absurdity of existence, and biological, social, and individual *limitations*; the American humanistic lineage, while acknowledging the former, tended to be more identified with life's *potentialities*—such as the abiding capacity for choice, for life-transformation, and for practical, embodied engagement with the world. By combining existential and humanistic elements then, early EH theorists attempted to meld the depth and sobriety of the European intellectual tradition with the "can do" pragmatism of the American psychological tradition and developed a sophisticated yet practical modality called "existential–humanistic" theory and practice (Bugental, 1978, 1987; May, 1983; May et al., 1958).

From EH to EI Therapy: Basic Principles

EH therapy embraces four basic principles. As intimated earlier, these begin with *presence,* or the holding and illuminating of that which is palpably significant within the client and between client and therapist. Presence, according to EH theorists, is both the ground and aim of effective therapy (Geller & Greenberg, 2012; Schneider & Krug, 2026).

Through presence, the therapeutic relationship is "held" in Rank (1924) and Winnicott's (1960) terms, such that the primal anxieties of groundlessness and helplessness can be encountered in a comparatively safe, loving, and understanding environment. Such an environment in turn supports the client to "drop into" both verbally and preverbally their most daunting dreads as well as dazzling desires, and through that process develop safer and more loving internalizations within themselves. These safer and more loving internalizations are not just intellectual or behavioral but manifest in one's "whole-body" experience of living. The result is a greater capacity to access and express the parts of oneself that were formerly blocked off and to live with more intentionality and depth in the here and now (May, 1981). By intentionality we echo May's (1969) definition of a whole-bodied orientation toward a given goal or direction. Intentionality is different than impulsiveness or whim because it draws on all possible modalities—for example, cognitive, affective, kinesthetic, and intuitive—to inform decision making. It is a manifestation of the freedom derived from presence, and the responsibility or "ability to respond" that is also a natural consequence of being more present and aware.

The second principle of EH therapy is *invoking the actual* or inviting and challenging clients to *become present* here and now (Schneider & Krug, 2026). Metaphorically, invoking the actual is akin to holding a mirror up to clients' *battle*—the part of clients that is attempting to break through and liberate themselves (e.g., a yearning to pursue a creative project) and the part of themselves that is attempting to hold themselves back and block what is attempting to break through. Invoking the actual often entails many revisitations to this battle before clients are capable of developing the tools to become more intentional about not only how they are currently living (and often "choked off") but how they are *willing* to live as the stakes in their battle become increasingly and palpably more evident. Therapists facilitate invoking the actual by calling attention to clients' *process* and not just words in their descriptions of their battles. By "process" we mean *how* clients describe their situations, not just the explanations they give or words they say. Thus noticing body language becomes critical at such times, such as the client's facial expressions, vocal fluctuations, position in their chairs, and other preverbal kinesthetic signs that indicate there is more going on than "reports" about a particular difficulty. If accurately sensed, each of these signs can be gateways to expanding and deepening clients' presence to their struggles, thereby "reoccupying"—both literally and figuratively—the parts they've blocked off.

While the above invitations to presence can be viewed as comparatively passive forms of mirroring, therapists' self-disclosures, such as "I feel a tightness in my stomach when you say that" or "I too once lost a sibling to gun violence," can be seen as comparatively active forms of mirroring. Most importantly, therapists' self-disclosures can, if artfully timed, significantly help deepen clients' self-exploration and thus integration of their anxieties. However, therapists need to be very discerning about such disclosures lest they overwhelm clients and trigger retraumatization (Meyers, 2020). The question therapists need to be mindful of throughout the therapy is: Will this disclosure or response serve to deepen *clients'* process of self-discovery, or will it serve someone else's agenda, such as the therapist themself?

The third principle of EH therapy, following organically on the heels of invoking the actual is *vivifying and confronting self-protections* (Schneider & Krug, 2026). Vivifying self-protections (or the defenses people use to stem reactivation of their core wounds) is the calling of attention to ways clients *stop* or block themselves from fuller self-presence. One example of vivifying a self-protection is for the therapist to note how a client felt deeply immersed in their sadness but then abruptly diverted from that sadness, for example, by talking about the weather or attempting to engage the therapist in a discussion about a new TV show. Through noting and tagging self-protections, therapists can help clients "see" closer and closer up how readily they cut themselves off from their immediate experience, and too frequently from living the fuller more liberating life they seek. While vivifying self-protections are much more common, the confrontation with self-protections is occasionally called for. Again, therapists' presence and whole-body experience of the client is a key guide as to when and how to confront (e.g., alarm) as distinct from vivify (e.g., alert) clients about their repeated avoidances. Confronting self-protections must be extremely selective because of the damage it can do if it fails to match clients' ability to stay present and work with a given core wound. A premature confrontation is often perceived as not only a breach of the supportive and understanding therapeutic relationship, but subconsciously perhaps as an attempt to thrust clients into the very places they've designed their lives around avoiding, and thus to annihilate them! In light of this awareness on the part of therapists, and in light of clients' palpable urgency albeit reluctance to change, therapists may "test the water" with a discerning confrontation like "Here we are again, with your staunch though tormenting decision to continue drinking—I wonder what that brings up for you right now?" Or "It really pains me to see how over and over again you keep yourself from really going out and living." On the even rarer occasions that a more direct confrontation may be warranted, it is even more imperative that it matches some impulse in the client to change, such as in cases of being physically or sexually abused, or edging dangerously close to self-destruction through drugs. At the same time, it is imperative at such points—as it is throughout the work—to continue holding the space for *clients'* sense of dignity and agency; otherwise, the therapeutic fulcrum switches to the therapist or some outside agency, which in subtle ways perhaps, fuels the very problem that brings clients to therapy in the first place.

The fourth and final principle of EH therapy is the *rediscovery of meaning and awe.* As clients are able to experience their battles closer and closer up, they optimally feel freer to weigh the priorities of their lives—how they're willing to live here and now. It is during this period that what Rank (1936) called the "counter-will" or Gestaltists such as Perls (1969) might have called "frustration" builds up to the point where, to put it bluntly, a person will not take it anymore. The individual refuses to live in the "safe" but miserable prison they have spent most of their lives in and they are not only ready for change, they are willing to carry out the change in their day-to-day lives. At first this change may take the form of a rediscovery and pursuit of meaning in their lives, whether that meaning pertains to a romantic relationship, a job, a creative project, or some other personally or socially substantive act. But the rediscovery of a particular meaning or goal in clients' lives may only be the beginning. On the heels of this rediscovery may be a whole new way of viewing life, an attitude or sensibility we call "awe" or the "awe toward all existence" (Schneider, 2023; Schneider & Krug, 2026). The awe toward all existence can be understood as the humility and wonder or sense of adventure that emanates from a whole-body experience of life. It is a distinct outgrowth of the EH practice supporting clients to move from positions of abject terror and paralysis to gradual, incremental intrigue, curiosity, and wonder about their own lives and the life and existence of all. To put it another way, clients at this point (usually toward the end of an intensive therapy) are increasingly able to experience what Schneider (2023, p. 2) called "life-enhancing anxiety" or the "capacity to live with and make the best of the depth and mystery of existence"; and this capacity typically leads to a sense of awe toward living, the capacity to experience one's smallness and fragility as well as vastness and possibility of a fuller, more conscious life. We can see the engagement of this sensibility in everyday walks in nature, in deeper more embodied experiences of intimacy, in the savoring of friendships or family relationships, or in the simple taste of foods and appreciation of each breath. Such a sensibility can also be seen in the exploration of a new travel destination or a work of art or science; its fruits—the fruits of a greatly enhanced inner (and outer) freedom are almost limitless. But those fruits are also invariably contextualized by limits, the interplay of which tends to accentuate the freedom (May, 1981).

EI Therapy: An Expanded Horizon of EH Practice

The EI approach to therapy is one way of understanding and coordinating a variety of bona fide (that is, evidence-based) practices within an overall existential or experiential context (Schneider, 2008). By *experiential* we mean an emphasis on the immediate, affective, kinesthetic or embodied, and profound or cosmic dimensions of living. The EI context, in other words, is roughly equivalent to that which is traditionally understood as the EH approach as a whole and draws on that lineage for its deepest level of contact within clients and between therapists and clients.

Like the EH format, the EI approach is grounded on and prioritizes therapeutic presence. However, in contrast to the EH format, the EI approach is much more explicit about presence as a guide or barometer to address two implicit and sometimes explicit questions that permeate the entire EI framework—How is the client *presently* living (e.g., What's really going on here)? And on the heels of that question—How is the client *willing* to live (that is, to respond to or take action on how they are presently living)? Within the EI approach a variety of bona fide modalities, such as medical-physiological, cognitive-behavioral, psychoanalytic-interpersonal, and ontological-experiential approaches, may be relevant for a given individual at a given point in time. The question as to modality is decided largely by clients' *desire and capacity for deeper or experiential change* and, of course phenomenologically, clients have a range of such desires and capacities.

Thus, through presence—the holding and illuminating of that which is palpably significant within clients and between clients and therapists—EI practitioners elucidate clients' capacities to explore how they are presently living (or as previously noted, their "battles") as well as their willingness to respond to or take action toward how they are presently living. Hence, presence becomes a guide or barometer by which EI therapists sense when and how to support clients given the personal, interpersonal, and cultural contexts within which they live. This means that sometimes relatively nonexperiential (e.g., medical, behavioral) interventions may be called for (e.g., to help a self-injurer), or semi-experiential approaches may be more relevant (e.g., cognitive, psychoanalytic) to work with clients who are more intellectualizing in their cognitive and emotional processing, or experiential (e.g., EH) approaches may be necessary to engage with clients who are more ready for and capable of preverbal–kinesthetic exploration. The key issue here, however, is the phenomenological attunement of the therapist with the client and the ability to collaborate in the context of that attunement (Schneider, 2008, 2015; Shumaker, 2012).

Schneider (2012) demonstrated this approach with "Allison," a 48-year-old cisgender female of European descent whose presenting problem was lack of assertiveness, particularly with her boss. While Schneider used cognitive-behavioral reframing to help Allison address her assertiveness with her boss, he first built a relationship with her and remained available to explore deeper issues, as they organically arose. Among these issues was Allison's ongoing struggle with core wounds she suffered from a severely abusive childhood, as well as intense yearnings to feel free in her life, not just with her boss. Thus, as Schneider stayed present to and invited Allison to become aware of feelings and body sensations, not just words, she gradually began to reveal dreams and fantasies that radically shifted her presenting problem of lack of assertiveness, to lack of freedom to live out her passions for a livelier, more expressive life. These steps in turn led to the engagement of an "embodied meditation" in the final session. In this session, Schneider invited Allison to identify sensations in her body that felt blocked or tense and to free associate to those sensations. The upshot of this engagement was that Allison was able to confront and work with a core wound that left her feeling like she was in a "black hole" for the majority of her life. Yet as she was able to stay with these sensations and "reoccupy" them with her "larger" or more adult self, she experienced herself emerging out of that darkness and into the light of a freer and more expressive self; this was a person who felt more connected to her grandchildren—and children in general—to yearnings for travel and the embrace of nature. In short, through an EI modality, Allison learned how to feel and not just cognize or behave in a more whole and vital fashion. She shifted from concern with being validated at work to concern with being validated in life; and from bettering her environment at work and among those she felt oppressed by to bettering her environment within, feeling "at home" within, and embarking on a vital new path toward the people and places she held dear (Schneider, 2012).

Next, we discuss a more recent horizon in EH and EI psychology, the impact of multicultural dimensions. It is clear that in order for EH and EI psychology to fulfill their foundational vision of what it means to be fully, experientially human and how that understanding impacts the vital and fulfilled life, they need to open to and be influenced by the many manifestations of that vision, both locally and globally.

MOBILIZING GLOBALLY: MULTICULTURAL TRENDS IN EH AND EI THERAPY

Multiculturalism is considered the fourth force in Western psychology, as it situates culture as central in the development of people's sense of self or identity formation across the lifespan. Culture is a way of being in the world that is evidenced by shared values, practices, beliefs, knowledge, and sense of belonging among groups of people (Birukou et al., 2013). "The central assertion of multicultural psychology is that all aspects of human behavior are learned and expressed in a cultural context and to comprehensively, and accurately understand a person's experience or behavior, it is necessary to understand the cultural context" (Hocoy, 2019, p. 19). In this framework, it is important to note that Western psychology is grounded in the culture of its founders, a Eurocentric worldview that is informed by such values as individualism (independence), dualistic thinking, mastery over nature, and competitiveness. Other cultural groups, including Native Americans, Americans of African ancestry, Americans of South Asian ancestry, and others, endorse a more collectivist worldview that values interconnectedness of all living beings (interdependence), child-centeredness, circular thinking, and spirituality (Koltko-Rivera, 2004), including the positioning of religion in one's reality and meaning making. Of course, there are variations within groups as to how these worldviews manifest, and the worldviews are not necessarily mutually exclusive as we consider the multicultural nature of humanity.

EH psychology, the third force (Hocoy, 2019), admirably expanded psychology's focus from the limitation of symptom reduction to the appreciation for a holistic approach to healing by considering the wholeness of the human experience and centering the client as the expert in their own lives (empowerment). However, it, too, is rooted in a Eurocentric worldview when considering the tenets of self-determination, self-actualization, and individual free will. EH psychology has been critiqued for its overemphasis on the individual, limited attention to the impact of culture on one's lived experiences, and its microscopic applicability in complex sociocultural situations, such as poverty (Berry Newton & Jackson, in press). Progressive EH scholar-practitioners have worked diligently to move the EH pendulum toward being culturally responsive (Diaz-Laplante, 2007; Hoffman et al., 2020; Johnson, 2001) and relevant in addressing the unique needs of diverse populations. For example, Granger (2020) has considered the impact of microaggressions in an EH schema; Spaeth (2020) explored how EH psychology can be used in the context of religious/spiritual diversity; Cleare-Hoffman and colleagues (2020) considered how to integrate cultural myths, rituals, and festivals in psychotherapy; and Sundararajan (2020) has explored the implications of Indigenous psychology for EH psychology.

Recently, there has been increased multidisciplinary (e.g., educational, commercial) attention to globalization, which can loosely be conceptualized "as a process of interaction and integration among the peoples, companies, and governments of different nations" (Chiu et al., 2011, p. 664). The field of psychology is beginning to make its contributions in understanding the psychology of globalization, particularly in terms of equity, diversity, and inclusion. There is much that EH psychology can offer when considering the emphasis on intercultural competence, "which is most often viewed as a set of cognitive, affective, and behavioral skills and characteristics that support effective and appropriate interaction in a variety of cultural contexts" (Bennett, 2009, p. 122). This conceptualization of intercultural competence can be a bit mechanistic if the primary objective is to replicate productive global persons. EH tenets of here-and-now, authenticity (especially when recognizing the interconnectedness of people; see Cleary, 2022), facing life directly, and others may afford deeper transformative change. There is more to simply ensuring that diverse faces are present; it is also necessary to embrace diverse ways of being and knowing (epistemological justice). Consider the following examples.

Situation A: I (Theopia Jackson) invite a multicultural group to my home for dinner, where I prepare some of my favorite southern cuisine, like fried chicken, collard greens seasoned with ham hocks, red beans and rice with smoked neckbones, sweet potato pie, and much more. As guests arrive, there is much chit chat getting to know one another. We move into the dining room, and I observe various levels of indulgence from those who are visually enjoying their meal to others who are barely eating. Upon inquiry, I embarrassingly discover that some are vegetarian or vegan or do not eat pork.

Situation B: Before guests arrive, I do my homework and realize the varied nutritional needs. The dinner options this evening still have some of my favorite southern cuisine, yet I have added certain choices like collards seasoned with smoked turkey, as well as vegan and vegetarian options. In doing so, my taste palate has discovered new treats, and I have expanded my culinary skills while ensuring that all who enter can leave fully satisfied.

These situations have implications for how EH psychology might approach the global dialogues in terms of engaging to identify the global synergies within the EH worldview, which is a viable approach. Specifically, Hoffman and colleagues' (2019) *Existential Psychology East–West* clearly delineated such connections, as well as missed opportunities or challenges. There is richness here yet there are also risks. If EH psychology interprets the global surge as bringing other groups into the fold, then unintentional colonization due to cultural blinders and assumed universality may occur (*intention vs. impact*). The second situation begs the question, can EH psychology engage in such dialogues not knowing the impact on the field itself or does it engage in conversations with the sole intention of impacting the other? Besides studying the worldview and/or cultural ways of being of its global counterparts, can EH psychology lean into the dialogues by letting go of what it knows and be open to new discoveries through theoretical self-reflection? Entering the dialogues for theoretical self-discovery or epistemological actualization should be the end goal in appreciating that EH psychology is still *becoming* while simultaneously moving EH tenets forward. This honors the realization that EH psychology has not finished its journey in promoting the fullness of humanity. Toward that end, a potential cultural blinder may be the preponderance of East–West dialogues in the absence or marginalization of North–South engagements for fully understanding Indigenous ways of being or science (Berry Newton & Jackson, in press). For instance, it may be beneficial for EI therapy, which emerged from EH psychology (Schneider, 2016), to move toward adding a "critical" component to the integration. As a critical integration, the integration moves beyond assimilation of other approaches, including cultural ones, into EH psychology with the assumption of it always being correct or dominant. Instead, it is allowing for the other approaches, especially cultural, to potentially change EH psychology and EI therapy in a bidirectional transformation.

When considering the budding global impact of EH psychology, Blommaer's observation may guide EH psychology well: "The global world has not become a village, but rather a tremendously complex web of villages, towns, neighborhoods, settlements connected by material and symbolic ties in often unpredictable ways" (as cited by Aristova, 2016, p. 154). As a tradition, EH psychology is uniquely positioned to significantly contribute to depth transformative change for the betterment of humanity. If not EH psychology, then who? The following recommendations are offered with this objective in mind, how EH psychology can be an influencer and global mobilizer in actualizing such a village:

1. EH psychology should engage in theoretical self-reflection to identify its cultural blinders and legacy of ethnocentric roots, as this is inherent in all theories yet has been particularly problematic from a multicultural standpoint in Western theories. Ethnocentrism is the tendency to organize the world intentionally or unintentionally through one's own cultural values, determining what is normal and what is not (Johnson, 2001). Ignoring, minimizing, or being oblivious to Indigenous or communal/community forms of healing and well-being may lead to unforeseen consequences and transubstantive errors, which are "the result of hegemonic predilection to use the principles of the dominant culture inappropriately to explain the behavior of other cultures both to others and to themselves in ways that are *inauthentic*" (Piper-Mandy & Rowe, 2010, p. 10) in practice.
2. EH scholars can approach global dialogues employing a cultural humility stance that requires comfort in the not knowing, empowering through relationship, self-critique/self-reflection, and a continued commitment to learning, growing, and *becoming* (Comas-Díaz, 2014; Tervalon & Murray-Garcia, 1998), as well as operationalizing cross-cultural empathy.
3. EH psychology should be intentional in explicitly denoting how it can be a *psychology for the people* (pushing back on the long-standing critique of privileging a specific socioeconomic class) with increased attention to understanding how culture and/or worldviews inform one's realities and to considering the value of social justice activism in clinical practice and scholarship.

Hoffman and colleagues (2016) summarized the problem well:

> Social justice issues often arise when groups, on a collective level, are forced to confront aspects of the givens of existence due to social structures or impositions. These can include threats to one's self or existence, being cut off from sources of meaning or relationship, or limitations being imposed on one's political freedom, which necessarily has implications for one's existential freedom. (p. 596)

In closing, EH psychology and EI therapy may be uniquely positioned to embrace the tenets recommended here. They have long had a liberatory framework, valued openness, and advocated for humility in the face of difference. However, they have not always actualized these intentionally within a cultural context. Extending these principles, with consideration to the recommendations above, will help EH psychology and EI therapy actualize their potential regarding multiculturalism, globalization, and social justice.

EH AND EI THERAPY APPLIED TO SOCIAL CRISES

As noted above, EH and EI therapy are now being applied to broader social issues. Given the rise in cultural and political divisiveness, climate change, violence, and wars, there has been an increasing realization that in order to more fully address the conditions for individual psychological disturbance one must look concertedly at its roots in collective contexts, and EI therapy is ideally suited for such a venture.

What follows is a brief sketch of key EH/EI applications to social challenges that impact both individual and collective dysfunction. One of the emergent demonstrations of these applications is the *experiential democracy dialogue* (EDD; Schneider, 2020). The EDD, which is a one-on-one approach to humanizing conversations between people with highly contrasting political and cultural backgrounds, derives from a hybrid of existential–phenomenological, psychodynamic, and couple-counseling principles of practice. It also draws from social psychological frameworks such as terror management theory and attachment theory (Bowlby, 1983; Schneider, 2013, 2020, in press; Solomon et al., 2015) as well as the "living room" style dialogues of grassroots organizations like Braver Angels (*www.braverangels.org*). Braver Angels is a conflict mediation organization that has over 12,000 members nationwide, providing depolarization workshops for self-identified liberals and conservatives in a wide range of community settings.

The EDD is a six-phase mediation approach that involves choosing a culturally or politically divisive topic; strict adherence to ground rules; visualizing what it might be like to engage with one's partner before starting the dialogue process; providing background on how each partner came to adopt their views; describing each partner's stance on the chosen topic; engaging in a stereotypes exercise where each partner describes stereotypes that have been imposed on them by people negative toward them, then identifies the false and misleading aspects of those stereotypes, and identifies nuggets of truth to the stereotypes; asking a question of each other from a place of genuine curiosity; and finally discussing what they discovered about themselves, each other, and the issue at hand.

Research suggests (*https://braverangels.org*), and personal experience has confirmed (Schneider, 2020) that these dialogues are rich and often surprising encounters with people who, on the surface, are on completely different sides of cultural or political issues. Not only do many of these same people end up feeling less estranged from and less angry with each other, they sometimes achieve common ground—even if it's a sense of resonance and friendliness.

Another application of EH/EI principles to social issues is the recent work of terror management theory (TMT), a social psychological perspective based on the work of Ernest Becker in his landmark book *The Denial of Death* (1973). Becker's thesis is that wide ranges of human destructiveness can be explained by what he viewed as death anxiety, or the "complex symbol" of death. To that effect, TMT theorists developed hundreds of experimental studies to investigate the validity of Becker's thesis. Through these studies they found that priming participants with death or death-like themes, such as photos of people in fatal accidents, or images of death in participants own lives, led to striking correlations with increased psychological rigidity, political conservatism, increased ethnocentrism, and increased identification with authoritarian leaders (Solomon et al., 2015). The significance of these findings, despite some controversy (e.g., see FeldmanHall & van Baar, 2022), cannot be underestimated, and have been used to understand the psychology of voting patterns in presidential elections, the bases for prejudice and bigotry, and the bases for terrorism among some fundamentalist sects (Solomon et al., 2015).

Another social application of EH/EI principles of practice has emerged with a new YouTube channel called the "Corps of Depth Healers" (*www.youtube.com/@CorpsofDepthHealers-ws9nq*; see also the related certificate program at *www.corpsofdepthhealers.com*). Developed by Kirk Schneider with the assistance of Tyler Gamlen, the Corps of Depth Healers is a resource for mental health providers who are concerned with fostering affordable and accessible therapeutic services, especially for underserved communities. These therapeutic services are focused on what Schneider and Gamlen (2023) have called *emotionally restorative relationships*, or relationships where people feel seen and heard and that get at the roots of their problems. Among these relationships are longer-term, in-depth psychotherapy, holistic life coaching, mentoring, and medical care; and bridge-building dialogues between diverse parties in communities, schools, businesses, and governmental settings.

Specifically, the Corps of Depth Healers YouTube channel provides video illustrations by leaders in a variety of mental health fields who apply depth-oriented principles of practice to a range of social conflicts. For example, there are video segments illustrating bridge-building dialogues between people on contrasting sides of political, ethnic, and religious conflicts. There are illustrations of experts on the application of existential and psychodynamic approaches to war and violence, the COVID-19 pandemic, cultural divides in organizations, and medical care among other critical societal problems. The aim of the Corps is to be a catalyst for providers who view the channel to extend the various examples of depth-oriented practices to their own work-settings, communities, and organizations. The long-term goal of the Corps is to mobilize a mass movement of depth healers to make available emotionally restorative relationships in the face of the growing contagion of emotionally impoverished relationships that are pervading nations across the world (Hoffman et al., 2020; Schneider & Gamlen, 2023).

Finally, there are a growing number of organizations and advocacy networks that are supporting depth and existential applications to social crises. PsiAN, or the Psychotherapy Action Network, is one such group (*https://psian.org*). Started about 10 years ago, PsiAN is a member-driven organization that advocates for therapies of depth, insight, and relationship (Michaels et al., 2023). These are therapies, such as relational psychoanalysis and EI approaches, that recognize the importance of the subconscious (or implicit) in the understanding and treatment of psychological disturbance. PsiAN also advocates for the availability and affordability of such approaches throughout the United States. With the support of its 5,000-plus members, PsiAN has contributed key legal, theoretical, and research reports on the value of depth-oriented therapy to such professional bodies as the American Psychological Association, relevant court proceedings (e.g., *Wit v. United Healthcare*), and credentialing boards (Michaels et al., 2023). In this light, PsiAN has become an important voice for upholding and extending the influence of depth-oriented therapies to a diverse clientele.

Another more recent advocacy organization is the Existential Movement (EM). The EM was initiated in 2023 by existential analyst Emmy van Deurzen, who assembled a bevy of like-minded practitioners to translate the riches of existential psychology into practical remedies for cultural and political upheaval. The EM has so far held several strategy sessions among its international advisors and has plans to sponsor public forums on topics such as managing contemporary anxieties and applying the EDD to address cultural and political divides (E. van Deurzen, personal communication, January 2024). Among the aims of the Existential Movement are

> to make existential ideas available to the wider public in order to help people achieve greater clarity in their reflection on human existence and in solving their personal and emotional problems. It seeks to create a safe space for this reflection and for the communal practice of a down to earth philosophical approach that brings wisdom to the international community. The mission of EM is to provide a broader base and a clearer perspective for people who wish to live their lives in a more reflective and meaningful way, without having to turn to existential therapy or counselling. (excerpt from the EM mission statement, *www.existential-movement.world/our-aims/*)

RESEARCH SUPPORT: EH AND EI PSYCHOTHERAPY AS AN EVIDENCE-BASED PRACTICE

The way research is used to support psychotherapy effectiveness has been evolving. Carl Rogers could be considered one of the founders, or at least first wave of researchers, investigating psychotherapy effectiveness research (Goldfried, 2007). Rogers used a variety of methods, most more qualitative in nature, to intensely examine the impact of psychotherapy interventions. Since Rogers, psychology has moved through multiple paradigms, including empirically supported treatment (EST), to the current modality of evidence-based practice in psychology (EBPP). As clarified by Wampold and colleagues (2007), *evidence* is an ambiguous term, which renders *evidence-based practice* somewhat ambiguous as well. Despite this, there have been many who have rushed to narrowly define EBPP in a manner that is similar to the previous EST approach. Sadly, this has been widely successful. However, returning to the seminal article in the *American Psychologist* by the American Psychological Association Task Force on Evidence-Based Practice (2006), it can be seen that research was one of three prongs of EBPP. Furthermore, within the research prong, research was intended to include multiple lines of investigation without privileging any method, including randomized clinical trials (RCTs), as the gold standard. The research should fit the research question instead of allowing the preferred or privileged method to determine the approach. With this broader, inclusive understanding of EBPP in psychology, it becomes evident that EH and EI psychotherapy are on solid ground (Hoffman & Bowers, 2016, Shahar & Schiller, 2016; Wampold, 2008).

Hoffman (2024; Hoffman et al., 2015) has advocated for a broad, inclusive approach to using research to investigate and support EH therapy. This broad approach encompasses: (1) investigating the different interventions that are part of EH therapy (i.e., authenticity, presence, genuineness, etc.); (2) investigating what aspects of EH therapy impact the client's well-being (i.e., meaning, the client's genuineness, self-acceptance, etc.); and (3) outcome studies. Ideally, this broad approach to investigating EH therapy includes both qualitative and quantitative methodologies. We advocate that this approach is superior to one that relies too heavily on any one strategy, including RCTs. A limitation of RCTs is that they typically rely upon strict adherence to a manualized approach. However, in the real world of psychotherapy, it is rare that therapists strictly adhere to a manualized approach—and for good reason. A manualized approach allows for limited ability to adapt to individual client needs and preferences, which is the third prong of EBPP. A multifaceted approach engaging research allows examination of the components of therapy in a manner that is more likely to relate to the manner in which therapy is typically practiced.

Hoffman (2024) noted, "If we reduce evidence-based practice to being about the modality, techniques, or objective and precise application of these, then we can be assured that a time is coming when AI [artificial intelligence] will replace counselors, psychotherapists, and other mental health professionals" (pp. 321–322). If this is the case, then therapists should be considering learning computer programing and/or prompt engineering (i.e., how one makes use of AI tools) alongside studying psychotherapy interventions. While AI therapy will likely have some benefits for mental health clients, there is a plethora of research and other evidence suggesting what Elkins (2015) referred to as the "human factors" of psychotherapy, and these are responsible for the bulk of psychotherapy change (see Elkins, 2015; Norcross & Lambert, 2019; Wampold & Imel, 2015). Comparatively, the specific modality and techniques contribute little to the overall change.

There is strong evidence for the various relational components that are at the foundation of EH and EI therapy (see Hoffman & Lac, 2025; Schneider & Hoffman, 2024). For example, there is consistent support for the effectiveness of therapeutic empathy (Elliott et al., 2018), genuineness (Kolden et al., 2018), positive regard (Farber et al., 2018), immediacy (i.e., here-and-now relational focus; Hill et al., 2018), presence (Geller & Greenberg, 2012), and meaning (Czekierda et al., 2017; Hoffman et al., 2015; Li et al., 2021; Tavernier & Willoughby, 2012; Vos, 2018). In addition to its direct effect on clients' therapeutic progress, a good therapeutic relationship can also enhance the effectiveness of other interventions, such as the integration of mindfulness, breathing techniques, somatic interventions, or even cognitive-behavioral interventions. Thus, the small amount of variance accounted for by technique becomes yet even smaller.

It could be argued that a weakness of EH therapy is the limited number of relevant outcomes studies; however, there remains relevant outcome research. Vos (2019) examined the outcome research on existential–phenomenological psychotherapy, finding general support. Similarly, Vos (2018) found strong support for meaning-centered therapies and interventions. While existential–phenomenological and meaning-centered therapies are different branches of existential therapy, these modalities are highly similar with more consistency between them than differences. Although it still would benefit EH therapy to have more direct outcome studies, these latter reviews of outcome research on existential therapies do provide some support.

While the research on the modality and interventions is important, Hoffman (2024) argued that, in accordance with the article by the American Psychological Association Task Force on EBPP, evidence should be rooted in the therapist as much as the modality. This assertion moves beyond a narrow understanding of science and research to recognize that psychotherapy effectiveness is rooted in a competent therapist. Or, as Hoffman argued, "EBPP is best understood as a competent therapist using a bona fide therapy vetted in the peer-reviewed literature and through practice-based evidence drawing from the best available research while adjusting for individual and cultural differences and preferences with appropriate cultural humility" (p. 319).

In accordance with this view, expecting EH and EI therapists to keep up with the relevant psychotherapy literature while learning to appropriately utilize and critique it is as important as having direct outcome studies. Therapies evolve and tend to use an integrative approach that (even if grounded in a particular modality) is adapted to the individual needs of the client. Doing this well improves the effectiveness of psychotherapy (Norcross & Wampold, 2019). Thus, therapists utilizing evidence-based strategies must be able to be informed, but nimble—adapting beyond what RCTs and many outcome strategies allow.

SUMMARY

In sum, EH therapy is now a multicultural, diagnostically diverse, and integrative perspective (Hoffman et al., 2020; Schneider & Krug, 2026; Shahar & Schiller, 2016). It is an evidence-based approach whose time has come (Wampold, 2008). Although there is much work to do to fulfill its potential as a foundational, intercultural paradigm, EH therapy is moving in that direction. As we have intimated in this chapter, if a paradigm that explores what it means to be fully, experientially human, and how that understanding impacts the vital life, cannot address our basic human challenges, what paradigm can? To this end, we hope we have provided readers with a rich glimpse of our practice world, and the urgency of its message.

REFERENCES

American Psychological Association Presidential Task Force on Evidence-Based Practice. (2006). Evidence-based practice in psychology. *American Psychologist, 6,* 271–285.

Aristova, N. (2016). Rethinking cultural identities in the context of globalization: Linguistic landscape of Kazan, Russia, as an emerging global city. *Procedia-Social and Behavioral Sciences, 236,* 153–160.

Becker, E. (1973). *The denial of death.* Free Press.

Bennett, J. M. (2009). Cultivating intercultural competence: A process perspective. In D. K. Deardorff (Ed.), *The SAGE handbook of intercultural competence* (pp. 121–140). Sage.

Berry Newton, M., & Jackson, T. (in press). Integrating multicultural perspectives. In L. Hoffman (Ed.), *APA handbook of humanistic and existential psychology.* American Psychological Association.

Birukou, A., Blanzieri, E., Giorgini, P., & Giunchiglia, F. (2013). A formal definition of culture. In K. Sycara, M. Gelfand, & A. Abbe (Eds.), *Models for intercultural collaboration and negotiation* (pp. 1–26). Springer.

Bowlby, J. (1983). *Attachment: Attachment and loss: Volume one.* Basic Books.

Bugental, J. F. T. (1978). *Psychotherapy and process: The fundamentals of an existential-humanistic approach.* Addison-Wesley.

Bugental, J. F. T. (1987). *The art of the psychotherapist.* Norton.

Chiu, C. Y., Gries, P., Torelli, C. J., & Cheng, S. Y. (2011). Toward a social psychology of globalization. *Journal of Social Issues, 67*(4), 663–676.

Cleare-Hoffman, H. P., Hoffman, L., & Perlstein, J. (2020). Cultural myths, rituals, and festivals. In L. Hoffman, H. P. Cleare-Hoffman, N. Granger, Jr., & D. St. John (Eds.), *Humanistic approaches to multiculturalism and diversity: Perspectives on existence and difference* (pp. 117–127). Routledge.

Cleary, S. (2022). *How to be authentic: Simone de Beauvoir and the quest for fulfillment.* St. Martin's Essentials.

Comas-Díaz, L. (2014). Multicultural psychotherapy. In F. T. L. Leong, L. Comas-Díaz, G. C. Nagayama Hall, V. C. McLoyd, & J. E. Trimble (Eds.), *APA handbook of multicultural psychology: Vol. 2. Applications and training* (pp. 419–441). American Psychological Association.

Czekierda, K., Banik, A., Park, C. L., & Luszczynska, A. (2017). Meaning in life and physical health: Systematic review and meta-analysis. *Health Psychology Review, 11,* 387–418.

DeRobertis, E. M., & Bland, A. M. (2020). Lifespan human development and "the humanistic perspective": A contribution toward inclusion. *Humanistic Psychologist, 48*(1), 3–27.

Diaz-Laplante, J. (2007). Humanistic psychology and social transformation: Building the path toward a livable today and a just tomorrow. *Journal of Humanistic Psychology, 47*(1), 54–72.

Elkins, D. N. (2015). *The human elements of psychotherapy; A nonmedical model of emotional healing.* American Psychological Association.

Elliott, R., Bohart, A. C., Watson, J. C., & Murphy, D. (2018). Therapist empathy and client outcome: An updated meta-analysis. *Psychotherapy, 55,* 399–410.

Fanon, F. (1963). *The wretched of the earth.* Grove Press.

Farber B., Suzuki, J., & Lynch, D. (2018). Positive regard and psychotherapy outcome: A meta-analytic review. *Psychotherapy, 55,* 411–423.

FeldmanHall, O., & van Baar, J. (2022). A tale of two perspectives: Reply to Schneider (2022). *American Psychologist, 77*(5), 712–713.

Geller, S. M., & Greenberg, L. S. (2012). *Therapeutic presence: A mindful approach to effective psychotherapy.* American Psychological Association.

Gerwig, G. (Director). (2023). *Barbie* [film]. Warner Bros.

Goldfried, M. R. (2007). What has psychotherapy inherited from Carl Rogers? *Psychotherapy: Theory, Research, Practice, Training, 44,* 249–252.

Granger, N., Jr. (2020). Microaggressions and humanistic psychology. In L. Hoffman, H. P. Cleare-Hoffman, N. Granger, Jr., & D. St. John (Eds.), *Humanistic approaches to multiculturalism and diversity: Perspectives on existence and difference* (pp. 63–75). Routledge.

Heidegger, M. (1962). *Being and time.* Harper & Row.

Hill, C. E., Knox, S., & Pinto-Coelho, K. G. (2018). Therapist self-disclosure and immediacy: A qualitative meta-analysis. *Psychotherapy, 55,* 445–460.

Hocoy, D. (2019). The challenge of multiculturalism to humanistic psychology. In L. Hoffman, H. P. Cleare-Hoffman, N. Granger, Jr., & D. St. John (Eds.), *Humanistic approaches to multiculturalism and diversity: Perspectives on existence and difference* (pp. 18–28). Routledge.

Hoffman, L. (2024). The possibilities and slippery slope of evidence-based practice in psychology: Why humanistic and existential psychologists must engage the conversation. *Humanistic Psychologist, 52*(3), 318–324.

Hoffman, L., & Bowers, V. (2016, March). *Existential-humanistic therapy and evidence-based practice in psychology: We are on solid ground.* Paper presented at the 9th Annual Conference of the Society for Humanistic Psychology, San Francisco, CA.

Hoffman, L., Cleare-Hoffman, H., Granger, N., & St. John, D. (Eds.). (2020). *Humanistic approaches to multiculturalism and diversity: Perspectives on existence and difference.* Routledge.

Hoffman, L., Granger, N., Jr., Vallejos, L., & Moats, M. (2016). An existential–humanistic perspective on Black Lives Matter and contemporary protest movements. *Journal of Humanistic Psychology, 56*(6), 595–611.

Hoffman, L., & Lac, V. (Eds.). (2025). *The evidence-based foundations of existential-humanistic therapy.* Amerinca Psychological Association.

Hoffman, L., Vallejos, L., Cleare-Hoffman, H. P., & Rubin, S. (2015). Emotion, relationship, and meaning as core existential practice: Evidence-based foundations. *Journal of Contemporary Psychotherapy, 45,* 11–20.

Hoffman, L., Yang, M., Kaklauskas, F. J., Chan, A., & Mansilla, M. (Eds.). (2019). *Existential psychology East–West* (Rev. & expanded ed.; Vol. 1, pp. 273–288). University Professors Press.

Janus, L. (2001). *The enduring effects of prenatal experiencing: Echoes from the womb.* Mattes Verlag.

Johnson, Z. (2001). Cultural competency and humanistic psychology. *Humanistic Psychologist, 29,* 204–222.

Kolden, G. G., Wang, C-C., Austin, S. B., Chang, Y., & Klein, M. H. (2018). Congruence/genuineness: A meta-analysis. *Psychotherapy, 55,* 424–433.

Koltko-Rivera, M. E. (2004). The psychology of worldviews. *Review of General Psychology, 8*(1), 3–58.
Kramer, R. (1996). *A psychology of difference: The American lectures of Otto Rank*. Princeton University Press.
Kramer, R. (2019). *The birth of relationship therapy: Carl Rogers meets Otto Rank*. Psychozocial-Verlag.
Kramer, R. (2023). Discovering the existential unconscious: Rollo May encounters Otto Rank. *Humanistic Psychologist, 51*(1), 15–35.
Li, J-B., Dou, K., & Liang, Y. (2021). The relationship between presence of meaning, search for meaning, and subjective well-being: A three-level meta-analysis based on the Meaning in Life Questionnaire. *Journal of Happiness Studies, 22*, 467–489.
Maslow, A. (1971). *The farther reaches of human nature*. Viking.
May (1969). *Love and will*. Norton.
May, R. (1981). *Freedom and destiny*. Norton.
May, R. (1983). *The discovery of being*. Norton.
May, R., Angel, E., & Ellenberger, H. (Eds.). (1958). *Existence: A new dimension in psychiatry and psychology*. Basic Books.
Merleau-Ponty, M. (1962). *The phenomenology of perception*. Routledge.
Meyers, D. (2020). What did Carl Rogers say about the topic of therapist self-disclosure?: A comprehensive review of his recorded clinical work. *Person Centered Journal, 25*(1–2).
Michaels, L., Woolridge, T., Burke, N., & Muhr, N. (2023). *Advancing psychotherapy for the next generation: Humanizing mental health policy and practice*. Routledge.
Norcross, J. C., & Lambert, M. J. (Eds.). (2019). *Psychotherapy relationships that work: Vol. 1. Evidence-based therapist contributions* (3rd ed.). Oxford University Press.
Norcross, J. C., & Wampold, B. E. (2019). Evidence-based psychotherapy responsiveness: The third task force. In J. C. Norcross & B. E. Wampold (Eds.), *Psychotherapy relationships that work: Vol. 2: Evidence-based therapist responsiveness* (3rd ed.; pp. 1–14). Oxford University Press.
Perls, F. (1969). *Gestalt therapy verbatim*. Bantam.
Piper-Mandy, E., & Rowe, T. D. (2010). Educating African-centered psychologists: Towards a Comprehensive Paradigm. *Journal of Pan African Studies, 3*(8).
Rank, O. (1924). *The trauma of birth*. Dover.
Rank, O. (1936). *Will therapy: An analysis of the therapeutic process in terms of relationship*. Norton.
Reuters. (2023, August 6). *Warner Bros movie "Barbie" ticket sales top $1 billion*. www.reuters.com/lifestyle/warner-bros-movie-barbie-ticket-sales-top-1-billion-2023-08-06/.
Rogers, C. (1961). *On becoming a person*. Houghton Mifflin.
Schneider, K. (2008). *Existential-integrative psychotherapy: Guideposts to the core of practice*. Routledge.
Schneider, K. (2009). *Awakening to awe: Personal stories of profound transformation*. Jason Aronson.
Schneider, K. (2012). The case of Allison: An existential–integrative inquiry into death anxiety, groundlessness, and the quest for meaning and awe. In P. Shaver & M. Mikulincer (Eds.), *Meaning, mortality and choice: The social psychology of existential concerns* (pp. 339–352). American Psychological Association.
Schneider, K. (2013). *The polarized mind: Why it's killing us and what we can do about it*. University Professors Press.
Schneider, K. (2015). Presence: The core contextual factor of effective psychotherapy. *Existential Analysis, 26*(2), 304–312.
Schneider, K. (2016). Existential–integrative therapy: Foundational implications for integrative practice. *Journal of Psychotherapy Integration, 26*(1), 49.ftext = Schneider, K. (2020). *The depolarizing of America: A guidebook for social healing*. University Professors Press.
Schneider, K. (2023). *Life-enhancing anxiety: Key to a sane world*. University Professors Press.
Schneider, K. (in press). Polarization and the experiential democracy dialogue. In L. Hoffman, X. Vallejos, D. Hocoy, P. Tummala-Narra, and E. DeRobertis (Eds.), *APA handbook of humanistic and existential psychology*. American Psychological Association Press.
Schneider, K., & Gamlen, T. (2023, November). Bridging the gap: Depth psychology and social healing. *Society for Humanistic Psychology Newsletter*.
Schneider, K., & Hoffman, L. (2024). Existential–humanistic and existential–integrative theory. In F. T. L. Leong, J. L. Callahan, J. Zimmerman, M. J. Consantino, & C. F. Eubanks (Eds.), *APA handbook of psychotherapy: Vol. 1. Theory-driven practice* (pp. 53–69). American Psychological Association.
Schneider, K., & Krug, O. (2026). *Existential–humanistic therapy* (3rd ed.). American Psychological Association.
Shahar, G., & Schiller, M. (2016). A conqueror by stealth: Introduction to the special issue on humanism, existentialism, and psychotherapy integration. *Journal of Psychotherapy Integration, 26*, 1–4.
Shumaker, D. (2012). An existential-integrative

treatment of anxious and depressed adolescents. *Journal of Humanistic Psychology, 52*(4), 375–400.

Solomon, S., Greenberg, J., & Pyszczynski, T. (2015). *The worm at the core: The role of death in life*. Random House.

Spaeth, D. (2020). Religious and spiritual diversity and humanistic psychology. In L. Hoffman, H. P. Cleare-Hoffman, N. Granger, Jr., & D. St. John (Eds.), *Humanistic approaches to multiculturalism and diversity: Perspectives on existence and difference* (pp. 203–214). Routledge.

Sundararajan, L. (2020). Indigenous psychology. In L. Hoffman, H. P. Cleare-Hoffman, N. Granger, Jr., & D. St. John (Eds.), *Humanistic approaches to multiculturalism and diversity: Perspectives on existence and difference* (pp. 193–202). Routledge.

Tavernier, R., & Willoughby, T. (2012). Adolescent turning points: The association between meaning-making and psychological well-being. *Developmental Psychology, 48*, 1058–1068.

Tervalon, M., & Murray-Garcia, J. (1998). Cultural humility versus cultural competence: A critical distinction in defining physician training outcomes in multicultural education. *Journal of Health Care for the Poor and Underserved, 9*(2), 117–125.

van Deurzen, E., Craig, E., Längle, A., Schneider, K., Tantam, S., & du Plock, S. (Eds.). (2019). *The Wiley world handbook of existential therapy*. Wiley.

Vos, J. (2018). *Meaning in life: An evidence-based handbook for practitioners*. Palgrave.

Vos, J. (2019). A review of research on existential-phenomenological therapies. In E. van Deurzen, E. Craig, A. Längle, K. J. Schneider, D. Tantam, & S. du Plock (Eds.), *The Wiley world handbook of existential therapy* (pp. 592–614). Wiley.

Wampold, B. E. (2008, February 6). Existential–integrative therapy comes of age. [Review of *Existential–integrative psychotherapy: Guideposts to the core of practice*]. *PsycCritique, 53*, Release 6, Article 1.

Wampold, B. E., Goodheart, C. D., & Levant, R. F. (2007). Clarification and elaboration on evidence-based practice in psychology. *American Psychologist, 62*, 616–618.

Wampold, B. E., & Imel, Z. E. (2015). *The great psychotherapy debate: The evidence for what makes psychotherapy work* (2nd ed.). Routledge.

Winnicott, D. (1960). The theory of the parent-child relationship. *International Journal of Psychoanalysis, 41*, 585–595.

Yalom, I. (1980). *Existential psychotherapy*. Basic Books.

CHAPTER 65

Courage amid Suffering

A Model of Existential Hope

Daryl R. Van Tongeren *and* Sara A. Showalter Van Tongeren

Suffering is a certainty. And because all people suffer, each person is exposed to the existential realities laid bare by the suffering. Adversity and trauma are stark reminders of the bounded nature of the human condition and the limitations each person faces when encountering ultimate concerns. Embracing an existential positive psychology approach to suffering, we posit that the human proclivity for meaning making predisposes humans to suitably navigate periods of suffering with resilience and hope. However, previous clinical approaches to suffering and theoretical accounts of hope have been limited and fail to appreciate the existential realities revealed in suffering. In this chapter, we examine suffering and highlight limitations of many clinical, therapeutic, and theoretical approaches to suffering. Understanding suffering as an existential issue, we describe various phases of suffering and the critical role of meaning in promoting flourishing amid such adversity (cf. Van Tongeren & Showalter Van Tongeren, 2020, 2021). Finally, we introduce a theoretical model for existential hope, which is grounded in the reality of ultimate concerns while being oriented toward an aspirational, participatory trust in an improved future.

AN EXISTENTIAL POSITIVE PSYCHOLOGICAL APPROACH TO SUFFERING

Psychological therapies have long sought to alleviate suffering and treat distress. And many of them have garnered considerable evidence for their efficacy in certain cases. However, we see many current predominant trends as limited when addressing suffering. Notably, we see at least three limitations. First, many approaches view suffering as *curable*. Insofar as many therapies have their roots in the medical model, we suspect they will be less effective. A central assumption in the medical model is the view that suffering is something to be fixed—it is often expressed in what are deemed as undesirable symptoms stemming from an unexpected or unwanted life situation. However, viewing suffering as an illness or disease is problematic. Because suffering is an inherent part of life, pathologizing suffering may exacerbate harm. Some research has suggested that in cases of severe grief or bereavement, some therapeutic approaches may actually worsen clinical outcomes (Jordan & Neimeyer, 2003). Because there is no cure for suffering, a "disease" model is insufficient. Treating it as such not only can invalidate the existential reality of the ubiquitousness of suffering, but also it fails to acknowledge the ways people are permanently affected by their suffering. When psychological and emotional pain are conceptualized as symptoms to be treated, addressed, and cured, it neglects to capture the persistent effects of suffering, rather viewing their lingering remnants as more evidence that there is something yet left to fix. It could very well be the case that such residual effects of suffering will always persist, and the person is fundamentally changed. No amount of treatment can "cure" some of these lingering aftereffects.

Second, many approaches are *prescriptive*. They suggest there is a "normalized" set of thoughts that accompany suffering and an acceptable timeline for metabolizing grief and loss. This is seen rather acutely in prolonged grief disorder (American Psychiatric Association, 2022). *Prolonged grief disorder* is defined as persistent feelings of grief and loss, including emotional pain and identity disruption, isolation, avoiding death reminders, and meaninglessness (all existential concerns), 1 year after the death of a loved one (or 6 months later for children or adolescents). Although nearly 10% of individuals will demonstrate persistent grief beyond the ascribed timeline, we wonder if this diagnostic criteria may be troublesome. Each person grieves on different timelines, and pathologizing longer grief trajectories may compound one's feelings of sadness and lead to stigmatization. Indeed, prior research has suggested that as many as 40% of individuals may experience significant and lasting changes as a result of their grief or loss (Neimeyer et al., 2002). Perhaps more critically, it strikes us as though many of the core expressions of prolonged grief are honest encounters of existential realities: confronting fears around identity, isolation, death, and meaninglessness. We caution against diagnosing the encounter of existential realities as problematic or disordered.

In the same way, cognitive-behavioral therapy (CBT) may be a less effective modality for people who are suffering when their heightened concerns and anxiety about threatening events are mischaracterized as delusions or polarized thinking. Many individuals who are suffering know firsthand the frailty of life and *rightly* embrace their finitude as they are aware of just how fragile life is. Someone with terminal cancer is not incorrect in thinking their life will end soon and their relationships will be rendered meaningless, which would naturally increase anxiety or distress. Here, there is no error in thinking to address; rather, they clearly see the existential realities that many others do not have to confront because their ongoing defenses protect them and they have not had the life experiences that thrust their salience into conscious awareness (Pyszczynski et al., 1997, 1999).

Finally, some approaches are *overly rigid*. There are concerns about the predominant narrative of CBT to which clients are expected to conform their thinking and behavior. The clinician is at a considerable privilege to craft a view of reality with which the client is expected to align. In cases of suffering, and especially among those who have been marginalized or had experiences that are less common among the general population, the clients' responses may be seen as problematic. Therapists working from a CBT-based orientation must caution against a proclivity of telling people what to think rather than exploring the legitimate reasons they may have for nondominant thoughts and behaviors. When applied overly rigidly, CBT runs the risk of invalidating the client. In many cases, people who are suffering are thinking quite clearly, having been disabused of many common positive illusions because of their suffering (Taylor, 1983). Similarly, people who are suffering are not engaging in catastrophic thinking, as might be miscategorized by CBT; rather, they have experienced extraordinary events that very well may be catastrophic, and their thinking accurately reflects the reality of their situation.

To clarify, CBT is highly effective with people who have anxiety for largely unrealized or unreasonable events. However, those experiencing suffering may be invalidated if their trauma-induced anxiety is labeled as a thinking error and they begin to doubt their own emotional and cognitive experiences. Indeed, their anxiety is a result of an actual threat. Over time, this can lead to confusion and disintegration, as people deny their experience in favor of conforming to an inaccurate label, only further exacerbating their suffering.

As an alternative, we approach suffering from an existential positive psychological framework. Existential positive psychology addresses suffering from an existential perspective that acknowledges human limitations, as well as the positive psychological perspective that human strengths and virtues can be cultivated to develop a meaningful, flourishing life (Van Tongeren & Showalter Van Tongeren, 2021; Wong, 2020). This orientation does two things. First, it buoys the potential for overwhelming despair and malaise that can arise from being mired in existential realities with a focus on the cultivation of virtues and strengths. Second, it grounds one in a full acceptance of ultimate concerns to avoid the potential for toxic positivity common with focuses solely on efforts for growth and resilience to the exclusion of accepting one's painful reality. The tension between the "positive and negative" or "light and dark" anchors people in a balanced state that more accurately reflects the difficulty of experiencing suffering. We briefly explain the tenets of this approach.

SUFFERING AS AN EXISTENTIAL ISSUE

All humans must come to terms with fundamental existential realities (Koole et al., 2006; Yalom, 1980). First, people bear the responsibility of making decisions in a chaotic and unpredictable world amid competing options. Second, people are phenomenologically isolated from one another, each subjectively experiencing the world in unique ways. Third, each person must come to terms with a changing identity over time. Fourth, people are forced to reconcile their own mortality, coming to grips with the reality that eventual death is the only certainty in life. Finally, freedom, isolation, unsure identity, and mortality often give rise to feelings of meaninglessness.

These existential realities have the potential to elicit a considerable amount of existential anxiety. To properly manage this terror, people construct and adhere to cultural worldviews, which are constellations of beliefs about oneself and the social world that answer these pressing questions and imbue life with order, permanence, and meaning (Pyszczynski et al., 2015). For example, religion is a common cultural worldview that mollifies these fears through the belief in a controlling, or guiding, God (or gods) that directs one's path, with whom one can connect in transcendent ways and who offers a clear sense of identity, grants their life meaning, and solves the problem of death through the promise of literal immortality (Van Tongeren, 2024). Given the psychological benefits of these cultural worldviews, people are motivated to defend them against threats and strive to uphold the integrity of their belief systems (Brandt & Van Tongeren, 2017). Both the content (i.e., what people believe) and the style (i.e., how they hold such beliefs) of one's worldview beliefs are critical in determining one's responses to life's adversities.

Worldviews are schemas, or cognitive frameworks for understanding human nature and how the world works. These assumptions become internalized expectations that provide order, stability, and predictability. However, suffering can violate these deeply held beliefs. If someone holds a belief that God is all-powerful, all-knowing, and all-loving, coupled with the belief that the world is fair and people get what they deserve (i.e., good things happen to good people), the experience of personal adversity, loss, or grief pressures these assumptions. The death of a loved one calls into question: Is God not powerful, unknowledgeable, or unloving? Or do I deserve this because I am not a good person? When the lived experience of suffering does not align with one's schematic understanding of the world, it feels like a threat to meaning that creates dissonance (Festinger, 1957; Park, 2010). Events that violate one's schema are either assimilated into the existing schema (i.e., revising the meaning of the event in a way that is consistent with one's worldview), or the schema is changed in order to accommodate this new information. The degree of the discrepancy between the events and one's worldview is related to the amount of distress one feels (Park, 2010). Suffering often shatters these worldview assumptions insofar as people are wholly unable to accommodate their suffering into their existing schemas, often leading to a disruptive shift in what, and often how, they believe. They then must find new ways to integrate their experience and metabolize their pain.

Despite its potential for disruption, suffering is an inescapable part of life. Everyone will one day suffer. Drawing from previous research (Van Tongeren & Showalter Van Tongeren, 2020, 2021), we define *suffering* as psychological or emotional pain that is relatively enduring or long-lasting (i.e., *chronic*) that violates one's long-standing beliefs about how the world operates (i.e., *cognitively threatening*), resulting in significantly altering one's life (i.e., *consequential*). In our view, suffering is an existential issue insofar as suffering lays bare core ultimate or basic concerns that every human faces in ways that one's worldview may be ill-equipped to address. Specifically, suffering is a violation of meaning that may shatter many of these assumptions or call into question one's worldview, often evoking a lengthy and painful process. Insofar as these worldviews are rendered inadequate or insufficient to address existential concerns, existential anxiety is significantly heightened. Thus, we view suffering as an existential issue. However, as one works toward accepting suffering as part of an inherent feature of being a bounded human, one is able to create meaning in the midst of one's suffering.

PHASES OF SUFFERING

Although each person's experience of suffering is unique, suffering may unfold in similar ways. We briefly describe different "phases" of suffering and the clinical priority during that phase (see Van Tongeren & Showalter Van Tongeren, 2020, for a fuller discussion). However, we provide a few nuances to this discussion. First, although we use the term *phase,* we do not imply that these are concrete periods of time, with rigid beginnings or endings; rather, these experiences likely blend into one another, and as someone experiences a new season in their suffering, remnants of the past extend into that one. Similarly, it is possible to reexperience aspects of previous phases or move through the phases in a different temporal pattern. Grief can linger and recur. Finally, there is no set amount of time someone should spend in any of these phases. People move through more quickly or slowly than others. Individual and contextual characteristics multiply determine one's progress. It is critical for clinicians to give leeway and follow the lead of their clients as they process their suffering. Finally, we note that in therapeutic work with clients who are suffering, clinicians may experience heightened existential anxiety. The discussion of these topics can be unsettling, so clinicians are encouraged to identify countertransference and use those emotional experiences as information to better shape their therapeutic approach.

Shock (Assess and Stabilize)

Often, the first pangs of suffering sting when the reality of one's suffering no longer aligns with one's cultural worldview. This discrepancy results in shattered assumptions about oneself (e.g., loss of perceived invulnerability, lack of perceived control), others (e.g., feelings of abandonment or loneliness), and the world (e.g., challenges to belief in a just world). As mentioned previously, the greater the discrepancy between the way people think the world should work and their experiences in it, the more distress and lost meaning they experience (Park, 2010). More significant or traumatic experiences elicit stronger and more painful reactions.

Clinically, therapists often begin with two goals. The first is to stabilize their client. In the midst of a sudden loss or unexpected adversity, clients may be feeling overwhelming grief, disorientation, and the numbness of emotional shock. Clinicians can provide a practical presence to their client, validate their experiences and shattered assumptions, provide them with some semblance of structure, and help them begin to build their distress tolerance for their negative emotions. The second goal is to begin to assess their meaning. Inquiring how their client is making sense of their life, the degree to which they feel like they matter, and if they feel like they have any purpose can be a good starting point. Asking questions about their worldview and doing so with the cultural humility that does not presuppose that any beliefs are inherently superior by adopting a posture of curiosity and learning, can help therapists understand where, and how severely, their clients' beliefs may be challenged (Hook et al., 2013). In addition, it can clarify from where a client is deriving meaning, and how difficult it might be for them to do so.

Grief (Acceptance)

Shortly after the initial sting of suffering subsides, most clients will feel a deep and profound sense of grief. Naturally, such grief is incredibly emotionally painful, and many clients will seek to avoid feeling the depths of this pain. Accordingly, some will engage in myriad avoidance techniques, though doing so often amplifies their emotional pain and leads to worse clinical outcomes (Chawla & Ostafin, 2007) and erodes meaning in life (Machell et al., 2015). This may look like avoidance-focused coping that is intended to direct their focus and attention away from the reality of their suffering or feelings of emotional discomfort.

There are therapeutic steps to overcome this default reaction of pain avoidance. Clinicians can help clients name their pain honestly. This candid acknowledgment often involves admitting their limitations as humans in the midst of real existential certainties. When clients downplay or minimize their suffering, it limits their abilities to navigate it in healthy ways and to make behavioral choices that lead toward flourishing. Conversely, accurately describing the depth of their pain and loss allows an authentic emotional process that can facilitate healing. Doing so may require helping teach clients how to overcome experiential avoidance through self-regulatory strategies, which can enhance meaning in life (Van Tongeren et al., 2018). Clients may get increasingly defensive as they move further into their emotional pain, so efforts to decrease client defensiveness and suppress the therapist's urge to rush their client through this phase are critically important—a process termed *integrative emotion regulation* (Roth et al., 2019). Ultimately, the clinical goal of this phase is acceptance: helping the client honestly embrace the full depth of their suffering and its existential implications.

Deconstruction (Active Questioning)

Although some people may stagnate after they accept their suffering, others find meaningful change by engaging in belief deconstruction. Deconstruction is marked by doubt, questioning, and struggling with one's strongly held beliefs (Van Tongeren, 2024). Given that many worldview beliefs are challenged and assumptions are shattered by suffering, many clients may be searching for meaning through the process of deconstructing their beliefs. The earlier in the process clients move toward a search for meaning, the better their longer-term trajectories tend to be (Silver & Updegraff, 2013). However, there are two caveats. A perpetual search for meaning that goes unsatisfied can lead to worse outcomes than never searching at all. Related, many of these core beliefs that are questioned are resistant to change. It can be difficult to chip away at one's deepest beliefs, because doing so undermines one's ability to address ultimate questions and exposes one to existential anxiety (Pyszczynski et al., 2015). Accordingly, this is a period of time when clients often feel the least amount of meaning.

Clinical support during this phase often looks like urging clients to go beyond their symptoms to get at the root beliefs that underlie their conceptualizations of the world that have been challenged by suffering. Once they do, therapists can facilitate existential questioning by linking the clients' unsettled beliefs to ultimate questions raised by their adversity. Thus, the goal in this phase is active questioning. This may also include gentle encouragement to curiously explore and seek out alternative ways of making sense of their suffering. Finally, because meaning often erodes during deconstruction, it is important to help support clients with psychoeducation in this process so that they do not get overwhelmed by nihilistic despair. Additionally, they can be encouraged to orient themselves in their actions and relationships that provide them with meaning.

Reconstruction (Autonomy)

Once a client's core beliefs have been laid bare and are sufficiently broken down and challenged, it is important to facilitate their reconstruction. Revision of one's worldview in alignment with the reality of one's suffering is the critical step in this phase. This may look different for each client. For some, it includes helping them eliminate some old beliefs and adopt new ones. It may mean abandoning the myth of greater meaning and the expectation that everything will make sense or serve some ultimate purpose (Baumeister, 1991). For many, it is helpful to see how their suffering fits into the narrative arc of their life story (White & Epson, 1990). Of course, their previous beliefs may continue to linger (e.g., Van Tongeren et al., 2021), which can make this an ongoing, iterative process.

The clinical goal of this phase is to build autonomy. Choosing one's set of worldview beliefs can be empowering, and therapists should prioritize an opportunity for revision and reconstruction. Many people will begin the therapeutic process not being aware of what worldviews have been violated. By encouraging them to engage in this process autonomously, they then are beginning to work through this new phase intentionally, which allows for recovering lost feelings of control and mastery. Part of this includes the therapist modeling intellectual openness, a sense of curiosity, and grace during this process. Motivational interviewing (Hettema et al., 2005) can help clients identify their core values and assemble a worldview consistent with such values. Ultimately, as clients reconstruct their beliefs, they will work toward (re)forming their identity in an authentic way. Helping them integrate their suffering into how they see themselves—not solely defined by adversity but incorporating it into their self-concept—can be valuable. This allows suffering to be appropriately metabolized into their sense of identity.

Moving Forward (Authenticity)

Ultimately, each client likely desires to live authentically. This is often marked by appropriately conceptualizing their suffering as something that has changed them, often indelibly, and allows them to engage in the world in a different way that is now consistent with their values and new way of understanding the world. Because suffering is likely to recur, it is critical to develop a sense of existential resilience (cf. Richardson, 2002). By this, we mean that people are able to cultivate a reliable resource of existential security from which they can draw when future adversity strikes. This resilient security can reduce defensiveness from future confrontations with existential reminders (Hart, 2014). Often, this co-occurs with intentional efforts to develop meaning through seeking coherence (i.e., making sense of their suffering and their place in it), significance (i.e., connecting with people and projects that provide mattering), and purpose (i.e., orienting oneself toward a larger goal beyond oneself).

To help clients develop authenticity, clinicians can focus on two goals. First, they can help their clients build existential resilience by allowing opportunities to engage with existential realities—and discuss their reactions to these ultimate concerns—within the therapeutic space. Through a kind of guided imagery, the repeated exposure to these reminders can help clients develop ready responses to managing their anxiety in productive, value-consistent ways. Second, they can help their clients cultivate vulnerable compassion, which is evidenced by an awareness and attunement with one's emotional state and a willingness to engage others who are hurting empathically and sympathetically (Van Tongeren & Showalter Van Tongeren, 2020). This can help people find another layer of meaning from their suffering, as they transform it into a gateway for interpersonal connection and empathic concern.

MEANING IS CRITICAL TO FLOURISHING IN SUFFERING

We see meaning as a critical vehicle by which individuals can flourish in the midst of suffering. Indeed, prior research has found that meaning-centered therapeutic approaches outperform standard "treatment-as-usual" modalities (Vos, 2016). Meaning has been defined as (1) the ability to make sense of one's life and social world (i.e., coherence), (2) feelings of worth and value (i.e., significance), and (3) being oriented toward something larger than oneself (i.e., purpose; George & Park, 2016; Martela & Steger, 2016). As we discussed, cultural worldviews are the primary sources of meaning that help people maintain a meaningful conceptualization of themselves and their world (Solomon et al., 2004). However, suffering often violates the assumptions of one's worldview, rendering them impotent to the critical meaning-making function necessary to manage existential anxiety and shield individuals from the impending terror of ultimate realities (Arndt et al., 2004). A primary outcome of suffering is meaninglessness (Van Tongeren & Showalter Van Tongeren, 2020).

Suffering may impair meaning in several ways. First, suffering is often seen as senseless, as people are unable to fit their negative experiences, grief, and loss into ways that fit with a predictable and coherent view of the world. Prior work has operationalized meaning as predicted associations or expected events (Heine et al., 2006; Heintzelman et al., 2013). Suffering is often sudden and unpredictable, and the more a situation violates expectations (e.g., the violent death of a child), the more senseless it is. Second, suffering robs people of their perceptions of worth and value. Suffering can be isolating, and people lose meaningful connections with others (including in the case of a loved one's death). The perception that one is not cared for or loved by a supernatural agent (such as God) who would allow this suffering to occur also undermines one's feelings of cosmic specialness or permanence. And to the degree that people hold just-world beliefs (Lerner & Lerner, 1980), they may question whether they are good and valuable when bad things are happening to them. Finally, suffering can disrupt people such that they lose their sense of purpose. For some, this is because their adversity has taken from them an ability to pursue goals they previously valued and that brought them meaning (e.g., no longer being able to complete triathlons because of a medical diagnosis). For others, the "fog" of grief and suffering disorients them from living a life oriented toward something larger than themselves; attending to their own needs is a necessary and adaptive response to suffering.

In our view, finding meaning in the midst of suffering allows people to flourish. The degree to which people are able to cultivate a lasting sense of meaning is central to the metabolizing of their suffering (Van Tongeren & Showalter Van Tongeren, 2020, 2021). Often, this occurs across the three levels of meaning. Cognitively, being able to make sense of one's suffering in a way that is coherent with one's worldview or fits within a broader narrative of one's life should enhance the felt sense of meaning. Relationally, when people feel deep connections with other people or with the sacred in the midst of their adversity or pain, they experience feelings of worth and value, perceiving their life as significant. Motivationally, when people are able to find a purpose that orients their actions to something larger than themselves—whether this is a result of, or in spite of, their suffering—they experience greater meaning. This enhanced meaning should provide a buffer from existential anxiety and help them better cope with their suffering (Haynes et al., 2017), and it should lead to greater flourishing.

FINDING FLOURISHING

This cultivation of meaning is critical for flourishing amid suffering. *Flourishing* has been defined as "doing or being well in the following five broad domains of human life: (i) happiness and life satisfaction; (ii) health, both mental and physical; (iii) meaning and purpose; (iv) character and virtue; and (v) close social relationships" (VanderWeele, 2017, p. 8149). In the context of suffering, we suspect this is expressed as the ability to integrate one's suffering in appropriate and whole ways. Specifically, this looks like recognizing one's suffering is one part of one's narrative story but not the complete story. It involves acknowledging the rightful place and size and impact of suffering in one's life as one pursues living in accordance with one's values. Individuals who can flourish in suffering are able to pursue well-being for themselves and others during, or as a result of, their suffering because they have accepted their suffering and integrated it into their sense of self.

Another expression of flourishing is value-aligned autonomy. A quote famously attributed to Viktor Frankl is "Between stimulus and response lies a space. In that space lie our freedom and power to choose a response. In our response lies our growth and our happiness." Consistent with that view, flourishing is a choice. After suffering, there is a felt sense that future changes or uncertainty nearly always give way to additional suffering. But flourishing requires that one acknowledges the anticipatory anxiety and still chooses to make a decision that is aligned with one's values in the midst of such emotions and cognitions. In this way, flourishing is not the absence of negative emotions or a strong emotional response to the trigger, but rather it is the autonomous decision in the midst of one's emotional reaction to traumatic triggers or eliciting events. Flourishing involves an existential awareness and acceptance.

The benefit of this view of flourishing is that it permits people to metabolize their suffering without needing to wait for the absence of emotional activation, which would likely rarely occur. Rather, flourishing occurs in making value-based decisions that promote well-being amid the strong emotional response that is shaped by one's prior (or current) suffering. This changes the metrics of flourishing to be more attainable. It is possible that people may have continued somatic and cognitive responses to triggers related to their suffering, and ridding themselves of this emotional response is likely an unreasonable requirement to flourish. Rather, flourishing involves becoming aware of one's behavioral and emotional tendencies and understanding such not as indicators of their regression or failure to heal, but rather as residual remnants of their suffering that will linger and as cues for one to autonomously choose one's desired outcome. Over time, this can allow for individuals to experience integration, as they integrate their negative and positive emotions into a coherent narrative, thereby reducing stigma by avoiding the dualistic thinking that suffering and flourishing are mutually exclusive. And quite possibly, it allows people to increase their authentic connections with others, through vulnerably sharing their experiences and compassionately seeing the pain of others. In this way, true flourishing extends beyond the self (VanderWeele, 2017).

TOWARD A MODEL OF EXISTENTIAL HOPE

Building on this existential positive psychological research of finding meaning amid suffering as the pathway toward flourishing, we propose a model of existential hope. We assert that an authentic, existential hope provides a strong framework for encountering and metabolizing suffering in healthy ways. Previous models of hope overemphasize pathways toward achieving one's goals and do not sufficiently consider existential realities (Synder, 2002). Accordingly, we see four primary limitations of current models of hope. First, hope can run the risk of becoming *delusional.* When people's sense of hope is misplaced well outside of reality and includes an expectation of impossible things, it can give way to delusion. The solution is a hope grounded in humility and honesty. Second, many accounts of hope are *diminished*; they conceptualize hope as goal pathways to achieve one's desired outcomes, and they more closely resemble self-efficacy. A broader view of hope requires optimistic expectation for something greater (i.e., improbable but not impossible). Third, many times hope is a *disengaged* anticipation. In this way, people hope that something good will happen and do little to help usher in that desirable reality. Rather, they wait for external forces to act to bring out their wishes. Authentic hope requires active participation. Finally, most views of hope *deny* existential realities. They ignore the ultimate concerns that every human faces. The remedy here is to include a consideration of existential realities and cultivate an appreciation for these truths.

Defining Existential Hope

Accordingly, we propose a framework for understanding hope from an existential perspective. Specifically, we view hope as (1) *humble*, honestly engaging with reality; (2) *optimistic*, anticipating a positive future outcome; (3) *participatory*, requiring personal involvement; and (4) *existential*, acknowledging the bounded limited nature of humanity. We expand on each necessary component in our HOPE model below.

• *Humble.* Unbridled hope can drift to positive illusions or fantasy-driven delusion. There is a difference between wishing for an impossible outcome and hoping for a better future that may realistically (even if improbably) come about. Existential hope is rooted in humility, which involves an accurate view of oneself and the world (Van Tongeren et al., 2019). In this way, it requires an honest evaluation of reality as it is, rather than distorting it to something that one wishes it was. This allows for an individual to properly identify the current status of aspects of their life they wish were different so they understand how great of a discrepancy there is between actuality and their hoped-for outcome.

• *Optimistic.* Hope is a longing for a better future. It involves the desire for one or more aspects of one's life or world to be changed in a way that is perceived as positive. It is more than merely identifying pathways to goals and having the means to reach those goals. It includes an ability to anticipate and imagine what that different future may be and motivates individuals toward that better future in real ways that affect one's emotional, cognitive, and behavioral processes. We might say that existential hope is the anticipation of a positive, if not unlikely or improbable, yet not impossible, future outcome.

• *Participatory.* Hope is active, requiring participatory involvement from individuals. It is not merely wishing for things to be different and doing nothing about it or relying on external agents or factors to bring about such change. Rather, it is a rightful understanding of what one can, and cannot, do to bring about one's desired future, and balancing the appropriate participation. Authentic, existential hope involves a degree of participation to achieve the desired future outcome.

• *Existential.* Hope requires an acknowledgment of human limitations and finitude. It is anchored in the acceptance of human boundedness and the pressing truth of the ultimate concerns that every human faces. Such hope can face the realities of groundlessness, isolation, identity, death, and meaninglessness, look into the existential chasm, and still choose to believe in something better, knowing full well the stakes of such belief.

There are considerable advantages to this view of existential hope. First, being grounded in humility and existential realities helps avoid the trappings for delusion or extreme cognitive distortions. Humble honesty means that people see the world *as it is* and still choose to hope anyway; yet this hope is contained within the realm of possible future outcomes. This helps protect people from the negative effects of delusional hope, which include defensiveness or denial of one's situation, or a wildly unsupported view of one's social world.

Second, a hope focused more on optimistic future outcomes rather than merely setting goals and the pathways to reach such goals, is necessary. Hope is more than self-efficacy and anticipating a future that is positive and good can be a strong motivation. It is bigger, bolder, and more open to radical new futures, yet anchored in requisite humility. It is marked by the expectation that despite the bounded nature of the human condition, an outcome can improve—or one may find a way forward toward flourishing in the midst of such limitations.

Third, it requires that people are actively involved in bringing about the change they desire to see, rather than simply wishing for some other, external agent or force to make their current or future life better. People become cocreators of this better future, actively engaging in the necessary work to bring it about. And while external forces (e.g., God, supernatural agents, governments, organizations) might be perceived as necessarily involved in such changes, the individual assumes their rightful amount of responsibility for bringing about this change.

Finally, this view of hope is rooted in the reality of existential concerns. Hope that denies such realities is merely defensiveness. Authentic hope is the choice to believe in a better future *while clearly accepting the existential realities of life.* Other instantiations of hope are incomplete or entail positive illusions that fail to appreciate the boundedness of the human condition. Taken together, *existential hope* is best expressed when individuals have a clear view of their smallness in this world, and in the light of existential realities, choose to believe that there is good in the world and a better future, and actively work toward bringing about that good new reality.

The Nature of Existential Hope

We further conceptualize existential hope as having cognitive, emotional, motivational, and behavioral expressions. Cognitively, it includes the intellectual assent for the legitimacy of existential realities, the view of such realities as truths rather than threats, and expectation for a better future outcome. Emotionally, we suspect it involves both positive and negative emotions: negative affect generated from the acknowledgement of ultimate concerns, as well as a willing choice to embrace joy and anticipatory happiness amid suffering. Motivationally, people are impelled to bring about the expected positive outcome for which they are hoping and may orient their lives toward this goal. Behaviorally, existential hope is expressed through the active engagement of actions designed to usher in the positive future, within the limits of what one realizes one can control and contribute.

Existential hope should be distinguishable from other adjacent constructs. Such hope is different from (1) cognitive delusions that presume an impossible (rather than improbable) future and lead toward emotional distress and increased anxiety and despair, (2) unfettered emotional optimism, wherein people only focus on the positive expected outcome without considering the likelihood for disappointment or a more emotionally varied reality, (3) amotivational fantasies that an external force will enact the hoped-for outcome, leading to a lack of perceived autonomy or willingness to act, and (4) a lack of participatory engagement in the behaviors necessary to bring about the desired outcome. Existential hope is rooted in the authentic acceptance of the existential realities, coupled with the active choice to believe something better will come and to actively work toward bringing that about to the degree that one has control, capacity, capability, and choice.

In addition, we suspect that existential hope is experienced as a state-like phenomenon. People may experience more or less existential hope depending on the nature of their suffering, their current belief system, the degree of discrepancy between their adversity and meaning-based expectations, and their cultural context. Perceptions of hope may fluctuate regularly, and some may be able to chronically experience state hope across time and situations, mirroring more "dispositional" proclivities toward existential hope. Yet we suspect that such hope may be cultivated, or developed, through intentional practice. To be sure, each of these theoretical claims are subject to empirical investigation and should warrant testing.

Two Organizing Hypotheses: Acceptance and Resilience

These theoretical assertions give rise to several empirically testable hypotheses. Specifically, we propose two organizing hypotheses that anchor our conceptual account. On the one hand, existential hope should be grounded in the acceptance of ultimate realities and fully embrace the boundedness of the human condition. Accordingly, the *hopeful acceptance hypothesis* assures that an authentic existential hope acknowledges and works toward accepting the truth of the core existential concerns. On the other hand, existential hope should also promote well-being in the face of adversity. Toward this end, the *hopeful resilience hypothesis* contends that existential hope provides meaning as a pathway to flourishing by expanding one's temporal orientation toward a more positive future beyond one's current suffering. We explicate these propositions below.

Hopeful Acceptance Hypothesis

First, based on our definition of existential hope, we propose the *hopeful acceptance hypothesis*. Namely, we predict that individuals demonstrating high levels of existential hope will more readily and easily accept the existential realities of the human condition, marked by a reduced defensiveness in light of making ultimate concerns cognitively salient. Prior research has demonstrated a host of defensive responses in reaction to reminders of existential concerns (e.g., see Pyszczynski et al., 2015; Van Tongeren & Green, 2010). Existentially hopeful individuals acknowledge existential realities as truths and not threats (cf. Van Tongeren & Showalter Van Tongeren, 2020) and thus should exhibit fewer defensive responses to existential reminders, such as mortality salience and meaninglessness. To the degree that such individuals have sufficiently embraced and integrated the inescapable fact of human mortality or the potential meaninglessness of life into their cultural worldviews, they should be less responsive to cues that make their finitude salient. At the very least, those individuals who can concede the legitimacy of such concerns, have dedicated sufficient cognitive and emotional processing to accepting their reality, and are not overly motivated to avoid contemplating such concerns should demonstrate attenuated negative responses to confronting existential realities. Of course, the defense against existential terror, such as the fear of death, occurs both consciously and nonconsciously (cf. Arndt et al., 2004), suggesting that some remnant of defensiveness may not only be a default, but also linger. Moreover, the content of one's cultural worldview may play a substantial role in how one responds to existential reminders (e.g., Pyszczynski et al., 2008). Still, cultivating an existential hope should mitigate such negative responses.

However, we hasten to clarify that an overemphasis on accepting existential dread without sufficiently building the meaning and permanence offered by cultural worldviews may undermine their security-providing function and render individuals with heightened anxiety. Because humans must balance demands for security amid motivations for growth (cf. Pyszczynski et al., 2003; Van Tongeren et al., 2016), holding one's beliefs too tentatively or being willing to revise one's core beliefs may erode well-being and leave individuals prone to the full terror of existential realities (Van Tongeren et al., 2023). Thus, a hopeful acceptance of existential concerns is anchored both by the humility garnered by embracing the limitations of the human condition *and* by the optimistic expectation that one may still flourish and grow in the midst of these constraints. It requires an honest acceptance and an expectant hope.

Some evidence has been garnered for this hypothesis. For example, belief in progressive hope—or the expectation that things will get better—has been shown to attenuate the negative responses to mortality salience (Rutjens et al., 2009). Other work has identified positive features of confronting existential concerns, such as mortality (Vail et al., 2012, 2015). For example, humility has been shown to mitigate negative responses to mortality salience (Kesebir, 2014). Consistent with this, research has demonstrated the benefits of embracing and accepting death as a reality, rather than denying it (e.g., Niemiec et al., 2010; Wong & Tomer, 2011). Future work should directly test the defense-reduction feature of existential hope in the wake of ultimate concerns.

Hopeful Resilience Hypothesis

A second testable hypothesis is that individuals high in existential hope demonstrate greater resilience and endurance in the midst of suffering, marked by greater meaning and well-being amid adversity. To the extent that existential hope includes an anticipatory expectation of a better future outcome, individuals are able to broaden their temporal perspective and avoid being overwhelmed by despair. This cognitive and emotional broadening enhances the availability of potential positive responses, such as drawing from one's character strengths or acting virtuously in the midst of suffering (see Fredrickson, 2001). Indeed, one's temporal perspective may play a role in how one responds to, or accepts, existential realities, such as death (Reed, 2025). When people embrace a belief that their life conditions will improve, suffering will not prevail, and their life will not be solely defined by suffering, they should report better well-being than those who feel overwhelmed by suffering, do not expect their life to improve, or expect that their identity will be defined exclusively by their suffering. One pathway to this enhanced well-being is the experience of meaning as an avenue toward flourishing.

We see several mechanisms by which existential hope may enhance meaning and promote flourishing. First, the active participation in bringing about a hopeful future outcome likely grants an individual a strong sense of purpose. Insofar as people are oriented toward a broader goal that is larger than themselves and motivated to act in ways that reach toward that self-transcendent goal, life often feels meaningful (George & Park, 2016; Martela & Steger, 2016). Second, reframing their experience of suffering as temporal, with the anticipation of improved life conditions, should provide a sense of coherence that helps people make sense of their suffering in light of the larger arc of their life, granting them a sense of meaning. Cognitively altering how one sees one's suffering can be powerful for making sense of one's seemingly senseless suffering, though therapists should caution against heavy-handed approaches that override the client's experiences or fall prey to unhelpful platitudes that "this, too, shall pass." Rather, clients should lead this coherence-driven experience as is helpful for their psychological processing of suffering. Third, when people see themselves as persistent and resilient amid the adversity of suffering—continuing to have positive experiences amid their distress—they may feel greater significance, worth, and value; despite the misfortune of life, they continue to endure. Some may see their mere existence as thus valuable and worthwhile, whereas others may perceive some divine or cosmic plan for their lives that imbues their daily existence with greater meaning, transforming their suffering into something they perceive as more noble or worthwhile. In sum, existential hope enhances meaning, which promotes well-being and flourishing.

There is some support for this hypothesis. Existential meaning has been linked with hope (Kuzendorf & Buker, 2008), and the relationship may be bidirectional (Mascaro & Rosen, 2005). To the extent that hope is associated with, or generates, existential meaning, and meaning helps facilitate flourishing in the midst of stressors or existential realities (Mascaro & Rosen, 2006), those high in existential hope should report better well-being and higher degrees of meaning amid suffering and adversity. Prior work has demonstrated the efficacy of meaning-focused therapeutic approaches in enhancing well-being (Vos, 2016), and spiritual meaning has been shown to be a buffer against the negative effects of adversity (Haynes et al., 2017). The predicted hope–meaning–flourishing causal chain deserves greater empirical attention.

Practical and Clinical Implications

In our view, the courage to suffer permits the development of existential hope. People who are able to understand suffering as an existential issue can honestly name and experience their pain, and who choose to cultivate meaning in the midst of their adversity may autonomously and authentically decide to invest in an existential hope in a flourishing future. Such a hope includes guardrails that protect from the hazards of delusion on one side and despair on the other. It is firmly grounded in an honest acceptance of the bounded limits of human nature and beckons an active participation in ushering in a positive future. Both theoretically and practically, this reconceptualizes hope as a virtue best expressed in the midst of adversity and suffering rather than a narrow goal pursuit or lofty belief in the impossible.

Clinically, this approach to hope permits clients to work toward integration of accepting the negative aspects of their suffering while simultaneously striving toward a different, better future. It avoids a false bifurcation of the exclusive expression of seemingly opposite emotional states (e.g., feeling either wholly negative or positive), empowers clients to appropriately make the changes they are in control of making without overclaiming responsibility or shirking accountability, and is anchored in an honest humility of a person's relative smallness in the vast scope of the universe. It grounds them into committing to hope as a choice amid improbable but not impossible odds and requires a full appreciation of the ultimate concerns. This can help allay depression and manage anxiety, while offering purpose and a deeper sense of meaning (cf. George & Park, 2016; Martela & Steger, 2016). In our view, the courage to hope is a tangible antidote to the inevitability of suffering: It helps clients make meaning as a pathway toward a flourishing life.

CONCLUSION

Suffering is as inescapable as death. Crucially, *how* one suffers matters greatly. We discussed advantages of adopting an existential positive psychological approach that conceptualizes suffering as an existential issue. By facing the existential terror engendered by confronting existential realities with the resolve and acceptance of existential hope, people can move toward making value-driven decisions to bring about a hoped-for, positive outcome in the future. Doing so does not necessarily alleviate one's suffering, but it is a way to act meaningfully and work toward experiencing flourishing, even amid adversity. Existential hope may serve as a motivating impetus to stay resilient in the darkest of hours, hoping for the light of days yet to come.

REFERENCES

American Psychiatric Association. (2022). *Diagnostic and statistical manual of mental disorders* (5th ed., text rev.).

Arndt, J., Cook, A., & Routledge, C. (2004). The blueprint of terror management. Understanding the cognitive architecture of psychological defense against the awareness of death. In J. Greenberg, S. Koole, & T. Pyszczynski (Eds.), *Handbook of experimental existential psychology* (pp. 35–53). Guilford Press.

Baumeister, R. F. (1991). *Meanings in life*. Guilford Press.

Brandt, M. J., & Van Tongeren, D. R. (2017). People both high and low in religious fundamentalism are prejudiced toward dissimilar groups. *Journal of Personality and Social Psychology, 112*, 76–97.

Chawla, N., & Ostafin, B. (2007). Experiential avoidance as a functional dimensional approach to psychopathology: An empirical review. *Journal of Clinical Psychology, 63*(9), 871–890.

Festinger, L. (1957). *A theory of cognitive dissonance*. Row, Peterson.

Fredrickson, B. L. (2001). The role of positive emotions in positive psychology: The broaden-and-build theory of positive emotions. *American Psychologist, 56*(3), 218–226.

George, L. S., & Park, C. L. (2016). Meaning in life as comprehension, purpose, and mattering: Toward integration and new research questions. *Review of General Psychology, 20*(3), 205–220.

Hart, J. (2014). Toward an integrative theory of psychological defense. *Perspectives on Psychological Science, 9*, 19–39.

Haynes, W. C., Van Tongeren, D. R., Aten, J., Davis, E. B., Davis, D. E., Hook, J. N., . . . Johnson, T. (2017). The meaning as a buffer hypothesis: Spiritual meaning attenuates the effect of disaster-related resource loss on posttraumatic stress. *Psychology of Religion and Spirituality, 9*(4), 446–453.

Heine, S. J., Proulx, T., & Vohs, K. D. (2006). The meaning maintenance model: On the coherence of social motivations. *Personality and Social Psychology Review, 10*(2), 88–110.

Heintzelman, S. J., Trent, J., & King, L. A. (2013). Encounters with objective coherence and the experience of meaning in life. *Psychological Science, 24*(6), 991–998.

Hettema, J., Steele, J., & Miller, W. R. (2005). Motivational interviewing. *Annual Review of Clinical Psychology, 1*(1), 91–111.

Hook, J. N., Davis, D. E., Owen, J., Worthington, E. L., Jr., & Utsey, S. O. (2013). Cultural humility: Measuring openness to culturally diverse clients. *Journal of Counseling Psychology, 60*(3), 353.

Jordan, J. R., & Neimeyer, R. A. (2003). Does grief counseling work? *Death Studies, 27*(9), 765–786.

Kesebir, P. (2014). A quiet ego quiets death anxiety: Humility as an existential anxiety buffer. *Journal of Personality and Social Psychology, 106*(4), 610–623.

Koole, S. L., Greenberg, J., & Pyszczynski, T. (2006). Introducing science to the psychology of the soul: Experimental existential psychology. *Current Directions in Psychological Science, 15*(5), 212–216.

Kunzendorf, R. G., & Buker, F. (2008). Does existential meaning require hope, or is interest enough? *Imagination, Cognition and Personality, 27*(3), 233–243.

Lerner, M. J., & Lerner, M. J. (1980). *The belief in a just world*. Springer.

Machell, K. A., Goodman, F. R., & Kashdan, T. B. (2015). Experiential avoidance and well-being: A daily diary analysis. *Cognition and Emotion, 29*(2), 351–359.

Martela, F., & Steger, M. F. (2016). The three meanings of meaning in life: Distinguishing coherence, purpose, and significance. *The Journal of Positive Psychology, 11*(5), 531–545.

Mascaro, N., & Rosen, D. H. (2005). Existential meaning's role in the enhancement of hope and prevention of depressive symptoms. *Journal of Personality, 73*(4), 985–1014.

Mascaro, N., & Rosen, D. H. (2006). The role of existential meaning as a buffer against stress. *Journal of Humanistic Psychology, 46*(2), 168–190.

Neimeyer, R. A., Prigerson, H. G., & Davies, B. (2002). Mourning and meaning. *American Behavioral Scientist, 46*(2), 235–251.

Niemiec, C. P., Brown, K. W., Kashdan, T. B.,

Cozzolino, P. J., Breen, W. E., Levesque-Bristol, C., & Ryan, R. M. (2010). Being present in the face of existential threat: The role of trait mindfulness in reducing defensive responses to mortality salience. *Journal of Personality and Social Psychology, 99*(2), 344–365.

Park, C. L. (2010). Making sense of the meaning literature: An integrative review of meaning making and its effects on adjustment to stressful life events. *Psychological Bulletin, 136*(2), 257.

Pyszczynski, T., Greenberg, J., & Goldenberg, J. L. (2003). Freedom versus fear: On the defense, growth, and expansion of the self. In M. R. Leary & J. P. Tangney (Eds.), *Handbook of self and identity* (pp. 314–343). Guilford Press.

Pyszczynski, T., Greenberg, J., & Solomon, S. (1997). Why do we need what we need?: A terror management perspective on the roots of human social motivation. *Psychological inquiry, 8*(1), 1–20.

Pyszczynski, T., Greenberg, J., & Solomon, S. (1999). A dual-process model of defense against conscious and unconscious death-related thoughts: An extension of terror management theory. *Psychological Review, 106*(4), 835–845.

Pyszczynski, T., Rothschild, Z., & Abdollahi, A. (2008). Terrorism, violence, and hope for peace: A terror management perspective. *Current Directions in Psychological Science, 17*(5), 318–322.

Pyszczynski, T., Solomon, S., & Greenberg, J. (2015). Thirty years of terror management theory: From genesis to revelation. In *Advances in experimental social psychology* (Vol. 52, pp. 1–70). Academic Press.

Reed, D. E. (2025). Future time perspective as an operationalization of existential concerns related to time. *Journal of Humanistic Psychology, 65*(1), 219–232.

Richardson, G. E. (2002). The metatheory of resilience and resiliency. *Journal of Clinical Psychology, 58,* 307–321.

Roth, G., Vansteenkiste, M., & Ryan, R. M. (2019). Integrative emotion regulation: Process and development from a self-determination theory perspective. *Development and Psychopathology, 31*(3), 945–956.

Rutjens, B. T., van der Pligt, J., & van Harreveld, F. (2009). Things will get better: The anxiety-buffering qualities of progressive hope. *Personality and Social Psychology Bulletin, 35*(5), 535–543.

Silver, R. C., & Updegraff, J. A. (2013). Searching for and finding meaning following personal and collective traumas. In K. D. Markman, T. Proulx, & M. J. Lindberg (Eds.), *The psychology of meaning* (pp. 237–255). American Psychological Association.

Snyder, C. R. (2002). Hope theory: Rainbows in the mind. *Psychological Inquiry, 13*(4), 249–275.

Solomon, S., Greenberg, J., & Pyszczynski, T. (2004). The cultural animal: Twenty years of terror management theory and research. In J. Greenberg, S. L. Koole, & T. Pyszczynski (Eds.), *Handbook of experimental existential psychology* (pp. 13–34). Guilford Press.

Taylor, S. E. (1983). Adjustment to threatening events: A theory of cognitive adaptation. *American Psychologist, 38*(11), 1161–1173.

Vail, K. E., III, & Juhl, J. (2015). An appreciative view of the brighter side of terror management processes. *Social Sciences, 4*(4), 1020–1045.

Vail, K. E., III, Juhl, J., Arndt, J., Vess, M., Routledge, C., & Rutjens, B. T. (2012). When death is good for life: Considering the positive trajectories of terror management. *Personality and Social Psychology Review, 16*(4), 303–329.

Van Tongeren, D. R. (2024). *Done: How to flourish after leaving religion.* American Psychological Association.

Van Tongeren, D. R., Davis, D. E., Hook, J. N., & Johnson, K. A. (2016). Security versus growth: Existential tradeoffs of various religious perspectives. *Psychology of Religion and Spirituality, 8,* 77–88.

Van Tongeren, D. R., Davis, D. E., Hook, J. N., & Witvliet, C. V. (2019). Humility. *Current Directions in Psychological Science, 28*(5), 463–468.

Van Tongeren, D. R., DeWall, C. N., Chen, Z., Sibley, C. G., & Bulbulia, J. (2021). Religious residue: Cross-cultural evidence that religious psychology and behavior persist following deidentification. *Journal of Personality and Social Psychology, 120,* 484–503.

Van Tongeren, D. R., DeWall, C. N., Green, J. D., Cairo, A. H., Davis, D. E., & Hook, J. N. (2018). Self-regulation facilitates meaning in life. *Review of General Psychology, 22,* 95–106.

Van Tongeren, D. R., & Green, J. D. (2010). Combating meaninglessness: On the automatic defense of meaning. *Personality and Social Psychology Bulletin, 36,* 1372–1384.

Van Tongeren, D. R., Severino, M., Kojima, Y., Miskowski, K., & Blank, S. (2023). Is there a dark side to humility?: Cross-sectional and longitudinal evidence for existential costs of humility. *International Journal for the Psychology of Religion, 33,* 136–150.

Van Tongeren, D. R., & Showalter Van Tongeren, S. A. (2020). *The courage to suffer: A new clinical framework for life's greatest crises.* Templeton Foundation Press.

Van Tongeren, D. R., & Showalter Van Tongeren, S. A. (2021). Finding meaning amidst COVID-19: An existential positive psychology model of suffering. *Frontiers in Psychology, 12,* Article 641747, 1–10.

VanderWeele, T. J. (2017). On the promotion of human flourishing. *Proceedings of the National Academy of Sciences, 114*(31), 8148–8156.

Vos, J. (2016). Working with meaning in life in mental health care: A systematic literature review of the practices and effectiveness of meaning-centered therapies. In P. Russo-Netzer, S. E. Schulenberg, & A. Batthyany (Eds.), *Clinical perspectives on meaning: Positive and existential psychotherapy* (pp. 59–87). Springer.

White, M., & Epston, D. (1990). *Narrative means to therapeutic ends.* Norton.

Wong, P. T. (2020). Existential positive psychology and integrative meaning therapy. *International Review of Psychiatry, 32*(7–8), 565–578.

Wong, P. T., & Tomer, A. (2011). Beyond terror and denial: The positive psychology of death acceptance. *Death Studies, 35*(2), 99–106.

Yalom, I. (1980). *Existential psychotherapy.* Basic Books.

Author Index

Subject Index

Note. *f*, *n*, or *t* following a page number indicates a figure, note, or table.